GYNECOLOGIC SURGERY

GYNECOLOGIC SURGERY

Edited by

William J. Mann, Jr., M.D.

Clinical Professor
Department of Obstetrics and Gynecology
Medical College of Virginia
Richmond, Virginia
Director of Medical Education in Obstetrics and Gynecology
Riverside Regional Medical Center
Newport News, Virginia

Thomas G. Stovall, M.D.

Associate Professor and Head
Section on Gynecology
Department of Obstetrics and Gynecology
Bowman Gray School of Medicine of Wake Forest University
Winston-Salem, North Carolina

Illustrated by Lydia V. Kibiuk, M.A.

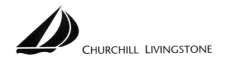

CHURCHILL LIVINGSTONE

New York, Edinburgh, London, Madrid, Melbourne, San Francisco, Tokyo

Library of Congress Cataloging-in-Publication Data
Gynecologic surgery / edited by William J. Mann, Jr., Thomas G.
   Stovall ; illustrated by Lydia V. Kibiuk.
      p. cm
   Includes bibliographical references and index.
   ISBN 0–443–08958–2
    1. Generative organs, Female—Surgery. 2. Urogynecologic surgery.
 I. Mann, William J., Date II. Stovall, Thomas G.
   [DNLM: 1. Genitalia, Female—surgery. 2. Urinary Tract—surgery.
 WP 660 G99725 1996]
 RG104.G955 1996
 618.1'059—dc20
 DNLM/DLC
 for Library of Congress   96–17726
                                                    CIP

Distributed in the United Kingdom by Churchill Livingstone, Robert Stevenson House, 1–3 Baxter's Place, Leith Walk, Edinburgh EH1 3AF, and by associated companies, branches, and representatives throughout the world.

Accurate indications, adverse reactions, and dosage schedules for drugs are provided in this book, but it is possible that they may change. The reader is urged to review the package information data of the manufacturers of the medications mentioned.

The Publishers have made every effort to trace the copyright holders for borrowed material. If they have inadvertently overlooked any, they will be pleased to make the necessary arrangements at the first opportunity.

Acquisitions Editor: *Jennifer Mitchell*
Assistant Editor: *Jennifer Hardy*
Production Editor: *Bridgett L. Dickinson*
Production Supervisor: *Laura Mosberg Cohen*
Cover Design: *Jeannette Jacobs*

Printed in the United States of America

First published in 1996   7 6 5 4 3 2 1

CONTRIBUTORS

Claudio A. Benadiva, M.D.
Center for Fertility and Reproductive Endocrinology, New Britain General Hospital, New Britain, Connecticut

Claire M. Carman, M.D.
Assistant Clinical Professor, Department of Surgery, Eastern Virginia Medical School Medical College of Hampton Roads; Breast Care Specialists, P.C., Norfolk, Virginia

Eva Chalas, M.D.
Associate Professor and Director, Division of Gynecologic Oncology, Department of Obstetrics and Gynecology and Reproductive Medicine, State University of New York at Stony Brook School of Medicine, Stony Brook, New York

Joel M. Childers, M.D.
Associate Professor of Clinical Obstetrics and Gynecology, Division of Gynecologic Oncology, Department of Obstetrics and Gynecology, University of Arizona College of Medicine, Tucson, Arizona

J. Lawrence Colley, M.D.
Vice President, Corporate Medical Policy, Trigon Blue Cross Blue Shield, Richmond, Virginia

Stephen H. Cruikshank, M.D.
Nicholas J. Thompson Professor and Chairman, Department of Obstetrics and Gynecology, Wright State University School of Medicine, Dayton, Ohio

Owen K. Davis, M.D.
Associate Professor, Department of Obstetrics and Gynecology, Cornell University Medical College; Attending Obstetrician and Gynecologist, Department of Obstetrics and Gynecology, The New York Hospital-Cornell Medical Center, New York, New York

Alan H. DeCherney, M.D.
Louis E. Phaneuf Professor and Chairman, Department of Obstetrics and Gynecology, Tufts University School of Medicine, Boston, Massachusetts

Albert Diket, M.D.
Associate Professor, Department of Obstetrics and Gynecology, Division of Maternal-Fetal Medicine, Louisiana State University School of Medicine in New Orleans, New Orleans, Louisiana

Thomas E. Elkins, M.D.
Abe Mickal Professor and Chairman, Department of Obstetrics and Gynecology, Louisiana State University School of Medicine in New Orleans, New Orleans, Louisiana

Denise M. Elser, M.D.
Assistant Professor, Department of Obstetrics and Gynecology, University of Illinois College of Medicine, Chicago, Illinois; Director of Urogynecology and Assistant Program Director, Department of Obstetrics and Gynecology, Christ Hospital and Medical Center, Oak Lawn, Illinois

Alan Garely, M.D.
Assistant Professor, Department of Obstetrics and Gynecology, Louisiana State University School of Medicine in New Orleans, New Orleans, Louisiana

Richard S. Guido, M.D.
Assistant Professor, Department of Obstetrics, Gynecology, and Reproductive Services, University of Pittsburgh School of Medicine; Director, Colposcopy Clinic, Department of Obstetrics, Gynecology, and Reproductive Services, Magee-Women's Hospital; Director, Gynecology Clinic, Department of Obstetrics, Gynecology, and Reproductive Services, Veterans Affairs Medical Center, Pittsburgh, Pennsylvania

Keith M. Harrigill, M.D., M.P.H./T.M.

Chief Resident, Division of Gynecologic Oncology, Department of Obstetrics and Gynecology, University of Arizona College of Medicine, Tucson, Arizona

Ken Hatch, M.D.

Professor and Chairman, Department of Obstetrics and Gynecology, University of Arizona College of Medicine, Tucson, Arizona

C. William Helm, M.D.

Director, Division of Gynecologic Oncology, Department of Obstetrics and Gynecology, Temple University School of Medicine, Philadelphia, Pennsylvania

Mitchel S. Hoffman, M.D.

Professor, Department of Obstetrics and Gynecology, University of South Florida College of Medicine, Tampa, Florida

Ronald E. Iverson, Jr., M.D., M.P.H.

Resident, Department of Obstetrics and Gynecology, Tufts University School of Medicine and New England Medical Center, Boston, Massachusetts

Lisa Jane Jacobsen, M.D., M.P.H.

Fellow, Department of Obstetrics and Gynecology, Tufts University School of Medicine, Boston, Massachusetts

John Jennings, M.D.

Associate Professor and Residency Program Director, Department of Obstetrics and Gynecology, University of Texas Medical Branch, University of Texas Medical School at Galveston, Galveston, Texas

Jacqueline C. Johnson, M.D.

Assistant Clinical Professor, Department of Obstetrics and Gynecology, Columbia University College of Physicians and Surgeons; Associate Director, Gynecologic Oncology, Department of Obstetrics and Gynecology, St. Luke's/Roosevelt Hospital Center, New York, New York

Isaac Kligman, M.D.

Assistant Professor, Department of Obstetrics and Gynecology, Cornell University Medical College; Assistant Attending Obstetrician and Gynecologist, Department of Obstetrics and Gynecology, The New York Hospital-Cornell Medical Center, New York, New York

Joseph J. Kryc, M.D.

Associate Professor of Clinical Anesthesiology, Departments of Anesthesiology and Obstetrics and Gynecology, and Vice Chairman, Department of Anesthesiology, University of Arizona College of Medicine, Phoenix, Arizona

Frank W. Ling, M.D.

Faculty Professor and Chairman, Department of Obstetrics and Gynecology, University of Tennessee, Memphis, College of Medicine, Memphis, Tennessee

William J. Mann, Jr., M.D.

Clinical Professor, Department of Obstetrics and Gynecology, Medical College of Virginia, Richmond, Virginia; Director of Medical Education in Obstetrics and Gynecology, Riverside Regional Medical Center, Newport News, Virginia

G. Rodney Meeks, M.D.

Director, Division of Gynecology, and Professor, Department of Obstetrics and Gynecology, University of Mississippi School of Medicine, Jackson, Mississippi

Thomas E. Nolan, M.D.

Associate Professor, Departments of Obstetrics and Gynecology and Internal Medicine, Louisiana State University School of Medicine in New Orleans; Director, Division of General Obstetrics and Gynecology, and Obstetric Intensive Care Unit Services, Department of Obstetrics and Gynecology, Louisiana State University Medical Center, New Orleans, Louisiana

Peggy A. Norton, M.D.

Associate Professor, Department of Obstetrics and Gynecology, University of Utah School of Medicine, Salt Lake City, Utah

Roger C. Odell, Electrical Engineer

President and CEO, Electroscope, Incorporated, Boulder, Colorado

Susan Pokorny, M.D.

Assistant Professor of Pediatrics and Obstetrics and Gynecology, Department of Obstetrics and Gynecology, Baylor College of Medicine; Director, Baylor Young Women's Clinic, Texas Childrens' Hospital, Houston, Texas

Robert F. Porges, M.D.

Professor and Vice Chairman, Department of Obstetrics and Gynecology, New York University School of Medicine; Director of Gynecology, Department of Obstetrics and Gynecology, New York University Medical Center, New York, New York

Clifford A. Rieders, J.D.

Partner, Law Firm of Rieders, Travis, Mussina, Humphrey & Harris; President of Central Pennsylvania Chapter of the Federal Bar Association; Board member and officer, Pennsylvania Trial Lawyers' Association, Williamsport, Pennsylvania

Deirdre Robinson, M.D.

Assistant Professor, Department of Obstetrics and Gynecology, Bowman Gray School of Medicine of Wake Forest University, Winston-Salem, North Carolina

Zev Rosenwaks, M.D.

Professor and Revlon Distinguished Professor of Reproductive Medicine, Department of Obstetrics and Gynecology, Cornell University Medical College; Attending Obstetrician and Gynecologist, Department of Obstetrics and Gynecology, The New York Hospital-Cornell Medical Center, New York, New York

Lee P. Shulman, M.D.

Associate Professor and Director, Division of Reproductive Genetics, Department of Obstetrics and Gynecology, University of Tennessee, Memphis, College of Medicine, Memphis, Tennessee

John T. Soper, M.D.

Professor, Division of Gynecologic Oncology, Department of Obstetrics and Gynecology, Duke University School of Medicine, Durham, North Carolina

Jana R. Spellman, R.N., C.N.O.R.

Nurse Manager, Trauma/Burn Surgical Services, Department of Trauma Administration, Regional Medical Center at Memphis, Memphis, Tennessee

John F. Steege, M.D.

Chief, Division of Gynecology, and Professor, Department of Obstetrics and Gynecology, University of North Carolina at Chapel Hill School of Medicine, Chapel Hill, North Carolina

Dale W. Stovall, M.D.

Assistant Professor, Department of Obstetrics and Gynecology, University of Iowa College of Medicine; Reproductive Endocrinologist, Department of Obstetrics and Gynecology, University of Iowa Hospitals and Clinics, Iowa City, Iowa

Thomas G. Stovall, M.D.

Associate Professor and Head, Section on Gynecology, Department of Obstetrics and Gynecology, Bowman Gray School of Medicine of Wake Forest University, Winston-Salem, North Carolina

Marc R. Toglia, M.D.

Assistant Professor, Department of Obstetrics and Gynecology and Reproductive Medicine, State University of New York at Stony Brook School of Medicine, Stony Brook, New York

Fidel A. Valea, M.D.

Assistant Professor, Division of Gynecologic Oncology, Department of Obstetrics and Gynecology and Reproductive Medicine, State University of New York at Stony Brook School of Medicine, Stony Brook, New York

Dimitri Voulgaropoulos, M.D.

Chief, Department of Anesthesiology, Carondelet St. Joseph's Hospital, Tucson, Arizona

ACKNOWLEDGMENTS

In order to obtain our goal of making this text state-of-the-art and all-inclusive of vaginal, abdominal, and laparoscopic surgery, it has been necessary to put unrealistic deadlines and burdens upon our authors. We wish to acknowledge their willing, cheerful, and able acceptance of these demands, and to thank them for complying in such an excellent manner.

We also wish to acknowledge and thank Jennifer Mitchell, Vice President, Professional and Reference Publishing, and Jennifer Hardy, Assistant Editor, of Churchill Livingstone. Their guidance, patience, and professionalism contributed significantly to our ability to successfully complete this effort.

CONTENTS

Section V Tubal and Ovarian Surgery

Section VI Urinary Tract Surgery and Repair of Fistulas

Section VII General Gynecologic Surgical Procedures

Section VIII Nonmedical Considerations

INTRODUCTION

WILLIAM J. MANN, JR.
THOMAS G. STOVALL

The discipline of gynecologic surgery encompasses the entire range of procedures on the internal and external female reproductive organs, as well as the procedures necessary to treat pathologic processes of these organs. This extends the domain of the gynecologist beyond that of the abdomen and its contents. Gynecologic surgery is an ever-evolving field, with changes occurring in indications for surgery, surgical techniques and methodologies, and in the outcome expectations of both patients and other health care providers. Questions are being asked by physicians, patients, and third-party payers (which includes state and federal government) as to what outcomes of a given procedure are appropriate, and as to what procedures can be shown to give the best outcome. This is complicated by disagreements over what constitutes the ''best'' outcome, and by a lack of past documentation on the efficacy of surgical procedures. The double-blind, randomized studies that we use to evaluate and compare medical therapies are problematic, if not impossible, to a large extent.

In the not too distant past, and even now, if a surgeon developed a new procedure or a variation of a known procedure, and successfully performed it with what the surgeon and patient believed was a good outcome, there was a considerable likelihood others would learn and attempt this innovation. Over time, as results accumulated, if the outcomes continued to be ''good,'' the procedure would become accepted and added to the gynecologist's armamentarium. Occasionally, as our knowledge of disease and physiology grew and new medical therapies became available, these procedures were found to be based on spurious assumptions or directed at final outcomes of pathologic procedures that could be reversed at an earlier stage. Then the procedure would be abandoned.

The recent explosion of laparoscopic surgery is following just such a course. New procedures and approaches to old problems are being developed rapidly, and nearly all procedures feasible by laporotomy are being attempted laparoscopically. Prospective, randomized studies of these methods are nearly impossible, but must be considered. As with other areas of medicine, hypothesis-driven research is important.

Modern times are also seeing an increased emphasis on cost, cost-effectiveness, and appropriateness of care. These ideas are clear in concept, but murky in application. Quality assessment, continual quality improvement, and outcomes analysis have become theoretical standards by which surgical results can be measured in theory. Yet the difficulty in separating cost considerations from quality outcome analysis—or even in agreeing as to how clear this separation must be—prevents easy application of these new ideas to gynecologic surgery.

To further complicate the situation, consumerism has entered medicine, and we now speak of ''health care providers'' and ''customers.'' Patient input, direction, and demand are even more important than in the past, and simultaneously, the public and government perception of ''runaway health costs'' has led to heated, extensive, and occasionally intelligent discussion of health care rationing. Gynecologists and their patients are no longer the sole determinants of whether an operation is performed, or even what operation will be performed. Preventive medicine is now recognized as the major necessary focus of health care, and it is closely tied to the concept of primary care. The notion of preventive surgery is seldom mentioned. Our specialty of obstetrics and gynecology has been influenced by this perceived need to become involved in primary care, and a significant amount of time in residency will be spent learning the role of the obstetrician and gynecologist as a primary care provider. Simultaneously, although residents must continue to be exposed to the subspecialties, less emphasis will be placed on them. There will be less time for our residents in the operating suite; more procedures and techniques for them to learn, and likely a marked reduction across the nation in the number of operative gynecologic procedures being done.

Rather than curse the darkness or retire into the woods, we have chosen to try to create a textbook that will address all of the above issues. We have selected active, working gynecologic surgeons who spend their days in the operating suite and who are recognized by their peers as experts, and we have asked them to share their skills with the reader. In doing so, we have asked them to include how they have adjusted to the factors mentioned above, that is, how have they changed or modified their indications for a given procedure, if at all, how do they deal with patients pre- and postoperatively in this environment of cost-effectiveness and continued quality assurance. For each open procedure, we have attempted to present the laparoscopic approach or if there is one and to offer a balanced discussion of which approach is best for a given patient. We have encouraged our authors to freely give their opinions as to what does and does not work, what is and is not important, and to tell us why they believe this. Much of gynecologic surgery today is based on common experience, but this area also is new and as yet unproven, or at least, in need of further evaluation.

In addition to specific procedures, we have attempted to present the pertinent anatomy for each section. Complications of specific procedures are given in the text along with the description of the operation, which we believe facilitates an understanding of what can go wrong and why. Furthermore, we have included sections on preoperative evaluation, nutritional support, and diagnostic studies.

This text is aimed at practicing gynecologic surgeons and residents in training who need a reference they can consult before entering the operating room and assisting at or performing a procedure. It is also meant to offer these more experienced surgeons a view of where given procedures fit into their practice today, and how working gynecologists have adapted their techniques to our time.

Just as our discipline of gynecologic surgery is evolving, so too must this text. Input from our readers will be greatly appreciated, and we apologize in advance to those who disagree with us, or who believe we have inappropriately emphasized or neglected a topic. Our authors have done their best to bring a hands-on feeling to the text, and to be authoritative and complete. Failure to do so reflects our editing of their work, not their enthusiasm for this project.

CHAPTER ONE

OPTIMIZATION OF THE PATIENT FOR SURGERY

THOMAS E. NOLAN

Informed Consent
Preoperative Testing
Bowel Preparations
Medical Stabilization
Cardiovascular
Assessment •
Pulmonary Assessment •
Renal Assessment • Fluid
Status • Diabetes Mellitus •
Hypertension • Hepatic
Disease • Colorectal
Cancer • Prophylactic
Antibiotics and Subacute
Bacterial Prophylaxis
Summary

In many cases, the patient who undergoes potentially complex surgery will have multiple medical problems. The time to address these problems is not as the complications arise in the postoperative period, but during the patient's preoperative evaluation. Many postoperative problems can be anticipated when taking the patient's history and administering the physical examination. In the hectic pace of a busy surgical practice, it is tempting to minimize the potential impact of a single symptom or disease. However, addressing these problems systematically in the preoperative evaluation may result in a shorter hospitalization with fewer complications. Patients with severe medical problems should cause the surgeon to rethink the aggressiveness and necessity of the planned operative procedure. Medical conditions can impact on the healing process. A basic understanding of the pathophysiology of a patient's particular disease may help prevent postoperative problems, and a current internal medicine textbook should be available to the surgeon for review of various disease processes, with an appreciation of the impact they may have on perioperative outcomes.

The ongoing demographic shift toward the elderly will impact the practicing gynecologist and make the issues raised in this chapter germane to most practitioners. Geriatric patients often have several physicians caring for them, and are receiving multiple medications. A careful survey for redundant and outdated medications is necessary, to formulate a consolidated medication schedule. Every medication must be reviewed for toxicity, interactions, and the drug's necessity given the patient's current condition. All the patient's other physicians should be informed of the planned procedure, and their recommendations for management sought.

In many cases, the patient's history should be corroborated by the family. This is critical in assessing alcohol use and the use of mood altering drugs. Memory problems or "sun-drowning" should be addressed and related to the nursing staff. Finally, nutritional support and home help should be arranged with the patient and her family preoperatively.

The purpose of this chapter is to introduce a current approach to managing intercurrent medical disease and the necessary preoperative workup. The chapter deliberately excepts diseases that may affect intraoperative and postoperative care; many of the disease entities and drugs mentioned may require additional reading and consultation. The operating surgeon has the responsibility to ensure that the consultants chosen are competent and appropriate. This chapter may be helpful in evaluating care rendered by other physicians. Many internists may not be familiar with operative gynecologic procedures and their impact on the patient. These guidelines will help, and will allow the gynecologist to better appraise the consultant and assist in determining the feasibility of performing surgery. This chapter is meant *to be only a starting point in the initial evaluation of patients for surgery.*

INFORMED CONSENT

A well-informed patient and family, preoperatively, can prevent possible misunderstandings and a litigation mentality postoperatively. "Informed consent is an ethical concept that has become integral to contemporary medical ethics and medical practice."[1] The issue of informed consent rose to prominence during the 1970s, as medical malpractice premiums and litigation increased dramatically.[2] In response to the monetary pressures of medical malpractice claims and liability, the insurance industry and hospital boards began to establish guidelines to educate physicians in informed consent—and hopefully to decrease their own liability.[3]

Prior to the 1970s, the physician acted for the benefit of the patient. Within this concept was some degree of physician-enforced destiny for the patient, which could be interpreted as paternalism. Since then, the concept of autonomy developed (i.e., the patient can participate in her own care). An outgrowth of autonomy is "informed consent" which, it was hoped, would correct physician paternalism and protect patient rights.

Several decision-making models have been advocated.[4] In the traditional model, the physician decides on a particular therapy and the patient, because of trust and confidence in the physician, agrees. Informed consent is an approach wherein the physician decides, but with the patient's knowledge, understanding, and agreement. Collaboration is when both individuals share in the decision-making process with alternative therapies being discussed. The final model is patient choice, wherein the patient makes the decision to proceed, with the physician's counsel. The model that best suits the patient will ultimately determine the nature of consent. Of interest, Green[4] states that most patients will choose the traditional model when asked to choose from these alternatives.

The experienced surgeon has learned that one of the most predictable aspects of surgery is the unpredictable nature of disease and its required operative solutions. Even though the patient may be young with a presumed single disease, additional complicating factors such as pelvic inflammatory disease, endometriosis, extensive cancer, and abdominal adhesions can have significant impact on the intraoperative management of a patient. When extensive disease is discovered during laparotomy, complications of surgery such as inadvertent enterotomy and injury to the urogenital system may lead to possible litigation. In the preoperative evaluation of the patient, dealing with these issue as part of informed consent is mandatory from both an ethical and a legal viewpoint. Despite the negative connotations of informed consent, especially discussing potential demise and injury, it is imperative that the surgeon approach patients in an open and direct fashion, discussing both the risks and benefits of the proposed procedure. Attitudes such as "Don't worry, I am competent enough to take care of this," or "Everything will be fine," may later lead to serious allegations if unexpected problems arise during surgery. In many studies, the proposed procedure was remembered by the patient, but potential complications and poor outcomes were not recalled immediately or at 6 months.[5,6] When possible, a colleague or nurse should be present during the discussion of informed consent to discourage later lapses of memory by well-intentioned families who have received legal advice. It is wise to document your discussion with the patient and the family.

In the event of an injury to the urinary tract or gastrointestinal system, the possibility of repair breakdown and other complications such as bowel obstruction and fistula formation are real. It cannot be overstated that the patient must understand before the surgery that complications are a part of operative intervention, regardless of how insignificant the procedure or how skilled and careful the surgeon. The prudent surgeon should spend enough time with the patient to give her an understanding of informed consent.

Although the most well-informed consent will probably not stop a lawsuit and does not divert responsibility for surgical error, it will result in less undue sympathy toward the plaintiff's allegation of surgical misconduct and provide an ethical basis for the surgeon. It also leads the patient to more honest expectations of her surgeon.

Hospitals have attempted many strategies when obtaining informed consent, such as taping conversations and documenting distribution of patient information pamphlets. Many lawsuits no longer allege problems with informed consent,

---

Informed Consent

A discussion of informed consent should include the following:

- Alternate methods of treatment, including medical if pertinent; also the consequences of declining medical or surgical care
- The dangers of surgery and anesthesia, which may—albeit rarely—result in death or neurologic crippling
- Injuries that can occur during surgery to anything within the abdomen, requiring subsequent repairs; special emphasis should be placed on colostomies and other disfiguring operations
- Complications, such as hemorrhage, infection, and the need for operative consult are possible, even during the best-planned surgery

but are concerned with operative technique and recognition of complications. In filing a malpractice suit, most plaintiffs will add as many potential allegations as possible, to hopefully find one that the jury will find sympathetic, and to ensure that no potential negligence is missed.

Surgeons should develop their own techniques for informing patients and documenting discussions. This author discusses the procedure with the patient and any family members the patient desires to bring along. The discussion is not limited to one encounter, but a second appointment is scheduled before hospitalization. If any questions arise between the initial encounter and the second, the patient is encouraged to write them down. When possible, a preoperative note lists the issues discussed with the patient before the planned admission and procedure. An introductory narrative includes indications for the procedure, further documenting the rationale for surgery, what the patient consented to have performed, and provides a history that may contribute to understanding why additional intraoperative procedures were needed. As stated previously, informed consent has become less important in litigation, but judicious attention to detail in the preoperative discussions may lessen potential liability.

PREOPERATIVE TESTING

Preoperative testing has undergone significant alterations recently. Formerly, many tests were ordered on a purely routine basis without justification, for the sake of "completeness." In the past decade, the use of many routine tests has been discontinued because of their lack of sensitivity and specificity in predicting poor outcomes or changing the surgical approach,[7] and, also to lower medical costs. If a normal test was performed in the previous year, and no obvious indication for retesting has occurred, duplication of tests has not been found useful.[8] By contrast, gynecologists are using imaging more frequently, to select patients who will not benefit from surgery or to obtain tissue for diagnosis of suspicious masses, so that they can better plan combined operative and adjunctive therapy. There has been no documentation that this increased reliance on imaging has improved patient outcomes.

Most schemes for preoperative testing attempt to stratify risk by using age and underlying disease as variables when ordering laboratory and imaging procedures. Routine chest radiographs are rarely useful in patients less than 60 years of age,[9] but the yield of significant lesions increases after age 60.[10] A commonly ordered laboratory test that has been repeatedly shown to not be cost effective is a so-called clotting profile consisting of a prothrombin time (PT), partial thromboplastin time (PTT), and fibrinogen.[11] An intravenous pyelogram (IVP) was a common preoperative imaging test for a pelvic mass prior to the mid-1980s. Most IVPs have been replaced by computed tomography (CT), with contrast

and ultrasound examination obtained for suspicious pelvic masses. The indications for IVP are now limited to cases where prior surgical procedures may have involved the ureter or where ureter entrapment may be present, such as with advanced cases of endometriosis and pelvic inflammatory disease.[12] A preoperative IVP does not prevent ureteral injury, and is not cost effective as a screening procedure. CT scans have commonly been used in workup of pelvic masses suspicious for malignancy and may be helpful in better evaluating disease sites outside of the true pelvis. Magnetic resonance imaging (MRI) is becoming more popular in defining disease spread and in evaluating lymph nodes that may require biopsy, and may change management options from surgery to radiotherapy and/or chemotherapy. Specialty imaging is evolving and is beyond the scope of this chapter. It is unclear, considering the increasing use of surgical staging for gynecologic cancers, whether these preoperative tests alter surgical management or change postoperative outcomes.

Routine chest radiographs in younger patients have been eliminated as have electrocardiograms (ECG). Evidence suggests that women under the age of 55 with no cardiac risk factors do not need a preoperative ECG.[13] Other age-related examinations have been eliminated, such as spirometry in patients over the age of 70 who have no history or risk factors for pulmonary complications.

Recently, physicians at Louisiana State University in New Orleans reassessed and limited preoperative testing to reflect conditions that may have an impact on operative approach or further evaluation before surgery. These recommendations reflect a common sense approach to most patients and are used by both the benign and oncology services.

Preoperative Laboratory Evaluation[a]

- Patients less than 40 years
  - Complete blood count (CBC), urine pregnancy test (UPT)
- Patients 40–60 years
  - CBC, electrocardiogram (ECG), electrolytes, creatinine, glucose (if on medication affecting potassium or glucose, diabetes type unimportant), chest radiograph (if history of pulmonary disease)
- Patients greater than 60 years
  - CBC, electrolytes, creatinine, glucose, ECG, chest radiograph

---

[a] Used at Louisiana State University at New Orleans.

Complete blood count (CBC) results obtained 3 weeks before surgery are acceptable while electrolyte, creatinine, and glucose testing is recommended 72 hours before surgery. Liver function testing should be limited to patients with suspected alcohol related diseases or suspected hepatitis. An ECG or chest radiograph can be done anytime in the 6 months before surgery, as long as the patient's clinical condition has not changed.

If the patient is less than 40 years old and healthy, a CBC within 2 to 3 weeks and a urine pregnancy test (UPT) within 1 week of her anticipated surgery is suggested. If the patient is bleeding or anemic, a CBC is ordered the day before surgery.

UPTs should be done on all menstruating women who have not undergone a sterilization procedure. The UPT should be done within 1 week of surgery. At some institutions, serum B-HCG can be performed more quickly and cheaply.

Type and screens for potential transfusion should only be drawn in open major cases. Laparoscopic cases, dilation and currettage (D&C), cone biopsies, and laser cases do not need a type and screen unless clinical judgment dictates a reasonable chance of transfusion. Type and screens are only good for 72 hours. In addition, it is uncertain whether these tests are helpful in the nonanemic patient prior to surgery.

A commonly ordered laboratory test that has been repeatedly shown to not be cost effective is a clotting profile consisting of a prothrombin time (PT), partial thromboplastin time (PTT), and fibrinogen. This should only be ordered if the patient has a suspicious history of bleeding disorders, has a known deficiency in clotting factors, or is currently on anticoagulants that affect the prothrombin or partial thromboplastin time. If evaluation is necessary, a bleeding time is probably a better screening test.

Electrolyte, creatinine, and glucose testing (CHEM 7 or SMA 7) should only be ordered on patients aged 40 to 60 if they take medications that effect renal function (e.g., potassium wasting diuretics). All patients over 60 years of age should have the test. The results are good for 72 hours.

Chest radiographs should be ordered on patients from 40 to 60 years old if they have pulmonary disease, and on all patients more than 60 years old if not performed in the previous 6 months.

ECGs should be ordered on all patients over 40 years of age and are good for 6 months.

Syphilis serology should be considered on all patients undergoing surgery, but is not mandatory. Human immunodeficiency virus (HIV) testing may also be appropriate in selected patients.

Medical consultation should be reserved for patients who have severe systemic diseases, especially if recently unstable. Medical consultation should be carefully considered and should ask specific questions, especially in regard to medication administration in the perioperative period and possible fluid problems. It is not appropriate to seek consultation for "medical clearance for surgery" in a patient with no defined medical problem.

Patients taking one or two antihypertensives with stable blood pressure do not generally require medical consultation. Patients with noninsulin-dependent diabetes (type II) with fasting blood sugars less than 200 mg/L do not require preoperative clearance. Patients who have a single medical problem that is stable should not receive routine medical consultation. However, medical consultation should be obtained for patients with unstable hypertension, a history of cardiovascular disease including myocardial infarction, a history of pulmonary edema, a history of severe steroid-dependent asthma, heavy cigarette use with suspicion of chronic obstructive pulmonary disease, and patients with connective tissue disease who are taking multiple medications.

Incentive spirometry should be encouraged preoperatively in patients with a greater than 40 packs per year history of cigarette use. It is no longer mandatory for patients over the age of 70. If incentive spirometry is taught to all patients before major procedures, the incidence of atelectasis or pneumonia may be reduced.

BOWEL PREPARATIONS

Most gynecologic surgery does not involve operative procedures on the bowel, but in some cases, the risk of unintentional injury to the bowel is high. During the evaluation of a case, an appraisal of the possibility of bowel surgery is appropriate and, if high, the gastrointestinal tract should be prepared. Proper bowel preparation will prevent fecal spillage into the peritoneal cavity and reduce the risk of infection or the need for colostomy. Many different approaches to bowel preparation are used and these usually reflect the experience and training of the surgeon. Effective bowel preparation should minimize patient discomfort and physiologic alterations, especially dehydration.

If a bowel preparation is performed, the assessment of fluid status prior to surgery should be considered (see the section on fluid status below). Electrolytes lost in bowel fluid approximate 0.5 normal saline. Fluid lost will be replaced by shifting fluid from the extracellular space into the intravascular space and then into the bowel lumen. This will result in fluid shifting from the intracellular space into the extracellular space. This will be reflected most often by a positive "tilt" test or a rising blood urea nitrogen (BUN), the net result being a decrease intravascular volume. Before anesthesia induction, hydration should aim to expand the diminished intravascular volume. Otherwise, the impact of intraoperative blood loss will be magnified.

Much of stool bulk is composed of live and dead bacteria. Normal bowel flora contains over 20 species of aerobes and over 50 species of anaerobes. *Escherichia coli* is the most common aerobe and *Bacteroides* spp. the most common anaerobe. These organisms are the most common contaminates

Indications for Bowel Preparation

- Potential for bowel resection is high (e.g., previous bowel surgery or ruptured appendix)
- History of advanced benign pelvic disease such as endometriosis or pelvic inflammatory disease
- "Frozen pelvis" on pelvic examination
- Disease has obliterated the rectal vaginal septum
- Suspected ovarian pathology or any suspicious adnexal mass, especially postmenopausal
- Possible bowel involvement on preoperative imaging
- History of diverticular disease
- History of pelvic radiation
- History of multiple pelvic surgeries or abdominal explorations
- Possible gastrointestinal involvement or colonic carcinoma
- Possibility of urologic pathology requiring conduit diversion

found in septic wounds after colon surgery. In the absence of antibiotic prophylaxis, wound infection rates range from 32 to 58 percent and infectious complications may be as high as 75 percent.[14] This suggests a need for antibiotic preparation combined with mechanical cleansing of the colon.

There are few contraindications for bowel preparation. The author and his colleagues have discontinued using osmotic high volume bowel preparations in patients undergoing repair of rectovaginal fistulas. Osmotic agents remain in the lumen for more than 12 hours and continue to drain once the patient is relaxed from anesthesia. This leads to continued fecal contamination during surgery. To avoid liquid stool in the operating field, only simple enemas are given the night before surgery. Other exclusion criteria include patients who cannot tolerate the mechanical aspects of the protocol, suspected bowel obstruction, ileus, and surgical emergency.[15]

Bowel preparation includes a mechanical cleansing of the bowel lumen to remove feces and reduce bacterial load. The ideal preparation should have a minimal alteration in the balance of body fluids and electrolytes with no significant alteration in nutritional and immunologic parameters. Patient acceptance and compliance should be sought by explaining the process and what the patient can expect to experience. Basic preparations use enemas, cathartics, liquid diets, and whole gut irrigation with a variety of solutions such as Ringer's lactate or normal saline, osmotics (e.g., mannitol), and nonosmotics (e.g., polyethelene glycol [Golytely, Braintree

Laboratories, Braintree, MA]).[16] Antibiotics are administered preoperatively either by mouth, enema, or parenterally, to reduce colony counts.

Extended preoperative diets of clear liquids are associated with a negative nitrogen balance unless low residue, nutritionally complete formulas are added. Unless the liquids are totally absorbed in the small bowel, any residue in the colon acts as bacterial media. Whole gut irrigation uses large volumes of electrolyte solutions through the gut. Volumes as high as 4 to 15 L have been used and were associated with significant sodium and fluid retention. Up to 2 L of free water can be absorbed. Symptoms vary from nausea to vomiting and abdominal pain, and present in 28 to 48 percent of patients.

Many early protocols to bowel preparation involved mannitol, an osmotically active agent commonly used during whole gut lavage. A significant problem with mannitol use is overgrowth of *E. coli*, which can contribute to sepsis. Most importantly, however, extracellular fluid was transferred from the bowel wall into the bowel lumen, leading to systemic dehydration.[17] These fluid shifts necessitated the addition of a balanced electrolyte solution to prevent dehydration and possible problems during the induction of anesthesia.

Preparations of polyethylene glycol in combination with a balanced electrolyte solution are currently the preferred bowel preparatory solution. These solutions may eliminate problems with whole gut irrigation. Polyethylene glycol acts as an iso-osmotic cathartic that is not absorbed from the gut and is nonfermentable by colonic bacteria, eliminating overgrowth of colonic bacteria. A sulfate group is substituted for a chloride in the preparation, which blocks the absorption of sodium and chloride cancelling the usual electrical and chemical gradient and preventing potassium exchange. These advantages result in minimal weight change with minimal alterations in water and electrolyte balance.[18] Disadvantages include nausea, a sensation of abdominal fullness, bloating, and a "salty taste," which may be improved by chilling. This can be done in an outpatient setting.

Controversy exists about whether oral or parenteral antibiotics given preoperatively are more effective in preventing postoperative infections. Neomycin, erythromycin, and metronidazole are the antibiotics must commonly used. Each of these antibiotics will lower colony counts of bowel flora. Neomycin is not absorbed from the gut, which limits its effectiveness in preventing sepsis; however, erythromycin and metronidazole are well absorbed and attain therapeutic serum levels. Erythromycin is associated with significant gastrointestinal discomfort. Because of the side effects and questions of efficacy, many surgeons have abandoned oral antibiotics for parenteral antibiotics.[19] Antibiotic regimens should be commenced before surgery to ensure adequate tissue levels (see below). The use of metronidazole or clindamycin alone is not effective because of poor gram-negative organism coverage. An aminoglycoside or third-generation cephalosporin should be added to metronidazole to broaden

Scheme for Preoperative Bowel Preparation

- Morning before surgery
  - Mix Golytely[a] solution and refrigerate
- Early afternoon before surgery
  - 4 L administered either orally or via a nasogastric tube over 3 hours (20–30 ml/min or 1.8 L/h)
  - Diarrhea usually begins within 40 minutes
  - Rectal effluent clears within 3 hours
- Evening of surgery (optional for elderly and admitted patients)
  - Begin intravenous fluids (5 percent dextrose with 0.5 normal saline and 20 mEq potassium chloride) at 75 to 125 ml/h (lower infusion rate in the elderly or in patients with left ventricular dysfunction)
- Morning of surgery
  - Begin intravenous fluids if not previously started
  - Administer antibiotics parenterally before induction of anesthesia
  - Suggested antibiotic regimen: third-generation cephlosprorin (cefotaxime, ceftizoxime) with either clindamycin 600 mg or metronidazole 500 mg

[a] Braintree Laboratories, Inc., Braintree, MA
(From Messing and Nolan,[15] with permission.)

coverage. Before surgery, the anesthesiologist should be appraised that a bowel preparation was performed and by which method. Perioperative fluid replacement may be affected by the type of bowel preparation.

If the bowel preparation is done on an outpatient basis, blood studies done the morning before surgery will demonstrate decreased intravascular volume. Intravenous hydration will help prevent intraoperative hypotension and oliguria, but require at least several hours of hospitalization.

MEDICAL STABILIZATION

Cardiovascular Assessment

The incidence of cardiovascular disease in the aging woman is currently being reassessed. Overall, cardiovascular disease affects one in four Americans.[20] Coronary artery disease is usually of later onset in women, but is responsible for almost 50 percent of all female cardiovascular events. Because the mortality is high, most testing has been directed toward identifying the patient at risk of coronary artery events. Additionally, because of an increase in the population over the age of 65 in the United States, the number of coronary events is projected to increase. It is estimated that the number of noncardiac surgical procedures will increase by 50 percent over the next 30 years,[21] and this increase will include the perioperative period. The number of patients undergoing noncardiac surgery with cardiovascular disease can be expected to double from 6 to 12 million during this time. Death from cardiovascular disease will remain a leading cause of postoperative mortality.[22]

Myocardial Ischemia

The incidence of intraoperative and postoperative ischemia and infarction is unknown. Perioperative ischemia may be induced by hypertension, anemia, hypoxemia, and tachycardia. Postoperative ischemia is thought to be silent and may occur up to 7 days after surgery.[23] The incidence of myocardial infarction in the general population is low (0.0 to 0.7 percent),[24] but increases to 1.8 percent in patients over the age of 40.[25] Factors that may contribute to perioperative ischemia/infarction include

1. Vasospasm secondary to release of stress-related humoral mediators[26]
2. Enhanced platelet aggregation due to changes in coronary artery perfusion due to vascular tone, blood pressure, and cardiac contractibility[27,28]

The difficulty in assessing any one of these variables as a single etiologic event is formidable. However, with existing coronary artery stenosis, any single factor could exacerbate already decreased flow, thereby inducing ischemia or infarction. Patient death from perioperative myocardial infarction ranges from 36 to 70 percent, underscoring the importance of recognition of risk factors in an attempt to limit these events.[25]

In the past 30 years, an increase in female cigarette smokers has resulted in a similar rise in overall cardiovascular risk and disease. Also, other medical conditions contribute to atherosclerotic heart disease and become more prevalent after age 40. Diabetes mellitus (both insulin and noninsulin dependent) and hypertension are both more common after age 40 and may contribute to atherosclerotic heart disease. Poorly controlled diabetes mellitus results in an unfavorable lipid profile, accelerating atherosclerotic deposition in peripheral and coronary arteries. Long-standing hypertension has been associated with coronary artery disease, as untreated hypertension may cause myocardial thickening, decreasing blood flow to the myocardium and resulting in ischemia.

The astute clinician will obtain a detailed history of chest pain and dyspnea, especially in women who have not received estrogen replacement therapy. A history of chest pain (regardless of how atypical) before any anesthetic will usually require preoperative cardiac testing. Atypical chest pain is usually defined as any chest pain syndrome that is not associated with exertion, stress, or radiation to the left arm or jaw. Dyspnea and cardiac insufficiency may be difficult to differentiate and usually require more involved workups, including spirometry and thallium scanning. Assessment of

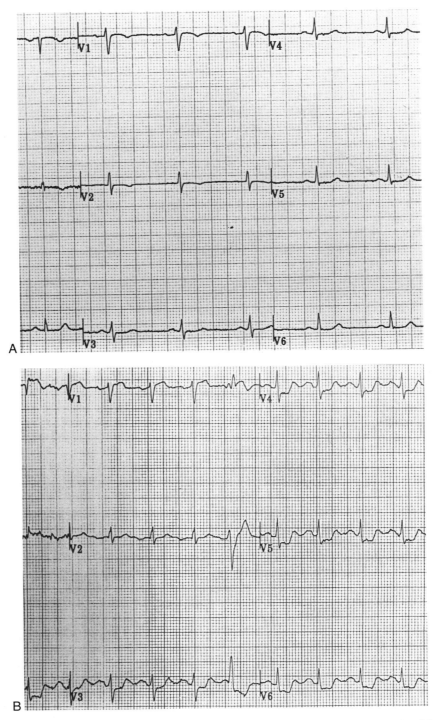

Fig. 1-1. Pre- and postexercise stress test. (**A**) In the pre-exercise electrocardiogram, note the levels of the ST segments. (**B**) After exercise, ST depression is obvious in the precordial leads, significant for anterior wall ischemia.

women for angina or cardiac insufficiency is made more difficult because of the relative lack of sensitivity and specificity of commonly used testing paradigms for coronary artery disease. This is especially true for resting ECGs and exercise stress testing (EST)[29] (Fig. 1-1). Due to the limited prognostic significance of EST in women, thallium scanning may have more utility. Thallium is a potassium analogue that is distributed through the myocardium and provides information concerning myocardial perfusion and viability. Thallium scanning is a dynamic representation of cardiac function with high sensitivity and specificity. A dynamic display of myocardial blood flow (or absence) and wall motion abnormalities suggests prior infarctions.[30] The major limitations of this test are expense and the difficulty of selecting patients who will benefit from the procedure. All abnormalities of myocardial perfusion or ventricular wall motion should be considered indications for cardiac catheterization.

Patients with stable angina are at no higher risk than other patients for anesthesia.[31] Stable angina occurs when the onset of chest pain is predictable, while unstable angina is unpredictable, with a changing pattern of frequency and/or intensity. Unstable angina, especially if occurring over several weeks, may herald an impending infarction. In a prospective study that attempted to predict perioperative complications in geriatric patients, the most important variable was the patients' ability to increase their heart rate above 99 beats/min.[32] Elderly patients who are unable to exercise may require a pharmacologic stress test using dipyridamole, a drug that causes maximum coronary vasodilation. This testing should be reserved for patients with a significant history of symptoms or prior cardiac disease.[32] The use of digitalis has decreased in recent years; however, patients on digitalis should have levels drawn preoperatively. Hypokalemia, which may result in terminal arrhythmia, must be avoided.

Patients who have a prior history of myocardial infarction should be closely assessed for myocardial dysfunction. Patients with normal ejection fractions and without histories of congestive heart failure (CHF) or pulmonary edema are at much lower risk of perioperative complications than patients that have been symptomatic. Goldman et al.,[33,34] in 1977, reported a classification of criteria for patients at high risk of major cardiopulmonary problems in the postoperative period. Patients with evidence of left ventricular failure manifested by gallop rhythms, CHF or pulmonary edema are at high risk.

Valvular Heart Disease and Cardiomyopathy

If valvular heart disease is suspected due to murmurs detected during the physical examination, an echocardiogram is valuable in the search for cardiomegaly or valvular disease. Echocardiography is less expensive than thallium scanning and produces information on cardiac wall dynamics,

---

Predictors of Perioperative Cardiac Morbidity

- Age
- Previous myocardial infarction
- Unstable angina
- Congestive heart failure
- Hypertension
- Diabetes mellitus
- Dysrhythmias
- Valvular heart disease
- Lipidemias
- Cigarette smoking
- Previous coronary artery surgery
- Sudden withdrawal of cardiac medications (β-blockers, nitrates, and calcium channel blockers)

---

ejection fraction, and potential valvular disease. Aortic sclerosis or stenosis (systolic murmur grade II or greater in the right second intercostal space, radiating to the neck) is the most common valvular lesion in the elderly, and should be evaluated by echocardiogram (Fig. 1-2). If any significant abnormalities are displayed in other preoperative testing or scanning, cardiac catheterization may be recommended. Cardiac catheterization remains the gold standard in assessing coronary arteries, wall function, ejection fraction, and valvular competence. Patients with significant coronary artery disease may require revascularization via coronary angioplasty before undergoing major surgery (surgery of significant duration and morbidity),[35] or coronary artery bypass grafting before noncardiac surgery,[36] and certainly, involvement of a cardiologist in the postoperative care.

Patients who have mild, stable cardiac symptoms and an ejection fraction of greater than 40 percent are usually not at significantly higher operative risk. Patients with ejection fractions of less than 40 percent should be considered (normal is 55 to 60 percent, determined by multiple gated acquisition [MUGA] scanning). A pulmonary artery catheter (PAC) is not mandatory in patients with ejection fractions between 30 and 40 percent but central vein access should be placed via either internal jugular or subclavian catheterization prior to surgery. The procedure is shown in detail in Figures 1-3 to 1-6 and is further described in other sources.[37] A patient with an ejection fraction of less than 30 percent is at high risk, and a PAC is strongly recommended. Judicious fluid management is of paramount importance in patients with any history of left ventricular dysfunction. Elderly patients with massive ascites from ovarian cancer and multiple risk factors for cardiovascular problems should also be considered for central access and a possible PAC, regard-

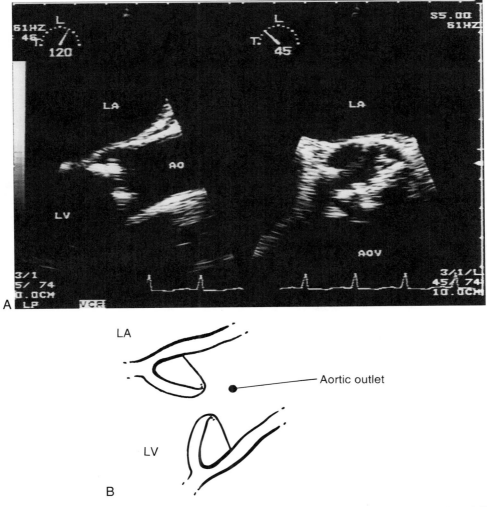

Fig. 1-2. **(A)** Echocardiogram of aortic stenosis with **(B)** explanatory drawing. An echocardiogram with calcified aortic valves from a bicuspid aorta. In normal individuals, uncalcified valves are not as well defined. LA, left atrial; LV, left ventricle; AO, aortic outlet; AOV,

less of the stability of their cardiac function, because of the extreme fluid shifts and intraoperative fluid needs. Patients who have ejection fractions of less than 20 percent should be considered only for emergency or lifesaving surgery, despite the nature of their complaints. If surgery needs to be accomplished in individuals with extremely low ejection fractions, a PAC is mandatory, as is close supervision during the perioperative period. Surgical procedures in these patients lasting more than 2 to 3 hours or procedures with potential fluid shifts (i.e., ovarian cancer with ascites) require a PAC.

Patients who have normal ejection fractions and minimal evidence of chamber enlargement or compromise may be best served by central venous access without a PAC. A bias of many cardiologists is that the induction of anesthesia and the immediate postoperative 12 to 14 hours is the critical time period for patients with ventricular wall abnormalities

and valvular disease. However, the period when third space mobilization of intraoperative fluids begins is 48 to 72 hours postoperatively, and is a time when the clinician should observe for late onset pulmonary edema. It is a mistake to remove both central lines and *access* 24 hours after the initial surgical event, to simplify care. Removal of the PAC is indicated because of the increased incidence of infections and other complications associated with it; however, central access should be used until approximately the third postoperative day. Central lines should be inserted only when you have determined they are needed; they should be removed only after the risk period has passed.

Perioperative Concerns

Chest pain evaluation should not be delayed. Historical aspects such as onset, duration of pain, and areas of radiation should be assessed. *It should never be assumed that chest*

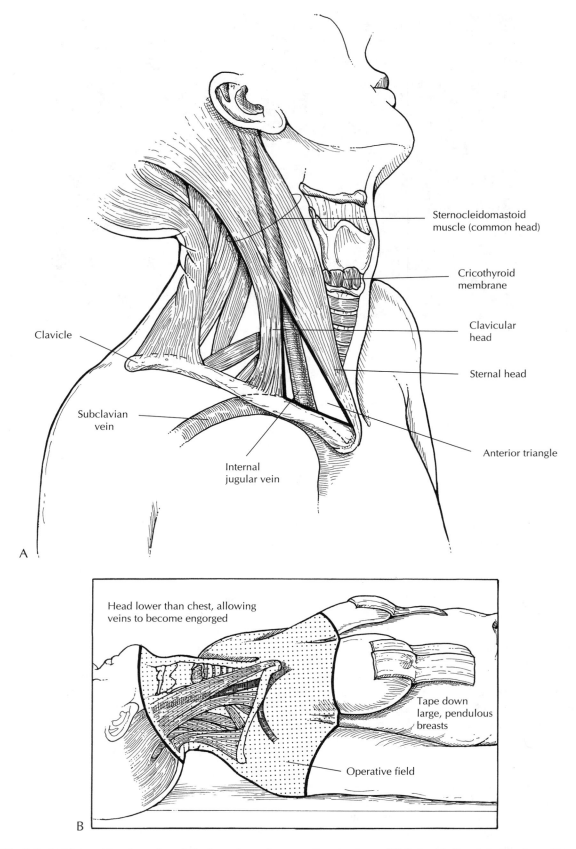

Sternocleidomastoid muscle (common head)

Cricothyroid membrane

Clavicular head

Clavicle

Sternal head

Subclavian vein

Anterior triangle

Internal jugular vein

A

Head lower than chest, allowing veins to become engorged

Tape down large, pendulous breasts

Operative field

B

Fig. 1-3. **(A)** Internal jugular vein, subclavian vein, and surrounding structures. **(B)** Patient in Trendelenburg's position for catheterization of either the internal jugular vein or subclavian vein.

pain is caused by gastrointestinal disease. After the history is taken the physical examination should be performed with special emphasis on neck vein distension (a common symptom of fluid overload or left ventricular dysfunction from ischemia) and gallop rhythms (suggestive of CHF). The chest examination should include close auscultation for rales in the posterior basilar region of the lungs, the most common site for pulmonary edema. Laboratory studies should include an arterial blood gas, ECG, and chest radiograph. Diabetics may have silent ischemia, and transfer to a cardiac care unit (CCU) may be warranted. Pulmonary embolism is the silent killer: any sudden onset of chest pain should be evaluated

with the above studies, blood gases, and a ventilation/perfusion scan or pulmonary angiogram as indicated. If the patient is hypotensive or has a change in vital signs, transfer to an intensive care unit (ICU) should be considered early in the course of evaluation. Consultation with an internist should never be delayed if myocardial infarction or pulmonary embolism is suspected. New onset congestive heart failure—especially if the patient has had no prior history of left ventricular failure—should be considered to be a myocardial infarction until that diagnosis is ruled out with a standard protocol (serial ECGs, serial enzymes, and telemetry monitoring).

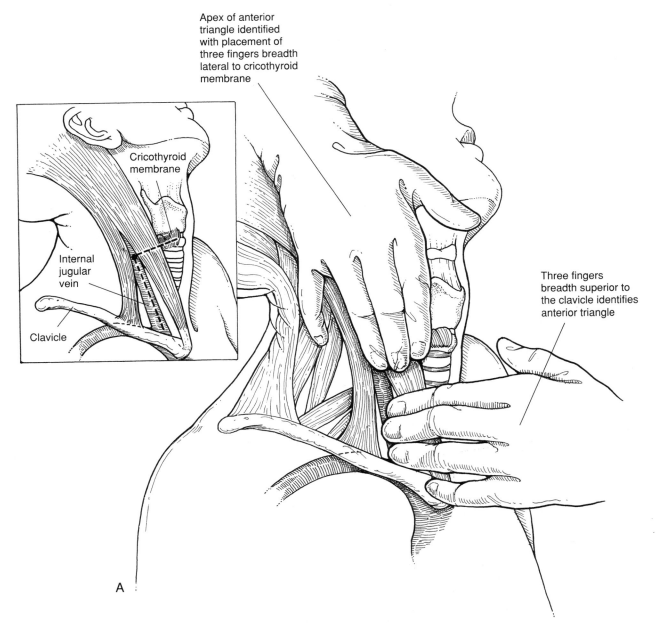

Apex of anterior triangle identified with placement of three fingers breadth lateral to cricothyroid membrane

Cricothyroid membrane

Internal jugular vein

Clavicle

Three fingers breadth superior to the clavicle identifies anterior triangle

A

Fig. 1-4. Internal jugular vein approach. **(A)** Careful palpation allows for proper needle placement. *(Figure continues).*

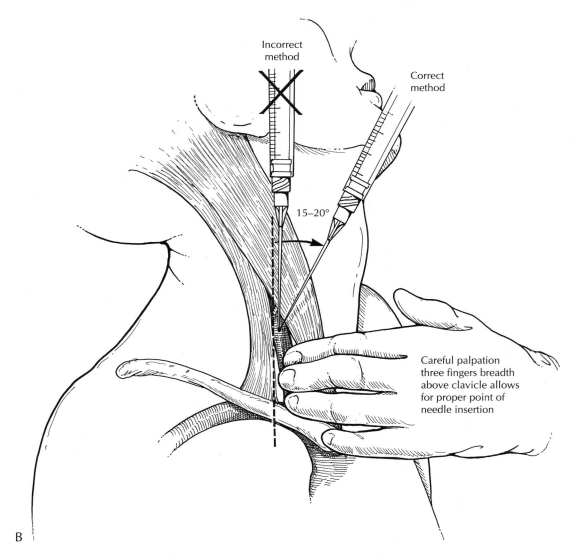

Incorrect
method

Correct
method

15–20°

Careful palpation
three fingers breadth
above clavicle allows
for proper point of
needle insertion

B

Fig. 1-4. *(Continued).* **(B)** Correct needle placement. The needle should *not* be parallel to the neck but should be at a 15- to 20-degree angle to the neck.

Fluid management is probably underappreciated by many gynecologic surgeons, because many of their patients are young. This thinking may change, especially with the increase in aggressive procedures for pelvic prolapse, incontinence, and oncology. Any abdominal procedure will have third spacing and the possibility of hemorrhage. The most difficult patients are those who undergo massive fluid shifts due to advanced ovarian cancer. Patients with ejection fractions of less than 30 percent may be extremely sensitive to salt-containing solutions. The patient with cardiomyopathy should be closely assessed to determine whether the risk/benefit ratio supports the performance of surgery. Stabilization of any additional medical conditions such as diabetes (osmotic diuresis) and introduction of new pharmaceutical agents should be evaluated before surgery. Most agents used in the care of these patients are available in both oral and parenteral forms; however, potency may vary with the route given.

The operating surgeon and internist/cardiologist should carefully design a fluid management and medication scheme before surgery. The anesthesiologist should also be included in the evaluation of these patients and overall supervision should be decided before the case begins. The needs of the anesthesiologist, surgeon, and cardiologist differ, and surgeons should have a very keen (and honest) appreciation of their limitations. If any conflicts or questions are raised preoperatively, these issues can be rectified before surgery. Accurate calculation of estimated blood loss and fluid needs should be documented and communicated during the case. Bowel preparations, the length of fluid restriction time, and agents that alter intravascular volume (diuretics) have to be appreciated when calculating fluid needs. Close assessment

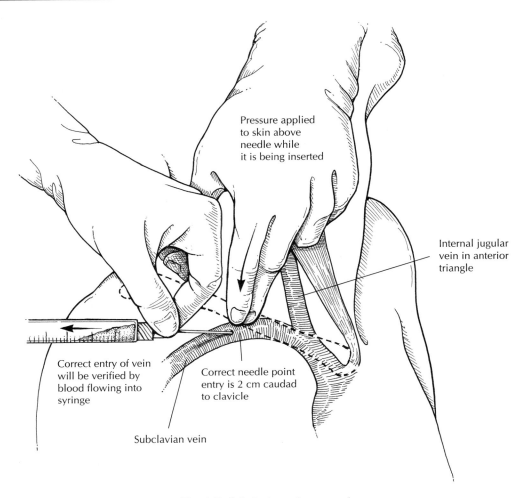

Pressure applied to skin above needle while it is being inserted

Internal jugular vein in anterior triangle

Correct entry of vein will be verified by blood flowing into syringe

Correct needle point entry is 2 cm caudad to clavicle

Subclavian vein

Fig. 1-5. Subclavian vein approach.

of intake and output is mandatory, especially during the first 12 hours. In many cases, the fluid needs of the patient are probably underestimated; however, in the elderly patient, in whom fluid needs are lessened, this may be less critical. The patient with low muscle mass and volume, especially the frail elderly patient, should not receive the standard 125 ml/hr of fluid. The urinary flow of these patients should be monitored closely and they should be started on 50 to 75 ml/hr. Patients over the age of 60 generally have reduced glomerular filtration rates of 60 to 75 ml/min. Drug excretion and fluid needs should be addressed immediately after surgery and on an ongoing basis during the postoperative period.

Finally, patients who are compromised by severe cardiovascular disease should be considered for immediate postoperative care in an intensive care environment. This is especially true in patients who have undergone long surgical procedures with blood loss in excess of 1,500 ml and/or who have received large volumes of intraoperative fluids, including blood products. Additionally, after prolonged procedures mechanical ventilation for the first 8 to 16 hours

postoperatively, with close monitoring via arterial line and pulse oximetry, may limit cardiopulmonary complications. Cases need to be considered individually; however, the prudent surgeon will evaluate the needs for monitoring and close nursing support in the postoperative period.

Pulmonary Assessment

Work of breathing is an important concept to understand when approaching problems in the perioperative patient. It is the summation of the actions of the thorax, diaphragm, intercostal muscles, accessory muscles, and expiratory muscles, which together effect oxygenation and ventilation. Elasticity and compliance of lung tissues require energy to overcome static forces and enact effective respiration. Underlying cardiopulmonary disease may be exacerbated by anesthesia and surgery. Lung capacities, the ability to ventilate and oxygenate, changing transairway and transpulmonary pressures are important variables that are altered when anesthesia and pain control are administered peri and postop-

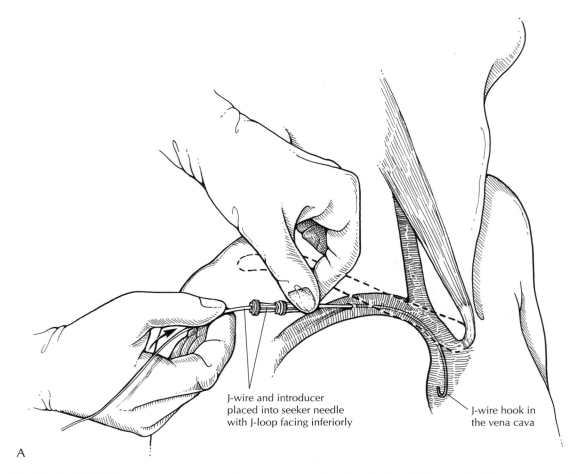

J-wire and introducer
placed into seeker needle
with J-loop facing inferiorly

J-wire hook in
the vena cava

A

Fig. 1-6. (A & B) Catheterization procedure after correct insertion of needle in subclavian vein. *(Figure continues).*

eratively. The patient with marginal pulmonary function or poor nutrition may decompensate by an inability to remove carbon dioxide because of the increased metabolic demands of major surgery.

Spirometric reports are complex, with multiple measurements, but only three are crucial in most cases: (1) spirometric standards vary for sex and height; (2) forced vital capacity (FVC) is the measure of a patient's ability to quickly expire as much air as possible with no time limitation; (3) the FEV_1 (forced expiratory volume at 1 second) is a segment of FVC measured during the initial second of expiration.

A low FEV_1 is consistent with obstructive airway disease or patient effort. Common etiologies are cigarette smoking that results in chronic obstructive pulmonary disease (COPD) or reversible bronchospasm (asthma). Chronic obstructive pulmonary disease is usually secondary to cigarette abuse and is an outflow obstruction of breathing. Patients commonly have dyspnea with minimal exercise (one to two flights of stairs) and pursed lip breathing. The FEV_1 may identify early, subtle clues of obstructive airway disease, but only when patient effort is good. Patients at high risk of perioperative complications should be considered for testing.

Limitations of spirometric testing derive from variation in patient morphologic characteristics. The ratio of FEV_1 to FVC was developed to compensate for these variables. The ratio of FEV_1 to FVC is a percentage useful in interpreting degrees of broncho-obstruction, with patients serving as their own standard. Values of 65 to 80 percent are consistent with mild obstruction; 55 to 65 percent is considered moderate obstruction; and less than 55 percent is severe obstruction. A normal 40-year-old woman who is 65 inches tall (165 cm) should have an FVC of 3.6 L and an FEV_1 of 2.8 L, which equals an $FEV_1/FVC\%$ of 77 percent. Patients with moderate to severe disease may require mechanical ventilation postoperatively, and an intensive care unit bed should be considered, with appropriate consultants available.

Arterial blood gases are an easy and quick measure of the ability to oxygenate and ventilate. Oxygenation, ventilation, and systemic acid-base balance are obtained. "Normal" values are age dependent, so older patients have different "normal" values than younger patients. Primarily, the ability to oxygenate decreases with age. A 60-year-old patient will have a normal PO_2 (partial pressure of oxygen) in the low 80s, while the 80-year-old patient may have a PO_2 as low as 60 to 65 mmHg (the rule of "60 = 80 and 80 = 60"). The most

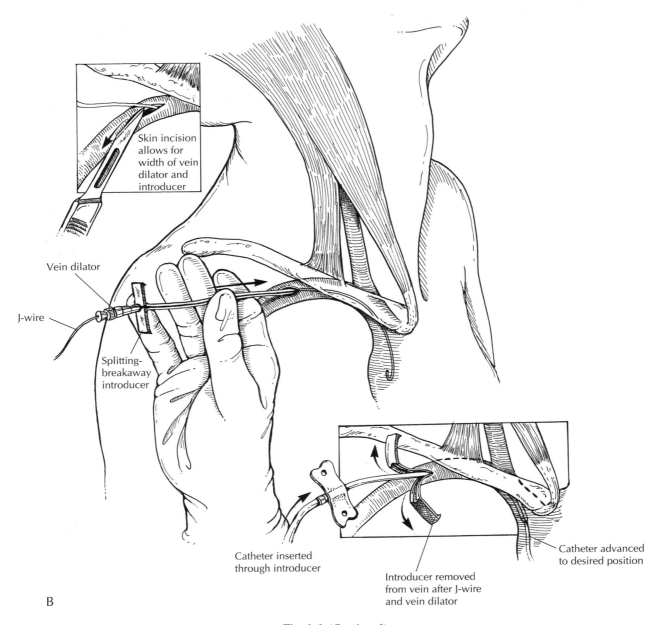

Skin incision allows for width of vein dilator and introducer

Vein dilator

J-wire

Splitting-breakaway introducer

Catheter inserted through introducer

Introducer removed from vein after J-wire and vein dilator

Catheter advanced to desired position

B

Fig. 1-6 *(Continued).*

important parameter on an arterial blood gas, however, is the PCO_2. Patients with PCO_2 higher than 45 mmHg, regardless of age, are at significant risk of postoperative problems.

Pulmonary conditions are becoming more prevalent in women over the past two decades as the incidence of cigarette smoking has increased. Patients with a greater than 40 pack year history of smoking should be considered for pulmonary function testing (PFT).[38] Other common indications for pulmonary testing are a history of asthma or any type of reversible bronchospastic disease. PFT should be performed with and without bronchodilators and also with a companion arterial blood gas. Age greater than 70 is no longer a criteria for pulmonary function testing. Any patients

with a history of dyspnea on exertion or chest pain syndrome should be considered for pulmonary function testing.[39]

Patients with a history suggestive of restrictive lung disease should also have pulmonary function testing. This is especially important in patients who have undergone radiotherapy or who give a history of sarcoidosis. Patients with central nervous system disorders that may affect respiratory drive, such as neuromuscular disease (e.g., multiple sclerosis and myasthenia gravis) should be tested. The immediate postoperative period, especially during the recovery from anesthesia, will require frequent monitoring. Close nursing and respiratory therapy support should be available during the first few days of the postoperative period.

Risk Factors for Postoperative Pulmonary Complications

- Age greater than 70
- Cigarette smoking (especially more than 40 pack years)
- Pre-existing pulmonary disease
- Excessive sputum production
- Obesity greater than 120 percent of expected weight
- Location of surgical procedure (upper abdomen > lower abdomen > vaginal incision)
- Neuromuscular disease (multiple sclerosis or myasthenia gravis)
- PCO_2 greater than 45 mmHg, PO_2 less than 70 mmHg on arterial blood gas
- Spirometric parameters
  - FVC of less than 50 percent after adjusting for age and sex
  - FEV_1/FVC of 65 to 75 percent equals mildly increased risk
  - FEV_1/FVC of 50 to 65 percent equals moderately increased risk
  - FEV_1/FVC of less than 50 percent equals markedly increased risk

Abbreviations: FVC, forced vital capacity; FEV_1, forced expiratory volume at 1 second.
(From Nolan,[81] with permission.)

Postoperative Concerns

The most common postoperative pulmonary problem is atelectasis. Individuals who are at high risk of postoperative atelectasis should receive instruction on the use of incentive spirometers preoperatively. If possible, cigarette smokers should stop smoking approximately 8 weeks before surgery and should be instructed on the use of incentive spirometers.[40] Goblet cells and ciliary cells may be damaged in smokers. Goblet cells are important because of a mucoid-like material they secrete that entraps foreign bodies and infectious agents. Ciliated cells protect the lower respiratory tract by moving secretions to the epiglottis, hypopharynx, and mouth, creating the mucociliary escalator. Endotracheal intubation and anesthetic gases impede the effectiveness of the mucociliary escalator and may contribute to postoperative pneumonias.

The primary function of the upper airways is to humidify and warm gases. In the immediate postoperative period, sup-plemental oxygen is given to prevent hypoxia from altered respiratory effort when recovering from anesthesia. If humidification and heat are not supplied by the nose, they are supplied by the mucosa and the mucosal blanket of the bronchotrachial tree. Inadequate humidification of inspired gases in the upper airway may cause lower airway problems such as blockages from retained, hardened secretions and mucus plugging. These secretions limit the natural ability to fight infections using the mucociliary tree. Figure 1-7 reviews the potential complications of retained secretions. Humidification is easily implemented by bubbling oxygen through water or the bubbling diffusion technique. These devices are adequate for the patient who is breathing spontaneously without an endotracheal tube. The intubated patient needs to have warmed air/oxygen mixtures because the upper airway is bypassed. The goals of bronchial hygiene are given in the boxed list below.

Important prognosticators for atelectasis and postoperative pneumonia are directly related to the surgical incision site. Upper abdominal incisions are associated with significantly more pulmonary problems than patients with lower abdominal or vaginal incisions.[41] The ability of the patient to cough and breathe deeply is compromised by upper abdominal incisions due to the pain and diaphragmatic dysfunction of altered phrenic nerve output.[42] Patients who have high incisions due to obesity, large masses above the umbilicus, or oncologic procedures should use incentive spirometers for at least 48 to 72 hours postoperatively. The use of intermittent positive pressure has fallen in disfavor and should be eliminated from practice. Blow bottles, a form of intermittent positive pressure in which fluid is pushed between two containers by blowing, were commonly used in the 1970s and early 1980s. Closed airways and alveoli were

Goals of Bronchial Hygiene Therapy

- Restore and maintain mucus blanket
- Hydrate dried, retained secretions
- Humidify inspired gases
- Promote expectoration
- Deliver aerosolized medications
- Prevent accumulation of bronchial secretions
- Promote mobilization of bronchial secretions
- Improve efficiency of distribution of ventilation by preventing atelectasis
- Optimize cough mechanism

(From Nolan and Gallup,[82] with permission.)

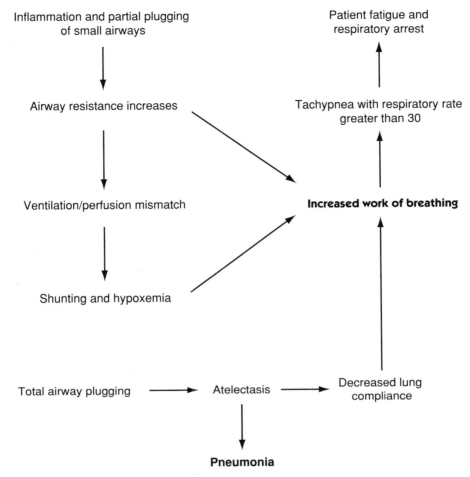

Fig. 1-7. Complications of retained respiratory secretions. (From Nolan and Gallup,[82] with permission.)

opened, but the positive pressure was transferred into the lower airways and secretions were retained. Incentive spirometry requires deep breathing and, when properly performed, opens lower air passages. Close supervision during initial use will facilitate proper usage.[43] Early ambulation, removal of nasogastric tubes, and judicious use of narcotics should be implemented postoperatively. The introduction of parenteral nonsteroidal agents should reduce narcotic needs in these patients. Elderly patients have greater pain tolerance than younger patients, and may only require benadryl and low doses of demerol (10 to 25 mg IM) for pain relief. Patient-controlled analgesics also may be helpful. The diagnosis of pneumonia should be considered when fever, a productive sputum, and a chest radiograph showing segmental infiltration are present.

Asthma

Asthma is a clinical syndrome of recurrent airway obstruction that either resolves spontaneously or with bronchodilator therapy. It is found in 1 to 5 percent of the adult population. Preoperative evaluation should include auscultation of

the lungs for wheezing and rales. Patients with evidence of bronchospasm on physical examination, or who require steroids several times each year, should be considered for preoperative steroids. Additionally, any patient who has received more than 7.5 mg/day of prednisone for more than 7 days in the previous year should be given perioperative steroids. A simple regimen of stress dosages for steroid replacement is found in the boxed list. Most bronchospasm occurring in the operating room is related to irritation from anesthetic agents, but occasionally, patients develop problems postoperatively.

In the operating room, ease of ventilation, arterial blood gases (ABGs), and pulse oximeters (to detect oxygen desaturation) are used to access the patient while under anesthesia. Acute bronchospasm in the perioperative state is easily recognized from patient complaints of dyspnea and difficulty with breathing and speaking. On physical examination, rhonchi, wheezes, and rales are heard and, occasionally, accessory muscles are used. Several parameters can be used to gauge the degree of bronchospasm present. Patients will often be sitting upright, perspiring, and anxious. Further testing is useful to determine whether transfer to an intensive

---

Stress Dose Replacement of Steroids

- Indication
  - Any patient who received more than 7.5 mg/day of prednisone for more than 5 days in the prior year
- Preoperative regimen
  - One hour before surgery
    100 mg hydrocortisone intravenously
- Postoperative regimen
  - Day 1: 100 mg hydrocortisone intravenously every 8 hours
  - Day 2: 100 mg hydrocortisone intravenously every 12 hours
  - Day 3: 100 mg hydrocortisone intravenously once in morning
- If patient begins oral feedings at any time: prednisone 20 mg the first day; decrease by 5 mg/day or until chronic dosage is reached

---

care unit is necessary. ABGs are the mainstay in assessing respiratory compromise. Pulse oximetry may be helpful. Asthmatics with high respiratory rates and ''normal'' PCO_2 values have significant air trapping and are prone to respiratory failure and/or arrest. A decrease in audible wheezes and rales in a cyanotic patient is a poor prognostic sign, signifying impending respiratory failure. Transfer to an ICU is indicated by (1) respiratory rates greater than 30 breaths/min with a PCO_2 greater than 40 mmHg and (2) hypoxia with PCO_2 levels of less than 60 mmHg. Placement of an arterial line and repeat ABGs should be considered on transfer for continued monitoring.

The usual therapy for acute attacks are primarily sympathomimetic drugs such as metaproterenol (Alupent; 0.3 ml of a 5-percent solution in 2.5 ml of saline, repeated every 4 hours as needed) or albuterol (Proventil; 0.5 ml of a 0.5 percent solution in 3 ml of saline, repeated every 6 hours as needed). If the patient is having a severe attack, or does not respond after one or two inhalation therapies, methylprednisone (Solu-medrol) should be given (1 to 2 mg/kg IV every 6 hours) until the patient can be placed on oral prednisone.

Pulmonary Infections

Antibiotic prophylaxis has become widespread in gynecologic surgery. Nosocomial pneumonias that develop during the postoperative period are, due to their rarity, probably best managed with an internist who is aware of pathogen trends within the hospital. There are increasing numbers of opportunistic infections, and resistant organisms are emerging with frightening regularity, especially in intensive care units. Anaerobic organisms are seen in elderly patients undergoing gynecologic surgery. The initial workup includes a posterior-anterior and lateral view chest radiograph. Most sputums obtained at the bedside are poor specimens unless induced by a respiratory therapist. If any respiratory compromise is evident, (especially a respiratory rate greater than 30 breaths/min), an ABG should be obtained and bedside pulse oximetry initiated. Patients who are septic, immunocompromised, or who have received large amounts of blood products may have early adult respiratory distress syndrome (ARDS). Finally, pulmonary embolism should be in the differential diagnosis of any postoperative gynecologic patient.

Deep Vein Thrombosis and Pulmonary Embolism Prophylaxis

The mortality of pulmonary embolus remains high and prevention continues to be the most effective treatment. Effective prevention in surgery has not changed since the publication of Vichow's classic description—stasis, intimal injury, and hypercoagulability (or alteration in the coagulation and fibrinolytic state).[44] Because most pulmonary embolisms arise from the lower extremity, most prevention schemes are targeted toward the legs. Practicing gynecologists should stratify risk factors and address the needs of each individual patient. Risk factors have been better defined over the past two decades.[45]

Conditions Associated With Venous Thromboembolism

- Prior history of deep vein thrombosis or pulmonary embolus
- Surgery greater than 30 minutes
- Extensive pelvic surgery
- Gynecologic malignancy, especially ovarian
- Hypercoagulable states (deficiency of antithrombin III, protein C, and protein S)
- Lupus anticoagulant/anticardiolipin syndrome
- Defective fibrinolytic system—defective tissue plasminogen activator (tPA) release or excessive release of tPA inhibitor
- Advanced age (greater than 40 and greater than 70)
- Obesity
- Medical conditions (nephrotic syndrome, sickle cell disease, hyperviscosity syndromes, and platelet abnormalities)
- Immobilization
- Indwelling central lines

Stratification of Risk

- Low risk: less than 40 years of age undergoing procedures lasting less than 30 minutes and with no other risk factors
- Moderate risk: age greater than 40 and procedure lasting more than 30 minutes
- High risk: history of prior deep vein thrombosis or pulmonary embolus greater than 40 years, with extensive surgery for malignancy[46]

Two major approaches to prophylaxis are available: non-pharmacologic and pharmacologic. The cost effectiveness of deep vein thrombosis (DVT) prophylaxis has been proved in multiple studies. Nonpharmacologic approaches are graduated compression stockings (GCS), intermittent pneumatic compression stockings (IPC), and, rarely, inferior vena cava interruption devices. Pharmacologic approaches include subcutaneous heparin (unfractionated), low molecular weight heparin, dextran, and very low dose warfarin.[47] Because of the rarity of use of low dose warfarin in gynecology, discussion is limited to the use of compression devices and heparin preparations.

GCS have varying compressions at different points in the stockings. Among low-risk general surgery patients, their use reduced venous thrombosis by 50 percent.[48] A major problem with GCS is that, when improperly worn (i.e., in the obese patient), the proximal portion may fall down and act like a tourniquet. Patients with low risk of venous thromboembolism may benefit from stockings until they are able to ambulate. IPCs may have two different benefits: (1) intermittent inflation prevents venous stasis and (2) stimulation of the endogenous fibrinolytic system.[49] IPCs have been successfully employed in gynecologic malignancies.[50] Many surgeons have combined these methods because of patients' perspiration discomfort from IPCs alone.

Low dose infractionated heparin has been used for years for prophylaxis. The usual dosage is 5,000 U subcutaneously 2 hours before surgery and then two to three times daily until the patient fully ambulates. In the obese patient, some clinicians increase the dose to 7,500 U administered three times daily until full ambulation is achieved. Low molecular weight heparins are becoming available and may offer some advantages:

1. Decreased bleeding
2. Daily dosage
3. Greater efficacy[51]

In moderate- to high-risk patients, a combination may be the best approach. Combined GCS and ICP with a heparin preparation may be efficacious.[52] In many patients, the use of GCS and ICP may be the only prophylaxis needed, but in high-risk patients, combination therapy may be justified. Problems with DVT and pulmonary embolus prevention continue to arise, due mostly to surgeons' inability to recognize and intervene preoperatively.

Respiratory Failure

Pulmonary failure fortunately is uncommon in the postoperative patient and a simplified classification is given in Table 1-1. The most common causes of respiratory failure arise from unrecognized chronic obstructive pulmonary disease. The most important preoperative prognosticators for eventual mechanical ventilation dependency are a PCO_2 of greater than 45 mmHg or a FVC of less than 1 L. Patients who do develop respiratory failure require special attention to the differing modes of ventilation and a pulmonary specialist should be consulted early. The other common cause of acute pulmonary failure is a pulmonary embolism. The obese patient, the cigarette smoker, and the patient who has recently undergone chemotherapy (which releases thromboplastins) are at high risk of pulmonary embolism. Pulmonary embolism is probably underrecognized in minor cases. It should be considered in any patient with tachycardia and chest pain. Any patient who complains of shortness of breath should undergo an ABG and chest radiograph to rule out pulmonary edema and infectious etiologies of respiratory failure. In patients at high risk of pulmonary edema, especially those with a history of CHF, postoperative oximetry at the bedside should be strongly considered. Finally, the obese patient with a history of snoring, inappropriate sleeping, and frequent headaches should be evaluated for sleep apnea, a syndrome of chronic intermittent obstruction of the upper respiratory tree. In the immediate postoperative period, these patients may have sudden epiglottic occlusion and respiratory arrest leading to death.

The clinical scenario for adult respiratory distress syndrome (ARDS) is classical in presentation, but unfortunately remains difficult to treat. Mortality rates continue to reach 70 percent. Usually, an initial insult is followed by progressive hypoxia and then respiratory failure. Despite our extensive descriptive knowledge of the presentation, little is known about prevention. The diagnosis is only made by exclusion and classical chest radiograph findings of hypoxia. No single etiologic substance or event is described, but the resulting physiologic cascade is well characterized. The clinician's role remains passive, primarily reacting to changing physiology with supportive therapy.

Patients in obstetrics and gynecology are at risk of the more common etiologies of ARDS. Sepsis is the most common predisposing factor for ARDS, with a mortality rate of 80 to 90 percent in most series.[53] Aspiration during general anesthesia was first described in gravid women at the time of cesarean section.[54] Massive transfusion from disseminated

Table 1-1. Clinical Causes and Types of Acute Respiratory Failure

Type	Mechanism	Causes	Clinical Conditions
Acute hypoxemia	↑ Ventilation/perfusion shunt	Airspace congestion	ARDS Pneumonia CHF Pulmonary edema
Hypoventilatory	↓ Respiratory drive	↓ CNS drive Neuromuscular dysfunction	End-stage asthma Drug overdose Myasthenia gravia
Postoperative	Atelectasis, mucus plugging	Functional residual capacity	Obesity Anesthesia Smoking
Shock states	Hypoperfusion	Sepsis Myocardial damage Hemorrhagic shock	Pelvic abscess Cardiomyopathy Postoperative hemorrhage

Abbreviations: ARDS, adult respiratory distress syndrome; CHF, congestive heart failure; CNS, central nervous system.
(Modified from Nolan and Hankins,[85] with permission.)

intravascular coagulation is classical for development of ARDS.[55] Gynecologic oncology is successfully using more toxic drugs and aggressive chemotherapeutic regimens that increase the number of patients susceptible to infection and sepsis.

The ARDS is a clinical syndrome resulting from increased microvascular and epithelial permeability at the alveolar level. The cardinal symptom is progressive dyspnea from hypoxia, due to extravasation of intravascular fluid across the capillary bed into the alveoli. This results in poor oxygen exchange at the level of the alveolus. Early physical findings include the following: (1) labored respiration, (2) tachycardia, (3) cyanosis, (4) rales, and (5) rhonchi. Early clinical markers are found in Table 1-2. The diagnosis is confirmed when arterial hypoxemia is present with a chest radiograph consistent with pulmonary edema, but without evidence of CHF. Very early in the clinical course, the chest radiograph may be confused with pneumonia. If the diagnosis is in doubt, a pulmonary artery wedge pressure of less than 18 mmHg will eliminate CHF as an etiology.

Multiple physiologic changes have been described in ARDS patients. These include

1. Rapid onset of disease, usually in the first 24 hours and no later than 72 hours from the inciting event
2. A decrease in PaO_2 while breathing room air, despite an increased ventilation rate
3. Severe refractory hypoxia, despite supplemental oxygen
4. Diffuse bilateral pulmonary infiltrates on chest radiographs, similar to the pattern seen with CHF
5. A capillary wedge pressure of less than 18 mmHg
6. A decrease of lung compliance
7. An increase in pulmonary vascular resistance[56]

Once the microvascular leak across capillary membranes begins, the ensuing physiologic cascade cannot be altered. The

Table 1-2. Early Clinical Markers in ARDS

Variable	Units	Normal	Early ARDS	Respiratory Failure
Respiratory rate	breaths/min	10–18	30–36	>30
PaO_2				
Room air	mmHg	>90	55–65	<55
Mask O_2	mmHg	>150	80–100	<60
$PaCO_2$	mmHg	36–42	32–45	>50
PaO_2/FIO_2	—	>350	200–350	<200
FEV_1	ml/kg	50–60	10–20	<10

Abbreviations: ARDS, adult respiratory distress syndrome; PaO_2, arterial partial pressure of oxygen; $PaCO_2$, arterial partial pressure of carbon dioxide; FIO_2, fraction of inspired oxygen; FEV_1, forced expiratory volume in 1 second.
(From Nolan and Hankins,[55] with permission.)

Gynecologic Etiologies of Adult Respiratory Distress Syndrome

- Direct injury
  - Trauma
- Filtration
  - Sepsis syndrome
  - Multiple transfusion
  - Fat embolism
  - Disseminated intravascular coagulation
- Drug reactions and overdosages
- Infectious agents
  - Viral, bacterial, fungal
  - *Pneumocystis carinii* pneumonia in susceptible hosts
- Idiopathic

provoking etiology should be treated (e.g., drainage of abdominal abscess, treatment of pneumonia) if possible. The only care is supportive, via oxygen therapy, mechanical ventilation and, if prolonged, nutrition. If the patient survives, however, normal pulmonary function usually returns. The most important aspects, of care for the gynecologist is recognition of the developing syndrome, timely transfer to an intensive care unit, and consultation with an internist or pulmonary medicine specialist for therapy.

Renal Assessment

Gynecologic patients with renal disease are uncommon in most practices. However, with the increasing availability of hemodialysis and renal transplantation, these patients are becoming more common.

The elderly patient with chronic hypertension and a preoperative BUN of greater than 20 mg/L or a creatinine of greater than 1.5 (1.0 in the thin, frail elderly patient) should be considered for renal assessment. A 24-hour urine sample for creatinine clearance, despite the difficulty in collection, is useful in detecting early renal insufficiency. Renal status is important to evaluate, especially in regard to drug metabolism and fluid management. Elderly patients are more likely to be on multiple medications that affect intravascular volume, and are susceptible to postoperative renal problems, especially acute tubular necrosis (ATN). Additionally, with the increased emphasis on preoperative imaging studies of pelvic masses, more studies using intravenous contrast agents are obtained. Patients with unrecognized renal insufficiency may develop contrast-induced nephropathy when challenged. Fortunately, most radiologists require a creatinine or BUN before imaging.

During the preoperative evaluation, the creatinine clearance will determine whether the patient has mild renal insufficiency (glomerular filtration rate [GFR] of greater than 50 ml/min), moderate renal insufficiency (GFR between 25 and 50 ml/min), advanced renal insufficiency (GFR of 10 to 25 ml/min) or severe renal insufficiency (GFR of less than 10 ml/min). Oliguria is defined as urine output of less than 400 ml/24 hr, while polyuria is greater than 3 L/24 hr. Surgical mortality in this group of patients is directly related to the degree of renal impairment, but has decreased to less than 4 percent.[57] Common problems encountered include infections, bleeding tendencies secondary to platelet dysfunction, anemia, and difficulties in nutrition and wound healing.

Hypertensive disorders are closely associated with renal insufficiency and may be related to the inability of the kidney to remove sodium and volume. Most patients with renal insufficiency will have hypertension and take various antihypertensive agents, including calcium channel blockers and diuretics. These agents, in combination with the underlying altered renin-angiotensin state, will result in some degree of intravascular depletion. During the induction of anesthesia, and the loss of blood inherent to surgery, volume shifts may occur. A simple tilt test (taking a blood pressure and pulse while the patient is lying down and repeating it after the patient stands for 5 minutes) assesses whether the patient is intravascularly depleted. A potentially avoidable complication of surgery is hypotension, which may result in acute tubular necrosis, further compromising renal status. Patients with advanced or severe renal insufficiency may require a PAC perioperatively to assess volume status. Additionally, they may require preoperative hemodialysis, especially with advanced disease.

Fluids and electrolyte balance are affected when the GFR decreases to 25 percent of normal levels (between 25 and 50 ml/min). Consultation with an internist or nephrologist should be considered at this level of renal impairment. Sodium retention begins at this time and may result in peripheral edema and hypertension. Fluid and sodium restriction should be instituted with good results but, in resistant cases, dialysis may be necessary perioperatively. If a bowel preparation is given, an additional 1 to 2 L of intake may be needed. When vomiting or diarrhea complicates the clinical situation, more fluids are needed and a PAC may be useful in the assessment of fluid status. It is important to replace fluids before administering an anesthetic, to avoid hypertension and possibly stroke. Replacement for third spacing in most procedures should be calculated into fluid requirements (e.g., approximately 300 to 500 ml of crystalloid for unusual losses). Patients having radical surgery or ovarian cancer may also be considered for central monitoring due to the multiple factors involved in fluid replacement. Fluid restriction in the postoperative state should be limited to 400 ml of fluid in addition to the normal calculated replacement.

As renal failure progresses, electrolyte abnormalities are common and, in some cases, require dialysis despite the absence of overt renal failure. Potassium disorders are frequently an indication for preoperative dialysis. Actually, hyperkalemia in levels of 5.5 mEq/L or greater can be treated with ion exchange resins such as Kayexalate, either orally or via an enema. Intravenous glucose and insulin with bicarbonate will shift potassium intracellularly, but the effect is short and should be used only in dire emergencies. ECG monitoring should be performed while the above infusions are being administered. After initial stabilization, dialysis may be considered before surgery. If patients receive dialysis before surgery, the potassium may be artificially low and will equilibrate over the subsequent 24 hours. Supplemental potassium should not be given in these situations.

Acidosis is common in patients with severe renal failure. Metabolic acidosis with pH levels of less than 7.25 percent should be corrected before surgery.[58] If the systemic pH is corrected too quickly, ionized calcium can drop acutely. Calcium-containing solutions, if needed, should be given with the gluconate salt. When administering any medication to patients with chronic renal failure (CRF), nephrotoxic drugs should be avoided. Doses of medications should be modified to reflect the degree of renal failure. Unless care is taken, CRF may become worse as a result of hypotension and medication, causing complete renal failure and requiring dialysis.

CRF has been associated with anemia, and hematocrits of 20 to 30 percent are commonly reported. The use of Epogen (Amgen Inc, Thousand Oaks, CA), a synthetic erythropoietin, has reversed the level of anemia in many patients. No particular level of preoperative anemia or hematocrit is an indication for transfusion before surgery. Patients with hematocrits of less than 20 to 25 percent and expected blood losses of greater than 500 to 1,000 ml intraoperatively should receive additional red cells. Packed red blood cells should be given during the preoperative dialysis to minimize potassium toxicity and increase intraoperative volume. Increased hematocrits of greater than 30 percent are associated with fewer bleeding problems; this is thought to be related to increased blood viscosity.[59] Uremia is associated with multiple bleeding problems. Platelet dysfunction is common in renal failure, especially when the serum creatinine is greater than 6 mg/L. Absolute platelet counts may be misleading, and a bleeding time is the proper test for evaluating patients. Because heparin is used in hemodialysis, surgery should be delayed for at least 2 hours after dialysis. If bleeding dysfunction persists despite frequent dialysis, cryoprecipitate should be given.[60] DDAVP (desmopressin) may also be given, and may potentiate von Willebrand factor, but only for the first several doses.[61]

Renal disease is associated with nutritional disturbances from malabsorption and anorexia. The patients diet should be assessed and modified in preparation for the expected catabolism and the need for additional protein. Vitamin and iron supplementation are necessary due to the loss of water-soluble vitamins during dialysis. Relative malnutrition is associated with immunocompromise and the use of prophylactic antibiotics is recommended.

CRF is associated with additional risk factors. Diabetes and uncontrolled hypertension are common etiologies for renal failure; however, these factors are also important for atherosclerotic cardiovascular disease. The underlying disease that led to the patient's renal failure should be stabilized. A targetted history for coronary artery disease should be obtained.

Patients who have undergone renal transplants and have a creatinine of less than 2 tolerate surgery very well. Due to the immunosuppressive drugs, they should be managed in close consultation with a nephrologist. Many of these patients are on maintenance prednisone and will require perioperative stress replacement doses. Additionally, due to the chronic immunosuppression, infection may be more difficult to diagnose. Therefore, any episodes of tachycardia or persistent low grade fever should be evaluated. A CBC with special attention to the differential count is important. The only manifestation of early sepsis may be a "shift to the left," manifested by band forms. Any abnormal parameter of vital signs should result in a fever workup. Additionally, even if the patient is anephric, residual infected urine may be found in the bladder. Bladder catheterization should be performed in addition to blood cultures.

Intraoperatively, hemostasis should be meticulously obtained. When positioning the patient on the operating table, special padding should be used to protect shunt sites and avoid unnecessary pressure. Intravascular volume must be maintained and adjusted for blood loss, but overhydration avoided. Postoperatively, early ambulation should be encouraged, and dialysis should be performed within 48 hours of surgery. Postoperative analgesics should be used as necessary, but closely monitored. Skin closure devices should be left in longer than usual, from 10 days to 2 weeks, because of delayed healing.

Fluid Status

Body fluids are arbitrarily divided into two compartments: intracellular (45 percent of body weight) and extracellular (20 percent of body weight). The extracellular compartment is further divided into two additional compartments: plasma and interstitial. Three normal sites are involved in fluid balance. The gastrointestinal tract processes 6 to 9 L every 24 hours, but ultimately loses 200 to 300 ml of fluid every 24 hours. Insensible losses are approximately 600 to 800 ml/24 hr and account for lung and skin losses. Renal losses reflect the hydration status of the body, but absolute loss is approximately 600 ml/24 hr. When calculating fluid losses, an additional 1,000 to 1,500 ml/24 hr may be necessary to compensate for these losses, and fluids needs may rise with increased body temperature and metabolic needs.

Acutely, surgery affects the plasma space; however, fluid shifts, especially free water, may take hours to equilibrate.

Sodium given in intravenous fluids may equilibrate within 30 minutes. Additionally, if dehydration is present from disease, exercise, or other causes, fluid may be removed from cells and may not reflect total body losses. Vasopressin release is altered with age, and the thirst mechanism is blunted. When replacing fluid, an important indicator is urine output. Despite an initial increase in urine flow when a fluid bolus is given (500 ml of normal saline, with appropriate potassium as needed over 20 to 30 minutes), larger quantities may be necessary over the next 12 to 24 hours to adequately replace total body stores. Finally, the possibility of concealed bleeding must be considered along with re-exploration as a potential therapeutic option.

Sodium balance requires replacement of 100 to 200 mg/day because of fixed losses from the skin and kidneys. Potassium losses are approximately 1 mg/kg of body weight. Replacement of sodium, potassium, and chloride are usually provided by balanced salt solutions. Additional potassium may be added in quantities up to 40 mEq/L in peripheral lines and 80 mEq/L in central lines. Potassium replacement should be gradual and requires larger quantities than expected due to the shift from the intravascular space to the intracellular space. Replacement should be monitored with electrolyte determinations, especially in the elderly and/or renally compromised. In patients with diarrhea, replacement should consist of equal volumes of 0.5 normal saline with 40 mEq/L of potassium. Gastrointestinal losses, usually from a nasogastric tube, should be replaced every 8 hours, milliliter for milliliter, with a solution of normal saline containing 40 mEq/L of potassium chloride. Magnesium deficiency, common in alcoholics and patients treated with cisplatin, should be treated with 1 of magnesium sulfate added to 1 L of balanced salt solution daily. Calcium deficiency should not be replaced acutely because of rapid equilibrium between the ionized and bound mineral.

The importance of preoperative fluid status is too often not recognized as a potential problem. Many surgeons tend to ''boilerplate'' postoperative fluid orders with 125 ml of a balanced salt solution given until clear liquids are tolerated. In most younger patients, this approach is tolerated, but in more complicated or elderly patients, this can result in pulmonary edema. Same day surgery admissions may hamper hydration before surgery, which may result in hypotension during the induction of anesthesia. The length of NPO status and febrile illness (e.g., a tubo-ovarian abscess) both increase fluid needs. Patients who live in southern environments during the summer may be admitted in a relatively dehydrated state. Elderly patients are known to have a decrease in vasopressin sensitivity and therefore may suffer from unrecognized decreased volume status. Bowel preparation and fistulas impact on fluid status and may result in greater fluid losses than is commonly appreciated. Medications for hypertension can affect vascular muscle tone, which may modify fluid requirements. Lastly, the immediate perioperative fluid management is controlled by the anesthesiologist. Some anesthesia personnel are reluctant to give large volumes of fluid. Fluid management is a joint responsibility and should not be automatically relegated to the anesthesia team.

Accurate assessment of intraoperative blood loss tends to be an ongoing debate in some operating suites. Arguments over 100 to 200 ml of blood loss are of little importance unless patient size (blood volume is 70 ml/kg of body weight), preoperative volume status, and other variables are calculated. Intraoperative ABG measurements now report hemoglobin values and may be used in emergencies. Vital signs are important to monitor, but will vary by anesthesia agent (muscle blockers and halogenated agents) and level of anesthesia (hypertension and tachycardia may reflect an underanesthetized patient). Urine flow continues to remain an important variable and represents an indirect measure of GFR and hence, hydration.

In the operating room, there is virtually no use for any fluid except for isotonic salt solutions. The type of fluid usually reflects the bias of the specialty: anesthesiologists and surgeons prefer lactated Ringer's solution, while the internist prefers normal saline. Lactated Ringer's solution consists of 130 mEq of sodium, 4 mEq of potassium chloride, 5 mEq of calcium chloride and 109 mEq of chloride. Additionally, lactated Ringer's solution contains 28 mEq of lactate (not lactic acid), which is converted to bicarbonate by the liver. The use of dextrose-containing solutions is usually a moot point, but is important in the diabetic patient because glucose will be readily provided for metabolism (see below). Solutions containing dextrose are used in the postoperative period to spare protein from glucogenesis. This may be of some importance in the elderly, who have reduced muscle mass.

Preoperative replacement of specific fluid losses should be performed over days, not hours. Diuretic usage, a common cause of hypokalemia, has decreased in the primary therapy of hypertension. The use of rapid fluid bolus for replacement of potassium has been commonly used, but does not replace total body loss of this important electrolyte. Patients taking diuretics should have their electrolytes checked at least 1 week before surgery. Ideally, potassium replacement should be done by supplementation with 40 mEq twice a day for 7 to 10 days in effervescent solutions, unless renal insufficiency is present.

Insensible losses and fluid replacement in the normal individual are approximately 600 to 1500 ml/day. The patient under 55 years of age having surgery should receive approximately 500 ml of fluid before the induction of anesthesia. If a bowel preparation is done, an additional 1,000 to 1,500 ml of gastrointestinal fluids can be lost. This fluid can be replaced intraoperatively or postoperatively. The author prefers intraoperatively. Blood loss is commonly replaced with 3 ml of crystalloid for every 1 ml of blood loss, but blood loss and crystalloid replacement calculations should be reviewed with anesthesia personnel before leaving the operating room. Also, urine output during the case is an important variable in assessing adequacy of volume replacement during surgery. If a retractor has been extensively used on the bladder, a short interval may be necessary before effective diuresis.

Absence of urinary flow should be systematically approached. The first and most important variable is ongoing blood loss, which is not recognized. A STAT hemogram or blood gas hemoglobin should be obtained prior to a fluid bolus. No amount of replacement therapy will reverse the absence of good hemostasis. Resuscitation and re-exploration should never be delayed, especially if vital signs are unstable. Once assessment of red cell status is obtained, fluid boluses of 250 to 500 ml of balanced crystalloid over 20 to 30 minutes should be initiated. The use of furosemide in the recent postoperative patient is to be discouraged, except in patients with overt pulmonary edema. If any questions exist, especially in the elderly or medically compromised (e.g., left ventricular dysfunction, renal insufficiency), a PAC should be considered. Furosemide is a "Doctor Feelgood" medicine; it will produce urine, but may exacerbate hypovolemia. In many cases, patients require 1 to 2 L of additional fluid to replace inordinate losses that were unrecognized before surgery. Once this limit has been reached, other etiologies should be sought.

For the patient who is medically compromised by heart disease and renal disease, accurate assessment of volume status becomes more important. In those individuals with relatively stable disease, prophylactic placement of PACs are initially unnecessary. However, if there is a reasonable chance that pulmonary artery catheterization may be used (e.g., the patient had prior pulmonary edema and ovarian debulking surgery with ascites) central access should be placed before surgery. A patient who becomes unstable during surgery represents the worst case for insertion of a central line. For this reason, central access should be maintained in the preoperative period so that quick conversion to a pulmonary artery introducer and catheter placement may proceed with minimal delay. If the patient can be admitted the day before surgery and pulmonary artery catheterization is needed, placement of the PAC the night before surgery with fluid challenges to characterize the vascular status may be helpful. In most cases, however, placement of the central line with judicious intraoperative fluid boluses may remedy the situation. In our current high-technology environment, we tend to forget that urine output, blood pressure, and pulse remain important physiologic parameters.

Indications for Pulmonary Artery Catheterization in Gynecologic Surgery

- Cardiac disease/dysfunction
  - History of pulmonary edema, congestive heart failure, or compromised left ventricular function (ejection fraction less than 40 percent)
  - Severe valvular heart disease (usually stenotic or atretic lesions)
  - Cardiomyopathy with ejection fraction less than 40 percent
- Pulmonary disease/dysfunction
  - Management of fluids with positive-end-expiratory pressure less than 15 mmHg in ARDS
  - Progressive pulmonary edema/hypoxemia
- Renal dysfunction
  - Persistent oliguria/renal failure despite volume challenge and afterload reduction (e.g., elderly patient after ovarian tumor reduction surgery)
- Sequelae of systemic infection
  - Septic shock, regardless of etiology, refractory to standard volume and pressor therapies

(Modified from Nolan et al,[83] with permission.)

Diabetes Mellitus

Diabetes mellitus affects nutritional status, electrolytes, intravascular volume status (osmotic diuresis), wound healing, and risk of infection. There are multiple preoperative regimens for control of insulin-dependent diabetes mellitus (IDDM), but none have proved superior to metabolic control.[62] Surgical stress releases high levels of circulating adrenal glucocortides and catecholamine, which may contribute to both hypoinsulin secretion and insulin resistance. A convenient model that characterizes the metabolic milieu of diabetes is to view insulin as an anabolic hormone and glucagon, cortisol, and growth hormone as counter-regulatory hormones.[63] Most patients with IDDM need approximately 0.75 to 1.0 U/hr of insulin in a normal fed state to maintain euglycemia. However, during the stress of surgery, more insulin may be required. Diabetic ketoacidosis (DKA) has been reported in 17 percent of patients with levels of glucose as low as 300 mg/dl.[64]

Before surgery, home glucose monitoring should be employed to normalize blood glucose. Preoperative laboratory studies should include a urine dipstick for protein. Some diabetic patients with advanced renal disease will have normal creatinine, but may be found to have proteinuria.[65] Admission 2 to 3 days before surgery, although ideal, is less common with the cost-containment policies currently in effect at most institutions. The diabetic patient should be the first case taken in the morning in order to limit the fasting interval. During surgery, fluids should contain 5 percent dextrose solution with 20 mEq of potassium, assuming normal renal function. Poorly controlled diabetics with high serum glucose may require more potassium, as extracellular potassium moves intracellularly with falling glucose levels. A commonly used protocol for insulin replacement is to give one-half of the usual morning dose of intermediate or long-acting insulin (NPH or lente) perioperatively. Intermittent boluses of regular insulin are given intraoperatively. The safest and most physiologic method is to give a constant infusion of low-dose insulin, but is time and labor intensive. Regular insulin at a dosage of 1 to 2 U/hr is given in response to the glucose level. More insulin is needed only rarely, unless the patient is infected or septic. Blood glucose determinations should be obtained before surgery, every hour during surgery, and every 2 to 4 hours in the first 24 hours after surgery. During surgery, a glucose level of 250 mg/L is acceptable because of an absence of reflexes to hypoglycemia under anesthesia. By contrast, the pre- and postoperative goal is to maintain normal glucose levels (70 to 140 mg/dl). Many medical consultants are not accustomed to seeking such "tight" glucose control.

Insulin has multiple endocrinologic functions, including moving glucose into cells, gluconeogenesis, glycogenolysis, ketogenesis in the liver, and regulating lipid and fat metabolism with lipoprotein lipase activity. A common mistake is to assume that when the patient is euglycemic, no insulin need be administered. If no insulin is given, alternative metabolic pathways are initiated. If a patient becomes hypoglycemic, *both* glucose and insulin must be administered. The rate of insulin infusion can be reduced to 0.1 U/hr *but never stop administering insulin*. Additionally, septic or infected patients may respond to insulin erratically until the infection resolves. These patients may run glucose levels of 200 mg/L or higher. All diabetics should be closely monitored for DKA in the first 48 hours after surgery. Altered breathing patterns and an increased respiratory rate may be the first indications of impending DKA. Respiratory rates greater than 24 to 28 breaths/min may represent respiratory alkalosis in response to early metabolic acidosis and DKA. Bicarbonate levels should be monitored daily for 2 to 3 days for the development of metabolic acidosis. An ABG is indicated in either clinical condition to better assess acid-base status. Gastroparesis may further complicate gut motility in the postoperative period, and metoclopramide may help abate nausea while stimulating the gut.[66]

Patients with NIDDM are far more common than those with IDDM and require minimal perioperative glucose control. The obese NIDDM patients have high serum glucose levels secondary to insulin resistance and dietary indiscretion. The thin NIDDM patient, however, will respond similarly to the IDDM patient. The vast majority of obese NIDDM patients, when hospitalized and placed on an ADA (American Diabetes Association) diet, will become euglycemic within 24 to 36 hours. Occasionally, certain stresses such as surgery and infection will result in NIDDM patients becoming ketotic and requiring insulin. A reasonable approach to replacing insulin during surgery (if required) is to add 10 U of regular insulin to 1 L of 5 percent dextrose solution and to infuse it at a rate of 125 ml/hr. In the postoperative period, many of these patients will not require additional insulin. Oral hypoglycemic agents should be restarted at discharge. Episodes of ketosis from surgery and infection do not change the primary physiology of altered insulin metabolism for a patient. Therefore, patients are not reclassified from NIDDM to IDDM if they become ketotic from surgical stress.

Hyperosmolar coma is different from DKA. Hyperosmolar coma is usually found in the elderly and is a result of either a stroke or an infection. These patients usually have NIDDM and have not maintained an adequate intake of fluids. Many of these patients present with serum glucose levels of 800 to 1,000 mg/dl, but without ketosis. The treatment is similar to DKA. The most pressing problem is fluid replacement, because these patients have total body deficiencies of 10 to 12 L. Two to three liters of normal saline is given initially over a 1- to 2-hour period and then reduced to 200 to 300 ml/hr to replace intravascular volume. This is followed by 0.5 normal saline with 20 mEq of potassium chloride (potassium is driven into cells with glucose under the influence of insulin) given at 200 to 300 ml/hr. Low doses of insulin (1 to 2 U/hr by constant infusion) or 5 to 10 U subcutaneously will help lower the glucose. Once the blood sugar reaches 200 mg/dl, then 5 percent dextrose solution of 0.5 saline with potassium at 125 ml is begun. Frequent blood electrolyte monitoring is necessary during the initial resuscitation. Once sensorium returns to normal, a regular diet and glucose lowering medications can be initiated.

Good perioperative glucose control has been correlated with better wound healing and a decreased evidence of infection. Animal studies suggest that tissue repair is poor because of altered collagen formation and because tensile strength is poor.[67] Patients with poorly controlled diabetes are compromised at different cellular levels such as bactericidal activity, phagocytosis, chemotaxis, and oponisation.[68] The use of prophylactic antibiotics may be reasonable in poorly controlled diabetics. Finally, a diabetic patient who presents with severe abdominal pain mimicking appendicitis or pelvic inflammatory disease with a ruptured tubo-ovarian abscess may actually have DKA. In one series, abdominal pain resolved in 63 percent of patients on normalization of blood sugar.[69]

Hypertension

Hypertension is more common in women than men after 50 years of age. Preoperative assessment of hypertensive patients should primarily focus on evidence of end-organ disease such as myocardial ischemia, peripheral vascular disease, and renal insufficiency. Significant levels of hypertension that may affect surgical outcome are a systolic pressure greater than 170 mmHg and a diastolic greater than 110 mmHg.[70] Despite preoperative control of blood pressure, up to 25 percent of patients with hypertension will have either a hypo- or hypertensive episode in the perioperative period. Postoperative problems noted with the hypertensive patient are either proximate to (within the first 48 hours) or distant to (up to 7 days after) surgery. Initially, hypoxia, fluid overload, and sympathetic stimulation from pain should be alleviated to minimize hypertensive events. Patients with altered left ventricular dynamics or renal insufficiency should be monitored closely at 36 to 48 hours, when mobilization of third space may result in pulmonary edema. The following discussion addresses specific agents and side effects that may affect perioperative management and outcome with management schemes.

Diuretics

Diuretics were once the mainstay of antihypertensive therapy. They are still commonly prescribed, but two major side effects have limited their usefulness. Hypokalemia is common with thiazide and loop diuretics, especially if they are not combined with a potassium-sparing agent. When diuretics are used, intravascular volume is "reset" at a lower level, leading to the common side effect of volume depletion. Decreased intravascular volume may be diagnosed preoperatively by performance of the tilt test and should not be limited to patients with hypertension, but also long-standing diabetics with possible autonomic dysfunction. Initially, blood pressure and pulse are measured in the supine position. The patient is then moved to the standing position for *5 minutes,* after which blood pressure and pulse are remeasured. A positive tilt test reflects an increase in pulse of 20 beats/min, or a drop in diastolic blood pressure of 20 mmHg. These patients are considered to be volume depleted. Volume replacement using balanced crystalloid solutions (i.e., normal saline or lactated Ringer's) should be initiated before induction of anesthesia. After 1 to 2 L of fluid are administered, the tilt test should be repeated. In the postoperative period, oliguria may be secondary to drug-induced volume contraction of altered vascular tone. Patients placed on diuretics for left ventricular dysfunction and pulmonary edema may require diuretics in the first 24 hours if progressive hypoxia by pulse oximetry or the physical examination suggests pulmonary edema (bibasilar rales, tachycardia, and S_3 gallop rhythm). These patients may require closer nursing supervision than may be available on the normal gynecology floor.

Calcium Channel Antagonists

First introduced as therapeutic agents for the treatment of supraventricular arrhythmias and angina pectoris, these medications have become extremely popular in antihypertensive therapy. As a group, they are exceptionally efficacious in black Americans and older patients who are resistant to β-blockers.[71] As longer acting formulations became available, their use in the treatment of hypertension increased for most groups of patients. (Since there are no intravenous formulations of this group of medications, longer acting formulations are useful when contemplating surgery.) The mode of action for these agents is by direct relaxation of vascular smooth muscle. If these medications are used accurately and intravascular volume is low, severe hypertension may result. Fortunately, this is rare. The major difference between the various agents in use is their effect on the AV node (Diltiazem has blocking effects). In the postoperative period, nitroprusside is usually substituted when acute blood pressure control is necessary.

Angiotensin-Converting Enzyme Inhibitors

The mode of action of angiotensin-converting enzyme (ACE) inhibitors is on the renin-angiotensin (vasoconstrictor) system, blocking the conversion of angiotensin I to angiotensin II. Because these agents have a long half-life and relatively few side effects, these drugs have become popular as first line agents in the treatment of uncomplicated hypertension. Originally, they were used for treatment of end-stage cardiomyopathies because of their ability to dramatically decrease preload and, therefore, unload the pulmonary system. If used acutely with diuretics, hypotension may result. Accordingly, diuretics should be stopped for 48 to 72 hours before initiation of the ACE inhibitors. Recently, an intravenous formulation for this group of medications has been introduced (analaprilate or Vasotec), which should allow for better control of patients perioperatively. The usual intravenous dose is 1.25 mg every 6 hours, and 5.0 mg is the maximum dose.

β-Blockers

β-Blockers have been available for 25 years and used successfully in the control of angina pectoris and hypertension. Due to multiple side effects such as constipation, sleep disorders in the elderly, and lethargy, they are currently used less often. β-Blocker preparations are either lipid or water soluble. The water-soluble group has a long half-life, making once-daily dosage available. Because of their long half-lives, they can be given preoperatively (atenolol and nadolol are commonly used formulations). Propranolol is lipid soluble and has been commonly used for years. Intravenous forms of β-blockers are available, but some are far more potent than the oral formulations. Propranolol is usually given in 1 to 2-mg doses intravenously rather than the usual oral dose of 20 to 40 mg. A serious side effect in cardiac patients is the β-blocker withdrawal syndrome.[72] In patients with clinically significant coronary artery disease, sudden withdrawal may result in unstable angina and myocardial infarctions.

Central Agents—Methyldopa and Clonidine

Methyldopa, commonly used in obstetrics, is rarely used because of side effects, which include taste and central nervous system dysfunction. Another central agent, clonidine, is also becoming less popular because of side effects such as the clonidine withdrawal syndrome. Eight to 24 hours after discontinuation of the medication, severe rebound hypertension may occur; however, it is usually observed only when the dosage is greater than 1.2 mg/day. Transdermal patches have been introduced, which are active for 7 days. Patches must be started 48 to 72 hours before surgery to reach satisfactory drug levels perioperatively.

Smooth Muscle Relaxants

Hydralazine is a vasodilator with a mechanism of action that directly relaxes arterial wall smooth muscle. Major side effects are headaches, tachycardia, and fluid retention. The addition of a β-blocker will limit tachycardia and headaches without compromising the blood pressure-lowering effects. Minoxidil is another commonly used drug in this class, but is of limited use to the gynecologist due to its side effects (beard growth) and potency. Patients receiving these medications usually have resistant hypertension and may require nitroprusside in the perioperative period to control blood pressure. Parenteral forms of hydralazine are available and very potent. The dosage for intravenous use is 0.5- to 1.0-mg increments every 15 minutes. (These patients are not pre-eclamptic and may go into shock if the dose is too high). The resulting tachycardia may be confused with hypovolemia in the immediate postoperative state.

α_1-Adrenergic blocking drugs have become popular due to their unique relationship with lipids. When used as single agents, total cholesterol and low-density lipoprotein cholesterol decrease while high-density lipoprotein cholesterol increases. The mode of action is to block postganglionic norephinephrine vasoconstriction in the peripheral vascular smooth muscle. Prazosin is considered a first line drug rather than a third step hypertensive drug found in older regimens (thiazides were the first step and β-blockers were the second step). These medications are not particularly potent and most patients can be observed and treated with other medications as indicated.

Intravenous Formulations

Certain time periods may be difficult for the hypertensive patient. Intubation can be worrisome due to the release of catecholamines with induction agents. Many of these patients can be treated with small intravenous boluses of nitroglycerine. In the immediate postoperative periods, nitroglyc-

erine or nitroprusside may be given for short intervals. Due to the potency of these agents and the rarity of their use in gynecologic practice, these patients may be better managed by the anesthesiologist and intensivist. The gynecologist should be aware of the side effects (usually tachycardia), which may be confusing in a postoperative time frame. Close observation of urine output and possibly more frequent measures of hemoglobin may help in evaluating volume status.

Hepatic Disease

Hepatic disease can be extremely subtle in recognition and workup. Alcohol use in women, although less prevalent than in men, still exists. A thorough history of alcohol abuse should be obtained at the time of preadmission and liver function ordered as appropriate. A potential group for unrecognized alcohol abuse is the elderly woman who has her evening sherry. Denial of alcohol abuse continues to be a problem in obtaining an accurate history. Subtle elevations in liver function studies may be the only clue to diagnosis. Other considerations for hepatic problems with elevated hepatic enzymes are carrier states for hepatitis. Patients who received blood transfusions before the late 1980s should be considered for hepatitis antigen screening, including hepatitis C antigen (formerly known as non-A, non-B hepatitis).

Colorectal Cancer

Colorectal cancer is the second most common cancer in the United Stated, with an estimated 160,000 new cases diagnosed each year and an annual mortality rate of 60,000. Although most patients are 50 years of age or older, 8 percent are discovered before age 40.[73] Years ago, it was axiomatic that colon cancer was prominently left sided; however, in the past several decades, the predominant site of origin has changed from the rectum to the proximal descending colon. A family history of any gynecologic cancer, prostate and bladder cancer, colorectal cancers, or a history of inflammatory bowel disease places a patient at higher risk of colon cancer. Additionally, any postmenopausal patient without a history of menometrorrhagia and iron-deficiency anemia should be considered at high risk of a carcinoma of the gastrointestinal tract, and this diagnosis should be made preoperatively.

Initial screening is done in two steps: (1) the rectal examination, or rectovaginal examination, and (2) the fecal occult blood testing (FOBT). FOBT is simple, inexpensive, and easily performed with the pelvic examination, but has become controversial as a cost-effective screening test.[74] Before age 40, there are many false-positive results to justify routine FOTB. The false-positive rate for FOTB in a normal population is approximately 6 percent.[75] False-negative results may reach as high as 50 percent due to the intermittent nature of bleeding in many lesions.[76] Prospective studies on the usefulness of FOBT testing are ongoing but at present it remains a valuable method.

Even though the normal workup of a positive screen for FOBT includes red meat-free diets when a patient is preoperative for pelvic surgery, further workup is indicated. Carcinoembryonic antigen (CEA) should not be ordered as a screening test or diagnostic test, but is only useful as a monitor of disease activity. Patients with lateral pelvic masses should be evaluated regardless of FOBT findings. Examination of the colon should be performed using radiographic techniques with flexible sigmoidoscope or by colonoscopy. Two radiographic techniques are available: (1) a single stream of barium that is easiest to perform and more comfortable for the patient; and (2) an air contrast technique that has greater sensitivity, but is time consuming and uncomfortable for the patient. Flexible sigmoidoscopy is also performed to examine at least the first 25 cm of the rectum (up to 60 cm is possible) and sigmoid, locations poorly imaged to the instilling catheter. If any suspicious lesion(s) is found, or the patient is at high risk of colorectal carcinoma, most internists and surgeons proceed to colonoscopy to evaluate the entire colon. Advantages of this procedure include direct visualization of lesions and the ability to biopsy and remove lesions for pathologic examination and therapy.

Prophylactic Antibiotics and Subacute Bacterial Prophylaxis

Antibiotic prophylaxis has been used for nearly two decades in obstetrics and gynecology. Many surgeries performed by gynecologists include removal of the cervix, therefore cutting across the vagina, an area rich in microbes. In the past, major morbidity of vaginal hysterectomies was postoperative cuff cellulitis and abscess. Since the introduction of antibiotic prophylaxis with vaginal surgery, a significant reduction in febrile morbidity has occurred. The role of antibiotic prophylaxis with abdominal hysterectomy, however, remains controversial.

Because the use of prophylactic antibiotics has become so prevalent, many younger gynecologists are unaware of the principles supporting the use of these medications. Antibiotics should be administered in the staging area of the operating room at the time that intravenous lines are started. This saves the patient the discomfort of an injection and will allow for observation of allergic responses before the induction of anesthesia.

The type of antibiotic administered inspired great debate in the 1980s, and the water was muddied further by the proliferation of cephalosporins. The pharmaceutical industry added to the confusion by multiple studies reaching the same conclusion: prophylactic antibiotics (except chloramphenicol)[78] given before the initiation of surgery decreased the number of immediate and late infections in vaginal hysterectomy. The author's choice for prophylaxis (the same for 15

Principles of Antibiotic Prophylaxis
• The incidence of postoperative infection in the planned procedure should be high enough to justify antibiotic use
• A high probability of microbial contamination should be present
• A proposed agent for prophylaxis should attack the microbes found in most infections, but not be routinely used for serious infections and should be
• Of low toxicity
• Safe
• Present, and reaching appropriate levels in tissues in the surgical field
• Administered for a short duration
• Of greater benefit than risk

(Data from Hamsell.[77])

years) is driven by cost and available data: 1 g of cefazolin as the intravenous lines are started. If the patient has had a severe reaction to penicillin (wheals, hives, respiratory distress), 900 mg of clindamycin is given. Clindamycin has aerobic capabilities that have been overlooked by most gynecologists.

Data for prophylactic antibiotics in abdominal hysterectomy is less compelling than with vaginal hysterectomy. Studies have reported reduced postoperative infections, while others show no difference in outcome between patients receiving antibiotics versus placebo.[77] Many of the studies have been small and with various biases introduced, such as the site of investigations. The use of prophylaxis should be individualized in these patients and be practice specific. A practitioner dealing with a low-risk group of patients may do well by not giving preoperative antibiotics, while in a large referral center, all patients should receive antibiotics. Clinicians at Charity Hospital in New Orleans use preoperative cefazolin 1 g IV just before surgery. A disproportionate number of the patients are obese, have a history of infertility (which is associated with pelvic inflammatory disease and endometriosis), longer operating times with residents in training, or significant nutritional and medical problems (e.g., diabetes). Cases should be considered individually, and preoperative antibiotics given to high-risk individuals. Because of the length and complexity of operations, gynecologic oncology cases should be considered high risk and prophylaxis strongly considered.

Heart disease currently affects 1 percent of women in their reproductive years, but with advancements in the medical and surgical therapy of congenital heart disease, this patient population should increase. Depending on the lesion, many of these patients are at risk of subacute bacterial endocarditis (SBE). An unfortunate statistic is the increasing number of women who are intravenous drug abusers, which accounts for an increased incidence of acquired cardiac lesions. Fortunately, the overall frequency of infective endocarditis has been low in women, but this factor may complicate minor or major gynecologic surgery, abortions, and outpatient procedures.

Subacute bacterial endocarditis involves "seeding" of abnormal cardiac anatomy with microorganisms indigenous to the operative site. The most common organisms are streptococcal and the duration of bacteremia is surprisingly brief (typically no longer than 15 to 20 minutes). Any manipulation of the integument, intestinal, lower urinary, and reproductive tracts can result in bacterium release leading to SBE. *Staphylococcus epidermidis* and *Streptococcus viridans* are the most common microorganisms cultured.

Conditions in Gynecology Requiring Prophylaxis

- Recommended
  - Urethral dilation
  - Urethral catheterization or urinary tract surgery if infection present
  - Incision and drainage of infected tissue
  - Vaginal hysterectomy
  - Abdominal hysterectomy in compromised host
- Not Recommended
  - In the absence of infection urethral catheterization, dilation and curettage, abortion, sterilization procedures, or insertion or removal of intrauterine devices

---

(Modified from Dajani et al,[79] with permission.)

Recommendations on Prophylaxis for Cardiac Condition

- Recommended
  - Prosthetic cardiac valves, including biosynthetic and homograft valves
  - Previous bacterial endocarditis, despite absence of heart disease
  - Most congenital malformations
  - Rheumatic and acquired valvular dysfunction despite repair
  - Hypertrophic cardiomyopathy
  - Mitral valve prolapse with regurgitation
- Not Recommended
  - Isolated secundum atrial septal defect
  - Surgical repair without residua beyond 6 months of secundum atrial or ventricular septal defect, or patient ductus arteriosus
  - Previous coronary artery bypass surgery
  - Mitral valve prolapse without regurgitation
  - Innocent or physiologic heart murmurs
  - Previous Kawasaki's disease or rheumatic fever without valvular dysfunction
  - Cardiac pacemakers and implanted defibrillators

(Modified from Dajani et al,[79] with permission.)

The incidence of rheumatic heart disease is decreasing in the United States but still accounts for 40 to 60 percent of infective endocarditis. Lesions most commonly associated with infection are tetralogy of Fallot, ventricular septal defect, patent ductus arteriosus, and valvular prostheses. Mitral valve prolapse (MVP) represents the most common congenital heart lesion, affecting 6 percent of the general population and up to 17 percent of women. Classically, the diagnosis has been made by auscultation of a midsystolic click with a late systolic murmur. Echocardiography should be used to confirm the diagnosis. Most individuals are asymptomatic but some patients experience chest pain and palpitations and report vague symptom complexes that characterize the "MVP syndrome." Mitral regurgitation is the most significant risk factor and requires antibiotic prophylaxis. Patients without mitral regurgitation have been eliminated from the group at risk of subacute endocarditis in the new recommendations of the American Heart Association (AHA).[79]

The new American Heart Association criteria, although extensive, are not intended to be comprehensive and deserve ancillary comments. Prophylaxis should be given perioperatively to those patients at risk of developing endocarditis and are undergoing procedures likely to result in significant bacteremia. As suggested by the authors, in the face of a given infection, the antibiotic of choice would be tailored to the specific organisms involved. In the case of a low-risk surgery, such as pelviscopy without hysterectomy, consider using standard prophylaxis.

Recommended Antibiotic Regimens in Gynecologic Procedures

- Ampicillin 2.0 g IV or IM 30 minutes before the procedure and followed by 1.0 g 6 hours after the initial dose. Gentamicin 1.5 mg/kg (less than 80 mg) 30 minutes prior to the procedure. Amoxicillin (1.5 g) may be given 6 hours after the initial oral dose. The second dose may be given intravenously as the clinical situation dictates.
- Penicillin-allergic patients should receive vancomycin 1.0 g IV over 1 hour with gentamicin 1.5 mg/kg (less than 80 mg) 30 minutes before the procedure. A repeat dose of gentamicin should be given 8 hours later.
- Consider clindamycin 900 mg IV in penicillin-allergic patients with gentamicin 1.5 mg/kg (less than 80 mg) 30 minutes before the procedure. A second dose of gentamicin may be given intravenously as the clinical situation dictates.
- Always individualize therapy where appropriate and use the above prophylaxis regimens as guidelines to therapy.

(From McCurdy and Nolan,[84] with permission.)

Fortunately, few cases of infectious complications appear in obstetric and gynecologic patients. Since 1940, 99 case reports of infectious endocarditis have been published in the English literature. Only 41 cases have been reported from 1960 to the mid-1980s, with a continued reduction in cases. Many of these cases were from criminal abortions, three were associated with intrauterine device placement, three were associated with dilation and curettage, and only one followed hysterectomy.[80]

SUMMARY

Preoperative assessment of the patient should be individualized and never "routine." The most serious traps most physicians fall into include the following:

1. Failing to check preoperative laboratory reports
2. Not performing a thorough physical examination
3. Not researching the effect disease entities will have on surgery
4. Minimizing patient symptoms and not prevailing with an appropriate workup or referral
5. Having minimal to no knowledge of drugs and their side effects outside the scope of gynecology
6. Assuming that medical complications are rare in gynecologic surgery

A well-thought out preoperative plan with an emphasis on intraoperative skills and close postoperative observation will elevate the good surgeon to a great one.

REFERENCES

1. ACOG committee on ethics. American College of Obstetricians and Gynecologists. Committee Opinion No. 108, 1992
2. Somers HM: The malpractice controversy and the quality of patient care. Milbank Q 55:193, 1977
3. Green J: The health care contract: key to minimizing malpractice. Insurance Corporation of America Professional Liability Newsletter 1, 1982
4. Green J: Minimizing malpractice risks by role clarification. Ann Intern Med 109:234, 1988
5. Priluck IA, Robertson DM, Buettner H: What patients recall of the preoperative discussion after retinal detachment surgery. Am J Opthalmol 87:620, 1979
6. Hutson MM, Blaha JD: Patients' recall of preoperative instruction for informed consent for an operation. J Bone Joint Surg 73A:160, 1991
7. Blery C, Charpak Y, Szatan M et al: Evaluation of a protocol for selective ordering of preoperative tests. Lancet 1:139, 1986
8. Macpherson DS, Snow R, Lofgren RP: Preoperative screening: value of previous tests. Ann Intern Med 113:969, 1990
9. Rucker L, Frye EB, Staten MA: Usefulness of screening chest roentgenograms in preoperative patients. JAMA 250:3209, 1983
10. Boghosian DH, Mooradian AD: Usefulness of routine preoperative chest roentgenograms in elderly patients. J Am Geriatr Soc 35:142, 1987
11. Rapaport SI: Preoperative hemostatic evaluations: which tests, if any? Blood 61:229, 1983
12. Simel DL, Matchar DB, Piscitelli JT: Routine intravenous pyelograms before hysterectomy in cases of benign disease: possibly effective, definitely expensive. Am J Obstet Gynecol 159:1049, 1988
13. Goldberger AL, O'Konski M: Utility of routine electrocardiogram before surgery and on general hospital admission. Ann Intern Med 105:552, 1986.
14. Condon RE, Nichols RL: Rational use of prophylactic antibiotics in gastrointestinal surgery. Surg Clin North Am 55:1309, 1975
15. Messing MJ, Nolan TE: Bowel preparation for gynecologic surgery. The Female Patient 18:15, 1993
16. Fleites RA, Marshall JB, Eckhauser ML et al: The efficacy of polyethylene glycol-electrolyte lavage solution versus tradi-

tional mechanical bowel preparation for elective colonic surgery: a randomized, prospective, blinded clinical trial. Surgery 98:708, 1985

17. Jagelman DG, Fazio VW, Lavery IC et al: A prospective, randomized, double-blind study of 10% mannitol mechanical bowel preparation combined with oral neomycin and short-term, perioperative, intravenous Flagyl as prophylaxis in elective colorectal resections. Surgery 98:861, 1985

18. Davis GR, Santa Ana CA, Morawski SG, Fordtran JS: Development of a lavage solution associated with minimal water and electrolyte absorption or secretion. Gastroenterology 78: 991, 1980

19. Panton ON, Atkinson KG, Crichton EP et al: Mechanical preparation of the large bowel for elective surgery: comparison of whole-gut lavage with the conventional enema and purgative technique. Am J Surg 149:615, 1985

20. Frye RL, Higgins MW, Beller GA et al: Task force III: major demographic and epidemiologic trends affecting adult cardiology. J Am Coll Cardiol 12:840, 1988

21. London MJ, Mangano DT: Assessment of perioperative risk. p. 53. In Stoelting RK, Barash PG, Gallagher TJ (eds): Advances in Anesthesia. Vol. 5. Year Book, Chicago, 1988

22. Mangano DT: Perioperative cardiac morbidity. Anesthesiology 72:153, 1990

23. Fegert G, Hollenberg M, Browner W et al: Perioperative myocardial ischemia in the noncardiac surgical patient, abstracted. Anesthesiology 69:A49, 1988

24. Tarhan S, Moffitt E, Taylor WF, Guiliani ER: Myocardial infarction after general anesthesia. JAMA 220:1451, 1972

25. Goldman L, Caldera DL, Nussbaum SR et al: Multifactorial index of cardiac risk in non-cardiac surgical procedures. N Engl J Med 297:845, 1977

26. Yasue H, Ogawa H, Okumura K: Coronary artery spasm in the genesis of myocardial ischemia. Am J Cardiol 63:29E, 1989

27. Fuster V, Steele PM, Chesebro JH: Role of platelets and thrombosis in coronary artery atherosclerotic disease and sudden death. J Am Coll Cardiol 5:175B, 1985

28. Conti CR, Mehta JL: Acute myocardial ischemia: role of atherosclerosis, thrombosis, platelet activation, coronary artery spasm, and altered arachidonic acid metabolism. Circulation, suppl. V, 75:V84, 1987

29. Osbakken MD: Exercise stress testing in women: diagnostic dilemma. Cardiol Clin 19:187, 1989

30. Zaret BL, Berger HJ: Nuclear cardiology. p. 1920. In Hurst JW, Schlant RC, Rackley CE et al (eds): The Heart. 7th Ed. McGraw-Hill, New York, 1990

31. Weitz HH: Noncardiac surgery in the elderly patient with cardiovascular disease. Clin Geriatr Med 6:511, 1990

32. Gerson MC, Hurst JM, Hertzberger VS et al: Cardiac prognosis in noncardiac geriatric surgery. Ann Intern Med 103:832, 1985

33. Goldman L, Caldera DL, Nussbaum SR et al: Multifactorial index of cardiac risk in non-cardiac surgical procedures. N Engl J Med 297:845, 1977

34. Goldman L: Cardiac risks and complications of noncardiac surgery. Ann Intern Med 98:504, 1983

35. Huber KC, Evans MA, Bresnahan JF et al: Outcome of noncardiac operations in patients with severe coronary artery disease successfully treated preoperatively with coronary angioplasty. Mayo Clin Proc 67:15, 1992

36. Boucher CA, Brewster DC, Darling RC et al: Determination of cardiac risk by dipyridamole-thallium imaging before peripheral vascular surgery. N Engl J Med 312:389, 1985

37. Nolan TE: Perioperative management of the surgical patient and central line placement techniques. p. 1. In Gallup DG, Talledo OE (ed): Atlas of Gynecologic Surgery. WB Saunders, Philadelphia, 1994

38. Jackson CV: Preoperative pulmonary evaluation. Arch Intern Med 148:2120, 1988

39. Tisi GM: Preoperative identification and evaluation of the patient with lung disease. Med Clin North Am 71:399, 1987

40. Torrington KG, Henderson CJ: Perioperative respiratory therapy: a program of preoperative risk assessment and individualized postoperative care. Chest 93:946, 1988

41. Ford GT, Whitelaw WA, Rosenal TW et al: Diaphragm function after upper abdominal surgery in humans. Am Rev Respir Dis 127:431, 1983

42. Dureuil B, Viires N, Cantineau JP et al: Diaphragmatic contractility after upper abdominal surgery. J Appl Physiol 61: 1775, 1986

43. Celli BR, Rodriguez KS, Snider GL: A controlled trial of intermittent positive pressure breathing, incentive spirometry, and deep breathing exercises in preventing pulmonary complications after abdominal surgery. Am Rev Respir Dis 30:12, 1984

44. Virchow R: Neuer fall von todlichen. Emboli der Lungerarterie. Arch Pathol Anat 10:225, 1856

45. Rossoff LJ: Diagnosis, treatment, and prevention of venous thromboembolism in women. Prim Care Update Ob/Gyn 1: 108, 1994

46. Goldhaber SZ, Morpurgo M: Diagnosis, treatment, and prevention of pulmonary embolism. JAMA 268:1727, 1992

47. Jeffery PC, Nicolaides AN: Graduated compression stockings in the prevention of postoperative deep vein thrombosis. Br J Surg 77:380, 1990

48. Merli GJ, Martinez J: Prophylaxis for deep vein thrombosis and pulmonary embolism in the surgical patient. Med Clin North Am 71:377, 1987

49. Knight MTN, Dawson R: Effect of intermittent compression of the arms on deep venous thrombosis in the legs. Lancet 2: 1265, 1976

50. Clarke-Pearson DL, Synan IS, Hinshaw WM et al: Prevention of postoperative venous thromboembolism by external pneumatic calf compression in patients with gynecologic malignancy. Obstet Gynecol 63:92, 1984

51. Verstraete M: Pharmacotherapeutic aspects of unfractionated and low molecular weight heparins. Drugs 40:498, 1990

52. NIH Consensus Conference. Prevention of venous thrombosis and pulmonary embolism. JAMA 256:744, 1986

53. Fein AM, Lippmann M, Holtzman H et al: The risk factors,

incidence, and prognosis of ARDS following septicemia. Chest 83:40, 1983

54. Mendelson CL: Aspiration of stomach content into the lungs during obstetrical anesthesia. Br J Obstet Gynaecol 52:191, 1946

55. Andersen HF, Lynch JP, Johnson TRB: Adult respiratory distress syndrome in obstetrics and gynecology. Obstet Gynecol 55:291, 1980

56. Nolan TE, Hankins GDV: Adult respiratory distress. p. 197. In Pastorek JG (ed): Infectious Disease in Obstetrics and Gynecology. Aspen Publications, Rockville, MD, 1994

57. Hampers CL, Rossier B, Zohlman R et al: Major surgery in patients on maintenance hemodialysis. Am J Surg 115:747, 1968

58. Burke JF Jr, Francos GC: Surgery in the patient with acute or chronic renal failure. Med Clin North Am 71:489, 1987

59. Livio M, Marclesi D, Remuzzi G et al: Uraemic bleeding: role of anemia and beneficial effect of red cell transfusion. Lancet 1:1013, 1982

60. Janson PA, Jubelirer SJ, Weinstein MJ et al: Treatment of bleeding tendency in uremia with cryoprecipitate. N Engl J Med 303:1318, 1980

61. Livio M, Mannucci PM, Vigano G et al: Conjugated estrogens for the management of bleeding associated with renal failure. N Engl J Med 315:731, 1986

62. Schade DS: Management of diabetes in the surgical patient. Med Clin North Am 72:1531, 1988

63. Hirsch IB, McGill JB, Cryer PE, White PF: Perioperative management of surgical patients with diabetes mellitus. Anesthesiology 74:346, 1991

64. Monro JF, Cambell IW, McCuish AG, Duncan LJP: Euglycemic diabetic ketoacidosis. BMJ 2:578, 1973

65. Mogensen CE, Christen CK, Vittinghas E: The stages in diabetic renal disease: with emphasis on the stage of incipient nephropathy. Diabetes, suppl. 2, 32:64, 1983

66. Snape WJ Jr, Battle WM, Schwartz SS: Metoclopramide to treat gastroparesis due to diabetes mellitus: a double-blind controlled trial. Ann Intern Med 96:444, 1982

67. McMurry JF Jr: Wound healing with diabetes mellitus: better glucose control for better wound healing in diabetes. Surg Clin North Am 64:769, 1984

68. Rayfield EJ, Ault MJ, Keusch GT et al: Infection and diabetes: the case for glucose control. Am J Med 72:439, 1982

69. Campbell EW, Duncan LJP, Innes JA et al: Abdominal pain in diabetic metabolic decompensations: clinical significance. JAMA 233:166, 1975

70. Goldman L, Caldera D: Risks of general anesthesia and elective operation in the hypertensive patient. Anesthesiology 50:285, 1979

71. Kiowski W, Bühler FR, Fadayomi MO et al: Age, race, blood pressure and renin: predictors for antihypertensive treatment with calcium antagonists. Am J Cardiol 56:81H, 1985

72. Frishman WH: Beta-adrenergic blocker withdrawal. Am J Cardiol 59:26F, 1989

73. Behbehani A, Sakwa M, Ehrlichman R et al: Colorectal carcinoma in patients under age 40. Ann Surg 202:610, 1985

74. Wagner JL, Herdman RC, Wadhwa S: Cost effectiveness of colorectal cancer screening in the elderly. Ann Intern Med 115:807, 1991

75. Simon JB: Occult blood screening for colorectal carcinoma: a clinical review. Gastroenterology 88:820, 1985

76. Winawer SJ, Schottenfeld D, Flehinger BJ: Colorectal cancer screening. J Natl Cancer Inst 83:243, 1991

77. Hamsell DL: Prophylactic antibiotics in gynecologic and obstetric surgery. Rev Infect Dis, suppl. 10, 13:S821, 1991

78. Goosenburg J, Emich JP Jr, Schwarz RH: Prophylactic antibiotics in vaginal hysterectomy. Am J Obstet Gynecol 105:503, 1969

79. Dajani AS, Bisno AL, Chung KJ et al: Prevention of bacterial endocarditis. JAMA 264:2919, 1990

80. Seaworth BJ, Durack DT: Infective endocarditis in obstetric and gynecologic practice. Am J Obstet Gynecol 154:180, 1986

81. Nolan TE: Surgery in the elderly: lowering risks by understanding special needs. Postgrad Med 91:199, 1992

82. Nolan TE, Gallup DG: The gynecologist and surgical respiratory care. The Female Patient 17:15, 1992

83. Nolan TE, Wakefield ML, Devoe LD: Invasive hemodynamic monitoring in obstetrics: a critical review of its indications, benefits, complications, and alternatives. Chest 101:1429, 1992

84. McCurdy CM Jr, Nolan TE: Review and update on prophylaxis in obstetrics and gynecology. The Female Patient 18:16, 1993

85. Nolan TE, Hankins GDV: Acute pulmonary dysfunction and distress. Emergency care of the obstetric patient. Clin Obstet Gynecol 22:39, 1995

NUTRITIONAL SUPPORT

JACQUELINE C. JOHNSON

Nutrition is often an overlooked factor in the care of the gynecologic surgery patient. Most women undergoing surgery for benign gynecologic conditions are otherwise healthy and well-nourished; however, a variety of chronic conditions or acute disease processes can adversely affect the patient's nutritional status and increase her risk of morbidity or mortality. It is important to screen for nutritional risk factors in the surgical patient and to have a working knowledge of nutritional support techniques and their complications.

RISK FACTORS

The gynecologic surgeon must be able to recognize patients who are at increased risk due to nutritional status and who would benefit from nutritional therapy. Patients who have chronic illnesses affecting their nutritional intake, such as inflammatory bowel disease, cancer, renal or hepatic failure, and intestinal fistulas or ileostomies are at increased risk of malnutrition and vitamin deficiencies. Patients who are elderly or poor or who suffer from depression, eating disorders, or drug and alcohol abuse, often have inadequate diets, as do patients who voluntarily restrict their dietary intake to certain foods or calorie ranges. Long periods of preoperative testing requiring bowel cleansing or fasting also affect nutrition, as do conditions such as ascites or abdominopelvic masses, which may prevent the patient from taking in a regular diet. Nausea, vomiting, and diarrhea are obvious nutritional issues that can cause serious metabolic disturbances if not addressed promptly.

MALNUTRITION AND ASSESSMENT

Two types of nutritional defects are well defined. A normal calorie intake with protein deficiency is known as *kwashiorkor;* a deficiency in both calories and protein is called *marasmus.* Although both types of nutritional deficiency are associated with perioperative complications, kwashiorkor is more often associated with a serious risk of poor outcome, including increased rates of sepsis and mortality.[1] Patients with kwashiorkor malnutrition may have depleted body protein, but their body weight is normal or increased, giving them a normal appearance. Kwashiorkor can develop over weeks or months and can most accurately be detected by measurement of serum proteins. Marasmus can be identified by weight loss indices. If the patient's weight has decreased to 80 to 90 percent of her ideal body weight, mild marasmus is evident; if the level is less than 70 percent, the defect is severe. In comparing the patient's weight to her usual healthy weight, a loss of 5 to 10 percent shows mild marasmus, while a loss of more than 20 percent of the patient's normal weight shows severe malnutrition.[2]

To date, there is no single method of accurately determining a patient's nutritional status. Measurement of the triceps skin fold with calipers has been used as an indication of total body fat stores, as 50 percent of fat is subcutaneous. The midarm muscle circumference has been used as an indicator of total body protein. These measurements are often inaccurate and have not been found to correlate well with nutritional status unless they are severely abnormal (i.e., less than the 10th percentile of normal individuals).[3]

The creatinine/height index is the ratio of the patient's 24-hour urinary creatinine excretion to normal excretion in height- and sex-matched controls. To obtain a true measurement, the patient must be on a meat-free diet, have normal renal function, and a normal state of protein metabolism. An index of 80 percent or less indicates a decrease in muscle mass. This index has not been shown to correlate well with clinical outcome and is difficult to accurately measure.[3]

Several plasma proteins are often measured as an indication of nutritional status. The most common of these are albumin, prealbumin, and transferrin. Albumin has a half-life of 18 to 21 days, is made by the liver, and functions as a transport protein. It is critical to the maintenance of oncotic pressure, and generalized edema results when albumin is severely depleted. Albumin levels of 2.8 to 3.2 mg/dl represent mild depletion, while severe depletion is present at levels of less than 2.1 mg/dl. Prealbumin is also a carrier protein with a serum half-life of 2 to 3 days. Changes in prealbumin levels can be seen within several days of nutritional changes. Levels of 10 to 15 mg/dl are indicative of mild deficiency, with less than 5 mg/dl showing severe deficiency. Transferrin is the transport protein that carries iron. Levels of transferrin can be altered by hormones, liver disease, and iron deficiency. It has a half-life of 8 days, and levels may respond to protein deficiency more acutely than do albumin levels. Transferrin levels of 150 to 200 mg/dl reflect mild protein deficiency, while levels under 100 mg/dl reflect severe depletion of the protein pool.[2,3]

Malnutrition affects the immune system adversely, and these changes can be measured in two ways. Total lymphocyte count has been used as an indicator of kwashiorkor. The total lymphocyte count is calculated by multiplying the percentage of lymphocytes in the differential by the total white blood cell count. Levels from 1,200 to 2,000 have been associated with mild protein depletion and less than 800 with severe malnutrition.[1,2] In malnutrition, the cellular immune system is affected earlier than humoral immunity and can be evaluated by skin testing. Common antigens such as mumps, *Trichophyton, Candida,* and tuberculin-purified protein derivative should elicit a skin response of 5 to 10 mm to at least one antigen. In severe malnutrition, this response is blunted or blocked due to poor cellular immunity. Multiple conditions can lead to abnormal skin testing, including human immunodeficiency virus infection, bacterial infections, cancer, trauma, hepatic or renal dysfunction, steroids, hemorrhage, general anesthesia, and a variety of medications—making skin testing of little clinical usefulness in surgical patients.[2,3]

Prognostic Nutritional Index

$$PNI = 158 - (16.6 \times ALB) - (0.78 \times TSF)$$
$$- (0.2 \times TFN) - (5.8\ ST)$$

PNI   prognostic nutritional index (used to calculate a percentage of risk)
ALB   albumin (g/dl)
TSF   triceps skin fold (mm)
TFN   transferrin (mg/dl)
ST   skin test (anergy panel) response

Skin test response values
   0 = no response
   1 = <5 mm induration
   2 = >5 mm induration

If PNI result is greater than 40 percent, the patient is at high risk.

Because no single test can accurately assess nutritional status, several combination indicators have been developed. The often-used prognostic nutritional index uses serum albumin, serum transferrin, triceps skin fold, and anergy panel testing to calculate a percentage of risk. A score of more than 40 percent was associated with a 6-fold mortality in one population of surgical patients.[4] The nutrition risk index has been used in cooperative group studies of nutrition in surgical patients. This index relies on serum albumin and weight change.[5]

These indices have not been shown to be superior to clinical assessment and largely reflect body size combined with serum proteins. Authors have shown that clinical impression of malnutrition by experienced evaluators or subjective global assessment (SGA) is as accurate as some combined indices.[2] Subjective global assessment ratings are based on clinical history and physical examination and place the patient into one of three groups: A, normal nutritional status; B, mild malnutrition; or C, severe malnutrition.

This rating system depends on recognition of clinical signs of malnutrition such as the loss of subcutaneous fat and muscle wasting that is characteristic of marasmus; or the generalized edema, ascites, loss of skin turgor, change in hair texture or color, hepatomegaly, and parotid gland enlargement characteristic of kwashiorkor.[2] In addition, the clinician must take into account a carefully obtained clinical history, looking for nutritional risk factors as outlined above. Past photos of the patient may be helpful in assessing weight loss and wasting.

In general, clinical information from the history and physical examination combined with serum protein measure-

Nutrition Risk Index

NRI = (1.591 × ALB)
    + (0.417 × current wt/usual wt) × 100

NRI   nutrition risk index
ALB   albumin (g/L)

If value is less than 100, the patient is considered malnourished.

(Data from Veterans Affairs Total Parenteral Nutrition Cooperative Study Group.[5])

ments can give a fairly accurate assessment of nutritional status. It is important for the surgeon to learn the signs and symptoms of malnutrition and to regularly look for them in the history and physical examination so that patients at risk can be readily identified and treated.

INDICATIONS FOR NUTRITIONAL SUPPORT

Although surgeons generally assume that well-nourished patients have fewer complications, clear guidelines for the use of nutritional support are difficult to discern from the literature. No large trials have been done in the gynecologic surgery population; however, data from the surgical literature can be useful and is reviewed here.

Death from starvation occurs when 30 to 40 percent of usual body mass is lost. A person maintained on a 5 percent dextrose intravenous solution postoperatively at 125 ml/hr receives 150 g or 510 kcal in glucose daily. In mildly stressed individuals requiring a baseline of about 2,100 kcal/day or more, a deficit is apparent. When the period of starvation is short, this is fairly well tolerated, although patients undergoing elective surgery may lose 10 percent of their total body nitrogen during the perioperative period. When the period without nutrition exceeds 5 to 7 days, severe depletion begins and, within weeks, death may ensue from starvation.[2]

It is well demonstrated in the surgical literature that malnourished patients have increased rates of surgical complications. Mullen[6] showed that for elective gastrointestinal surgery, surgical complications were increased in patients who had lower albumin levels, decreased subcutaneous fat, decreased transferrin, or impaired anergy testing. Multiple studies have shown increased perioperative complications in malnourished patients, yet the literature defining appropriate

patients for nutritional support is inconclusive. One large cooperative group trial that randomized patients undergoing major abdominal surgery to pre- and postoperative total parenteral nutrition (TPN) versus no TPN showed no significant difference between the two groups in major complications or postoperative mortality.[5,7] They did note a higher rate of infectious complications in the TPN group among patients who were borderline or mildly malnourished, a group that demonstrated no benefit from TPN. Severely malnourished patients, however, had a decrease in noninfectious complications compared to controls, and no increase in infectious complications. The study concluded that perioperative TPN should be used only in severely malnourished patients as assessed by global nutritional assessment. It is important to note that TPN actually increased complications in the patients who were not severely malnourished.

A review of 20 studies in the surgical literature regarding perioperative nutritional support was published by Campos and Meguid.[8] These authors found that 7 to 15 days of preoperative nutrition in malnourished patients decreased postoperative complications and that enteral nutrition was equivalent to TPN for preoperative nutritional supplementation. This review also found that for postoperative nutrition, ad lib oral intake, TPN, or total enteral nutrition (TEN) were equally effective. Early enteral nutrition in patients undergoing abdominal operations decreased the incidence of sepsis and decreased weight loss and hospital stay. Shorter preoperative supplementation was not associated with improvement in postoperative complications.

In a randomized study of postoperative TPN in patients undergoing major general surgical procedures, Sandstrom et al[9] could not show a clear benefit to postoperative TPN in unselected patients who were able to resume adequate oral intake by 8 to 9 days postoperatively. The need for prolonged support of 14 days or more was associated with increased morbidity and mortality. Based on a number of assessment criteria, they were unable to identify preoperatively which patients would require prolonged TPN and would benefit from an early start of nutritional support.

Askanazi et al[10] showed with a randomized study in patients undergoing radical cystectomy that the hospital course could be shortened from an average of 24 to 14 days by immediate postoperative intravenous nutrition over 5 percent dextrose. No difference, however, was seen in mortality or complication rates for this extensive pelvic procedure. The authors postulate that increased muscle strength and healing allowed for earlier ambulation and discharge. More studies using current discharge criteria, including cost analysis, are needed before a case can be made that TPN speeds recovery and discharge in the gynecologic patient population.

Several recommendations for gynecologic surgery patients can be made from the above studies. It seems clear from the surgical literature that patients who can be identified by clinical parameters to be severely malnourished will benefit from preoperative nutritional enteral or parenteral supplementation. The period of preoperative support that has been shown to be beneficial is 1 to 2 weeks—a few days has not been shown to be beneficial. In some elective surgical procedures, time will allow for this preoperative period; however, in many cases, surgery cannot be safely delayed. Further studies are needed to demonstrate a benefit of perioperative TPN in the well-nourished or borderline malnourished gynecologic surgery patient.

Patients undergoing surgery who can be expected to return to a full diet within 5 to 9 days do not benefit from TPN unless severely malnourished preoperatively. However, when it becomes clear that the period without nutrition will be longer than 7 to 9 days, nutritional supplementation should be started as soon as possible. The preferred route of supplementation is enteral when the gut is functional. Candidates for enteral feedings would be patients with a functioning and accessible gut who are intubated for respiratory failure, cardiac failure, or sepsis, or patients who are anorexic or unable to swallow. When malfunction of the gut—such as prolonged ileus, partial bowel obstruction, or extensive gastrointestinal surgery—is the reason for continued starvation, TPN is indicated.

Other indications for TPN or TEN in the gynecologic surgery patient include

1. Toxicity to the gastrointestinal tract secondary to chemotherapy
2. Severe cases of hyperemesis gravidarum
3. Severe pelvic infection or sepsis with prolonged ileus
4. Postoperative bowel obstruction or ileus
5. Respiratory failure requiring intubation
6. Inflammatory bowel disease or short bowel syndrome
7. In select cases, gynecologic cancer

Patients with short bowel syndrome may require lifelong parenteral nutritional support. When these patients require gynecologic surgery, consultation with a nutrition team and the patient's gastroenterologist or general surgeon is recommended, as a variety of metabolic disturbances can be encountered in such patients.[11,12] Patients with malignant, inoperable bowel obstruction secondary to gynecologic malignancies can be managed at home with palliative TPN support. It has been shown that in the case of gynecologic malignancies, patients can survive from 10 to 77 days at home on TPN, with an average survival for patients with ovarian cancer of 39 days.[13] In this study, 9 of 10 patients and families believed that home parenteral nutrition was either beneficial or very beneficial during the terminal phase of the illness.

PHYSIOLOGY OF STARVATION

When the body's exogenous fuel supply is limited, many mechanisms come into play to increase survival. Death from starvation occurs in about 60 to 70 days when the body has lost one-third to one-half of its total protein. Body protein has no storage form. All protein is in use, either circulating (40 percent) or in skeletal muscle (60 percent), and catabolism of body protein will eventually be fatal to the organism. Survival mechanisms in starvation are aimed at protecting the body's protein component for as long as possible.[14]

A variety of hormone responses occur during starvation. Catecholamines are increased by 10 percent after uncomplicated elective surgery to an over 50 percent increase in trauma or peritonitis. Glucocorticoids are released in increased amounts. These in turn act to increase glycogenolysis, the release of stored glycogen from muscle and liver. The stored glycogen in liver and skeletal muscle, approximately 900 kcal, is usually metabolized in less than 24 hours. Lactate and pyruvate, are produced by the metabolism of glucose and can be converted back to glucose through the Cori cycle in the liver and kidney. Other tissues such as cardiac muscle can use lactate directly as fuel.[2,14]

The body then turns to catabolism to create fuel. Insulin levels drop and glucagon levels increase. Lipolysis is stimulated and fat stores are tapped, releasing triglycerides that, in turn, are broken down into free fatty acids and glycerol. Ketones are produced and can be used by some tissues directly for fuel. Heart muscle, skeletal muscles, and renal cortex, can use alternate fuel sources such as fatty acids and ketones when glucose is not available.[15,16] Other tissues—such as brain, renal medulla, bone marrow, red and white blood cells, nerves, and tissues involved in repair (such as macrophages and fibroblasts)—are wholly dependent on glucose. In the central nervous system, which consumes 100 to 150 g/day of glucose, profound hypoglycemia can induce coma and neurologic damage over a period of minutes. Free fatty acids cannot be converted to glucose to meet this demand; however, glycerol can be converted to glucose. Glycerol makes up only 10 percent of triglycerides and is only a limited source of glucose.[2,14]

Glucocorticoids, glucagon, and catecholamines also act to stimulate release of amino acids from muscle and promote gluconeogenesis. Gluconeogenesis is the process by which amino acids are processed into glucose for fuel. Different amino acids are used in different ways. Branched chain amino acids can be used directly by skeletal muscle for fuel. These amino acids are also metabolized to alanine, which is the major substrate for gluconeogenesis in the liver. Alanine also can be derived from pyruvate, a by-product of muscle function, to serve as fuel for gluconeogenesis in the liver. In later starvation, renal gluconeogenesis increases and amino acids released from muscle are converted to glutamine, which is used make glucose in the kidney. Some amino acids are transformed into acetyl-CoA, which enters the Krebs cycle. Others are converted to various substrates along the cycle itself to produce energy.[2,14]

In the acute phase of fasting, a healthy person may lose up to 1 g/kg/day of body nitrogen (or 6.25 g/kg/day protein). After 5 to 7 days of starvation, mechanisms take place to adapt to long-term starvation and to spare body protein further. The brain adapts to using ketones as a fuel source, lipolysis is further increased, and gluconeogenesis from protein breakdown is relatively suppressed. The body's activity and metabolism are slowed to conserve remaining resources. Once all fat stores have been used, the body begins to rely on its structural protein as a fuel source, and catabolism is active. Use of amino acids for glucose production, as described above, results in loss of lean body mass that is fatal if starvation continues.

COMPONENTS OF NUTRITIONAL SUPPORT

Nutritional support is aimed at the conservation of protein and the replacement of essential substances to maintain homeostasis. This goal is accomplished by assessing the patient's protein, calorie, fluid, and electrolyte needs and supplying them enterally or parenterally. Providing adequate protein and calories, along with other essential elements, provides the patient with a fuel and nitrogen source that conserves body mass when normal food intake is not possible or is limited. The adequacy of nutrition can be ensured by calculating the patient's nitrogen balance. This ratio of nitrogen supplied to nitrogen excreted can give important information about the patient's nutritional status and is described in detail in the sections to follow.

Nutritional support can also be used to replenish patients deficient in one or more nutrients. Each component of nutritional support is discussed below, followed by recommendations on order-writing and follow-up of nutritional support.

Calories

A major goal of nutritional support is to provide adequate calories to patients who are unable to take in sufficient calories to meet the body's daily requirements. Intravenous 5 percent dextrose solutions or a clear liquid diet provide about 500 kcal (170 kcal/L) while the average daily caloric intake for a 70-kg individual is about 2,700 kcal/day. Well-nourished individuals may tolerate this level for 5 to 7 days, but poorly nourished patients and those who remain on limited diets for longer than 7 days require caloric supplementation.

The amount of fuel required under various conditions can be estimated by the Harris-Benedict equation. In unstressed

Table 2-1. Adjustments to Resting Metabolic Expenditure

Clinical Status	Stress Factor
Well nourished, unstressed	1.0
Hospitalized, bed rest	1.2
Hospitalized, ambulatory	1.3
Fever	$1 + .13/°C$
Peritonitis	1.2–1.37
Sepsis, acute	1.4–1.8
Sepsis, hypotensive	0.5
Septic, recovering	1.0
Heavy exercise	6.3

starvation or with hypotension, requirements decrease; when illness or the stress of surgery is present, requirements increase. This equation gives an estimate of fuel requirements in unstressed, trained persons who are inactive after a 12-hour fast and may therefore not be applicable to the typical hospitalized elderly patient who develops a small bowel obstruction after hysterectomy. To compensate for various clinical states, a system of stress factors was introduced (Table 2-1). They are multiplied by the resting metabolic expenditure (RME) to determine the adjusted value for a particular clinical situation.

Although the Harris-Benedict equation, adjusted by stress factors, can be used to calculate caloric requirements in the surgical patient, this author and colleagues have found a simpler system to be clinically useful[2] (Table 2-2). Rarely in the gynecologic surgery patient are more than 40 kcal/kg/day needed or tolerated. These estimates are practical and useful in the gynecologic patient population.

The major caloric source in enteral nutrition formulas is carbohydrates in the form of cornstarch, sucrose, lactose, maltodextrin, wheat starch, corn syrup, tapioca starch, or a variety of other agents. Fat calories are also supplied in various forms and are discussed in the section on fats below. Parenteral nutrition uses glucose (dextrose) as its major calorie source. It is known that for optimal nitrogen balance, 150 to 200 kcal are needed for each gram of nitrogen given. The protein/calorie ratio must be calculated to avoid excess or inadequate calories.[1,17] In the calculation of calories in TPN, protein calories are not counted. Instead, grams of protein

Harris-Benedict Equation for Women

Resting metabolic expenditure =
$$655.1 + (9.56 \times wt\ [kg]) + (1.85 \times height\ [cm]) - (4.68 \times age\ [yr])$$

Table 2-2. Alternative System for Determining Caloric Requirements

Stress Level	Caloric Requirement (kcal/kg/day)
No stress, minimal activity	28
Mild stress	30
Moderate stress	35
Severe stress	40

(6.25 × grams of nitrogen) are balanced with kilocalories from glucose and fat sources. For dextrose, a monohydrate solution of glucose, a variety of solutions are available. The most commonly used for full nutritional support are 50 percent dextrose, which provides 1.7 kcal/ml, and 70 percent dextrose (2.38 kcal/ml) for use in more concentrated forms of TPN. A well-tolerated glucose infusion level is about 5 mg/kg/min or 504 g/day (1,713.6 kcal/day) for a 70-kg individual, or around 1 L of 50 percent dextrose solution (just over 24 kcal/kg/day). Higher infusion rates (up to 20 mg/kg/min) have been used, but side effects such as hyperglycemia will be significant at this level.[18]

Complications of excessive glucose administration include glucose intolerance with hyperglycemia and osmotic diuresis. Levels that cause more than 2+ glycosuria will cause osmotic diuresis, which can lead to hyperosmolar nonketotic coma. This condition has a mortality of 40 to 50 percent.[2] In addition, excess glucose will likely be converted to fat, which may be deposited in the liver, causing hepatic steatosis. This condition is increased in TPN when fats are not added as an additional calorie source. Liver enzymes may become elevated, as well as alkaline phosphatase. Cholestasis and bile plugging may occur. Approximately one-half of patients on TPN for 4 to 6 weeks develop gallbladder sludge. These changes are usually reversible when TPN is discontinued. A balance of 10 to 30 percent of nonprotein calories such as fats can avoid some hepatic complications and increase calorie levels appreciably.[19]

High glucose solutions will generate high levels of carbon dioxide, which may precipitate respiratory distress in patients with underlying pulmonary compromise. Patients being weaned from mechanical ventilation require calories to assist their muscles with the work of breathing. High glucose loads in these patients may cause failure to wean because of the patient's inability to handle increased carbon dioxide production. TPN mixtures of 50 percent fat and 50 percent carbohydrate calories may be appropriate for patients with underlying pulmonary disease.[1]

Due to the possible complications of hyperglycemia, patients begun on TPN should have their glucose monitored closely. Usually the infusion of high-concentration glucose TPN is begun slowly, at 50 ml/hr and increased by 25 ml/hr every 12 hours as the patient tolerates until the desired level is reached. During this time, frequent fingerstick glucose (every 4 to 6 hours) and daily serum glucose levels should be measured. Glucose levels should be maintained between 100 and 180 mg/dl. Levels over 200 mg/dl should be treated by decreasing the rate of infusion or by adding appropriate insulin to the TPN mixture as described below. Urine should be monitored for more than 2+ glycosuria to avoid osmotic diuresis. Once patients are clinically stable and have equilibrated on a TPN formula, less frequent monitoring may be appropriate. It should be noted that patients stable on their TPN formulas who develop sudden glucose intolerance are often septic, and appropriate workup should be done.[17,18]

Protein

A major goal of nutritional support is preserving body nitrogen stores. Protein has no storage form in the body, and all protein is in use either as circulating serum protein or as structural protein such as muscle. Any use of the body's protein for fuel is a loss of functional protein mass. Death from depletion of body nitrogen occurs after about 60 days of starvation. In highly catabolic states such as trauma, extensive surgery, burns, or acute sepsis, depletion can occur much more quickly.

The minimum protein requirement for maintaining body mass in a resting state in normal individuals has been found to be 0.43 g/kg/day of dietary protein. This may be as high as 0.6 g/kg/day in elderly patients. For estimates of protein amounts in formulation of nutritional support, the values in Table 2-3 can be used.[2]

In postoperative patients, positive nitrogen balance can usually be achieved with 1.3 to 1.5 g/kg/day of protein. Enteral preparations use a variety of protein sources such as egg albumin, soy protein, caseinate, hydrolyzed casein, and mixtures of select amino acids based on formula needs.[20] Parenteral protein sources are varied, based on certain disease states. The most common are 8.5 and 10 percent amino acid solutions. A variety of brands are available and differ from institution to institution. This section describes requirements in terms of percent solutions. Readers are advised to compare these to specific formulations available through their own hospital pharmacies.

When using enteral feeding formulas, the measurement of protein and calories is simplified by the packaging. One can give enough of the solution—which is already balanced—to provide the amount of protein and calories desired, as tolerated by the patient. In parenteral solutions, calories from amino acids are not included in the calculation of calories. The grams of protein desired are calculated and, using the standard solutions, can be added to the TPN mixture to provide the desired protein requirements.

For a 70-kg patient requiring 1.5 g/kg/day of protein, 105 g of protein are required. This translates through the formula

Table 2-3. Protein Estimates in Formulation of Nutritional Support

Stress Level	Protein Requirements (g/kg/day)
No stress	0.7–0.8
Mild stress	0.8–1.0
Moderate stress	1.0–1.5
Severe stress	1.5–2.0

below using an 8.5 percent amino acid solution to 1,235 ml/day:

Amino acid volume

$$= \frac{Wt\ (kg)\ \times\ protein\ requirement\ (g/kg/day)}{amino\ acid\ solution\ (\%)} \times 100$$

This 105 g of protein is equivalent to 16.8 g nitrogen (105/6.25 = 16.8 g) and requires 150 nonprotein calories per gram nitrogen × 16.8 g nitrogen or at least 2,520 kcal of nonprotein calories to be metabolized properly and to attain positive nitrogen balance.

Nutrition adequacy is measured by nitrogen balance, which is calculated when the patient is stable on TPN. A 24-hour urine collection is made to measure total urine urea nitrogen (UUN) or nitrogen excretion. This measurement is used to determine whether the calories and grams of nitrogen being supplied are adequate (accounting for losses in stool and insensible losses) to provide for muscle rebuilding and conservation of body protein. This is the major goal of nutritional supplementation—to avoid catabolism of body proteins and avert starvation. In patients who are not in positive nitrogen balance, increased protein or nonprotein calories, or both, may be required. Some authors have shown that a positive nitrogen balance can be achieved by increasing the dextrose intake alone or by adding insulin to maintain blood sugar levels at less than 150 g/dl. In addition, other elements of the TPN should be adjusted so that electrolytes are normal and phosphorus, magnesium, calcium, and trace elements are balanced.[14]

Special formulations rich in branched chain amino acids are available for use in hepatic failure. These amino acids can provide energy for skeletal muscle, heart, and brain when gluconeogenesis mechanism is faulty in liver failure. They can also compete with aromatic amino acids for transport across blood-brain barrier and help to increase hepatic protein synthesis, thus decreasing the concentration of aromatic amino acids that contribute to hepatic encephalopathy.[16,21] In renal failure as well, specialized amino acid solutions are available, containing essential amino acids exclusively or in high concentrations. Patients on dialysis can bear a higher protein load, and 50 percent essential amino acid solutions can be used, as protein will be lost with dialysis. In patients in whom dialysis is not feasible at the present time, small amounts of essential amino acids can be given with restricted fluid volumes until dialysis is possible.[22]

In patients with hepatic or renal failure, consultation with nutritionists and a gastroenterologist or nephrologist is recommended for assistance with nutritional management. Many hospitals now have a multidisciplinary nutrition team or TPN support team that consults on all patients on TPN or TEN and makes recommendations for treatment and evaluation of nutritional therapy.

Fat

Fat added to enteral or parenteral feeding solutions provides a way to increase calories significantly, as fat contains 9 kcal/g as compared to carbohydrate's 3.4 kcal/g. Fat is usually added to enteral formulas in the form of safflower oil, corn oil, coconut oil, sunflower oil, milk fat, or medium chain triglyceride oil.[20] Medium chain triglycerides do not require breakdown by the intestinal mucosal enzymes and are easily absorbed through the intestinal cells and into the portal vein.[2] They are useful when the absorptive capacity of the gut is compromised. Essential fatty acids (linoleic, linolenic, and arachidonic acid) are those which cannot be synthesized in the body. All enteral formulas (except those that are fat free) contain adequate levels of linoleic acid from which arachidonic acid can be made, and will prevent essential fatty acid deficiency. Enteral feeding formulas are mixed to avoid fat-related complications that are noted with the parenteral administration of fat.

Fat is necessary to prevent essential fatty acid deficiency and can greatly increase the caloric intake of patients on TPN. High glucose levels can prevent breakdown of fat stores in the body, providing access to essential fatty acids, even if body stores of these are adequate. It has been shown that 500 ml of 10 percent lipid solution given two to three times weekly will prevent fatty acid deficiency in patients on TPN. If used as a calorie source, fat infusions can be given daily or mixed in some TPN solutions.

The lipid dose can be calculated by determining how many fat calories are needed and determining the lipid grams needed by the formula in the boxed list (p. 42). Lipid solutions commonly are available in 10 or 20 percent solutions providing 1.1 and 2.0 cal/ml, respectively. They use soybean and safflower oil and contain high levels of linoleic acid,

---

Nitrogen Balance Calculation to Determine Nutritional Adequacy

Nitrogen balance = N in − N out

N in = protein intake in g/6.25 = grams of N in the protein given

N out = urine urea nitrogen (UUN) mg/100 ml ×

$$\frac{urine\ vol\ (L/day)\ +\ 20\%\ of\ UUN^a\ +\ 2\ g}{100}$$

---

[a] 20 percent of UUN is added as insensible loss and 2 g for loss through the stool.

Formula to Determine Amount of Lipid Solution

Lipid grams = fat kilocalories needed/9 kcal/g
Lipid volume (ml)
= lipid grams/% lipid solution × 100

---

the primary essential fatty acid.[20] It is recommended that no more than 30 to 60 percent of nonprotein calories be supplied as fat in TPN. Higher fat concentrations will provide more calories; however, clearance of fat from the bloodstream—which occurs similar to clearance of chylomicrons in dietary fat—may be overwhelmed by high fat loads. High-fat blood levels may cause decreased platelet adhesiveness and have rarely been implicated in pulmonary dysfunction, possibly by decreasing diffusion capacity.[16] Initial or rapid infusions of intravenous lipids can cause nausea, vomiting, fever, chills, and back or chest pain, which resolve with slower infusion rates. Mild elevations of liver enzymes can also be seen. Most adults can tolerate dosages up to 2,000 ml of 10 percent solution daily without complications. Lipids can be especially useful as a calorie source in patients who show evidence of glucose intolerance.

Deficiency of fat is characterized by manifestations of essential fatty acid deficiency, dry skin, hair loss, and scaly dermatitis. These signs are not clinically apparent for 1 to 2 months of deficiency, but may appear sooner in patients on TPN because access to fat stores is blocked by increased insulin levels due to high blood glucose levels.

Fluids

The body is made up of 55 percent water, which forms an important element in providing total nutrition. Too much or too little total body water can cause serious metabolic consequences. Most patients can tolerate and will require 2,000 to 3,000 ml/day of fluid parenterally and the same amount of enteral feedings. Patients with cardiac, renal, or hepatic decompensation will require decreased fluid volumes, depending on their clinical status. Septic or febrile patients may require more fluids but, as noted above, some patients in sepsis have decreased calorie requirements, calling for more dilute feeding solutions. The formulas in the box titled Fluid Balance Management are helpful in the management of fluid balance.

Dehydration can be evident by hypernatremia. Serum sodium is elevated 3 mEq/L for each liter of water deficit and blood urea nitrogen (BUN) increases 3 mg/dl for each liter of water deficit. If a deficit of water is detected, one-

---

Fluid Balance Management

Water deficit

Water deficit (L) = 0.6 × wt (kg)
(1 − 140/serum sodium)

Fluid requirements equal

1,500 ml × body surface area (m²)

where body surface area can be obtained from nomograms using height and weight.

Or

Fluids equal

100 ml/kg for first 10 kg body weight + 50 ml/kg for the next 10 kg body weight + 25 ml/kg for each kg over 20

---

half of the calculated deficit should be replaced over 8 hours with isotonic solution or .45 percent saline. With adequate renal function, sodium will be excreted appropriately. Dextrose in water should not be used to expand body fluid volume.

Likewise, overhydration can be detected by a dilution of BUN and serum sodium. It is marked by increased body weight and increased urine output. Restriction of free water is the treatment for overhydration, and hypertonic salt solutions (e.g., 5 percent sodium chloride) are only used in emergency situations where serum sodium is under 120 mEq/L with acute brain swelling, seizures, and coma.[2]

Normal urinary excretion of solute requires 1,200–1,500 ml/day and normal insensible losses, 500 to 1,000 ml/day. Patients undergoing extensive catabolism will produce 350 to 500 ml/day of water from the breakdown of fat and muscle. Patients reaching positive nitrogen balance may require up to 500 to 800 ml/day of extra fluid to build new cells and to replace water not released by breakdown of body tissues. Two methods for calculating maintenance fluid requirements are given in the box titled Fluid Balance Management.[2]

Fluid balance should be monitored by renal function, urine output, and daily weight. Patients should be watched for signs of fluid overload, particularly pulmonary edema. Total body peripheral edema is often a sign of poor nutritional status and, in the absence of other signs of fluid overload, should not be treated with diuretics. An attempt to move the patient into positive nitrogen balance and improve serum protein status will be more likely to improve peripheral edema.

Electrolytes and Acid-Base Status

Electrolytes

Requirements for electrolytes can vary from patient to patient, with renal and cardiac function, and other disease states. Renal compromise from sepsis, hypotension, age, chronic illness, or prior chemotherapy or drug toxicity can influence electrolyte balance. In addition, patients who have been severely malnourished for a long period may experience refeeding syndromes. Huge body deficits of potassium and phosphorus may be present and these become evident as ions shift into cells with refeeding or restoration of fluid status. These deficits must be replaced, requiring twice-daily monitoring and aggressive treatment of electrolyte disturbances. This refeeding syndrome is thought to be one of the reasons why survivors of the concentration camps in World War II died after being rescued and receiving nutrition.[14]

Enteral feeds are balanced with needed electrolytes, and specific deficits such as potassium or calcium can be addressed with intravenous supplementation or by adding supplements to the feeding formula. Recommendations for electrolytes for patients on TPN comprise wide ranges, and electrolytes should be checked daily when TPN is started until the patient is stable on a formula, then two to three times weekly.

Suggested levels used in parenteral nutrition formulas are listed in Table 2-4. These levels are suggested ranges and must be carefully adjusted to each patient's clinical status. Patients with normal renal function and normal electrolytes preinfusion can be started on a mixture of electrolytes in the mid- to high range of the requirements. It is important to note that the table contains total *daily* requirements. Patients receiving 180 mEq/day of sodium will receive 60 mEq in each 1-L bag of their daily 3 L of TPN.

In patients with normal renal function on appropriate volumes of intravenous fluids, sodium rarely becomes a serious problem. Hyper- and hyponatremia are signs more indicative of abnormal fluid status than of body sodium deficit. The required amount of sodium should be given daily (Table 2-4) and fluid balance evaluated as described above. Hyponatremia can result from overly aggressive diuresis with loop diuretics in the absence of adequate sodium supplied by TPN solutions.[14]

Table 2-4. Recommended Daily Mineral/Electrolyte Requirements for Intravenous Supplementation

Mineral/Electrolyte	Requirement (mEq)
Sodium chloride	60–180
Potassium chloride	60–120
Magnesium sulfate	8–24
Potassium phosphate	15–45 mmol phosphate
Calcium gluconate	10–20

Potassium levels can drop as malnourished patients are re-fed, due to the shift of potassium into cells. Wide shifts in potassium can occur as hemodynamics stabilize in the septic patient, as acute renal failure resolves, or as postoperative fluid shifts and diuresis occurs. Potassium should be supplied in amounts above the midlevel of the recommended range in patients who have normal renal function, and adjusted as needed with daily monitoring of potassium levels. Patients with compromised renal function can develop high levels of potassium on TPN, which can lead to fatal cardiac arrhythmias. These patients may need very little or no potassium added to their TPN solutions. Potassium should be carefully monitored in all patients on intravenous fluids and should not be added to any parenteral fluids until renal function is known to be adequate and baseline serum potassium has been measured.

Calcium, when supplied in adequate amounts, is rarely a problem in patients on TPN, but should be monitored along with electrolytes. Patients who have bleeding disorders or hemorrhage require calcium as a cofactor for clotting factors and may need extra supplementation. Hypocalcemia can produce weakness, tetany, arrhythmias, or seizures. Hypercalcemia can produce weakness, nausea, constipation, lethargy, and coma and can be a severe problem in cancer patients with metastatic bone disease. Serum calcium measurements should be adjusted to account for albumin levels seen in malnourished patients by adding to the measured serum calcium the corrective factor of 0.8 (4.0 − serum albumin). This will give the true calcium level in hypoalbuminemic patients.[2]

Magnesium should be supplied as recommended above in TPN solutions. It serves as a cofactor in many enzyme systems. A deficiency of magnesium can cause cardiac arrhythmias, muscle weakness or fasciculations, tremors, nausea, and vomiting. Magnesium also affects the balance of phosphorus, calcium, and potassium, and should be monitored with the same frequency. One may find it difficult or impossible to correct abnormal levels of these without also correcting a low magnesium level.[18] As obstetrician/gynecologists are well aware, magnesium can be given in intramuscular or intravenous doses of up to several grams, as is done in the treatment of pre-eclampsia. To avoid the necessity of such large doses, magnesium should be supplemented daily in TPN solutions. Patients with renal failure may develop serious hypermagnesemia and may not require daily magnesium supplementation. Magnesium should be measured with electrolytes in patients on TPN.

Acid-Base Status

The acid-base status of patients on TPN can be affected in two ways that can be prevented by adjustment of TPN solutions. Gastrointestinal suction may remove stomach acid containing hydrochloric acid in large amounts, thus removing chloride ions. This can lead to metabolic alkalosis, which can require supplemental acid to be added to TPN solutions. Sodium chloride should be supplied in TPN in adequate amounts to prevent chloride ion deficit.

Frequently with TPN solution, chloride ions will be given in excess as sodium, and potassium and sometimes calcium are given as chloride salts. Care should be taken to avoid too high a chloride load. Potassium can be supplied not only as chloride, but also as phosphate, which is an important nutritional component of TPN. One milliliter of potassium phosphate solution supplies 4.4 mEq/ml of potassium and 3 mmol of phosphate. Extremely low levels of phosphate (less than 0.3 mmol/L) can cause respiratory arrest, seizures, and coma. Low but not critically low levels of phosphate can cause muscle weakness and respiratory distress. Severe hypophosphatemia can occur when malnourished patients are begun on TPN as phosphate shifts into cells.[18]

Phosphate must be given slowly to avoid precipitation of calcium phosphate into the bloodstream. Supplemental phosphate can be given to patients with critically low phosphate levels at a rate of 0.08 to 0.16 mmol/kg over 6 hours.[14] Care should be taken to measure phosphate levels daily when patients are begun on TPN, as it is much simpler to provide the nutrient in high amounts in TPN than to replace a serious phosphate deficit once it develops.

For patients with a tendency towards acidosis with low serum bicarbonate, additional buffering capacity can be provided by replacing sodium or potassium as acetate ions. This will also help to avoid hyperchloremic states. In general, sodium and chloride should be given in a 1:1 ratio. If additional potassium is needed, the phosphate or acetate salts can be used. Patients with hyperchloremic acidosis should receive a portion of their sodium requirements through sodium acetate.

Trace Elements

Trace elements are substances that are present in very small quantities in the body. Nine have been identified as essential in humans. These are iron, zinc, chromium, copper, iodine, manganese, molybdenum, selenium, and cobalt. Others such as arsenic, nickel, and fluorine have not been shown to be essential.[15] Patients who require short-term TPN are unlikely to need supplementation of these elements; however, most are nontoxic and easy to supply in parenteral feedings. Most enteral feeding formulas contain a mixture of trace elements. Many hospital pharmacies use a commercial mixture of trace elements that is mixed into 1 L of the patient's TPN daily. If a mixture is not available, elements can be added in the amounts noted in Table 2-5.

Iron

Iron is provided in most enteral nutrition formulas. The addition of iron to TPN is controversial. It has been shown in a number of studies that bacteria thrive in an iron-rich environ-

Table 2-5. Trace Element Daily Supplementation

	Oral	Intravenous
Zinc	10–15 mg	2.5–5.0 mg
Copper	1.2–3 mg	0.5–1.5 mg
Chromium	50–290 μg	10–15 μg
Manganese	0.7–5 mg	0.15–0.8 mg
Iodine	150 μg	1.2–3.0 μg
Selenium	50–200 μg	40–120 μg
Iron (women)	18 mg	1–10 mg
Molybdenum	45–500 μg	20–120 μg
Cobalt	2 μg	Given as vitamin B_{12}

ment, that iron may decrease the bacteriocidal activity of leukocytes, and that TPN solutions containing iron may increase a patient's risk of sepsis.[2,15,23–25] Patients who have required transfusion may not need iron supplementation, as they have received a large bolus of iron in the form of hemoglobin, which will be broken down and added to body iron stores. Although anemic patients may benefit from iron supplementation, some studies have shown that TPN alone may enable patients to mobilize body iron stores without exogenous iron administration.[26] Iron can be provided as iron dextran if needed in patients on long-term TPN to prevent anemia. The risk is allergic reaction. Iron deficit can be calculated (see box titled Iron Deficit Calculation) and the milligrams of iron given as iron dextran in 1,000 ml of D_5W in severely iron-deficient patients.[2] In general, in patients on short-term TPN or in patients at high risk of infection, iron supplementation is best avoided.

Zinc

Zinc is needed for wound healing and as a component of numerous metalloprotein enzyme systems in the body. Increased intestinal losses can be significant in patients with diarrhea or ileostomies and should be replaced. Increased supplementation of 2 mg/day is indicated in highly stressed catabolic patients.[4] Zinc deficiency is marked by dermatitis, alopecia, abnormal immune response, and poor wound healing due to decreased collagen synthesis.[2,15] Zinc is nontoxic in normal doses.

Iron Deficit Calculation

Iron (mg) needed =

$$0.3 \, (\text{wt [lb]}) \times \frac{(100 - \text{Hb} \times 100)}{14.8}$$

Chromium

Chromium is essential for proper glucose metabolism and is involved in amino acid metabolism and protein synthesis. Deficiency of chromium leads to glucose intolerance. Patients on high-carbohydrate diets, like those on parenteral nutrition, may become chromium deficient, leading to altered insulin function and glucose intolerance. Toxicities of chromium are not known.[2,14,15]

Copper

Copper is also a component of metalloprotein enzyme systems and patients on long-term TPN can become deficient. Copper is involved in normal central nervous system function and in the function of cytochrome oxidase and superoxidase dismutase enzymes. Deficiency can result in microcytic anemia and leukopenia. Supplemental doses are not likely to lead to toxicity. However, as excess copper is eliminated in the liver, it should not be added to TPN in patients with severe liver or biliary tract disease.

Iodine

Iodine is important in normal thyroid function, which is necessary for proper response to stress and metabolic regulation. Iodine is absorbed through the skin and, in patients who have catheter care or other procedures involving skin preparation with povidone-iodine solutions, adequate amounts of iodine may be obtained through this route. Toxicity is not seen with doses recommended for supplementation, and iodine may be a component of mixed trace element solutions.[2,15]

Manganese

Manganese is required in extremely small amounts as a cofactor in some enzyme systems. A deficiency syndrome has been described with dermatitis, slow growth, weight loss, and hypocholesterolemia. Manganese is primarily involved in metabolic systems, possibly in insulin function. Toxicity also has been described in persons working in manganese mines, with a syndrome similar to Parkinson's disease. Normal supplemental levels are nontoxic, and supplementation is required for proper metabolic function of patients on TPN. Manganese is eliminated by the liver and should be decreased in patients with hepatobiliary disease.[2,14,15]

Molybdenum

Molybdenum deficiency has been described in a patient on long-term TPN who developed evidence of enzyme deficiencies associated with molybdenum as a cofactor, xanthine oxidase, and sulfite oxidase.[27] This syndrome included neurologic abnormalities and resolved with molybdenum administration. Supplementation is recommended in patients on long-term TPN. Molybdenum is renally excreted.

Selenium

Selenium is required for proper function of the glutathione peroxidase enzyme, which is involved in the metabolism of peroxides. Lack of selenium may result in impaired granulocyte function and impaired immunity. T-lymphocyte function can also be impaired. The inactivation of free radicals may be impaired by selenium deficiency, and in rats, selenium deficiency increased lung damage when animals were exposed to 100 percent oxygen.[14] Selenium may play an important role in protecting cells from free radical damage.

Cardiomyopathy on short-term TPN associated with selenium deficiency has been described.[28,29] Muscle cramps and proximal muscle weakness have also been described as symptoms of selenium deficiency. A syndrome called Keshan's disease has been known for years in one area of China (which has very low soil selenium levels), consisting of a fatal cardiomyopathy from selenium deficiency.[30] Selenium should be routinely supplied to patients on TPN. Toxicity, which can cause dermatitis, nail and hair loss, nausea, and fatigue is not usually seen at the recommended doses. Selenium is renally excreted and high levels may develop with supplementation in patients with renal failure. Toxicity is augmented in patients with hypoproteinemia or vitamin E deficiency.[2,15]

Cobalt

Cobalt is required in humans as cyanocobalamin, vitamin B_{12}. No supplementation of cobalt in TPN solutions is needed if vitamin B_{12} is provided in adequate amounts.

Vitamins

Vitamins are required as cofactors in enzyme systems, and are important in the metabolism of other nutrients. Most enteral feeding formulas contain vitamin mixtures and little additional supplementation is required. Patients receiving TPN require vitamins, particularly water-soluble vitamins, which are not stored in the body. Commercial vitamin mixtures are available, which can be added to TPN daily and are designed to meet American Medical Association Nutrition Advisory Group guidelines.[14] Certain clinical conditions will alter metabolism of some vitamins, and some patients may come to surgery with vitamin deficiencies that will not be corrected with standard vitamin solution. These situations require specific vitamin therapy.

Fat-Soluble Vitamins

Fat-soluble vitamins A, D, E, and K are stored in the body and deficiency is unusual. Parenteral feeding may block access to fat stores and may precipitate fat-soluble vitamin deficiency states. Fat- and water-soluble vitamins should be supplied during feeding with TPN.

Vitamin K depends on gut flora for its synthesis. Patients who have had changes in gut flora due to antibiotics or mechanical bowel preparations (which decrease gut flora) may be vitamin K deficient. Patients on parenteral nutrition should be supplemented with 10 mg/wk of vitamin K given intramuscularly.[2] Intravenous vitamin K can cause anaphylaxis. Patients on warfarin anticoagulation should not be given supplements, as vitamin K administration will counteract warfarin. In addition, patients on enteral feedings or on regular diets may require supplementation of vitamin K if liver disease is present. Vitamin K can correct mild abnormalities in coagulation profiles in patients whose liver disease results in decreased synthesis of vitamin K-dependent coagulation factors.

Vitamin E may also be deficient in patients with liver disease and require additional supplementation. Vitamin E is an antioxidant important in stabilizing cell membranes and limiting damage by free radicals in the tissues. Vitamin E deficiency has been thought to increase thrombotic complications. Deficiency is likely in patients who are severely malnourished or who have increased fat excretion in the stool (steatorrhea). These patients may need extra supplementation. No toxicities have been described. The recommended daily intravenous dose is 10 IU.[2,14,15]

Vitamin D can cause toxicity in excess amounts.[18] Vitamin D toxicity can cause nausea, headache, weakness, decreased serum magnesium, osteoporosis with increased serum calcium and phosphorus, and deposition of calcium deposits in the kidney, heart, and lungs. Likewise, deficiency of vitamin D, known as rickets in children, can cause osteomalacia in adults, with low serum calcium and phosphorus levels.[2,31] The recommended daily dose in TPN solutions is 200 IU.[14]

The recommended dose of vitamin A is 3,300 IU/day in a TPN solution. Normally it is derived from dietary carotenes. Patients with intestinal conditions causing diarrhea or malabsorption may be vitamin A deficient. Vitamin A is stored in the liver and toxic effects can include jaundice and liver enlargement. Other symptoms of toxicity are epistaxis, fatigue, lethargy, increased intracranial pressure, headaches, dry skin, and brittle nails. These symptoms usually resolve when intake of the vitamin is stopped.

Symptoms of vitamin A deficiency are night blindness, dermatitis, leukopenia with increased susceptibility to infection, and decreased endogenous steroid production.[2] Vitamin A is particularly important in patients receiving systemic steroids or radiotherapy, as it may improve wound healing in these patients.

Water-Soluble Vitamins

The water-soluble vitamins must be supplied daily, as they are not stored in the body. They are rapidly excreted and toxicity is not a concern. A critical B vitamin in patients on TPN is thiamine, vitamin B_1. Deficiency of thiamine can cause beriberi, a high output cardiac failure, and Wernicke's encephalopathy. High-carbohydrate TPN solutions increase the need for thiamine and exaggerate the deficiency. Thiamine deficiency is particularly important in alcoholic patients.[2,15] Requirements for thiamine are also increased in pregnancy and it should be well supplied to patients on TPN for hyperemesis gravidarum. The daily intravenous dose is 3.0 mg; however, much higher initial doses (up to 100 mg) may be needed in patients who are thiamine deficient.[14,24] No toxicities have been described.

Vitamin B_2, or riboflavin, deficiency can cause scaly skin, itching and dryness of eyes, redness of the tongue or lips (cheilosis), and angular stomatitis. Deficiency is seen in patients with diarrhea, liver disease, or alcoholism.[31] The recommended daily dose in TPN is 3.6 mg. Riboflavin is required for function of the electron transport chain and other enzymes of respiration.[2]

Niacin is another B vitamin required by respiratory enzyme systems. Deficiency of niacin results in pellagra, and is found in populations for whom corn is the major dietary component. Deficiency can cause stomatitis, glossitis, and neurologic symptoms. Nausea and severe diarrhea with ulceration may occur.[31] It is recommended that TPN solutions be supplemented with 40 mg of niacin daily.

Vitamin B_6, pyridoxine, is a cofactor for several metabolic enzyme systems. Deficiency is marked by personality changes, depression, acneform rash, and peripheral neuropathy.[2,31] The recommended supplementation in TPN solutions is 4.0 mg daily.

Vitamin B_{12} is stored in the liver and deficiencies are uncommon, except in patients with malabsorption due to lack of intrinsic factor or to resection of the terminal ileum where the vitamin is absorbed. A megaloblastic anemia known as *pernicious anemia* may develop in severely deficient patients. Neurologic symptoms are common due to the need for the vitamin in myelin synthesis. Paresthesias, unsteadiness, and central nervous symptoms such as confusion, agitation, and psychosis can develop in patients with severe deficiency.

Cyanocobalamin, vitamin B_{12}, represents the body's requirement for the trace element cobalt. Recommended doses of 5.0 μg daily in TPN solutions are recommended, but very high doses of 1,000 μg can be given as single intramuscular doses for patients with severe deficiency. In patients on long-term TPN, it is recommended to provide 1,000 μg/mo IM. No toxicity is known. Vitamin B_{12} requirements are increased in pregnancy.[31]

Folate is required for normal cell growth and function, and requirements are increased in pregnancy and for conditions of increased red blood cell turnover, such as hemolytic anemia. Alcoholic patients are often folate deficient and require additional supplementation. Megaloblastic anemia is the major sign of folate deficiency and can be corrected with adequate supplies of the vitamin. Glossitis and stomatitis may also occur.[2,31] The daily recommended dose for TPN solutions is 400 μg.[14]

Biotin deficiency has been described with paresthesias, depression, irritability, total body alopecia, and erythematous skin eruptions. Biotin is active in the metabolic pathways of the Krebs cycle and in folate metabolism.[2,15,31] The recommended dose in daily TPN solutions is 60 μg.

Pantothenic acid functions as coenzyme A in metabolic pathways. No deficiency syndrome has been described. It has been described as a treatment for ileus, but is unproven. Excess levels can cause diarrhea, but no toxic effects have been reported. Supplementation of 15 mg/day has been recommended in TPN solutions.[2,14]

Vitamin C (ascorbic acid) is important in wound healing and collagen formation. It is also involved in the electron transport chain. Deficiency of vitamin C is known as scurvy. Symptoms include weakness, irritability, myalgia, spontaneous hemorrhages, poor wound healing, and bleeding gums. Intravenous supplementation of 100 mg/day in TPN solutions is recommended for normal patients. Higher doses are rarely toxic and can be useful in patients who are deficient or when wound healing is a prime concern. High doses may interfere with heparin and warfarin anticoagulation, and may cause high urinary oxalate levels, leading to urinary stones.[2,14,31]

ADMINISTERING NUTRITIONAL SUPPORT

Enteral Feeding

The best route for nutritional support, if feasible, is the functioning gut.[32] It has been shown that use of the gastrointestinal tract in the early postoperative period can reduce the incidence of infection.[33] This is because the gut, if bypassed, begins to atrophy. Intestinal crypts flatten and the normal IgA antibody secretion is decreased. The walls become more permeable to bacteria and bacteria enter the system, leading to sepsis. In addition, the normal acids produced in the upper gastrointestinal tract are decreased, often by antacids or nasogastric suction, and this barrier to infection is lowered.

For patients whose gut is accessible and functional, this should be the route of nutritional support. Nutritional support can also be extra calories and nutrients given to patients who are taking an oral diet but do not have the appetite to take in enough normal food. In these cases, liquid supplements are available that are flavored and contain sufficient calories, protein, vitamins, and minerals to totally replace the oral diet. Patients may continue taking an ad lib diet, but do not need to force more intake if they are receiving adequate amounts of the supplements as determined by their calculated protein and calorie needs. One benefit in patients who are undergoing preoperative bowel preparation or preparation for bowel testing such as barium enemas, is that low-residue liquid nutrition formulas can be used with a clear liquid diet to supplement nutritional status without leaving fecal residue in the colon.[20]

For patients such as those intubated for respiratory failure, tube feeding is appropriate. The gut is functional and can be accessed with a thin feeding tube placed through the nose into the gastrointestinal tract. Nasogastric tubes can be used to infuse enteral feedings; however, due to the possibility of large residual volumes in the stomach, this route is not recommended. Aspiration of tube feedings is a serious complication that can be fatal, and the possibility of gastric distension and large residual volume increases this risk. Nasogastric tubes can be used for feeding, providing that residual volumes are checked frequently and conditions such as sepsis, respiratory distress, and electrolyte imbalance (which may increase gastric atony) are not present. Percutaneous gastrostomy feeding tubes can also be placed.[14]

Placement of a small bore (8–12 French) feeding tube into the duodenum by gravity is preferred. Tubes are available with a weighted end, which assists in placement past the pylorus, decreasing the risk of large residual volumes in the stomach and aspiration. Residuals can still occur in the stomach and should be monitored. In addition, a nasogastric tube for stomach decompression may be necessary if gastric atony is present. Tubes can also be placed surgically into the jejunum, decreasing the risk of aspiration, but delivering a high osmotic load directly to the small bowel.[15]

Calculation of the patient's protein, calorie, and fluid needs is done as described above. Many varieties of enteral feeding solutions are available, from solutions that can be given orally to elemental diets that require minimal gut function for absorption. Special mixtures high or low in protein, osmols, fiber, branched chain amino acids, and other special requirements are available. Low-glucose formulas are available for patients with underlying pulmonary disease, and special mixtures exist for patients with renal or hepatic failure. Data suggest that specialized formulas that are high in glutamine may be beneficial in critically ill patients, to maintain the immune function of the gastrointestinal mucosa and decrease the incidence of sepsis.[7]

After choosing a route of administration and a formula appropriate for the patient, the volume/day needed to supply adequate nutrition is calculated. Hyperosmolar enteral solutions are diluted initially to one-half or one-third strength. Isotonic products may not need to be diluted. In patients in whom fluid overload is a concern, lower infusion rates of full-strength solution are appropriate.

The position of the tube to be used for feeding is checked with a radiograph before beginning the infusion. The infusion is begun slowly—20 to 50 ml/hr with the head of the bed elevated 30 degrees at all times during infusion. Infusion rates should be pump controlled if possible. If the patient is tolerating the feedings well, the infusion rate can be increased by 10 to 25 ml/hr or the concentration can be increased to three-quarters of full strength every 12 to 24 hours. Do not increase strength and concentration at the same time.

The tube position should be checked throughout the day to watch for displacement. The stomach should be aspirated for residual volumes every three to four hours initially, then, if the feeds are tolerated well and the patient's clinical condition is unchanged or improving, every 12 to 24 hours. Residuals over 100 ml at initial infusion rates or 150 to 200 ml at full infusion rates are an indication to stop feedings and recheck in 1 hour. If the residual is gone, feeds may be started at a slower rate. If high residuals persist, parenteral feeding may be necessary. If signs of intolerance are present after a rate or concentration change (such as abdominal distension, nausea, or severe diarrhea) the patient should be given the previously tolerated level for 24 hours.[14,15]

Patients on tube feedings should be monitored the same as patients on parenteral nutrition. Initially, electrolytes should be checked daily to assist with fluid and electrolyte balance, and twice weekly once the patient is stable. Weight and urine testing for glycosuria should be taken daily, and measurements of intake and output to check fluid status and to prevent osmotic diuresis. Weekly liver function testing, blood counts, and coagulation profiles assist in monitoring the patient's status.

Complications of enteral feedings include aspiration (as discussed above), diarrhea with dehydration, and inability to tolerate feeding. Initial diarrhea after starting tube feedings is an osmotic diarrhea resulting from failure of the gut to absorb the nutrients provided. Bacterial depletion from broad spectrum antibiotics can also cause diarrhea. Osmotic diarrhea can be resolved by decreasing the concentration of the feeds or by using elemental formulas that easily pass through the walls of the intestine. Lactose intolerance can be avoided by using lactose-free solutions. Antidiarrheals and stool bulking agents or increased fiber in the solution may also be helpful, but must be monitored carefully to avoid ileus or obstructive symptoms.

If diarrhea does not appear to be osmotic and does not respond rapidly to changes in feeding administration, stool should be tested for *Clostridium difficile* toxin and white blood cells, to rule out pseudomembranous colitis—which can be fatal if untreated. Treatment with oral metronidazole or, in resistant cases, vancomycin can avoid serious complications. Postoperative patients treated with broad-spectrum antibiotics, which diminish normal gut flora, are at increased risk of this condition.

Fluid and electrolyte imbalance can usually be corrected by adjustments in the volume of feedings. Occasionally, intravenous fluids are required. Potassium, calcium, and magnesium supplements can be added to feeding solutions or can be supplemented intravenously. Patients with diarrhea will require extra fluids in one form or another. With enteral feeding solutions at appropriate doses, no supplementation of vitamins or trace elements is needed. Vitamin K supplementation of 10 mg/wk IM may be required if gut flora is depleted. Adequacy of nutrition provided can be assessed by nitrogen balance as described above.

Parenteral Nutrition Methods

Peripheral TPN

There are theoretically two routes of administration for TPN: peripheral vein and central vein. Peripheral parenteral nutrition requires low glucose concentrations because of the high osmolality of TPN solutions. The peripheral formulas must be lipid-based to provide adequate calories without high osmolality, which is destructive to peripheral veins. Lipid solutions and dextrose/amino acid solutions must be run concurrently to avoid damage to peripheral veins.

Peripheral TPN is limited in calories, more expensive than central TPN, and solutions are more complex in design. It is not useful in patients who are unable to tolerate high fat loads. It was used in the past to avoid complications associated with central line placements in critically ill patients, in patients with limited central access, and as a temporizing measure for patients expected to require intravenous feedings for a short time or until central access could be established.

In view of the recent improvement in peripherally placed central venous access devices and their low complication rate, very little use is currently seen for peripheral TPN. Peripherally inserted central lines can now be placed sterilely at the bedside or in an office setting, into the large central veins. These devices can be accessed easily, left in place for several weeks, and changed easily in the event of septic complications. They do not require tunneling and are easy to maintain. This technique is recommended over peripheral TPN administration.

Central TPN

Central TPN must be administered through a dedicated, newly placed, clean line to avoid infectious complications. Care of TPN lines is discussed fully in the following sections.

A typical TPN formulation for a moderately stressed postoperative patient weighing 134 lb is shown in Figure 2-1. TPN is formulated by selecting the desired fluid volume, which, in this case, is 2,000 ml of TPN and 500 ml of a 10 percent lipid solution daily—well above the fluids required as calculated based on body weight by the equation in the box titled Fluid Balance Management. TPN is formulated by calculating the patient's calorie and protein requirements and translating these into appropriate volumes of amino acid and dextrose solution, taking into account the 550 calories from 500 ml lipid infusion.

In this case, the patient requires 35 kcal/kg/day or 2,135 calories daily and 1.3 g/kg/day of protein. In the planned mixture, she will receive 500 ml of 50 percent dextrose in each of 2 L of TPN daily, giving a total of 1,700 carbohydrate calories. Thus, with 500 ml of 10 percent lipid solution daily, 24.4 percent of the patient's daily calories are from fat, a well-tolerated level. This level could be increased if the patient were carbohydrate intolerant. The patient will also receive 1,000 ml of 8.5 percent amino acid solution or 85 g of protein. For this patient weighing 61 kg, this amount provides 1.39 g/kg/day, or just above the chosen protein requirement.

To calculate whether calories are adequate for the nitrogen given, we find that 85 g of protein equals 13.6 g of nitrogen. At 150 to 200 kcal/g of nitrogen required, this amount of protein requires 2,040 to 2,720 kcal/day. The patient with the regimen above will receive 2,250 kcal, well within the range.

The amino acid and dextrose solutions are divided between 2 L, adding electrolytes according to the recommendations in Table 2-4. Sodium chloride is added at 40 mEq/L, potassium phosphate at 20 mmol/L of phosphate (29 mEq of potassium), magnesium sulfate at 10 mEq/L, and calcium gluconate at 10 mEq/L. Potassium chloride is needed because potassium requirements are higher than the 58 mEq provided by potassium phosphate. To balance the chloride ions in the potassium chloride with sodium, 20 mEq/L of sodium acetate is added. This is particularly important in patients with hyperchloremic acidosis, as discussed above.

Trace elements and multivitamins are added using commercial solutions, one solution to each liter in standard doses.

It is best not to mix vitamins and trace elements in the same mixture. Electrolytes are monitored daily initially and electrolyte concentrations adjusted accordingly.

Some have advocated using 1,000 U/L of heparin to maintain vein patency. This was used in peripheral TPN and may be helpful if small-bore peripherally inserted lines are used. It is not needed in TPN given through a large-gauge central venous line.

Insulin may be required in patients on TPN due to the high glucose loads. Most patients will tolerate the infusion rates of glucose as noted above. However, patients who develop hyperglycemia over 180 mg/dl or patients with 2+ or greater glycosuria are at increased risk of complications. Insulin should be mixed directly into the TPN solution. When glucose intolerance is seen on fingerstick testing, coverage with subcutaneous doses of insulin on a sliding scale may be used as needed until a new TPN solution containing insulin can be mixed. The dose of insulin required during the previous 24 hours can be added to the next day's TPN solution. Some insulin has been reported to adhere to plastic tubing and bags, but response to the added dose will be a result of insulin that reaches the patient, and following glucose levels will be adequate to monitor dose. No extra insulin should be added in because of adherence to plastic.

If high levels of insulin are required in a nondiabetic patient, calorie requirements and the glucose/fat ratio should be reexamined to avoid overfeeding, which will lead to increased fat deposits. Insulin can also shift potassium into

---

Patient 134 lb (61 kg); moderately stressed, normally nourished preoperatively

Patient requirements
  Fluids

$$100 \text{ ml} \times 10 \text{ kg} = 1,000 \text{ ml}$$
$$+ 50 \text{ ml} \times 10 \text{ kg} = 500 \text{ ml}$$
$$+ 25 \text{ ml} \times 41 \text{ kg} = \underline{1,025 \text{ ml}}$$
  Total fluids $= 2,525 \text{ ml}$

Calories (moderate stress requires 35 kcal/kg/day and 1.0–1.5 g/kg/day protein)

$$35 \text{ k cal} \times 61 \text{ kg} = 2,135 \text{ kcal}$$
$$1.3 \text{ g/kg/day} \times 61 \text{ kg} = 79.3 \text{ g}$$
$$79.3 \text{ g protein} / 6.25 \text{ g nitrogen} = 12.68 \text{ g nitrogen}$$

Need 150–200 kcal/g nitrogen = 1,902–2,536 kcal (1 g protein = 6.25 g nitrogen)

TPN plan
  2,000 ml/day crystalloid TPN over 24 hours and 500 ml/day 10% lipid solution over 12 hours

A

Fig. 2-1. (A & B) Sample TPN calculation. See text for details. *(Figure continues.)*

Sample TPN solution

	Liter 1	Liter 2
50% Dextrose solution	500 ml	500 ml
8.5% Amino acid solution	500 ml	500 ml
Sodium chloride	40 mEq/L	40 mEq/L
Potassium phosphate	20 mmol (29 mEq K)	20 mmol (29 mEq K)
Potassium chloride	20 mEq/L	20 mEq/L
Sodium acetate	20 mEq/L	20 mEq/L
Magnesium sulfate	10 mEq/L	10 mEq/L
Calcium gluconate	10 mEq/L	10 mEq/L
Multivitamins	1 dose	— 1 dose
Trace elements	—	

Totals

50% Dextrose solution	1,000 ml
8.5% Amino acid solution	1,000 ml
Sodium	120 mEq/day
Chloride	120 mEq/day
Potassium	98 mEq/day
Phosphate	40 mmol/day
Acetate	40 mEq/day
Magnesium	20 mEq/day
Calcium	20 mEq/day
Multivitamins	1 dose/day
Trace elements	1 dose/day
As a separate solution	500 ml 10% lipid solution

This solution supplies	2,500 ml/day
Fluids	
Calories	1,700 kcal/day (1 L 50% dextrose solution at 1,700 kcal/L)
Carbohydrate	85 g/day (1,000 ml 8.5% amino acid solution)
Protein	13.6 g/day (85 g protein/6.25 g nitrogen/1 g protein)
Nitrogen	550 kcal/day (500 ml/day 10% lipid solution at 1.1 kcal/ml)
Fat calories	

Total fat and carbohydrate calories

2,250 kcal/day = 550 + 1,700 (percentage fat calories = 24.4%)

$$\frac{2,250 \text{ kcal/day}}{13.6 \text{ g nitrogen/day}} = 165.44 \text{ kcal/g nitrogen}$$

For our patient

$$\frac{2,250 \text{ kcal/day}}{61 \text{ kg}} = 36.8 \text{ kcal/kg/day}$$

$$\frac{85 \text{ g/day protein}}{61 \text{ kg}} = 1.39 \text{ g/kg/day protein}$$

B

Fig. 2-1 *(Continued).*

cells and hypokalemia may result. Strict attention should be paid daily to potassium levels in the TPN solutions of patients on insulin.[2]

Hypoglycemia can occur if TPN is abruptly discontinued, due to high endogenous insulin levels. TPN that is being stopped after a number of days of continuous infusion should be gradually reduced in rate and replaced with 10 percent dextrose before stopping the infusion completely.

TPN bags should be ordered daily and, in the first week of therapy, should be adjusted based on the patient's daily laboratory values. It is important to note that the volumes ordered in liters may be exceeded by the actual volumes in each TPN bag by a small amount, due to the addition of electrolytes or vitamin solutions. In addition, rates of infusion may be slightly less than expected, owing to dressing or tubing changes or a delay in bag changes. In this situation, a buildup of ordered TPN may occur.

When ordering TPN, it is important that each liter ordered be consecutively numbered and that daily checks be performed to determine that each day's ordered TPN has been administered. If this is not monitored, it is possible after several days to find that a patient has several bags waiting that were ordered the day or days before. This is not only expensive, but it causes a delay in changes in electrolytes, which are ordered in response to laboratory values that day, while the patient is receiving TPN ordered 2 days ago.

Newer formulations of TPN allow lipid solutions to be mixed directly into amino acid and carbohydrate solutions. If lipids cannot be mixed in a single bag system, they can be given through a Y-connector over 6 to 24 hours along with the TPN infusion, to minimize side effects. Care should be taken that the total fluid volume per hour given during combined infusion is tolerated by the patient.

Cyclic TPN

Home infusion of TPN is indicated in several instances discussed in the indications section above. It is convenient for the patient receiving home TPN to have the infusion at night over 12 to 16 hours and to be disconnected from the intravenous apparatus during the day to allow free ambulation. In addition, a cyclic pattern of TPN administration mimics normal eating, in that there is a prolonged period of fasting each 24-hour period. Although no differences in nutritional benefit have been found in studies of cyclic TPN, patient convenience is maximized. Little reactive hypoglycemia is seen with even a short 1-hour taper at the end of the infusion. Home infusion companies can now provide programmable pumps that can increase and decrease infusion rates over several hours at the start and end of the infusion to minimize complications.

Complications

The metabolic complications of TPN and its components have been discussed thoroughly in the sections above. The major complications seen in TPN administration are related to central line placement and maintenance. It is imperative that experienced personnel insert or supervise the insertion of such lines. A description of line insertion is beyond the scope of this chapter.

One line or lumen of a sterilely placed line should be dedicated to TPN. The line used for TPN infusion should not have been placed under emergent conditions. It should be newly inserted when TPN is begun and inserted under strict, sterile conditions. Subclavian, internal jugular, or femoral lines can be used for TPN administration. Their position in a large central vein should be confirmed by radiograph prior to using the line. As described above, peripherally inserted central venous lines can also be considered.

No blood draws or other infusions are allowed through a dedicated TPN line. The tubing used in TPN administration should be changed daily. Dressing changes should be done sterilely. The frequency of dressing changes varies with the hospital policy. A clear dressing allows visualization of the catheter entry site and, if the dressing is sealed and the site clean, it may be left in place for several days. If a gauze dressing is used, it should be changed daily so the site can be visualized. Use of povidone iodine ointment is preferred by some authors because of its broad bacteriocidal spectrum and its decrease of fungal colonization of the site. Antibiotic ointments have been shown to increase the risk of fungal colonization.[2]

In the presence of fever, a workup to determine its source is initiated. If an obvious source is found, such as pneumonia or urinary tract infection, antibiotic treatment is begun and the catheter is left in place. If blood cultures are negative and the infection resolves, the catheter may safely remain in place. If the catheter is the suspected source or if no obvious source can be found, blood cultures should be drawn and

---

Possible Complications of Central Line Insertion

- Pneumothorax
- Hemothorax
- Hematoma with tracheal compression
- Arterial puncture
- Laceration of the thoracic duct
- Cardiac arrhythmias
- Inability to insert the line
- Death

the catheter removed. The patient should be treated and, when the episode is resolved and the patient afebrile, a new catheter is inserted and TPN restarted. A new site should be chosen. If fungal infection is suspected, the TPN should be stopped immediately and the catheter removed. Fungemia is a life-threatening emergency and fungal growth is increased in the presence of high-glucose TPN solutions.

Thrombosis of the major vessel around a central catheter requires removal of the catheter and often will require heparinization and long-term anticoagulation. Vascular surgery consultation is recommended in this situation, which can have serious consequences. Long-term anticoagulation may be indicated.

SUMMARY

Multiple methods of nutritional support are available to the surgeon. It is important to attempt preoperatively, through clinical evaluation, to identify patients who are at risk of increased morbidity due to their nutritional status. Severely malnourished patients will benefit from preoperative support, either oral or parenteral. Well-nourished patients who are unable to resume a regular dietary intake by 7 to 9 days after surgery will require nutritional support.

Nutritional support can be maximized through the use of formulas to determine the patient's requirements and by nitrogen balance measurements to assure adequate nutrition. Careful monitoring of electrolytes and clinical status can avoid metabolic imbalances, while proper catheter insertion and care can avoid the more common septic complications.

REFERENCES

1. McClave SA, Short AF, Mattingly DB, Fitzgerald PD: Total parenteral nutrition, conquering the complexities. Postgrad Med 88:235, 1990
2. Grant JP: Handbook of Total Parenteral Nutrition. WB Saunders, Philadelphia, 1992
3. Smith LC, Mullen JL: Nutritional assessment and indications for nutritional support. Surg Clin North Am 71:449, 1991
4. Schlag P, Decker-Baumann C: Strategies and needs for nutritional support in cancer surgery. Recent Results Cancer Res 121:233, 1991
5. Veterans Affairs Total Parenteral Nutrition Cooperative Study Group: Perioperative total parenteral nutrition in surgical patients. N Engl J Med 325:525, 1991
6. Mullen JL: Consequences of malnutrition in the surgical patient. Surg Clin North Am 61:465, 1981
7. Hehir DJ, Gorey TF: Intravenous nutritional support and the surgeon: where next? Ir J Med Sci 161:401, 1992

8. Campos ACL, Meguid MM: A critical appraisal of the usefulness of perioperative nutritional support. Am J Clin Nutr 55:117, 1992
9. Sandstrom R, Drott C, Hyltander A et al: The effect of postoperative intravenous feeding (TPN) on outcome following major surgery evaluated in a randomized study. Ann Surg 217:185, 1993
10. Askanazi J, Hensle TW, Starker PM et al: Effect of immediate post-operative nutritional support on length of hospitalization. Ann Surg 203:236, 1986
11. urdum PP, Kirby D: Short-bowel syndrome: a review of the role of nutritional support. J Parenteral Enteral Nutr 15:93, 1991
12. Dudrick SJ, Latifi R, Fosnocht DE: Management of short bowel syndrome. Surg Clin North Am 71:625, 1991
13. August DA, Thorn D, Fisher RL, Welchek C: Home parenteral nutrition for patients with inoperable malignant bowel obstruction. J Parenteral Enteral Nutr 15:323, 1991
14. Schilchtig R, Ayres SM: Nutritional Support of the Critically Ill. Year Book Medical Publishers, Chicago, 1988
15. Silberman H: Parenteral and Enteral Nutrition. p. 81. Appleton & Lange, E. Norwalk, CT, 1989
16. Baue AE: Nutrition and metabolism in sepsis and multisystem organ failure. Surg Clin North Am 71:549, 1991
17. Robison RJ, Madura JA: Total parenteral nutrition: indications and techniques. Indiana Medicine May:359, 1984
18. Ladefoged K, Jarnum S: Metabolic complications to total parenteral nutrition. Acta Anaesthesiol Scand 29:89, 1985
19. Baker AL, Rosenberg IH: Hepatic complications of total parenteral nutrition. Am J Med 82:489, 1987
20. Hui YH: Handbook of Enteral and Parenteral Feedings. p. 205. John Wiley & Sons, New York, 1988
21. Latifi R, Killam RW, Dudrick SJ: Nutritional support in liver failure. Surg Clin North Am 71:567, 1991
22. Compher C, Mullen JL, Barker CF: Nutritional support in renal failure. Surg Clin North Am 71:597, 1991
23. Ward CG: Influence of iron on infection. Am J Surg 151:291, 1986
24. Bothe A, Benotti P, Bistrian BR, Blackburn GL: Use of iron total parenteral nutrition. N Engl J Med 93:1153, 1975
25. Weinberg ED: Iron and susceptibilty to infectious disease. Science 184:952, 1974
26. Stead NW, Curtas S, Grant JP: Enhanced mobilization of iron from body stores in malnourished patients during intravenous support. Surg Gynecol Obstet 154:321, 1982
27. Abumrad NN, Schneider AJ, Steel D, Rogers LS: Amino acid intolerance during total parenteral nutrition reversed by molybdate. Am J Clin Nutr 34:2551, 1981
28. Levy JB, Jones HW, Gordon AC: Selenium deficiency, reversible cardiomyopathy and short term intravenous feeding. Postgrad Med J 70:235, 1994
29. Reeves WC, Marcuard SP, Willis SE, Movahed A: Reversible cardiomyopathy due to selenium deficiency. J Parenter Enteral Nutr 13:185, 1989

30. Brown MR, Cohen HJ, Lyons JM et al: Proximal muscle weakness and selenium deficiency associated with long term parenteral nutrition. Am J Clin Nutr 43:549, 1986

31. Berkow R: The Merck Manual of Diagnosis and Therapy. Merck & Co., Inc., Rahway, NJ, 1982

32. Moran BJ, Jackson AA: Perioperative Nutritional Support. Br J Surg 80:4, 1993

33. Moore FA, Feliciano DV, Andrassy RJ et al: Early enteral feeding, compared with parenteral reduces postoperative septic complications. Ann Surg 216:172, 1992

CHAPTER THREE

ELECTROSURGERY: BIOPHYSICS, SAFETY, AND EFFICACY

ROGER C. ODELL

Electrosurgical energy is the most commonly used energy source in the discipline of surgery. In open laparotomy, the surgeon has a better vantage point for controlling bleeding and dissection and has more options to complement the surgical technique. In laparoscopy and other closed procedures, delivering electrosurgical energy is a requirement for optimizing surgical outcome. With the recent shift to minimally invasive techniques comes quite an array of marketing and sales presentations that further complicate a topic that was not clearly understood from the start. This chapter should provide a better understanding of the biophysics involved in electrosurgery, to enhance safety and efficacy during minimal-access surgery. See Appendix 3-1 for a glossary of key terms.

Electrosurgical energy in laparoscopy dates back to the mid-1960s, when gynecologists began performing total desiccation (coaptation) through a channel within the laparoscope (single-puncture technique). During the course of performing such procedures electrosurgically, a number of misadventures occurred.[1] Investigations of incidents, such as arcing of electricity with resulting bowel injury, led to concerns regarding the use of monopolar electrosurgery. Consequently, monopolar electrosurgery was discouraged in laparoscopic procedures for two decades. This chapter reviews these complications, explains the physics of how they

occurred, and discusses ways of minimizing and eliminating these hazards in the future. First however, the biophysics of electrosurgical energy for dissection, fulguration, and desiccation are discussed.

BACKGROUND

The use of high-frequency electrical energy for surgical application dates back nearly a century. *Electrosurgery* is the generation and delivery of radio frequency current between an active electrode and a dispersive electrode in order to elevate the tissue temperature for the purpose of dissection, fulguration, and desiccation. In contrast to electrocautery, the electric current actually passes through the tissue. In 1927, Harvey W. Cushing, M.D., with the assistance of William T. Bovie, Ph.D., provided the first in-depth documentation of the principles of the art as well as the biophysics of electrosurgery. Cushing's publications and surgical demonstration of this energy source popularized its use and acceptance. These early documents detailed his appreciation of Bovie's device and his promotion of the versatility of this energy source. By no means did Cushing and Bovie invent electrosurgery; the Germans and French had documented the biophysics of electrosurgical currents in the late 1800s

(D'Arsonval, Jacques 1891). William L. Clark a general surgeon in Philadelphia, documented the removal of large benign and malignant growths of the skin, head, neck, and breast with electrosurgery in 1910. But it was truly Cushing's and Bovie's documentation that changed the course of neurosurgery and other surgeons' views of the potential uses of electrosurgical energy.

ELECTRICAL ENERGY AND TISSUE TEMPERATURE

Energy cannot be created or destroyed; rather, it is converted to another form of energy. In the case of electrosurgery, electrical energy is converted into heat at the active electrode target site for the purpose of vaporizing (cutting) and coagulation. Table 3-1, on the relationship of temperature rise and tissue condition, will help in the later discussion specific to electrosurgical modalities and their effect on tissues and vessels.

The three electrical elements that figure into temperature rise are *current* (I), *voltage* (V), and *resistance (impedance)* (R).

To help simplify the complexities of electrical theory, a direct analogy to a water or hydraulic energy source is made. The water tower in Figure 3-1 presents a hydraulic energy source for the purpose of performing work. Figure 3-2 shows an equivalent electrosurgical "tower" with the electrical terms *current, voltage,* and *resistance* inserted. This direct relationship is important in overcoming the mystique of electrosurgical modalities. The reader should note that both the water tower and the electrosurgical energy sources are operating with thousands of feet of head pressure and thousands of volts. The potential for extremely high voltage—the height of the water tower—is a key element in the design of an electrosurgical unit (ESU). While water towers typically are 100 feet or so above the ground, and household appliances operate off 120 volts, the voltages amassed by the electrosurgical generator must exceed 5,000 to 10,000

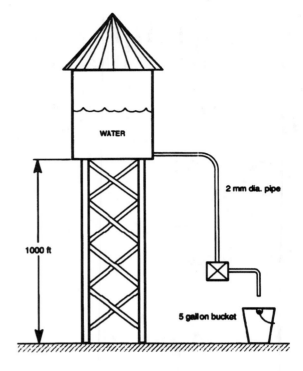

Fig. 3-1. Schematic of hydraulic energy source. (Courtesy of Electroscope, Inc., Boulder, CO.)

volts peak to peak to be effective in all aspects of electrosurgery.

The relationship between the elements of electrosurgical energy is demonstrated by *Ohm's law:*

$$I = V/R$$

The *power formula* is valuable in understanding how the waveforms of the modalities (cut, fulgurate, and desiccate) compare in the performance of various therapeutic maneuvers:

$$W = V \times I$$

Table 3-1. Affect of Temperature on Tissue Condition

	Temperature (°C)					
	34–44°	44–50°	50–80°	80–100°	100–200°	>200°
Effect						
Visible	None	None	Blanching	Shrinkage	Steam "popcorn"	Carbonization cratering
Delayed	Edema	Necrosis	Sloughing	Sloughing	Ulceration	Larger crater
Mechanism	Vasodilation, inflammation	Disruption of cell metabolism	Collagen denaturation	Desiccation	Vaporization	Combustion of tissue hydrocarbons

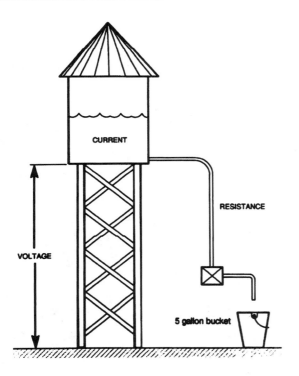

Fig. 3-2. Hydraulic energy source with electrical equivalents terms. (Courtesy of Electroscope, Inc., Boulder, CO.)

where W represents energy in wattage. The ratio of voltage to current is primarily responsible for the tissue effects observed when time and electrode size are kept equal.

Power density is the relationship of the size of active electrode in contact with the tissue to its effect on the tissue at a given energy setting:

$$\text{Power density} = (\text{current density})^2 \times \text{resistivity}$$

In noncontact modalities (i.e., cutting and fulguration) this would be equivalent to the sparking area between the active electrode and the tissue. Only in desiccation is the exact surface area of the electrode in contact with the tissue of importance when calculating power density. During fulguration and cutting, the electrode is not in contact; therefore, the power density can only be approximated. During cutting and fulguration, the electrode is in motion. Therefore, the exact energy in joules is difficult to calculate at a given point as compared to static application. These concepts are expanded in the next section.

In general, the larger the electrode surface area, the lower the power density; and the smaller the electrode surface area, the higher the power density.

The element of *time* is the primary component for controlling the depth and degree of tissue necrosis at a given energy setting. Many other considerations are also relevant, but time is particularly important, as is demonstrated in the following sections.

Energy (calculated in joules) is equivalent to wattage × time:

$$E = W \times T$$

Therefore, the longer the electrosurgical energy is applied, the higher the temperature rise and the greater the volume of tissue destroyed. The temperature within the tissue (surgical target site) is directly proportional to wattage × time.

THERAPEUTIC ELECTROSURGICAL MODALITIES

Electrosurgical energy affords the surgeon three distinct therapeutic effects on tissue: dissection, fulguration, and desiccation. Unfortunately, most ESUs are simply labeled ''cut'' and ''coag,'' terms that do not dispel the present confusion pertaining to the optimal use of electrosurgical energy. In open procedures its optimal use was frequently overcome because the surgeon had direct access to the surgical site and could use hemostats and sutures as needed. This is not the case in laparoscopy and may result in far more severe complications as a result of operating outside the body.

Dissection

Dissection is a high-current, low-voltage (continuous) waveform that elevates tissue temperature rapidly (100°C or more), producing vaporization or division of tissue with the least effect of lateral thermal spread (coagulation) to the walls of the incision (Figs. 3-3 and 3-4). During optimal electrosurgical cutting, the current travels through a steam bubble between the active electrode and the tissue. It is important to recognize that electrosurgical cutting is a *noncontact* means of dissection. The electrode floats through the tissue and there is very little tactile response transmitted to

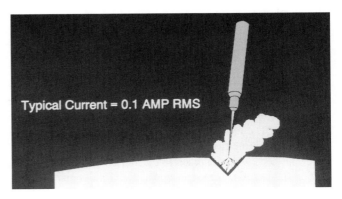

Fig. 3-3. Electrosurgical cutting, Electrode not in contact with tissue. (Courtesy of Electroscope, Inc., Boulder, CO.)

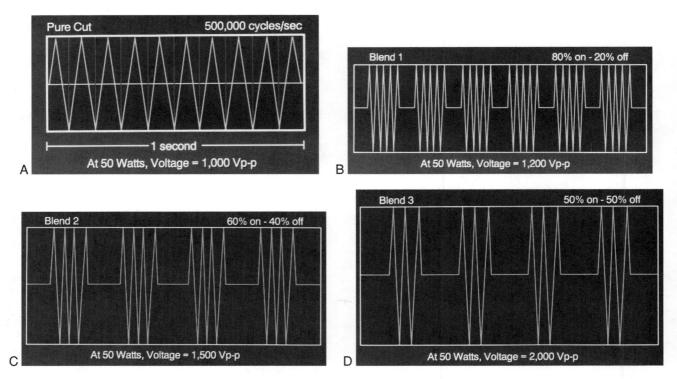

Fig. 3-4. (A) Cut waveform. **(B)** Blend 1. **(C)** Blend 2. **(D)** Blend 3. (Courtesy of Electroscope, Inc., Boulder, CO.)

the surgeon's hand. The dynamics or velocity of the electrode, as well as the waveform, determine the depth and width of necrosis of the incision. Necrosis depths of under 100 μm are attainable with electrosurgical energy during dissection. The continuous waveform is analogous to the garden valve shown in Fig. 3-1, which delivers a constant, even flow of water. Due to the constant flow of current and the lowest possible voltage required to dissect, the width and depth of necrosis to the walls of the incision are minimal. Therefore, the ratio of high current to low voltage within the waveform produces less necrosis or coagulation when desired. If the electrode is allowed to remain stationary or is slowed, the maximum temperature attained is increased, as is the depth and width of thermal damage to the walls of the incision.

Fulguration

Fulguration is a high-voltage, low-current, noncontinuous waveform (highly damped), which is designed to coagulate by means of spraying long electrical sparks to the tissue (Fig. 3-5). The most common use of fulguration is to arrest oozing emanating from a large area, (such as in a capillary or arteriole bed), where a discrete bleeder cannot be identified.

Cardiovascular, urologic, and general surgeons have relied on fulguration for their most demanding applications (i.e., hepatic resections, bleeding from a bladder tumor resection, and surface bleeding on the heart). With fulguration, a

very superficial eschar is produced; therefore, the depth of necrosis is minimal as a result of the defocusing of the power density. By drawing the electrode away from the tissue, the power density goes down, defocusing the energy or current. A great deal of the energy is dissipated in heating the air between the electrode and the tissue through which the current must pass. Fulguration, as well as electrosurgical cutting, are noncontact modalities. Fulguration can be initiated in two ways:

1. By slowly approaching the tissue until a spark jumps to the tissue, whereby a raining effect of sparks will

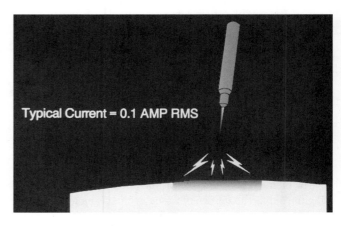

Fig. 3-5. Fulguration, Electrode not in contact with tissue. (Courtesy Electroscope, Inc., Boulder, CO.)

be maintained until the electrode is withdrawn or the tissue is carbonized to the point where the sparks cease

2. Bouncing the electrode off the tissue so as to create a raining effect of sparks to the tissue, without the painstaking effort of approaching the tissue until a spark jumps without touching

Electrosurgical fulguration is the most effective means of arresting capillary oozing or bleeding. Before fulgurating, it is important to evacuate blood or saline fluid from the target site. Sparking to blood or saline wastes time and energy. Evacuating the field or diluting it with nonisotonic solutions such as calycine or sterile distilled water can serve to clarify the target site and optimally deliver the current to stop the bleeding most efficiently.

The depth of necrosis is in the range of 0.5 to 2 mm, depending on how long the surgeon sparks the target site. The key is to stop the moment the bleeding has stopped to minimize the depth of necrosis.

Desiccation

Any waveform will desiccate due to the electrode being in contact with the tissue (Fig. 3-6). Regardless of the current/voltage ratio, the electrode surface area in contact with the tissue and the wattage times the time are the determining factors in regard to the volume of tissue necrosis. Desiccation is another form of coagulation. Most surgeons do not distinguish between fulguration and desiccation, but refer to both as coagulation. The application of electrosurgical current by means of direct contact with the tissue will result in all of the energy delivered by the ESU being converted into heat within the tissue. By contrast, with both cutting and fulgurating, a significant amount of the electrical energy converts to heat that goes into the atmosphere between the electrode and the tissue. Therefore, with contact coagulation/

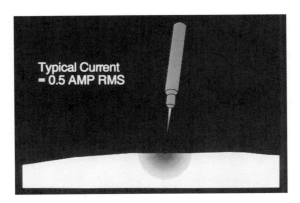

Fig. 3-6. Desiccation, Electrode in contact with tissue (no sparking between electrode and tissue) (Courtesy of Electroscope, Inc., Boulder, CO.)

desiccation, the increased energy delivered into the tissue results in deep necrosis (as deep as it is wide), as observed on the surface where the electrode makes contact (Fig. 3-6).

The most common need for desiccation is when a discrete bleeder is encountered. In that scenario, a hemostat is applied to the vessel and the electrosurgical energy is applied to the body of the hemostat (or coagulation forceps used to grasp the vessel). Consequently, the current must pass through the instrument into the tissue grasped by the jaws and back to the patient via the return electrode. The coaptation of vessels was documented as producing a collagen chain reaction resulting in a fibrous bonding of the dehydrated denatured endothelial cells.[2] Because the electrode is in good electrical contact with the tissue, the voltage/current ratio is not nearly as important as in cutting and fulgurating. In practical application, the cut/blend waveforms are superior to the fulguration waveform when desiccation is desired. The primary reason is that the fulguration waveform will tend to spark through the coagulated tissue, resulting in voids at the end of the vessel. Also, when sparks occur at the contact point of electrode to tissue, heating the metal will result in tissue adhering to the electrode when drawn off the target site. Bleeding will continue each time the eschar is pulled off due to adhesion from heat within the electrode.

In bipolar desiccation, the waveform plays a far more important role. Today, for the most part, the manufacturers have incorporated a continuous low-voltage, high-current waveform in the bipolar output to maximize the effect on desiccation. In the older models, the manufacturer allowed the surgeon to select either a continuous cut, blend, or fulguration waveform when bipolar desiccation was needed. A lack of physician understanding in combination with vague literature on tissue effects when bipolar desiccation was performed with these waveforms, led to a number of documented problems.[3] Therefore, at this time, the generally accepted waveform for bipolar desiccation is a continuous low-voltage, high-current waveform. When bipolar desiccation is critical, the author recommends that a newer model ESU with a dedicated continuous bipolar waveform be utilized. If an ESU that allows selection of both cut/blend and fulguration (coagulation) bipolar waveforms must be used the pure cut (continuous) waveform should be used first for best results. When performing desiccation, patience is the key to good results. Typically, the power density is much lower when desiccating. The physical size of the active electrodes is therefore larger. The larger electrode or contact area to tissue will require longer activation times to attain the desired therapeutic effect. Speeding up the desiccation process with higher energy levels will most likely be counterproductive, increasing the temperature to the tissue adjacent to the electrode(s) and potentially forcing the current to spark through the necrosis. This will result in fulguration rather than desiccation. Fulguration or sparking immediately stops the deep-heating process and starts to carbonize the surface of the tissue only. Therefore when sparking is observed in the process of desiccating, one should stop, reduce the power, or pulse the current by keying the ESU on and off to overcome this natural tendency for sparking to occur at high wattage levels. Sparking is not needed or wanted when desiccating. It causes tissue sticking, creates uneven necrosis, and may compromise the effort to coapt the vessel. To assist the surgeon when desiccating, an ammeter (End Point Monitor, EM-2, Electroscope, Inc., Boulder, CO) may be used to determine end point coagulation/desiccation. This will assist in confirming the visual effect as seen by the surgeon, which is accompanied by the end point of current flow on the monitor. The ammeter provides both visual and audible indicators of current flow and, when the electrolytic fluid within the tissue is dehydrated, the meter will show no current flow. Total or complete desiccation occurs after dehydration has taken place.

INHERENT RISKS

Since the inception of monopolar electrosurgery, three potential sites for patient burns due to electrosurgical current have been identified, one intended and two unintended.

The intended site is at the active electrode where the unit is used to cut, fulgurate, or desiccate the tissue in surgery. By design, the active electrode has a high-power density and heats tissue rapidly. This electrode can burn the patient severely if not kept in control at all times. Therefore, the author strongly recommends that when not in use, the active electrode be stored in an insulated holster or tray and placed on top of the Mayo stand. The draping material alone in no way acts as a suitable insulator to protect the patient from inadvertent activation.

The first unintended burn site is a consequence of current division to alternate ground points to the patient, which can only occur on a ground-referenced ESU. The second is due to a fault (i.e., a partial detachment or a manufacturing defect) at the site of the patient return electrode that forces the current to return to the ESU via a high-current density. The patient return electrode (ground plate) has an approximate surface area of 20 in.[2] or more when properly applied. Therefore, very little temperature rise occurs at this site under normal conditions.

Within the last two decades, potential burn risks have been overcome by the development of isolated ESU outputs and contact quality monitors. These safety features are available on most units sold within the past 15 years. Isolated ESU outputs were introduced in the early 1970s. The primary purpose of their introduction was the prevention of alternate ground site burns due to current division (i.e., burns to electrocardiographic electrodes and small point contact between the patient body and metal points to the operating room table). Today, the number of alternate site burns (as a direct result of current division) is essentially zero because of the introduction of isolated ESUs. There is a small percentage of hospitals that utilize ground-reference ESUs. Therefore, it would be wise to determine the type of ESU that is in service at your hospital.

Contact quality monitoring circuits were introduced in the early 1980s. They were introduced to prevent burns at the patient return electrode site. The contact quality monitor incorporates a dual section patient return electrode and circuit for the purpose of evaluating the total impedance of the patient return electrode during surgery. Therefore, if the patient return electrode became compromised in the course of surgery, the contact quality circuit would inhibit the electrosurgical generator's output based on this dual section patient return electrode and circuit combination. This feature essentially eliminated burns at the site of the patient return electrode.

These two technological advancements truly reduced the potential for patient burns during classical open electrosurgical procedures. They are featured in ESUs manufactured by Aspen, Birtcher, and Valleylab.[4]

LAPAROSCOPIC ISSUES

The use of electrosurgery in laparoscopic surgery has primarily been limited to bipolar modalities.[5] With the recent shift to laparoscopy for general, urologic, and other surgical disciplines, apprehension arose as to whether monopolar electrosurgical energy could be safely used in laparoscopy, as compared to other energy sources. The more common misconceptions in using electrosurgery in laparoscopy are addressed in the next section.

There are three potential hazards in the use of electrosurgical energy during laparoscopy: insulation failure (which poses the greatest risk to the patient), capacitive coupling, and direct coupling. All three of these hazards can be classified as stray energy out of the view of the laparoscope that may result in unintended burns to nontargeted tissue. These alternate site burns can be severe and may damage vital internal structures. The burns are particularly dangerous to hollow organs such as the bowel, as they may lead to unrecognized perforation, subsequent infection, and possibly death.[6] The three potential hazards are a direct result of two factors: trocar cannulas used to introduce instruments and the limited field of vision provide by the laparoscope.

There is also the potential for unintended thermal burns as a result of stray energy out of view of the surgeon. These burn injuries are difficult to diagnose because they are delayed in presentation. The reporting of actual injuries is low, as a result of medicolegal implications.[7]

Insulation Failure

Most laparoscopic accessories are approximately 35 cm long. The laparoscopic images on the monitor display typically less than 5 cm of the distal end of the device. The

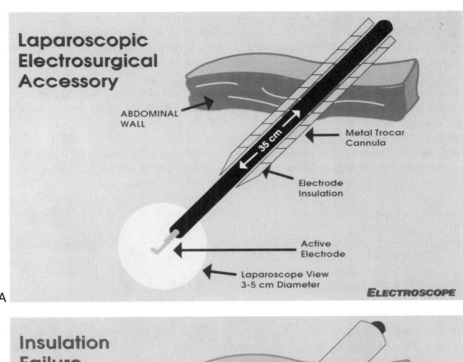

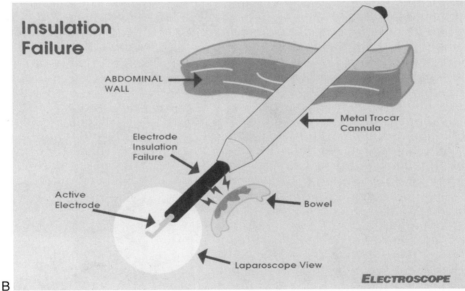

Fig. 3-7. (A) Full view of electrosurgical accessory into the peritoneal cavity. (B) Full view of electrosurgical accessory with insulation failure. (Courtesy of Electroscope, Inc., Boulder, CO.)

active electrode used for the delivery of the electrosurgical energy has insulation covering most of the electrode (Fig. 3-7A). Unfortunately, 90 percent or more of this insulated portion of the electrode is beyond the viewing image seen on the monitor. Consequently if the insulation breakdown occurs on the shaft of the electrode, out of view of the operator, a severe burn may occur to the bowel or other organs near or touching the electrode at this site (Fig. 3-7B). Insulation failures can occur for several reasons, including normal wear, handling in central supply, sharp edges on the trocar cannula, and coronal heating as a result of the high-voltage

frequency product (resulting in the melting of the instrument's insulation). It is most important for surgeons to closely examine or have these biomedical staff routinely inspect these electrodes. This will minimize but not eliminate this hazard. A common misconception suggests that disposable devices will eliminate insulation failure the quality of insulation typically found on disposables may, however, be of a lower quality than that of reusable instrumentation.[7a] Mechanical damage to shaft insulation can occur during the first use of the electrode and may present a risk to the patient.

Capacitive Coupling

The second hazard results from capacitive coupling of energy into other metal laparoscopic instruments or trocar cannulas. The principle of capacitance in electrical physics is beyond the scope of this chapter, but 5 to 40 percent of the power that the electrosurgical unit is set to deliver can be coupled or transferred into a standard 5-mm (10 cm long) trocar cannula. The energy in itself may not be dangerous, providing it is allowed to pass through a low-power density pathway, such as an all-metal (conductive) trocar cannula

inserted into the abdominal wall, and returned to the patient return electrode.

Capacitive coupling becomes a problem when this energy is allowed or made to pass through a high-power density pathway (Fig. 3-8). This can happen when partially plastic (nonconductive) and partially metal (conductive) trocar cannulas are utilized. Some trocar manufacturers supply a plastic thread to the metal cannula tube to help hold the cannula in the abdominal wall when the laparoscopic electrode is positioned in and out of the cannula port (Fig 3-8). The use of *all metal* or *all plastic* trocar cannulas is highly recom-

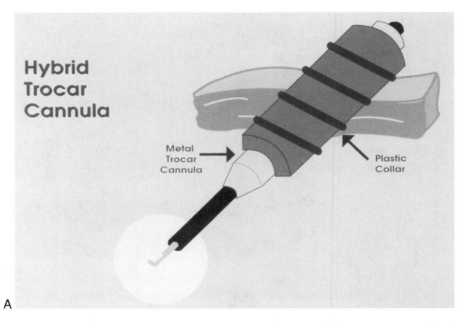

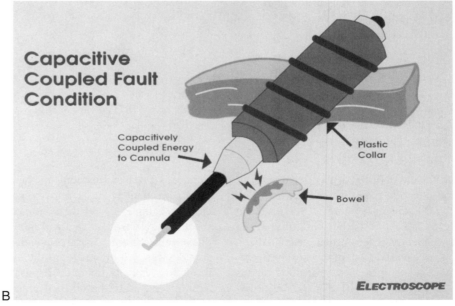

Fig. 3-8. (**A**) Hybrid trocar cannula that blocks the capacitive current from the abdominal wall. (**B**) Capacitive coupling with dangerous stray pathway back to patient return electrode. (Courtesy of Electroscope, Inc., Boulder, CO.)

mended to avoid this hazard. Capacitive coupling may also occur when suction-irrigation devices are used.[8] Up to 80 percent of the energy was shown on commercially available devices. Capacitive coupling to a lesser degree can occur when crossing another laparoscopic instrument with the electrosurgical laparoscopic electrode within the peritoneal cavity (i.e., traumatic grasper). The energy transfer between these instruments can range from 1 to 10 percent of the power set on the ESU. Some caution should be taken under this condition, especially during long activation times.

The issue of capacitive coupling was first detected in operative, single-puncture, laparoscopic procedures.[9] The laparoscope used in these procedures have an operating channel (30 to 40 cm) through which to pass various instruments. It was observed that when a plastic 10- to 12-mm cannula was used to pass the operating laparoscope, the distal end of the metal laparoscope could deliver a portion (40 to 80 percent) of the power set on the ESU, and burns to adjacent tissue were documented. Therefore, during single-puncture operative laparoscopy where electrosurgery may be used, only all metal trocar cannulas should be used to pass both the laparoscope and electrosurgical electrode into the peritoneal cavity. A strong recommendation was made by the Food and Drug Administration (FDA) to this effect.[10]

Direct Coupling

The third potential hazard associated with the use of monopolar energy occurs when the electrode tip is accidentally touched to the laparoscope or other conductive instruments (Fig. 3-9) such as traction/countertraction devices during activation. If all metal trocar cannulas are used, the energy will pass into the abdominal wall via a low-power density pathway. This will minimize the potential for injury. If plastic cannulas are used, the current may exit to the bowel or other organs touching the laparoscope or other device, out of view of the monitor. This is because the plastic cannula blocks (insulates) the directly coupled energy from the abdominal wall and prevents it from returning to the patient return electrode. Therefore, it is strongly recommended to always use metal cannulas for the laparoscope port and other ports into which conductive instruments are inserted. In the event of accidental activation and touching of the tip to the laparoscope or other instrument, one should stop; pan the instrument back, view the anatomy that it is laying across, and look for tissue discoloration before proceeding.

Active Electrode Monitoring

To eliminate the first two hazards—insulation failure and capacitive coupling—in the delivery of monopolar energy, industry introduced *active electrode monitoring* (AEM) systems in 1991. These perform a similar function to the contact quality monitors. Both systems monitor potential

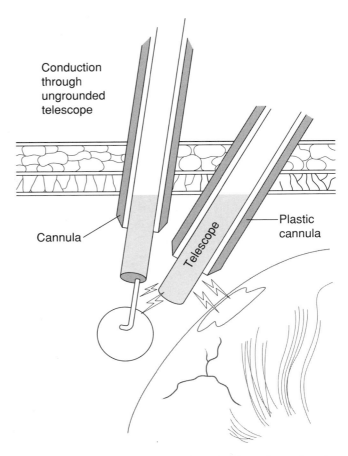

Fig. 3-9. Direct coupling occurs when the electrode touches the laparoscope or other conductive instruments within the peritoneal cavity.

burn sites that are not in the view or control of the surgeon. AEM was designed to actively monitor for insulation failure and excessive capacitive coupling out of the view of the laparoscope. The Electroshield AEM* system features either a reusable adaptive shield to the hospital's existing dissecting and coagulating laparoscopic electrodes (Fig. 3-10A) or a line of totally integrated 5 and 10 mm instruments (Fig. 3-10B) with the conductive shield integrated into the device. These instruments are reusable or limit use in design to help keep device cost low. The Electroshield Monitor EM-2 dynamically detects (Fig. 3-11) insulation faults that may occur during surgery and shields against capacitive coupling.[11] If an unsafe condition exists, the Electroshield system automatically signals the ESU to deactivate before a burn can occur. This fail-safe technological advancement allows the surgeon to use monopolar electrosurgical energy in laparoscopic pro-

---

*Electroshield AEM is a registered trademark of Electroscope, Inc., Boulder, CO and is distributed by Valleylab, Inc. of Boulder, CO.

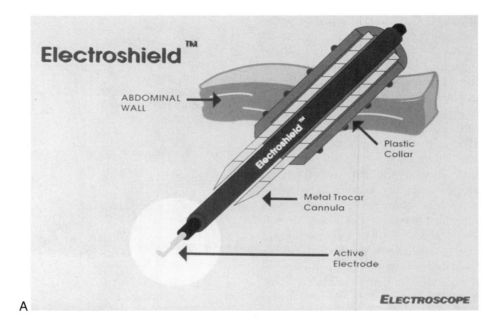

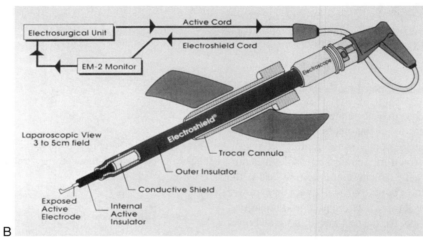

Fig. 3-10. (**A**) Electroshield: a conductive shield that surrounds existing laparoscopic electrosurgical instruments. (**B**) Integrated Shielded Electrode Diagram. (Courtesy of Electroscope, Inc., Boulder, CO.)

cedures with the same degree of confidence as in open procedures. The shielding system controls the potential hazard of stray energy out of the view of the laparoscope, which is the fundamental difference in the delivery of this energy in laparoscopy as compared to open laparotomy. The Emergency Care Research Institute (ECRI), a nonprofit health organization that performs an advisory role on the matters of clinical engineering, publishes *Health Devices,* which is subscribed to by most hospitals in the United States and has provided the most comprehensive analysis to date for the need and efficacy of AEM in laparoscopy when monopolar electrosurgery is utilized.[12] The author strongly recommends reading the entire issue cited in reference 12.

MISCONCEPTIONS

There are two misconceptions that need to be addressed in regard to the delivery of monopolar electrosurgical energy during laparoscopy.

The first misconception is that electrosurgical current, when delivered at the target site, behaves differently in laparoscopy versus open surgical procedures. In reality, the biophysics are identical in regard to the current path taken enroute to the patient return electrode in open versus laparoscopic application (which is commonly understood as the path of least resistance).

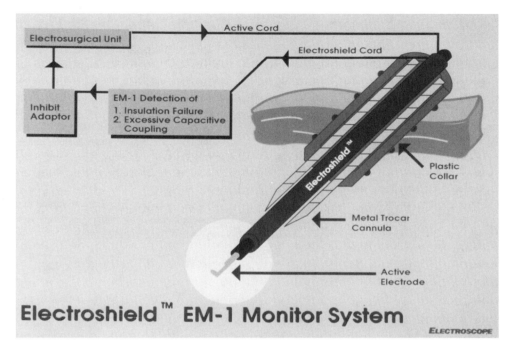

Fig. 3-11. Electroshield monitoring system. This system dynamically detects any insulation faults and shields against capacitive coupling. (Courtesy of Electroscope, Inc., Boulder, CO.)

Complications have been reported in both open and laparoscopic applications of monopolar energy where a pedicel of tissue is created by stretching or otherwise, and the current is reconcentrated through this narrowing cross section of tissue, resulting in temperature rise to the tissue at that point. This condition is true for both open as well as laparoscopic procedures. Better surgical techniques could prevent these complications if surgeons have a better understanding of the biophysics in the delivery of the energy. A case in point that is worth reviewing is female laparoscopic sterilization.[1]

The second misconception is that sparking cannot be controlled when monopolar current is utilized. Sparking has been defined as follows by the medical community: "In a closed peritoneal cavity, the humidity level and other factors suggest that uncontrollable sparks may occur (as compared with open procedures). Monopolar current is therefore not suitable for laparoscopy."

The voltages necessary to perform monopolar (coagulation) electrosurgery are known to be on the order of 3,000 to 5,000 volts peak at maximum control settings (120 watts). Normal operating settings in the range of 20 to 50 watts, coagulation mode, or control settings of 3 to 5, may produce voltages between 1,500 to 3,000 volts peak. It takes 30,000 volts to spark 1 in. in air under the best conditions.[13,14] In carbon dioxide, it takes roughly 30 percent more voltage to spark 1 in., or 39,000 volts compared to normal air. Humidity levels do not play a significant factor. Sparking from the active tip of the electrode can therefore be controlled better in laparoscopy versus open procedures.

SUMMARY

The use of monopolar electrosurgical energy has been the gold standard for the past 50 years.[15] Its utility has the most diverse capabilities (fulguration, precise vaporization [dissection], coaptation of large vessels) of surgical energy sources Technological advances in performance and safety have positioned this device as one of the most useful tools in a surgeon's armamentarium.[12] The adaptation of active electrode monitoring for stray energy as a result of insulation failure or capacitive coupling and the use of all metal trocar cannulas will increase the confidence of the surgeon and the safety of the patient. Its use will again prove itself in laparoscopy. As with any surgical tool or energy source, education and skill are required. This introduction to the principles of the biophysics of electrical energy on tissue and corresponding safety considerations is a first step toward furthering one's understanding of this powerful surgical tool.

REFERENCES

1. Engel T: Electrosurgical dynamics of laparoscopic sterilization. J Reprod Med 15, 1975
2. Sigel B, Dunn MR: The mechanism of blood vessel closure by high frequency electrocoagulation. Surg Gynecol Obstet 121:823, 1965
3. Rioux JE: Laparoscopic tubal sterilization: sparking and its control. La Vie Medical au Canada Farancais 2:760, 1973

4. Contact quality monitoring. Health Devices, February 1985

5. Corson SL: Electrosurgical hazards in laparoscopy. JAMA 227:1261, 1974

6. Willson PD, McAnena OJ, Peters EE et al: A fatal complication of diathermy in laparoscopic surgery. Minimally Invasive Surgery March:19, 1994

7. Soderstrom RM: Bowel injury litigation after laparoscopy. J Am Assoc Gynecol Laparosc 1(1):74, 1993

7a. Grosskinsky CM, Hulka JF: Unipolar electrosurgery in operative laparoscopy: capacitance as a potential source of injury. J Reprod Med 40:549, 1995

8. Voyles CR, Tucker RD: Unrecognized hazards of surgical electrodes passed through metal suction devices. Surg Endosc 8:185, 1994

9. Soderstrom RM: Hazards of laparoscopic sterilization. p. 33. In Sclarra JW (ed): Gynecology and Obstetrics. Vol. 6. Harper & Row, New York, 1982

10. Federal Registry 45:12701, February 26, 1980

11. Tucker RD, Voyles CR, Silvis SE: Capacitive coupled stray currents during laparoscopic and endoscopic electrosurgical procedures. Biomed Instrum Technol 25:303, 1992

12. Sacks E: Clinical perspective: the risks of laparoscopic monopolar electrosurgery. Health Devices/ECRI 24(1):1, 1995

13. Gallagher TJ: High Voltage Measurements Testing and Design. John Wiley & Sons, New York, 1983

14. Pearce JA: Electrosurgery. John Wiley & Sons, New York, 1986

15. Voyles CR, Tucker RD: Education and engineering solutions for potential problems with laparoscopic monopolar electrosurgery. Am J Surg 164:57, 1992

GLOSSARY OF KEY TERMS

Active electrode monitoring (AEM)   A technique of placing a sleeve around the electrode to detect stray energy. Stray energy generally occurs due to breaks in insulation or to capacitive coupling.

Bipolar electrosurgery   Electrosurgery in which current flows between two bipolar electrodes that are positioned around tissue to create a surgical effect (usually desiccation). Current passes from one electrode, through the desired tissue, to another electrode—thus, completing the circuit without entering any other part of the patient's body.

Capacitance   The property of an electrical circuit that enables it to transfer an electrical charge from one conductor to another, even when separated by an insulator.

Capacitive coupling   Occurs when electrical current is transferred from one conductor (the active electrode), through intact insulation, into adjacent conductive materials (tissue, trocars).

Capacitor   Created when two conductors are separated by air or an insulator (nonconductor).

Circuit   The path along which electricity flows.

Coagulation   The clotting of blood or destruction of tissue with no cutting effect. Electrosurgical coagulation incorporates intermittent bursts of high-voltage low-current electricity.

Coaptation   The sealing of a vessel with heat energy.

Current   The number of electrons moving past a given point each second, measured in amperes. Electrons flowing in one direction is a direct current. An electron flow that reverses direction at regular intervals is an alternating current.

Current Density   The electric current per unit area of conductor perpendicular to the direction of flow.

Cutting   Occurs when intense sparks focus the energy and volatilize the tissue. It results from high-current density in the tissue, causing cellular fluid to burst into steam and disrupt the structure. Voltage is low and current flow is high.

Damped   As in "damped waveform"; the transformation of a continuous cut waveform to a pulsed, damped train of energy packet to enhance the electrosurgical coagulation. See Figure 3-4 for further clarification.

Desiccation   The electrosurgical effect of tissue dehydration and destruction caused by direct contact between the electrosurgical electrode and tissue.

Direct coupling   Occurs when electrical current is transferred from one conductor included in the circuit (the active electrode) to another conductor outside of the circuit (scopes, graspers) as a result of direct contact.

Electroshield   Patented protective sheath used in conjunction with a monitoring device to prevent stray electrosurgical energy from burning a patient at an unintended site out of view of the laparoscope.

Electrosurgery   The passage of high frequency electrical current through tissue to create a desired clinical effect.

Fulguration   The electrosurgical effect of tissue coagulation using electrical arcs (sparks) that jump through the air from the electrode to the tissue.

Impedance   Opposition offered by an electric circuit to the flow of an alternating current, measured by the ratio of the effective applied voltage to the effective current.

Insulation failure   Occurs when the insulation barrier is breached, allowing current to travel outside of the intended circuit.

Necrosis   The death of a piece of animal tissue from burning, loss of blood supply, and so forth.

Power   The energy produced or delivered over a period of time (measured in watts).

Resistance   The opposition offered by a substance (e.g., a conductor) to the flow of electrons (current) along the circuit (measured in ohms).

Unipolar (monopolar) electrosurgery   Electrosurgery in which current flows into the patient and is concentrated by the active electrode to create a surgical effect. The current then travels through the patient's body and returns to the generator via the return electrode.

Voltage   The force that drives the electrons (current).

Volt   Unit of energy used to move 1 ampere of current across 1 ohm of resistance.

CHAPTER FOUR

OVERVIEW OF LASERS

THOMAS G. STOVALL

> **Laser Energy**
> **Carbon Dioxide Laser**
> **Neodymium: Yttrium-**
> **aluminum Laser**
> **Argon Laser**
> **Laser Safety**

LASER ENERGY

The use of laser energy in gynecologic surgery allows the surgeon to produce tissue effects under certain circumstances that cannot be as easily or efficiently produced using electrical energy. However, in current practice, electrosurgery has replaced many of the applications for which lasers have been used. Like many other surgical techniques and instruments, the laser and its associated energy have a defined place in the armamentarium of the gynecologic surgeon.

Laser is an acronym for *l*ight *a*mplification by *s*timulated *e*mission of *r*adiation. A wide variety of lasers have been developed, only a few of which are applicable for use by the gynecologic surgeon. The output from any laser is an electromagnetic wave, and the characteristics of these waves are major determinants of the properties that a particular laser possesses. The properties of laser radiation are outlined in the box of that title. These properties are of paramount importance to the gynecologic surgeon, because they allow a particular laser to have reproducible affects on various tissue types.[1,2]

A laser produces its energy through excitation of an atom from its normal energy state to a higher energy level through absorption of thermal, electrical, or optic energy. When the atom returns to its normal energy state, there is spontaneous emission of radiation, which releases the energy that has been previously absorbed. For gynecologic surgery, the most common lasers used include the carbon dioxide (CO_2), neo-dymium:yttrium-aluminum garnet (Nd:YAG), argon, and potassium titanyl-phosphate (KTP). A comparison of the various lasers is outlined in Table 4-1.

Lasers create their tissue effect by heating the tissue, which is a result of the tissue absorbing the energy produced by the laser. If the laser energy is not absorbed by the tissue, it has no effect or, if it is scattered over a broad surface area, the effect becomes more diffuse. When the tissue is heated to about 60°C, protein denaturation and coagulation occur. At temperatures above 100°C, intracellular water begins to evaporate, causing tissue vaporization. The tissue burns and/

Properties of Laser Radiation

- Monochromatic: all of the produced waves have essentially the same wavelength and the same energy
- Collimated: all waves travel in the same direction and are parallel to each other; thus, even over long distances, the laser beam diverges only slightly
- Coherence: all waves are in phase with each other in both space and time; there is a fixed time relationship for amplitude and phase between any two points on the wave

---

Table 4-1. Comparison of Laser Properties for Commonly Used Lasers

	CO$_2$	Argon	Nd:YAG/KTP
Type	Gas	Gas	Solid
Wavelength	10,600 nm	500 nm	532/1,064 nm
Spectrum	Infrared	Visible	Infrared
Aiming beam	HeNe	Argon	HeNe
Absorption	Water, glass	Hemoglobin	Proteins
Penetration	0.1 mm	2 mm	4–6 mm
Delivery	Rigid mirrors	Fiber	Fiber
Coagulation	+	+ +	+ + +
Excision	+ + +	+	+

Abbreviations: CO$_2$, carbon dioxide; Nd:YAG/KTP, neodymium:yttrium-aluminum garnet/potassium (itanyl-phosphate).

Table 4-2. Tissue Effects at Different Power Densities

Power Density (W/cm^2)	Tissue Effect
0.5	Warming
5–300	Superficial contraction/coagulation
300–1,200	Excisional vaporization
1,200–15,000	Incisional vaporization
15,000–100,000	Rapid incision

CARBON DIOXIDE LASER

The CO$_2$ laser is the most commonly used laser in gynecologic surgery. It is most often used for treatment of genital tract dysplasia and condyloma, as well as intra-abdominally for vaporization or excision of endometriosis. This laser operates in the far infrared portion of the electromagnetic spectrum and is therefore invisible. Because of this property, the laser beam must be aimed concurrently with a helium-neon laser. As the laser energy is absorbed, the water in the tissue is heated to boiling and the tissue is vaporized. This vaporization results in smoke production, which must be evacuated so that it does not interfere with the laser beam.

A variety of delivery systems are available depending on the type and site of surgery that is to be performed. The laser can be coupled to an operating microscope or colposcope, used with a handheld delivery system, coupled to a wave guide or fiber, or coupled to a laparoscope. It can also be directed through a separate trocar site. Because this laser beam can be reflected, it is necessary to use specialized instrumentation to absorb the laser beam. This reflective property can also be used as an advantage in areas that are difficult to reach, such as the lateral vaginal side walls or the undersurface of the ovaries. In these instances, the laser beam can be reflected using mirrors or other shiny surfaces.

This laser system is activated by depressing a foot pedal and can be delivered using several modes. The continuous mode releases energy until the foot pedal is released, whereas the single or repeat pulse mode delivers either one burst of energy or repeated bursts of energy at various time intervals. The laser energy can also be pulsed using a com-

or carbonizes. The ultimate effect on a particular tissue is determined by the power density of the laser[3] (Table 4-2). That is, the concentration of energy is greatest at the focal point of impact of the laser beam:

$$PD \ (W/cm^2) = \frac{(power \ in \ watts) \times 100}{(spot \ diameter \ in \ mm^2)}$$

Thus, the power density (PD) is inversely proportional to the square of the impact area. Therefore, if the laser's spot size (size of impact) is doubled, the power delivered is reduced by one-fourth.

The focal length of the laser refers to the distance from the focusing lens at which the concentration of power is greatest. The focal length of a laser depends on the lens, the delivery system being used, and the type of laser. The tissue damage is greatest at the focal length of the laser (although a diffuse beam could cause damage). If the beam is defocused, the area of impact is greater and the tissue damage is decreased at the same power or energy level (Fig. 4-1).

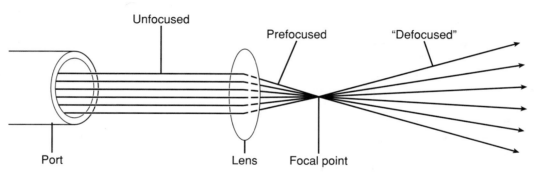

Fig. 4-1. Demonstration of focal point.

puter to control the firing of the laser. These modes are referred to as superpulse, chopped pulse (Sharplan Lasers, Israel), Ultrapulse (Coherent, Inc. USA), and Powerpulse (Surgilase, Inc., USA).

NEODYMIUM: YTTRIUM-ALUMINUM LASER

The Nd:YAG laser emits energy near the visible infrared portion of the electromagnetic spectrum. The laser energy is delivered using quartz fibers, which can be focused more precisely using sapphire tips. This laser is poorly absorbed by water and blood, and thus, has relatively deep tissue penetration that may not be visible to the operator. Because it is not absorbed by water or blood, it is a commonly used laser for hysteroscopic surgery,[4] whereas the CO_2 laser has virtually no use in hysteroscopic surgery. Tissue penetration using a bare fiber results in tissue penetration of 3 to 4 mm deep. With the addition of fiber tips, the depth of penetration is only 0.1 to 0.3 mm, a depth that is only slightly deeper than the CO_2 laser. The shape of the various tips determines the zone of impact and the thermal effect of the laser (Fig. 4-2). The use of the tips also makes intra-abdominal use of this laser more practical. This laser produces little smoke, an advantage for laparoscopic surgery.

ARGON LASER

The argon laser emits energy in the visible blue-green spectrum. Like the Nd:YAG laser, this laser can be transmitted by a flexible fiber. This laser has limited use in gynecology, but has the advantage of being preferentially absorbed by red (blood). For example, endometriotic implants absorb the beam while nonred tissue allows for passage or reflection of the beam.[5,6]

POTASSIUM TITANYL-PHOSPHATE LASER

The KTP laser is a frequency-doubled YAG laser that uses a KTP crystal in the path of a Nd:YAG beam. With this laser, tissue penetration is only 0.5 to 2 mm, or just slightly deeper than the CO_2 laser. Like the argon laser, this laser frequency is preferentially absorbed by red (hemoglobin). Also like the argon and Nd:YAG laser, the KTP laser is delivered using a flexible fiber.[7]

LASER SAFETY

The specific safety measures that must be taken depend on the type of laser being used, the delivery system, and the surgical site. Laser safety is not only the responsibility of the manufacturer, but also the responsibility of the entire surgical team.

Eye protection is required for all lasers and, because each laser has a specific wavelength, different types of eyewear are necessary. The CO_2 laser requires the use of clear plastic or glass eyewear, and should be equipped with side shields. If the laser is attached to the laparoscope, it is not necessary to wear glasses. The Nd:YAG laser requires eyewear that will stop a wavelength of 1,060 nm (green tint), while protective eyewear for the argon and KTP lasers must stop a wavelength of 488 to 532 nm (orange tint). The patient should also be given protective eyewear or alternatively, the patient's eyes can be taped closed.

If vulvar or cervical surgery is performed or if a handheld delivery system is used, moistened cloth towels should be used to avoid an accidental fire. When surgery is performed near the rectum, a moistened sponge should be placed inside the rectum to avoid the possibility of a methane gas explosion. The risk of the laser plume is uncertain, and probably

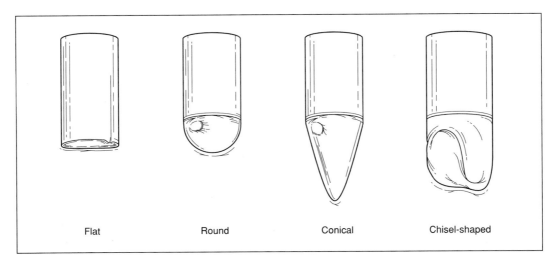

| Flat | Round | Conical | Chisel-shaped |

Fig. 4-2. Variety of sapphire tips available.

presents little risk. However, it only makes practical sense to avoid the plume if at all possible.[8]

REFERENCES

1. Baggish MS (ed): Basic and Advanced Laser Surgery in Gynecology. Appleton-Century-Crofts, E. Norwalk, CT, 1985
2. Keye WR: Laser Surgery in Gynecology and Obstetrics. 2nd Ed. Year Book Medical Publishers, Chicago, 1990
3. Martin DC: Tissue effect of lasers. Semin Reprod Endo 9:127, 1991
4. Loffer F: Hysteroscopic endometrial ablation with the Nd:YAG laser using a nontouch technique. Obstet Gynecol 69:679, 1987
5. Keye WRJ, Kixon J: Photocoagulation of endometriosis by the argon laser through the laparoscope. Obstet Gynecol 62:383, 1983
6. Diamond MP, DeCherney AH, Polan ML: Laparoscopic use of the argon laser in nonendometriotic reproductive pelvic surgery. J Repro Med 31:1011, 1986
7. Daniell JF, Miller W, Tosh R: Initial evaluation of the use of the potassium-titanyl-phosphate (KTP/532) laser in gynecologic laparoscopy. Fertil Steril 46:373, 1986
8. Wisniewshi PM, Warhol MJ, Rando RF et al: Studies on the transmission of viral disease via the CO_2 laser plume and ejecta. J Repro Med 35:1117, 1990

CHAPTER FIVE

OVERVIEW OF LAPAROSCOPIC SURGERY

THOMAS G. STOVALL

In recent years, the use of the laparoscope has proliferated as an essential diagnostic and operative tool. Probably no single method or surgical technique has received as much attention from the medical and lay communities as has laparoscopic surgery. This chapter does not deal with the specific surgical procedures that can be performed by laparoscopy, but rather with the broader issues related to laparoscopy and the surgical techniques that are common to many endoscopic procedures.

ROLE OF LAPAROSCOPY IN GYNECOLOGIC SURGERY

Kelling[1] described the first diagnostic laparoscopy in 1901. However, as early as 1806, Bozzini and Lichtlerter[2] attempted urethroscopy using a tube and candlelight, and in 1865, Desormeaux[3] presented the first description of cystoscopy. Jacobaeus[4] first referred to the word *laparoscopy* when he published his report of peritoneal, thoracic, and pericardial inspection.[4] Although most of the early development of the technique occurred in Germany, the first American description of laparoscopy was by Bernkeim[5] in 1911. The first laparoscopic tubal sterilization was reported by Anderson[6] in 1937, but advances in instrumentation and technique have allowed a greater number of procedures to be performed and the technology has rapidly moved into an outpatient setting.

The most recent membership survey of the American Association of Gynecologic Laparoscopists reported 80,031 procedures performed by 1,205 physicians,[7] an increase in the number of procedures reported in the 1988 survey.[8] It is difficult to make direct comparisons between surveys, since the surveys were not identical in terms of the type of procedures reported and the method for collection of complications.

Despite the widespread use of this technology, little data has been generated to show that these procedures are efficacious and offer significant advantages over laparotomy. The potential advantages cited by most authors of laparoscopy over laparotomy include shorter operative time, faster recovery, decreased adhesion formation, and decreased cost.[9–11] Although a few randomized clinical trials are available, none of these have the power to draw firm conclusions. Most of the current literature consists of case series that are primarily descriptive study designs. Differences between actual costs and charges for laparoscopic equipment makes economic evaluation difficult. Thus, no definitive conclusions can be made regarding the preferability of laparotomy or laparoscopy.

Laparoscopic surgical procedures are usually done in an effort to replicate procedures that have been found successful at laparotomy. Once described they tend to proliferate very rapidly. Still other procedures are designed out of a need for treatment of a specific gynecologic disorder. These procedures are usually described in small case series and, if successful, tend to be adopted very quickly. This is contrary to what happens when a new medical treatment is described or drug discovered: multiple, randomized, double-blind, controlled trials are required before the new drug is approved for use. This appears to be a double standard. It also does not seem to be the most prudent method by which to introduce a surgical technique for our colleagues or our patients. If the ''best'' drug or operation is not provided, it may be very costly to our patients and to the medical community. It would seem to be more prudent to conduct multicenter, collaborative clinical trials using standardized protocols and outcome measures, once the feasibility of a surgical procedure has been established. In other words, just because a procedure *can* be preformed using 1 to 5 small incisions through a laparoscope connected to a video monitor does not necessarily mean that it *should* be, and publicity in lay press or media is not equivalent to refereed publication in medical journals. Despite these issues, laparoscopic surgery has made an impact on gynecologic surgery like no other surgical technique. Its future impact can only be imagined.

PATIENT POSITIONING

The patient is placed in a supine position and kept flat until general anesthesia has been administered. The patient is then placed in Trendelenburg's position (20- to 45-degree angle) to assist with displacement of the bowel. The patient can then be transferred to a dorsal lithotomy position using candy-cane type stirrups or kept flat and placed in Allen stirrups (Edgewater Medical Systems, Mayfield Heights, OH). Operator preference and the scope of intended procedure determine the optimal position.

INSTRUMENTATION

Laparoscopic instrumentation has made remarkable progress over the past 20 years. As a general statement, almost all instruments that are available for laparotomy are now available for use at laparoscopy. However, because the instruments must fit through a 3- to 20-mm port and must be of sufficient length to reach the pelvis, there are currently limitations on the types of instruments that can be used.

Virtually all instruments are available in a reusable, disposable, or hybrid form (part of the instrument is disposable and part is reusable). It is generally accepted that the cost of the disposable instrumentation makes their use less cost-effective, although they do have the advantage of always being available and their cutting edges are always sharp. The instrumentation discussed is available from a variety of manufacturers.

Telescopes

Telescopes for laparoscopy are of two basic types, those with and those without an operative channel (Fig. 5-1). They range in size from 3 to 12 mm, and have straight or angled lenses. The 0-degree lens provides a panoramic view of the pelvis and is preferred by most gynecologic surgeons, although angled 30-, 45-, and 135-degree lenses assist in evaluating the anterior abdominal wall or working around masses. The choice of telescopes is generally based on operator preference. The larger the caliber of the telescope, the greater the number of fiber bundles contained therein, and the higher the quality of the video picture. Telescope warmers are available and are used by some surgeons to reduce

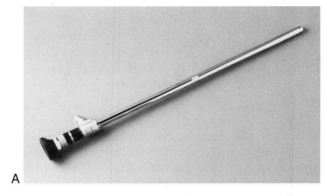

A

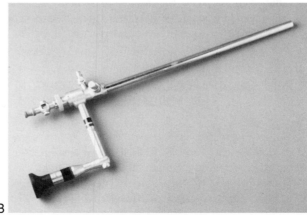

B

Fig. 5-1. (A) Straight diagnostic laparoscope with zero-degree lens. **(B)** Operating type laparoscope with zero-degree lens.

fogging during the procedure. Antifog solutions are also very successful. Three-dimensional systems are under evaluation.

Light Source

The application of fiberoptic technology has allowed a greater intensity of light to be delivered to the laparoscope and into the abdomen. Light transmission is improved as the number of fibers increases, as the size of the cable increases, and as the power of the light source increases. Illumination is reduced at each junction in the system, such as the use of a beam splitter or when there is an operating port. Transmission is also reduced if the optic cables are damaged or broken.

Cannulas and Trocars

Cannulas are available in all diameters ranging from 3 to 12 mm to accommodate laparoscopes and instrumentation of all sizes (Fig. 5-2). Cannulas are equipped with either a trumpet valve or flapper valve to prevent gas leakage. Trocars have either a pyramidal or conical tip, and should be sharp enough to produce the force necessary to penetrate the abdominal wall. Most trocars are constructed with a hollow channel, having openings at the tip as well as at the top of the instrument. This creates a rush of gas when the peritoneal cavity is penetrated by the trocar. When this occurs, the instrument does not need to be passed further into the abdomen. Blunt trocars and transparent tips that allow visualization during insertion have recently been developed, but experience with them is limited.

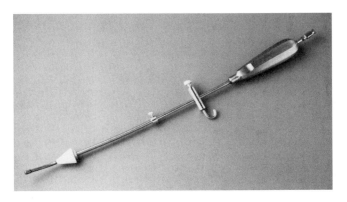

Fig. 5-3. Cohen cannula used for uterine manipulation.

Uterine Cannula

A uterine cannula is used to facilitate most gynecologic laparoscopies. A cannula is not used when (1) the uterus is absent, (2) anomalies exist that prevent exposure of or access to the cervix, (3) the patient is a prepubescent female, (4) an intrauterine pregnancy is suspected, or (5) the procedure planned includes oocyte recovery. The uterine cannula is used to manipulate the uterus and thereby facilitate visualization of and access to pelvic structure. Also, most cannulas permit injection of a dye solution (chromopertubation) to assess tubal patency. A variety of uterine manipulators are available. The most widely used are the Cohen cannula (Fig. 5-3) and the Hulka uterine manipulator (Fig. 5-4).

Pneumoperitoneum Needle

Several types of pneumoperitoneum needles are available. The one most frequently used is the Veress needle (Fig. 5-5). This needle has two working parts: an outer needle with a

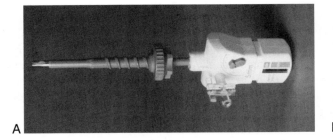

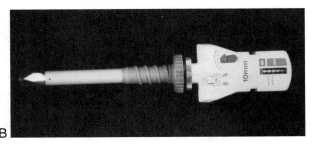

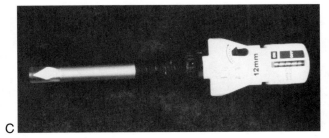

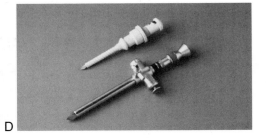

Fig. 5-2. Disposable laparoscopic cannula and trocars with fascial screws: **(A)** 5 mm, **(B)** 10 mm, **(C)** 12 mm. **(D)** Nondisposable laparoscopic cannula and trocar (5 mm, 10 mm).

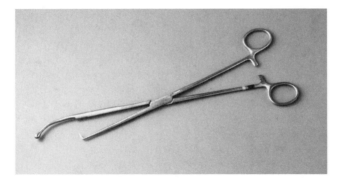

Fig. 5-4. Hulka uterine manipulator. This type of uterine manipulator does not allow for injection of dye.

sharp beveled edge, and an inner, spring-loaded, retractable blunt shaft that extends beyond the end of the needle point. As soon as the peritoneum is penetrated, the blunt shaft is propelled forward by the spring-loaded mechanism beyond the sharp tip, thus making the instrument a blunt-tipped instrument.

Grasping Instruments

Grasping forceps have been designed for tissue manipulation and have grasping ends. Some are broad and flat, while others are finer and made for delicate tissue handling (Fig. 5-6). Toothed forceps are also available for traction on tissue that is to be removed. These forceps are most commonly used for grasping ovarian cyst and leiomyoma. Forceps with pointed ends are also available for tissue dissection and surgical plane development (Fig. 5-7).

Scissors

Scissors are available with varying size blades. Hook scissors (Fig. 5-8), curved-blade scissors, and scissors with straight blades or with teeth can also be used. Monopolar current can be attached to scissors. Other methods available for cutting include various types of laser energy and electrosurgical needle tip electrodes. A bipolar instrument is also available that combines both tissue desiccation and cutting in one instrument.

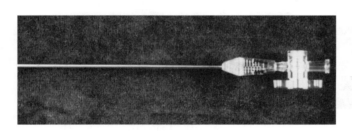

Fig. 5-5. Veress type pneumoperitoneum needle.

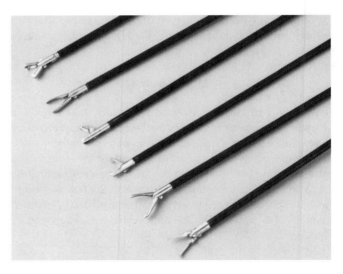

Fig. 5-6. Laparoscopic instruments used for tissue grasping; tissue biopsy, and manipulation.

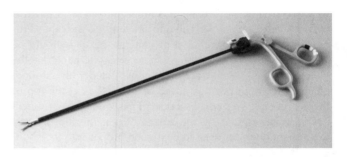

Fig. 5-7. Laparoscopic instrument used for tissue dissection.

Suturing

Instrumentation is available for both extracorporeal and intracorporeal knot-tieing. Tissue can be reapproximated using either a straight or curved needle (Fig. 5-9). The needle is first placed down the trocar and grasped with a laparoscopic needle holder. The needle is then passed through the

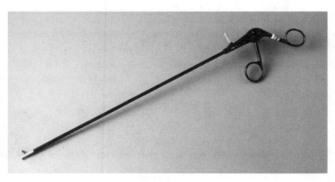

Fig. 5-8. Laparoscopic scissors.

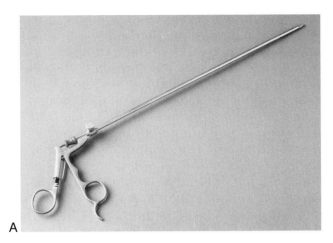

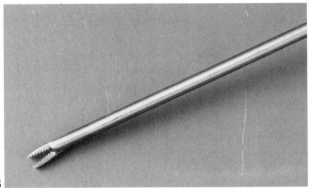

Fig. 5-9. (A) Laparoscopic needle driver and **(B)** holder.

tissue that is to be approximated, grasped, and brought out through the trocar. A simple half-hitch knot is then created, and pushed into place with a knot-pusher (Fig. 5-10). A square knot is then made by using another half-hitch down to secure the knot in place (Fig. 5-11). Figure 5-12 outlines one of several methods that can be used to create a surgical knot using an intracorporeal suturing technique.

Pre-tied surgical loops (Fig. 5-13) are designed to be placed over structures with pedicles and then tightened in place. These are especially useful for removal of the ovary or fallopian tube. Once in place, the suture tag is cut and, most commonly, a second loop is placed to secure hemostasis.

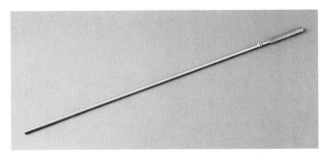

Fig. 5-10. Laparoscopic knot-pusher.

Staples

Stapling has been widely used during laparotomy, especially in bowel reanastomosis and resection and to obtain hemostasis of bleeding vessels. Clip appliers containing both absorbable and nonabsorbable staples are available for laparoscopy (Fig. 5-14). An endoscopic stapler is available that places six rows of titanium staples, 3.0 cm in length, and simultaneously divides the stapled tissue. The staples compress the tissue to either 1.5 mm or 1.0 mm, depending on the cartridge selected (Fig. 5-15). All currently available instruments are disposable. Stapling as a laparoscopic surgical technique can be used for a variety of procedures such as hysterectomy, oophorectomy, and appendectomy.

Suction/Irrigation

Suction and irrigation are important for all types of laparoscopic surgery. Irrigation is used for removal of char or for visualization when bleeding is encountered. Irrigation can also be used for hydrodissection and creation of tissue planes. A variety of suction instruments have been designed. All these are adequate for removal of irrigation fluid. A large-bore device is best for removal of blood clots when brisk bleeding is encountered or most commonly for ectopic pregnancy rupture and also for passing laser fiber. Suction/irrigation devices are also available, which offer a combination of cautery or needle tip electrodes (Fig. 5-16).

Video

The use of video monitors allows the surgeon and the remainder of the operating team to visualize the procedure. The camera is attached to the telescope and white-balanced before being placed into the abdominal cavity. Earlier cameras used beam splitters to allow the surgeon to look down the telescope as well as operate from the video monitor. This is really not necessary and decreases the quality of the picture obtained. Generally, two monitors are used for pelvic laparoscopy, with one video being placed at the foot and the second placed across the operating table from the surgeon. Whether a permanent videotaped copy of the procedure should be made is controversial. Some surgeons prefer to provide a copy to the patient while others believe that it is not necessary and potentially increases the surgeon's liability.

TISSUE REMOVAL

Tissue morcellators are used for reduction of large masses into smaller fragments to assist with tissue removal. Tissue bags can be used for tissue isolation before or after morcellation (Fig. 5-17). The bags can be removed through a secondary trocar. Tissue dilators are available for stretching a 10-

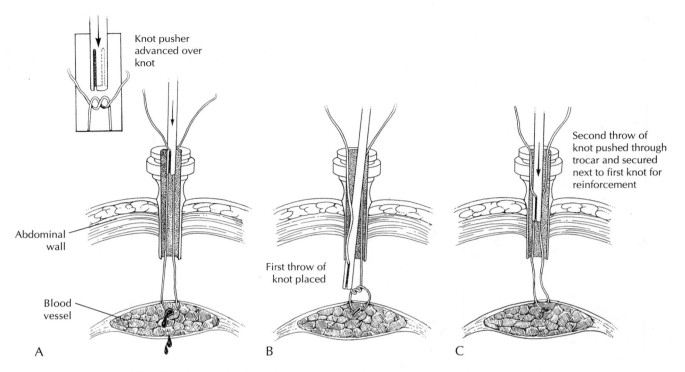

Fig. 5-11. **(A–C)** Creation of an extracorporeal knot using a laparoscopic knot-pusher.

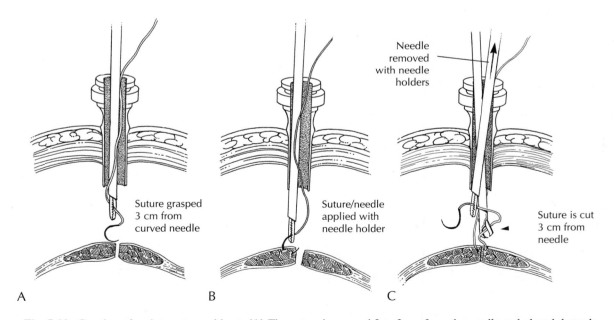

Fig. 5-12. Creation of an intracorporeal knot. **(A)** The suture is grasped 2 to 3 cm from the needle and placed through the trocar into the abdominal cavity. **(B)** The needle is passed through the two tissues to be reapproximated. **(C)** The suture is cut and the needle is removed from the abdomen. *(Figure continues.)*

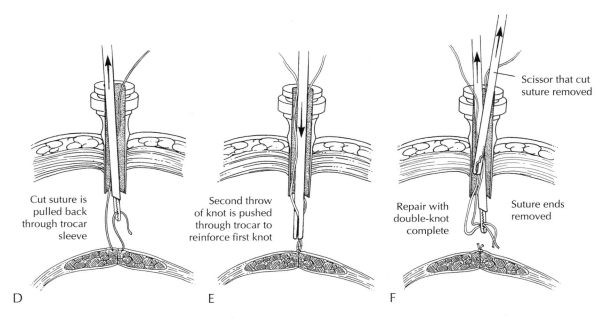

Cut suture is pulled back through trocar sleeve

Second throw of knot is pushed through trocar to reinforce first knot

Scissor that cut suture removed

Repair with double-knot complete

Suture ends removed

D   E   F

Fig. 5-12 *(Continued).* **(D&F)** The cut end is pulled through the trocar sleeve and an extracorporeal knot tied.

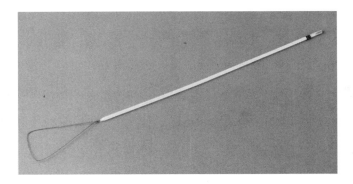

Fig. 5-13. Pre-tied surgical loops.

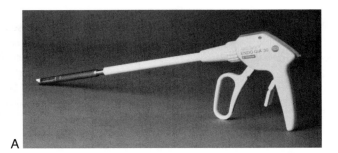

A

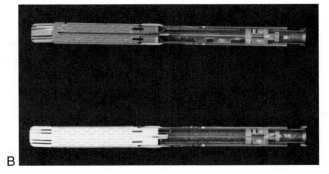

B

Fig. 5-15. **(A)** Endoscopic stapling device and **(B)** replacement staple cartridges.

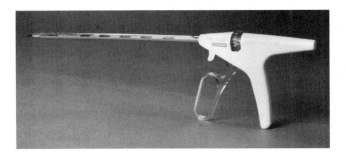

Fig. 5-14. Disposable type clip applicator.

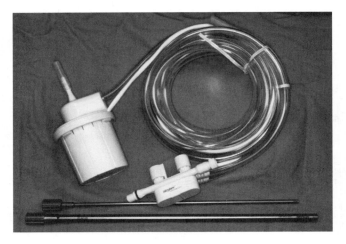

Fig. 5-16. Suction/irrigator used for laparoscopic surgery.

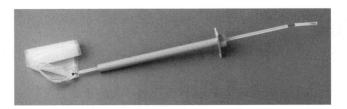

Fig. 5-17. Tissue bag used for removal of tissue fragments, ovarian masses, or fallopian tubes.

mm port to a 20-mm port. This technique can be very helpful for tissue removal. A colpotomy incision can also be used as an alternative to tissue removal through a secondary trocar. This technique is very helpful for removal of larger tissue pieces or for larger ovarian masses. A corkscrew device is screwed into myomas and these can be removed through a colpotomy incision or through a minilaparotomy incision.

PLACEMENT OF THE VERESS NEEDLE

The Veress needle is usually placed intraumbilically but may be introduced in the area located midway between the pubic symphysis and the umbilicus; immediately supraumbilically at the midline, the lateral border of the rectus muscle at either the left or right McBurney's point; or at the lateral border of the rectus muscle two finger breadths below the left costal margin. It has also been used transfundally[12] and through the posterior vaginal fornix.[13] To place the Veress needle, a small incision is made just large enough to accommodate the needle and the principal trocar and cannula. The sacral promontory and aorta are palpated, and the length of needle necessary to reach the peritoneal cavity is estimated. The Veress needle is grasped between the finger and thumb of the right hand. The surgeon's right hand is rested on the

patient's abdomen and the tip of the needle inserted through the skin incision. The left hand can then grasp the lower abdomen and elevate the tissue. The Veress needle is advanced at a 45-degree angle toward the hollow of the pelvis and, as it penetrates the peritoneum, the displaced hub of the needle will click against the top, indicating that penetration of the peritoneum has occurred. Two ''pops'' occur: first, the fascia and second, the peritoneum. To confirm proper placement, a 10-ml syringe containing 4 ml of normal saline is connected to the Veress needle. The plunger is withdrawn to make sure that no blood appears in the needle, indicating a vessel injury, and that no bowel contents are obtained, suggesting a bowel injury. The saline is then injected. If the needle is correctly positioned, there will be no recovery of saline on aspiration and the plunger will snap when it is released, due to the negative pressure created. An alternative method is referred to as the hanging drop method. A drop of saline is placed at the open end of the needle and the abdomen is then elevated; the negative pressure created should cause the drop of water to be sucked in to the abdominal cavity.

INSUFFLATION

The gas line is connected and the gas turned on after verification that the pneumoperitoneum or primary trocar is intraabdominal. The pressure should not be greater than 15 mmHg. If this is the case, the abdominal wall should be grasped and gently elevated. This will dislodge any omentum that has lodged against the needle opening. The angle of the needle, if used, should be increased and the needle rotated to free the opening. If none of these maneuvers reduces the increased pressure to an acceptable level, the needle should be removed and replaced. If gas pressures are normal at 1 L/min, liver dullness to percussion will be lost after 45 to 60 seconds. Once liver dullness disappears, the rate of gas flow can be increased. Typically, 2 to 4 L of gas will be required, with the volume necessary somewhat dependent on the depth of anesthesia and the patient's size. When the abdomen has been sufficiently insufflated, the flow of gas is stopped and the pneumoperitoneum needle removed.

TROCAR PLACEMENT

Primary Placement

Before insertion, the appropriate trocar for the laparoscope size should be chosen. The trocar should be grasped with the third finger placed against the shaft of the trocar for better control. The trocar and cannula are introduced subcutaneously for a distance of 2 to 3 cm. The angle of introduction is increased to 45 degrees towards the hollow of the sacrum. Proper depth of insertion is identified when a rush of gas from the peritoneal cavity is heard. Once placed, the trocar is retracted and the cannula advanced for 1 to 2 cm to ensure that it is adequately placed within the peritoneal cavity. The trocar is removed and the telescope introduced. Direct trocar insertion is another method that can be used. The insertion technique is the same, except that the pneumoperitoneum needle is not used and no gas is insufflated until after the intra-abdominal location has been identified.

Multiple studies have been done comparing direct trocar insertion with the use of a Veress needle followed by trocar insertion (indirect method). The results of these studies suggest that both methods are equally safe in terms of bowel and major blood vessel injury. In some studies, the number of injuries when using the pneumoperitoneum needle are higher as the result of injuries directly related to placement of the needle. The use of the direct entry method has been shown to decrease the amount of intra-abdominal gas required and reduces operative time with laparoscopic sterilization.[14–21]

Secondary Placement

The secondary trocar should be placed under direct visualization. A suprapubic trocar can be placed centrally about two finger breadths above the symphysis pubis. Before this trocar is placed, the bladder should be emptied. The author prefers to leave a bladder catheter in place throughout the surgical procedure. Lateral lower pelvic ports are helpful in many cases. The trocar should be placed lateral to the deep inferior epigastric vessels. Transillumination of the abdominal wall will often identify these superficial vessels and aid in trocar placement. Again, these trocars should be placed under direct visualization. If bleeding is encountered, a variety of suture passers have been devised to aid with suture ligation of these vessels.

In patients with known extensive adhesions, or if abdominal insufflation cannot be accomplished through the umbilicus, Veress needle insertion can be done in the left ninth intercostal space, anterior axillary line. The trocar is then inserted at the left costal margin in the midclavicular line.

CLOSURE OF TROCAR INCISION

Although not a ''new'' complication, incisional bowel herniation after laparoscopy is receiving more discussion. Whether the incidence of this complication is increasing is uncertain; it may be more common as a result of the type of operative laparoscopic procedures that are being done. These more complicated procedures require multiple ancillary ports and larger diameter ports for specimen removal and operative instrumentation, such as staples. Increased operative times and greater tissue manipulation may lead to

fascial weakening, and the use of fascial screws increases the incision size and may result in greater fascial tissue damage. Because of these factors, many surgeons have suggested that the fascial defects created at laparoscopy should be reapproximated. However, multiple studies have shown that closure of the fascial defect does not in and of itself guarantee that a hernia will not form.

The first case of bowel herniation through a laparoscopy incision was first described by Fear[22] in a patient who coughed as the laparoscope was being removed at the completion of the procedure. Subsequently, Schiff and Naftolin[23] were first to report a small bowel herniation postoperatively.

Montz et al[24] surveyed members of the American Association of Gynecologic Laparoscopists. In this report, 933 hernias were reported from an estimated 4,385,000 laparoscopic procedures, for an incidence of 21 per 100,000 procedures. Of these 933 hernias, 167 (17.9 percent) were reported to have occurred despite fascial closure. Similar results were reported by Boike et al.[25] In their multicenter retrospective review, 19 herniations were identified. An attempt to close the fascia at the initial surgery was reported in 9 of 19 (43 percent) of cases. Yet another multicenter report of 3,560 operative laparoscopies found six incisional hernias (0.17 percent).[26] It appears that the risk of herniation is greater for extra umbilical sites and is greater with the use of 12-mm trocar (3.1 percent) than with a 10-mm trocar (0.23 percent).

Most authors suggest that the fascial defect should be closed if an extra umbilical port greater than 10 mm is used. Fascial reapproximation may be accomplished in a variety of ways. The fascia may be directly visualized using army-navy or similar type retractors. When possible, the fascia can be grasped with an Allis or Kocher clamp and sutured. A number of specialized instruments have been devised and include the Grice suture needle (Ideas for Medicine, Clearwater, FL), the Carter-Thomason needle-point suture passer (Advanced Surgical Education, San Clemente, CA), the EndoClose instrument (U.S. Surgical Corporation, Norwalk, CI), and the Reverdin suture needle (Aesculap, Tuttlingen, Germany).[27,28] Despite these instruments and techniques, it is probably not possible to eliminate the complication completely.

COMPLICATIONS

As the type and extent of surgical procedures that can be done laparoscopically expands, the number of complications that occur is bound to increase as a result of the procedures' complex natures. The number of complications also appears to be related to the surgeon's experience and the number of procedures performed. See and colleagues[29] surveyed 181 urologic surgeons at 3 months and 12 months following completion of a laparoscopy course that included didactic lectures, live case presentations, simulator training, and a live-animal laboratory. At 3 months, surgeons who performed procedures without additional training were 3.39 times more likely to have at least one complication compared with those surgeons who sought additional training. At 12 months, surgeons who received no additional training were 4.85 times more likely to have had a complication. In addition, those surgeons in a solo practice or those with a variable surgical assistant were 7.74 and 4.80 times more likely to have had a complication. Thus, although formal training and didactic lectures are important, these do not substitute for continued operating room experience with a more experienced laparoscopist.

Vascular Injury

The most common site of vascular injury is the inferior epigastric vessels that are punctured during secondary trocar placement. These vessels can generally be avoided by placement of the secondary trocar lateral to the rectus muscles and/or by transillumination of the lower abdominal wall. Hurd et al[30] described the abdominal wall vasculature using computed tomography (CT) and suggested that the lateral trocar should be placed approximately 8 cm from the midline and at least 5 cm above the symphysis to minimize the risk of vessel injury. When perforated, a variety of techniques have been described for suture ligation of the bleeding vessels. The most common techniques include using fascial closure needles under laparoscopic guidance to pass the suture lateral and medial to the vessels. Trying to cauterize these vessels is usually ineffectual.

Perforation of the aorta or vena cava is a well-known and life-threatening event that fortunately is very rare. Baadsgard et al[31] reviewed 16 reported cases of great-vessel injury. Two of the 16 patients died, with the remaining 14 requiring immediate surgical repair. Fourteen of the 16 injuries resulted from Veress needle injury. Hurd et al[32] evaluated the abdominal wall anatomy of 33 women by computed tomographic scan and magnetic resonance imaging to determine the best placement of the Veress needle and primary trocar to avoid injury to the retroperitoneal vessels. They found that, for the nonobese patient, the needle could be inserted at a 45-degree angle through the base or lower margin of the umbilicus with little risk of major vessel injury. In the obese patient, however, the trocar could be inserted at 45 degrees, but placement should begin through the base of the umbilicus. In another study, Hurd and colleagues[33] found that the umbilicus was located at or cephalad to the aortic bifurcation, and to the bifurcation where the left common iliac vein crosses the midline.

Bowel Injury

Injury to the bowel can occur as a result of electrosurgical injury or injury as a result of the pneumoperitoneum needle or when the laparoscopic trocar is placed. Cases of injury resulting from the pneumoperitoneum needle can be managed conservatively and generally do not require any treatment. By contrast, the vast majority of trocar punctures require suture reapproximation, while burn injuries require resection of 1 to 2 cm of viable tissue around the injury site to ensure that the area represents tissue that has not been damaged.[34–40] In some clinical situations, the use of free intra-abdominal air demonstrated on an upright abdominal radiograph is used to diagnosis a ruptured intraperitoneal viscus. This radiographic sign is generally not helpful after laparoscopic surgery. Farooqui and Bazzoli[41] reported that 38.5 percent of patients had more than 2 cm^2 of free air at 24 hours postlaparoscopy, despite any clinical evidence of bowel perforation. Thus, this complication must be suspected based on clinical presentation in the patient with increased pain or fever following laparoscopy.

Urinary Tract Injury

During laparoscopy, injury to the urinary tract occurs most commonly at the bladder during secondary trocar insertion. This injury can be minimized by placement of the secondary trocar under direct visualization and by making certain that the bladder is emptied before trocar placement. Thermal injury to the bladder generally results from dissection during laparoscopic hysterectomy or with dissection and destruction of endometriosis.[42–45] As with bowel injuries, if the bladder is punctured with a pneumoperitoneum needle, no treatment is generally required. In the case of a trocar injury, however, the perforation should be sutured if recognized at the time of the initial surgery. If unrecognized, the patient generally presents with urinary ascites, abdominal pain, and distension. This can be accompanied by fever, chills, nausea, and vomiting, and most patients give a history of oliguria. These patients will have markedly elevated blood urea nitrogen (BUN) and creatinine concentrations and respond to aggressive hydration and bladder drainage. Cystoscopy is rarely indicated; these types of injuries will heal spontaneously and do not require surgical repair.

Ureteral injury is becoming more common as a result of increasing numbers of laparoscopic-assisted vaginal hysterectomies being performed, although ureteral injury can occur during other operative laparoscopic procedures as well.[46–49] Delayed fistulas have been seen, presumably due to thermal injury.

CREDENTIALING

Credentialing or approving a surgeon to perform a particular surgical procedure is not new and has been discussed in a variety of forums since laparoscopy became commonplace. Credentialing involves a review of the procedures performed, the quality of the procedures, as well as the indications and patient selection criteria that the surgeon uses. Interest in credentialing comes from residency programs, malpractice insurance companies, third-party payers, government health agencies, and consumer advocacy groups. How this process is to occur is also of great debate. In the future, it might be possible to use computer models or interactive computers along with laboratory exercises. However, at the present, these technologies are not widely available for laparoscopic techniques.

Numerous pitfalls can occur during the credentialing process. Who is the first to be credentialed? How often will it take place? Will credentialing be procedure specific or technique driven? What will be done with the surgeon who is currently performing the procedures but does not pass the credentialing process? What are the acceptable rates of complications for the various operative procedures? These are but a few of the questions that must be answered.

Most recently, the Society of Reproductive Surgeons has published credentialing guidelines for laparoscopic surgery.[50,51] Stratification of laparoscopic procedures has been proposed by the Society of Reproductive Surgeons and the American Fertility Society. Again, these guidelines can be

Principles of Credentialing for Laparoscopic Surgery

- Member in good standing with institution
- American Board of Obstetrics and Gynecology certified (or eligible)
- Privileges granted in all prerequisite procedures
- Ability to perform prerequisite procedures safely, efficiently, and effectively
- Individual procedures granted
  - Specific endoscope
  - Specific energy source/modality
  - Specific skill level
- Training for a procedure must include
  - Formal didactic course[a]
  - Supervised laboratory experience[a]
  - Observation by an experienced surgeon[a]
  - Supervision by previously credentialed surgeon
- Periodic review of newly granted privileges (recertification)

---

[a] A letter from the director of an approved residency training program can be substituted when appropriate. (Data from Keye.[50])

Stratification of Laparoscopic/ Hysteroscopic Procedures

Laparoscopic Procedures

- Level I. Procedures not requiring additional training
  - Laparoscopic sterilization
  - Needle aspiration of simple cysts
  - Ovarian biopsy
  - Minor adhesiolysis
  - Partial salpingectomy for ectopic pregnancy
  - Linear salpingostomy for ectopic pregnancy
  - Endoscopic surgery for the American Fertility Society (AFS) stage I and II endometriosis
- Level II. Procedures requiring additional training
  - Laparoscopic division of uterosacral ligaments
  - Adhesiolysis for moderate and severe adhesions or adhesions involving bowel
  - Laser or diathermy drilling to ovaries for polycystic ovarian syndrome
  - Neosalpingostomy for hydrosalpinx
  - Salpingectomy or salpingo-oophorectomy
  - Endoscopic management of endometrioma and ovarian cystectomy
  - Laparoscopic-assisted vaginal hysterectomy
  - Endoscopic surgery for AFS stage III and IV endometriosis
  - Appendectomy
- Level III. Procedures requiring significant additional training
  - Pelvic lymphadenectomy
  - Extensive pelvic side wall dissection
  - Presacral neurectomy
  - Dissection of an obliterated pouch of Douglas
  - Bowel surgery
  - Retropubic bladder neck suspension
  - Hernia repair
  - Ureteral dissection

Hysteroscopic Procedures

- Level I. Procedures not requiring additional training
  - Diagnostic hysteroscopy
- Level II. Procedures requiring additional training
  - Endometrial resection/ablation
  - Division or resection of uterine septum
  - Endoscopic surgery for Asherman syndrome
  - Myoma resection
  - Fallopian tube cannulation

(Data from society of Reproductive Surgeons, The American Fertility Society.[51])

used as a recourse for individual institutions to use in establishing their own quality assurance and credentialing processes.

REFERENCES

1. Kelling G: Uber Oesophagoskopie, Gastroskopie, and Zolioskopie. Munch Med Wochenschr 49:21, 1902

2. Bozzini P, Lichtleiter: Eine Erfindung zur Anschauung innerer Teile and Krankheiten. J fur Praktische Heilkunde 24:107, 1896

3. Desormeaux AJ: Del'Endoscopieet de ses Applications au Diagnostic et au Traitement des Affections de l'Uretre et de la Vessie Bailliere, Paris, 1865

4. Jacobaeus JC: Uber due Moglichkeit die Zystoskopie bei Untersuchlung seroser Hohlungen anzerwerden. Munch Med Wochenschr 57:2090, 1910

5. Bernkeim BM: Organoscopy: cystoscopy of the abdominal cavity. Ann Surg 53:764, 1911

6. Anderson ET: Peritoneoscopy. Am J Surg 35:36, 1937

7. Levy BS, Hulka JF, Peterson HB, Phillips JM: Operative laparoscopy: American Association of Gynecologic Laparoscopists, 1993 membership survey. J Am Assoc Gynecol Laparosc 1: 301, 1994

8. Peterson HB, Hulka JF, Phillips JM: American Association of Gynecologic Laparoscopists' 1988 membership survey on operative laparoscopy. J Reprod Med 35:587, 1990

9. Azziz R, Steinkampf MP, Murphy A: Postoperative recuperation: relation to the extent of endoscopic surgery. Fertil Steril 5:131, 1989

10. Lundorff P, Thorburn J, Hahlin M et al: Adhesion formation after laparoscopic surgery in tubal pregnancy: a randomized trial versus laparotomy. Fertil Steril 55:911, 1991

11. Levine RL: Economic impact of pelviscopic surgery. J Reprod Med 30:655, 1985

12. Morgan HR: Laparoscopy: induction of pneumoperitoneum via transfundal puncture. Obstet Gynecol 54:260, 1979

13. Neely MR, McWilliams R, Makhlouf HA: Laparoscopy: pneumoperitoneum via the posterior fornix. Obstet Gynecol 45:459, 1975

14. Borgatta L, Gruss L, Barad D, Kaali SG: Direct trocar insertion vs. Verres needle for laparoscopic sterilization. J Repro Med 35:891, 1990

15. Poindexter A, Ritter M, Fahim A, Humphrey H: Trocar introduction performed during laparoscopy of the obese patient. Surg Gynecol Obstet 165:57, 1987

16. Byron JW, Markenson G, Miyazawa K: A randomized comparison of Verres needle and direct trocar insertion for laparoscopy. Surg Gynecol Obstet 177:259, 1993

17. Kaali SG, Bartfai G: Direct insertion of the laparoscopic trocar after an earlier laparotomy. J Repro Med 33:739, 1988

18. Saidi MH: Direct laparoscopy without prior pneumoperitoneum. Obstet Gynecol 31:684, 1986

19. Saali S, Bartfai G: Direct insertion of the laparoscopic trocar after an earlier laparotomy. J Repro Med 33:739, 1988

20. Copeland C, Wing R, Hulka JF: Direct trocar insertion at laparoscopy: an evaluation. Obstet Gynecol 62:655, 1983

21. Jarrett JC: Laparoscopy: direct trocar insertion without pneumoperitoneum. Obstet Gynecol 75:725, 1990

22. Feear RE: Laparoscopy: a valuable aid in gynecologic diagnosis. Am J Obstet Gynecol 31:297, 1968

23. Schiff I, Naftolin F: Small bowel incarceration after uncomplicated laparoscopy. Obstet Gynecol 43:674, 1974

24. Montz FJ, Holschneider CH, Munro MG: Incisional hernia following laparoscopy: a survey of the American Association of Gynecologic Laparoscopists. Obstet Gynecol 84:881, 1994

25. Boike GM, Miller CE, Spirtos NM et al: Incisional bowel herniations after operative laparoscopy: a series of nineteen cases and review of the literature. Am J Obstet Gynecol 172: 1726, 1995

26. Kadar N, Reich H, Liu CY et al: Incisional hernias after major laparoscopic gynecologic procedures. Am J Obstet Gynecol 168:1493, 1993

27. Berguer R: A technique for full thickness closure of laparoscopic trocar sites. J Am Coll Surg 180:227, 1995

28. Carter JE: A new technique of fascial closure for laparoscopic incisions. J Laparoendosc Surg 4:143, 1994

29. See WA, Cooper CS, Fisher RJ: Predictors of laparoscopic complications after formal training in laparoscopic surgery. JAMA 270:2689, 1993

30. Hurd WW, Bude RO, DeLancey JOL, Newman JS: The location of abdominal wall blood vessels in relationship to abdominal landmarks apparent at laparoscopy. Am J Obstet Gynecol 171:642, 1994

31. Baadsgaard SE, Bille S, Egeblad K: Major vascular injury during gynecologic laparoscopy. Acta Obstet Gynecol Scand 68:283, 1989

32. Hurd WH, Bude RO, DeLancey JOL et al: Abdominal wall characterization with magnetic resonance imaging and computed tomography: the effect of obesity on the laparoscopic approach. J Repro Med 36:473, 1991

33. Hurd WW, Bude RO, DeLancey JOL, Perl ML: The relationship of the umbilicus to the aortic bifurcation: implications for laparoscopic technique. Obstet Gynecol 80:48, 1992

34. Roopnarinesingh S, Raj-Kumar G, Woo J: Laparoscopic trocar point perforation of the small bowel. Int Surg 62:76, 1977

35. Milliken RA, Milliken GM: Gastric perforation: rare complications of laparoscopy. NY State J Med Jan:77, 1975

36. Endler GC, Moghissi KS: Gastric perforation during pelvic laparoscopy. Obstet Gynecol 47:40, 1976

37. Esposito JM: Hematoma of the sigmoid colon as a complication of laparoscopy. Am J Obstet Gynecol 117:581, 1973

38. Birns MT: Inadvertent instrumental perforation of the colon during laparoscopy: nonsurgical repair. Gastrointest Endosc 35:54, 1989

39. Thompson BH, Wheeless CR Jr: Gastrointestinal complications of laparoscopy sterilization. Obstet Gynecol 41:669, 1973

40. Shell JH Jr, Myers RC: Small bowel injury after laparoscopic sterilization. Am J Obstet Gynecol 115:285, 1973

41. Farooqui MO, Bazzoli JM: Significance of radiologic evidence of free air following laparoscopy. J Reprod Med 16:119, 1976

42. Georgy FM, Fetterman HH, Chefetz MD: Complication of laparoscopy: two cases of perforated urinary bladder. Obstet Gynecol 120:1121, 1974

43. Homburg R, Segal T: Perforation of the urinary bladder by laparoscope. Am J Obstet Gynecol 130:597, 1978

44. Deshmukh AS: Laparoscopic bladder injury. Urology 19:306, 1982

45. Sherer DM: Inadvertent transvaginal cystotomy during laparoscopy. Int J Gynaecol Obstet 32:77, 1990

46. Grainger DA, Soderstrom RM, Schiff SF et al: Ureteral injuries at laparoscopy: insights into diagnosis, management, and prevention. Obstet Gynecol 75:839, 1990

47. Gomel V, James C: Intraoperative management of ureteral injury during operative laparoscopy. Fertil Steril 55:416, 1991

48. Woodland MB: Ureter injury during laparoscopic-assisted vaginal hysterectomy. Am J Obstet Gynecol 167:757, 1992

49. Kadar N, Lemmerling L: Urinary tract injuries during laparoscopically assisted hysterectomy: causes and prevention. Am J Obstet Gynecol 170:47, 1994

50. Keye WR: Hitting a moving target: credentialing the endoscopic surgeon. Fertil Steril 62:1115, 1994

51. Society of Reproductive Surgeons, The American Fertility Society: Guidelines for attaining privileges in gynecologic operative endoscopy. Fertil Steril 62:1118, 1994

CHAPTER SIX

LAPAROSCOPIC TROUBLESHOOTING

JANA R. SPELLMAN

Becoming actively involved in a laparoscopy program, whether large or small, can either be gratifying or extremely frustrating. If the laparoscopy program is not set up and conducted in a proactive manner by the surgeon and operating room staff, every laparoscopic procedure performed in the operating suite can be a "zoo."

Unfortunately, this environment is familiar to all who have participated in any type of laparoscopic procedure in an operating room. Dr. Kurt Semm demonstrated operative laparoscopy for many years, which he referred to as "pelviscopy." Once it caught the attention of others, it spread rapidly.[1] With the advances in technology, the list of laparoscopic procedures has lengthened as this technology has been incorporated into many specialties.

In the early 1970s, sterilization, lysis of mild adhesions, and fulguration of endometriosis were basically the only three procedures performed through the laparoscope. By the late 1980s and early 1990s, a new era of sophisticated surgical procedures had been developed. A number of abdominal gynecologic procedures had been mastered through the laparoscope, resulting in conversion from inpatient procedures to an outpatient surgery setting.[1]

Laparoscopic surgery is complicated and intensely technological, so it should and must proceed smoothly and efficiently. Due to the increased demand for specialized endoscopy instrumentation, manufacturers have custom instrumentation available for every possible use. Nothing is more unnerving than a laparoscopic procedure with faulty or incomplete equipment. There still seems to be a mindset that laparoscopy is a minor procedure. For this reason, inexperienced personnel are often given the responsibility of caring for the delicate instrumentation. Many times the operative procedure is delayed, or even abandoned, due to the ignorance of operating room staff or surgeon.[1] Many hours of operating room time, anesthesia time, and personnel downtime are wasted, due to the lack of responsibility, familiarity, and accountability for laparoscopic instrumentation. Not only is this very costly to the hospital in replacing laparoscopic equipment, but it can be very costly to the patient as well.

In order for a laparoscopy program to be successful, regardless of the size of the hospital or operating room, there must be dedicated personnel who are responsible for caring for and maintaining this equipment. The only alternative—continuous replacement of instrumentation that has been abused and neglected—is very costly to the hospital.

A standardized inventory and checklist of all laparoscopic equipment and instrumentation that the physician has deemed necessary to perform each laparoscopic procedure must be maintained and checked on a daily basis. There should never be a time when, after trocar insertion, the surgeon is notified that no clips or scissors are available, or the Fallope ring applicator is out for repair. There can be a tremendous difference between a capable laparoscopist and a superb laparoscopist, depending on their exhaustive knowledge of what laparoscopic equipment is available.

Diagnostic and Operative Laparoscopy Equipment

- Basic laparoscopy equipment
    12-mm operating telescope (laser compatible)
    10-mm operating telescope
    10-mm double-puncture telescope
    12-mm trocar and sheath
    10-mm trocar and sheath
    8-mm trocar and sheath
    5-mm trocar and sheath
    Verres needle (long and short)
    Sealing caps for 12-mm, 10-mm, 8-mm, and 5-mm trocars
    5-mm reducing sleeve
    Light cord (2)
- Sterilization equipment
    Single-puncture Fallope ring applicator
    Cohen uterine manipulator (small and large tips)
    Kleppinger biopolar cautery forceps (single and double puncture)
    Monopolar cautery cable (2)
    Bipolar cautery (2)
- Instrumentation
    Suction/irrigator probe (single and double puncture)
    Hulka uterine manipulator
    Hook scissors, 5 mm (single and double puncture)
    Standard biopsy forceps, 5 mm (single and double puncture)
    Semm biopsy forceps, 5 mm (double puncture)
    Grasping forceps with teeth, 5 mm (single and double puncture)
    Atraumatic grasping forceps (single and double puncture)

- Needle coagulator (single and double puncture)
    Knife coagulator (single and double puncture)
    Probe with centimeter markings, 5 mm (single and double puncture)
    Aspiration needle probe, 5 mm (single and double puncture)
    Morcellator with 10-mm trocar and sheath
    Peritoneal scissors straight with serrated edges (single and double puncture)
    Fibroid grasper (Semm) claw forceps
    Needle holder, 3 mm (for use with 3–0 chromic endosuture)
- Miscellaneous equipment
    Aquapurator or disposable Gyneflo irrigator/aspirator
    Suction/irrigator probe and tubing, 5 mm
    Endoloops
    Knot guide
    High flow automatic insufflator with tubing (7 to 9 L/min)
    Sony 19-in UL monitor (2)
    Endovision video camera with 38-m endocoupler
    Video cart (2) with mount on arm (closed with lock)
    Panasonic half-inch VHS videocassette recorder
    Video light source
    8-ft liquid light cable
    35-mm camera
    Electrosurgical unit (mono- and bipolar)

A list of the diagnostic and operative laparoscopy instrumentation needed for most gynecologic procedures is provided in the box. This list can be adapted to one's specific needs.[2]

With the growth in sophisticated procedures and equipment, the expertise required of the operating room staff has likewise increased. The need to create laparoscopic surgery teams is now vitally important.[3]

ACCOUNTABILITY

It also is important that the responsibilities of the nurse and of the surgeon be well defined. This provides for a means of continuity and accountability.

Nurse's Responsibility

The team should consist of at least one nurse who has been fully trained and has received in-service education on the total purchase, care, and maintenance of laparoscopic instrumentation and equipment and who will be actively involved in the surgical procedure. Depending on the number of laparoscopic setups, the number of surgeons, and the number of laparoscopic procedures performed, there may need to be a division of instrumentation between two or more nurses. This may warrant the establishment of more than one laparoscopic surgical team. Regardless, each nurse should have specific responsibilities and should be held accountable for the care and maintenance of the designated instrumentation. In turn, the nurse should maintain a close working relationship with the surgeon(s). Due to the technological explosion in laparoscopy, the laparoscopic instrumentation inventory will need to be updated or adapted periodically to accommodate new laparoscopic procedures.

Physician's Responsibility

The physician must supply the appropriate nurse(s) with a list of the instrumentation, equipment, and supplies needed to perform each laparoscopic procedure. The equipment will

---

Procedure: Laparoscopy (operative)
Surgeon:
Glove size:

Supplies	Instruments
Peri/Gyn pack	All instrumentation on the laparoscopy cart
Prep pan set	Scopes
Raytex	Cords
Towels	Instruments
Gloves	Video carts (2)
Lap sheet	
16 F French red catheter	Suture
10 ml syringe	3–0 or 4–0 A CE-4 (subcuticular)
#11 Blade	
Gowns ×4	Irrigation
Extra prep sticks	Normal saline
	Dressing
	Bandaid

Helpful Hints
1. Soak cords and scopes in Cidex for 20 minutes.
2. Steam autoclave the instrumentation.
3. Will position in knee stirrups (laparoscopy cart) padded with sheets.
4. Place on prep table: side open speculum, Tenaculum, Cohen cannula, French catheter (will put in when they prep).
5. Will position both video monitors at the foot of the table after draping.
6. Please have diagnostic and operative laparoscopy instrumentation available.

Fig. 6-1. Example of a surgeon's preference card.

not be there unless requested. In coordination with the operating room supervisor, it must be determined what equipment is already available, what equipment can be adapted, and what equipment must be purchased. One must be very careful in mixing and matching laparoscopic instrumentation and equipment from different manufacturers. In many instances, an actual decrease in the intensity of light and poor video quality may result from the mixing of instrumentation. Most sales representatives will give clinicians the instrumentation on a trial basis before the purchase is made, allowing time for problems to be worked out. One should request feedback from the operating room supervisor regarding the anticipated date of availability. Each surgeon should have a set of preference cards noting supplies, instruments, equipment, suture, irrigation solution, and dressing needed for all procedures performed in that particular operating room (Fig. 6-1). During the initiation of a new procedure, the surgeon should arrive a few minutes early to survey the back table and make last-minute adjustments. Communication between surgeons and nurses and accountability are the keys to successful surgical teams.

Another important aspect of a successful laparoscopic program is the provision of ongoing in-service training of the nursing personnel and the operating laparoscopist.[4] This in-service training should be mandatory. The surgeon should be willing to provide hands-on instruction to the nursing personnel. It is rarely difficult to find appropriate training—either within the hospital or in the immediate area—for the operating room staff and physicians.

After the nursing personnel and the surgeon have received adequate training in the use of laparoscopic instrumentation and equipment, rules for the maintenance and use of equipment must be established.

IMPACT ON VARIOUS DEPARTMENTS

Many challenges have been confronted by the operating room staff and central supply and purchasing departments as a result of the increased number of endoscopic procedures. There has been a growing concern regarding the cleaning and sterilization of rigid and flexible endoscopic instruments. Gynecologic surgeons are now being joined in the endoscopic revolution by other specialists, particularly general surgeons. Because the lines of authority and responsibility may cross between several clinical departments, nurses, physicians, and the hospital administrative staff must remain sensitive to the needs of everyone involved with endoscopy. Equipment purchased for one service, but needed by another, must be made accessible to everyone. Duplicate sets are likely to be needed.

The decontamination, cleaning, and sterilization of rigid endoscopic instruments have received an increasing amount of attention. Similarly, the care of handheld instrumentation has received an enormous amount of consideration. The cus-

Rules For Maintenance and Use of Equipment

1. Equipment should not be dismantled during cleansing unless the person cleaning is fully informed on how to reassemble it.
2. Each endoscope set should be labeled. (As yet, there is no standard among different companies; models change and fittings may have to be coordinated.) One must be sure that the labeling tape will not interfere with the moving parts of the endoscope.
3. The maintenance program should be ongoing, with continued and repeated surveillance of the equipment and a backup for each item. When a piece becomes worn, a replacement should be ordered early. (Most companies do not have loan sets, and if one item is missing, the entire endoscopy set may be worthless.)
4. Every effort should be made to avoid dropping or bending any pieces of equipment. A dropped endoscope will jar the lens loose. If an operating tool (e.g., the cautery device) is bent, it will not pass smoothly through the sleeve.
5. Each item should be labeled properly so that the surgeon is handed the appropriate instrument. A cutting scissor instead of a grasping forcep will result in a cut and bleeding vessel instead of a cauterized one.
6. *If in doubt, do not steam autoclave endoscopy equipment.*

(Modified from Soderstrom,[1] with permission.)

tom design and shape of endoscopic instruments have been considered excessively costly and difficult to maintain. If laparoscopic instrumentation is handled properly, these concerns are unfounded.

Surgeons should be familiar with the standards that have been established by the Association of Operating Room Nurses (AORN)[5] (Table 6-1).

RECOMMENDED PRACTICES FOR CARE OF INSTRUMENTATION

The recommended practices presented in Table 6-1 were developed by the AORN Recommended Practices Coordinating Committee and have been approved by the AORN

Table 6-1. Recommended Practices For Care of Instruments, Scopes, and Powered Surgical Instruments

Recommended Practice	Rationale/Description
An instrument should be used only for the specific purpose for which it was designed	Proper use of instruments will ensure their effectiveness. Instruments that function ineffectively can delay the surgical procedure and increase the risk of infection and patient injury
Instruments should be kept free of gross soil during surgical procedures	Inadequate removal of dried blood and secretions from instruments may result in possible concealed organisms. Corrosion, rusting, and pitting occur when blood and debris are allowed to dry in or on surgical instruments. Instruments with lumens may become obstructed from organic material. Irrigating with sterile water removes residue and prevents tissue damage. Saline cause deterioration of instrument surfaces
Decontamination of instruments should occur immediately after completion of the surgical procedure	Instruments are considered contaminated as the presence of pathogens may not be known at the time of surgery. Immediate decontamination of instruments is necessary for the protection of personnel and to prevent transmission of pathogens. The decontamination process for surgical instruments involves four steps: prerinsing, washing, rinsing, and sterilizing. Soaking and prerinsing instruments in an enzymatic detergent solution for a minimum of 2 minutes effectively removes all visible debris except for ointment, thus proving to be an acceptable alternative to manual cleaning. Delicate instruments are usually washed manually. Adherent particles of tissue, bone, and blood may resist cleaning in the automated cleaner and can cause instrument corrosion. An enzymatic soaking solution may be useful for these and other hard-to-clean instruments. Abrasives damage the protective surface of the instruments, contribute to corrosion, and impede sterilization
Following initial decontamination by manual or automatic decontamination. Instruments should be processed in an ultrasonic cleaner	Instruments are processed in an ultrasonic cleaner to remove small particles of debris from the crevices. Instruments must be rinsed to remove surface suspended particles. Dissimilar instruments (e.g., copper, brass, stainless steel) should not be combined in an ultrasonic cleaner. Ultrasonic cleaning of dissimilar metals causes ion transfer resulting in etching and pitting. Chrome-plated instruments may be damaged by mechanical vibrations that cause flaking. The use of recommended detergents is important to the overall performance of an ultrasonic system. Ultrasonic cleaning can prolong the life of instruments
Instruments with movable parts should be lubricated after every cleaning and according to the manufacturers' written instructions	The ultrasonic cleaner removes all lubricant from instruments. The lubricating solution should not be rinsed or wiped off of the instruments. The lubricating solution must be water soluble to allow steam penetration; oily solutions cannot be penetrated. Instrument lubrication (1) protects against rusting, staining, and corrosion, (2) improves instrument function, (3) lessens the growth of bacteria, and (4) allows penetration of steam
Instruments should be inspected and prepared for storage and/ or sterilization following the cleaning process	Inspection provides evidence of thorough cleaning and proper functioning of all instruments. Instruments in poor working condition are hazardous to personnel and patients perioperatively. Instruments must be thoroughly dried before storage to prevent rust formation. Proper storage provides protection from damage. The sterilizing agent must contact all surfaces to ensure sterilization. Instrument trays are designed for effective sterilization and provide space for orderly arrangement of instruments. Damage to delicate and sharp instruments can render them ineffective
Flexible ad rigid endoscopes should be inspected, tested, and processed according to design and type and manufacturers' written instructions	Use of damaged instruments may increase the risk of tissue trauma, infection, and the length of the operative procedure. The removal of dried secretions and organic material is imperative for cleaning, disinfection, or sterilization. Cleaning and drying of the endoscopes and accessories is essential to reduce gross soil and minimize dilution of the disinfectant solution. Tap water may contain a variety of microorganisms; rinsing should not recontaminate equipment. Moisture retained in channels will create a reservoir for microbial growth. Medical devices with multiple pieces, such as endoscopes, or that have crevices, joints, and channels are more difficult to disinfect than a flat surface because problems may arise in the penetration of a chemical germicide to all parts of the equipment. Removing the gross soil from narrow structures such as channels and lumens is difficult. Sterilization of all parts and accessories of endoscopes should be processed according to manufacturer's written instructions. Immediately before use, the disinfected endoscopes should be rinsed with sterile water

(From The Association of Operating Room Nurses,[5] with permission.)

board of directors. These practices are believed to be an optimal, achievable level of practice. The recommended practices provide guidelines to assist the perioperative nurse in the decontamination, cleaning, maintenance, handling, storage, and sterilization of surgical instruments, endoscopes, and powered surgical instruments. All participants should be cognizant of this information so that a safe environment can be provided for the patient. The appropriate committees in the practice setting should review all practices related to care and handling of instruments, endoscopy equipment, and powered surgical instruments (Table 6-1). Additional guidelines should be followed for the disinfection of laparoscopic instruments. For example, when using high-level disinfection, the chemical germicide should not damage the equipment. The level of disinfection is influenced by the (1) amount of organic soil present, (2) type of microbial contamination, (3) concentration of chemical germicide, and (4) duration of exposure to the chemical germicide. An automated cleaner may be used in place of manual cleaning.[5]

TROUBLESHOOTING TIPS

When a problem occurs, one should first the power switch on all equipment in use is turned "on." If there is still a problem, ensure that one should begin by checking the equipment and working in toward the field. Many times when problems are detected at the field, it is because the instrumentation is not connected to the equipment. If the problem continues after the power has been turned on and everything is connected, the actual cart electrical supply source might not be plugged in, a common mistake that renders the electrical current nonaccessible. It is very important to note that after the initial setup of new laparoscopic equipment, a large majority of the problems reported to biomedical engineering or the manufacturer is due to "user error." Untrained personnel manipulating equipment of which they lack adequate knowledge are a common source of problems. The biomedical engineering department and the manufacturer should always be available to provide assistance.

Mobile Cart with Articulating Arm and Locking Doors

All equipment and instrumentation should be stored in a multishelved mobile cart. The life of the equipment is extended if placed in a dust-free environment. With this cart, all instrumentation and equipment can be kept together, as opposed to being stowed in drawers in a storage room. The security of the equipment is maintained by locking front and rear doors. Keeping the rear door locked will aid in preventing connection tampering, which can result in inoperable equipment.

Wiring/Isolation Transformer

An isolation transformer is intended for use with all nonmedical-grade equipment and reduces microampere leakage below 10 μA. When the laparoscopy equipment is assembled on the cart, it may be helpful to have a diagram of the actual setup and connections, from the back of the machine (e.g., how the videocassette recorder [VCR] is connected to the video monitors). For example, every "video out" must go to a "video in." The equipment should be assembled as follows: camera wired to VCR wired to video printer wired to monitor source. The video light source does not need to be connected to any other equipment. *Untrained, inexperienced personnel should not attempt to redirect wiring unless absolutely sure of the correct setup.* One cord plugged into the wrong outlet or piece of equipment may shut down the entire system. Wire redirection is better left to the biomedical engineering department or the company representative. The diagram should be completely individualized to the particular video system. The local sales representative or biomedical engineering department can send someone to the operating room to assist with the completion of this diagram.

Light Source

Halogen and Xenon are the two light sources most widely used. A halogen light source is generally not used for video laparoscopy, due to its yellow color and 150-watt capacity. Xenon light sources are recommended for video laparoscopy because they have 300-watt availability. If the light does not come on when ignited, one should attempt to reignite. If the light still does not come on or goes out during the procedure, it is usually because the bulb has burned out. A Xenon light source bulb will range in price from $650 to $700. Only an experienced user should change bulbs on this equipment. Due to the risk of electrical shock, the manufacturer's manual should be consulted. Both old and new bulbs must be handled with a pad, to prevent burning of fingers when removing the old bulb. Also, keeping the oils of the hands off the glass may extend the life of the new bulb. If changing both of the bulbs does not work, then the light source should be checked out by the biomedical engineering department, since the problem is probably due to a short in the circuit.

Insufflators

Usually, nothing goes wrong with the insufflators. If it does, the insufflator tank(s) is usually empty or the valve is in the "off" position. If there is an internal tank and an external tank, the internal tank must be filled manually by the circulating nurse periodically throughout the procedure. The internal tank should always be checked first, then the external tank. The most common problem is not filling the internal tank completely. There must be a regulator on the external tank. High-flow insufflators (6 to 15 L/min) usually do not have an internal tank. The gas goes directly from the external tank, through the insufflator, and into the patient. Also, there may be a kink in the actual tubing, either going from the field to the insufflator or from the insufflator to the external tank. If the pressure reading is above 20 mmHg while insufflating, something is wrong. The stopcock might inadvertently have been closed. At different times during the procedure, there may be an escape of carbon dioxide or other preferred insufflating gas around the trocar site, which may prohibit the insufflator from insufflating at a higher rate than the gas escaping. Always be sure the tank is shut off at the conclusion of a case. There is a growing trend of using inline filters between the insufflator and the patient, which prohibits debris from passing through the insufflator tubing.

Video Camera (Control Box, Camera Cable, and Camera Head)

Most of the time, camera problems are related to fogging. Every part must be antifogged with a sterile antifogging agent. If the antifogging agent is not used correctly, usually 15 to 30 minutes after the laparoscopy has begun, the coupler will have to be disassembled and any condensation that has accumulated must be dried. The accumulation of condensation is thought to be from the change in the temperature of the telescope. Many times the problem related to the video camera is in the cable itself. If the picture is blank or "fuzzy," wiggling the cord at the camera control unit (equipment) or at the head of the camera (where it attaches to the scope) may correct the problem. If wiggling the camera cord corrects, re-enacts, or enhances the problem, the camera cord should be replaced. Often touching the lens to bowel will clear the picture. Wiping the lens with a warm saline-soaked gauze, although time consuming, also works well. Antifog solutions, of dubious value, are commercially available. Due to the delicacy of the video camera, each member of the operating team must handle it very carefully. If dropped or physically abused, the video camera is very expensive to replace. Another common mistake made by operating room personnel is not soaking the camera cord with the protective cap in place. This allows the disinfecting agent to penetrate around the connection, which may leave the camera inoperable. Often while soaking the cameras, the gasket between the camera coupler and the camera head can get moisture in it. This can be repaired by replacing the actual coupler gasket and not the more costly camera gasket.

Videocassette Recorder

When there is a problem with the VCR, it is usually because there is no tape inside or the tape has not been rewound. Many VCRs, when turned on, will display "line" or "auxiliary." If it displays channel 1 or channel 2, it usually will not work. If, while viewing the recorded tape, the picture is fuzzy, the tape heads may need to be cleaned. A VCR head cleaner may be used or the biomedical engineering department notified. There will be no display on the video monitor when the VCR is on. The only assurance that the VCR is working is the display "record" on the face of the VCR.

Color Video Printer

Most of the time, a problem with the color printer is a ribbon error or a paper jam. There are two sensors that detect the start of the ribbon. One roll usually contains 100 prints (100 paper/100 ink). The paper and the ink should be changed at the same time to ensure equal availability. If a problem other than this is encountered the biomedical engineering department should be notified.

Electrosurgical Generators and Cords

Staff must always ensure that the patient is grounded. If the coagulator is not working, the cord in use might not be the correct cord for that particular instrument. If it is the correct cord, many times there is a bad connection at the instrument itself. Cautery cords should always be examined for broken wires or frayed edges. If detected, the damaged cord should be removed immediately from the field and sent to be repaired. All cautery instruments should be tested before the start of the procedure. Another common problem is "not enough juice." Before asking the circulator to increase power, connections should be checked, along with making sure that the current is not grounding somewhere else.

Video Monitor

A 19-inch monitor is usually preferred because of its larger image. On the front of most video monitors, there will be a red button labeled "reset." If this button is pushed, this will return the settings of the video monitor back to the factory specifications. If video monitor problems are encountered during the procedure, the problem should be isolated to the individual video monitor. All connections and settings for that particular monitor should be checked. If unsure of the particular settings for that monitor, the reset button can be pushed and held until the red light stops blinking. When the red light stops blinking, the video monitor has been set back to the original factory specifications.

35-mm Camera

A 400-speed high-quality film such as Kodak Ektachrome or Fuji Velvia should be used. An adaptor attaches the camera to the endoscope. If using an Olympus camera and Olympus light source, a connecting cable will be needed for proper light exposure.[6]

CO₂ Laser

The most common problem with the CO_2 laser is related to maintenance. Before beginning the procedure, both gas tanks should be checked and replaced if needed. The laser should always be test fired before the procedure. The laser should always be put on "standby" when not in use, and nonreflective instruments used. Problems associated with the smoke evacuator usually involve the filter. If the suction is not sufficient, the filter should be checked to ensure that tissue is not obstructing the tubing. The lens, microslad, or coupler should never be autoclaved. If no He-Ne beam is being emitted, the mechanical shutter is probably closed, and should be opened. If the beam is dim or flickering, the machine should be run on standby for 10 to 15 minutes. If there is no laser output when the footswitch is depressed, it is probably because the footswitch is disconnected or the system is not in an operating mode.

Laparoscopes, Hysteroscopes, and Cystoscopes

Endoscopes should never be steam autoclaved.[1] Heat greater than 100°F will damage the seal on the lens and the view will appear cloudy or "bubbly." To check to see whether the optic fibers are intact in an endoscope, the eyepiece should be held up to a light while looking at the distal end of the scope. Broken fibers can be detected because they will not transmit light. Darkened areas appear where the lumen of the fibers should be. The laparoscopy insufflator should never be used for hysteroscopy.

Endometrial Rollerball Resectoscope

The resectoscope must be assembled carefully and accurately. The resectoscope loop must be inspected to ensure that it is intact. This will inhibit a smooth resection. If using a rollerball, it should be inspected to be sure that it rolls freely and the wire is intact. Many times, when assembling the resectoscope, the electrode is not secure. This may result in the inability to conduct the electrical current. If dextran is used as a distension media, all instruments must be thoroughly cleaned. If the dextran is allowed to dry, it may render the instrument inoperable.

Rigid Hand Instruments

Instruments that have cracked or broken insulation should never be used. All instruments must be inspected for performance, missing parts, burrs, or bends. If an instrument will not transmit an electrosurgical current, replace the cord first, then the instrument.

Light Cords

Light cords should never be steam autoclaved.[1] In trying to determine whether a light cord is defective, one should hold one end of the light cord up to a light and look at it. If over 50 percent of the light fibers are darkened, the cord should be discarded as it is beyond repair. Due to the increase in the number of laparoscopic procedures being done and competition between manufacturers, light cords are extremely inexpensive and a replacement is usually cheaper and more cost-effective than attempting to repair the damaged light cord. Only in isolated situations can these light cords actually be repaired.

Trocars

Reusable trocars must be kept sharp, which is difficult. For this reason, disposable trocars are popular. Reusable trocars must be disassembled, cleaned, and lubricated following each case. All trocars and sleeves should be inspected before the procedure for burrs and bending at the end. If the valve does not work freely, it has not been sufficiently lubricated.

Stirrups

Stirrups must always be secured firmly to the operating room table. In addition, one must be sure that the proper stirrup holders are attached to the operating table. Many stirrup holders are incompatible with stirrups, which may result in injury to the patient. The patient is inspected closely before placing drapes, to avoid pressure areas and incorrect anatomic positioning. Posterior tibial and dorsalis pedal pulses must be checked after placement in the stirrups.

SUMMARY

With the growing demand and adaptable technology, gynecologic laparoscopy is here to stay. Important aspects of a successful laparoscopy program include dedicated personnel, standardized inventory, and ongoing in-service training. The physician and nurse must realize their individual responsibilities and establish accountability. The formation of laparoscopic surgery teams is vital to a successful laparoscopy program in any setting. All members of the operating team must realize the importance of providing high-quality, safe, and efficient care for their patients. Adequate instrumentation—both primary and backup—must be made available. The use of disposable instrumentation, as primary or backup, will depend on the individual needs of the physician or hospital.

The medical literature is very limited in information on troubleshooting laparoscopic instrumentation. This chapter can be easily shared with operating room personnel, and is intended to be used as a guide for problem solving, as well as a guide for the care of these delicate instruments. With the concern and cooperation of all members of the operative team, the goal of performing a laparoscopy with the appropriate equipment present, sterilized, and in working condition before trocar insertion, does not seem all that unreasonable.

REFERENCES

1. Soderstrom RM: Operative Laparoscopy: The Masters' Techniques. Raven Press, New York, 1993

2. Spellman JR: Regional Medical Center at Memphis. Diagnostic and Operative Laparoscopy Instrumentation Inventory.

3. Semm K: Operative Manual for Endoscopic Abdominal Surgery. Year Book Medical Publishers, St. Louis, MO, 1987

4. Sanfilippo JS, Levine RL: Operative Gynecologic Endoscopy. Springer-Verlag, New York, 1989

5. American Association of Operating Room Nurses: AORN Standards and Recommended Practices for Perioperative Nursing 1995. Association of Operating Room Nurses, Denver, CO, 1995

6. Laparoscopic Surgery Update. 1:58, 1993

CHAPTER SEVEN

ANESTHETIC CONSIDERATIONS

DIMITRI VOULGAROPOULOS
JOSEPH J. KRYC

PREOPERATIVE EVALUATION: THE ANESTHESIOLOGIST'S PERSPECTIVE

An evaluation of the patient before the administration of an anesthetic is extremely important to the anesthesiologist. The information obtained during this visit will assist in the selection of anesthetic agents and techniques, and identify potential problems before the administration of anesthesia.

The best time for the patient to be seen by the anesthesiologist is several days before the intended procedure. This allows the anesthesiologist time to review the surgeon's evaluation, laboratory data, radiographs, and other information regarding the patient. If abnormalities are detected and further evaluation is required, there is time to discuss these findings with the surgeon and order additional studies with minimal disruption to the patient. In the past, the preoperative visit was routinely performed the night before surgery. As same-day surgery and ambulatory surgery increased in popularity, the opportunity for the anesthesiologist to evaluate the patient in the hospital decreased. In response to changing practice patterns, anesthesiologists have developed a variety of methods to obtain the information required for the administration of a safe anesthetic, including preoperative assessment clinics, questionnaires, telephone interviews the night before surgery, and computer-assisted information gathering systems. The end result is the same: the acquisition of information and the development of a patient-physician relationship.

History and Physical Examination

The main objectives of the history and physical examination are to establish a relationship with the patient, become familiar with the patient's present illness and past history, identify any areas of potential concern, evaluate the general physical condition of the patient, and identify those conditions that may be improved before surgery (Table 7-1).

History

The process begins with a history of the chief complaint and present illness. The nature of the disease, the acuity of the illness, and the extent of organ system involvement are all important to the appropriate selection of an anesthetic technique. Allergic reactions to medications used in the past are important to identify if complications are to be avoided intraoperatively. Patients will frequently state that they are allergic to a particular drug; however, on more detailed questioning, they often describe a variety of symptoms such as nausea and vomiting, constipation, and dizziness. True allergic reactions are associated with pruritic rashes, difficulty breathing, swelling about the head and neck, and hypotensive episodes. If these symptoms are obtained from a patient, the possibility of a previous allergic reaction is high and the drug should be avoided during the administration of anesthesia.

Preoperative Visit

A properly conducted preoperative visit includes the following:

- A thorough history and physical examination
- A review of the old chart
- A discussion of the anesthetic options available to the patient
- A discussion of the risks and complications associated with the intended anesthetic
- An opportunity for the patient to ask questions
- The prescription of preoperative medication, if necessary

Medication

A detailed history regarding the current use of medications is important if potential drug interactions during anesthesia are to be avoided. Unknown medications may potentiate the depressant effects of many anesthetic agents and adversely affect patient outcomes. Special attention should be directed toward medications that a patient is taking for the control of chronic medical conditions such as hypertension, congestive heart failure (CHF), cardiac arrhythmias, angina, diabetes, and respiratory disorders. These patients often become *physiologically* dependent on these medications and if they are abruptly discontinued a variety of problems may ensue. It is best to continue these medications up to and including the day of surgery. Exceptions include antiplatelet medications (i.e., aspirin and nonsteroidal anti-inflammatory drugs [NSAIDS]), anticoagulants (i.e., heparin and warfarin), and monoamine oxidase inhibitors (MAOIs).

Aspirin and NSAIDs interfere with platelet function by inhibiting cyclo-oxygenase, an enzyme within the platelet that converts arachidonic acid to thromboxane A_2 (TxA_2). Thromboxane A_2 is a prostaglandin that activates platelets and causes platelet aggregation and intense vasoconstriction at the site of vascular damage. Aspirin irreversibly inhibits platelet cyclo-oxygenase.[1] Because this enzyme is not regenerated, one aspirin tablet may affect platelet function for as long as 1 week. Other drugs (NSAIDs, vitamin E, dipyridamole, steroids, tricyclic antidepressants) do not inhibit cyclo-oxygenase irreversibly. As a result, these agents interfere with platelet function for a shorter period (i.e., 24 to 48 hours).[1] If possible, these drugs should be discontinued before elective surgery if platelet transfusions are to be avoided.

Heparin is an anticoagulant that forms a complex with circulating antithrombin III and potentiates the ability of this

Table 7-1. Preoperative Evaluation

A. History
  1. History of present illness and chief complaint
  2. Allergies
  3. Current medications
  4. Past medical history
    a. Cardiovascular
      i. Palpitations, arrhythmias, angina, chest pain
      ii. Dyspnea, orthopnea, shortness of breath
      iii. Exercise tolerance
      iv. Hypertension, myocardial infarction
    b. Pulmonary
      i. Shortness of breath, difficulty breathing, hemoptysis
      ii. Productive/chronic cough
      iii. Asthma/bronchospastic component
    c. Endocrine
      i. Diabetes mellitus
      ii. Thyroid disorders
    d. Neuromuscular
      i. Seizures, strokes, loss of sensation
      ii. Muscle disorders
    e. Gastrointestinal
      i. Heartburn ulcers
      ii. Hepatitis or other liver dysfunction
    f. Hematologic
      i. Prolonged bleeding during menopause, dental extractions or injuries
      ii. Easy bruising, petechiae
      iii. Blood transfusions (how many, when)
    g. Genitourinary
  5. Past surgical history
    a. Previous procedures, dates, types of anesthetics
    b. Complications associated with previous surgery/anesthesia
  6. Family history associated with anesthetics
  7. Tobacco (number of packs per day, number of years)
  8. Ethonol consumption
  9. Substance abuse
  10. Dentures, loose teeth, teeth in poor condition, caps, permanent bridges, etc.
  11. Contact lenses, glasses, hearing aids, etc.
B. Physical examination
  1. Evaluation of head and neck
    a. Movement of the neck (rotation, flexion and extension)
    b. Ability to open mouth
    c. Ability to visualize posterior pharynx
    d. Distance from mandible to larynx
    e. Evaluation of dental hygiene
  3. Heart
    a. Rhythm, heart sounds, murmurs
  3. Pulmonary
    a. Auscultation and percussion of lungs for presence of rales, rhonchi, wheezes, effusions, etc.
  4. Neurologic
    a. Mental status, neurologic deficits
C. Review of laboratory data
D. Informed consent: description of intended anesthetic technique(s), risks, and complications
E. Preoperative medication orders (if needed)
F. American Society of Anesthesiologists (ASA) physical status

compound to inhibit the formation of thrombin. This prevents the conversion of fibrinogen to fibrin and is best measured with an activated partial thromboplastin time.[2] Because there is no specific chemical assay for heparin, the half-life of its clinical effects has been used to determine treatment. Based on this, the half-life of heparin appears to be dose-dependent and ranges from 30 minutes to approximately 3 hours. Heparin is often administered at 4- to 6-hour intervals, and clotting studies are usually obtained before the next dose. In most clinical situations, withholding treatment for 6 to 8 hours results in a normal coagulation profile. If necessary, heparin reversal can be achieved more rapidly with the administration of protamine, a specific reversal agent. Protamine binds with the heparin molecule and prevents its interaction with antithrombin III, thereby limiting its anticoagulant effects.

Warfarin is an oral anticoagulant that inhibits the hepatic production of vitamin K-dependent clotting factors (factors II, V, IX, and X). As these clotting factors have relatively long half-lives, it takes some time for the maximal effect of this agent to be apparent. In addition, there is a longer time associated with reversal.[3] Warfarin therapy is best measured using the prothrombin time, which is dependent on the concentration of factors II, V, IX, and X. For patients scheduled to undergo elective surgery, anticoagulant therapy should be discontinued 48 to 72 hours before surgery. The anticoagulant effects of warfarin can be reversed more rapidly with the administration of vitamin K; however, reversal is dependent on the production of new clotting factors and may take at least 24 hours before the prothrombin time returns to normal. Immediate reversal can be achieved with the intravenous administration of fresh frozen plasma.

Monoamine oxidase inhibitors are a heterogenous group of drugs used to treat severe forms of depression. They prevent the metabolism of monoamines and result in an increase in the intraneuronal concentrations of the amine neurotransmitters, including dopamine, norepinephrine, epinephrine, and serotonin (5-hydroxytryptamine). Adverse effects associated with the use of these agents have limited their clinical use. The most commonly encountered problems are associated with (1) the consumption of foods containing tyramine (i.e., cheeses, wines), which precipitates a severe hypertensive crisis; (2) the administration of opioids, which can cause hypertension, hypotension, tachycardia, diaphoresis, respiratory depression, hyperthermia, seizures, and coma; and (3) the administration of anesthesia as stimulation of the sympathetic nervous system, which under these conditions, can result in severe hypertension and cardiac arrhythmias.[3] The MAOIs produce long-lasting, irreversible enzyme inhibition that is unrelated to the duration of treatment. When the drug is discontinued, regeneration of monoamine oxidase may take as long as 2 to 3 weeks. The anesthetic management of patients receiving MAOIs is controversial. The current recommendation is to discontinue the drug for at least 2 weeks before surgery; however, this recommendation is based on limited data and no controlled studies.[4,5] More recent information questions the need to discontinue these agents preoperatively, as only a few potent drug interactions have been described. Those drugs associated with complications include opioids that release catecholamines (meperidine) or histamine (morphine) and indirect acting sympathomimetic agents (ephedrine), and should be avoided during the administration of anesthesia.[6]

Cardiovascular Disorders

Information pertaining to the patient's past medical and surgical history is particularly important to the anesthesiologist. Of special concern are problems involving the heart and lungs. From the anesthesiologist's point of view, it is important to optimize any cardiovascular condition prior to an elective procedure. Hypertensive disease that is untreated or poorly controlled preoperatively is often associated with wide fluctuations in blood pressure during the operation. It is also associated with (1) an increase in systemic vascular resistance, (2) decreased intravascular volume, (3) an exaggerated pressor response, and (4) edema. Hypertension is also an important marker as a risk factor for congestive heart failure and ischemic heart disease. Patients with untreated or poorly controlled hypertension prior to surgery often experience exaggerated responses to laryngoscopy and intubation. In addition, there is an increase in the incidence of transient myocardial ischemia. Approximately 75 percent require treatment with a vasodilator. In addition, there is evidence indicating that this group of patients has a higher incidence of postoperative complications such as hypertension due to an increase in circulating endogenous catecholamines and an increase in the incidence of congestive heart failure and myocardial ischemia.[7] Poor outcomes can also be expected in patients with untreated mild hypertension if associated with other disorders such as angina, obesity, smoking, and previous myocardial infarctions.[8]

Angina, if treated and stable, is not a contraindication to surgery. However, the development of unstable angina or angina at rest, symptoms suggestive of congestive heart failure, diaphoresis, or progressive orthopnea requires a more thorough investigation before proceeding with elective surgery. Patients who have experienced a myocardial infarction in the past have a higher incidence of perioperative infarction with subsequent operative procedures. The overall risk is approximately 5 percent. If the infarct is recent (i.e., within 3 months), the perioperative risk for reinfarction is 15 to 30 percent. This decreases to 10 to 15 percent if surgery is performed between 3 and 6 months postinfarction, and declines to less than 5 percent if surgery is performed after 6 months. The mortality associated with a perioperative reinfarction is very high and varies from 50 to 70 percent.[9] Therefore, the best time for elective surgery is at least 6 months after a myocardial infarction. The highest incidence of perioperative reinfarction in these patients occurs with procedures involving the thoracic cavity, great vessels, and the upper abdomen. Patients who have had coronary artery bypass grafts are not at increased risk if they are asymptomatic at the time of surgery.[10]

Invasive cardiac monitoring is often used in patients with cardiac disease who are considered to be high risk, to prevent the deleterious effects of myocardial ischemia (i.e., pulmonary edema, hemodynamic instability, arrhythmias, and myocardial infarction). Although not proved, it has been suggested that early recognition of myocardial ischemia leads to earlier treatment, which theoretically would prevent additional complications.[11] For those patients with ischemic cardiac disease, the intraoperative period is associated with the lowest number of ischemic episodes as compared with the pre- and postoperative periods. Although there is no one best indicator of intraoperative myocardial ischemia, the use of multiple monitoring devices will assist in the early detection of ischemic events.

Depending on the severity of the process, any patient with a history of cardiac disease who is scheduled for an elective procedure should be evaluated by an internist or a cardiologist prior to surgery. In emergency situations it may be impossible to maximize the patient's preoperative condition; however, it is important to obtain as much information as possible before the induction of anesthesia if patient outcomes are to be optimized.

Respiratory Disorders

The respiratory system may be affected by a wide variety of disease states that are of particular interest to the anesthesiologist. Patients with a history of asthma, chronic obstructive disease, smoking, and other pre-existing pulmonary disorders have a higher incidence of ventilation/perfusion abnormalities intraoperatively and during the immediate postoperative period that may result in oxygen desaturation and hypoxemia.[12] If a patient complains of a chronic cough, dyspnea, hemoptysis, or the production of purulent sputum, a preoperative pulmonary evaluation and chest radiograph is warranted. A more extensive workup is indicated in patients presenting with moderate to severe pulmonary disease. In these patients, the initial studies should include pulmonary function tests with and without bronchodilators and arterial blood gas determination on room air. A more detailed evaluation can proceed based on the results of these tests. Preoperative treatment with antibiotics, steroids, bronchodilators, and chest physiotherapy should be considered in any patient who is symptomatic before surgery.[13]

Particular attention should be directed to asthmatic patients who have received steroid therapy within the past year. The normal adrenal gland secretes approximately 200 mg/day of cortisol. During periods of extreme stress (i.e., surgery) secretion may increase to as high as 500 mg/day. Because acute adrenal insufficiency is a life-threatening process and there is little risk in treating patients for the short

term with steroids during isolated periods of stress, supplemental steroids should be empirically administered to all patients who have received daily steroid treatment for at least 1 week during the year before surgery. The most common form of steroid coverage during the intraoperative period is to administer hydrocortisone 200 to 300 mg/70 kg of patient weight in divided doses on the day of surgery. This can be easily accomplished by administering 100 mg of hydrocortisone intravenously in the preoperative holding area; intraoperatively; and in the postanesthesia care unit. Patients receiving steroids at the time of the preoperative visit should receive their usual dose of steroids on the morning of surgery and supplemental steroids as previously described. Patients with evidence of intense bronchospasm within the past month will benefit from the use of supplemental steroids in this manner, as this will help attenuate the intense bronchospasm that is sometimes experienced at the time of endotracheal intubation.

Upper respiratory infections (URIs) that occur in the preoperative period are considered a contraindication to surgery if the onset is recent, the patient is febrile, there is an associated leukocytosis, and the intended operative procedure is long and complex. If the infection is near the end of its course and the procedure is short or performed on an outpatient basis, surgery may be allowed to proceed, as there is no increase in the incidence of pneumonia in these patients.[14]

Hepatic Disorders

Hepatic disorders are important to the anesthesiologist because many of the anesthetic agents used are metabolized in the liver. In addition, acute fulminant and chronic hepatic disorders are often associated with coagulopathies due to a decrease in the production of vitamin K-dependent coagulation factors (II, VII, IX, and X) and an increase in platelet destruction. The administration of anesthesia to patients with unsuspected hepatic disease or acute viral hepatitis is associated with a mortality rate of 10 to 70 percent.[15] If abnormal liver function studies are detected preoperatively, it is best to delay elective surgery and perform a more detailed evaluation of the patient. In patients with a history of hepatitis there is often an association with substance abuse and other viral infections such as acquired immunodeficiency syndrome (AIDS). This knowledge is helpful in the prevention of disease transmission to the anesthesiologist and other hospital personnel.

Endocrine Disorders (Diabetes Mellitus)

The most common endocrine disorder encountered in the surgical patient is diabetes mellitus. Prior to surgery, the anesthesiologist should determine the patient's insulin requirements and verify that the blood glucose is well controlled. If the fasting blood sugar (FBS) is greater than 300 mg/dl, surgery should be rescheduled and the patient managed medically. Many patients with diabetes develop end organ pathology, including

1. Cardiovascular complications—coronary artery disease, hypertension (occurs in 30 to 60 percent of patients with diabetes), cardiac autonomic neuropathy (results in degeneration of the afferent and efferent components of the sympathetic and parasympathetic nervous system and is associated with silent myocardial ischemia and infarction), and impaired ventricular function (caused by an idiopathic cardiomyopathy associated with diabetes)
2. Renal disorders—acute and chronic renal failure
3. Gastrointestinal disorders—delayed gastric emptying, which increase the risks of aspiration pneumonitis[16]

The perioperative management of diabetes is an art. Although many regimens have been described, the object is to maintain glucose homeostasis throughout the course of surgery. Despite the known advantages of tight control in the chronic diabetic state, there are no studies that document improved outcomes when the blood glucose is kept at near normal levels during the perioperative period. The concept of tight control is not appropriate to the perioperative period, as attempts to maintain blood glucose in the normal range may lead to episodes of hypoglycemia. This is of major concern to the anesthesiologist, as there are no reliable signs or symptoms to diagnose this condition when the patient is anesthethized.[17] Maintaining perioperative blood glucose levels in the range of 100 to 200 mg/dl will effectively control the catabolic response to surgery and stress and should be used as a guideline when preparing patients for surgery.

For patients with insulin-dependent diabetes mellitus (IDDM) undergoing minor surgical procedures and expected to resume oral intake shortly after surgery, the following routine is often adequate: On the morning of surgery, a blood glucose is obtained and an intravenous infusion of 5 percent dextrose started. One-half of the usual morning dose of intermediate-acting insulin is administered subcutaneously. Blood glucose levels should be monitored every 1 to 2 hours throughout the intraoperative period and during the immediate postoperative period. Additional insulin requirements should be managed with a sliding scale of regular insulin.[16]

In the ambulatory setting, patients with insulin-dependent diabetes should be instructed to withhold treatment until arrival at the facility. This will prevent the development of hypoglycemia if surgery is delayed or other problems arise.

For insulin-dependent patients undergoing major surgical procedures, a more comprehensive regimen is recommended. The main objective in these patients is to maintain glucose homeostasis during the procedure. This can easily be accomplished with a constant infusion of glucose and insulin. On admission to the holding area, blood for a fasting blood sugar and potassium measurement is drawn with im-

mediate results requested. A 5 percent dextrose intravenous solution is started and infused at 50 ml/hr/70 kg body weight. A separate insulin solution (50 U regular insulin in 250 ml 0.9 percent sodium chloride) is connected to an infusion pump and piggybacked into the dextrose infusion. The rate of insulin infused is calculated by the following equation: insulin (U/hr) = plasma glucose (mg/dl)/150 and guided by hourly blood glucose determinations.[16] Intraoperative fluid requirements are managed through a separate intravenous site. The infusion can be maintained as long as the patient remains NPO (nothing by mouth) and is commonly discontinued within 24 to 48 hours after surgery.

Hematologic Disorders

Hematologic abnormalities represent a major concern to the anesthesiologist. Two conditions that are particularly important are pre-existing coagulopathies and anemias. Coagulopathies are frequently identified by obtaining a detailed hematologic history. Bleeding gums, petechiae, easy bruising, excessive bleeding during menstruation, and prolonged bleeding following dental extractions or other surgical procedures are often indicative of a bleeding diathesis. If the history is suggestive of a bleeding disorder, a thorough evaluation of the coagulation system is indicated and includes the following: prothrombin time, partial thromboplastin time, fibrinogen, fibrin-split products, platelet count, bleeding time, and possibly a thromboelastogram.[18] If the coagulopathy is severe, regional anesthesia and surgery are often contraindicated until the disorder is corrected.

Anemia, from whatever cause, is associated with a decrease in oxygen delivery to the tissues. To compensate for this, cardiac output increases proportionately. Tissue hypoxia results when oxygen demand is greater than oxygen supply. This condition may develop in anemic patients who are anesthetized, as increases in cardiac output are often limited due to the depressant nature of anesthetic agents. Until recently, guidelines suggested that the minimum hemoglobin level prior to elective surgery should be 10 g/dl (hematocrit 30 percent). This practice is controversial as the risk of blood-borne infections associated with transfusion therapy is probably greater than the risk associated with a low hemoglobin. A hematocrit of 25 to 30 percent is now viewed as adequate for many surgical procedures if the anemic process is diagnosed preoperatively and is chronic in nature, the patient is hemodynamically stable, the potential for major blood loss during the procedure is minimal, and the risk created by delaying surgery is greater than the risk associated with the use of blood.[19] In the gynecologic patient, acute anemia is most commonly the result of active bleeding. In this situation, transfusion therapy is indicated if the patient is hemodynamically unstable. However, if bleeding is controlled immediately, hemodynamic stability may be achieved with the use of crystalloids and/or colloids rather than blood or blood products, thereby reducing the risks associated with transfusion therapy.

Approximately 1 to 2 percent of all pregnant women will require some form of surgery and anesthesia during their pregnancy. Although fetal abnormalities have not been associated with the administration of anesthesia during the first trimester, the incidence of spontaneous abortions is somewhat higher in this group of patients and appears to be related to the site of surgery and not to the anesthetic agents. Until this issue is resolved, it is important to identify those women who are pregnant and, if possible, delay surgery until the second trimester.

Finally, it is important for the anesthesiologist to determine the presence of any familial conditions that may cause complications during the intraoperative period. Malignant hyperthermia (MH) is an uncommon inherited disorder of skeletal muscle that has traditionally been associated with the administration of general anesthetics and is characterized by a rapid increase in temperature and a high mortality rate (more than 70 percent).[20] Malignant hyperthermia is due to an acute loss of control of intracellular calcium, which triggers uncontrolled muscle contractions and initiates a hypermetabolic response that is characterized by an increase in carbon dioxide production and oxygen consumption. As a result of these changes, tachycardia, arrhythmias, tachypnea, acidosis, rhabdomyosis, hyperkalemia, and myoglobinuria are often seen.[20] Although an elevated temperature is a common finding in patients with malignant hyperthermia, it is often a late sign and generally not very useful in establishing the diagnosis. The incidence varies from 1 per 62,000 to 1 per 250,000 administrations of anesthesia. Treatment involves the removal of the offending agent (usually a volatile agent such as halothane and drugs such as succinylcholine), hyperventilation, cooling the patient, and the administration of dantrolene, which inhibits the release of calcium from the sarcoplasmic reticulum. Since the introduction of dantrolene, the mortality associated with this disorder has decreased to less than 10 percent.[21]

Succinylcholine is a depolarizing muscle relaxant that is frequently used to optimize intubating conditions during the induction of anesthesia. It has a rapid onset and short duration of action, which makes it an ideal drug for this purpose. It is metabolized by plasma pseudocholinesterase, an enzyme manufactured in the liver. A small number of patients exhibit a genetic deficiency of this enzyme and are susceptible to prolonged neuromuscular blockade when succinylcholine is administered. Treatment involves sedation and ventilatory support until the drug is metabolized.

Physical Examination

During the physical examination the anesthesiologist inspects the head and neck to determine whether any impairment exists to motion or position. The anatomy of the mouth and oral pharynx are evaluated and abnormalities recorded.

Physical aspects that suggest a difficult intubation include a small mouth, a narrow and receding mandible, an overbite, a large tongue, a short distance between the chin and larynx, and a soft palate and uvula that are difficult to visualize.[22] An evaluation of the lungs consists of auscultation for evidence of rales, rhonchi, wheezes, and prolonged expiratory phase of respiration. Percussion is used to identify dullness in the thoracic cavity suggestive of pleural effusions. The heart is evaluated with the patient in the sitting and lying position for evidence of heaves, thrusts, arrhythmias, murmurs, and clicks. It is important for the anesthesiologist to perform a brief neurologic examination and document any physical impairments before surgery so that proper precautions can be instituted to protect these structures during surgery.

Laboratory Testing

The use of routine preoperative laboratory tests for all patients is questionable and has recently come under scrutiny. An abnormal test is uncommon if the history and physical examination are negative.[23,24] In addition, it has been shown that abnormal results obtained from routine laboratory testing are often ignored and do not alter the course of anesthesia or surgery.[25] Preoperative laboratory testing should be based on the patient's disease process, age, proposed operation, current medications, and the type of anesthetic that is being considered (i.e., regional). Specific tests should be used to evaluate those organ systems that are identified as potential problems during the history and physical examination. The objective of this type of testing is to clarify the extent of disease and determine the possibility for improvement before surgery.[26,27]

Is there an age when routine preoperative testing should be performed? There is no definitive answer to this question; however, many institutions have developed guidelines regarding the use of these tests (Table 7-2).

Choice of Anesthetic Technique

In many situations, a variety of options exist regarding the type of anesthetic employed for a given surgical procedure. If options are available, it is the responsibility of the anesthesiologist to describe the techniques, risks, and complications associated with each of these procedures. The choice of a particular technique is made by the patient. At times, the choice of techniques may be limited due to complications associated with the patient's illness, the position of the patient during surgery, or concerns of the surgeon. If at all possible, the patient's request should be honored. It is therefore important that open communication be maintained between the surgeon, anesthesiologist, and patient if the best possible conditions are to exist at the time of the operation.

Table 7-2. Guidelines for Preoperative Laboratory Testing for Elective Surgical Procedures

Laboratory tests tequired when minimum blood loss anticipated

Age (yr)	Male	Female
<40	None	Hemoglobin/hematocrit
40–60	Electrocardiogram	Electrocardiogram
	Blood urea nitrogen	Blood urea nitrogen
	Glucose	Glucose
		Hemoglobin/hematocrit
>60	Electrocardiogram	Electrocardiogram
	Chest radiograph	Chest radiograph
	Hemoglobin/hematocyte	Hemoglobin/hematocrit
	Blood urea nitrogen	Blood urea nitrogen
	Glucose	Glucose

Laboratory tests required when blood loss is anticipated
  Hemoglobin/hematocrit on all patients
  Blood for type and screen (or type and cross)
  Transfusion consent
  Additional laboratory tests, radiographs, and electrocardiograms as dictated by patient's age and condition

Serum potassium determined in all patients on chronic diuretic therapy or dialysis

Blood glucose determined in all patients with diabetic mellitus immediately before surgery

Serum pregnancy test on all females of childbearing age unless waived by the patient or patient has had a previous surgical procedure that precludes pregnancy

Urine drug screen immediately before surgery in patients suspected of substance abuse before admission

Risks of Anesthesia

It is difficult to assess the risks associated with the administration of anesthesia as it is intimately involved with and influenced by the surgical procedure. Several studies have attempted to identify the risk by reviewing adverse outcomes during or after surgery. Difficulty arises when comparing these studies, as there are differences in definitions, anesthetic techniques, and time periods used to identify the perioperative period.[28]

In 1977, the French Health Ministry performed a nationwide survey of major intraoperative and postoperative complications occurring within 24 hours of surgery. They reported a mortality of one death for every 13,000 operations.[29] A second study reviewed over one million surgical procedures performed in the United Kingdom and examined anesthetic-related deaths or postoperative deaths occurring within 6 days of surgery. They reported that the anesthetic-related mortality was one death for every 10,000 operations. Additional reports from New South Wales and the United States have indicated similar mortality rates.[29] A common finding in these studies is that many anesthetic-related deaths

are preventable and are associated with an inappropriate application of knowledge, a poor standard of practice, a lack of experience, and equipment failure.

Although the inherent risks associated with anesthesia are small, patients that are very young or very old and those with multiple organ disease are at much greater risk.[30] When discussing the risks of anesthesia with a patient, it is beneficial to describe these risks in relation to something common and familiar to the patient, such as the concept of flying from coast to coast. On many occasions, an individual can fly from New York City to Los Angeles without a problem. However, infrequently, there are mechanical problems that delay the flight and rarely, there are problems encountered during flight that can be life-threatening. It appears that there is a better understanding regarding the low incidence of problems associated with anesthesia when described in these terms.

Unfortunately, there are very little data available that describe the likelihood of developing other complications associated with the administration of anesthesia, such as pulmonary embolism, stroke, and renal failure. In 1986, Cohen and Collins reported that approximately 18 percent of all patients experienced some form of complication following the administration of anesthesia. Most of these were considered minor in nature. Nausea and vomiting were the most common problems, occurring in more than 50 percent of the patients. The second most frequent complication was a sore throat related to endotracheal intubation.[29]

The risks associated with any operative procedure depend on a number of variables such as the age of the patient, the health of the patient, the skill of the surgeon, the type and duration of surgery, and the anesthetic agents and techniques employed. In 1940, the American Society of Anesthesiologists (ASA) developed a physical status classification that was designed to give anesthesiologists the ability to compare outcomes in similar patient populations within their own institutions and between institutions.[30] Except for a minor modification in 1961, this classification system has remained unchanged for approximately 50 years (Table 7-3). This classification is used to determine the physical status of the patient. It is not a risk scoring system. Several studies have explored the possibility of using this system as a predictor of anesthetic risk; however, no correlations have been identified.[31]

Preoperative Medication

Many patients are extremely apprehensive before surgery. The preoperative visit by the anesthesiologist is extremely helpful in alleviating a significant amount of anxiety and fear.[32] Despite adequate psychological preparation, some patients will require additional support on the day of surgery. In this situation, the use of pharmacologic agents is indicated. Preoperative medication is most often used to induce seda-

Table 7-3. American Society of Anesthesiologists (ASA) Physical Status

ASA Status	Description
I	Healthy patient
II	Mild systemic disease that is generally well controlled
III	Severe systemic disease that is not incapacitating but is poorly controlled or not controlled
IV	Severe systemic disease that is a constant threat to life
V	Moribund (not expected to live 24 hours irrespective of surgery)
VI	Organ donor
E	Emergency patient

tion, produce amnesia, and relieve anxiety and fear. However, additional goals and therapeutic effects may be desired.

There is no general consensus regarding the use of preoperative medication or the choice of a particular agent. This aspect of anesthetic care is cloaked in tradition. The selection of drugs is often based on physician bias and previous experience and is, therefore, more empiric than scientific. There are many drugs available for use in the preoperative period. The choice of an agent should be individualized for each patient with respect to age, the surgical procedure, the desired effects of the medication, and the association of any chronic medical disorders that may prolong or alter the effects of these drugs.

Hypnotics and Sedatives

Hypnotics are drugs that produces a sleep-like state, whereas sedatives decrease activity and produce a calming effect. Both groups of drugs are also capable of producing widespread central nervous system (CNS) depression and, in the preoperative period, are used primarily to induce drowsiness

---

Goals For Preoperative Medications

- Decrease anxiety
- Produce sedation and amnesia
- Produce analgesia
- Decrease anesthetic requirements and facilitate induction
- Dry airway secretions
- Decrease gastric fluid and pH

---

and produce sleep. The most commonly prescribed hypnotics and sedatives include benzodiazepines, barbiturates, and chloral derivatives such as chloral hydrate. At the present time, the benzodiazepines are the most widely used as preoperative medications.

Benzodiazepines

As a group, the benzodiazepines exhibit similar pharmacologic effects. In the CNS, γ-aminobutyric acid (GABA) is an inhibitory neurotransmitter. The benzodiazepines augment or facilitate this neurotransmission, which produces amnesia, sedation, muscle relaxation, and anticonvulsant activity and decreases anxiety.[33] Although amnesia is usually dose-dependent, it does not always correspond to the level of sedation. Preanesthetic doses are associated with minimal effects on the respiratory and cardiovascular system. However, when administered in conjunction with other depressants (i.e., opioids) or in larger doses, they cause profound depression. Major disadvantages identified with benzodiazepines are the absence of intrinsic analgesia and the patient variability in response. Elderly patients are particularly sensitive to these agents and may experience agitation rather than sedation, due to hypoxia associated with respiratory depression.

The commonly used benzodiazepines include diazepam (Vallium), lorazepam (Ativan), and midazolam (Versed) (Table 7-4). Until recently, diazepam was the most commonly used agent for premedication. It is a long-acting agent that effectively produces sedation, anxiolysis, and amnesia. When used intravenously or intramuscularly, it is associated with phlebitis and pain due to the organic solvents in the vehicle. Hepatic metabolism results in the production of an active metabolite with an extremely long elimination time (21 to 37 hours), which is responsible for the prolonged clinical effects associated with this drug.[33] Diazepam is often used as an oral preparation preoperatively because of unpredictable uptake after intramuscular injection and pain associated with parenteral administration.

Lorazepam is an intermediate-acting agent with effects similar to the other benzodiazepines. Despite a short half-life, lorazepam is associated with a long latency period (approximately 2 hours) and prolonged sedation, due to its binding characteristics with the benzodiazepine receptor.[34] Because of these characteristics, lorazepam has had limited use in the ambulatory setting. However, it is extremely useful for inpatients undergoing major operative procedures.

Midazolam is a short-acting drug that is water soluble and rapidly metabolized. It is not associated with pain on injection and is capable of producing extensive retrograde amnesia that helps the patient to forget events preceding surgery. Because of an increased affinity for the benzodiazepine receptor, midazolam is two to three times more potent than diazepam and has been associated with a number of respiratory arrests following rapid injection.[35] When used in

Table 7-4. Comparison of Benzodiazepines

Medication	Route of Administration	Dose	Time to Peak Effect (hr)	Elimination Half-Time (hr)	Active Metabolite	Comments
Diazepam (Vallium)	Oral	5–20 mg	1–1.5	20–40	Yes	Pain with parenteral use
	IV	0.1–0.2 mg/kg	Immediately–0.5			Phlebitis with IV use
Midazolam (Versed)	IM	0.07–0.08 mg/kg	0.5	1–4	No	Respiratory arrest with IV use
	IV	Titrated to effect (1–2.5 mg/ dose)	Immediately			Retrograde amnesia
Lorazepam (Ativan)	Oral	2–4 mg	2	12–18	No	
	IM	1–4 mg	2–4	10–20	No	Painful with IM injections
	IV	1–4 mg	1–1.5	10–20	No	Profound amnesia

areas other than the operating room, extreme caution is advised and emergency airway management equipment should be immediately available.

Flumazenil (Romazicon) is a new benzodiazepine antagonist. It reverses the clinical effects of the benzodiazepines by interfering with their ability to bind with the receptor. It is associated with a rapid onset of action (approximately 5 minutes) and short duration (approximately 1 to 3 hours).

Opioids

Opioid is a word used to describe all compounds with morphine-like actions. Opioids are a large class of drugs that comprises natural alkaloids (morphine), semisynthetic derivatives (codeine), and synthetic derivatives (fentanyl). As a group these agents cause mild sedation and potent analgesia and are frequently used in anesthesia for a variety of reasons, including pain relief, premedication, and supplementation of general and regional anesthesia.

The discovery of opioid receptors by several independent investigators in 1973 provided the framework that led to the identification of endogenous opioid peptides by Beaumont and Hughes in 1976.[36–38] Following the discovery of endogenous opioid peptides, differences were observed in their activity when compared to morphine in certain bioassy systems. The differential ordering of activity across several tissue types led to the identification of multiple opioid receptors in the CNS (Table 7-5). The pharmacologic effects of the opioids are due to complex interactions of a specific drug with a specific receptor. Based on receptor specificity, opioids can be classified according to their primary site of action. Opioids such as morphine, meperidine (Demerol), and fentanyl bind exclusively with the mu (μ) receptor. These drugs are known as pure agonists and are associated

with euphoria, physical dependence, respiratory depression, and analgesia. Opioids such as butorphanol (Stadol) and nalbuphine (Nubain) are compounds that can bind with more than one type of opioid receptor (μ and kappa [κ]). These agents are known as agonists-antagonists. At the κ-receptor, these drugs are pure agonists and cause analgesia, sedation, and miosis; at the μ-receptor, they are competitive antagonists and produce no pharmacologic effect when bound with this specific receptor.

Table 7-5. Opiate Receptor Classification and Actions of Agonets and Agonists/Antagonists

Receptor Type	Effects	Drug/Action
μ_1	Supraspinal analgesia Dependence	Morphine/agonist Meperidine/agonist Fentanyl/agonist
μ_2	Respiratory depression Decrease gastrointestinal Euphoria	Butorphanol/no effect Nalbuphine/antagonist Naloxone/antagonist
Delta (Δ)	Spinal analgesia	None
Kappa (κ)	Spinal analgesia Sedation Miosis	Morphine/agonist Meperidine/agonist Fentanyl/agonist Butorphanol/agonist Nalbuphine/agonist Naloxone/antagonist
Sigma (σ)	Dysphoria Hallucinations	Butorphanol/agonist Nalbuphine/agonist Naloxone/antagonist

In the preoperative setting these agents are frequently prescribed if the patient is experiencing moderate to severe pain before surgery or if invasive procedures are anticipated before the induction of anesthesia (i.e., placement of an arterial or central venous catheter). The administration of these drugs can be associated with respiratory and cardiovascular depression, as well as hypotension. As with the benzodiazepines, these effects are more profound when administered to the debilitated or elderly patient or in combination with other depressant drugs. In addition, these agents decrease gastrointestinal motility and delay gastric emptying, which increases the risk of aspiration prior to the induction of anesthesia. Due to stimulation of the chemotactic trigger zone, nausea and vomiting are common side effects associated with the administration of these drugs. For this reason, opioids are frequently administered with phenergan or vistaril to counteract these effects.

Aspiration Pneumonitis Prevention

Any patient scheduled for surgery must be considered at risk of aspiration pneumonitis. The incidence is higher in patients scheduled for emergency procedures and in those with a history of hiatal hernia, diabetes, gastroesphogeal reflux, and obesity.[39] Studies by a number of authors indicate that, in adults, there is a potential risk of aspiration if the volume of gastric fluid is 25 ml or greater and the pH of this fluid is 2.5 or less.[40] In healthy adult populations scheduled for elective surgery the potential risk of aspiration has been estimated to be as high as 40 to 80 percent. However, in actuality, the incidence of aspiration is extremely low. In addition, several recently performed studies have suggested that gastric emptying is enhanced by clear fluid intake prior to surgery.[41,42] The low incidence of gastric aspiration and enhanced gastric emptying by clear fluids has resulted in a re-evaluation of the concept of a preoperative fast. Many institutions continue to recommend an NPO status for at least 6 hours before surgery. However, they also allow patients to consume clear liquids (4 to 5 oz) and to take oral medications 3 to 4 hours preoperatively.[39]

Pharmacologic agents that alter gastric volume and pH are also used to decrease the risk of aspiration pneumonitis. Anticholinergic agents such as atropine and glycopyrrolate are used for their antisialagogue and vagolytic properties. They are also capable of decreasing gastric volume and increasing gastric pH; however, these effects are transient and not important clinically. In addition, the anticholinergic agents have been shown to relax the gastroesophageal sphincter, which would, theoretically, increase the risk of aspiration. Although used clinically for other reasons, these agents are not useful in preventing aspiration pneumonitis.

Histamine receptor antagonists (H$_2$ blockers) have the ability to block the histamine-induced secretion of gastric acid. As a group these drugs have relatively few side effects and are extremely effective in decreasing the risk of aspiration. They are most beneficial when used in a multiple dose regimen at least 24 hours before surgery. Recent studies have also demonstrated their clinical effectiveness when administered at least 30 to 60 minutes preoperatively. Cimetidine was the first H$_2$ blocker available for clinical practice. It has a short half-life and requires frequent dosing. Cimetidine has been implicated in altering the metabolism of other drugs and elevating blood levels by inhibiting hepatic cytochrome P450 oxidation.[43] The drugs most commonly influenced in this manner include the local anesthetics, anticoagulants, some β-blockers, benzodiazepines, and theophylline.

Ranitidine was the second H$_2$-receptor blocker introduced. It has a longer duration of action and subsequently requires less dosing during the day. It too has been associated with the inhibition of metabolism of other drugs but to a lesser degree than cimetidine.[43]

Famotidine is the latest drug of this class to be introduced into clinical practice. However, unlike the previous agents, this drug is not associated with hepatic enzyme inhibition. If possible, it is best to administer these drugs the night before and the morning of surgery if optimal results are to be realized.[43]

Antacids are commonly used to neutralize gastric pH. This group of drugs is inexpensive and effective if administered 15 to 30 minutes before the induction of anesthesia. Particulate antacid suspensions were initially used for the prevention of aspiration. However, it was quickly appreciated that these compounds, if aspirated, produced a syndrome as severe as that associated with gastric acid. If indicated, nonparticulate mixtures are the antacids of choice.

Dopamine antagonists, as characterized by metaclopramide, increase gastroesophageal sphincter tone, enhance gastric emptying, and are effective antiemetics. By promoting gastric emptying and decreasing gastric volume, these drugs can be used to decrease the risk of aspiration in high-risk patients. Metaclopramide effectively crosses the blood-brain barrier and has been associated with extrapyramidal effects (that respond to droperidol) and stress-induced tachycardia.

ANESTHETIC TECHNIQUES AND AGENTS

Ensuring that a patient is comfortable for surgery entails the use of anesthesia at one of three sites. At the incision, local anesthetic can be infiltrated by the surgeon. Alternatively, anesthetic agents can be introduced into the epidural or subarachnoid space to provide regional anesthesia of the lower half of the body by actions at the level of the spinal cord and adjacent nerve roots. Finally, general anesthesia provides complete hypnosis, amnesia, and analgesia for those procedures that cannot be performed by one of the other approaches.

Monitored Anesthesia Care

The least invasive anesthetic option, monitored anesthesia care (MAC), consists of (1) infiltration of local anesthetic by the surgeon, (2) monitoring of vital signs, and (3) intravenous sedation. Historically, it has been indicated in the medically complicated patient for whom monitoring requires the undivided attention of an individual specifically trained to manage abnormalities of either the pulmonary or cardiovascular system. The second indication is to ensure analgesia and/or amnesia for the patient when placement of the block may be painful or complete anesthesia cannot be obtained by local infiltration. With recognition that pain need not be a part of the perioperative experience, MAC is being used with increasing frequency for many surgical procedures previously done as a "straight local."

The major advantage of MAC, especially in the fragile patient, is that it is minimally invasive in terms of cardiopulmonary perturbations. Assuming adequate analgesia can be provided by local anesthesia, it will be the least stressful way to conduct the surgical procedure. Linked to good intraoperative analgesia is the fact that the block will probably be more effective than one supplementing a general anesthetic because it has been tested by the surgical procedure itself and augmented as necessary. If long-acting local anesthetic agents are used, then analgesia will last 4 to 6 hours into the postoperative period, allowing the patient to obtain needed pain medication and to situate themselves at home while free of discomfort.

Agents

Agents used to provide sedation for MAC include the previously described benzodiazepines and opioids as well as ketamine, barbiturates, and propofol. No single agent is the perfect intravenous sedative. Rapid onset and brief duration of action characterize all the intravenous anesthetic agents, and is a function of their high-lipid solubility. Redistribution from the central compartment into the less well-perfused periphery accounts for termination of effect, not hepatic metabolism.

Ketamine

Ketamine is a potent analgesic agent with a completely unique side-effect profile that accounts for a different spectrum of clinical use. It rapidly produces anesthesia by disruption of neural transmission between the spinal cord and higher cortical structures. A patient may appear to be awake, but will remain unresponsive to painful stimuli. One advantage of ketamine is that it is a water-soluble compound that is painless to administer intramuscularly or intravenously. Very analgesic, even at subhypnotic doses, it preferentially blocks pain of somatic origin.[44] It has been widely utilized on burn units for dressing changes and wound debridement.

There is minimal depression of laryngeal or airway reflexes and respiratory drive is preserved.

Several disadvantages preclude the regular use of ketamine. At anesthetic doses, it is frequently associated with emergence delirium that may be as minor as visual and auditory illusions during arousal from anesthesia to morbid hallucinations that can persist beyond the perioperative period. This problem is more common in older patients, females, and individuals without prior exposure to the drug.[45] Prior administration of benzodiazepines appears to reduce the incidence of severe reactions. Through stimulation of the sympathetic system, both heart rate and blood pressure increase. The patient with compromised coronary circulation or elevated intracranial pressure could be adversely affected. For these reasons, routine employment of ketamine for conscious sedation cannot be advocated. Analgesia can be achieved with ketamine by incremental intravenous doses of 0.2 to 0.4 mg/kg.

Barbiturates

Barbiturates rapidly induce general anesthesia lasting 5 to 10 minutes. The brief periods of unconsciousness allow painless placement of regional blocks, cardioversions, and electroconvulsive therapy. Barbiturates are not appropriate for conscious sedation. That loss of consciousness is brief does not negate the fact that all protective airway reflexes are lost, and a period of apnea necessitating assisted ventilation may ensue. Barbiturates have no intrinsic analgesic effect and may lower the pain threshold, causing increased discomfort and anxiety rather than sedation. Despite the short duration of action, patients are often left with a "hangover."

Propofol

Propofol offers many advantages over the agents discussed above. It is used as an intravenous sedative, an induction agent, and a maintenance anesthetic. The drug has a rapid rate of onset and dissipation of effects with no persistent sedation or psychomotor depression. For the purpose of conscious sedation, propofol can be administered as small boluses or as an infusion. Its high rate of clearance means that a steady plane of sedation can be achieved and maintained for hours with no accumulation. It also has mild analgesic and amnestic properties following hypnotic doses. Most patients describe it as a very soothing, relaxed state. Pleasant dreams on arousal are common. At subhypnotic doses, propofol also appears to have antipruritic and antiemetic effects. As little as 10 to 20 mg have been used to treat opioid side effects.[47] Propofol is painful to inject, although this can be attenuated by using a freely flowing intravenous catheter in a large vein and pretreatment with intravenous lidocaine. The dose for conscious sedation is 25 to 50 µg/kg/min.

Monitoring Requirements

Monitoring of the patient undergoing a procedure under MAC should include attention to the central nervous, respiratory, and cardiovascular systems. At a minimum, vital information can be obtained by talking with the patient and intermittently monitoring the pulse and blood pressures. Most of the agents discussed above cause CNS depression. Furthermore, the injection of local anesthetics into the surgical field may produce high plasma levels. Medications should be titrated so that the patient remains communicative, reporting symptoms of local anesthetic toxicity such as ringing in the ears, numbness around the mouth, or lightheadedness. Signs of CNS excitation occur at lower plasma levels than CNS or cardiovascular depression. Most sedatives decrease the respiratory drive, resulting in hypoxia and hypercarbia. Although widely used, it must be recognized that pulse oximetry is a monitor of oxygenation, not ventilation. Patients receiving supplemental oxygen may have considerable elevations in arterial carbon dioxide before oxygen saturation falls, thereby highlighting the limitation of pulse oximetry.

Side Effects

Patients must be committed to being awake and capable of managing their mental stress and anxiety, and the procedure must be one for which a local anesthetic block will provide good relief. Heavy sedation is not a reasonable substitute. Without the benefits of a regional anesthetic, greater sedative requirements may obtund protective airway reflexes, increasing risk.

Regional Anesthesia

Regional anesthesia provides complete anesthesia at the surgical site, obviating the need for supplemental sedation. This may be beneficial in the elderly patient, who might demonstrate prolonged recovery. As discussed above, the awake patient assumes some of the monitoring role with regard to adequacy of cardiopulmonary function. The stress of endotracheal intubation is avoided, there is less respiratory compromise, and there is more complete ablation of the hormonal response to surgery. As compared to general anesthesia, various studies have demonstrated decreased catabolism, improved pulmonary function, and a decreased incidence of myocardial ischemia. Rheologic changes confer an advantage with regard to perioperative blood loss and thrombosis, and decreased immunocompetence at the cellular level.

The two commonly used regional techniques for gynecologic surgery are spinal and epidural anesthesia. Performance of a spinal anesthetic requires that the needle traverse the skin and subcutaneous tissues, the supraspinous and interspinous ligaments, the ligamentum flavum, the epidural space, the dura mater, and the arachnoid membrane (Fig. 7-

1). The needle is introduced at an interspace between L2 and S1, well below the usual termination of the spinal cord. Free flow of cerebrospinal fluid (CSF) indicates correct placement, and then one of the above agents is introduced into the CSF.

Anesthetic considerations with spinal anesthesia include attention to patient position, equipment used, and agents injected. A midline insertion is usually easier, and is less traumatic because it avoids the tender paraspinous muscles and the epidural blood vessels that tend to lie laterally in the epidural space. In the sitting patient, the midline can be ascertained with greater certainty, especially in obese or scoliotic individuals, and improved lumbar flexion opens up the interspaces, making needle placement easier. Use of the atraumatic whiteacre or sprotte needle prevents postdural puncture headaches. Theoretically, spreading dural fibers rather than cutting them means that when the needle is removed, the dural fibers reapproximate, reducing CSF leak. In the high-risk obstetric population (e.g., the patient with a history of previous headaches and the outpatient whose readmission for treatment of a postdural puncture headache would be onerous) an atraumatic needle should be employed.

From the patient perspective, there is little difference between the performance of a spinal and an epidural anesthetic, and with respect to patient position and angle of approach, the procedural considerations are similar as well. The major difference is that instead of penetrating the dura mater, the potential epidural space is found by a loss of resistance technique using constant pressure on either an air- or saline-filled syringe (Fig. 7-2). When the epidural space is found, medication can be injected or a catheter can be inserted and secured for later injection.

Agents

Commonly used agents for injection into the epidural or subarachnoid space are local anesthetics, opioids, and adrenergic agonists. As a general rule, the subarachnoid dose is 10 to 20 percent of the epidural dose. Local anesthetics exert their effect on nerve roots passing through the epidural or subarachnoid space, blocking impulses from reaching the spinal cord. Spinal anesthesia is conducted with lidocaine 5 percent, bupivacaine 0.75 percent, and tetracine 1 percent. The addition of dextrose makes these formulations hyperbaric, allowing gravity to determine the height of the block by influencing spread within the CSF. There is considerably greater choice regarding agents used in the epidural space, since the blood-brain barrier is not compromised. However, when an agent is selected for epidural use, one must consider the possibility that it may accidently enter the subarachnoid space, resulting in neurologic problems. An example is the epidural use of 2-chloroprocaine (Nesacaine). Neurologic deficits such as cauda equina syndrome and adhesive arachnoiditis may follow accidental subarachnoid administration.

In contrast to local anesthetics, opioids diffuse to neurons within the substance of the spinal cord, inhibiting transmis-

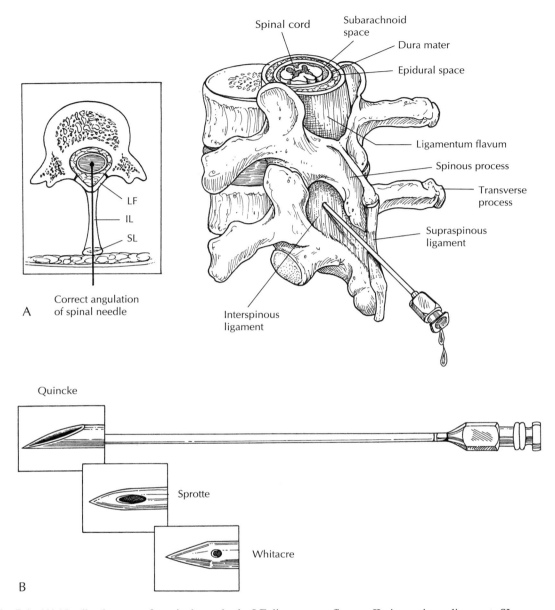

Fig. 7-1. (A) Needle placement for spinal anesthesia. LF, ligamentum flavum; IL, interspinous ligament; SL, supraspinous ligament. (B) Spinal needles.

sion of pain stimuli centrally. Preservative-free morphine (Duramorph) was the first opioid to be used routinely, but because of delayed onset and long duration, it is primarily employed for postoperative pain relief. The speed of onset of sufentanyl and fentanyl makes them useful for augmenting intraoperative anesthesia, especially the visceral pain associated with peritoneal traction mediated by the vagus nerve. Meperidine has intrinsic local anesthetic properties, and an intrathecal dose of 50 to 100 mg will provide surgical anesthesia in patients allergic to both classes (amide and ester) of local anesthetics. By activity at α_1-receptors, epinephrine, and phenylephrine produce vasoconstriction that reduces uptake and removal of local anesthetics by the vascular system.

Stimulation of α_1-receptors has a direct analgesic effect. Epidural clonidine, the α_1-agonist, has been investigated quite extensively, and significantly reduces anesthetic requirements. However, hypotension remains the major side effect.[47]

Spinal Versus Epidural Anesthesia

There are several reasons why a spinal anesthetic may be preferred to an epidural anesthetic. The former is faster to perform and the concrete end point of CSF ensures a higher degree of success. In patients with a previous history of back surgery, obliteration of the epidural space with scar tissue

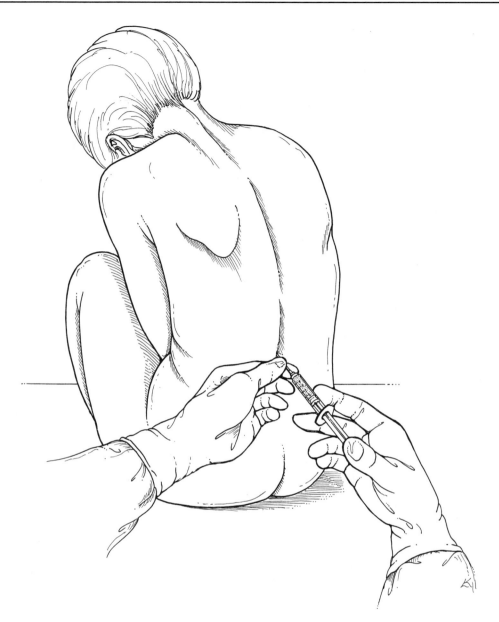

Fig. 7-2. Sitting position for epidural anesthesia.

may make epidural anesthesia problematic. The incidence of inadvertent dural punctures will be higher and anesthesia may be poor because of suboptimal spread of local anesthetic solution. In general, there is a perceived higher quality of anesthesia with spinal versus epidural techniques, and this is confirmed by measurements of spinal cord-evoked potentials, which demonstrate more complete interruption of ascending neural pathways during spinal anesthesia.[48]

The major limitation of a spinal anesthetic is the duration of the medications administered. Effective surgical anesthesia time is defined as the length of time a surgeon can operate and still expect the patient to remain comfortable. For lidocaine and bupivacaine, the duration of surgical anesthesia

above the umbilicus is 1 and 2 hours respectively. By contrast, epidural anesthesia is usually performed as a continuous technique. Incremental dosing via a catheter allows one to obtain a specific anesthetic level. Patients with severe cardiac or pulmonary dysfunction might not tolerate the sudden and unpredictable onset of a single-shot spinal and the associated hemodynamic compromise or pulmonary dysfunction. The block can also be extended as needed both anatomically and temporally. A continuous technique can also be performed, thereby combining the certainty of spinal anesthesia with the flexibility of a catheter. However, the Food and Drug Administration (FDA) discouraged employment of small bore catheters following a series of reports of persistent neurologic deficits following their use. If an epidural needle and catheter is used, there is a much greater chance of a postdural puncture headache. Only in the medically compromised patient would the benefits outweigh the risks. There is minimal risk of a postdural puncture headache following an epidural anesthetic, since the dura is not intentionally penetrated, and consequently, it remains the most commonly used continuous technique. Furthermore, an epidural catheter can be left in place to provide postoperative analgesia.

Monitoring Requirements

Prior to initiation of a block, a noninvasive blood pressure cuff and electrocardiograph should be placed, as hypotension often results from the induced sympathectomy. If a block extends to the thoracic level, inhibition of cardiac accelerator fibers may result in bradycardia and a decrease in cardiac output. Following the anesthetic level alerts the anesthesiologist of the potential for cardiac or respiratory embarrassment as the block extends. Pulse oximetry is helpful in assessing adequacy of ventilation, especially in a patient with underlying pulmonary disease. Mental status should be monitored as well by conversing with the patient and inquiring about symptoms of local anesthetic toxicity. A review of closed claims of deaths during spinal anesthesia strongly suggest that respiratory insufficiency, most likely as a result of oversedation, probably was a major contributing factor to the poor outcome following cardiorespiratory arrest.[49]

Side Effects

The most common side effects are cardiovascular hypotension, tachycardia, and occasionally bradycardia with a high level. Rarely, ''total spinals'' have been described, in which unconsciousness is induced, presumably as a result of central hypotension or local anesthetic migration to supraspinal levels. This latter entity is usually seen with the accidental subarachnoid injection of larger epidural doses of local anesthetic. Central ischemia is the presumed etiology for nausea and vomiting. Intravascular injection with associated neurologic and cardiovascular toxicity is possible with the higher doses used during epidural anesthesia. CNS symptoms of ringing in the ears, numbness around the mouth, or abnormal taste occur at the lowest doses. At higher serum levels, seizures may be induced, and cardiovascular collapse has occurred with the use of bupivacaine.

General Anesthesia

The third technique for providing intraoperative comfort during gynecologic surgery is general anesthesia. It provides complete hypnosis, amnesia, and analgesia without noxious interventions while the patient is awake. The anesthesiologist can manipulate ventilation, circulation, and muscle tone to optimize surgical conditions. Procedures performed in the extreme lithotomy or prone position are difficult for an awake patient to endure for extended periods and a regional anesthetic may not provide complete anesthesia for procedures involving the upper abdomen.

Agents

In adults, induction of general anesthesia is usually accomplished with either pentothal or propofol. Traditionally, in the hemodynamically compromised patient, ketamine has been the agent of choice because of the sympathetic stimulation it triggers. An alternative that is devoid of the psychological side effects associated with ketamine is etomidate, also notable for its remarkable hemodynamic stability. All these agents are similar in providing rapid induction of general anesthesia, minimizing the period between loss of consciousness and the point at which intubation can be achieved. When an intravenous induction is not possible, such as in the pediatric patient, a mask inhalational induction can be performed.

Once the patient is asleep and the airway is secured, general anesthesia is maintained with either a volatile agent or an intravenous agent, or most commonly, a combination of both. All volatile agents decrease cerebral metabolism, cause vasodilation and bronchodilation, and reduce myocardial contractility. Their effect on blood pressure and organ-specific blood flow is a complex interplay of multiple factors. Halothane is the oldest and least expensive agent, and is characterized by a sweet smell that is less pungent than enflurane or isoflurane, making it appropriate for inhalational inductions. Two new agents recently introduced into clinical practice, sevoflurane and desflurane, provide much more rapid inductions and arousals than the other agents in clinical use. This may translate into more efficient utilization in the outpatient setting.

One alternative to a pure volatile technique is the nitrous-narcotic technique. Nitrous oxide is required because opioids alone do not guarantee amnesia. Nitrous oxide is not potent enough to serve as a sole anesthetic like the volatile agents described above. However, similar to sevoflurane and desflurane, it has a very low solubility that translates to a rapid onset and offset of anesthetic effects. The major concern with use of nitrous oxide is the potential for gastrointestinal dilation that may compromise surgical exposure. Brief procedures limited to the pelvis are unlikely to be affected, but the more extensive and prolonged the surgery, the greater the risk of hindering surgical progress. As stated above, the usual approach is a ''mixed'' technique in which some opioids are administered to provide postoperative analgesia, and a volatile agent with or without nitrous oxide is administered. In the outpatient undergoing laparoscopic procedures where postoperative nausea is often seen, a propofol infusion provides a more pleasant arousal, with significantly less nausea than any other technique.

Airway Management

General anesthesia is induced with the patient in the supine position. If surgery is performed in either the prone or lateral decubitus position, the airway is secured first, and then the patient is repositioned. For short procedures in which a patient may breathe spontaneously, mask ventilation with or without an airway may be appropriate. Intubation is indicated if the patient is considered to have a full stomach, the airway will not be readily available once the patient has been positioned for surgery, or the procedure is quite prolonged. Two alternate methods for airway management are the laryngeal mask (LMA) and transtracheal jet ventilation (Fig. 7-3). The LMA is being used increasingly in place of mask ventilation because it ensures greater airway patency and protection from oral secretions. The LMA does not stimulate the trachea, eliminating the coughing that may occur during arousal. A lighter plane of anesthesia can be used, which results in faster arousal. Insertion of the LMA does not require muscle relaxation, thereby avoiding the additional risks associated with use of muscle relaxants. However, the LMA is not a substitute for endotracheal intubation when indicated to secure the airway. Furthermore, an endotracheal tube allows for the provision of positive pressure ventilation, prevents insufflation of the stomach, and helps ensure adequate ventilation in the patient with decreased lung compliance due to either intrinsic lung disease or obesity. When a patient cannot be intubated or ventilated, the traditional approach would be an emergency cricothyrotomy, which requires skill and entails a risk of bleeding. A less traumatic and more easily mastered alternative is transtracheal jet ventilation. Transtracheal jet ventilation entails insertion of a needle through the cricothyroid membrane, which is then attached to a jet ventilator. Intermittent insufflation with oxygen at 30 PSI will inflate the lungs, oxygenating the patient; passive recoil results in exhalation of carbon dioxide.

Monitoring Requirements

Since the anesthesiologist assumes more complete control of normal physiologic processes in the patient under general anesthesia, monitoring assumes even greater importance. Life-preserving interventions such as intubation have the potential to cause mortal injury if not performed properly. Anesthetic agents chosen because of their salutary effects likewise have harmful side effects that the anesthesiologist must watch for vigilantly. As with all anesthetic techniques, the ASA standards for intraoperative monitoring require continual evaluation of the adequacy of the patient's oxygenation, ventilation, circulation, and temperature. At a minimum, this entails proper use of and attention to an oxygen analyzer in the breathing circuit, pulse oximetry, a carbon dioxide monitor in the expiratory limb in the intubated patient, an electrocardiogram, and an available temperature probe. The patient should also be observed clinically by noting proper chest excursions, auscultating breathing sounds, observing skin color, and intermittently checking the blood pressure and pulse. Anesthetic agents are capable of dramatic and sudden alterations in cardiopulmonary function that must be anticipated and treated appropriately.

Side Effects

The common side effects of general anesthetics are postoperative nausea and vomiting, and blunted sensorium. Succinylcholine may result in muscle aches and pains. Patients may complain of blurred vision, a sore throat, or low back pain, depending on the specific technique used. Although usually minor, nausea and vomiting is one of the leading causes of unanticipated admissions following outpatient surgery.[50] There are more serious problems with general anesthesia. The fundamental problem is that an asleep patient is unable to serve as a monitor of physiologic well-being. This may be as simple as ensuring that limbs are properly positioned to avoid nerve damage or as profound as detecting the inadequacy of cerebral or coronary perfusion.

POSTOPERATIVE CARE

The two major areas of concern with regard to care of the patient in the postoperative period are management of postoperative pain and recognition of anesthetic complications. For a variety of reasons, the anesthesiologist may not be as intimately involved in the patient's care, but prompt recognition of patient needs and problems is more likely to ensure that the patient is attended to properly.

Pain Management

Tissue injury triggers postoperative pain that is directly related to the extent of injury. For example, severe pain may last 4 to 5 days following nephrectomy or thoracotomy versus 1 to 2 days after hysterectomy, and a transverse abdominal incision is less painful than a vertical incision crossing several dermatomes. Cellular injury also releases noxious compounds that sensitize peripheral nociceptive receptors. Similar amplification occurs in the spinal cord when afferent stimuli initiate positive feedback loops that increase neuronal excitability in the dorsal horn. The increased level of excitability may induce skeletal muscle spasm, which increases pain. When the afferent stimuli reach the brain, painful emotion and conscious awareness of the nature of the injury result.

Unpleasant as this response may be, it represents a signaling mechanism designed to avoid further injury. In fact, the

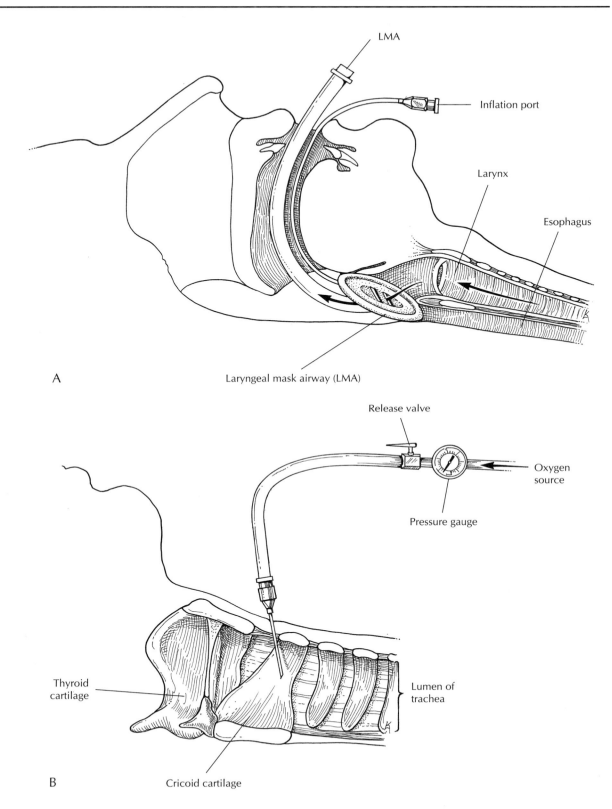

Fig. 7-3. (A) LMA ventilation. **(B)** Transtracheal jet ventilation.

silent physiologic responses to injury are more likely to harm the fragile patient undergoing major surgery. Referred to as the stress response to surgery, major endocrinologic and metabolic changes are triggered that tax multiple organ systems. Effective analgesia not only improves the patient's mental state of being, but also may reduce the stress response, thereby reducing the morbidity associated with major surgery. Both local anesthetics administered by the surgeon during MAC cases or a regional anesthetic would obtain this benefit. In fact, any agent that interferes with transmission and processing of noxious afferent stimuli along nociceptive pathways has potential utility, such as nonsteroidal agents like ketorolac, opioids, and α_2-agonists.

Parenteral Techniques

The traditional approach for the treatment of postoperative pain has been intramuscular narcotics. Other modalities currently employed include nonsteroidal agents, patient-controlled analgesia (PCA), epidural narcotics and/or local anesthetics, and intrathecal narcotics.

Intramuscular Narcotics

When administered intramuscularly, narcotics such as morphine and meperidine attain peak serum levels in 45 minutes (range 15 to 106 minutes) and are effective for 75 to 90 minutes. The major advantage is low cost, both of drug and equipment. For this reason, it is widely available, and most medical personnel are familiar and comfortable with their administration. The major disadvantages are that it is painful to administer, and often results in inadequate pain relief. This is both a result of the pharmacologic profile (i.e., long time to onset and short duration) and underprescribing. Inadequate prescribing is often due to an incomplete knowledge regarding the pharmacologic actions of the agents, a fear of addiction, and great interindividual variability. For example, opioids are routinely administered every 4 hours on a PRN basis. This is not pharmacologically sound, since the half-life of morphine is considerably shorter (about 2 or 3 hours). Individuals can vary by several hundred percent in narcotic needs. Once in pain, the patient must wait the specified interval before alerting the nurse, who then checks the orders and administers the appropriate dose. Then the patients waits for relief. To hasten onset and prolong effectiveness, larger than optimal doses are often administered. Consequently, patients go through periods of pain, relief, oversedation, and then recurrent pain.

Patient-Controlled Analgesia

PCA is specifically designed to avoid the cyclic nature of intramuscular opioid administration in which a patient may spend more time in periods of pain and oversedation than with optimum relief. It is based on the concept that adequate pain relief can be attained with a constant serum level of opioids. The appropriate serum level lies within a narrow range that is patient specific; too low and the patient suffers pain, too high and the patient experiences unwanted side effects. The drug is administered by a device that allows the patient to self-administer small amounts at set time intervals. The total amount is limited by a 4-hour cap that is set by the prescribing physician. Theoretically, the dose should be adequate to offer some relief, but not overwhelm the patient. The lockout interval prevents the patient from administering another dose until the desired effects are dissipated.

The advantages are obvious: opioids are obtained in a more timely fashion and constant serum levels are achieved, rather than the cyclic pattern of intramuscular administration. Of all modalities available, patients select PCA as their favorite. They believe that it provides the greatest control over their postoperative pain. Gratification is instantaneous, and they can weigh whether the benefit of additional pain relief outweighs the side effects of additional opioids. The major disadvantage is the cost of the apparatus. At present, opioids administered by PCA must either be purchased in special vials or individually mixed by the hospital pharmacy. Cost/benefit studies that explore the reduced workload for the nursing staff have not been undertaken. Unfortunately, in many institutions in which PCA has been introduced, it has been subjected to close scrutiny and required the institution of formalized patient observation forms to document analgesia and incidence of side effects. The result is probably increased nursing paperwork in those units in which PCA is used. Furthermore, since intramuscular administration has been almost universally characterized by inadequate dosing, there is a mistaken perception that PCA is riskier because of associated cases of respiratory depression. This is borne out by standard PCA protocols that limit its use in so-called high-risk patients such as elderly or obese patients. On the contrary, an appropriate PCA regimen is probably *safer* in these patients than intramuscular dosing if the goal is equivalent pain relief.

Any opioid can be used with a PCA device, but fentanyl, morphine, and meperidine are most commonly employed, at concentrations of 0.01, 1, and 10 mg/ml, respectively, which allows a standard 1- to 2-ml incremental demand dose to be used safely. The lockout interval is the time after dosing that a patient must wait before the device will allow additional dosing. In theory, it should be related to the time between administration and penetration of the CNS with resultant analgesia and respiratory depression. This would be 5 to 10 minutes for fentanyl, 10 to 15 minutes for morphine, and 8 to 12 minutes for meperidine. However, since any single dose is very unlikely to pose a significant risk, the lockout interval is usually set for much less than would be suggested by the pharmacologic action. As long as dosing is impeded, the safety of this modality will be preserved. In general, PCA devices are set up to run in a purely demand mode where the patient must request each dose, or a continuous mode in which the patient receives a continuous infusion. In the latter, 25 to 50 percent of total anticipated need is administered as a continuous infusion, with the remainder available on demand. The advantage of a continuous mode in the sleeping patient is that serum opioid levels are maintained, avoiding episodes of severe pain on arousal. In the patient with severe pain or high opioid requirements (or both), it allows the patient to more easily achieve appropriate serum levels. With continous modes, there is a potential for overdose, should opioid requirements change as a result of the natural healing process or the inadvertent coadministration of other respiratory depressants.

Nonsteroidal Preparations

In addition to added cost, PCA administration may also be associated with any of the opioid side effects such as dizziness, nausea, vomiting, pruritus, somnolence, urinary retention, inhibition of bowel function, and respiratory depression. Nonsteroidal compounds can be used to avoid the adverse effects of opioids. Oral formulations are quite effective, but their application in the perioperative period is problematic. Some success has been achieved with rectal administration of indomethacin. With the development of the parenteral formulation ketorolac, prostaglandin inhibitors can now be used to treat perioperative pain in the NPO patient. Ketorolac 30 mg is equivalent to morphine 12 mg. As with other prostaglandin inhibitors, it has the potential to cause transient platelet dysfunction (with potential bleeding complications), gastric upset, and renal insufficiency, although clinically significant problems have only appeared in rare case reports.[51,52]

Initial studies explored the substitution of ketorolac for opioids, and found that following intramuscular administration onset, duration and analgesia were similar. Patients receiving ketorolac also had less nausea, earlier return of bowel function, and less pain with activity. In these studies, patients received opioids intraoperatively, and it was believed that ketorolac was not adequate for severe pain.[53,54] Coadministration of ketorolac with other analgesics could reduce opioid requirements, and hence side effects. As a supplement to either PCA or epidural postoperative pain regimens, ketorolac does have an opioid-sparing effect.[55,56] Less postoperative emesis, earlier return of bowel function, and decreased incidence of bladder spasm was counterbalanced by increased surgical drainage. Furthermore, the benefit of ketorolac appears to fade after the first postoperative day. Although approved only for intramuscular administration, many studies have been done utilizing the intravenous route. The half life is 5 hours for either route of administration, suggesting that dosing intervals should be similar.[57]

Epidural Analgesia

Epidural anesthesia is also commonly used for postoperative pain relief. Three modalities have been employed: intermittent boluses, continuous infusions, and patient-controlled ep-

idural analgesia (PCEA). Each has advantages and disadvantages, and the choice is a function of the agent selected as well as patient needs and operator preference. Analgesia can be provided with opioids or local anesthetics, or both. Local anesthetics provide superior analgesia, but at the expense of a motor block that can restrict activity and produce hypotension. Epidural opioids do not cause motor weakness or hypotension, but are associated with typical opioid side effects. Duramorph has a uniquely long duration of activity in the epidural space, and bolus administration can be as infrequent as once every 12 to 24 hours. Often dilute concentrations of both opioids and local anesthetics are combined as a continuous infusion, thus minimizing the side effects encountered when these drugs are used independently. The advantages of PCA opioids described above also apply to PCEA, and drug usage may be up to one-third less than that of a continuous infusion. There are also epidural-specific theoretical advantages to PCEA. Since part of the activity of epidurally administered drugs is achieved at CNS sites, bolus administration may allow greater CNS penetration. Spread within the epidural space is probably superior with boluses.

One of the concerns raised in the case of narcotic-only infusions is whether epidural catheters are simply glorified intravenous administration devices. This question is justifiably raised when pharmacologic studies show no significant difference in plasma levels after 15 minutes when morphine is given to parturients either by intravenous or epidural routes.[58] Similar findings have been seen with epidural infusions of both sufentanyl and fentanyl in a variety of different procedures. Pain relief and reduction in stress hormones also appear to be equivalent.[59] Of even more concern is the lack of a consistent reduction in narcotic side effects such as altered bowel function. When opioid infusions have been demonstrated to provide superior pain relief, often side effects requiring treatment, such as nausea, pruritus, bladder spasm, and respiratory depression, are increased.[60]

In the high-risk surgical patient with underlying cardiopulmonary disease, a risk/benefit analysis may support the use of epidural analgesia for postoperative pain. The potential for superior analgesia, earlier extubation, improved pulmonary toilet, and more aggressive ambulation may reduce perioperative complications. In the complicated patient, the minor side effects of epidural opioids are outweighed by the benefits of reduced perioperative morbidity. In fact, since the goal is to reduce the stress response as much as possible, and opioids alone do not ablate this response as effectively as local anesthetics, these are the very patients that would benefit from combinations of local anesthetics and opioids. Analgesia is superior with the combination, but motor weakness and hypotension may entail greater limitations on ambulation and require more intensive nursing care. In the typical patient undergoing extensive surgery with the expectation of severe postoperative pain, epidural opioids will probably provide pain relief superior to parenteral regimens, but at the expense of greater side effects. In most other cases, it is difficult to justify the additional risk and cost of epidural analgesia when patients state a preference for PCA because of the greater autonomy it affords them in their pain management.

Intrathecal Opioids

One further choice with regard to postoperative analgesia is intrathecal opioids. In the patient undergoing a procedure under regional anesthesia, it is possible to inject preservative-free morphine into the subarachnoid space: 0.1 to 0.5 mg will peak in about 60 minutes, and can last from 18 to 24 hours, providing complete analgesia in the immediate postoperative period. The primary limitation is that it is a one-shot technique, and duration can only be extended by increasing the dose. In fact, when first introduced, significantly larger doses were used, and analgesia lasting 2 or 3 days was not uncommon. However, the incidence of side effects, most importantly respiratory depression, also increased to an unacceptable level. The second limitation has been that only patients undergoing the procedure under spinal anesthesia were candidates. This is no longer absolutely necessary. With the development of the "atraumatic" spinal needles, it is feasible to perform surgery under general anesthesia, and then inject preservative-free morphine at the conclusion of surgery, prior to arousal.

Somewhat more controversial is the concept of preemptive analgesia. When pain stimuli enter the CNS, they generate positive feedback loops that amplify the perceived pain stimulus and lower the response threshold for future pain stimuli. As a result, the perception of pain is greater and persists longer than accounted for by the injury per se. The underpinning of preemptive analgesia is that blocking of pain stimuli from entering the CNS interrupts this remodeling of neural pathways. Less pain is perceived and it is easier to treat.

Complications

The second major postoperative concern is recognition of anesthetic complications. Although minor complications are common, serious complications can occasionally become major injuries if not recognized early and treated appropriately. Often a patient may first complain to a nonanesthesiologist, and it is prudent for all caregivers to be aware of the potential kinds of anesthetic complications so that proper therapy can be instituted in a timely fashion.

Regional Anesthesia

Complications commonly seen after regional anesthesia are backache and persistent paresthesias. Backache may result from localized needle trauma and usually will resolve within a few days. Ligamentous sprain may last 1 to 2 weeks and responds to heating pads and anti-inflammatory agents. It is caused by the loss of the lumbar lordosis following muscle relaxation by a regional anesthetic or the use of muscle relaxants during general anesthesia. A major aggravating factor is performance of the procedure in the lithotomy position. Significant paresthesias rarely persist beyond 6 months.[61] However, any documented nerve deficit warrants a full neurologic examination to establish the extent and site of injury, and determine whether further investigation is warranted.

With spinal and, occasionally, epidural anesthesia, a patient may develop a postural headache referred to as a postdural puncture headache. These headaches normally resolve spontaneously, but can be quite painful. The bifrontal or bioccipital headache intensifies on assuming an upright position and is ameliorated by recumbancy. They usually occur 24 to 48 hours after the dural puncture, but may occur weeks after the anesthetic. In the case of a "wet tap" with an epidural needle, they may occur immediately, illustrating that the probability and severity of a postdural puncture headache is also related to the caliber of the needle. Although the headache usually resolves without treatment within a few days, and almost always within the week, they may persist for weeks to months.[62] The incidence is higher in females and younger patients.

Conservative therapy is usually all that is required and consists of hydration to increase CSF production, avoidance of strenuous activity, and administration of analgesics. However, severe headaches may progress to more serious problems such as cavernous sinus thrombosis and subarachnoid hemorrhage. Patients may occasionally present with other symptoms, for example, blurred vision or decreased hearing. Despite the absence of headaches, these symptoms are even more alarming because they indicate cranial nerve irritation. Permanent nerve injury may result if the condition is not treated appropriately. A good rule of thumb is that if a patient presents with a mild headache that persists beyond 2 weeks, an incapacitating headache, or evidence of cranial nerve pathology, epidural blood patching should be performed as soon as possible. Usually curative, a second or third patch is occasionally needed. Other than minor aggravating back pain and a low grade fever, it is a relatively innocuous procedure.

Severe complications of regional anesthesia are fortunately quite rare, with an incidence of 1 in 10,000 to 1 in 50,000. Direct needle trauma during placement of an anesthetic may cause transient nerve paresthesias. There may be chemical irritation from talc or detergents left after improper cleansing of reusable equipment. Finally, there may be direct nerve toxicity, either from high concentrations of local anesthetics or preservatives added to the local anesthetic solution. The time course of injury is a useful way to characterize the neurologic deficits. Injury present immediately on resolution of the anesthetic could be a nerve root myelopathy or anterior spinal artery syndrome. The former diagnosis is suggested by the presence of a discrete neurologic injury that follows a dermatomal distribution. Anterior spinal artery syndrome presents as flaccid paralysis with intact sensory function. The mechanism of injury is ischemia limited to the anterior portion of the spinal cord. The thoracolumbar enlargement is most at risk because of the tenuous blood supply provided by the artery of Adamkiewicz. The syndrome is frequently associated with hypotension and severe blood loss, and it is hypothesized that pressure from injected local anesthetic solutions further compromises spinal cord perfusion. Neither injury is amenable to treatment.

Injuries that develop during the first 24 hours after surgery are amenable to treatment that can dramatically alter the patient's course. Epidural hematomas may result from trauma to epidural veins, but the majority are spontaneous and occasionally associated with anticoagulant therapy. The patient presents with back pain. There may be localized tenderness at the site. Radiculopathy and paresis are slowly evolving signs. Surgical incision and drainage can prevent permanent neurologic deficit if performed within 12 hours. Septic meningitis usually presents within 24 hours, a time course more prolonged than epidural hematomas, but the symptoms are similar, with the addition of nuchal rigidity. In addition, there are signs of infection; the patient may be febrile and PMNs and bacteria will be present in the CSF. Treatment is with antibiotics. Epidural abscess is the slowest progressing of the three lesions. Contrary to expectations, most abscesses are due to hematogenous spread, although direct infection from a regional anesthetic is possible in a very ill, immunocompromised individual who has had an indwelling epidural catheter for prolonged periods. There are also symptoms of fever, severe back pain, nuchal rigidity, and localized tenderness. Treatment is surgical drainage and antibiotic therapy.

In addition to these three medical emergencies in which early intervention can dramatically improve prognosis, there are three additional complications that are less amenable to therapy: aseptic meningitis, cauda equina syndrome, and adhesive arachnoiditis. Compared to septic meningitis, aseptic meningitis is less acute in onset. The patient may also present with nuchal rigidity and headache, temperature, and PMNs in the CSF. However, the CSF will be culture negative, and spontaneous recovery within 1 week is the norm. Cauda equina syndrome is a mild form of acute myelopathy affecting the smaller nerve fibers of the cauda equina. The symptoms are urinary and fecal incontinence and lower extremity paresis and perineal hypesthesias. Onset is usually rapid and recovery, if it occurs, is usually within days to weeks. Occasionally, any of the acute deficits described above can lead to adhesive arachnoiditis. This disorder is characterized by proliferation of the pia-arachnoid, which can obliterate the subarachnoid space. An arteritis may be present, hindering cord blood supply. Onset is gradual, on the order of weeks to months, and may lead to chronic progressive sensory loss and paresis of lower extremities. The combination of an arteritis and the development of scar tissue encasing the spinal cord can cause severe permanent damage that extends far beyond the initial area of the inciting injury.

General Anesthesia

Intubation

Dental injuries account for the most anesthesia-related malpractice claims. Incidence varies from 1 in 150 to 1 in 1,000.[63] Risk factors include poor dentition, primary teeth, recent removal of orthodontic braces, and caps and bridges. Dislodged teeth can be reimplanted if saved in moist guaze. More rarely, manipulation of the head can result in cervical cord injury in the patient with acute cervical fractures, rheumatoid arthritis, Down syndrome, and Arnold-Chiari malformations. Laryngeal and tracheal injury may also occur. An examination of 1,000 patients following routine intubation demonstrated hematomas of the vocal cords and supraglottic region, as well as a 1- to 5-percent incidence of lacerations of the vocal cord mucosa.[64] Tracheal injury may occur from oversized tubes, overinflation of the cuff, and the use of stylets and tube changers.

Failure to secure an airway in a timely fashion is much more serious. The delay may result in transient hypoxia and, possibly, permanent neurologic deficits. The unprotected airway is at risk of aspiration with resultant pulmonary injury. In animals, the extent of pulmonary injury is a function of both the volume of gastric aspirate inhaled and the acidity of the fluid. This was the major impetus for the development of standards limiting oral intake for all patients undergoing anesthesia. Unrecognized esophageal intubation, usually a catastrophic event, is decreasing as a cause of injury, probably in large part because of the development and implementation of practice standards that mandate the use of pulse oximetry and strongly encourage the use of capnography.

Anesthetic Overdose

Anesthetic overdose is most likely to present intraoperatively, with respiratory insufficiency if the patient is breathing spontaneously, or cardiovascular collapse. It may be due to inappropriate selection of anesthetic depth by the anesthesiologist or equipment malfunction. Awareness during surgery associated with postoperative recall is usually a problem caused by inadequate anesthesia. With the widespread use of muscle relaxants as a means to achieve optimal surgical relaxation, it is possible that a patient may be fully paralyzed and awake during a procedure, secondary to inadequate anesthesia, and be unable to communicate that fact. Should the patient report intraoperative awareness, it is important that this belief not be summarily dismissed, but rather acknowledged as a real possibility and explored. It is rare that a patient will have been in pain as well; usually anxiety results from misunderstood memories that perpetuate themselves in nightmares the patient cannot explain.

Positioning Complications

As the individual responsible for rendering the patient insensible to pain during operative procedures, responsibility for ensuring that the patient is safely cared for rests with the anesthesiologist. Surgical exposure may require relatively unanatomic positioning that may result in pressure necrosis of unpadded weight-bearing areas; injury to protuberant structures such as the breasts, the nose, and the ears; blindness from pressure on the eyes; and bald spots from pressure on the scalp. The patient may suffer thermal injury from warm fluids and heating blankets, and electrical burns from improperly grounded equipment. Poor positioning may result in nerve injury, especially of the brachial plexus from hyperextended shoulders, femoral and peroneal nerve injuries from being in the lithotomy position, and ulnar and radial nerve palsies from misuse of armboards or inadequate protection from mechanical injury. In general, these injuries are not permanent but the pace of recovery can be quite prolonged. Complete explanation of the etiology of the injury and assurance to the patient that healing will take place is important.

REFERENCES

1. Granlee G: Interaction of systems: drugs and coagulation. ASA Annual Refresher Course Lectures, Lect 512, 1994

2. Wood A: Drugs and the coagulation system. p. 597. In Wood, Wood (eds): Drugs and Anesthesia: Pharmacology for Anesthesiologists. 2nd Ed. Williams & Wilkins, Baltimore, 1944

3. Stoelting RK, Dierdorf SF, McCammon RL: Psychiatric illness. p. 720. In: Anesthesia and Co-Existing Disease. 2nd Ed. Churchill Livingstone, New York, 1988

4. Hirshman CA, Lindeman K: MAO inhibitors: must they be discontinued before surgery? JAMA 260:3507, 1988

5. Wells DG, Bjorksten AR: Monamine oxidase inhibitors revisited. Can J Anaesth 36:1, 1989

6. Lawson NW: Autonomic nervous system physiology and pharmacology. p. 319. In Barash P, Culen B, Stoelling R (ed): Clinical Anesthesia. 2nd Ed. JB Lippincott, Philadelphia, 1992

7. Barash P: The high risk patient for non-cardiac surgery: preoperative evaluation. ASA Annual Refresher Course Lectures, Lect 231, 1993

8. Madhavan S, Alderman MH: The potential effect of blood pressure reduction on cardiovascular disease. Arch Intern Med 141:1583, 1981

9. Goldman L: Cardiac risks and complications of noncardiac surgery. Ann Intern Med 98:504, 1983

10. Akl BF, Talbor W, Neal JF, Havens D: Noncardiac operations after coronary revascularization. West J Med 136:91, 1982

11. Barash PG: The high risk patient for non-cardiac surgery: preoperative evaluation. ASA Annual Refresher Course Lectures, Lect 522, 1994

12. Tisi GM: Preoperative evaluation of pulmonary function. Ann 119:293, 1979

13. Stein M, Cassara EL: Preoperative pulmonary evaluation and therapy for surgery patients. JAMA 211:787, 1970

14. Roizen MF: Preoperative evaluation. p. 743. In Miller RD (ed): Anesthesia. 3rd Ed. Churchill Livingstone, New York, 1990

15. Brown BR: Anesthetic management of the patient with abnormal liver function. ASA Annual Refresher Course Lectures. Lect 241, 1993

16. Roizen MF: Perioperative management of the diabetic patient. ASA 1993 Annual Refresher Courses, Lect 164, 1993

17. Ammon JH: Perioperative management of the diabetic patient. ASA Annual Refresher Course Lectures, Lect 144, 1994

18. Wallerstein RO Jr: Laboratory evaluation of a bleeding patient. West J Med 150:51, 1989

19. Kowalyshyn TJ, Prager D, Young J: A review of the present status of preoperative hemoglobin requirements. Anesth Analg 51:75, 1972

20. Rosenberg H: Malignant hyperthermia. ASA Annual Refresher Course Lectures, Lect 225, 1994

21. Kaplan RF: Malignant hyperthermia. ASA Annual Refresher Course Lectures, Lect 522, 1993

22. Benamof JL: Management of the difficult airway: the ASA algorithm. ASA Annual Refresher Courses, 1993

23. Tunbull JM, Buck C: The value of preoperative screening investigations in otherwise healthy individuals. Arch Intern Med 147:1101, 1987

24. Korvin CC, Pearce RH, Stanley J: Admissions screening: clinical benefits. Ann Intern Med 83:197, 1975

25. Kaplan EB, Sheiner LB, Boeckmann AJ et al: The usefulness of preoperative laboratory screening. JAMA 253:3576, 1985

26. Muskett AD, McGreevy JM: Rational preoperative evaluation. Postgrad Med J 62:925, 1986

27. Moorman JR, Hlatky MA, Eddy DM et al: The yield of routine admission electrocardiogram. Ann Intern Med 103:590, 1985

28. Goldstein A, Keats AS: The risk of anesthesia. Anesthesiology 33:130, 1970

29. Derrington MC, Smith G: A review of anaesthetic risk, morbidity and mortality. Br J Anaesth 59:815, 1987

30. Saklad M: Grading of patients for surgical procedures. Anesthesiology 2:281, 1941

31. Vacanit CJ, VanHouten RJ, Hill RC: A statistical analysis of the relationship of physical status to postoperative mortality in 68,388 cases. Anesth Analg 49:564, 1970

32. Egbert LD, Battit GE, Turndorf H, Beecher HK: The value of the preoperative visit by an anesthetist. JAMA 185:553, 1963

33. Wood, Wood: Intravenous anesthetic agents. p. 196 Drugs and Anesthesia: Pharmacology for Anesthesiologists. 2nd Ed. Williams & Wilkins, Baltimore, 1990

34. Ameer B, Greenblatt DJ: Lorazepam: a review of its clinical pharmacological properties and therapeutic uses. Drugs 21:161, 1981

35. Reves JG, Fragen RJ, Vinik HR, Greenblatt DJ: Midazolam: pharmacology and uses Anesthesiology 62:310, 1985

36. Pert CB, Snyder SH: Opiate receptor: demonstration in nervous tissue. Science 179:1001, 1973

37. Beaumont A, Hughes J: Searching for the endogenous analgesic (editorial). Lancet 2:665, 1976

38. Beaumont A, Hughes J: Biology of opioid peptides. Annu Rev Pharmacol Toxicol 19:245, 1979

39. Kallar SK, Everett L: Potential risks and preventive measures for pulmonary aspiration: new concepts in preoperative fasting guidelines. Anesth Analg 77:171, 1993

40. Robert RB, Shirley MA: Reducing the risk of acid aspiration during cesarean section. Anesth Analg 53:859, 1974

41. Maltby JR, Sutherland AD, Sole JP, Shaffer EA: Preoperative oral fluids: is a five hour fast justified prior to elective surgery? Anesth Analg 65:112, 1986

42. Hutchinson A, Maltby JR, Reid CRG: Gastric fluid volume and pH in elective patients. Part I: coffee or orange juice vs. overnight fast. Can J Anaesth 35:16, 1988

43. Wood, Wood: H_1 and H_2 receptors, 5-HT, kinins, cardinoid syndrome. p. 611. In Wood, Wood (eds): Drugs and Anesthesia: Pharmacology for Anesthesiologists. 2nd Ed. Williams & Wilkins, Baltimore, 1990

44. Sadove MS, Shulman M, Hatano S, Fevold N: Analagesic effects of ketamine administration in subdissociative doses. Anesth Analg 50:452, 1971

45. White PF, Way WL, Trevor AJ: Ketamine-its pharmacology and therapeutic uses. Anesthesiology 56:119, 1982

46. Borgeat A, Wilder-Smith OHG, Suter PM: The nonhypnotic therapeutic applications of propofol. Anesthesiology 80:642, 1994

47. Motsch J, Graber E, Ludwig K: Addition of clonidine enhances postoperative analgesia from epidural morphine: a double blind study. Anesthesiology 73:1067, 1990

48. Lund C, Selmar P, Hansen OB et al: Effect of epidural bupivacaine on somatosensory evoked potentials after dermatomal stimulation. Anesth Analg 6:34, 1987

49. Caplan RA, Ward RJ, Posner K, Cheney FW: Unexpected cardiac arrest during spinal anesthesia: a closed claims analysis of predisposing factors. Anesthesiology 68:5, 1988

50. Gold BS: Unanticipated admission to the hospital following ambulatory surgery. JAMA 262:3008, 1989

51. Fleming BM, Coombs DW: Bleeding diathesis after peri-operative ketorolac (letter). Anesth Analg 73:235, 1991

52. Steinberg RB, Tessier EG: Gastrointestinal bleeding after administration of ketorolac (letter). Anesthesiology 79:1146, 1993

53. Gin T, Kan AF, Lam KK, O'Meara ME: Analgesia after cesarean section with intramuscular ketorolac or pethidine. Anaesth Intens Care 21:420, 1993

54. Rice ASC, Lloyd J, Miller CG et al: A double blind study of the speed of onset of analgesia following intramuscular administration of ketorolac tromethamine in comparison to intramuscular morphine and placebo. Anaesth 46:541, 1991

55. Parker RK, Holtmann B, Smith I, White PF: Use of ketorolac after lower abdominal surgery. Anesthesiology 80:6, 1994

56. Grass JA, Sakima NT, Valley M et al: Assessment of ketorolac as an adjuvant to fentanyl patient-controlled epidural analgesia after radical retropubic prostatectomy. Anesthesiology 78:642, 1993

57. Peirce RJ, Fragen RJ, Pemberton DM: Intravenous ketorolac tromethamine versus morphine sulfate in the treatment of immediate postoperative pain. Pharmacotherapy 10:111s, 1990

58. Zakowski M, Ramanathan S, Sutin KM et al: Pharmacokinetic profile of morphine in parturients following intravenous or epidural administration. Reg Anesth 19:119, 1994

59. Camu F, Debuecquoy F: Alfentanil infusion for postoperative pain: a comparison of epidural and intravenous routes. Anesthesiology 75:171, 1991

60. Allaire PH, Messick JM, Oesterlin JE et al: A prospective randomized comparison of epidural infusion of fentanyl and intravenous administration of morphine by PCA after radical retropubic prostatectomy, Mayo Clin Proc 67:1031, 1992

61. Vandam LD, Dripps RD: Long term follow-up of patients who received 10,098 spinal anesthetics. JAMA 172:1482, 1960

62. Parris WCV: Use of the epidural blood patch in the treatment of chronic headaches. Anesthesiology 65:344, 1986

63. Lockhart P, Feldbau EV, Gabel RA et al: Dental complications during and after tracheal intubation. JAMA 112:480, 1986

64. Kambic V, Radsel Z: Intubation lesions of the larynx. Br J Anaesth 50:587, 1978

CHAPTER EIGHT

CLINICAL ANATOMY OF INCISIONS

G. RODNEY MEEKS

Abdominal wall incision and closure are among the most frequently performed surgical procedures. Often, the time spent fashioning an incision exceeds the time required for the primary surgical procedure. Complications associated with the incision may occur more frequently and may be more serious than those associated with the surgical procedure. Yet many surgeons regard an abdominal incision only as access for the planned surgery and give minimal forethought to the abdominal wall structures that may be damaged at laparotomy. In reality, the incision is an additional major operation on a second organ system and deserves an equal measure of planning. This chapter reviews pertinent abdominal wall anatomy, discusses common incisions and closure techniques, outlines the process of wound healing, and details the prevention and management of complications.

ABDOMINAL WALL ANATOMY

The abdominal wall is a functional unit composed of marvelously integrated components. It provides containment of visceral structures, protection of vasculature, structural sta-

bility, and a mechanism to control intra-abdominal pressure and motion of the trunk on the pelvis. The general size and shape of the abdomen are defined by the bony pelvis below, the costal margin above, and the lumbar spine, which joins the thorax to the pelvis.

Integrity of the anterior abdominal wall is dependent primarily on the rectus abdominis muscles, the flank muscles, and the conjoined tendon of the flank muscles, which form the rectus sheath. These muscles assist with respiration, and control the expulsive efforts of urination, defecation, coughing, and parturition. They work with the back muscles to flex and extend the trunk at the hips, rotate the trunk at the waist, and protect viscera by becoming rigid.

Contour of the abdomen is dependent on age, muscle mass and tone, obesity, intra-abdominal pathology, parity, and posture. These factors may significantly alter topography and become a major obstacle to proper incision selection and placement. Knowledge of the layered structure of the abdominal wall permits efficient and safe entry into the peritoneal cavity. The principal structures from exterior to interior are skin, subcutaneous tissue, muscles with aponeuroses, bony pelvis to which other structures are attached, transversalis fascia, properitoneal fat, and peritoneum. Nerves, blood vessels, and lymphatics are present throughout. The surgeon must be completely familiar with anterior abdominal wall anatomy and topography before an intelligent decision regarding incision selection can be made.

Skin

Simple skin punctures with round needles produce elliptical holes, because tension on the cut edges is not the same in all directions. The distance between the sides of the ellipse reflects the degree of tension on skin edges and varies in different regions. Skin lines of approximately equal tension are known as Langer's lines.[1] Across the lower abdomen, these lines are oriented in a predominately transverse direction with a gentle cephalic concavity (Fig. 8-1).

If an incision is placed parallel to lines of tension, minimal forces pull the skin edges apart. Conversely, if an incision is perpendicular to lines of tension, the skin edges tend to be pulled apart. Transverse incisions seem to heal with a narrower, more cosmetic scar because they are parallel to Langer's lines and have less tension. Longitudinal or oblique incisions heal with a broader scar because they cut across lines of tension.

Subcutaneous Tissue

Subcutaneous tissue is predominately globules of adipose and can be separated into layers based on the presence of superficial and deep fibrous tissue matrices. The more super-

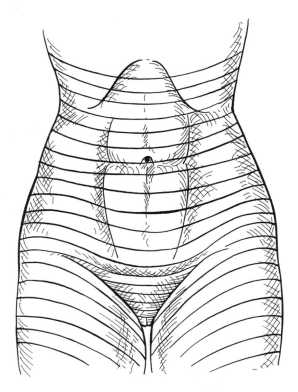

Fig. 8-1. Langer's lines. The lines of skin tension in the lower abdomen are transverse, with a gentle cephalic concavity.

ficial layer is called Camper's fascia.[2] This fibrous layer is poorly defined, and fatty tissue predominates. The deeper layer, which is more well defined, is called Scarpa's fascia. This fibrous layer is membranous and elastic. Because Scarpa's fascia is best defined laterally, it is often seen in transverse incisions but may not be identified easily in longitudinal incisions.[3] In reality, although they are called fascia, neither is particularly well defined or strong, and both are more like fibrous networks.

Muscles

Posterolateral, lateral, and anterior portions of the abdominal wall are composed of three paired broad flat muscles: the external obliques, the internal obliques, and transversus abdominis. Each has an aponeurosis or tendon. The aponeuroses fuse at the midline with opposite side counterparts to form a sheath that surrounds the rectus abdominis and pyramidalis muscles.

External Oblique Muscle

The external obliques are the most superficial of the flank muscles. They originate as digitate processes on the outer and caudal borders of the lower eight ribs of the thorax. The muscles course diagonally in a caudal and medial direction. The posterior portion of the muscle inserts onto the external lip of the iliac crest. The remainder of the muscle forms a broad aponeurosis that passes over the rectus abdominis muscle. It fuses with its counterpart at the linea alba and forms a portion of the rectus sheath. The most inferior portion of the aponeurosis is attached to the anterior superior iliac spine and to the public tubercle. Between these bony points the aponeurosis turns back on itself to form the J-shaped inguinal ligament. The external inguinal ring is superior and medial to the pubic tubercle. Fibers of the aponeurosis encircle the round ligament as it passes through the ring. These fibers are then called the external spermatic fascia (Fig. 8-2).

Internal Oblique Muscles

The internal oblique muscles originate on the thoracolumbar fascia, the intermediate line of the interior two-thirds of the iliac crest, the lateral inguinal ligament, and adjacent iliac fascia. The portion of the internal oblique that originates on the thoracolumbar fascia courses diagonally in a cephalic and medial direction to insert on the lower three ribs of the thorax and xiphoid process. The portion arising on the iliac crest courses cephalad and medial and forms an aponeurosis. The aponeurosis then splits into two lamellae. One passes anterior and the other posterior to the rectus muscle above the semilunar line of Douglas (arcuate line). Below the arcuate line, the entire aponeurosis passes anterior to the rectus

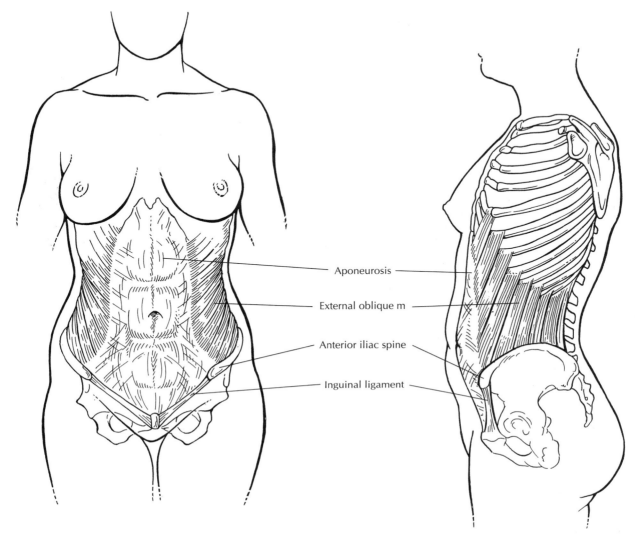

Fig. 8-2. External oblique muscles. The muscle fibers run in a caudal and medial direction. The muscle changes to an aponeurosis approximately at a vertical line through the superior anterior iliac spine.

muscles. The lower, most internal oblique muscle arises on the inguinal ligament and passes medially and slightly caudal where it fans out over the round ligament. Most of the internal oblique fibers are perpendicular to the external oblique muscles, except for the lowest fibers, which are almost parallel. The internal oblique aponeuroses fuse at the linea alba (Fig. 8-3).

Transversus Abdominis

The innermost flank muscles are the transversus abdominis. They originate on the costal cartilage of the lower six ribs, the thoracolumbar fascia, the internal lip of the iliac crest and iliac fascia, and the lateral inguinal ligament. The muscles course medially and form an aponeurosis at the lateral edge of the rectus muscle. They fuse at the linea alba. The

upper two-thirds of the aponeurosis—like that of the posterior lamellae of the internal oblique—passes behind the rectus above the arcuate line. The lower one-third below the arcuate line passes anterior to the rectus. The fibers of the caudal internal oblique and transversus abdominis are fused. This explains why only two layers are discernible in the lateral pole of a transverse lower abdominal incision. The superficial layer is the external oblique aponeurosis, and the deep layer is the fused internal oblique and transversus abdominis aponeuroses (Fig. 8-4).

Rectus Abdominis Muscles

The rectus abdominis muscles arise on the crest of the pubic symphysis and course directly cephalad, where they insert on the costal cartilage of the fifth, sixth, and seventh ribs

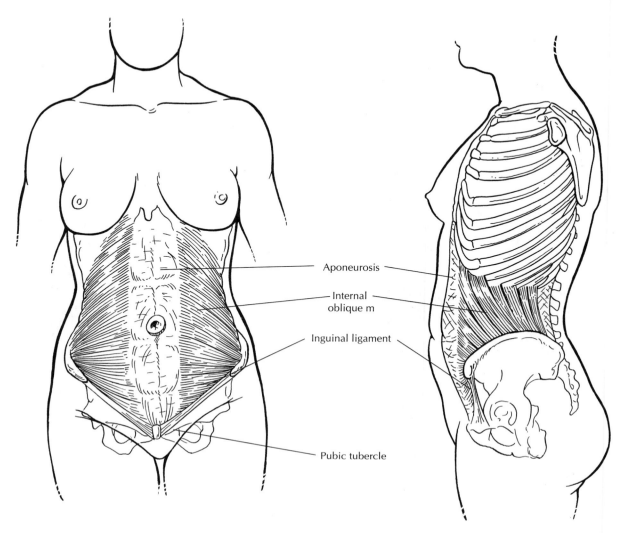

Fig. 8-3. Internal oblique muscles. The muscle fibers run in a cephalic and medial direction. The fibers are perpendicular to the external oblique muscles and form an aponeurosis approximately at a vertical line through the pubic tubercle.

and the xiphoid process. They are enclosed in an aponeurotic sheath that comprises the aponeuroses of the external oblique, internal oblique, and transversus abdominis muscles. The rectus muscles are firmly attached to the rectus sheath, especially at the linea transversus, which are normally confined to the region above the umbilicus.[4] If present below the umbilicus, great difficulty is encountered in separating the anterior sheath and rectus muscle. If this muscle is cut, it heals by forming a transverse fibrous band (Fig. 8-5).

Pyramidalis Muscles

The pyramidalis muscles are small, triangular-shaped muscles that are also contained in the rectus sheath. They arise on the pubic bone and insert on the linea alba several centi-

meters above the symphysis. Although these have only minimal function, they assist in locating the midline.

Rectus Sheath

The rectus sheath is composed of the broad sheet-like aponeuroses of the flank muscles. The aponeuroses unite with the corresponding members of the opposite side to form a dense white covering of the rectus abdominis and the pyramidalis muscles. This covering is sometimes improperly called rectus fascia.

The anterior sheath from the xiphoid to one-half the distance from the umbilicus to the pubis, consists of the external oblique aponeurosis and the anterior lamellae of the internal oblique aponeurosis. The posterior sheath consists of the posterior lamellae of the internal oblique aponeurosis and the

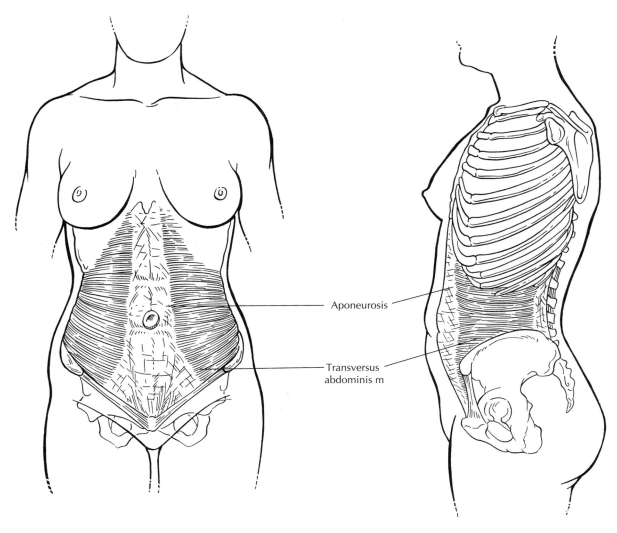

Fig. 8-4. Transversus abdominis muscles. The muscles are perpendicular to the midline. The aponeurosis fuses with the aponeurosis of internal oblique muscles.

transversus abdominis aponeurosis. The crescentic border of the arcuate line is formed by the termination of the posterior sheath. Below the arcuate line, all aponeuroses pass anterior to the muscles. Only the transversalis fascia, extraperitoneal fat, and peritoneum are posterior. Medial to the rectus muscles, the aponeuroses of all three flank muscles fuse to form the linea alba. Cranial to the arcuate line, the anterior and posterior sheaths are fused at the linea alba (Fig. 8-6).

The line of demarcation between the external oblique muscle and its aponeurosis is a vertical line through the anterior superior iliac spine. Fibers of the internal oblique and transversus abdominis muscles extend farther toward the midline and become aponeurotic at an imaginary line drawn through the pubic tubercle. Muscle fibers of the internal oblique lie under the aponeurosis of the external oblique.[5] Lateral to the rectus abdominis, the aponeuroses are separable, but they fuse as they reach the midline. At the lateral

poles of the incision, the aponeuroses may be incised separately (Fig. 8-6).

Transversalis Fascia

Transversalis fascia is a fibrous layer that covers the inner surface of the transversus abdominis muscles. It is contiguous with the fascia of the iliac bone, the diaphragm, the fascia of the parietal pelvic floor muscles, the thoracolumbar fascia, and contralateral transversalis fascia. Although it may be visible beneath the rectus abdominis muscle, this fascia is generally weak and insignificant. However, it is stronger in certain specialized areas near the esophageal hiatus and in the inguinal regions. It may be separated from the peritoneum by a layer of fat. It is frequently incised off the bladder when the peritoneal cavity is opened. The transversalis fascia

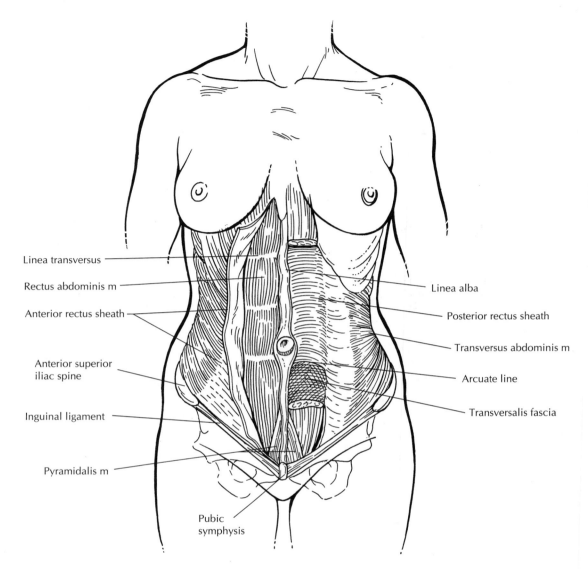

Linea transversus

Rectus abdominis m

Anterior rectus sheath

Anterior superior
iliac spine

Inguinal ligament

Pyramidalis m

Pubic
symphysis

Linea alba

Posterior rectus sheath

Transversus abdominis m

Arcuate line

Transversalis fascia

Fig. 8-5. Rectus abdominis muscles. These muscles form two broad straps, which arise on the pubic symphysis and insert on the ribs.

should not be confused with the transversus abdominis aponeurosis.

Peritoneum

The peritoneum is a single layer of serosa that lines the abdominal cavity. It is supported by a thin layer of connective tissue. Five vertical folds are formed by underlying ligaments or vessels that converge at the umbilicus. The reflection of the bladder on the abdominal wall is triangular and its apex fuses into the urachus, a remnant of the embryonic allantois. The single middle umbilical ligament is created by the urachus as it courses from the bladder to the umbilicus. Lateral to this are the paired medial (previously known

as lateral) umbilical ligaments, which are remnants of the obliterated umbilical arteries. They course from the internal iliac arteries to the umbilicus. The most lateral folds are the lateral umbilical ligaments and are associated with the deep inferior epigastric vessels.

Vasculature

The abdominal wall contains a rich vascular arcade, which is divided into a superficial and a deep plexus.[6] The superficial blood vessels supply tissues above the external oblique aponeurosis and anterior rectus sheath, while the deep vessels supply the muscles and tissue below. The superficial inferior epigastric, the superficial circumflex iliac, and the

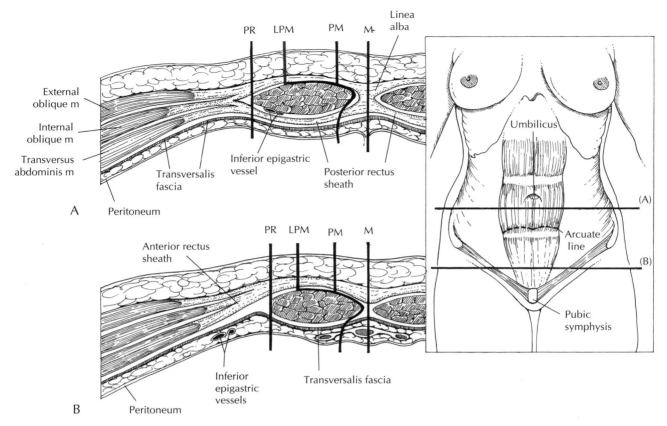

Fig. 8-6. Cross section of the lower abdominal wall. The rectus sheath is formed by fusion of the aponeurosis of the flank muscles. **(A)** The anterior sheath of the rectus abdominis muscle is formed by the aponeurosis of the external oblique muscle and the split aponeuroses of the internal oblique muscle. The posterior sheath is formed by aponeurosis of transversus abdominis muscle and posterior lamellae of internal oblique muscle. **(B)** Below the arcuate line, the posterior sheath is absent and all aponeuroses pass anterior to the rectus muscle. Transversalis fascia and peritoneum are the only posterior layers. M midline; PM, paramedian; LPM, lateral paramedian; PB, pararectus.

external pudendal vessels are located in the subcutaneous tissues. Superior and inferior deep epigastric vessels are present in the musculofascial layers, as are the deep circumflex iliac and the musculophrenic vessels. All of the abdominal wall, except the linea alba, has an excellent blood supply (Fig. 8-7).

Inferior Deep Epigastric Arteries

The inferior deep epigastric artery branches from the external iliac artery as it passes under the middle of the inguinal ligament. It ascends medial to the inguinal ring and superficial to the transversalis fascia. It proceeds toward the umbilicus and crosses the lateral border of the rectus muscle at the arcuate line where it enters the posterior rectus sheath. Once the artery enters the sheath, it branches extensively. The angle between the vessels and lateral border of the rectus

forms the apex of the inguinal (Hasselbach's) triangle, the base of which is the inguinal ligament.

The inferior deep epigastric vessels are bounded only by loose areolar tissue below the arcuate line. Trauma to this portion of the inferior deep epigastric artery may result in considerable hemorrhage. Because hematomas commonly dissect into the retroperitoneal space, large quantities of blood may be lost before outward evidence of hematoma is detectable.

Superior Deep Epigastric Arteries

The superior deep epigastric artery is a branch of the internal thoracic artery. It enters the rectus sheath at the seventh costal cartilage and descends on the posterior surface of the rectus muscle. The superior and inferior deep epigastric arteries freely anastomose with one another to provide a gener-

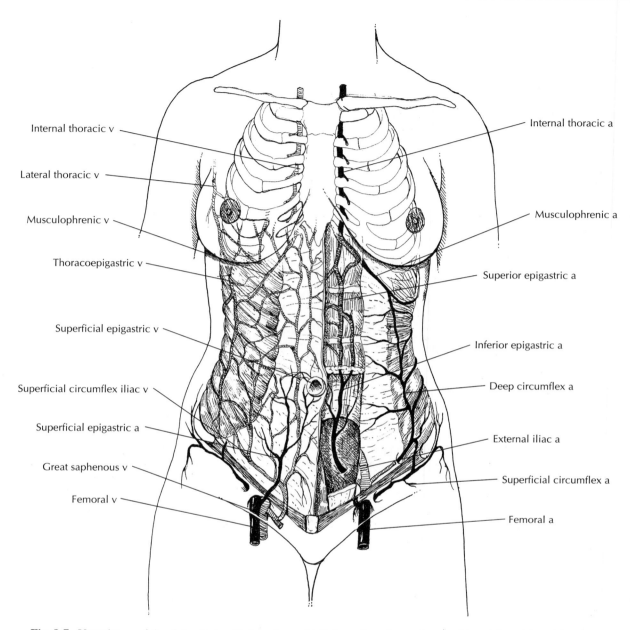

Internal thoracic v

Lateral thoracic v

Musculophrenic v

Thoracoepigastric v

Superficial epigastric v

Superficial circumflex iliac v

Superficial epigastric a

Great saphenous v

Femoral v

Internal thoracic a

Musculophrenic a

Superior epigastric a

Inferior epigastric a

Deep circumflex a

External iliac a

Superficial circumflex a

Femoral a

Fig. 8-7. Vasculature of the abdominal wall. Superior and inferior epigastric arteries provide a rich arcade, arising from the internal thoracic artery superiorly and the external iliac artery inferiorly. The musculophrenic artery and deep circumflex iliac artery supply the lateral abdominal wall. The superficial vessels follow a pattern similar to the deep vessels, with the exception that there is no superior epigastric counterpart and the superficial epigastric veins and the superficial iliac veins often arise from the great saphenous vein.

ous collateral circulation between the subclavian and external iliac arteries.

A common pathway between these vessels is not present in some individuals. However, obstruction of the aorta or iliac artery results in considerable collateral circulation through the epigastric vessels. If they are ligated, ischemia of the lower extremity may result. Therefore, it is important to palpate the dorsal pedis pulse following temporary occlusion before transection of these vessels is contemplated.

Deep Circumflex Iliac Arteries

The deep circumflex iliac artery also branches from the external iliac artery or, less frequently, from a common root including the inferior epigastric artery. Its course is lateral and vertical behind the inguinal ligament. It then turns medially at the iliac crest where it pierces the transversus abdominis muscle. Between the transversus abdominis and internal oblique muscles, numerous connecting branches supply the lower and lateral abdominal wall. Anastomoses with the intercostal and lumbar vessels supply branches to all the flank muscles.

Musculophrenic Arteries

The musculophrenic artery is also a branch of the internal thoracic artery. It lies behind the costal cartilage to supply the intercostal spaces and upper abdominal wall. Anastomoses from intercostal and subcostal vessels to the deep circumflex iliac vessels occur in the deep layer.

Superficial Vessels

The superficial inferior epigastric vessels run diagonally in the subcutaneous tissues from the femoral artery toward the umbilicus. They can be identified on a line between the palpable femoral pulse and umbilicus just superficial to Scarpa's fascia. As they approach the umbilicus, the arteries branch extensively.

The external pudendal arteries have a medial and diagonal course from the femoral artery and supply the region of the mons pubis. These vessels branch extensively as they approach the midline. Bleeding is typically heavier here than in other subcutaneous areas of the abdomen.

The superficial circumflex iliac vessels proceed from the femoral vessels to the flank. The superficial vessels follow the general pattern of the deep vessels and arise from the iliac or femoral vessels. The exception is that the superficial inferior epigastric have no superior counterparts.

Veins and Lymphatics

For the most part, veins follow arteries and there is no need for further description. The only exception would be when the veins are enlarged. Veins may be dilated in patients with obstructed blood flow through the liver and porta hepatus. They may also be engorged in patients with large pelvic masses.

Lymphatics follow the course of the veins. Normally, above the umbilicus, they drain to the internal mammary chain and to the subclavian vessels. Below the umbilicus, they drain to the external iliac vessels.

Nerves

The intercostal and lumbar nerves enter the abdominal wall between the transversus abdominis and internal oblique muscles and run in a generally caudal and medial direction. Each nerve innervates a dermatome, although some overlapping function is seen. Although technically not classified as nerves of the abdominal wall, the femoral nerve, the lateral femoral cutaneous nerve, and the genitofemoral nerve are

discussed because they might be damaged during abdominal surgery (Fig. 8-8).

Intercostal Nerves

The 7th through the 12th intercostal nerves innervate the abdominal wall. Because of overlapping dermatomes, the fifth and sixth intercostal nerves might also contribute. The intercostal nerves divide into lateral cutaneous branches and anterior branches.

The anterior branch continues medially—after giving rise to a lateral cutaneous branch—to innervate the internal oblique and transversus abdominis muscles. After entering the rectus sheath, they innervate the rectus abdominis along its lateral border. Terminal intercostal branches penetrate the anterior rectus sheath as cutaneous nerves to supply the subcutaneous tissues and skin. The seventh intercostal nerve innervates the level of the xiphoid. The 10th nerve supplies the region of the umbilicus. The anterior branch of the 12th nerve innervates the pyramidalis muscles and the skin just above the mons.

With the exception of the 12th nerve, the lateral cutaneous branches have anterior and posterior divisions. The lateral cutaneous branch of the 12th nerve does not divide but passes over the iliac crest behind the anterior superior iliac crest. It provides sensation to the gluteal skin.

Iliohypogastric Nerves

The 12th intercostal and the first lumbar nerves form the iliohypogastric nerve, which passes medial to the anterior superior iliac spine. It provides motor fibers to external oblique, internal oblique, and transversus abdominis muscles and provides sensory fibers to the skin of the mons pubis. The anterior cutaneous branch of the iliohypogastric nerve provides sensory innervation to the skin of the upper and lateral thigh.[7] It communicates with the ilioinguinal nerve and provides sensory fibers to the skin overlying the external inguinal ring and symphysis.

Ilioinguinal Nerve

The ilioinguinal nerve is formed by the combination of the first and second lumbar nerves and passes medial to the superior anterior iliac spine to supply the lower abdominal wall. A branch of the ilioinguinal nerve accompanies the round ligament as it passes through the inguinal canal. It exits the canal at the external inguinal ring and provides sensory fibers to the labia majora and the upper aspect of the medial thigh.[7]

Lateral Femoral Cutaneous Nerve

The second and third lumbar roots give rise to this nerve, which crosses the psoas muscle slightly above the femoral nerve. It exits the abdomen near or through the inguinal

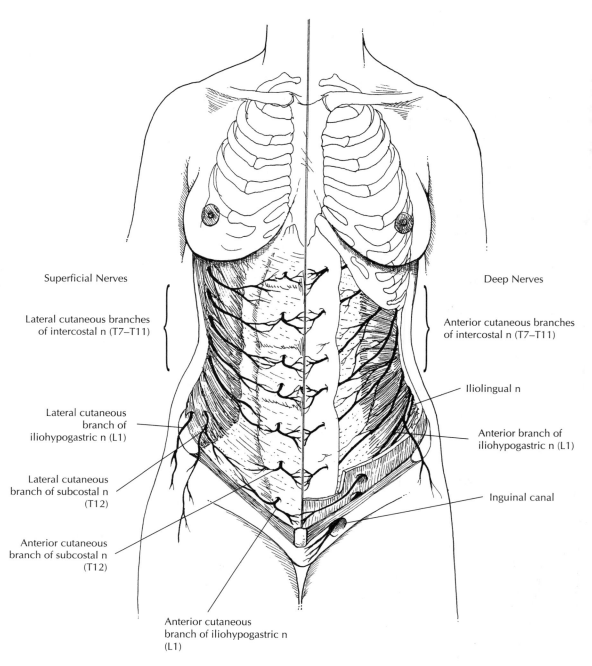

Superficial Nerves

**Lateral cutaneous branches
of intercostal n (T7–T11)**

**Lateral cutaneous
branch of
iliohypogastric n (L1)**

**Lateral cutaneous
branch of subcostal n
(T12)**

**Anterior cutaneous
branch of subcostal n
(T12)**

**Anterior cutaneous
branch of iliohypogastric n
(L1)**

Deep Nerves

**Anterior cutaneous branches
of intercostal n (T7–T11)**

Iliolingual n

**Anterior branch of
iliohypogastric n (L1)**

Inguinal canal

Fig. 8-8. Nerves of the abdominal wall. The anterior abdominal wall is innervated by the lower six intercostal nerves, the iliohypogastric nerves, and the ilioinguinal nerves.

ligament. Sensory innervation is provided to the anterior and lateral thigh.[8]

Femoral Nerve

The femoral nerve receives fibers from the second, third, and fourth lumbar roots. The nerve travels in the psoas muscle and then runs in a groove between the psoas and the iliacus muscles. It emerges under the inguinal ligament and

terminates as motor and sensory branches. Motor fibers to the quadriceps femoris are responsible for leg extension, and those to the sartorius and pectineus are responsible for flexion and outward rotation of the thigh.[9]

Genitofemoral Nerve

The genitofemoral nerve has fibers from the first and second lumbar nerves and rests on the psoas muscle lateral to the external iliac artery. The genital branch provides sensation to the mons pubis and labia majora. The femoral branch provides sensation to the femoral triangle.[10]

ABDOMINAL WALL INCISIONS

A well-planned incision has four essential elements: accessibility, extensibility, preservation of function, and security. The incision must provide ready access to anticipated pathology and adequate exposure, since operating through an inadequate incision is not only difficult but potentially dangerous. The incision must be extensible if the scope of operation needs to be increased. The incision should interfere minimally with abdominal wall function by preserving important abdominal structures. It should heal with adequate strength to reduce the risk of wound disruption and incisional hernia. Other considerations for incision selection include (1) need for speed of entry, (2) certainty of the diagnosis, (3) the body habitus, (4) the presence of previous scars, (5) potential problems with hemostasis, and (6) cosmetic outcome.

General Considerations

Lighting

Illumination is critical to the success of any procedure. Shadow-free illumination, which is brighter than the ambient light of the operating theater, should be provided for the entire length of incision. Normally, overhead surgical lamps are adequate. Supplemental illumination may be provided by headlight, flexible surgical light, or combination devices that provide irrigation, suction, and illumination.

Skin Preparation

Removing dirt and contaminants by physical means and reducing skin bacterial concentration are the goals of skin preparation. Typically, skin preparation is accomplished in stages. The first is a general shower to remove dirt. Next, in the operating theater, immediately before surgery, the application of a bacteriocidal soap removes body oil and skin debris and dilutes the bacteria concentration. Finally, the application of a long-acting bacteriocidal agent kills bacteria pushed to the surface from skin pores during surgery. This should be applied in concentric circles away from the operative site, from xiphoid to symphysis, and laterally well beyond the iliac spines. Some surgeons omit the preoperative application of soap, preferring only to apply the long-acting bacteriocidal solution by swabbing or spraying the solution onto the skin. The umbilicus needs specific attention to remove debris.

A bacteriostatic occlusive drape may be applied after skin preparation. In theory, these provide antisepsis for the duration of the surgery. However, by causing increased perspiration, more bacteria may be pushed to the surface. Increased heat and moisture may promote bacterial growth. Over time, the drape might come loose as moisture collects. Because of these negative aspects, the author no longer uses occlusive drapes.

Numerous antiseptics are available, each with its own characteristics. Alcohol is the standard against which others are judged. It has immediate activity against both gram-positive and gram-negative bacteria. Although alcohol is not sporicidal, it is active against many fungi, some viruses, and mycobacteria.[11] Ethanol, normal propyl alcohol, and isopropyl alcohol are all effective in 70 percent concentration. A 1-minute alcohol scrub is as effective as a 4- to 7-minute scrub with other agents. Complete air drying of skin, bedding, and drapes is mandatory, especially if laser or electrosurgery will be used, because of flammability. Because it causes desiccation of the skin and is combustible, the practicality of alcohol is limited.

Povidone-iodine is a combination iodine and high molecular weight water-soluble polymer. It was developed to prevent the skin reaction commonly seen with iodine-alcohol solutions. The slow release of iodine creates bacteriocidal activity against most organisms. Iodophors, however, lose some antimicrobial activity with drying. Chlorhexidine is relatively more effective against gram-positive than gram-negative organisms and has poor activity against tubercle bacteria and viruses. Its utility is that it remains chemically effective for more than 5 hours.[12] Studies have shown that the rate of wound infection is similar regardless of which of these antiseptic solutions is used for skin preparation.[13]

Preparation of skin may include hair removal. However, the contribution of body hair to infection is debatable. If necessary, hair should be removed immediately before surgery by clipping, since shaving may damage the skin and increase the chance of infection.[14] In many instances, hair removal is not needed. It is the author's practice to remove a minimum of body hair and then only immediately before skin preparation in the operating theater.

Incision Placement

An appropriately placed incision of adequate length is enhanced by minimal tissue trauma, complete hemostasis, adept use of retractors and packs, correct posture of the patient on the operating table, and efficient illumination. The use of a sharp scalpel to make a single, clean incision through skin and into the subcutaneous tissues provides a clean edge that is easy to close. The scalpel will also cleanly transect small superficial vessels, producing spasm and preventing immediate bleeding. If the subcutaneous tissue is incised to the rectus sheath with as few scalpel strokes as possible, tissue trauma will be minimized. Electrocautery tends to produce relatively larger zones of injury and increased infections, although the improved hemostasis obtained with cautery may be of some benefit.[15]

Small bleeding vessels in the subcutaneous tissues can be occluded with well-directed cautery or ligation with fine suture. Pinpoint cautery using the spark rather than direct contact will prevent excessive devitalization of tissue, and fine suture should be used to reduce inflammation. Isolation of larger vessels is best accomplished by dissection with a hemostat and suture ligation, which minimizes tissue necrosis.

Once the incision is completed, any adhesions that are present should be lysed to allow full exploration of the abdomen and to allow placement of a self-retaining retractor. Adhesions can be taken down sharply by elevating the peritoneal edge with hemostats and identifying avascular cleavage planes. Especially during long cases, the cut edges of the subcutaneous tissue should be protected to prevent desiccation of the tissue. This may be accomplished by placing moist towels at the incision edges or suturing the peritoneum to the skin. The author prefers suturing the peritoneum to the skin. It protects the subcutaneous tissues, and unlike moist laparotomy packs or towels, does not have the bulk that sometimes limits access through the incision.

When the self-retaining retractor is put in place, the surgeon must protect the nerves on the psoas muscle. The nerves are often compromised when the lateral retractor blade compresses them against the psoas muscle. This risk is reduced by using lateral blades of appropriate length. Elevating the retractor with towels will prevent excessive pressure on the nerves. Excessive pressure on the inguinal ligament may also compromise the nerves.

The bowel is next packed into the upper abdomen with two or three laparotomy pads to allow adequate exposure of pelvis contents. If packing is excessively tight, venous return may be compromised, producing hypotension, and terminal nerve endings in bowel may be unduly traumatized, resulting in a prolonged ileus. Use of Trendelenburg's position will help to secure the bowel in the upper abdomen, but the position should not be too steep, because pulmonary function will be compromised. Gentle extension of the torso may enhance exposure, especially with transverse incisions. Patients must, however, be returned to a neutral position to eliminate undue tension on the suture line when the fascia is closed.

Incision Selection and Placement

Numerous longitudinal, transverse, and oblique incisions have been described. They may be placed in an infraumbilical or supraumbilical location. Most are identified by their location on the abdominal wall. Some, especially transverse incisions, are identified by the name of the surgeon who described or popularized the incision. Few longitudinal incisions are known by eponyms. Each has vocal proponents.

Longitudinal Incisions

Longitudinal incisions were preferred during the earliest days of surgery for laparotomy because the linea alba is relatively avascular and because of the belief that transecting the rectus muscle would result in its atrophy. Terminal branches of the nerves are present near the linea alba, but only small branches cross the midline. Longitudinal incisions therefore cause minimal denervation or vascular injury. As incisions are placed more laterally and are made longer, the risk of denervation increases considerably and limits the utility of lateral incisions. The risk of encountering the epigastric vessels also increases. Longitudinal skin incisions are usually made from just below the umbilicus to a point just caudal to the symphysis, and the incision on the rectus sheath should be extended to the symphysis. If these steps are not taken, exposure may be limited, as the lower pole of the wound is pulled into the field when the lateral skin edges are retracted.[16] The incision may be shortened or extended above the umbilicus. The subcutaneous tissue is incised to the rectus sheath. If the sheath is incised over the rectus muscle belly, usually a single layer is encountered. Lateral to the muscle and in a plane through the pubic tubercle, the anterior sheath has two layers.

The peritoneum is opened longitudinally for all longitudinal incisions. It may be in close attachment to the posterior rectus sheath and the two may be opened together. The peritoneum is elevated with forceps. The author prefers to pick up and drop the peritoneum at least three times with the help of an assistant, so that bowel and omentum have a chance to fall away. The peritoneum is opened as cranially as possible by pushing a scalpel against the peritoneum (not slicing or using scissors). Once a small opening is created, air enters the peritoneal cavity and breaks the surface tension, which allows the bowel to fall away further. It is important to use a finger to explore for adhesions that may be present if the patient has had previous surgery. The bladder can be identified because of its opaqueness and markedly increased vascularity. Since the bladder is highest in the midline, and because the urachus may communicate with the bladder, care should be taken to incise the peritoneum slightly off the midline. This will reduce the risk of bladder injury, eliminate the risk of urine leaking from an incised urachus, and provide better exposure. Alternatively, the urachus can be incised and ligated[17] (Fig. 8-9).

Midline Incision

This universally applicable incision is the most commonly employed incision worldwide because of its simplicity and because it can provide exposure to any viscus and all areas of the retroperitoneum. The incision may be extended from symphysis to xiphoid without disrupting nerves, muscle fibers, or blood vessels.[18] The only caution is to avoid the ligamentum teres. Extension of the incision around the umbilicus is usually made to the left, since the ligamentum teres

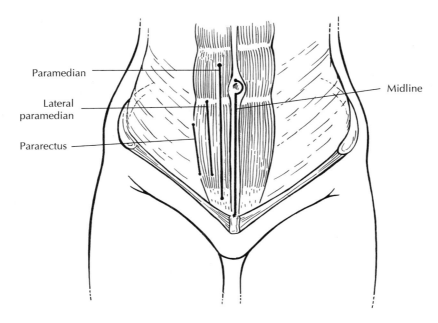

Fig. 8-9. Longitudinal skin incisions: midline; paramedian; lateral paramedian; pararectus.

rests on the right. The incision may also be extended directly through the umbilicus[19] (Fig. 8-10).

In the subumbilical area the linea alba tends to be more narrow than in the upper abdomen, but the midline is normally easy to identify in parous women who have at least a small diastasis recti. The linea alba is incised between the muscles. If the midline is not obvious, identification of the pyramidalis may be helpful, since it inserts on the linea alba. If the rectus sheath is inadvertently opened slightly off the midline, it is of no consequence. Sometimes the muscle must be dissected laterally to allow identification of the posterior sheath, especially if diastasis recti is not present. Above the arcuate line, the posterior rectus sheath can be incised in the midline. The transversalis fascia and peritoneum are also incised in midline. The author prefers to use the scalpel for the entire entry process.

The greatest advantages of the midline incision are that it provides the quickest entry, which is especially important if the patient is unstable or seriously ill, and the best exposure and extensibility, which are of particular importance if diagnosis is uncertain. Because deep tissue planes are not opened, it may be ideal for patients who are anticoagulated, who have enlarged epigastric vessels from any cause that may be injured, or who have intra-abdominal infection.

Paramedian Incision

A paramedian incision may be made 2 to 5 cm to the left or right of the midline. The rectus sheath is incised over the rectus muscle and dissected free from the medial muscle edge. Once the anterior sheath is separated, the muscle is retracted laterally to reveal the posterior sheath. The posterior sheath is not adherent to the rectus muscle and is of course absent below the arcuate line. It can be incised the entire length of the incision and later will be covered with rectus muscle. An alternative is to split the muscle at its inner one-third and outer two-thirds junction. Splitting the muscle causes some weakness because nerves to the inner one-third of the muscle are severed. The peritoneum is then incised longitudinally (Fig. 8-11).

Advantages of a paramedian incision are ease of entry, good extensibility, excellent exposure, and secure healing. Some claim that it is stronger than the midline because it avoids the avascular lines alba, and that the frequency of incisional hernia is reduced.[20] These claims have not been substantiated. Like the median incision, the paramedian avoids the rectus muscle innervation because nerves enter the muscle from a lateral direction. However, more vessels are encountered and it requires slightly longer to complete. Access to the contralateral pelvis may be somewhat limited unless the incision is very long.

Subsequent median and contralateral paramedian incisions must be avoided, since reduced blood supply may lead to necrosis or delayed healing and risk of infection. Re-entry of a paramedian incision almost always requires a transrectus approach, because the muscle becomes densely adherent to the rectus sheath, making separation of the two virtually impossible.

Lateral Paramedian Incision

A lateral paramedian incision is placed at junction of the outer one-third and inner two-thirds of the rectus muscle.[21] The sheath may consist of the two layers here. After the sheath is incised, the muscle is retracted laterally as in the conventional paramedian incision. The posterior sheath and

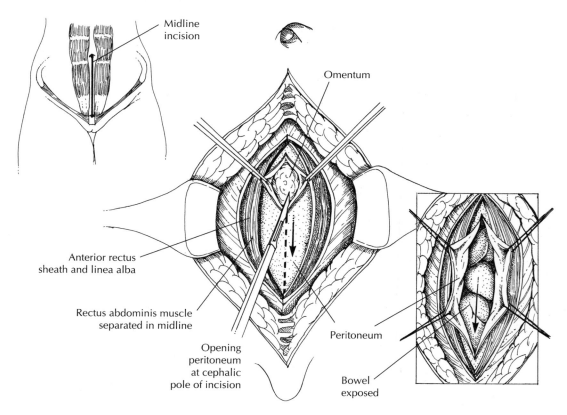

Fig. 8-10. Midline incision. The linea alba is incised and muscles separated in the midline. The peritoneum is opened at cephalic pole of incision. The peritoneal incision is expanded longitudinally, slightly off midline to avoid urachus.

peritoneum are incised under the rectus muscle, in the same plane as the anterior sheath incision.

The advantage is less risk of dehiscence or incisional hernia because a wide shutter mechanism is provided by the intact rectus muscle.[22] It requires more time to complete and to close than the midline incision. Access to the contralateral pelvis may be restricted unless the incision is very long. The potential for injury to the inferior epigastric vessels is increased. Mass closure is relatively more difficult.

Pararectus Incision

A pararectus incision, sometimes called Battle's incision, is placed at the lateral border of the rectus muscle, which is retracted medially. This infrequently utilized incision is primarily heralded for appendectomy or drainage of pelvic abscess.[23] It causes denervation of the rectus, resulting in paralysis and, ultimately, atrophy of the muscles. The length of

this incision must be restricted to no more than two dermatomes, to prevent serious weakness of the abdominal wall.

Transverse Incisions

Efforts to prevent evisceration and incisional hernia led to the development of transverse incisions.[24] It was initially feared that routine use of transverse incisions would cause atrophy of the rectus muscle distal to an incision. This was based on the mistaken belief that a transverse incision transecting the muscle belly would allow the cut edge to retract and damage the nerves of the caudal muscle. Unlike the biceps muscle, which undergoes atrophy, the rectus does not. Few if any nerves are sacrificed, because the path of the nerves is parallel to a transverse incision. The muscles are firmly attached to the rectus sheath and retract minimally, provided that they are not separated excessively. An additional concern was injury to vessels. In reality, nerve or ves-

Fig. 8-11. Paramedian incision. **(A)** The anterior rectus sheath is opened for the full length of the incision 2 to 3 cm from the midline. The rectus muscle is retracted laterally and the posterior sheath is incised longitudinally under the muscle bed. **(B)** The lateral paramedian incision is placed near the lateral border of the rectus. When the muscle is retracted laterally, the inferior deep epigastric artery is seen. Finally, the posterior sheath is closed.

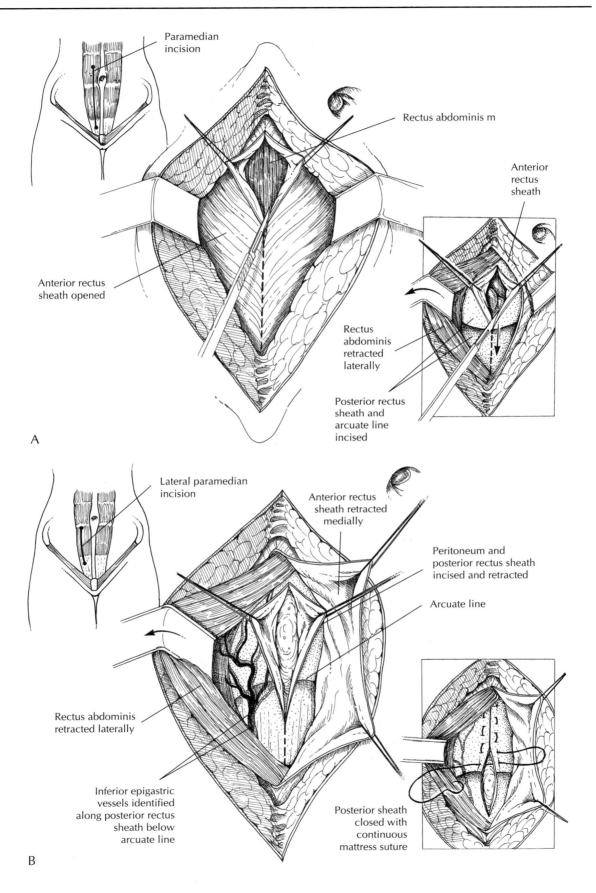

Paramedian incision

Rectus abdominis m

Anterior rectus sheath

Anterior rectus sheath opened

Rectus abdominis retracted laterally

Posterior rectus sheath and arcuate line incised

A

Lateral paramedian incision

Anterior rectus sheath retracted medially

Peritoneum and posterior rectus sheath incised and retracted

Arcuate line

Rectus abdominis retracted laterally

Inferior epigastric vessels identified along posterior rectus sheath below arcuate line

Posterior sheath closed with continuous mattress suture

B

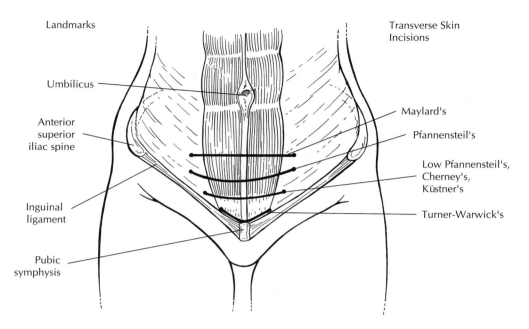

Landmarks

Umbilicus

Anterior
superior
iliac spine

Inguinal
ligament

Pubic
symphysis

Transverse Skin
Incisions

Maylard's

Pfannensteil's

Low Pfannensteil's,
Cherney's,
Küstner's

Turner-Warwick's

Fig. 8-12. Transverse skin incisions.

sel injury is rare, except when the incisions extend very widely into the internal oblique and transversus abdominis muscles.

All of these procedures begin with a transverse skin incision centered above the symphysis pubis. The incisions are distinguished by their distance above the symphysis. They may range from a few centimeters in length to more than 15 cm. They may be straight or have a gentle curve with cephalic concavity. Several vertical marks can be placed across the incision line to aide in symmetrical reapproximation. This is especially helpful if the incision is curved. Placing the incisions in the pubic hair line or in a natural skin crease may enhance the cosmetic result. The incision should not, however, be placed in a deep skin fold of a large panniculus, where maceration of the skin may increase the risk of infection. The subcutaneous tissue is initially incised transversely with all approaches. Transverse skin incisions should result in narrower scars because they follow Langer's lines. The limited access to the upper abdomen afforded by transverse incisions must be considered.

Transverse incisions are usually separated into four categories. Pfannenstiel's incision is a muscle-separating operation. Cherney's incision is a tendon-detaching operation. Maylard's incision is a true muscle-cutting incision. Finally, Küstner's incision is a median incision using a transverse skin incision (Fig. 8-12).

Pfannenstiel's Incision

Pfannenstiel's incision, the most popular transverse incision, is placed 2 to 5 cm above the symphysis, but usually well below the superior anterior iliac spines.[25] Incision of the rectus sheath is oriented in a transverse direction, often at the apex of the pyramidalis muscles. A slight upward concavity may enhance exposure. The lateral aponeurosis is comprised of two layers, the external oblique aponeurosis and the fused aponeuroses of the internal and transversus abdominis muscles. These should be incised separately.

Sharp dissection is usually necessary to separate the anterior and posterior rectus sheaths at the linea alba. The anterior sheath should be separated from rectus muscles superiorly to the umbilicus and inferiorly to the symphysis. If a smaller incision is contemplated, the sheath may be dissected to a lesser extent. In general, for optimal exposure, it is recommended that the sheath be dissected for a distance at least equal to the transverse length of the incision.

The pyramidalis muscles should not be separated from the inferior rectus sheath to which they are usually adherent. If they remain on the rectus, they can be separated in the midline along with the rectus muscles. The midline raphe of rectus is identified and separated down to the transversalis fascia. This may be done bluntly or sharply, except at attachment of pyramidalis, which must be done sharply. The posterior sheath and peritoneum are opened vertically. The peritoneum should be incised as high as possible initially and slightly off center, to minimize the risk of injury to bladder and urachus.

The Pfannenstiel incision provides excellent access for local gynecologic conditions such as cesarean birth and pelvic surgery. Urologists use this incision for retropubic access to the prostate gland. Postoperative strength is excellent. The skin incision leaves an almost imperceptible scar, because it is often hidden in the pubic hairline or obscured by a skin crease.

The four points that limit exposure are the lateral poles

of the fascia and the superior and inferior extent of dissection. The incision in the aponeuroses may be extended to the iliac crest. Other limits are the symphysis and umbilicus. If greater exposure is needed, the rectus tendons may be incised. The rectus muscles should not be transected because they have already been separated from the rectus sheath.

Since exposure is limited and there is minimal opportunity to extend the incision, this incision should be used only when pathology is confined to the pelvis. Of historical interest is that Pfannenstiel did not advocate hysterectomy with this incision because of the limited exposure. Opening and closing the wound takes longer than longitudinal incisions. Because more tissue planes are opened, the chance of seroma and hematoma formation is increased, and vulnerability to infection may also be greater. Indeed, because of these considerations, it is relatively contraindicated in the presence of active abdominal infection or if speed is of the essence. The incidence of inguinal hernia with the Pfannenstiel incision, at least in men, may actually be increased when the incision is close to the external inguinale ring[26] (Fig. 8-13).

Cherney's Incision

The Cherney incision is similar to the Pfannenstiel incision, with the exception that the skin incision is slightly lower.[27] Many surgeons dissect the upper aponeurosis minimally, although it may be dissected exactly as in a Pfannenstiel incision, if necessary for exposure. The rectus sheath is elevated from the rectus muscles inferiorly until pubic symphysis is reached. Leaving the pyramidalis muscles attached to the sheath minimizes bleeding.

The transversalis fascia is perforated lateral to muscles but medial to inferior epigastric vessels in Hesselbach's triangle. The recti tendons and lower muscle bellies of the recti are isolated from the underlying bladder and vesicouterine peritoneum by blunt dissection. The tendons are cut above the periosteum of the pubis. Bleeding is uncommon, since the tendons are relatively avascular. However, by leaving a 0.5-cm segment of tendon on the symphysis, bleeding can be controlled with simple sutures if necessary. This is not possible if the tendons are cut directly on periosteum. If tendons are underdeveloped, this incision is contraindicated, because

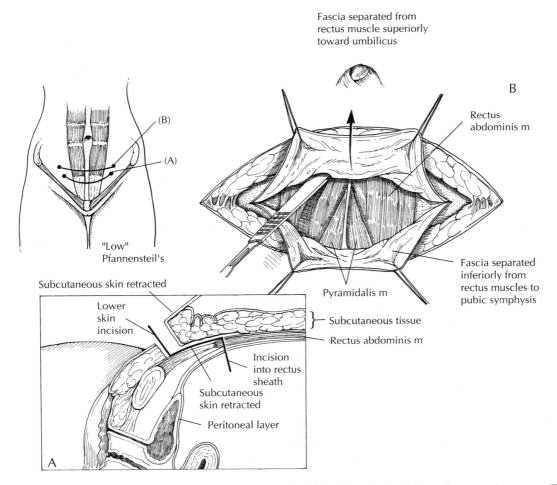

Fig. 8-13. Pfannenstiel's incision. **(A)** "Low Pfannensteil: the skin incision is placed lower for cosmetic reasons. The subcutaneous tissues are dissected to allow standard placement of rectus sheath incision. **(B)** Fascia is separated from rectus muscle superiorly and inferiorly. *(Figure continues.)*

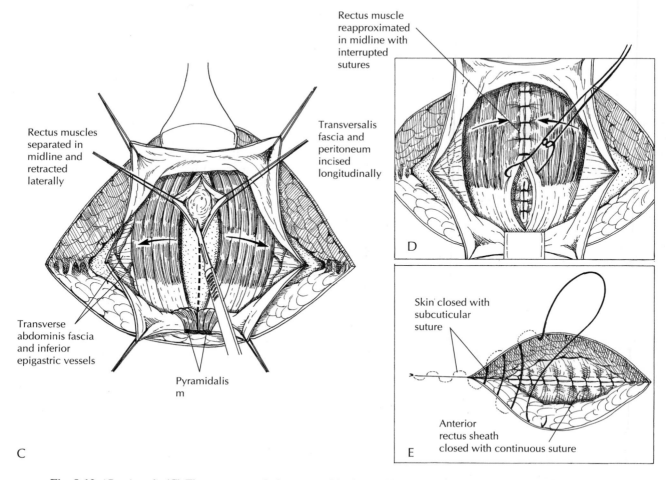

Rectus muscle reapproximated in midline with interrupted sutures

Rectus muscles separated in midline and retracted laterally

Transversalis fascia and peritoneum incised longitudinally

Transverse abdominis fascia and inferior epigastric vessels

Pyramidalis m

Skin closed with subcuticular suture

Anterior rectus sheath closed with continuous suture

C

D

E

Fig. 8-13 *(Continued)*. **(C)** The rectus muscle is separated in the midline and the peritoneum is incised longitudinally. **(D)** Sutures may be placed in the rectus muscle to close a rectus diastasis. **(E)** Sheath is closed with continuous suture. Skin is approximated with a subcuticular suture.

the muscle must be transected.[28] The tendinous portion of the muscle is retracted upward, much like a window shade. The peritoneum is incised longitudinally.

Cherney's incision is less time-consuming than the Maylard. Exposure to the retropubic space of Retzius is excellent and is particularly well suited for all types of retropubic urethropexy. The aponeuroses can be opened to the iliac crest to enhance exposure. Healing is secure and few technical problems interfere with success. The risk of hematoma and seroma are similar to a Pfannenstiel incision because the same tissue planes are opened (Fig. 8-14).

Maylard's Incision

The Maylard incision is also known as the Mackenrodt incision and may be used at any level of the abdomen.[29,30] When placed at the level of the anterior superior iliac spine and with a gentle cephalad concavity, it gives excellent exposure to the pelvis and is especially well-suited for iliac node dissection. The aponeurosis is incised to a point about 2 to 3 cm

medial to the superior anterior iliac spine. The aponeurosis incision may be extended above the iliac spine to enter the upper abdomen.

The rectus muscles are incised transversely with a scalpel, electrocautery, or surgical stapling device. The muscles should be separated from the aponeurosis as little as possible. Because there is no posterior sheath, the muscle may retract. To prevent retraction, the cut edge of muscle may be sutured to the anterior sheath with mattress sutures of 0-caliber absorbable material.

The deep inferior epigastric vessels will be seen near the lateral margin of the rectus muscles and are buried in properitoneal fat. These are usually sacrificed to prevent accidental injury, although some surgeons believe this is not necessary. A clamp is used to isolate the vascular bundle, which is then transected and doubly ligated. The epigastric vessels near the umbilicus may divide into many small branches that must be ligated individually.

Hemostasis should be complete before opening the peritoneum. The peritoneum is incised transversely, and the mid-

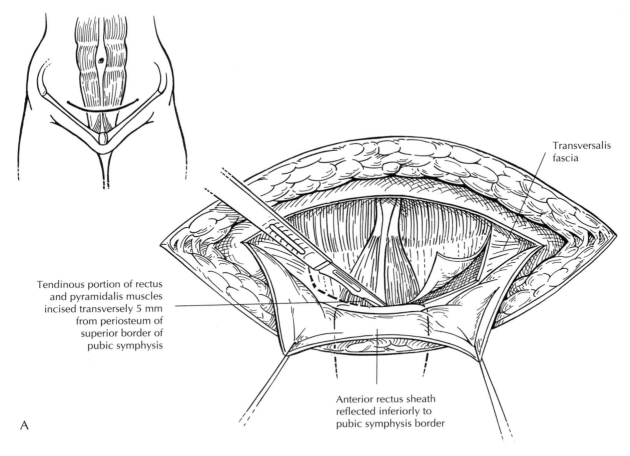

Transversalis fascia

Tendinous portion of rectus and pyramidalis muscles incised transversely 5 mm from periosteum of superior border of pubic symphysis

Anterior rectus sheath reflected inferiorly to pubic symphysis border

A

Fig. 8-14. Cherney's incision. **(A)** Transverse incision of rectus sheath. *(Figure continues.)*

line urachus should be ligated. The lateral umbilical ligaments that represent the obliterated umbilical arteries are cut. Normally, minimal lateral retraction is necessary. Prolonged lateral retraction may lead to femoral nerve injury. The nerves of the rectus muscles are not disturbed.

The Maylard requires additional time when compared to other transverse incisions, but offers better exposure. If the aorta or iliacs are obstructed from coarctation or atherosclerosis, the epigastric vessels may be a major source of collateral circulation for the lower extremity. Care must be taken when ligating the epigastric vessels, because ligation of the vessels may cause ischemia of the lower extremity. To ensure that ligation will not produce ischemia, the dorsal pedis pulse may be palpated after temporarily occluding the vessel. If pulses diminish, the vessels should not be ligated[31] (Fig. 8-15).

Küstner's Incision

Küstner's incision is initiated with a transverse skin incision approximately 5 cm above the symphysis.[32] Subcutaneous adipose is then separated from the rectus sheath in a vertical plane to reveal the linea alba. Numerous small branches of the superficial epigastric plexus of vessels may be encoun-

tered and must be ligated to prevent excess oozing. Because of the need for extensive hemostasis, this incision tends to be very time-consuming. Care must be taken to dissect only enough to expose the linea alba and not to separate the subcutaneous tissue too far laterally. A vertical median incision is then made in the linea alba. The procedure for the median incision is then followed.

This incision seems to combine the disadvantages of both median and transverse incisions and therefore has limited utility. Collection of blood and serum increases the risk of infection and may necessitate drainage. It affords less exposure than the Pfannenstiel, and it affords almost no extensibility. This incision was developed to reduce the risk of evisceration; however, the incidence of herniation is similar to midline incisions. It is sometimes called a modified Pfannenstiel incision, but incorrectly so. The author normally uses this incision only when reoperation is necessary. Even then a simple median incision may be preferred, except for the minor risk of an intersecting skin incision (Fig. 8-16).

Turner-Warwick's Incision

Turner-Warwick's skin incision is centered 2 to 3 cm above the symphysis and is placed within the lateral borders of the rectus muscles.[33] The subcutaneous tissue is incised to the

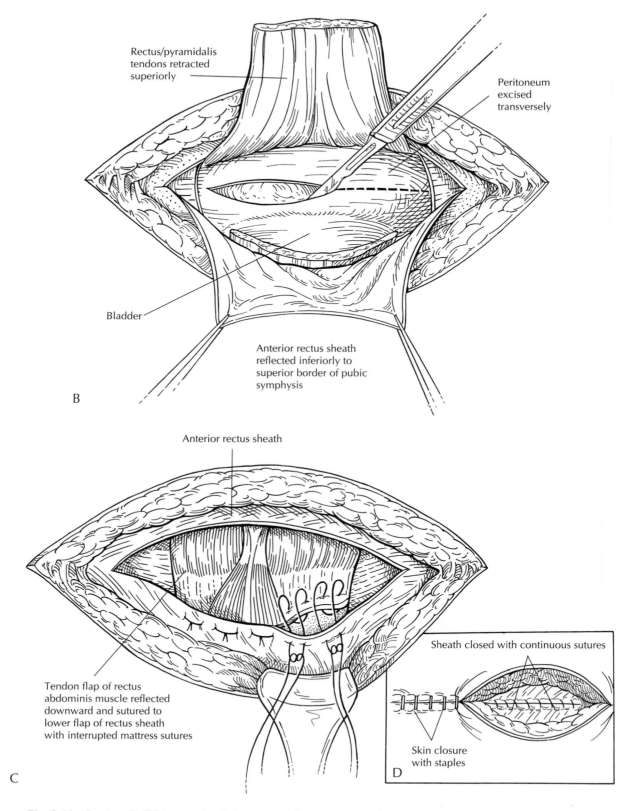

Rectus/pyramidalis
tendons retracted
superiorly

Peritoneum
excised
transversely

Bladder

Anterior rectus sheath
reflected inferiorly to
superior border of pubic
symphysis

B

Anterior rectus sheath

Tendon flap of rectus
abdominis muscle reflected
downward and sutured to
lower flap of rectus sheath
with interrupted mattress sutures

Sheath closed with continuous sutures

Skin closure
with staples

C

D

Fig. 8-14 *(Continued).* **(B)** Lower sheath is separated from rectus muscles. Tendons are exposed and incised 0.5 cm above periosteum of symphysis. **(C)** Tendons are sutured to lower rectus sheath above symphysis with permanent suture material. **(D)** Sheath is closed in a continuous manner.

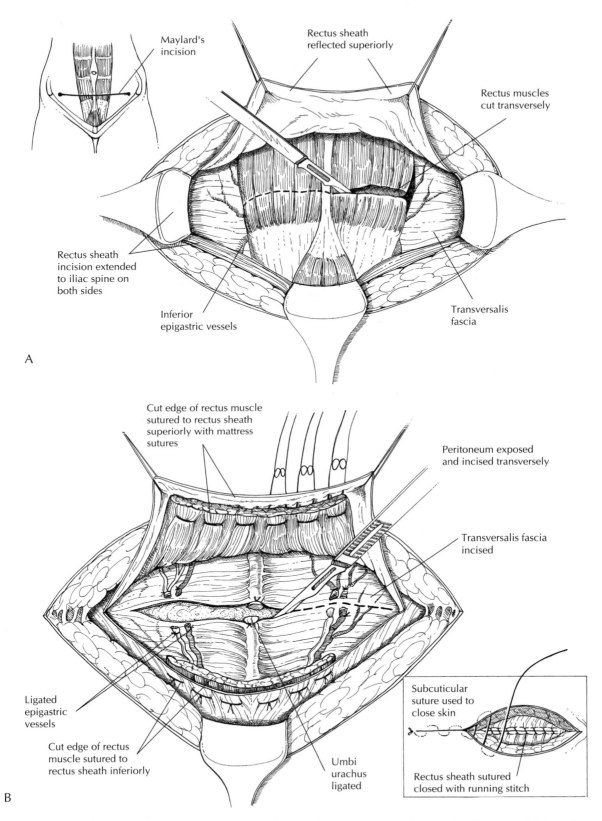

Fig. 8-15. Maylard's incision. Transverse muscle-cutting incision. **(A)** Incision of rectus sheath is extended laterally to iliac spine to expose rectus muscle. Rectus muscles are cut transversely. **(B)** Cut edges of muscles are sutured to the rectus sheath. Ligated epigastric vessels and exposed transversalis fascia. Transversalis fascia and peritoneum are incised transversely. Urachus is ligated.

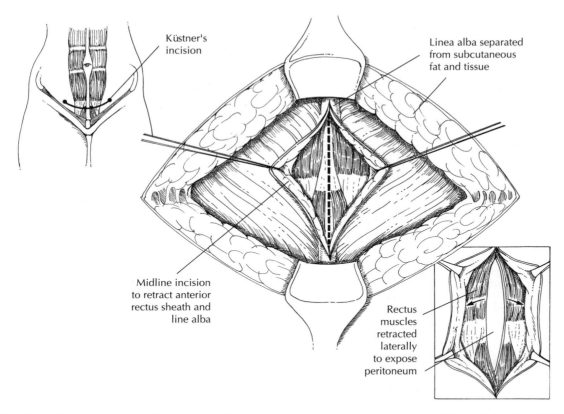

Fig. 8-16. Küstner's incision. Transverse incision to sheath, subcutaneous tissue separated from linea alba. Midline incision in linea alba.

rectus sheath and then in the lower pole is separated from the rectus sheath to below the symphysis. The aponeurosis incision is usually 2 cm below the symphysis and 4 cm across. The rectus sheath incision is angled upward to the lateral border of the rectus, but remains medial to the internal oblique and transversus abdominis muscle bellies. A Kocher clamp can be placed on the aponeurosis for traction as it is separated from the muscle by blunt and sharp dissection. The pyramidalis muscles usually remain attached to aponeurosis. The rectus muscles are separated from the transversalis fascia. The peritoneum is incised in the midline. The Turner-Warwick incision provides excellent exposure to the retropubic space, but upper pelvis and abdominal exposure is severely limited (Fig. 8-17).

Oblique Incisions

McBurney's Incision

The gridiron incision of McBurney is a muscle-splitting incision.[34] It is initiated with an oblique skin incision, which runs in a caudal and medial direction. It is centered over a point midway from the umbilicus to the superior anterior iliac spine (McBurney's point). Length may range from 3 to 12 cm or more.

The skin and subcutaneous fat are incised to the external oblique aponeurosis, which is opened parallel to the direction of their fibers. This reveals the underlying internal oblique and transversus abdominis aponeurosis, which are usually fused. These muscles are also separated parallel to the direction of its fibers. Generally, the direction of the fibers is perpendicular to those of the external oblique aponeurosis.

Retractors may be used to stretch the incision for better exposure. If exposure is still not adequate, the incision may be first expanded laterally and upward, and then medially if necessary. Lateral extension may be made following the fibers of the external oblique muscle. Further medial access can be obtained by incising the anterior rectus sheath and rectus muscle. The epigastric vessels should be identified and possibly ligated to avoid bleeding.

The transversus abdominis muscle is dissected from the properitoneal fat and peritoneum. The peritoneum is elevated with forceps and incised with a scalpel. The cecum is very close to and fixed near the site of entry, and care must be exercised to avoid injury.

McBurney's incision provides excellent access for an appendectomy or extraperitoneal drainage of pelvic abscess. In the case of an abscess, the incision needs to be lower than with an appendectomy. It is easily expanded and cosmesis is excellent.[35] Although it is usually oblique, it may be

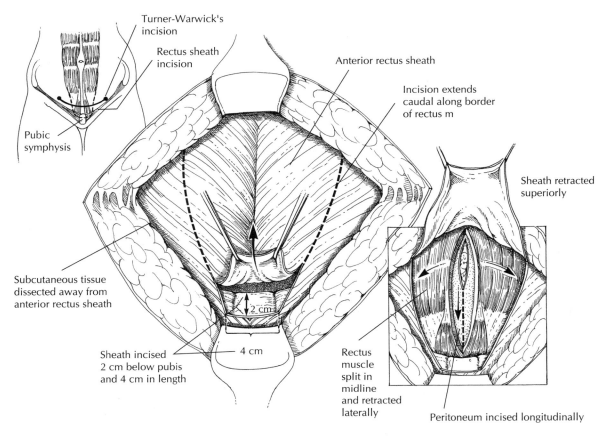

Fig. 8-17. Turner-Warwick's incision. Transverse skin incision. Subcutaneous tissue is dissected from the anterior sheath to a point at least 2 cm below the pubis. The sheath is incised 2 cm below the pubis and at least 4 cm in length. The incision is extended cephalad along the borders of the rectus muscles. Peritoneum is incised longitudinally.

placed in a transverse direction or in skin crease, or made lower to promote an improved cosmetic result. A left-sided incision may also be made for abscess drainage.[36]

When the incision is placed transversely between the junction of the lower and middle third of a line from the superior anterior iliac spine to the umbilicus and the lateral border of the rectus abdominis muscle, it is sometimes known as a Rockey-Davis incision or Elliot incision. The aponeurotic layers are opened in a fashion similar to McBurney's incision. The incision may be made on the left. Exposure is excellent to the ipsilateral lower quadrant. It may be made lower to gain better access to a pelvic abscess (Fig. 8-18).

Re-entry Incisions

Whenever possible, re-entry of the abdomen should be performed through the previous incision. A second incision, especially if heavily undercut, may compromise the blood supply, leading to necrosis at points of intersection of the incisions or at skin bridges between incisions. Anytime there has been previous surgery, the possibility of bowel adhesions must be remembered.

PRINCIPLES OF WOUND CLOSURE

Wound Healing

Wound healing is a balance between tissue damage during an operation and the body's ability to decontaminate and repair it. The process is identical regardless of the tissue involved. The resultant scar depends on the severity of tissue trauma, the foreign body used to repair the wound, and the presence of factors that may delay the process or reduce tensile strength of the final scar. The process of wound healing is separated into four areas: inflammation, epithelialization, fibroplasia, and maturation for the purpose of discussion. However, these are somewhat arbitrary divisions, as they occur simultaneously.

Inflammation

The inflammation phase of healing is sometimes called the lag phase, because wound strength does not begin to return immediately. It is under the direction of the inflammatory response. Key components of this phase are hemostasis, vascular permeability, and cellular recruitment. Vasoconstric-

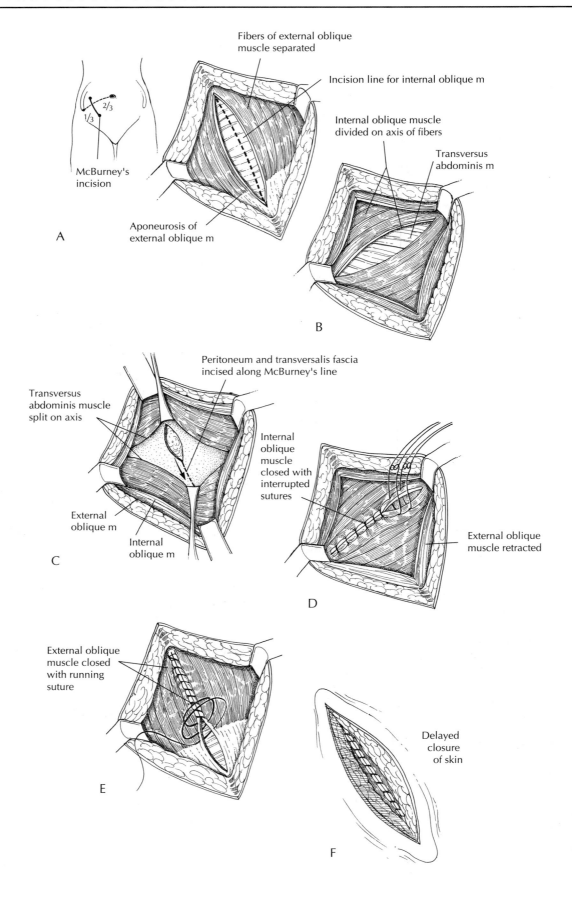

Fibers of external oblique
muscle separated

Incision line for internal oblique m

Internal oblique muscle
divided on axis of fibers

Transversus
abdominis m

McBurney's
incision

Aponeurosis of
external oblique m

A

B

Peritoneum and transversalis fascia
incised along McBurney's line

Transversus
abdominis muscle
split on axis

Internal
oblique
muscle
closed with
interrupted
sutures

External
oblique m

Internal
oblique m

External oblique
muscle retracted

C

D

External oblique
muscle closed
with running
suture

Delayed
closure
of skin

E

F

tion follows initial injury and provides at least a measure of hemostasis for 5 to 10 minutes. Platelets aggregate in severed vessels and capillaries. Exposure of platelets to connective tissue triggers the clotting cascade. Wandering tissue macrophages orchestrate subsequent events.[37] Mononuclear leukocytes accumulate and are transformed into macrophages. Mast cells degranulate, releasing histamine and other mediators of vasodilation and cellular migration. Chemotaxis results in a concentration of polymorphonuclear leukocytes that digest bacteria, foreign debris, and necrotic tissue with lysosomal enzymes. Small vessels become permeable to molecular and cellular mediators of the inflammatory response. This accumulation of plasma and cellular elements is noted clinically as edema and swelling. Except in the presence of infection, this is completed within 3 days.

Epithelialization

Epithelialization (also called migration) includes basal cell proliferation and epithelial migration.[38] The fibrin bridgework within a clot allows migration of epithelial cells. The basal cells enlarge, divide, and migrate. Proliferation continues until individual cells are surrounded by cells of similar type. In a clean surgical wound, the epithelial cells migrate downward to meet in the depths of the dermis. Migration ceases when the layer is rejuvenated; this is normally completed by 48 hours. The superficial layer of epithelium is very thin, easily traumatized, and gives little tensile strength, but it does creates a barrier to the bacteria and other foreign bodies. Myofibroblasts, which are present in the wound by the fifth day, produce contractile proteins. These pull the edges of the wound together but are dependent on tissue mobility.

Fibroplasia

Fibroblast proliferation, collagen production, and accumulation of ground substance are features of fibroplasia. Fibroblasts are transformed from local mesenchymal cells, are usually present in the wound within 24 hours, and by day 10, predominate.[39] They attach to the fibrin matrix of the clot, multiply, and produce glycoprotein and mucopolysaccharides, which make up the ground substance. Fibroblasts synthesize collagen, the primary structural protein of the body. On the second day, collagen production begins, but it is secreted as an amorphous gel devoid of strength. Maximum collagen production begins around day 5 and continues for at least 6 weeks.[40] The collagen matrix stimulates angio-

genesis. Collagen and capillaries together form granulation tissue.

Maturation

Key elements of maturation include collagen cross-linking, collagen remodeling, and wound contraction. Initially, a triple helix, tropocollagen, is formed by three protein chains. Two are identical α_1 protein chains and the third is an α_2 protein. Bundles of tropocollagen combine to form collagen. Five types of collagen have been identified. Types I and III predominate in the skin and aponeurotic layers. Tensile strength of the wound is directly proportional to the amount of collagen.[41] As disorganized collagen is degraded and reformed, covalent cross links are formed that enhance tensile strength. Maximum strength depends on the interconnection of collagen subunits. Although the diameter and morphology of collagen fibers do not have the appearance of normal skin until 180 days, approximately 80 percent of the original strength is obtained by 6 weeks.[42] During the immediate postoperative period, rest and immobility are important for successful healing to occur. During the maturation phase, appropriate patient activity with concomitant stresses and strains is essential to increasing tensile strength by remodeling, which may continue for many years.

Incision Closure

The ideal abdominal wound closure should be easy to perform quickly, reasonably comfortable for the patient, and leave an aesthetic scar. Ideally, the abdomen will be as strong after the operation as before and have a low risk of infection, incisional hernia, and wound disruption. The purpose of sutures is to approximate and splint opposite edges of the incision until the collagen matures. Suture materials are reviewed and each layer of the abdominal wall is then discussed in regard to wound closure.

Suture Materials

Perhaps the greatest development in wound closure is the choice of suture materials now available (Table 8-1). Polymer chemistry and wire technology have provided synthetic and metallic alternatives to natural fibers. In vivo degradation time has classically provided a general classification system for suture. Nonabsorbable sutures typically maintain tensile strength for more than 60 days, while absorbable sutures lose tensile strength in less than 60 days. Synthetic

Fig. 8-18. McBurney's incision. (**A**) Incision through McBurney's point. (**B**) Fibers of exterior oblique separated. Internal oblique muscle split. (**C**) Peritoneum and transversalis fascia incised. (**D**) Internal oblique closed with interrupted suture. (**E**) External oblique closed with running suture. (**F**) Delayed closure of skin.

Table 8-1. Classification of Common Suture Materials

Type	Generic Name
Absorbable	
Natural fibers	Plain catgut
	Chromic catgut
Synthetics	Polyglycolic acid (Dexon)
	Polyglactin (Vicryl)
	Polydioxane (PDS)
	Polyglyconate (Maxon)
Permanent	
Natural fibers	Cotton
	Linen
	Silk
Synthetics	Polyamide (Nylon)
	Polypropylene (Prolene)
	Polybutester (Novafil)
	Polyester (Mersilene)
	Coated polyester (Ti-cron, Tevdek)
Metal	Stainless steel (Flexon)
	Silver

sutures are more uniform and provide support to the healing wound for a longer period than natural fibers. They may be monofilament or multifilament, which is twisted or braided. The coefficient of friction may be reduced by the application of silicone, polytetrafluoroethylene (PTFE, Teflon), or various other coatings.

Common permanent synthetics fibers are derived from polyamide (Nylon), polyester (Dacron), polypropylene (Prolene), and polybutester (Novafil). A significant limitation of metallic suture is that it requires special instruments to tie or twist a knot and to cut. Metallic sutures are made from silver or stainless steel wire. These permanent sutures lose minimal tensile strength. Nonabsorbable sutures of natural origin, such as cotton, silk, and linen, in theory remain permanently in the incision. In reality, they gradually lose tensile strength and may disappear. If identified during a subsequent incision, these sutures of natural origin often have

become so disintegrated that they have no ability to support tissues[43,44] (Table 8-1).

Absorbable sutures are generally degraded in anywhere from a few days to a few weeks. A newer designation, delayed absorbable synthetic sutures, retain tensile strength for up to 60 days. The in vivo half-life for tensile strength is approximately 1 week for chromic catgut, 2 weeks for polyglycolic acid (Dexon) and polyglactin 910 (Vicryl), approximately 3 weeks for polyglyconate (Maxon), and 6 weeks for polydioxanone (PDS).[45]

Suture properties to be considered are knot security, tensile strength, tissue reaction, and wound security (Table 8-2). Knot security describes the suture's ability to maintain a knot without slippage, is best with multifilament sutures. Monofilament sutures with a high memory are more likely to slip or become untied. Tensile strength is a measure of the force necessary to break a suture strand, and increases with suture caliber. However, tensile strength varies from one suture type to another. The synthetic materials are stronger than natural fibers on a caliber per caliber basis. Sutures are usually weakest at the knot, although square knots seem to maintain the greatest tensile strength. If suture breaks at a site remote from the knot, damage is often iatrogenic because of inadvertent crushing of the suture. Monofilament synthetics are especially prone to damage because any crack in the outer coat may lead to failure.

The inflammatory tissue reaction is similar the first 7 days, regardless of the suture material. The chronic inflammatory reaction is dependent on suture type. Natural fiber sutures create a more intense reaction than synthetics. One aspect of tissue reaction is creation of a protein-rich exudate. Excess production may predispose to infection. Because increased tissue reaction to suture may be associated with sepsis and produce delays in healing, sutures with minimal reaction and risk of infection are best for wound closure. Tissue reaction is a function of suture material and caliber rather than the number of knots, although excessive knots are not justified.[46] Continuous closure techniques allow a minimum of knots.

Wound security assesses the entire healing process and

Table 8-2. Characteristics of Sutures

Material	Knot Security	Tensile Strength	Tissue Reaction	Wound Security (Days)
Plain gut	+	+	+ + + +	5
Chromic gut	+ +	+ +	+ + + +	14
Polyglycolic acid	+ + + +	+ + +	+ +	21
Polyglactin	+ + +	+ + +	+ +	30
Polydioxanone	+ +	+ + + +	+ +	60
Polyglyconate	+ +	+ + + +	+ +	60
Polyamide	+	+ + +	+	300
Polyester	+ + + +	+ + + +	+ +	300 +
Polypropylene	+ + +	+ + + +	+	300 +
Stainless steel	+ + + +	+ + + +	+ +	300 +

specifically, the strength imparted by suture. It reflects the original tensile strength and absorption or digestion of the suture materials. Synthetic sutures and natural sutures have recently been studied in a comparative fashion and synthetics seem to be superior.[47]

Another feature of suture is its ability to stretch. Most synthetics have very little ability to stretch; however, those with this ability, such as Polybutester (Novofil), may stretch up to 30 percent. Tissue edema may stress sutures by 10 to 15 percent immediately following surgery.[48] If the suture has some ability to stretch, the likelihood of the suture cutting through the tissue may be reduced.

To determine the risk of infection for different sutures, sutures have been implanted in subcutaneous tissue and then inoculated with staphylococcus. Synthetic nonabsorbable monofilament sutures of nylon, wire, and polypropylene were associated with less serious infection than were multifilament and natural fiber sutures.[49] A second way to evaluate the risk of infection is to place sutures into solutions containing bacteria and then quantify the number of bacteria that each absorbs. Both braided silk and nylon absorb similar numbers of bacteria, while monofilament sutures absorb significantly less.[50] Braided polyglycolic acid absorbs an intermediate number of bacteria. This implies that some compounds associated with sutures may reduce the rate of bacterial absorption and proliferation.[51]

Peritoneum

Many surgeons believe closure of the peritoneum is needed to prevent adhesions by covering denuded surfaces; to prevent bowel from pushing against the suture line and between suture loops; to increase the tensile strength of the wound; and to enhance the speed of healing. Unlike skin, peritoneal mesothelium does not heal from side to side, but regenerates from the exposed connective tissue bed with extraordinary rapidity.[52] If underlying tissue is not damaged, mesothelium regeneration is normally complete by 48 to 72 hours, and adhesions do not form. No difference has been shown in the bursting strength of laparotomy incisions in dogs when these wound are closed identically, except for peritoneal closure.[53] In humans, the incidence of wound dehiscence and incisional hernia was no different when wounds were closed identically, except for peritoneum.[54] Therefore, there seems to be little reason to suture the peritoneum itself. This author makes no effort to approximate either the visceral or parietal peritoneum in most situations.

Fascia (Rectus Sheath)

The fascia is the most critical layer in wound closure. Since successful healing is primarily dependent on adequate approximation of fascial edges, the best method of fascia closure has generated long-standing debate. The debate centers on whether to use a continuous running suture technique or interrupted suture technique. Whether to use a layered closure or mass closure is a second critical issue. Discussion of the healing process in regard to fascia may help to provide a rationale for choice of suture material and suturing techniques.

The inflammatory process at the wound edge produces collagenase, which assists digestion of necrotic debris but also results in lysis of collagen and partial digestion of fascia.[55] Collagenolytic activity peaks on the fifth postoperative day and extends up to 1 cm from the incision edge.[56] During these first few postoperative days, tensile strength of the sutured wound may actually decline by as much as 50 percent before a slow increase in tensile strength begins.[57]

Wounds have less than 5 percent of the tensile strength of unwounded tissue in the first postoperative week, and wound security is dependent solely on suture that has been secured in strong healthy tissue for support. Maximum strength rarely, if ever, exceeds 80 to 90 percent. Fortunately, only 15 to 20 percent of maximum strength is necessary for normal daily activities.[58] Since return of tensile strength can take more than 70 days, sutures that maintain their strength for at least this length of time are preferred. Therefore, most surgeons select a delayed absorbable or nonabsorbable suture for abdominal wall closure.

Tensile strength of a wound follows a characteristic nonlinear pattern and depends on the synthesis of new connective tissue by fibroblast. Adequate blood supply is critical to supply nutrients and oxygen. The fascia edge should be approximated without undue tension, which may disrupt microvasculature and limit perfusion. If ischemia is severe, necrosis may develop and prolong healing. A comparison of tightly tied suture versus those tied only tightly enough to approximate edges demonstrated that loosely tied sutures produce stronger wounds.[59]

Simple interrupted or figure-of-eight sutures were practical when most sutures were placed using individually threaded sutures. They have the advantage of not relying on a single knot or suture strand for security. Unfortunately, the inherent tendency is to pull the tissue tightly together to ensure that secure knots are tied. This may cause ischemia.

Historically, surgeons expressed concern that suture failure would allow wound disruption if a continuous technique were used. This concern is now moot, since modern suture materials rarely fail. The helical nature of the continuous running suture evenly distributes tension along the entire length of the incision.[60] The continuous suture technique allows superior tissue perfusion.[61] Continuous closure can result in significant time-saving, since fewer knots need to be tied.[62] It is also less tedious to tie three square knots precisely than to tie many knots.

Meticulous layer-by-layer anatomic closure with closely spaced fine suture was a surgical tenet for many years. Introduction of the Smead-Jones mass closure, where sutures are placed 1 cm from the incision edge and passed again near the edge in a mattress fashion, significantly reduced the inci-

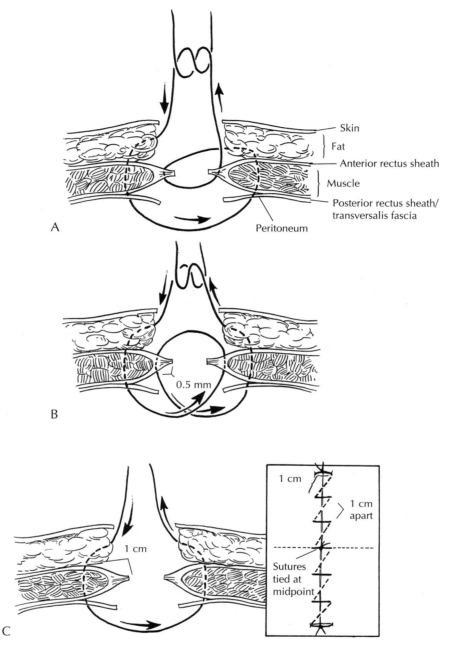

Fig. 8-19. Mass closure. **(A)** Smead-Jones closure. Suture passes laterally through rectus sheath and peritoneum and adjacent fat. The suture crosses midline to pick up medial edge of fascia on opposite side of incision. **(B)** Alternative closure (the author's preference). The far bite is 1 to 1.5 cm away from the edge. The near bite is 5 mm from the edge. **(C)** Running mass closure. Two sutures are used, beginning from each pole of the incision. Sutures are 1 cm away from edge and 1 cm apart. The sutures are tied at the midpoint of the incision.

dence of wound dehiscence.[63] Distributing suture tension between two points by placing far-near or near-far bites seems to give a stronger closure, because two points must rupture before sutures tear out of tissue.[64] Often Smead-Jones is modified to exclude peritoneum, which is closed separately or not at all (Fig. 8-19).

Recently, use of continuous mass closure with permanent suture has been proven equally effective to the interrupted technique and requires less time.[65] Suture should be placed 1 cm away from the incision edge and 1 cm apart, with the total suture length being approximately four times the length of incision.[66] Mass closure techniques incorporate the transversalis fascia and posterior sheath. Peritoneum does not need to be included, but often is. Large studies have now demonstrated the safety of this closure method, and in view of shorter operating time, it would seem to be an obvious choice[67] (Fig. 8-19).

Subcutaneous Tissue

Suturing Camper's fascia may prevent scar depression and ultimately, an unsightly scar.[68] There is some question about whether closure of the subcutaneous fascial layers adds tensile strength to the incision during layered closure.[69] The author's experience does not support these contentions, and the author makes no effort to close the subcutaneous tissue layer except when included as part of mass closure.

Skin

The author prefers to use a primary subcuticular closure for all primary incisions. Transverse re-entry incisions can be closed with subcutaneous sutures because of reduced skin tension. Recently, a subcuticular stapling device using absorbable staples has been introduced. It has the advantages of speed and that nothing needs to be removed. Do not scrimp during skin closure, because this is one of the primary methods by which the patient assesses the surgeon's skill.

Unique Aspects of Closure Based on Incision Type

Longitudinal Incision Closure

The omentum should be placed beneath the incision. The peritoneum may or may not be closed. With the layered technique, the posterior sheath should be closed, and this may include the peritoneum. Including the posterior sheath during layered closure seems to give a stronger tensile strength. Mass closure can be accomplished with a continuous or interrupted technique. If interrupted sutures are placed, the Smead-Jones far-near suture technique should be employed. The far portion should be placed at least 1 cm away from the edge and the near bite approximately 2 to 3 mm from the edge.

When the continuous mass closure is employed, it is helpful to include the posterior sheath. The suture length should be at least four times the incision length. Peritoneum may or may not be included. The skin may be closed by staples, fine suture, or a subcuticular suture. The subcuticular closure is more difficult in the vertical incision (Fig. 8-19).

This author does not close the peritoneum; enough data exist to recommend continuous suture technique without regard to layered or mass technique. The fascia is closed with a running suture of permanent material. The author begins a suture at each pole of the incision and ties them where they meet in the middle of the fascia. The sutures are placed

at least 1 cm from the edge and 1 cm apart and the length of suture is estimated at four times the incision length. This author normally uses a general closure one-half round needle; if the incision is primary, subcuticular closure for the skin; and because the incisions are irregular with re-entry incisions, staples.

Transverse Incision Closure

Pfannenstiel and Cherney Incisions

The Pfannenstiel and Cherney incisions are closed in a similar manner. Closure of peritoneum may be omitted. The rectus muscles will usually approximate themselves but if rectus diastasis is present, the muscles can be pulled to the midline with several loosely tied absorbable sutures. The aponeurosis is closed with interrupted or continuous suture. Both absorbable and nonabsorbable sutures have been described for closure. Skin can be closed by any method, but a subcuticular technique is easily performed, since the edges are easily approximated. The only difference for the Cherney incision is the need to reattach the tendons. They are attached to the lower aponeurosis of anterior rectus sheath rather than to the periosteum of the symphysis directly (Fig. 8-14).

The author prefers to leave the peritoneum unsutured because it does not add strength to the wound, and to close the aponeurosis with an absorbable running suture of 2–0 caliber, because the risk of hernia or dehiscence is exceedingly small. Subcuticular skin closure with 4–0 suture gives a satisfactory result and no sutures need to be removed. This may be especially helpful, since many patients are discharged before it is time to remove skin sutures or staples. The author uses horizontal mattress sutures of 2–0 permanent suture material to attach the tendons to the lower aponeurosis when closing the Cherney incision. The use of delayed absorbable sutures is an alternative.

Maylard's Incision

Oozing from the cut muscle and extensive tissue fluid collection may be significant enough to warrant removal by a closed suction drainage system, which is placed under the fascia. The fascia may then be closed with interrupted or continuous sutures, usually of 1 or 0 suture caliber. Permanent or delayed absorbable suture is preferred. A mass closure technique can be used.

The author closes the fascia with running permanent suture of 0 caliber in a mass technique, and closes the skin using a subcuticular technique with absorbable 4–0 suture.

Oblique Incision Closure

Because oblique incisions are muscle-splitting, the muscles are approximated by their own contraction when anesthetic paralysis resolves. The wound would likely heal with skin closure only. Simple closure is, however, recommended. The peritoneum may be closed with pursestring suture or not at all. The internal oblique and transversus abdominis should be approximated with loosely tied absorbable sutures. The external oblique aponeurosis may be closed with interrupted or continuous absorbable sutures. The skin may be closed with interrupted fine nylon sutures, subcuticular sutures, or skin staples. Because these incisions are often used when intra-abdominal infection is present, delayed primary closure should be considered[70] (Fig. 8-18).

The author prefers to leave the peritoneum unsutured and to use loosely tied interrupted absorbable sutures spaced 1 cm apart in the internal oblique layer. Often this requires only 1 or 2 sutures. The external aponeurosis is closed with absorbable 2–0 suture in a running fashion. The skin is closed with staples so that the incision can be reopened if necessary.

Needles

Although a myriad of needles are available, most are designed for very special suturing needs. Most surgeons use and need to be familiar with relatively few types of needles. Needles are classified in terms of shape, caliber, degree of curvature, type of point, and how suture is attached (swaged or threaded).

Needles may be curved or straight. Straight needles are used primarily for skin closure. They are of the cutting variety and are designed to be handheld. Curved needles require a needle driver. They are characterized by the diameter of their arc, degree of curvature, and caliber. Degree of curvature is one-fourth, three-eighths, one-half, and five-eighths circles. Selection of size and curvature depends on the tissue to be sutured and the depth of dissection. The greater the curvature, the easier it will be to manipulate the needle in deep or confined spaces.

Needles are also judged on the diameter of the body of the needle. Caliber is dependent on the wire diameter from which the needle is made. These are defined as fine, medium, and heavy. The medium ones, which are sometimes called general closure needles, have utility in most tissues. They are especially useful for pedicles and fascia. The fine needles are sometimes called intestinal because of their frequent use in gastrointestinal surgery. They are commonly used for delicate or thin tissue, small pedicles, and blood vessels. The heavy needles are often referred to as hernia needles. They are designed for use on fascia and ligaments and other dense tissues.

Taper point needles are atraumatic. They create the smallest holes because the tissues are stretched and can retract around the suture. These are the most commonly employed and have utility in all tissues except skin. Cutting needles have at least two honed edges and are used in dense or scarred tissue. The conventional cutting needle has three sharpened edges on its concave surface. It cuts tissue easily

in the direction of the pull of the needle. A reverse cutting needle has a cutting edge on its convex surface. It generally cuts tissue away from the pull of the needle and may prevent accidentally cutting through the tissue edges. Reverse cutting needles produce larger holes. Care must be taken with cutting needles to prevent laceration of tissue and accidental cuts to surgical personnel.

A free needle must be threaded though an eyelet. Swaged needles are a single unit with the suture attached directly. The swaged sutures may have the sutures attached to needles permanently or in a way to allow the needle to be pulled off with a gentle tug. The latter ones are know as control release or "pop-off" needles and may save time when numerous interrupted sutures are necessary. Because they are smaller and always remain sharp, swaged needles cause less trauma to tissues. Since they are disposable, there is less chance of metal fatigue. Reduced handling and manipulation may reduce glove punctures and needle sticks.

Most abdominal incisions can be closed with one-half or five-eighths circle, taper point, general closure needles. Hernia needles may be used if the fascia is thickened or scarred. Rarely, a cutting needle is necessary for standard closures. Needles used to place retention sutures are usually the reverse cutting variety.

Glove punctures and finger sticks with surgical needles account for up to 80 percent of the accidental exposure to body fluids.[71] Blunt needles offer surgical personnel a degree of protection from exposure to blood-borne pathogens because even when penetration of gloves occurs, penetration of the skin is less likely.[72] This benefit did not cause significant problems and penetration of the fascia was possible with minimal increase in force.

The author's experience with blunt needles is that they may be used to close fascia satisfactorily. Because of the blunt tip, they do not immediately pierce the tissue and extra concentration is necessary to ensure proper needle positioning. A second minor problem is that significantly greater effort is necessary when suturing, especially in an old suture line. There may be times that require that the surgeon to change to a traditional taper point or even a cutting needle (Fig. 8-20).

Knots

Most suture failures occur at the knot as opposed to the other portion of suture. Thus, secure knots are critical for a strong closure. Either the square knot or the surgeon's knot (a double loop on the first throw) are recommended. The primary benefit of a square knot is that it becomes even tighter when the limbs of the suture are pulled. Other types of knots typically loosen and may give way when the limbs of suture are pulled.[73] Each suture material has a recommended number of throws that yield adequate knot security. In general, a surgeon's throw followed by three squared throws (2 = 1

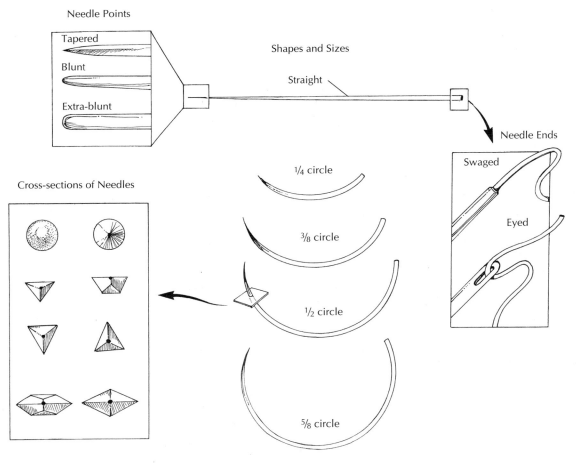

Fig. 8-20. Needles characteristics.

= 1 = 1 knot) gives the best tensile strength.[74] Although knots are the weakest part of the suture, square knots maintain 90 percent of the tensile strength of untied sutures.

Early attempts to exploit greater tensile strength of nonabsorbable sutures were thwarted by the frequency of suture sinuses when multifilament natural fiber sutures were used. Knots always provide space in which bacteria can become enmeshed and are thus the most common site of sinus formation. The risk may approach 80 percent if a contaminated wound is closed with natural suture.[75] Excision of the sinus tract and suture are required to cure the problem. Use of both monofilament permanent and absorbable suture reduces the frequency of sinus formation even if the wound is contaminated.[76] Use of absorbable suture may eliminate palpation of the knot, a distressing problem in thin women (Fig. 8-21).

Drains

What are now considered the tenets of surgical drainage have evolved since the middle of the 19th century. Although drainage of abscess, seroma, hematoma, and fistula is ac-

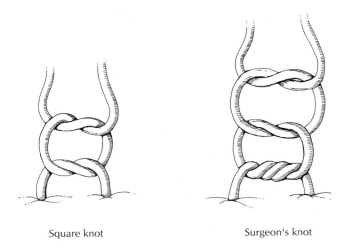

Fig. 8-21. Knots. **(A)** Square knot and **(B)** surgeon's knot.

cepted, controversy is focused on prophylactic drainage to inhibit accumulation of tissue fluids and to reduce the incidence of wound infection. Many current applications of drains are based less on scientific evidence of benefit than on strongly held opinion.

Drains are categorized as passive or active. Passive drains rely on gravity to be effective. The Penrose drain, which is made of latex, is the most widely used passive drain. It is available in varying diameters and its main benefit is to keep a drainage pathway open. The cigarette drain, a Penrose drain stuffed with gauze, in theory wicks fluid away from a wound, but in practice has no real advantage over simple drains. Other passive drains include the Foley catheter, the Word catheter, and the Malecot catheter. Two-way flow of fluid may occur in passive drains as Valsalva maneuvers, coughing, and compression alter pressure dynamics. Passive drains should be advanced slightly each day.

Application of negative pressure to drains eliminates their dependency on gravity. These active drains may be open systems, referred to as *sump drains,* or completely closed systems. Sump drains, the most popular of which is the Salem sump, are double-lumen tubes. Patency is maintained by applying continuous suction to the larger outside lumen and allowing ambient air to enter the smaller inner lumen. Because low pressure prevents fluid accumulation and causes minimal tissue injury, suction for sump drains is best kept in the 30 to 40 mmHg range (''low Gomco''). The system may be converted to a closed system by clamping the smaller lumen. Double-lumen drains have several drawbacks. Airborne bacteria may contaminate the tubing. The outside diameter of the tube is relatively large and rigid, which may cause pressure necrosis or pain, limiting patient mobility.[76a]

A closed system consists of a single-lumen tube to which suction is applied and is effectively unidirectional. Most surgeons now prefer a closed drainage system with a flattened, soft, pliable silicone rubber tube, rigid enough to maintain patency, and with a self-contained portable source of suction. Numerous systems are available and the Jackson-Pratt Drain is perhaps the most popular (Fig. 8-22). Optimal suction for a closed system is 10 to 30 cm of water. The closed system also allows accurate measurement of drainage. A drawback to closed drains is that they may become clogged with tissue.[76b]

Currently available drains may be fashioned from latex, red rubber, silicone rubber, and polyvinyl chloride. Silicone is an excellent material because it is hypoallergenic, soft enough to prevent tissue necrosis, and rigid enough to maintain patency when suction is applied. Latex produces an intense tissue response and may stimulate an inflammatory exudate in the drain tract itself. Because latex drains collapse, suction is not normally applied. Polyvinyl and red rubber have intermediate characteristics of both silicone rubber and latex.[76c]

Perhaps the best documented benefits of drainage in gyne-

cology are reduced incidence of lymphocyst, hematoma, and urinary fistula following radical hysterectomy with pelvic lymphadenectomy and para-aortic node dissection.[76d] T-tube drains placed in the vaginal cuff following hysterectomy prevent febrile morbidity, but are really no better than prophylactic antibiotics.[76e] Another potential advantage is elimination of dead space by removal of tissue fluid, which may allow better apposition of wound edges. Closed drains facilitate healing, especially when large skin flaps are involved as with groin node surgery and radical vulvectomy.[76f]

The benefits of draining abdominal incisions are more controversial. Traditional indications for prophylactic drainage of an abdominal incision include obesity, entry into the space of Retzius, and muscle-splitting incisions. Patients who are very obese may have a large collection of tissue fluid. Because fat has a very poor blood supply, its bacterial resistance is limited. Muscle-splitting incisions and entry into the space of Retzius are often associated with a large collection of blood and serum (Fig. 8-23).

Complement concentrations fall in stagnant fluid within 24 hours. Because complement is necessary for opsonization of bacteria, a low complement concentration may allow bacteria to multiply, which in turn may lead to infection of the abdominal incision. Theoretically, if collections of serum and blood can be removed from the subcutaneous tissue by a drain, the incidence of wound infection should be reduced.[76g]

In practice, the concept of prophylactic drainage to prevent infection, at least in contaminated incisions, may be ill-conceived. Animal studies have shown that wounds inoculated with bacteria and then drained with either active or passive drains actually have a greater risk of infection than when drains are not used.[76a] Passive drains were associated with an infection rate in excess of 90 percent and active drains with an infection rate of less than 20 percent.[76h] Passive drains would therefore seem to have few indications.

Draining clean abdominal incisions with a closed system and using prophylactic systemic antibiotics seem to work equally well in preventing febrile morbidity and wound infection. Therefore, choosing between drainage and prophylactic antibiotics poses a therapeutic dilemma. The author prefers to use prophylactic antibiotics, which have systemic benefits, as opposed to drains, which have only local benefits. Use of both prophylactic drainage and prophylactic antibiotics is not normally recommended because normal flora may be reduced, leading to a wound contaminated with antibiotic-resistant organisms.[76i]

The drain may be used to irrigate the wound with antibiotic or debridement solutions. Irrigation of wounds with antibiotics may lower the incidence of wound infections.[76j] However, antibiotic solutons may be toxic to the cellular elements necessary for healing. For this reason delayed primary closure of an abdominal incision may be an alternative to drainage. The author now uses antibiotic irrigation only in vulvar abscesses in diabetic patients in whom prolonged or recurrent infections and even necrotizing fasciitis is possible.

Complications of drains include infection, hemorrhage, kinking, and hernia. The drain must exit through a separate stab wound and not via the incision because infection may occur at the drain site, especially with passive drains. If a stab wound is placed laterally, injury to the epigastric vessels may result in significant hemorrhage. The drain should have a direct path to prevent kinking and subsequent obstruction. A stab wound involving the rectus sheath must be adequate to prevent kinking of the drain and to allow its removal, but not so large that a hernia may form. Normally, an incision greater than 5 mm but less than 10 mm is ideal. Since closed suction systems require smaller incisions, herniation is uncommon.

The author does not use a drain routinely for any abdominal incision. However, if drainage is clinically indicated, drains of soft nonreactive materials that allow patient movement but maintain patency are preferred. The author believes the Jackson-Pratt drainage system is best. The drain is placed through a separate stab wound and removed as soon as possible.

Experimental and clinical experience suggest that drains should be used sparingly because ingress of bacteria may occur via the drain itself and the drain is a foreign body. Indeed, some studies show that wounds that do not require drains have the lowest rate of infection. Clinical judgment must be used to determine whether the risk of abscess formation or wound failure justifies use of a drain. Multiple factors must be considered, the most important of which is the accumulation of significant fluid. If drainage is deemed necessary, closed systems are preferred. However, drains are not a substitute for good surgical technique. Indeed, contemporary surgical management, adequate hemostasis, elimination of dead space, and use of prophylactic antibiotics may obviate the need for drains.[76k]

WOUND COMPLICATIONS AND MANAGEMENT

Many potential pitfalls await the surgeon making an abdominal incision. These include hematoma, seroma, sepsis, neural injury, incisional hernia, and wound dehiscence. Complications range from minor annoyances to those with serious morbidity and life-threatening conditions. Complications associated with the incision are more common and often more serious than with the primary surgical procedure. Over one-half of patients who have a serious complication have had previous surgery.

Hematoma and Seroma

Hematoma formation is a common complication that is seen more often in transverse than in longitudinal incisions. Anticoagulated patients are at greater risk. However, most hematomas occur in nonanticoagulated patients and proba-

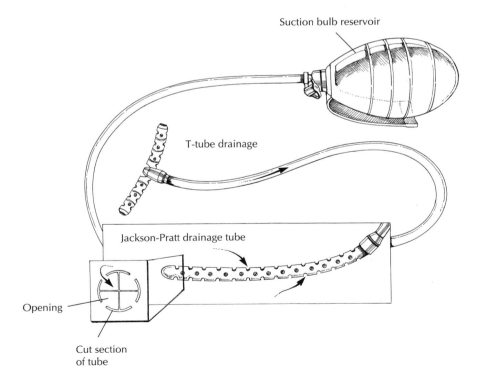

Suction bulb reservoir

T-tube drainage

Jackson-Pratt drainage tube

Opening

Cut section of tube

Fig. 8-22. Closed suction drainage systems. Many sizes are available.

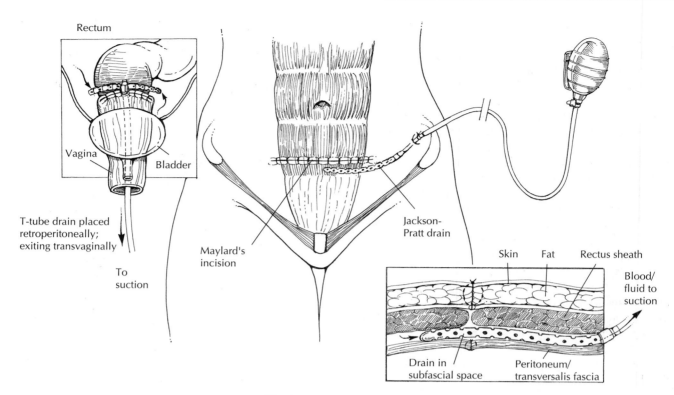

Fig. 8-23. Placement of drain.

bly represent failure of primary hemostasis. Small hematomas can be managed expectantly. Larger ones may need drainage. Ultrasound may help with diagnosis. Fortunately, there is rarely a significant volume of blood lost in the wound.

Seromas are uncommon in gynecologic incisions except for those associated with lymphadenectomy. Small ones will disappear. Larger ones require drainage. Injection of Evan's sky-blue dye in the web of the toes will stain lymphatic channels. This may allow identification and ligation of channels feeding the lymphocyst.[77]

Collections of serum and blood will push the incision apart and will significantly slow approximation of tissues. Collections of serum or blood also predispose to wound infection since bacteria can multiply without inhibition in the stagnant fluid. However, a drain is also a foreign body and provides an avenue for ingress of bacteria.[78] Drains are best limited to very select patients with significant risk of hematoma or seroma, even if the patient is obese. A closed suction drainage system through a separate incision is preferred (Figs. 8-22 and 8-23).

Nerve Injury

Neural injury is a distressing complication that may result in an unexpected conclusion to an otherwise successful operation. Three types of injury occur. First, the incision may

transect nerves. Second, closure of fascial layers may result in nerve entrapment, leading to dysfunction or pain. Third, a retractor used during operation can compress nerves, a common source of injury to the intraabdominal nerves.

Longitudinal incisions that spare the rectus muscle by retracting it laterally or that transect it at its inner one-third result in only minor paresthesias and rectus muscle paralysis because only the most terminal portions of the nerves are damaged. Loss of skin sensation in the immediate proximity of the scar can be annoying. However, because of overlapping dermatomes, loss of sensation is not a serious problem. This is true even if the incision is extended above the umbilicus.

Likewise, transverse incisions that are placed within the borders of the rectus muscles and 3 cm above the symphysis have minimal loss of neural function because the incisions are parallel to the nerves. Dissection of the anterior rectus sheath—as required for the Pfannenstiel incision and the Cherney incision—stretches the terminal sensory nerve fibers, which typically follow perforating branches of the vessels. Because efforts to maintain hemostasis may injure the accompanying nerve, perforating vessels should be cut and ligated only if necessary to control bleeding. Numbness above the incision usually has a triangular distribution with the apex toward the umbilicus.

Wide incisions into the muscle belly of the internal oblique place the iliohypogastric and ilioinguinal nerves at greater risk of injury.[7] An attempt should be made to identify and avoid nerves that may be visible at the lateral edge of incision. Very low placement of an incision may put the femoral nerve and other nerves that pass through the inguinal ligament at risk of injury.[79] A neuroma may form at the transected edge of a nerve and be quite painful.

Nerve entrapment is likely in all the same situations in which nerves are in danger of being transected. Entrapment may result in complete loss of function or, more commonly, in partial loss. Entrapped motor fibers lead to weakness because not all muscles fibers can be recruited. Pain receptors, which are nonadaptive to repeated stimulation, have very low excitation thresholds when stimulated continuously as by nerve entrapment.[80] If entrapment is believed to be the cause of dysfunction, suture removal should be considered. Entrapment of iliohypogastric or ilioinguinal nerves in lateral poles of transverse incisions may cause pain in the lower abdomen and groin.[81] Some have recommended suturing only the external oblique aponeurosis to prevent nerve injury; however, deep sutures may still entrap nerves. If the incision must be extended laterally, injury to the lateral femoral cutaneous nerve may be recognized from numbness of the anterior thigh.

Nerves may be compressed by the lateral retractor blades of a self-retaining retractor (which places pressure on the psoas muscle) or by extreme flexion of the hip in lithotomy position. The lateral blades press on the femoral nerve as it emerges from the border of psoas muscle before exiting the pelvis at the inguinal ligament. Femoral neuropathy is surprisingly common and may occur in 10 percent of patients who undergo laparotomy.[82] It is manifest by anesthesia of the anterior thigh and weakness in the quadriceps muscles. Most femoral neuropathies resolve spontaneously. If they do not, significant disability may occur with weakness of leg extension and inability to climb stairs.[83]

A similar compression mechanism seems to produce neuropathy of the genitofemoral nerve and lateral femoral cutaneous nerve, which lie on the psoas muscle belly. Genitofemoral neuropathy causes anesthesia or paresthesia of the labia majora and upper medial thigh without motor deficits.[10] Injury to the lateral cutaneous nerve causes numbness to the anterior and lateral thigh.[8] These nerves are not palpable, but they are in the psoas muscle lateral to external iliac vessels. Retractor blades must be elevated away from this area to protect the nerves. Thin women seem to be at higher risk.

Wound Infection

Wound infection may occur in up to 4 percent of patients with clean wounds and 35 percent of patients with grossly contaminated wounds. Infectious complications can be traced to failure of the healing process to eliminate bacteria that are invariably introduced into the wound. Infection may be initiated by direct inoculum of bacteria from the patient's or surgeon's skin; by contamination from infected abdomi-

nal contents; or by opening a viscus that may have bacteria (e.g., the urinary tract, large bowel, or vagina). Hand preparation of the surgeon is especially important, since at least 20 percent of gloves are punctured during the course of surgery.[84]

However, it is a misconception that infectious complications are primarily related to breaches of sterile technique.[85] Injection of vasoconstrictive agents may reduce the initial outpouring of factors that initiate the inflammatory response. This creates a time period for bacteria to multiply without inhibition and thus overwhelm the host defense.[86] Avoiding excessive tissue damage that may lead to necrosis and suturing techniques that cause ischemia is key to prevention of infection.

Diagnosis

Low-grade fever associated with mild erythema, induration, and tenderness is a common manifestation of infection. Separation of the incision edges and purulent drainage are later signs. These may be obscured if a subcuticular suture skin closure was used.

A dishwater-like drainage from the incision is typical of necrotizing fasciitis, a potentially lethal process. The edges of the incision become dusky and pale and have a devitalized appearance. An obvious line of demarcation between viable and nonviable tissue is often present. Tissue, especially the subcutaneous adipose, becomes mushy and easily fractured. A striking feature is the rapidity of progression that seems to advance before one's eyes. Necrotizing fasciitis is a surgical emergency. Delay of even a few hours can lead to fatal progression of the disease.[87]

Treatment

The benchmark of therapy is drainage and debridement. The wound will not heal as long as purulent material separates the edges. The wound must be opened to allow drainage and cultures should be obtained. The wound is irrigated to remove most of the exudate. Some degree of disagreement centers on what irrigating solution should be used. Some use hydrogen peroxide or iodophors to remove necrotic debris and sterilize the wound. Although these solutions help with debridement and decontamination, they are also toxic to the cellular elements of healing. Because of this toxicity, others advocate saline only for irrigation. Without regard to irrigation, mechanical debridement with a scalpel or scissors must be performed until all devitalized tissue and infectious material are removed. The wound is then packed with gauze, which is changed three to four times daily. Devitalized tissue and infected tissue must be removed whenever present. A bed of granulation tissue will usually form within 2 to 4 days.

Secondary intention is a tried and true method to allow the wound to heal. Prolonged disability in excess of 6 weeks and loss of protein via the wound are well-documented draw-backs. Recently, secondary closure after formation of a bed of granulation tissue has been shown to be effective.[88] The edges of the incision may be approximated with sutures or with an adhesive nonocclusive bandage. Reclosure should be preformed as soon as the granulation tissue begins. Otherwise, wound contraction begins making the edges rigid and somewhat more difficult to pull together. Also, granulation tissue is rich in capillaries and may bleed because the fresh bed of capillaries is quite fragile. This could cause a hematoma to form in the wound and compromise healing. Secondary closure may be accomplished without general anesthesia, on the patient care unit or in the office following discharge. Less than 5 percent of wounds will become reinfected and require re-exploration.

Prevention

Surgeons may modify rates of infection by altering the management of abdominal incisions.[14] Since devitalized tissue may be associated with poor healing, the surgeon should attempt to minimize tissue trauma by using a sharp scalpel with a minimum of cutting strokes.[89] Hemostasis is best achieved with precise cautery or fine nonreactive suture. Copious irrigation may dilute the inoculum of bacteria, remove fat globules, and eliminate bits of free tissue. If oozing cannot be controlled, or if collection of tissue fluid is excessive, a wound drain may be considered.[90] Delayed primary closure or secondary intention may be alternatives in very high-risk patients. Closure on day 4 greatly reduces the chance of infection, and it may be considered in patients at risk of poor healing or infection and when the wounds are contaminated.[91]

Antibiotics given during the immediate preoperative period have been shown to reduce febrile morbidity in some surgical procedures. Although evidence is less clear-cut for wound infection, patients who have abdominal hysterectomy may benefit from prophylactic antibiotics.[92] Prophylactic antibiotics are given in one dose immediately before surgery. Many regimens and classes of antibiotics have been used. Prophylactic antibiotics prevent postoperative infection. This author prefers a first-generation cephalosporin given 30 minutes before incision.[93]

Fascial Disruption

Failure of the fascia to heal properly leads to dehiscence, which is perhaps the most serious wound complication. Dehiscence is separation of the layers of the abdominal incision and may be partial or complete. Complete dehiscence is marked by separation of all layers. This may have a disastrous outcome in the form of evisceration. A less critical but still serious problem is wound dehiscence without evisceration. Both are surgical emergencies. An annoying problem

is wound hernia, which is defined as separation of muscle and fascia while peritoneum, subcutaneous tissue, and skin remain intact.[94] It can be corrected on an elective basis.

Incidence

The reported incidence of fascial dehiscence ranges from 0.4 to 5.8 percent.[95] A significant problem in interpreting these figures is accurately defining the patient population that is being reported. This complication is now thought to occur in approximately 1 percent of all surgeries and in less than 0.4 percent of gynecologic surgery patients.[96,97]

Incisional hernia is common too. It develops in approximately 1 percent of uncomplicated surgical cases, 10 percent of patients with wound infection, and 30 percent of patients following repair of dehiscence.[98] Over one-half appear within 6 months of original operation, approximately three-quarters are present by 2 years, and 97 percent are present by 5 years.[99]

Etiology

Wound disruption is ultimately due to intra-abdominal pressure or abdominal wall muscle tension overcoming suture strength, knot security, and tissue strength or holding power. What enables mature collagen to stretch and allow incisional hernia after apparent adequate healing remains obscure. Problems with slow or delayed healing are rare in young

---

Conditions Associated With Increased Risk of Fascial Disruption

- Age
- Poor nutrition
- Pulmonary disease
- Cardiovascular disease
- Obesity
- Diabetes
- Radiation therapy
- Infection
- Vomiting
- Distension
- Anemia
- Alcoholism
- Vitamin deficiencies
- Mineral deficiencies
- Emaciation
- Cancer
- Steroids
- Ascites
- Coughing

and healthy patients; however, a number of systemic factors contribute to the problem of fascial failure in other patients. Several factors may simultaneously impede wound healing. Often no obvious cause or precipitating factors are identified. We must also consider epidemiologic features, mechanical factors, medical illnesses, choice of incision, type of suture, and method of closure.

Patient Characteristics

Dehiscence is more common in patients more than 60 years old.[100] The male/female ratio is 3.0:1. Stretching of the wall with pregnancy may afford a measure of protection, while the greater muscle mass in men may place them at increased risk.[101] Patients who are obese are more likely to experience dehiscence.[102] One-half of all dehiscences may occur in patients with malignancy.[103]

Mechanical Factors

Vomiting, hiccups, coughing, and bowel distension may seriously stress the freshly repaired wound. These factors may lead to suture failure or, more likely, to suture pulling through tissue.[104] Postoperative ileus and chest infection seem to have a particular association with wound dehiscence.[105]

Mechanical factors should be prevented or treated aggressively if present. Appropriate use of antiemetics will reduce vomiting, as will adequate analgesia. Nasogastric suction is appropriate to reduce postoperative distention, as is attention to operative packing and serum electrolyte concentration. Hiccups may respond to phenothiazines. Chronic chest problems are best treated during the preoperative period. Preoperative teaching will greatly enhance patient compliance with postoperative pulmonary therapies such as deep breathing and use of incentive spirometry.

Medical Problems

Impairment of nutrition, serious metabolic dysfunction, and medical illnesses have been associated with poor wound healing. Vitamin C is essential for collagen synthesis; it is depressed in patients who have hemorrhage severe enough to warrant transfusion. This may account for the increased risk of abdominal wound dehiscence in patients having surgical hemorrhage.[106] Furthermore, chronic anemia is associate with an increased incidence of wound dehiscence.[107]

Patients who develop postoperative uremia have a high incidence of wound dehiscence as do patient who require peritoneal dialysis.[108,109] Poor healing may be caused by limited proliferation of fibroblasts and subsequent reduction in collagen.[110] Patients who are jaundiced have a fourfold increase in the incidence of wound disruption.[111] Obstructive jaundice is associated with delays in fibroplasia and angiogenesis, as well as reduced tensile strength.[112] Other factors associated with poor healing are listed in the boxed list.

Obesity is associated with increased rates of infection and with technical difficulties in closure, and is often cited as a major causative factor for dehiscence.[113] Nutritional deficiencies that are severe enough to produce hypoalbuminemia result in weakened wounds, probably because of reduced protein precursors and vitamin deficiencies. Cachexia associated with malignancies commonly leads to a severe malnourished state.[114] Diabetics have more than five times the risk of infections as nondiabetics.[14] Reduced ability of polymorphonuclear leukocytes to phagocytize bacteria may be one explanation, especially for those diabetic patients in poor control. Perioperative control of glucose concentration in the diabetic patient reduces wound problems and improves overall outcome.[115] Pancreatitis is also associated with poor wound healing.[116]

Steroids given in physiologic doses seem to minimally decrease tensile strength and probably have little effect on dehiscence. Glucocorticoids, when administered in pharmacologic doses, interfere with function of both polymorphonuclear neutrophils and macrophages and are associated with reduced wound strength.[117]

Incision Type

The midline incision is denigrated as the incision with the highest risk of dehiscence and incisional hernia. Because the clinical impression of many surgeons have supported these beliefs, oblique or transverse incisions have been advocated on the grounds that they are stronger and less likely to experience wound disruption and herniation. These virtues supposedly mitigate the fact that these incisions are more time-consuming and more tedious to perform than longitudinal incisions. Rarely included in the discussion are the facts that midline incisions are often required when there is great urgency, as in cases of hemorrhage, trauma, or sepsis; are made in patients with serious medical illnesses; and are often placed through previous incisions. The more sophisticated incisions tend to be used in selective, more healthy patients, but are not free of complications.

A tenet of surgery has been that incisions heal side-to-side. However, tension on an incision is proportional to its length.[118] Use of the lateral paramedian incision has been shown to lower the incidence of incisional hernia from 10 to 1 percent.[119,120] With this exception, prospective studies have shown little if any difference in dehiscence and hernia formation between midline, paramedian, and oblique or transverse incisions.[121,122] Wound hernias have a similar association. Herniation is more common when the incision is in excess of 18 cm.[123]

Suture Type, Suturing Techniques, and Knots

The main causes of wound failure are failure of suture to remain anchored in the fascia, suture breakage, and knot failure. Therefore, suture selection may affect the rate of dehiscence.[124] Absorbable suture material has an increased risk of dehiscence because up to 80 percent of tensile strength is lost within 2 weeks.[125] Chromic catgut suture closure of the fascia is associated with an 11 percent dehiscence rate.[126] No improvement is demonstrated when catgut was used in layered fashion or mass closure.[127] Use of retention sutures when fascia is closed with chromic catgut reduced the incidence of dehiscence, but only to the same reduction as was seen when nylon was used without retention sutures being placed.[128] Because of the rate of dehiscence, there appears to be no place for catgut suture on the fascia. Polyglycolic acid and polyglactin 910 seem to give better results than catgut and similar to permanent sutures in healthy patients who have no unusual risk of dehiscence. In high-risk patients, polyglycolic acid and polyglactin remain inferior to nylon.[129]

If the suture and knot are intact, dehiscence associated with nonabsorbable suture is most commonly the result of suture cutting through softened tissue.[104] In up to 90 percent of abdominal wound dehiscences the knots are intact. However, the sutures have cut through the tissue in a postage-stamp fashion, due to pressure necrosis resulting from sutures being placed too close to the wound edge or from weakened tissue associated with medical illness, wound infection, or pressure necrosis.[130]

Most dehiscences do not occur immediately, but 4 to 8 days after surgery when the tissue is weakest.[131] The farther from the incision edge the suture is placed, the greater the distance of fascia through which the sutures have to tear, thus leading to a more secure incision.[132] Since tissue is weak 1 cm from the incision, sutures should be placed more than 1 cm from the wound edge to ensure that the tissue is strong enough to hold the suture.

Suture failure is uncommon, especially with permanent sutures. Although the suture may fracture if it is not strong enough for the task it is asked to perform, the smallest suture caliber that will adequately support the fascia should be selected. Selection of a suture with tensile strength far in excess of the tissue it supports has no rationale. The suture may be weakened if it is frayed during tying or if the monofilament suture is grasped with an instrument that may fracture the surface.[133] Adherence to proper surgical technique will prevent fraying, which may weaken the suture. The knot may become loose. Always tying square knots should minimize knot slippage. If prolonged healing is anticipated, such as in an infected wound, monofilament synthetic nonabsorbable suture is the best choice.[134]

At-risk patients need permanent sutures, which give long-term support to the incision. Herniation seemed higher in wounds with absorbable sutures than in those closed with permanent sutures.[135] Permanent sutures had one-third less incisional hernias as compared to absorbable sutures. Use of monofilament sutures is recommended for closure of most longitudinal incisions. Monofilament synthetic nonabsorbable sutures thus seem to have qualities nearest to ideal.[136]

Diagnosis

Many patients who have a complete dehiscence have a sense of something "popping" or "giving way." Profuse drainage of serosanguinous fluid from the incision is common and bowel often rests immediately under the skin incision. Prompt recognition allows placement of an abdominal binder that may protect the patient from evisceration.

A bulge that increases with the Valsalva manuever almost always indicates an incisional hernia. Small hernias commonly go unnoticed and are seen only at the time of provocative maneuvers. At the other extreme, they present as a large (often enlarging) bulging mass that may be associated with abdominal wall weakness. The fascial defect is often palpable. The size may be a cosmetic problem and embarrassing. Small neck hernias are associated with strangulation of bowel or omentum. Pain is evidence of incarceration. Large hernias are rarely associated with incarceration, although skin necrosis, intestinal fistulae, and evisceration have been reported.

Therapy

When complete dehiscence is suspected, wound exploration must be accomplished with adequate anesthesia under sterile conditions. Once opened, the wound should be thoroughly debrided. This is best accomplished mechanically, since it appears that many solutions used for irrigation may delay the healing process. Fascia may be closed with permanent suture in a mass fashion or with retention sutures, which should be left in place for at least 21 days. Retention sutures may be placed perpendicular to the wound or parallel to the edge. The perpendicular sutures are the most commonly employed. The parallel ones require two sutures placed 2 cm away from the edge then pulled together with a third suture.[137] If this author suspects complete dehiscence, the patient is returned to the operating room on an urgent basis for exploration and debridement. The author prefers retention sutures for reclosure, and closes the skin when granulation tissue is present.

Repair of hernia is usually elective. Small hernias do not require repair, unless there is evidence of incarceration. Large or disfiguring ones deserve repair both for cosmetic appearance and for return of full strength of the abdominal wall. The old scar is excised. Hernia sac is isolated with meticulous dissection. Fascial edge should be widely exposed and then repaired with suture alone, with synthetic mesh, or with pants-over-vest technique. Recurrent hernias and attenuated tissues will do best with mesh. Wire was at one time the suture of choice, but it now seems to offer no advantage over permanent monofilament suture.

Prevention

In patients at especially high risk, one must opt for the most secure closure possible, even if it requires more time.[138,139] The most secure closure is through-and-through retention

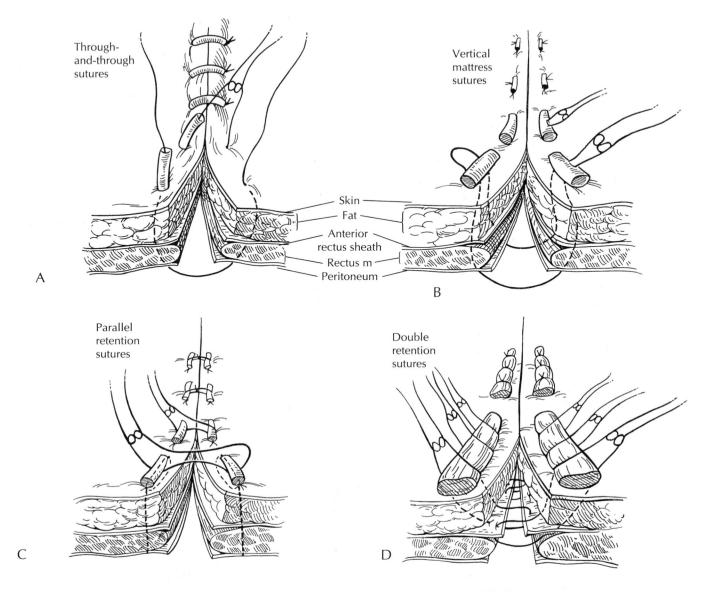

Fig. 8-24. Retention sutures. **(A)** Through-and-through closure of wound dehiscence. **(B)** Mattress retention sutures. **(C)** Parallel retention sutures using a third suture for wound closure. **(D)** Retention sutures that pull the fascial edge to the opposite skin.

sutures, which includes all layers, including peritoneum and skin. Retention sutures will decrease the number of wound dehiscences but not eliminate them entirely.[140] Normally, number 2 caliber suture or larger is used. Retention sutures are placed 2 cm or more from the edge of the incision and 1 cm apart. Retention sutures may be used to re-enforce standard closures (Fig. 8-24).

A running mass closure, Smead-Jones technique, or placement of retention sutures are options. Mass closure with continuous permanent sutures is one of the most significant advances in preventing dehiscence. A key element is placement of suture bites 1.5 to 2 cm from the incision edge. No advantage to layered closure has been demonstrated. Like-

wise, no advantage to interrupted mass closure has been shown. Under most circumstances, the author's preference is mass closure without external retention sutures, because the external retention sutures may be uncomfortable and may leave large scars.

Mortality From Burst Abdomen

Historically, complete abdominal wound dehiscence has been associated with a mortality rate as high as 30 percent. Less than 10 percent is quoted today and is likely lower in gynecology patients who tend to be healthy.[100,101,103,140] It likely is not that dehiscence itself is so lethal, but rather that it so often occurs in an elderly patient who is chronically ill with devastating medical problems or major traumatic injuries.

SPECIAL SITUATIONS

Massive Obesity

Obesity complicates the selection of the incision, because exposure is limited, operating may be difficult, and wound healing may be compromised. Obesity is associated with an increased incidence of wound infection and hematoma formation, and the potential for ventral hernia. Morbid obesity is defined as twice ideal body weight; often, this degree of obesity leads to panniculus formation. A large protruding panniculus of the lower abdomen wall presents an especially difficult technical dilemma. Topography of the abdominal wall is distorted, since the umbilicus is displaced so far caudally that it no longer approximates the location of the sacral promontory and bifurcation of the aorta.

Two decisions must be made regarding patients with a panniculus. The first is placement of the incision. Whether a transverse or longitudinal incision is superior in the obese patient remains a controversial issue. Some patients who are very obese with a large hanging panniculus have very little fat directly over the symphysis. A transverse incision may be made with minimal technical difficulty. An increased risk of infection is a drawback to placing a incision in this deep skin crease, which is often macerated. To avoid the deep crease of the panniculus and the risk of infection, the incision may be placed in a periumbilical transverse direction.[141] The panniculus may be pulled down and a subumbilical longitudinal midline incision made, but the panniculus may be buttonholed.[142] If the panniculus is very low-hanging, a supraumbilical incision may be made. The entire panniculus is retracted below the level of the symphysis, placing the incision over the pelvis. The Bookwalter retractor may aid with the exposure and is rigid enough to hold the abdominal wall in places[143] A traditional midline incision can also be made and extended around the umbilicus[144] (Fig. 8-25).

The second decision is whether to perform a panniculectomy. Panniculectomy was initially described to alleviate problems of surgical exposure and to reduce postoperative

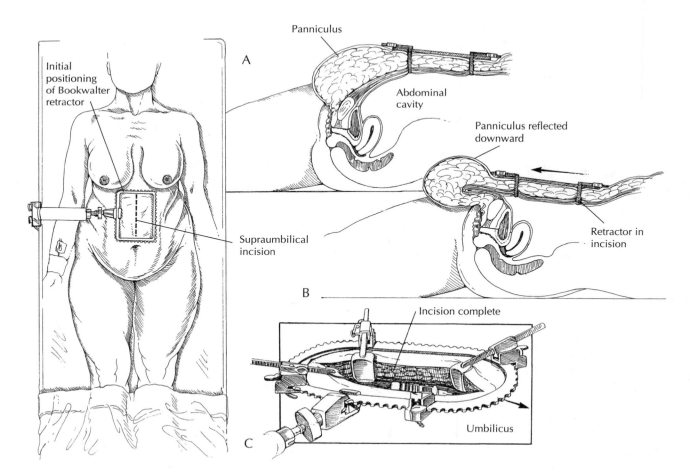

Fig. 8-25. (A) Bookwalter retractor placement. (B) Panniculus retracted caudad and a supraumbilical incision made. (C) Bookwalter retractor and accessory retractors in place.

problems with wound healing.[145] However, at least one-third of patients still have significant morbidity, which may involve cardiopulmonary compromise, sepsis, and anesthesia problems.[146] With better monitoring of postoperative patients and improved anesthetic techniques, a resurgence of interest in panniculectomy and abdominoplasty has occurred.

No absolute indications exist for panniculectomy. When the adipose tissue is so thick that even the longest instruments can not reach the pelvis, panniculectomy may facilitate surgery. Obesity to an extent that the abdomen hangs down over the symphysis and onto the thighs is also an indication, because of compromised healing. A large diastasis recti that needs to be repaired may also be an indication.

Two techniques of panniculectomy are commonly employed (Figs. 8-26 and 8-27). In the first, a transverse elliptical incision is made over the abdomen. The upper incision is made from one lateral lumbar region and extended to the opposite side, 3 to 4 cm above the umbilicus. The inferior incision is made from the lateral abdomen through the crease of the panniculus. The umbilicus can be saved by transplantation to the upper abdominal skin. The underlying fat is cut deeply and beyond the skin incision edges, so that the panniculus can be removed. Although meticulous hemostasis is mandatory, excessive cautery must be avoided. The angles must be incised in a V shape to remove redundant skin and to eliminate bunching of tissue. This makes a Y

incision on the skin closure. After removal of the panniculus, a vertical or transverse incision can be made. If plication of the rectus muscle and fascia is needed, a median incision is best.[145]

The second technique begins with a W incision in the lower abdomen.[147] The incision begins over the symphysis in the midline at the pubic hairline. The incision is extended downward and laterally to the inguinal ligament near the external ring. The incision is then extended upward and laterally to the iliac crest and parallel to the inguinal ligament. The upper margin is made above the umbilicus in the redundant adipose tissue. An upper flap is developed to the costal margin and the panniculus is excised. If a thin layer of adipose is left attached to the fascia, tissue fluid can be reabsorbed more readily. The umbilicus is saved and placed in the upper skin flap.

When closing the abdominal wall, the linea alba is plicated. Multiple sutures are used to anchor the upper flap to the fascia. Suction drainage is necessary to prevent excessive accumulation of tissue fluids. Skin closure may require a jackknife position.[143] Skin staples or interrupted 3–0 nylon sutures may be used to close the skin. A pressure dressing is necessary to minimize serum collection. Some make a padded plaster mold of the abdomen and use it for pressure to prevent seroma and hematoma formation. Others merely apply an elastic tape dressing (Fig. 8-28).

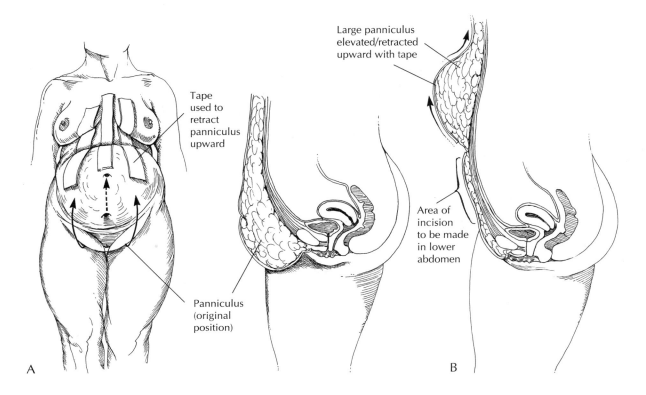

Fig. 8-26. (**A**) Panniculus retracted upward and held by wide tape. (**B**) Subumbilical incision is made.

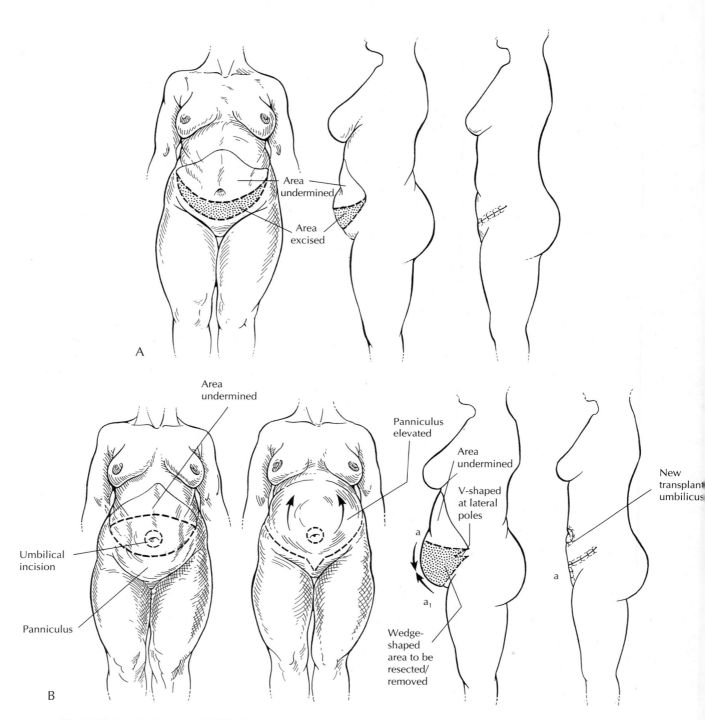

Fig. 8-27. Panniculectomy. **(A)** Elliptical transverse incision extending from one flank to the other below the umbilicus. **(B)** Elliptical transverse incision extending from one flank to the other above and below the umbilicus with V-shaped lateral poles.

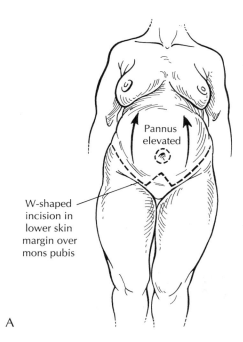

Pannus
elevated

W-shaped
incision in
lower skin
margin over
mons pubis

A

Fig. 8-28. (A) W-shaped incision made beneath the panniculus and umbilicus incised and preserved. *(Figure continues.)*

Cancer and Irradiated Surgical Fields

Cancer itself probably has little direct effect on wound healing or fascial disruption. However, many associated factors do have an impact. Poor nutrition resulting from limited intake or compromised bowel function may slow the healing process. Cancer patients are more likely to have a contaminated wound from an opened viscus or intraabdominal abscess. Postoperative ileus or collection of ascites may stress the fresh wound. The incision often must be placed in a previously irradiation field.

Because surgery and radiation are complementary treatments for many gynecologic cancers, tissue healing after operating in an irradiated field and the effects of radiation on a maturing incision are critical in regard to wound management. Much of our knowledge regarding the effects of radiation on surgical incisions has been derived from otolaryngeal surgery, which is frequently performed following primary radiotherapy. A second source is radiotherapy for treatment of keloids. Radiation effects may be divided into acute and chronic reactions.

The acute reaction consists of rapid cessation of mitotic activity, followed by cellular swelling. Edema develops in the walls of small vessels. Connective tissue becomes edematous and congested because of dilated and engorged lymphatic channels and small vessels. Radiation inhibits differentiation of fibroblast from mesenchymal cells and proliferation of endothelial cells into vascular buds. If the injury is lethal, cellular dissolution and focal necrosis may be seen.

Chronic radiation injury is caused by a progressive endar-

teritis. Endothelial swelling narrows the vessel lumen, which restricts blood flow and may even cause thrombosis. Similar effects occur in lymphatic channels. The supply of oxygen and nutrients is reduced to critical concentrations. The humoral and cellular immune defense systems function inefficiently. Proliferation of fibrous tissue causes the abdominal wall to lose suppleness, harden, and become shiny. The skin becomes pigmented and telangiectasias develops.[148] These changes, which are especially common with orthovoltage, are progressive, and many years are required for them to stop. Newer high-energy sources are relatively skin-sparing.

As with other insults, a window of vulnerability exists in regard to receiving radiotherapy. If 250 R is given 24 hours before wounding, little effect is seen on repair. The same dose administered 36 hours after wounding will maximally retard neovascularization and normal tissue contraction. Radiation effects are far more deleterious to an open wound than a closed wound. The effect is reduced to a minimum at 5 to 7 days after the incision is made. Thus, a securely healing wound that has completely epithelialized and has no serum or blood collection can be irradiated 1 week postoperatively without deleterious effects. However, radiotherapy in the face of sepsis is doomed to failure with formation of a chronic radiation ulcer.

Incision placement and timing may be modified to reduce the risk of wound complications. If surgery is performed 4 to 6 weeks after radiotherapy, healing will progress relatively normally because the severe inflammation is subsiding and blood supply is still good. As more time passes, microcirculation is diminished and long-term irradiation effects develop, presenting obstacles to incision healing. The risk of surgery rises logarithmically as the dose of irradiation increases. Sometimes incisions may be placed to avoid the irradiated field. Radiation has minimal effects on a mature wound. However, if adhesions limit peristalsis, significant bowel injury may occur.

Irradiated tissue may have insufficient blood supply to withstand an incision without necrosis. Therefore, skin incisions must never be crossed or made parallel in a field of irradiated tissue, because of significantly increased risk of necrosis, poor healing, and infection. Pain in irradiated wounds may be from ischemia. Because of susceptibility to any type of injury, any insult may trigger a cycle of necrosis and infection.

Radiation ulcers require extraordinary measures to heal completely. Daily exposure to oxygen at three atmospheres of pressure may allow spontaneous closure of a wound. Hyperbaric oxygen appears to overcome the deficient microvascular circulation. New circulation can be obtained by surgery to create pedicle flaps of skin or muscle. Pedicle grafts of omentum have been used to fill large tissue defects.[149]

Patients who have undergone preoperative radiation have delayed healing, reduced tensile strength, and increased risk of infection. The increased risk of dehiscences warrants a closure technique that provides long-lasting support to the incision. Permanent suture materials have been shown to

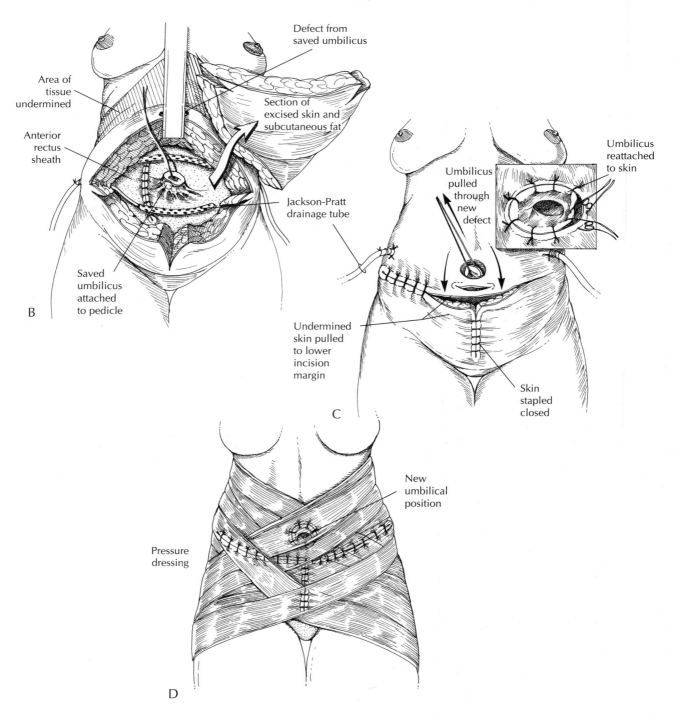

Fig. 8-28 *(Continued).* **(B)** Undermined skin is pulled to the lower incision and excess skin excised. **(C)** Umbilicus repositioned in upper flap and W incision closed. **(D)** Pressure dressing applied.

reduce wound complications.[142] Delayed absorbable synthetic suture also may be appropriate for some patients.[150] The author believes that an abdominal wound in an irradiated field should always be closed with some form of retention suture and recommend a running mass closure with monofilament synthetic sutures.

SUMMARY

Success of any operation depends on a wisely chosen incision based on sound anatomic principles, and on meticulous closure with a technique that will result in a secure wound. The gynecologic surgeon has the responsibility of deciding which abdominal incision is best suited for a surgical procedure and which closure technique will provide adequate security. Selection of an incision that provides optimal access to the surgical field is critical because limited exposure will make the procedure more difficult and harbors potential dangers. Because wound complications may have no obvious cause, and because recognizing high-risk patients is not always possible, many advocate using the most secure closure possible in all patients. Closure techniques that use a continuous monofilament permanent synthetic suture and wide bites reduce the incidence of dehiscence. Because many pitfalls await the unsuspecting surgeon, care must be taken to guard against habit and to select an incision and closure appropriate to the task. In an effort to avoid the inherent risk of abdominal incisions, minimally invasive procedures such as operative laparoscopy have been developed and alternative approaches, such as vaginal hysterectomy, have been advocated. Both may have an expanded role in the future.

REFERENCES

1. Langer K: Cleavage of the curia (the anatomy and physiology of the skin). Presented at the Meeting of the Royal Academy of Sciences, April 25, 1861. Clin Orthop 91:3, 1973

2. Tobin CE, Benjamin JA: Anatomic and clinical re-evaluation of Camper's Scarpa's and Colles' fascia. Surg Gynecol Obstet 88:545, 1949

3. Forster DS: A note on Scarpa's fascia. J Anat 72:130, 1937

4. Milloy FJ, Anson BJ, McAfee DK: The rectus abdominis muscle and the epigastric arteries. Surg Gynecol Obstet 110: 293, 1960

5. Anson BJ: An Atlas of Human Anatomy. p. 241. WB Saunders, Philadephia, 1950

6. Nahai F, Brown RG, Vasconez LO: Blood supply to the abdominal wall as related to planning abdominal incisions. Am Surg 42:691, 1976

7. Sippo WC, Burghardt A, Gomez AC: Nerve entrapment after Pfannensteil incision. Am J Obstet Gynecol 157:420, 1987

8. Schneiderman BI, Bomze E: Paresthesias of the lateral cutaneous nerve after pelvic surgery. Am Surg 33:84, 1967

9. Kvist-Poulsen H, Borel J: Iatrogenic femoral neuropathy subsequent to abdominal hysterectomy: incidence and prevention. Obstet Gynecol 60:516, 1982

10. Stulz P, Pfeiffer KM: Peripheral nerve injuries resulting from common surgical procedures in the lower abdomen. Arch Surg 117:324, 1982

11. Laufman H: Current use of skin and wound cleansers and antiseptics. Am J Surg 157:359, 1989

12. Peterson AF, Rosenberg A, Alatary SO: Comparative evaluation of surgical scrub preparations. Surg Gynecol Obstet 146: 63, 1978

13. Berry AR, Watt B, Goldacre MJ et al: A comparison of the use of povidone-iodine and chlorhexidine in the prophylaxis of post operative wound infection. J Hosp Infect 2:55, 1982

14. Cruse PJE, Ford R: The epidemiology of wound infection: a 10-year prospective study of 62,939 wounds. Surg Clin North Am 60:27, 1980

15. Madden JE, Edlich RF, Custer JR et al: Studies in the management of contaminated wounds. IV. Resistance to infection of surgical wounds made by knife, electrosurgery and laser. Am J Surg 119:222, 1970

16. Christopherson WA: Surgical incisions and their anatomic basis. p. 29. Buchsbaum HJ, Walton LA (ed): Strategies in Gynecologic Surgery. Springer-Verlag, New York, 1986

17. Everett HS, Mattingly RF: Urinary tract injuries resulting from pelvic surgery. Am J Obstet 71:702, 1956

18. Ellis H: Midline abdominal incisions. Br J Obstet Gynaecol 91:1, 1984

19. Paes TR, Stoker DL, Ng T, Morecroft J: Circumbilical versus transumbilical abdominal incision. Br J Surg 74:822, 1987

20. Cox PJ, Ausobsky JR, Ellis H, Pollock AV: Towards no incisional hernias: lateral paramedian versus midline incisions. J R Soc Med 79:711, 1986

21. Guillou PJ, Hall TJ, Donaldson DR et al: Vertical abdominal incisions: a choice? Br J Surg 67:395, 1980

22. Calahane MJ, Shapiro ME, Silen W: Abdominal incision: decision or indecision. Lancet 1:146, 1989

23. Skandalakis JE, Gray SW, Rowe JS: Anatomical Complications in General Surgery. McGraw-Hill, New York, 1983

24. Speert H: Obstetric and Gynecologic Milestones. p. 630. Macmillan, New York, 1958

25. Pfannenstiel J: Ueber die Vortheile des suprasymphysaren Fascienquerschnitts für die gynäkologischen Koliotomien zugleich ein Beitrag zu der Indikationsstellung der Operationswege. Samml Klin Vortr (Leipzig) 268:1735, 1900

26. Griffiths DA: A reappraisal of the Pfannenstiel incision. Br J Urol 48:469, 1976

27. Cherney LS: A modified transverse incision for low abdominal operations. Surg Gynecol Obstet 72:92, 1941

28. Brand E: Letter to the editor. Am J Obstet Gynecol 165:235, 1991

29. Mackenrodt A: Die Radikaloperation des Gebärmutterscheidenkrebses mit. Ausräumung des Becken. Verh Dtsch Gynäkol ix:139, 1901

30. Maylard, AE: Direction of abdominal incisions Br J Med 2: 895, 1907

31. Krupski WC, Sumchai A, Effeney DJ, Ehrenfeld WK: The importance of abdominal wall collateral blood vessels. Arch Surg 119:854, 1984

32. Küstner O: Der suprasymphysare kreuzschnitt, eine methode der coeliotomie bei wenig umfanglichen affectioen der weiblichen beckenorgane. Monatsschr Geburtsh Gynäkol 4: 197, 1896

33. Turner-Warwick R, Worth P, Milroy E, Duckett J: The suprapubic V incision. Br J Urol 46:39, 1974

34. McBurney C: The incision made in the abdominal wall in cases of appendicitis, with a description of a new method of operating. Ann Surg 20:38, 1894

35. Delaney HM, Carnevale NJ: A ''bikini'' incision for appendectomy. Am J Surg 132:126, 1976
36. Hajj SN, Mercer LJ, Ismail MA: Surgical approaches to pelvic infections in women. J Repro Med 33:159, 1988
37. Leibovich SJ, Ross R: The role of macropaghes in wound repair. Am J Pathol 78:71, 1975
38. Odland G, Ross R: Human wound repair. I. Epidermal regeneration. J Cell Biol 39:135, 1968
39. Ross R, Everett NB, Tyler R: Wound healing and collagen formation. VI. The origin of the wound fibroblast studies in parabiosis. J Cell Biol 44:645, 1970
40. Doillon CJ, Dunn MG, Bender E, Silverr FH: Collagen fiber formation in repair tissue: development of strength and toughness. Coll Relat Res 5:481, 1985
41. Haukipuro K: Synthesis of collagen types I and III in reincised wounds in humans. Br J Surg 78:708, 1991
42. Howes EL, Harvey SC: The strength of the healing wound in relation to the holding strength of the catgut suture. N Engl J Med 200:1285, 1929
43. Douglas DM: Tensile strength of sutures: less when implanted in living Tissue. Lancet 2:499, 1949
44. Moloney GE: The effect of human tissues on the tensile strength of implanted nylon sutures. Br J Surg 48:528, 1961
45. Bourne RB, Bitar H, Andreae PR et al: In-vivo comparison of four absorbable sutures: Vicryl, Dexon plus, Maxon, and PDS. Can J Surg 31:43, 1988
46. van Rijssel EJC, Brand R, Admiraal C et al: Tissue reaction and surgical knots: the effect of suture size, knot configuration and knot volume. Obstet Gynecol 74:64, 1989
47. Sanz LE, Patterson JA, Kamath R et al: Comparison of Maxon suture with Vicryl, chromic catgut, and PDS sutures in fascial closure in rats. Obstet Gynecol 71:418, 1988
48. Rodeheaver GT, Borzelleca DC, Thacker JG, Edlich RF: Unique performance characteristics of Novafil. Surg Gynecol Obstet 164:230, 1987
49. Alexander JW, Kaplan JZ, Altemeier WA: Role of suture material in the development of wound infection. Ann Surg 165:192, 1967
50. McGeechan D, Hunt D, Chadhuri A, Rutter P: An experimental study of the relationship between synergistic wound sepsis and suture materials. Br J Surg 67:636, 1980
51. Thiede A: Controlled experimental histological and microbiological studies on the inhbition of infection by polyglycolic acid. Chirurg 51:35, 1980
52. diZerega GS: The peritoneum and its response to surgical injury. p. 1. In diZerega GS, Malinak LR, Diamond MP, Linsky CB (eds): Treatment of Post Surgical Adhesions. Wiley-Liss, New York, 1990
53. Karipineni RC, Wilk PJ, Danese CA: The role of peritoneum in the healing of abdominal incisions. Surg Gynecol Obstet 142:729, 1976
54. Tulandi T, Hum HS, Gelfand MM: Closure of laparotomy incisions with or without peritoneal suturing and second look laparoscopy. Am J Obstet Gynecol 158:536, 1988
55. Adamsons RJ, Musco F, Enquist IF: The chemical dimensions of a healing incision. Surg Gynecol Obstet 123:515, 1966
56. Grillo HC, Gross J: Enzyme found in healing wound. Medical World News 6:38, 1965
57. Foresman AF, Edlich RF, Rodeheaver GT: The effect of new monofilament absorbale suture on healing of muscular aponeurotic incisions, gastrostomies, and colonic anastomosis. Arch Surg 124:708, 1989
58. Douglas DM: The healing of aponeurotic incisions. Br J Surg 40:79, 1962
59. Bartlett LC: Pressure necrosis is the primary cause of wound dehiscence. Can J Surg 28:27, 1985
60. Fagniez PL, Hay JM, Lacaine F, Thomsen C: Abdominal midline incision closure: a multicentric randomized prospective trial of 3,135 patients, comparing continuous vs. interrupted polyglycolic acid sutures. Arch Surg 120:1351, 1985
61. Poole GV, Meredith JW, Kon ND et al: Suture technique and wound bursting strength. Am Surg 50:569, 1984
62. Orr JW, Orr PF, Barrett JM et al: Continuous or interrupted fascial closure: a prospective evaluation of No. 1 Maxon suture in 402 gynecologic procedures. Am J Obstet Gynecol 163:1485, 1990
63. Jones TE, Newell ET, Brubaker RE: The use of alloy steel wire in the closure of abdominal wounds. Burg Gynecol Obstet 72:1056, 1941
64. Larsen JS, Ulin AW: Tensile strength advantage of the far-and-near suture technique. Surg Gynecol Obstet 131:123, 1970
65. Kirk RM: Effect of method of opening and closing the abdomen on incidence of wound bursting. Lancet 2:352, 1972
66. Leaper DJ, Pollack AV, Evans M: Abdominal wound closure: a trial of nylon, polyglycolic acid and steel sutures. Br J Burg 64:603, 1977
67. Gallup DG, Talledo EO, King LA: Primary mass closure of midline incisions with a continuous running monofilament suture in gynecologic patients. Obstet Gynecol 73:674, 1989
68. Chez RA, McDuff HC: The Pfannenstiel incision. Contemp Ob-Gyn 7:55, 1976
69. Del Valle GO, Combs P, Qualls C, Curet LB: Does closure of Camper's fascia reduce the incidence of post-cesarean superficial wound disruption Obstet Gynecol 80:1013, 1992
70. Gottrup F, Fogdestam I, Hunt TK: Delayed primary closure: an experimental and clinical review. J Clin Surg 1:113, 1982
71. Marcus R: Surveillance of health care workers exposed to blood from patients infected with the human immunodeficiency virus. N Engl J Med 319:1118, 1988
72. Montz FJ, Fowler JM, Farias-Eisener R: Blunt needles in fascial closure. Surg Gynecol Obstet 173:147, 1991
73. van Rijssel EJC, Trimbos JB, Booster MH: Mechanical performance of square knots and sliding knots in surgery: a comparative study. Am J Obstet Gynecol 162:93, 1990
74. Tera H, Aberg C: Strength of knots in surgery in relation to type of knot, type of suture material and dimension of suture thread. Acta Chir Scand 143:75, 1977

75. Cutler EC, Dunphy JE: The use of silk in infected wounds. N Engl J Med 224:101, 1941

76. Usher FC, Allen JE, Crosthwait RW, Cogan JE: Polypropylene monofilament: a new biologically inert suture for closing contaminated wounds. JAMA 179:780, 1962

76a. Magee C, Rodeheaver GT, Golden GT et al: Potentiation of wound infection by surgical drains. Am J Surg 131:547, 1976

76b. Dougherty SH, Simmons RL: The biology and practice of surgical drains. Part I. Curr Probl Surg 29:559, 1992

76c. Dougherty SH, Simmons RL: The biology and practice of surgical drains. Part II. Curr Probl Surg 29:635, 1992

76d. van Nagel JR, Schiwietz DP: Surgical adjuncts in radical hysterectomy and pelvic lymphadenectomy. Surg Gynecol Obstet 143:735, 1976

76e. Wijma J, Kauer FM, Van Saene HKF et al: Antibiotics and suction drainage as prophylaxis in vaginal abdominal hysterectomy. Obstet Gynecol 70:384, 1987

76f. Abitbol MM: Carcinoma of the vulva: improvement in the surgical approach. Am J Obstet Gynecol 117:483, 1973

76g. Alexander JW, Korelitz J, Alexander NS: Prevention of wound infections: a case for closed suction drainage to remove wound fluids deficient in opsonic proteins. Am J Surg 132:59, 1976

76h. Raves JJ, Slifkin M, Diamond DL: A bacteriologic study comparing closed suction and simple conduit drainage. Am J Surg 148:618, 1984

76i. LaBlanc KA, Tucker WY: Prophylactic antibiotics and closed tube thoracostomy. Surg Gynecol Obstet 160:259, 1985

76j. Farnell MB, Worthington-Self S, Mucha P et al: Closure of abdominal incisions with subcutaneous catheters. A prospective randomized trial. Arch Surg 121:641, 1986

76k. Platt R, Zaleznik DF, Hopkins CC et al: Perioperative antibiotic prophylaxis for herniorrhaphy and breast surgery. N Engl J Med 322:153, 1990

77. Piver MS, Malfetano JH, Lele SB, Moore RH: Prophylactic anticoagulation as a possible cause of inguinal lymphocyst after radical vulvectomy and inguinal lymphadenectomy. Obstet Gynecol 62:17, 1983

78. Magee C, Rodehaever GT, Golden GT et al: Potentiation of wound infection by surgical drains. Am J Surg 131:547, 1976

79. Hudson AR, Hunter GA, Waddell JP: Iatrogenic femoral nerve injuries. Can J Surg 22:62, 1979

80. Sippo WC, Gomez A: Nerve-entrapment syndromes from lower abdominal surgery. J Fam Pract 25:585, 1987

81. Grosz CR: Iliohypogastric nerve injury. Am J Surg 142:628, 1981

82. McDaniel GC, Kirkley WH, Gilbert SC: Femoral nerve injury associated with the Pfannenstiel incision and abdominal retractors. Am J Obstet Gynecol 87:381, 1963

83. Vosburg LF, Finn WF: Femoral nerve impairment subsequent to hysterectomy. Am J Obstet Gynecol 82:931, 1961

84. Cole WR, Bernard HR: Inadequacies of present methods of skin preparation. Arch Surg 89:215, 1964

85. Condie JD, Ferguson DJ: Experimental wound infections: contamination versus surgical technique. Surgery 50:367, 1961

86. Stevenson TR, Rodeheaver GT, Golden GT et al: Damage to tissue defenses by vasoconstrictors. J Am Coll Emerg Phys 4:532, 1975

87. Cederna JP, Davies BW, Farkas SA et al: Necrotizing fasciitis of the total abdominal wall after sterilization by partial salpingectomy. Am J Obstet Gynecol 162:138, 1990

88. Dodson MK, Magann EF, Meeks GR: A randomized trial of secondary wound closure and closure by secondary intention in superficial wound dehiscence. Obstet Gynecol 80:321, 1992

89. Lyon JB, Richardson AC: Careful surgical technique can reduce infectious morbidity after cesarean section. Am J Obstet Gynecol 157:557, 1987

90. Moss JP: Historical and current perspectives on surgical drainage. Surg Gynecol Obstet 152:518, 1981

91. Loudon MA, Barua JM: A novel and convenient method of delayed primary skin closure for grossly contaminated abdominal wounds. J R Coll Surg Edinb 39:47, 1994

92. Hemsell DL, Hemsell PG, Heard Ml, Nobles BJ: Preoperative cefoxitin prophylaxis for elective abdominal hysterectomy. Am J Obstet Gynecol 153:225, 1985

93. Mamsen A, Hansen V, Moller BR: A prospective randomized double-blind trial of ceftriaxone versus no treatment for abdominal hysterectomy. Eur J Obstet Gynecol Repro Biol 47:235, 1992

94. Guiney EJ, Morris PF, Donaldson GA: Wound dehiscence: a continuing problem in abdominal surgery. Arch Surg 92:47, 1966

95. Banerjee SR, Daoud I, Russel JC, Becker D: Abdominal wound evisceration. Curr Surg 40:432, 1983

96. Baggish M, Lee W: Abdominal wound disruption. Obstet Gynecol 46:530, 1975

97. Pratt J: Wound healing: evisceration. Am J Obstet Gynecol 132:165, 1973

98. Ellis HY, Gajraj H, George C: Incisional hernias: when do they occur? Br J Surg 170:290, 1983

99. Akman PC: A Study of five hundred incisional hernias. J Int Coll Surg 37:125, 1962

100. Tweedie FJ, Long RC: Abdominal wound disruption. Surg Gynecol Obstet 99:41, 1954

101. Penninckx FM, Poelmans SV, Kerremans RP, Beckers JP: Abdominal wall dehiscence in gastroenterological surgery. Ann Surg 189:345, 1979

102. Pitkin RM: Abdominal hysterectomy in obese women. Surg Gynecol Obstet 143:532, 1976

103. White H, Cook J, Ward M: Abdominal wound dehiscence: a ten year survey from a district general hospital. Ann R Coll Surg Engl 59:337, 1977

104. Bartlett L: Pressure necrosis is the primary cause of wound dehiscence. Can J Surg 28:27, 1985

105. Daveson B, Landers D: Physiological advantages of the transverse incision in gynecology. Obstet Gynecol 17:305, 1961

106. McGinn FP, Hamilton JC: Ascorbic acid levels in stored

blood in patients undergoing surgery after blood transfusion. Br J Surg 63:505, 1976

107. Nayman J, McDermott FT, Gurr GW: Wound dehiscence in acute renal failure. Med J Aust 1:799, 1969

108. Androulakakis PA: Uraemia and wound healing. Br J Surg 67:380, 1980

109. Moffat FL, Deitel M, Thompson DA: Abdominal surgery in patients undergoing long-term peritoneal dialysis. Surgery 92:598, 1982

110. Colin JF, Elliot P, Ellis H: The effect of uraemia upon healing: an experimental study. Br J Surg 66:793, 1979

111. Armstrong CP, Dixon JM, Duffy SW et al: Wound healing in obstructive jaundice. Br J Surg 71:267, 1984

112. Bayer I, Ellis H: Jaundice and wound healing: an experimental study. Br J Surg 63:392, 1976

113. Pasulkas P, Bistrian B, Benoitti P, Blackburn G: The risks of surgery in obese patients. Ann Intern Med 104:540, 1986

114. Alexander HC, Prudden JF: The causes of abdominal wound disruption. Surg Gynecol Obstet 122:1223, 1966

115. Goodson HIW, Hunt TK: Wound healing and the diabetic patient. Surg Gynecol Obstet 149:600, 1979

116. Trapnell J: Management of the complications of acute pancreatitis. Ann R Coll Surg Engl 49:361, 1971

117. Oxlund H, Fogdestam I, Viidik A: The influence of cortisol on wound healing of the skin and distant connective tissue response. Surg Gynecol Obstet 148:876, 1979

118. Sloan GA: A new upper abdominal incision. Surg Gynecol Obstet 45:678, 1927

119. Donaldson DR, Hegarty JH, Brennan TG et al: The lateral paramedian incision: experience with 850 cases. Br J Surg 69:630, 1982

120. Grenall MJ, Evan M, Pollock AV: Midline or transverse laparotomy? A random controlled trial. Part I: influence on healing. Br J Surg 67:188, 1980

121. Sanders RJ, DiClemente D: Principles of abdominal wound closure. II. Prevention of wound dehiscence. Arch Surg 122:1188, 1977

122. Ellis H, Coleridge-Smith PD, Joyce AD: Abdominal incisions—vertical or transverse? Postgrad Med J 60:407, 1984

123. Ellis H, Bucknall TE, Cox PJ: Abdominal incisions and their closure. Curr Probl Surg 22:4, 1985

124. Greenburg G, Saik RP, Peskin GW: Wound dehiscence: pathophysiology and prevention. Arch Surg 114:143, 1979

125. Herrmann JB: Changes in tensile strength and knot security of surgical sutures in vivo. Arch Surg 106:707, 1973

126. Goligher JC, Irvin TT, Johnston D et al: A controlled clinical trial of three methods of closure of laparotomy wounds. Br J Surg 62:823, 1975

127. Leaper DJ, Rolenberg IL, Evans M, Pollock AV: The influence of suture materials on abdominal wall healing assessed by controlled clinical trials. Eur Surg Res 8:75, 1976

128. Tagart REB: The suturing of abdominal incisions: a comparison of monofilament nylon and catgut. Br Med J 54:952, 1967

129. Bucknall TE, Ellis H: Abdominal wound closure: a comparison of monofilament nylon and polyglycolic acid. Surgery 89:672, 1981

130. Alexander HC, Prudden JF: The causes of abdominal wound disruption. Surg Gynecol Obstet 122:1223, 1966

131. Wolff WI: Disruption of abdominal wounds. Ann Surg 131:534, 1950

132. Tera H, Aberg C: Tissue strength of structures involved in musculo-aponeurotic layer sutures in laparotomy incisions. Acta Chir Scand 142:349, 1976

133. Masterson BJ: Selection of incisions for gynecologic procedures. Surg Clin North Am 71:1041, 1991

134. Bucknall TE: The effect of local infection upon wound healing: an experimental study. Br J Surg 67:851, 1980

135. Pollock AV: Laparotomy. J R Soc Med 74:480, 1981

136. Postlethwaite RW: Five year study of tissue reaction to synthetic suture. Ann Surg 190:54, 1979

137. Rappaport W, Allen R, Chvapil M et al: A comparison of parallel versus perpendicular placement of retention sutures in abdominal closure. Am Surg 56:618, 1990

138. Higgins GA, Antkowiak JG, Esterkyn SH: A clinical and laboratory study of abdominal wound closure and dehiscence. Arch Surg 98:421, 1969

139. Wallace D, Hernandez W, Schlaerth JB et al: Prevention of abdominal wound disruption utilizing the Smead-Jones closure technique. Obstet Gynecol 56:226, 1980

140. Poole G Jr: Mechanical factors in abdominal wound closures: the prevention of fascial dehiscence. Surgery 97:631, 1985

141. Krebs HB, Helmkamp BF: Transverse periumbilical incision in the massively obese patient. Obstet Gynecol 63:241, 1984

142. Morrow CP, Hernandez WI, Townsend DE, Disaia PJ: Pelvic celiotomy in the obese patient. Am J Obstet Gynecol 127:335, 1977

143. Greer BE, Cain JM, Figge DC et al: Supraumbilical incisions for pelvic surgery in the morbidly obese patient. Obstet Gynecol 76:471, 1990

144. Gallup DG: Modifications of celiotomy techniques to decrease morbidity in obese gynecology patients. Am J Obstet Gynecol 150:171, 1984

145. Kelly HA: Excision of the fat of the abdominal wall: lipectomy. Surg Gynecol Obstet 10:229, 1910

146. Pratt JH, Irons GB: Panniculectomy and abdominoplasty. Am J Obstet Gynecol 132:165, 1978

147. Reginault P: Abdominoplasty by the W technique. Plant Reconstr Surg 55:265, 1975

148. Telok HA, Mason ML, Wheelock MD: Histopathologic study of radiation injuries of skin. Surg Gynecol Obstet 90:335, 1950

149. Grillo HC, Potsaid MS: Studies in wound healing. IV. Retardation of contraction by local X irradiation and observations relating to the origin of fibroblastic repair. Ann Surg 154:471, 1961

150. Hoffman MS, Villa A, Roberts WS et al: Mass closure of abdominal wound with delayed absorbable suture in surgery for gynecologic cancer. J Repro Med 6:356, 1991

CHAPTER NINE

GYNECOLOGIC SURGICAL INSTRUMENTS

JOHN JENNINGS

Surgical Knives
Needle-Holders
Forceps
Hemostatic Clamps
Hysterectomy Clamps
Scissors
Retractors
Suction Devices
Cervical Dilators
Ligature Carriers
Stapling Devices
Laparoscopic
  Instruments

It has been said that "a good carpenter knows his tools." In the same manner, skilled surgeons must know the applications and limitations of the instruments they regularly use. Novice surgeons usually select instruments according to the advice and habits of their surgical mentors. Personal experience modifies and often limits the selection of instruments eventually used by the advanced surgeon. The economic forces at work to standardize operative costs may further limit the choice of instrumentation. Surgical instruments are in many ways simply extensions of the human hand. There is inevitably a "feel" for different instruments designed to accomplish the same purpose. This chapter is an effort to familiarize the reader with basic gynecologic surgery instrumentation and advantages of individual instruments. The chapter is in no way intended as an endorsement of any particular manufacturer or supplier; the author has made a conscientious effort to state certain preferences for instrumentation based on experience but with the recognition of satisfactory alternatives.

SURGICAL KNIVES

The exposure and conduct of a surgical procedure depends on the use of sharp cutting instruments that are properly chosen to accomplish a specific task. The traditional surgical scalpel, available in a variety of sizes and shapes, is adequate for most gynecologic procedures. Electrosurgical cutting instruments are certainly the preference of some surgeons, and it is a matter of some fact and much opinion, whether there is a significant difference in outcome with use of either instrument.[1]

Blades are firmly attached, usually with a needle-holder, to the scalpel handle. The Bard-Parker handle has a general utility, and all blades that are commonly used during gynecologic surgeries will fit this handle. The length of the knife handle to be used depends on the surgical task. Shorter handles are easier to control and are best used for making skin incisions and for working in shallow incisions. Longer handles are particularly useful in a deep pelvis. Resting the operating hand on the abdominal wall or against a self-retaining retractor can improve the surgeon's control of the knife (Fig. 9-1).

Scalpel blades have been designed in various sizes and shapes to accommodate special purposes. Abdominal incisions are best made with either a #20 or a #22 Bard-Parker blade. The #22 is the most versatile; this blade can be used through the fascial incision and to open the peritoneum. (There is no evidence to show that it is necessary to have a separate "skin knife" and "deep knife."[2]) The #15 blade has a small cutting area, which increases safety when a scalpel is used in a tight operative field. This #15 blade is also useful for making small skin incisions that are necessary for laparoscopic procedures, postpartum sterilizations, and drain incisions. The #11 blade is ideally suited for incision and drainage procedures. Its sharply pointed design both defines and limits its use. An angled scalpel handle, which has this spear-pointed design, is frequently used for cold knife cervical conization[3] (Fig. 9-2).

Disposable surgical knife blades are uniformly very sharp. They will dull when incising rigid abdominal scar tissue or if inadvertently scraped against a metal surface such as previously placed wire suture material. A dull blade can be hazardous because it may require the surgeon to sacrifice control by varying the pressure applied to the knife to accomplish the desired cut. It is possible to carefully use the knife handle for blunt dissection, but the cutting edge of the blade must be directed away from all hands in the operative field.

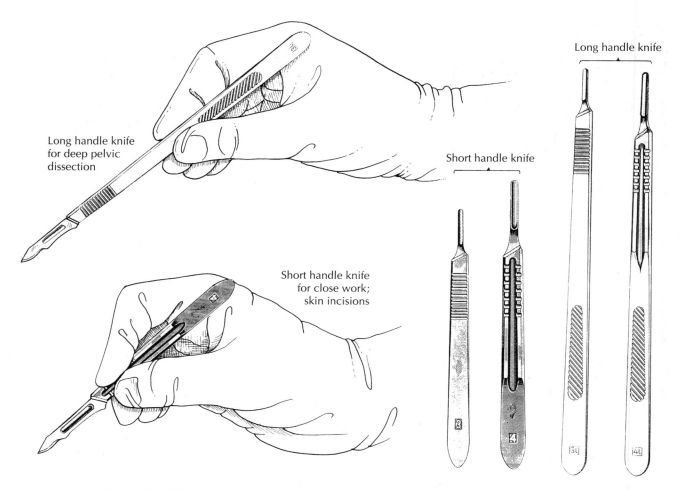

Fig. 9-1. Knife handles are manufactured in varying lengths and grips for different surgical tasks.

If unintentional injury to the patient or to the surgical assistants is to be avoided, the sharpness of the surgical knife must be constantly respected. After use, the knife should be given handle-first to the scrub assistant. A knife should never be in the surgical field unless it is in the control of the surgeon's hand, and should never be laid on the drapes of the operative field.

The use of electrosurgical cutting instruments requires an understanding of the physics of electricity, which are no less complicated than those of the laser.[4] The current waveform can be modified to facilitate either a cutting or a coagulation mode. Current waveforms can also be blended for simultaneous cutting and coagulation. A cutting current can be applied to a knife, a wire, a band loop, a snare, a microneedle, or energized scalpels or scissors (Fig. 9-3).

Regardless of the form of the electrode, the surgeon must consider the intensity of the current as well as the output impedance of the generator. It must be recognized that the current density on the contact surface of the cutting instrument will determine the depth of tissue damage that will occur. Surgery is not a barbecue, and the goal of the use of electrosurgical incision should be to inflict minimal tissue

trauma while simultaneously providing hemostasis.[5] Electrosurgical cutting instruments, when properly used, may add dimension to the surgeon's technique but should not be considered to be an absolute replacement for the traditional, nonelectrified scalpel. Most gynecologic patients have good small vessel hemostatic mechanisms that do not require the surgeon's attention. An incision made with a sharp scalpel with electrocoagulation or suture ligature of larger vessels may still be the least traumatic to tissue.[6]

NEEDLE-HOLDERS

The surgical needle-holder's purpose is to firmly hold a curved surgical needle as it is passed through tissue, to easily release the needle, and then to easily regrasp the needle. Much effort has been directed to the design of needle-holders, because the accurate placement and recovery of the needle can be critical in preventing unnecessary bleeding and tissue damage.[7] Ideally, the needle-holder should be designed to firmly grasp the needle without flattening or bending it or damaging the suture material.[8] The jaws of most

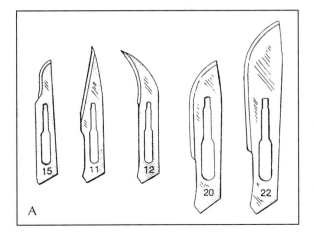

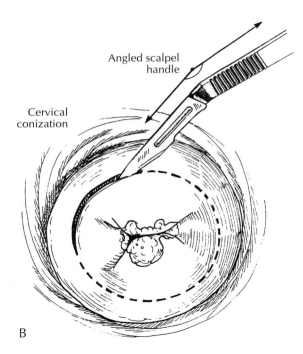

Fig. 9-2. (A) Scalpels most commonly used by gynecologic surgeons. (B) The angled scalpel is useful in performing cervical conization.

needle-holders are flat and have the potential to bend smaller radius or smaller caliber needles.[9] In gynecologic surgery, much of the critical placement of sutures requires only one or two passes through tissue. Consequently, the ability of the needle-holder to accurately drive the needle through tissue is more important than its damage to a needle that will be discarded.[10] It is not unusual for a surgeon to use a larger caliber needle during pelvic surgery. The needle-holder should have jaw strength that is sufficient to hold these needles without springing. Smaller radius needles can be protected from bending with the use of a needle-holder with

a narrower jaw; however, this will sacrifice some of the holder's firmness of grasp and decrease the needle's potential to roll, depending on the tissue resistance.

The quality of needle sharpness is important to the performance of the needle-holder. A sharp needle causes less tissue trauma and requires less force to pass through tissue. Additionally, there is reduced tendency for needles to bend or break if the needle is optimally sharp. Currently, surgical needles are manufactured to resist breakage,[11] but the improper use of the needle-holder and a poor choice of needle can lead to an unpleasant, painstaking, and sometimes futile search for a retained broken needle. Although it is scientifically possible to reduce needle bending and breakage by matching strengths of needle-holders and needles,[12] the same needle-holder is usually used for multiple needle types during the same procedure.

For gynecologic surgery, needle-holders must be available in short, medium, and long lengths. In some cases, only long instruments can be used for safe suture placement. However, for most gynecologic cases, the 8-in. needle-holder is adequate. The straight-jawed needle-holder (Fig. 9-4) has the most utility in pelvic surgery. The exit of the needle from the tissue is predictable, and there is less tendency for the needle to roll in firm tissue. The straight needle-holder is also more forgiving when regrasping needles, because the functional length of the jaws is longer than that of curved needle-holders. Some gynecologic surgeons prefer a curved needle-holder, such as the Heaney design (Fig. 9-5A), for use in vaginal surgery.[13] There is a reasonable argument that this type of needle-holder allows easier visualization of needle placement, although possibly at the expense of more difficult visualization of needle exit. A double-curved Stratte needle-holder (Fig. 9-5B) has a distinct advantage in the tight confines of the retropubic space during urethral or paravaginal suspension procedures: the unique curvature of this needle-holder can allow the operator to effectively place the sutures without the hand obscuring visualization.

Needle-holders are generally designed with a locking mechanism that requires an opposite action for locking and unlocking.[3] For a right-handed surgeon, this motion becomes very natural and is easy to master, because the thumb of the right hand can easily produce the motion to lock or unlock the needle-holder. Left-handed surgeons may have less difficulty with an offset locking mechanism that requires only a push-push or squeezing motion to lock and unlock the needle holder[14] (Fig. 9-6). Regardless of the type of locking mechanism, the surgeon's own experience is the most important factor in preventing poorly timed needle release.

FORCEPS

Surgical forceps serve as an extension of surgeon's thumb and index finger. The design of all forceps is very similar except for differences in the length, width, and type of sur-

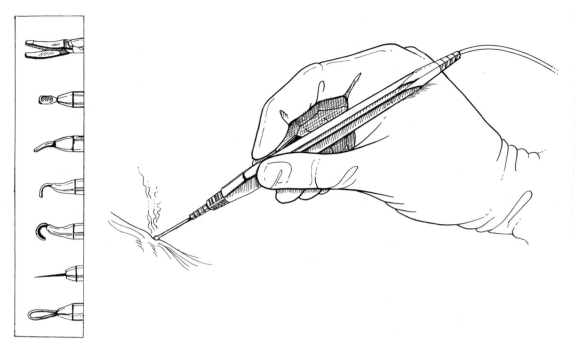

Fig. 9-3. Electrosurgical cutting instruments come in a variety of designs useful for both open laparotomy and laparoscopic procedures.

face that grips the tissue.[3] The colloquial term ''pickup'' that is used interchangeably with ''forceps'' implies a limited function that is not accurate. Surgical forceps are, in reality, quite satisfactory transmitters of most functions that are performed by the thumb and index finger, and enable these functions to be performed in limited spaces with limited areas of grasp. Variations of the widths and textures of the grasping surfaces and the lengths of the shafts have widened the range of surgical needs that forceps can meet. Notably, forceps do not substitute for the tactile sensation of the surgeon's fingertips. (This is one area in which laparoscopic surgery is at a disadvantage—the complete use of instruments prohibits being able to ''just see what it feels like.'')

Knowledge of how to handle forceps has become increasingly important. Transmission of disease by body fluids can be reduced by decreased direct tissue handling and by keeping hands out of surgical fields where sharp instruments are being passed through tissue.[15] Needle-stick injuries can be reduced significantly with the proper handling of tissue with forceps. Most novice surgeons tend to use their hands to reload needles on holders outside of the surgical site. Obstetricians and gynecologists are likely to develop this bad habit when repairing episiotomies without assistance. The proper selection and use of forceps is a good demonstration of a surgeon's experience; it reflects consideration for the gentle handling of the patient's tissue, minimizes risk of needle sticks, and facilitates better visualization of the operative field.

Tissue forceps are tissue forceps. They are not designed

to handle metal instruments or needles; they are designed to handle tissue. Although the tensile strength of most forceps is such that considerable trauma is required to damage them, it is possible to ''spring'' the forceps or change the alignment of the grasping surface with improper use. Retrieving needles with forceps is sometimes necessary and expeditious. Ideally, the forceps should be used to grasp the tissue through which the needle is to be passed and to hold the tissue until the needle has completed its arc and has been regrasped by the needle-holder. Repositioning of the needle on the needle-holder is sometimes necessary with this technique; it is possible to perform this maneuver with minimal stress on the forceps and little risk of damage to the instrument.

Gynecologists, like other surgeons, tend to develop individual prejudices for certain types of forceps. Most can readily defend their choices, if for no better reason than it is ''what I am accustomed to using.'' Adson forceps and the Brown-Adson modification are commonly used for handling the skin. Brown-Adson forceps seem to be somewhat superior because the design of the jaws allows easy manipulation of skin (Fig. 9-7). The texture of fascial tissue requires the grasping design of instruments such as the Martin forceps (Fig. 9-8A), Bonney forceps (Fig. 9-8B), Russian forceps (Fig. 9-8C), or the Potts-Smith forceps with teeth (Fig. 9-8D). Many obstetricians and gynecologists learn to use the Russian forceps when doing cesarean sections and subsequently transfer this habit to gynecologic procedures. These forceps have a rather large grasping surface and are particu-

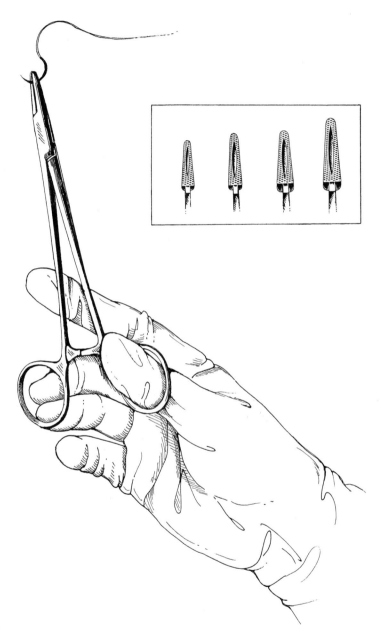

Fig. 9-4. Straight needle-holder. Needle-gripping surfaces are pictured in the inset.

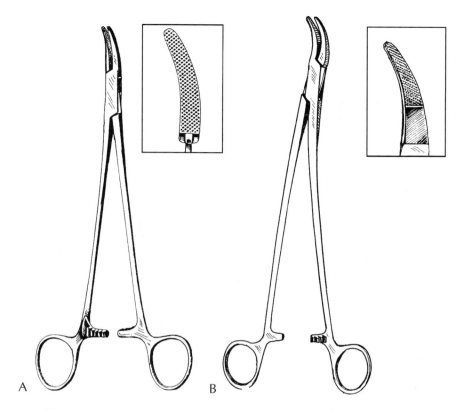

Fig. 9-5. **(A)** Heaney needle-holder. **(B)** Double-curved Stratte needle-holder.

larly suitable for use in closure of the uterus at cesarean. If it is necessary to grasp with tension, a rather wide bite of tissue is required. Martin forceps have two teeth and a serrated grasping surface that will firmly hold tissue. Bonney forceps have multiple smaller teeth and may be less traumatic without sacrificing grasping efficiency. The Potts-Smith forceps with teeth have a smaller grasping surface, but the teeth are large enough to effectively grasp tissue and hold tension. There are no clear advantages of any one of these forceps types in handling fascial tissue, but this author has the least preference for the Russian forceps and the most preference for the Potts-Smith forceps.

Forceps that are used within the peritoneal cavity should inflict minimal tissue trauma. Because of the delicate nature of visceral tissue, it is not desirable to apply firm tension. The forceps that have already been mentioned can be quite useful in the peritoneal cavity. A general thumb forceps with a cross-serrated grasping surface without teeth can be used for minimally traumatic handling of tissue. Evans pelvic tissue forceps in the 10-in. length or longer can also be useful in the deep pelvis. Adson bayonet forceps have a design that can displace the hand from potential obstruction of the field of view (Fig. 9-9). The selection of forceps with grasping teeth for use in the pelvis is acceptable but with the recognition that the teeth can be traumatic to vasculature. Whenever possible, the tissue within the peritoneal cavity should be

handled with the least traumatic tissue forceps that will effectively grasp the tissue. An atraumatic grasping instrument, such as the Babcock clamp, is useful for grasping rounded structures such as the fallopian tubes (Fig. 9-10). For most experienced surgeons, the selection of forceps for a particular surgical maneuver is almost a reflex based on the thickness of the tissue to be grasped and on the countertraction that is required.

HEMOSTATIC CLAMPS

In a surgical catalog, the instruments that surgeons commonly refer to as "hemostats" are labeled "forceps." The colloquial term "clamp" is almost universally used to refer to the group of ratchet-design hemostatic forceps. In a single instrument catalog, there are as many as 100 different types of hemostatic forceps. This discussion is limited to five different clamps that incorporate the basic design that is common to all hemostats.

The Halsted mosquito forceps come in curved and straight patterns with horizontal serrations (Fig. 9-11). These are delicate hemostats and are designed to specifically grasp the vessel below the point of severance. Applying the hemostat to a large wad of tissue surrounding the bleeding point leads to excessive tissue necrosis either from ligature constriction

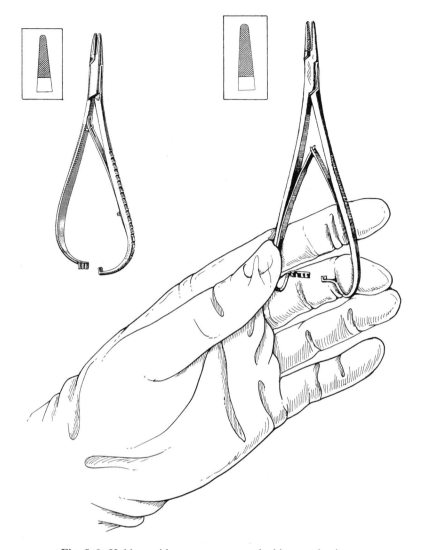

Fig. 9-6. Holders with squeeze-squeeze locking mechanisms.

or cauterization of a larger-than-necessary amount of tissue. Kelly clamps (Fig. 9-12) are larger curved instruments and are frequently the favorite hemostats of gynecologic surgeons. The tonsil forceps (Fig. 9-13A) have a longer-shaft and a fine grasping surface that is particularly useful to the pelvic surgeon. Kocher or Rochester-Ochsner clamps (Fig. 9-13B) are other gynecologic favorites because of their tooth design, which can grasp the opened vaginal cuff firmly. The Mixter forceps (Fig. 9-14), commonly called a right-angle forceps, and their modifications can be used for passing a ligature around a clamped pedicle as well as for hemostasis. The narrow tip of these forceps and the right-angle curve can simplify the clamping of smaller, difficult-to-isolate vessels.

Hemostats are multiuse instruments to the surgeon and consequently have been subjected to a variety of abuses that can effectively ruin their clamping surfaces. It is quite frustrating to isolate a vessel with difficulty, clamp it, loosen the grasp of the hemostat, and then find that the clamping tips are bent or worn from improper usage. Hemostats can satisfactorily substitute for almost any tissue-grasping instrument. They are not intended to serve as pliers to loosen wing nuts on self-retaining retractors or to cut wire.

HYSTERECTOMY CLAMPS

The premier operation of the gynecologic surgeon is the hysterectomy. Whether this operation is performed through the abdominal or vaginal route, it is necessary to effectively control the rich vascular supply until the very last pedicle is ligated. A variety of specialized clamps have been designed to accomplish this purpose.

The ideal hysterectomy clamp should maintain a secure purchase on tissue without an excessive crushing force.[16] A hysterectomy, no matter how carefully performed, is a traumatic procedure. The vascular supply is extensive and

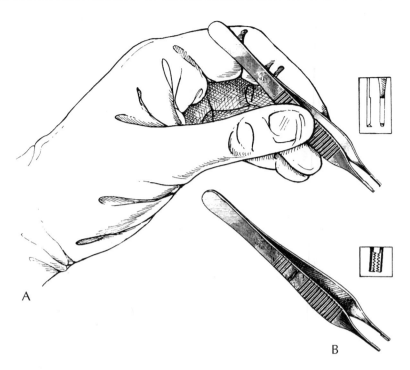

Fig. 9-7. Notice the gripping mechanism of (**A**) the Adson forceps versus (**B**) the Brown-Adson forceps.

well collateralized, and in the paracolpos and parametria, the vessels are surrounded by dense supporting structures. The hysterectomy clamp must be able to firmly grasp and hold these structures until the pedicles are severed and secured by suture. When tissue slips from the clamp, there is inevitably unnecessary bleeding that may be difficult to control and will potentially increase the risk of damage to the urinary tract or larger vessels. The relative safety of this operation is largely based on the design and efficiency of use of the hysterectomy clamp.[17]

Hysterectomy clamps are designed with a total length of 8 to 9 in. and may have either a curved or straight tip. The grasping surface can have either oblique, longitudinal, or horizontal serrations. The curve of the hysterectomy clamp should be gentle enough to avoid forcing the bite of tissue laterally. The Heaney clamp (Fig. 9-15A) and its curved Ballentine modification (Fig. 9-15B) have radii that make them useful throughout the hysterectomy procedure, particularly by the vaginal route. The straight Ballentine clamp (Fig. 9-16A) is most suited for use in clamping the cardinal ligament complex in the abdominal approach because without detachment of the uterosacral ligament, a curved clamp is more awkward to apply. The serrations on the Heaney clamp are oblique, and the grasping tip may have either a single or double tooth. The coarseness of the serration pattern on the Heaney clamp can also be varied to increase the strength of the tissue grip. The Heaney-Ballentine or curved Ballentine has longitudinal serrations that may be preferable because this design will minimize the risk of lateral slippage

of tissue from the clamp. The Garland hysterectomy forceps (Fig. 9-16B) are angled, not curved, and have longitudinal serrations similar to the Ballentine clamp.

It would be difficult to argue that hysterectomy clamps are anything but crushing clamps. There is no reason to apologize for the tissue trauma that these clamps inflict. Needless to say, large-bite hysterectomy clamps should not be placed across tissue where the surgeon desires to maintain viability. The vascular supply to the uterus must be ligated during hysterectomy, and any tissue that is distal to a hemostatic ligature will be nonviable. A hysterectomy performed with atraumatic small bites is likely to have just as much nonviable tissue distal to the ligatures as a procedure performed with a larger clamp. It is for this reason that gynecologists are likely to continue using these same hysterectomy clamps or a similar variation for both vaginal and abdominal cases.

SCISSORS

It has been said by some surgeons that "scissors are for paper dolls; a *real* surgeon uses a scalpel." This rather narrow-minded statement does not take into account that the specialized design and construction of surgical scissors make their use efficient and safe. Scissors are not meant to replace the scalpel. They are designed to be used when the scalpel is impractical or even hazardous.

Scissors are designed with either straight or curved blades. They may have sharp-sharp points, blunt-blunt points, or

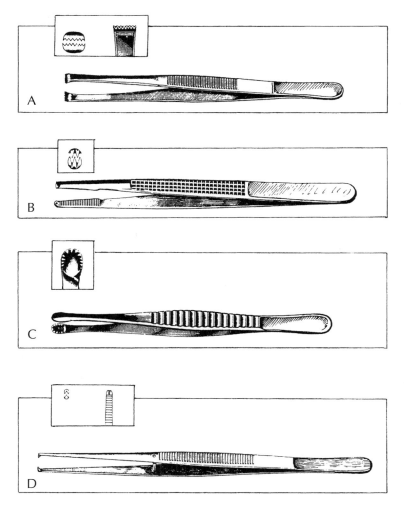

Fig. 9-8. **(A)** Martin tissue forceps have a broad tooth-gripping surface. **(B)** The Bonney tissue forceps have horizontal serration and sharp teeth. **(C)** The unique design of the Russian tissue forceps allows for easy handling of both tissue and surgical needles. **(D)** The Potts-Smith tissue forceps have horizontal serration and a small tooth grip.

blunt-sharp points. The Mayo dissecting scissors (Fig. 9-17A) have rounded tips that reduce inadvertent puncture of tissue and can have either beveled or rounded cutting blades. In varying lengths, the Mayo scissors can be useful for surgery in the pelvis and abdomen. Metzenbaum scissors (Fig. 9-17B) have shorter blades proportionate to the shafts than Mayo scissors and are more suitable for delicate tissue dissection. The versatility of these two types of scissors has resulted in their widespread popularity among gynecologists.

Other specially modified scissors have useful functions in gynecologic surgery. Jorgenson scissors (Fig. 9-18) have very sharply curved blades that can be placed into the opened vagina and can circumferentially cut the vagina at the level of the vaginal fornices. Excision of the cervix in this manner preserves vaginal length and provides a smoothly cut edge for easy suturing of the vaginal cuff. Iris scissors (Fig. 9-19) with sharp-sharp points are frequently used by plastic surgeons because of their delicate blades and resultant preci-

sion cuts. These scissors can be very useful in vaginal repair work when tissue is scarred, as might be found with a repeat anterior colporrhaphy. The points of these scissors are advantageous because of their delicate cut, but they can penetrate the urinary bladder if used carelessly.

RETRACTORS

All retractors have the same basic function of providing exposure in the surgical field. Knowledge and appropriate selection of retractors can simplify a procedure. Conversely, inadequate exposure can create difficulties in an otherwise easy operation. When complications arise and a surgeon calls for help from a surgical consultant, a frequent first step is the improvement of exposure by either repositioning or changing retractors. This is an obvious testimony to the need for wisely choosing and positioning retractors. Handheld re-

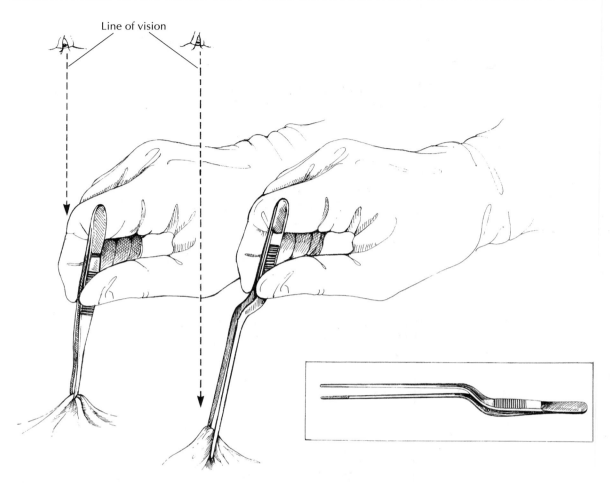

Line of vision

Fig. 9-9. The Adson bayonet forceps (on right) can provide a better line of vision (as opposed to straight forceps).

tractors have been designed for almost every conceivable need; by necessity this discussion must be limited to those instruments most frequently used by the gynecologist. Self-retaining retractors are almost universally used in gynecologic laparotomies and have been adapted for maximizing pelvic exposure. The use of retractors, either handheld or self-retaining, will be significantly biased by the surgeon's experience and opinion.

The Heaney retractor is a right-angled vaginal retractor that is found on almost every vaginal surgery setup (Fig. 9-20). This retractor will easily extend to the depth of the cervix in most patients and can be useful for exposure of the cervix, vaginal fornices, and the vaginal approach to the peritoneal cavity. The long blade on the large Heaney retractor has the disadvantage of sometimes pushing the operative site away from the surgeon, particularly when the vaginal mucosa is intact. A smaller version of the Heaney retractor has been manufactured for circumstances in which a shorter blade is more desirable. The abrupt bend of the retractor can occasionally interfere with visualization at the introitus; other retractors with a rounded curvature are more appropriate when this happens.

The Breisky-Navratil retractors are widely used for vaginal exposure among European gynecologic surgeons but are less popular in the United States[13] (Fig. 9-21A). These retractors have the advantage of a curve that will allow a lateral, superior, or inferior tow on the vaginal tissue without the assistant's hand drifting into the operator's field of view. These retractors come in a variety of lengths and widths that expand the usefulness of the basic design. The design of the Deaver retractor (Fig. 9-21B) has also been modified in varying lengths and widths to make it useful in both vaginal and abdominal surgeries. If the Deaver retractor is placed too deeply, the assistant's hand and the bulge of the retractor's curve may limit the operator's vision. It is not unusual to use several different handheld retractors during the course of an operation. The surgeon should direct the positioning of the retractors by the assistants and choose the most appropriate retractor for the particular surgical step.

The Richardson retractor (Fig. 9-22A) and its Eastman modification (Fig. 9-22B) are favorites of gynecologic surgeons. These designs are useful in both abdominal and vaginal operations. They are beneficial in opening and closing incisions when it is desirable to directly visualize the fascial

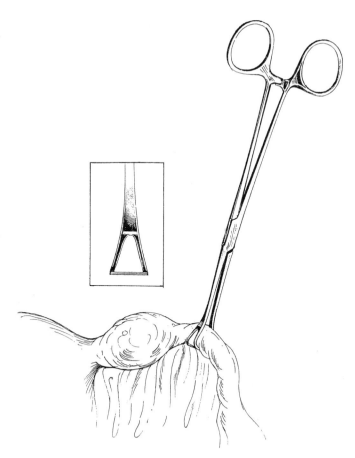

Fig. 9-10. The rounded grasp of the Babcock clamp is useful for handling of the fallopian tube.

surface. They can also be useful for lifting the abdominal wall or enhancing exposure in the pelvis. The curved tip of the blade favors the traction on tissue but is capable of damage by digging into tissue if too much force is applied.

The Auvard weighted speculum and its modifications (Fig. 9-23A) are essentials for many types of vaginal surgery. Some models are manufactured with suction channels that may be connected to standard operating room suction equipment. The blades have also been modified to accommodate the variations in vaginal size and the curvature of the sacrum. The shorter-blade weighted speculum is multipurposed but is ideal for uterine dilation and curettage, cervical conization, and other vaginal procedures. The longer-blade weighted specula, including the duck-billed variation, are most useful when a posterior colpotomy has been performed (Fig. 9-23B).

Although many gynecologic operations require only the use of well-positioned handheld retractors, self-retaining retractors facilitate continued operative exposure with fewer hands in the operative field. The Rigby vaginal retractor (Fig. 9-24A) and the Gelpi perineal retractor (Fig. 9-24B) are useful for vaginal procedures. Among gynecologists, the most popular self-retaining abdominal retractors are the Bal-

four retractor (Fig. 9-25) and the O'Sullivan-O'Connor retractor (Fig. 9-26). The Balfour can be modified with either solid or fenestrated side blades of varying sizes and with different designs of center blades. The retractor bar can be either smooth or ratcheted. An extension can be added to the Balfour retractor to accommodate an upper abdominal blade.[18] The O'Sullivan-O'Connor has two smaller side blades and upper and lower center blades providing a four-quadrant retraction configuration. This retractor has less versatility than the Balfour because the side blades are not detachable. Because it is easily placed and the upper abdominal blade can aid in keeping the bowel out of the pelvic operative site, the O'Sullivan-O'Connor is the preference of many gynecologists. The Franz retractor (Fig. 9-27) is frequently used for tubal infertility surgery.[19] This retractor has the advantage of easy placement in smaller incisions while providing retraction in four directions. It also has interchangeable blades of various sizes that make it useful even in overweight patients.

Self-retaining retractors can be disadvantageous if improperly used. The variations in blade size bespeak the fact that one size does not "fit all." Improper size of blades and poor retractor placement not only do not give the expected exposure, but can lead to serious injury to vasculature, nerves, intestines, and muscles.[20] Self-retaining retractors should be intermittently released during prolonged surgical procedures to avoid sustained pressure from the blades. Upper abdominal blades combined with firm packing can compress the vena cava and contribute to postoperative adynamic ileus. Bruising of the rectus muscles from self-retaining retractors can significantly contribute to postoperative discomfort. The Bookwalter retractor is a favorite of gynecologic oncologists because of the versatility of the blade application (Fig. 9-28). Careful selection and proper placement of the self-retaining retractor can avoid the potential problems with its use and can provide the necessary operative exposure.

SUCTION DEVICES

Many specialized suction devices have been designed for specific surgical procedures. Variations of the Yankauer tonsil suction are most commonly used by gynecologic surgeons (Fig. 9-29). The tips of this suction tube are rounded and therefore reasonably atraumatic. The device may be equipped with a shutoff valve or with a finger hole to control suction use. Disposable variations have been designed with irrigation capability and light attachments. The tonsil-type suction with controlled suction can be used as a retracting device and for gentle blunt dissection. The original Yankauer suction has a major disadvantage: the screw-on tip sometimes loosens and falls into the surgical wound. The relatively small holes in the suction tip are capable of concentrating significant suction force that may catch and firmly hold

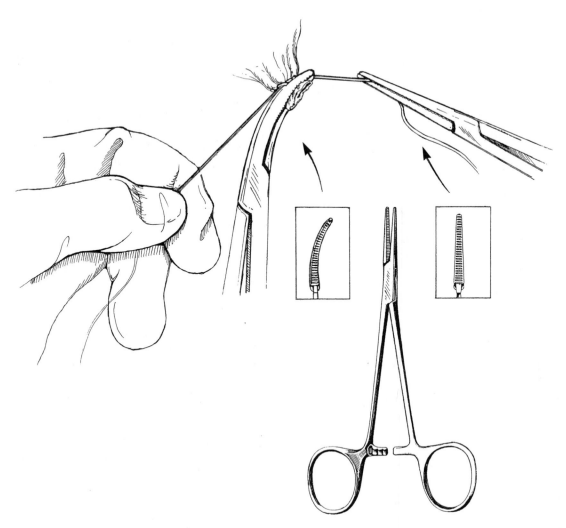

Fig. 9-11. Curved and straight Halstead mosquito forceps have multiple uses.

tissue even after the negative pressure is released. A double-lumen Poole suction (Fig. 9-30) is useful for evacuating blood from the deep pelvis or abdominal ''gutters'' but does not have as much utility as other devices do for tissue retraction. The proliferation of disposable suction-irrigation devices has made the selection of these instruments one of individual preference and operating room supply.

CERVICAL DILATORS

There are three commonly used types of cervical dilators, none of which have distinct advantages over the others beyond the surgeon's personal preference.[21] The Hanks uterine dilator (Fig. 9-31A) has a collar that theoretically will gauge and control the depth of penetration into the uterine cavity (Fig. 9-31B). Hegar dilator (Fig. 9-32A) may come as either a single- or double-ended instrument and has a smaller curvature than the Hanks dilator. The Pratt dilator is double-

ended with a longer midshaft (Fig. 9-32B). Some gynecologists prefer a Wylie- or Goodell-type dilator (Fig. 9-33), but these instruments are more prone to tear the cervix because their dilating force is concentrated in two directions rather than circumferentially. Safe cervical dilation is always preceded by evaluation of the direction and depth of the uterine cavity by sounding with a malleable, calibrated sound (Fig. 9-34).

LIGATURE CARRIERS

The management of vaginal vault prolapse by sacrospinous ligament suspension has prompted the design and modification of ligature carriers for the specific purpose of safely penetrating and retrieving a suture in this location. This procedure was originally performed using Deschamp aneurysm needle (Fig. 9-35A), but there can be considerable difficulty in ligature retrieval with this instrument.[13] The

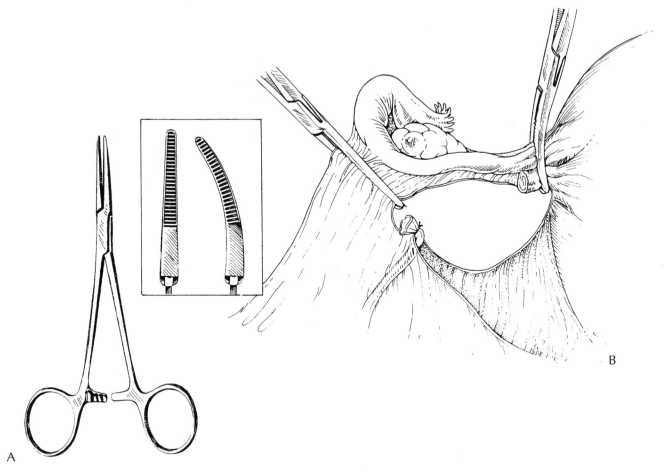

Fig. 9-12. Application of **(A)** the straight Kelly clamps and **(B)** the curved Kelly clamps.

Miya Hook and its accompanying grooved retractor further simplified the procedure (Fig. 9-35B). More recently, a modification of the Shutt suture punch, originally an orthopaedic instrument, has been successfully used for sacrospinous ligament suspension[22] (Fig. 9-36). Exposure of the sacrospinous ligament surface is critical to the successful, uncomplicated completion of this procedure. Any of the above mentioned instruments are capable of safe passage of the ligature throughout the sacrospinous ligament and use is a matter of personal preference.

STAPLING DEVICES

To use or not use stapling devices has been a source of debate among gynecologic surgeons. There is very little argument among gynecologists that skin closure staples (Fig. 9-37B) are a satisfactory alternative to suturing techniques.[23] The debate continues to center around the intra-abdominal or intravaginal uses of stapling devices.[24] The widespread acceptance of staples in gastrointestinal surgery has occurred because of significant time saving along with technical equality to suture techniques. Gynecologic surgeons have generally been a "hard sell" for most stapling devices because the time reduction is not as great and the cost-effectiveness is either marginal or unacceptable.

The development of lactomer copolymer absorbable staples (Fig. 9-37A) has made their use acceptable for vaginal closure because nonabsorbable sutures are capable of causing dyspareunia.[25] Staples offer the advantage of a reduction in blood loss at the time of vaginal cuff closure and the possibility of a decrease of granulation tissue formation. The tight closure of the vaginal cuff accomplished by staples has the disadvantage of potentially restricting spontaneous, dependent drainage from the hysterectomy site, although arguably, this same phenomenon will occur with suture closure. Placement of the staple line at the vaginal cuff requires vaginal dissection beyond the cervix to create enough surface to allow adequate tissue approximation. This can be limited by a large or abnormally configured cervix and therefore will negate the use of the stapler in many cases. Lactomer polymer staples have also been used successfully for

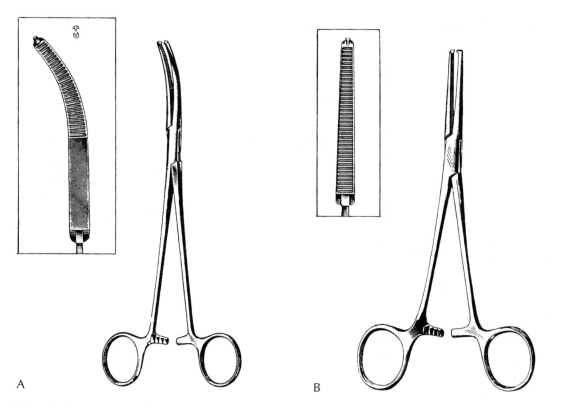

Fig. 9-13. **(A)** Hemostatic tonsil forceps have a small tooth grip. **(B)** Rochester-Ochsner forceps have a large tooth and horizontal serration.

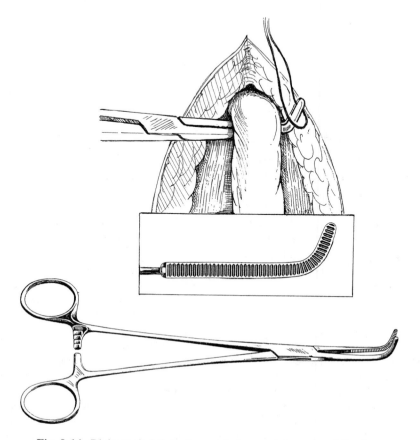

Fig. 9-14. Right-angle Mixter forceps being used for a vessel ligation.

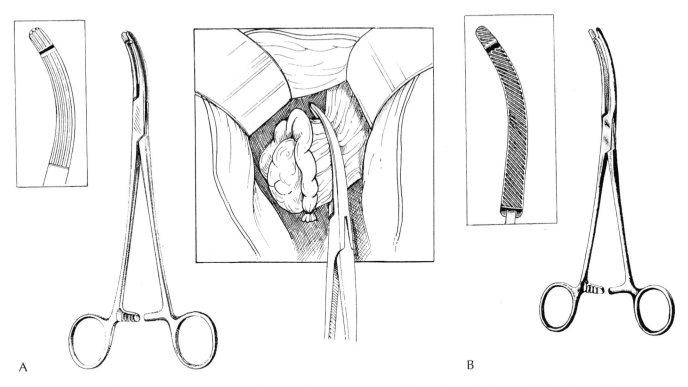

Fig. 9-15. (A) Heaney clamp with longitudinal serration contrasted with **(B)** serration of the Heaney-Ballantine modification.

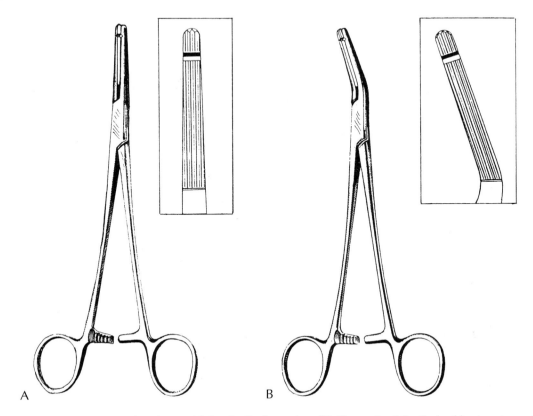

Fig. 9-16. (A) Straight Ballantine clamp with longitudinal serration. **(B)** The angle of the Garland hysterectomy clamp is preferred by some surgeons.

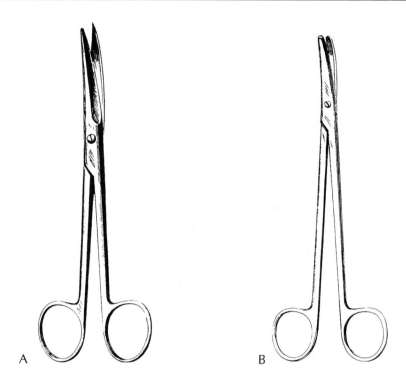

A   B

Fig. 9-17. **(A)** Blunt-sharp version of the Mayo dissecting scissors. **(B)** Note the blunt-blunt tips of the Metzenbaum dissecting scissors.

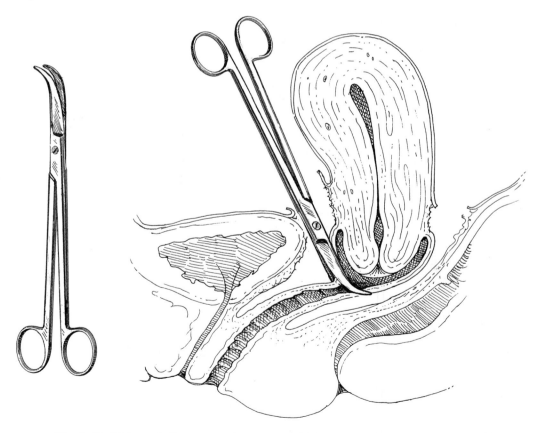

Fig. 9-18. Right-angle Jorgenson scissors are useful in cervical dissection and removal.

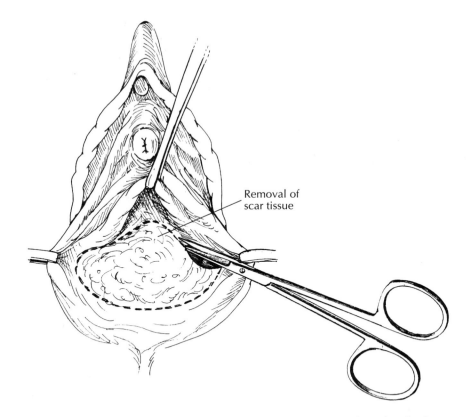

Removal of scar tissue

Fig. 9-19. Sharp, pointed, fine Iris scissors during a repeat anterior colporrhaphy.

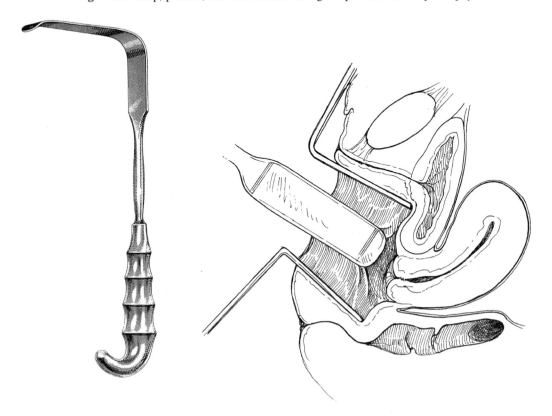

Fig. 9-20. Right-angle Heaney retractor is especially designed for vaginal exposure.

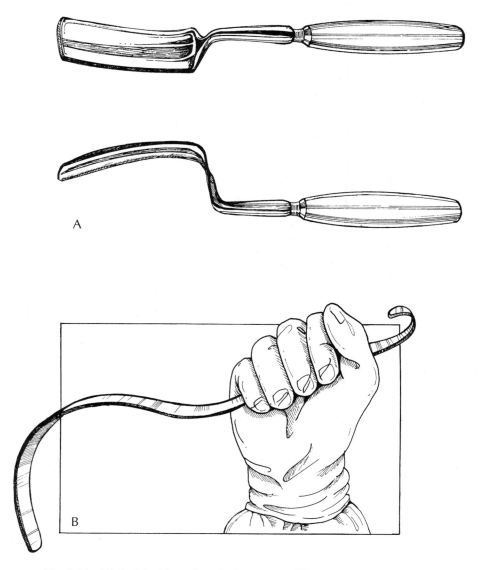

Fig. 9-21. **(A)** Breisky-Navratil vaginal retractors. **(B)** Narrow Deaver retractor.

closure of the uterine incision at the time of cesarean section.[26]

Stapling devices for other aspects of hysterectomy have been used more in European countries than in the United States.[24] Several manufacturers now produce stapling devices that are quite satisfactory for ligation of the attachment structures of the uterus (Fig. 9-37B). These devices are technically easy to use, particularly if the pelvic anatomy is not distorted. A potentially life saving use of a stapling device in pelvic surgery has been the control of bleeding from the presacral veins.[27] The most common indications for hysterectomy in the United States are uterine leiomyoma and endometriosis, both of which are likely to be accompanied by considerable alteration in pelvic anatomy.[28] Continued improvement in staple technology and reduction in cost are likely to increase the use of these devices in the future.

LAPAROSCOPIC INSTRUMENTS

Gynecologic surgeons are the pioneers of minimally invasive surgery. Laparoscopic tubal sterilization procedures were the first widely used endoscopic procedures. The long history of laparoscopic gynecologic surgery has logically led to a long list of instruments.[29] It is impossible to include within the confines of a single chapter the extensive advances in instrumentation for gynecologic laparoscopy. The basic instrument design has remained remarkably consistent, even with the many varieties of disposable instruments that are now available. This discussion is directed at the laparoscopic instruments that are tried and proven and with which gynecologic laparoscopists should universally be familiar.

Insufflation of the abdomen is a necessity of safely performed laparoscopic surgery. The Verres needle (Fig. 9-38)

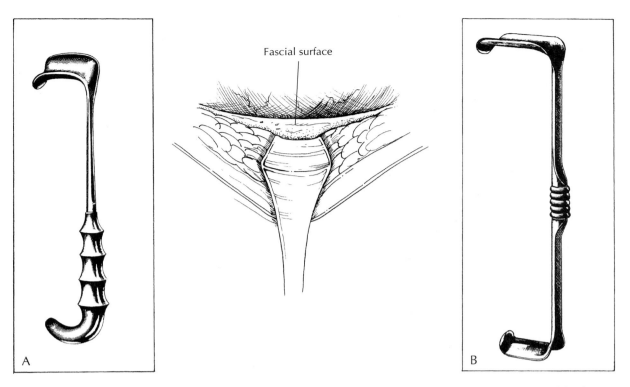

Fig. 9-22. (A) Richardson retractor as it exposes the fascial surface. **(B)** Eastman modification of the Richardson retractor.

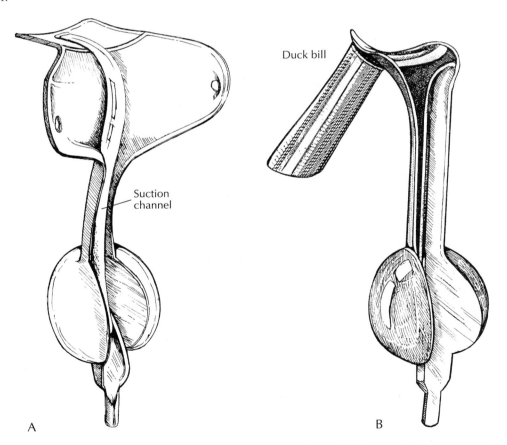

Fig. 9-23. (A) Auvard weighted speculum with a suction channel. **(B)** Duck-billed weighted retractor, which can be inserted into the opened posterior cul-de-sac during vaginal hysterectomy.

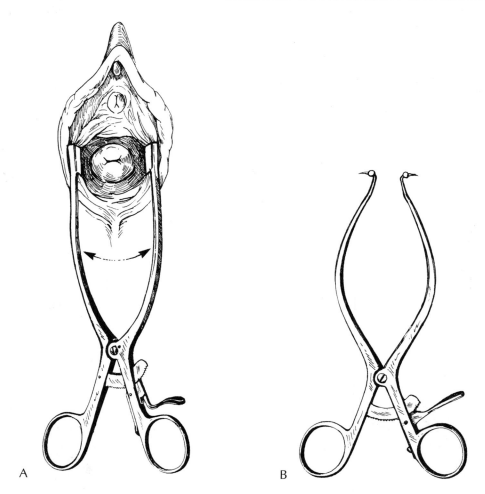

Fig. 9-24. (A) Rigby vaginal retractor positioned for vaginal exposure. **(B)** Gelpi retractor tips are designed to limit penetration.

is designed to primarily penetrate the abdominal wall with minimal risk of injury to abdominal contents.[30] The spring-loaded blunt stylet is designed to shield the sharp needle point from tissue once the needle has entered the abdominal cavity. Before insertion of the Verres needle it is extremely important to examine the function of this spring mechanism. If the needle shaft is even slightly bent, the blunt stylet may not snap properly and the Verres needle becomes a dangerously sharp instrument that is blindly inserted. Some surgeons have advocated discarding use of the Verres needle in favor of direct trocar insertion, legitimately arguing that patient injuries are fewer or equal and that operative time is reduced.[31] The mechanism of the Verres needle does produce a very distinct end point when the peritoneal cavity is entered. Positioning of the needle can be confirmed by demonstration of generated negative pressure by lifting the abdominal wall or freely injecting saline.[32] Preperitoneal insufflation of gas will distort the abdominal cavity and pelvic structures and may make operative laparoscopic procedures

prohibitively difficult or impossible. Therefore, proper placement of the Verres needle can be the most important aspect of a laparoscopic procedure.

The laparoscopic trocar (Fig. 9-39), in varying sizes, is used for both visual and operative port sites. The trocar may have either a conical tip or a pyramidal tip, the choice of which is a matter of surgeon's preference. The trocar must be sharp to render maximum safety on insertion. The risk of injury to abdominal wall vessels is not totally avoidable.[33] The nondisposable trocar sleeve is equipped with a trumpet-type valve that allows easy insertion of the laparoscope or instruments with minimal loss of pneumoperitoneal gas. Disposable trocars (Fig. 9-40) have the advantage of consistent sharpness and the added safety feature of a spring-operated protective sheath that shields the trocar tip after the peritoneal cavity is entered. The additional cost per case can be significant if multiple puncture sites are all made with disposable trocars. The safety features of the disposable trocar are most useful when performing the initial, blind insertion.

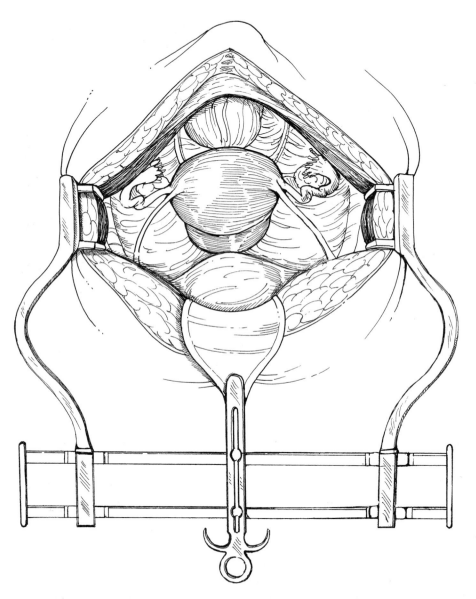

Fig. 9-25. The Balfour abdominal retractor is self-retaining and is shown in its common placement.

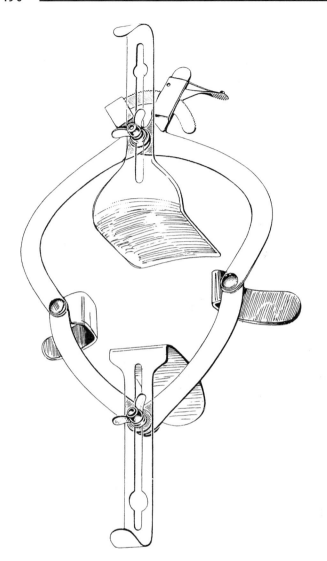

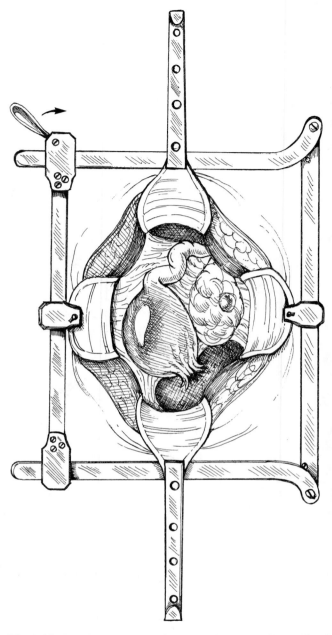

Fig. 9-26. The O'Sullivan-O'Connor retractor has an adjustable bladder blade and an adjustable upper abdominal blade.

The diameter of the trocar sleeve aperture can be modified by converters to accommodate varying sizes of instruments and still maintain effective gas seal.

A laparoscopic operation begins with a thorough inspection of the pelvic structures. This may require mobilization of tissue, indirect palpation with instruments, and aspiration-irrigation capability. The Modified Frangenheim instrument set can facilitate these functions with a dual puncture (Fig. 9-41). The aspirator-irrigator is Luer-locked and calibrated and may be equipped with a self-filling syringe. A probe needle, or grasper, can also be inserted through the 5-mm second puncture site. This type of instrument set will function for most diagnostic laparoscopy and is useful in the initial steps of any operative laparoscopic case.

Laparoscopic tubal sterilization is the most frequently performed laparoscopic operation. The Kleppinger forceps (Fig.

Fig. 9-27. The Franz abdominal retractor is shown with its wider side blades.

9-42) are commonly used for tubal coagulation. They have either a scissor-style or a syringe-style handle and may be electrosurgically equipped either in unipolar or bipolar fashion. The jaws of these forceps are designed to not only coagulate the tubal structure but also disrupt the vascularity of the mesosalpinx supplying the coagulated tubal segment. The Hulka clip, made of plastic jaws and a gold-plated stainless-steel spring, is applied with a special applicator[34] (Fig. 9-43). The instrument is relatively simple to operate and the Hulka clip is effective for sterilization when the tubal anatomy is normal and the vascularity of the tube is included

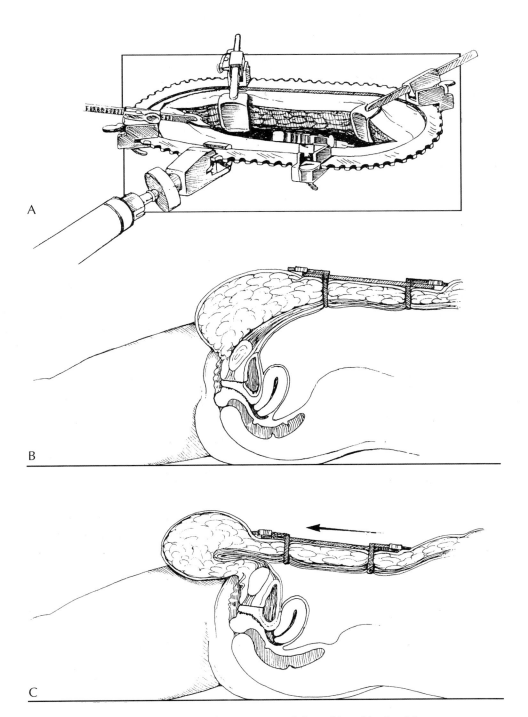

Fig. 9-28. **(A–C)** Bookwalter retractor as it is positioned in the abdomen.

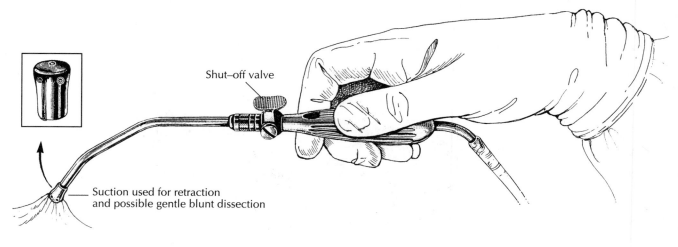

Fig. 9-29. Yankauer suction has an easily accessible shutoff valve.

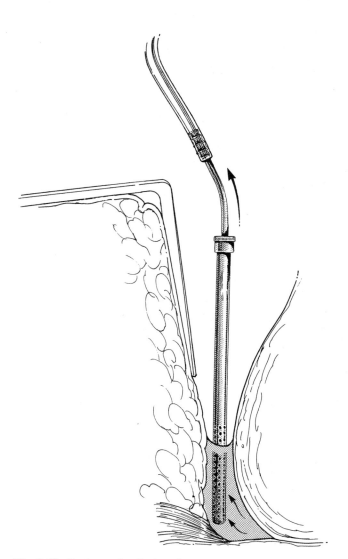

Fig. 9-30. Poole suction limits adherence to tissue surfaces.

in the clip.[4] The advantage of this system is the potential reversibility. The Falope ring, like the Hulka clip, avoids potential complications of tubal coagulation, but does not have the same reversibility potential because it inflicts damage to a longer segment of a fallopian tube[4] (Fig. 9-44). The high elasticity of the silicone Falope ring and the relative ease of use of the applicator have contributed to its popularity.[4]

Atraumatic tissue-grasping instruments designed for laparoscopic use have double action and curved jaws and are operated by either a scissors or a spring handle (Fig. 9-45). A disposable Babcock-type atraumatic grasper with a ratcheted scissors handle can be particularly useful in handling adnexal structures. Biopsy forceps can double as grasping instruments but can be traumatic to the tissue. Biopsy forceps are not designed for cutting functions. For most cutting needs, hooked scissors[35] are a very practical instrument because the jaw is designed to hold tissue until the cut is made. Sawtooth scissors hold tissue in a similar manner but have no particular advantage over the hooked scissors (Fig. 9-45B). Scissors can be equipped with cautery, either unipolar or bipolar, providing hemostasis without changing instruments. The unipolar J-hook electrode and the hook electrode are also useful cutting instruments and are each designed with an irrigation/suction tube that adds to their versatility (Fig. 9-46). Laparoscopic scalpels resemble a small # 11 scalpel and may be inserted through either a primary or a secondary operative port. The scalpel can be attached to unipolar cautery.[30]

Suturing techniques using laparoscopic instrumentation are in principle the same as those in open laparotomy. The needle and tissue graspers are, by necessity, small enough to fit through the operative ports. Needle-holders are designed with locking jaws and are controlled by either an axially aligned or a spring-assisted scissors handle (Fig. 9-47A). The jaws of the needle-holder are strong and their

(Text continues on p. 205.)

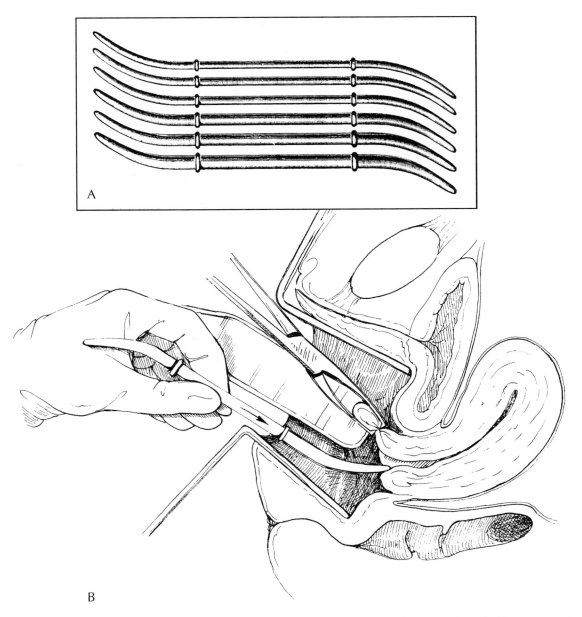

Fig. 9-31. (A) Hanks uterine dilators are sized for progressive cervical dilation. (B) The cuff on the Hanks dilator is designed to limit uterine penetration.

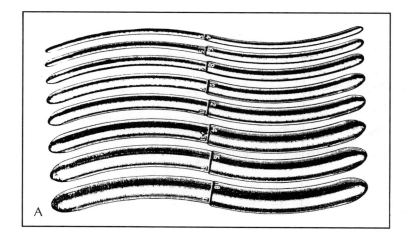

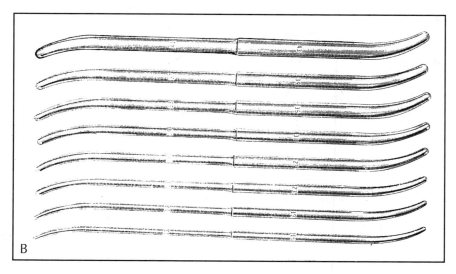

Fig. 9-32. **(A)** Hegar uterine dilators are double-ended and are of progressive sizes. **(B)** Pratt uterine dilators are more satisfactory for uteri.

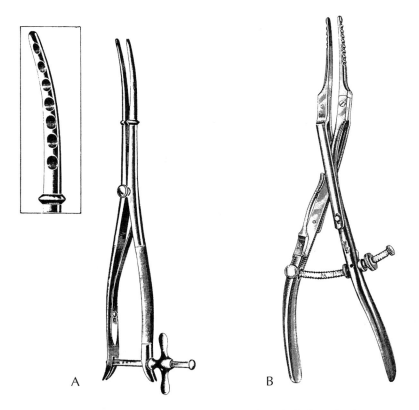

Fig. 9-33. (A) Wyliet or **(B)** Goodell-type dilator is a single insertion instrument.

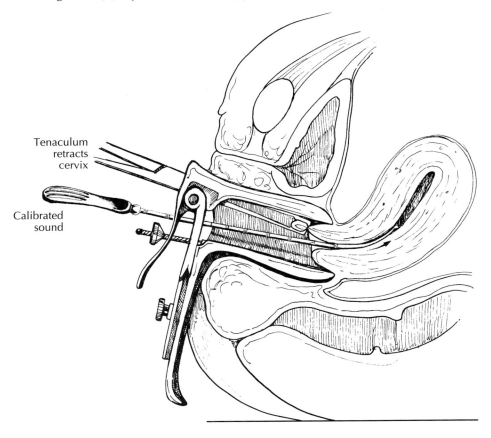

Tenaculum
retracts
cervix

Calibrated
sound

Fig. 9-34. Uterine sounding shown with a malleable, calibrated Simpson uterine sound.

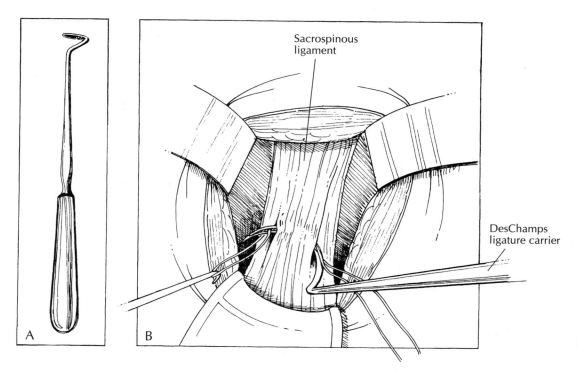

Fig. 9-35. **(A)** Deschamp aneurysm ligature carrier. **(B)** The Deschamp aneurysm ligature carrier shown piercing an exposed sacrospinous ligament.

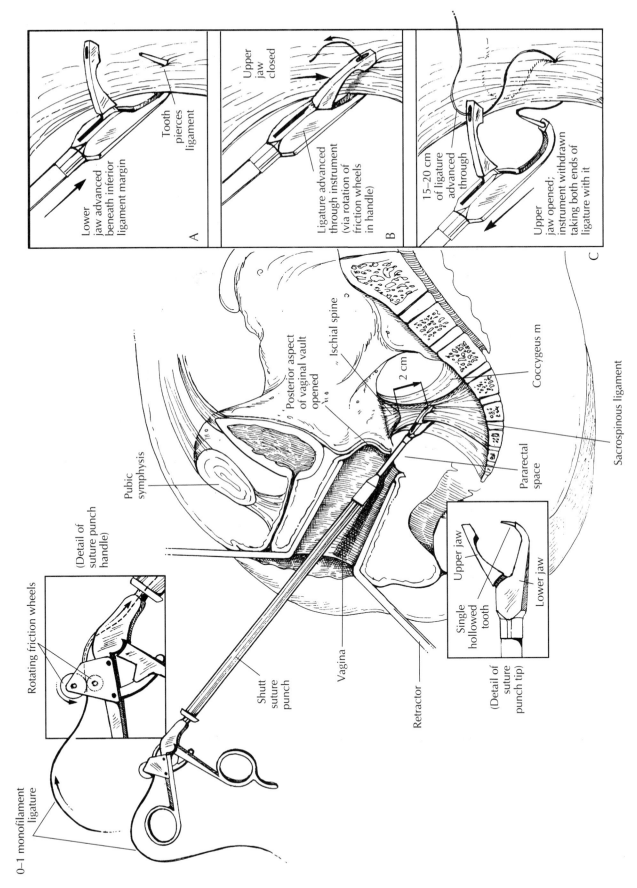

0–1 monofilament ligature

Rotating friction wheels

(Detail of suture punch handle)

Pubic symphysis

Posterior aspect of vaginal vault opened

Ischial spine

2 cm

Coccygeus m

Pararectal space

Sacrospinous ligament

Shutt suture punch

Vagina

Retractor

Upper jaw

Lower jaw

Single hollowed tooth

(Detail of suture punch tip)

A Lower jaw advanced beneath inferior ligament margin — Tooth pierces ligament

B Ligature advanced through instrument (via rotation of friction wheels in handle) — Upper jaw closed

C 15–20 cm of ligature advanced through — Upper jaw opened; instrument withdrawn taking both ends of ligature with it

Fig. 9-36. Shutt suture punch, originally designed for orthopaedic surgery, is proficient in sacrospinous ligament suspension.

197

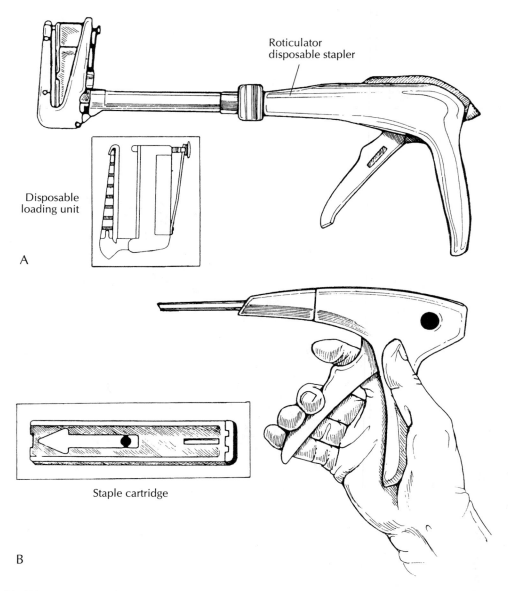

Roticulator
disposable stapler

Disposable
loading unit

A

Staple cartridge

B

Fig. 9-37. **(A)** Roticulator disposable surgical stapler with disposable loading unit. **(B)** Skin staple gun and cartridge.

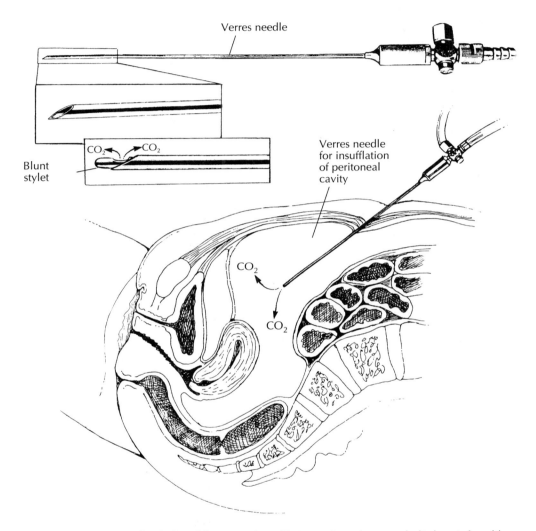

Verres needle

Blunt stylet

CO_2 ← → CO_2

Verres needle for insufflation of peritoneal cavity

CO_2

CO_2

Fig. 9-38. Verres needle, designed for protection of inner peritoneal organs, in its inserted position.

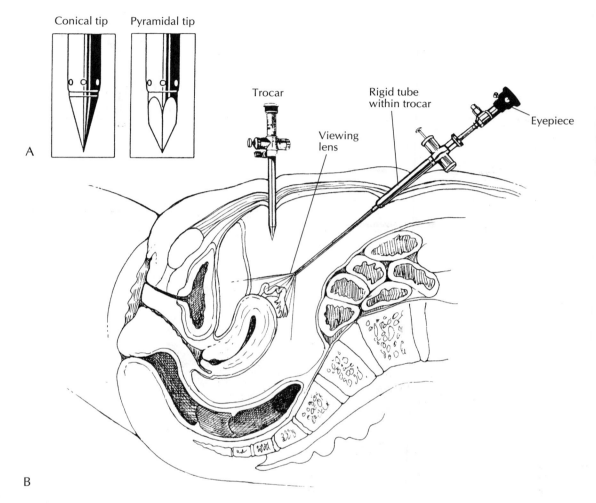

Conical tip   Pyramidal tip

A

Trocar

Rigid tube within trocar

Viewing lens

Eyepiece

B

Fig. 9-39. **(A)** Trocar tips and **(B)** trocar with the stylet in place and an instrument inserted.

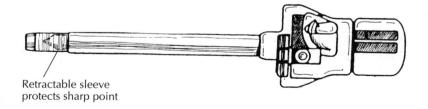

Retractable sleeve protects sharp point

Fig. 9-40. Disposable, surgical port with a protective sleeve over the sharp point.

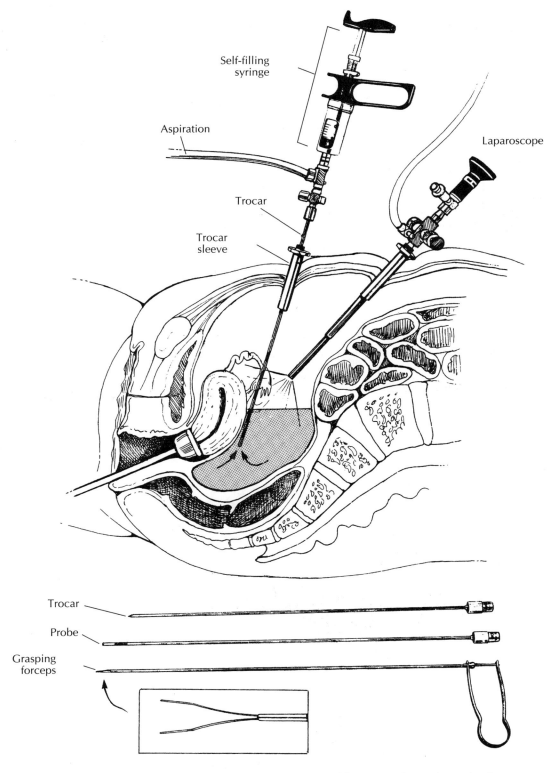

Self-filling syringe

Aspiration

Laparoscope

Trocar

Trocar sleeve

Trocar

Probe

Grasping forceps

Fig. 9-41. Wolf Modified Frangenheim set for laparoscopy with trocar probes and grasping forceps.

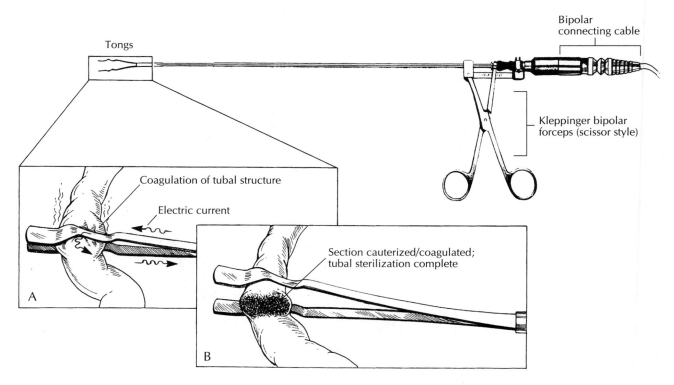

Fig. 9-42. (A & B) Wolf-Kleppinger forceps grasp and cauterize a fallopian tube for sterilization.

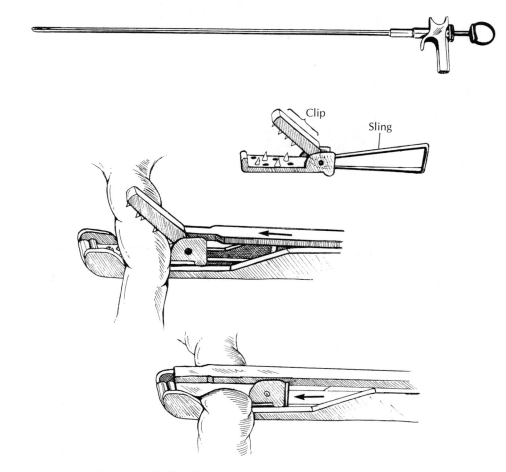

Fig. 9-43. Wolf-Hulka clip applicator positioned to release the clip.

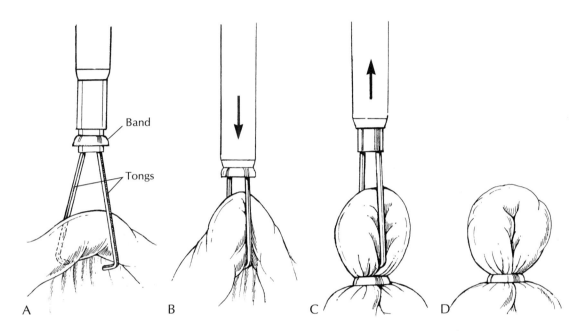

Fig. 9-44. (A–D) Grasping of the tube and application of the Falope ring.

Disposable atraumatic graspers

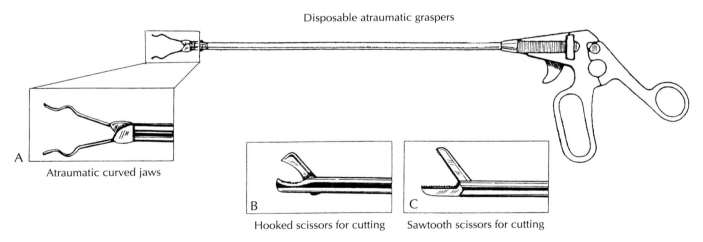

Atraumatic curved jaws

Hooked scissors for cutting

Sawtooth scissors for cutting

Fig. 9-45. (A) Ratcheted atraumatic endo-Babcock. **(B)** Hooked scissors with tapered jaw. **(C)** Sawtooth scissors.

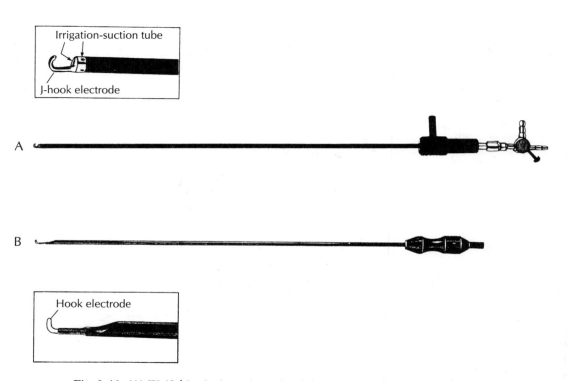

Fig. 9-46. **(A)** Wolf J-hook electrode suction irrigation tube and **(B)** hook electrode.

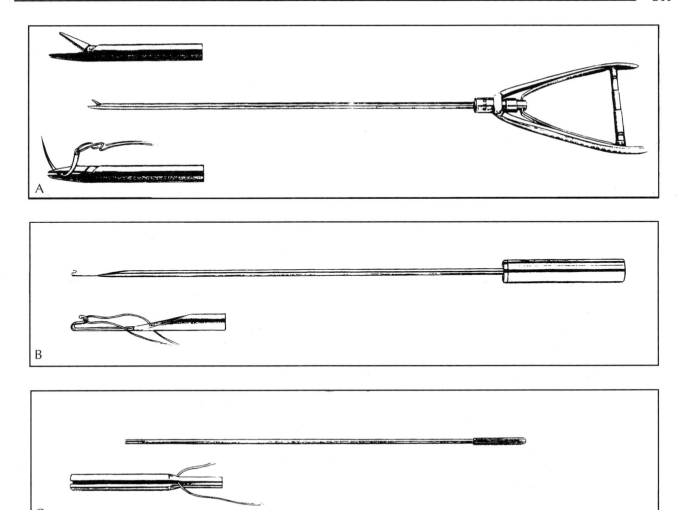

Fig. 9-47. (A) Wolf endoscopic needle-holder. **(B)** Wolf laparoscopic suture manipulator. **(C)** Wolf knot-pusher.

approximation is exact to allow the instrument to be used for intracorporeal knot-tying.[36] A suture manipulator is useful in the proper placement of the suture (Fig. 9-47B). Knot-pushers are designed for both extracorporeal and intracorporeal knot-tying (Fig. 9-47C). Use of these instruments requires a hand-eye coordination that can only be made efficient with practice; the instrument manufacturers have designed training devices for this purpose.

Operative laparoscopy requires attention to detail. The surgeon is responsible for the electrosurgical equipment, laser equipment, and all instrumentation used. The rapid advances in operative laparoscopy are a tribute to the ingenuity of the laparoscopic surgeon and require a constant re-education as new developments occur.[37] This is an area where the surgeon must know the appropriate instrumentation and its use because the best surgical instrument of all, the surgeon's hand, cannot get directly into the surgical field.

There are many surgical catalogs with thousands of instruments, many of which have gynecologic application. An in-

dividual surgeon cannot possibly know and be proficient in the use of all of these instruments. The redeeming fact, particularly in gynecologic surgery, is that it is possible to become very knowledgeable and efficient in the use of a select number of instruments that are commonly used in surgery of the female reproductive tract.

REFERENCES

1. Hemsell DL, Hemsell PG, et al: Abdominal wound problems after hysterectomy with electrocautery vs. scalpel subcutaneous incision. Inf Dis Obstet Gynecol 1:27, 1993

2. Hasselgren P-O, Hagbert E, Malmer H et al: One instead of two knives for surgical incision. Arch Surg 119:917, 1984

3. Malt RA: The Practice of Surgery. WB Saunders, Philadelphia, 1993

4. Semm K: Operative Manual for Endoscopic Abdominal Surgery. Year Book Medical, Chicago, 1987

5. Sowa DE, Masterson BJ, Nealon N, von Fraunhofer JA: Effects of thermal knives on wound healing. Obstet Gynecol 66:436, 1985

6. Hambley R, Hebda PA, Abell E et al: Wound healing of skin incisions produced by ultrasonically vibrating knife, scalpel, electrosurgery, and carbon dioxide laser. Dermatol Surg Oncol 14:1213, 1988

7. Chen NC, Towler MA, Moody FP et al: Mechanical performance of surgical needle holders. J Emerg Med 9:5, 1991

8. Stamp CV, McGregor W, Rodeheaver GT et al: Surgical needle holder damage to sutures. Am Surg 5:300, 1988

9. Towler MA, Chen NC, Moody FP et al: Biomechanics of a new atraumatic surgical needle holder. J Emerg Med 9:477, 1991

10. Corson SL, Sedlacek TV, Hoffman JJ: Greenhill's Surgical Gynecology. 5th Ed. Year Book Medical, Chicago, 1986

11. Abidin MR, Thacker JG, Lombardi SA et al: Needle holder damage to surgical needles. Am Surg 55:681, 1989

12. Edlich RF, Towler MA, Rodeheaver GR et al: Scientific basis for selecting surgical needles and needle holders for wound closure. Clin Plast Surg 17:583, 1990

13. Nichols DH: Instruments and sutures. p. 120. In Nichols DH (ed): Gynecologic and Obstetric Surgery. Mosby–Yearbook, St. Louis, 1993

14. Bernstein G: Needle holders—an instrument especially for the left-handed surgeon. J Dermatol Surg Oncol 14:505, 1988

15. Bennett NT, Howard RJ: Quantity of blood inoculated in a needle stick injury from suture needles. J Am Coll Surg 178:107, 1994

16. Masterson BJ, Sullivan TG, Townsend PR: Development of a noncrushing vascular clamp for pelvic surgery. Am J Obstet Gynecol 132:113, 1978

17. Masterson BJ: Selecting instruments for gynecologic surgery. Contemp Ob/Gyn 12:31, 1978

18. Gershenson DM, DeCherney AH, Curry SL: Operative Gynecology. WB Saunders, Philadelphia, 1993

19. Hunt RB: Atlas of Female Infertility Surgery. 2nd Ed. Mosby–Year Book, St. Louis, 1992

20. Applegate WV: Abdominal cutaneous nerve entrapment syndrome. Surgery 71:118, 1972

21. Smith MF, Stehn JL: Basic Surgical Instrumentation. WB Saunders, Philadelphia, 1993

22. Sharp TR: Sacrospinous suspension made easy. Obstet Gynecol 82:873, 1993

23. Barnhill DR, Park RC: Latest on stapling. Contemp Ob/Gyn 39:19, 1994

24. Beresford JM: Automatic stapling techniques in abdominal hysterectomy. Surg Clin North Am 64:609, 1984

25. Stovall TG, Summitt RL, Lipscomb GH, Ling FW: Vaginal cuff closure at abdominal hysterectomy: comparing suture with absorbable staples. Obstet Gynecol 78:415, 1991

26. Villeneuve MG, Khalifé S, Marcoux S, Blanchet P: Surgical staples in cesarean section: a randomized controlled trial. Am J Obstet Gynecol 163:1641, 1990

27. Hill ADK, Menzies-Gow N, Carzi A: Methods of controlling presacral bleeding. J Am Coll Surg 178:183, 1994

28. Wilcox LS, Koonin LM: Hysterectomy in the United States, 1988–1990. Obstet Gynecol 83:549, 1994

29. Rock JA, Warshaw JR: The history and future of operative laparoscopy. Am J Obstet Gynecol 170:7, 1994

30. Rock JA, Murphy AA, Jones HW (eds): Female Reproductive Surgery. Williams & Wilkins, Baltimore, 1992

31. Byron JW, Markenson G, Miyazawa K: A randomized comparison of Verres needle and direct trocar insertion for laparoscopy. Surg Gynecol Obstet 177:259, 1993

32. Mattingly RF, Thompson JD: Te Linde's Operative Gynecology. 6th Ed. JB Lippincott, Philadelphia, 1985

33. Hurd WW, Pearl ML, DeLancey JO et al: Laparoscopic injury of abdominal wall blood vessels: a report of three cases. Obstet Gynecol, suppl. 82:673, 1993

34. Hulka JF: Studies in simpler tubocclusion methods. Obstet Gynecol 122:337, 1978

35. Sotrel G (ed): Tubal Reconstructive Surgery. Lea & Febiger, Philadelphia, 1990

36. Koninckx PR: An improved needleholder for endoscopic knot tying. Fertil Steril 58:640, 1992

37. Hatlie MJ: Climbing 'the learning curve.' JAMA 270:1364, 1993

CHAPTER TEN

EXAMINATION UNDER ANESTHESIA

WILLIAM J. MANN, JR.

The technologic developments relating to various imaging techniques that can be applied to the female pelvis and abdomen have led to the mistaken idea that the history and physical examination are less important than in the past. Often clinical experience and physical findings are trusted less than the ''shades of gray'' printed out from a video terminal or ultrasound screen. But this unrealistic reliance on computed tomography, magnetic resonance imaging, and ultrasound misses the point. The correct and desired approach is to accumulate clinical experience by comparing the results of patient evaluation with laboratory and imaging results, and to correlate all of these with pathologic findings at surgery. This slow, thoughtful review of preoperative evaluation in all of its many dimension will lead the gynecologic surgeon to a more reasoned decision-making process by which to decide when and what surgical intervention is appropriate.

To improve one's examining skills, the young surgeon must take every opportunity to palpate an abnormal finding, particularly when visual confirmation can be immediately attained at surgery. There is no better way to learn the intricacies and complexities of the pelvic and abdominal examination than to perform a thorough examination under anesthesia in the operating room, immediately before beginning the surgical procedure.

With surgeries such as dilation and curettage or surgical conization, the examination under anesthesia offers the best means of determining the axis of the cervical canal and the position of the uterus, to avoid perforation of the fundus or inadvertent entry into the peritoneal cavity. In patients scheduled for laparotomy, the decision to make a vertical or transverse incision, or even the choice of a vaginal versus an abdominal approach, can be made more precisely based on findings during pelvic examination under anesthesia.

TECHNIQUE

Palpation of the Supraclavicular Areas

After adequate induction of anesthesia, this surgeon palpates the supraclavicular areas, both axilla, and the breasts, looking for previously undetected adenopathy or masses. The abdomen is then inspected, with particular attention paid to the umbilicus to look for previously unknown umbilical hernia, and to previous incision sites for potential areas of fascial separation. The liver edge is then percussed out and gentle palpation attempted. Unsuspected hepatomegaly is of particular importance when upper abdominal laparoscopy ports are planned, and occasionally, even the umbilical port may lie over an enlarged liver. The entire abdomen is then palpated, and if masses are found, a careful estimate of their size and consistency is made and compared to subsequent laparotomy findings. The presence of an omental cake and fixation of the umbilicus—signs of advanced intraperitoneal disease—may be detected more easily under anesthesia. If ascites is present or suspected, a fluid wave can be percussed and palpated. Masses not felt in the ascitic abdomen when the patient is awake may be more easily felt when anesthesia has reduced abdominal wall muscle tone. Finally, the ingui-

207

nal areas are inspected and palpated prior to placing the patient in the lithotomy position, or ''frog-legging'' her.

Pelvic Examination

The pelvic examination under anesthesia proceeds as any examination with inspection, then palpation. Skin lesions over the vulva and inner thighs, as well as any abnormalities of the vagina or cervix, can be examined with a bright light or with a colposcope. Under anesthesia, the vagina can be manipulated with retractors to allow complete visualization, which often cannot be done in an awake patient without considerable discomfort. Any visible abnormalities can be palpated to assess consistency, mobility, and relation to adjacent structures. Presumably, all patients will have had a speculum examination prior to surgery; however, occasionally patients cannot tolerate this and anesthesia allows the only opportunity to visualize the vagina and cervix, and obtain cytology.

Bimanual Examination

A bimanual examination can then be performed. When an abnormal finding is present, such as a mass, there is a tendency to focus on this abnormality to the exclusion of other findings that may also be present. To prevent this, it is necessary to have a set procedure that is followed in each patient, to ensure thoroughness. For example, this author first palpates the labia, looking for Bartholin's cysts or

other cutaneous abnormalities. Next, the undersurface of the urethra is milked, looking for pus in the urethra, a diverticulum, or Skene's glands. The texture of the vagina is palpated, looking for nodules such as condyloma, lateral vaginal cysts, or palpable abnormalities of the cervix and/ or fornices. Two fingers are then introduced, and the lateral aspects of the cervix and then the uterus are carefully palpated. Patients usually void subsequent to coming to the operating suite, but if a full bladder is palpated, it is drained and a catheter left in, if needed for planned surgery. The right and then left adnexae are palpated next. Then an examining finger is introduced into the rectum and the bimanual examination is again repeated going first midline, right, and then left.

Medical students and young house staff often first palpate a normal ovary or nulliparous uterus during these examinations under anesthesia, allowing them to improve and better perform pelvic examinations elsewhere. Similarly, parametrial nodularity is difficult to describe, but easy to recognize once felt.

ADVANTAGES

The value of the examination under anesthesia as a teaching tool is self-evident. Its clinical value may be less apparent, particularly to surgeons who rush to the scrub sink while operating room personnel position, prepare, and drape the patient. This is a mistake. This author has seen pelvic masses

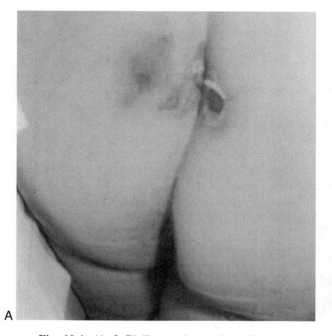
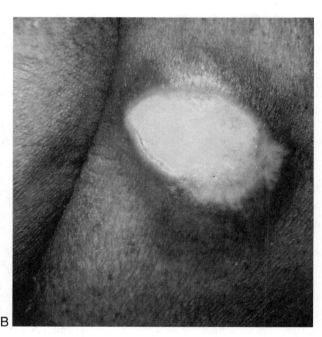

A   B

Fig. 10-1. (A & B) Two patients who suffered severe chemical burns from iodine preparatory solutions that were allowed to puddle beneath their buttocks while they were in the dorsal lithotomy position.

disappear with catheterization; previously unsuspected abdominal masses change incision selection, and parametrial findings lead to oncology consultation. In addition, patient positioning—if done poorly—can lead to pressure necrosis and neuropathy, areas of grave medicolegal concern to the surgeon, which are not appropriately delegated to others. Prone patients need to be positioned to prevent their heels from contacting hard surfaces, and if an arm is to be placed at the side, it must be done carefully. In lithotomy, the hips must be carefully flexed and supported, and the hips, knees, posterior thigh, and heels padded. Knees must be carefully flexed, or if placed in under the knee stirrups, adjusted so that tissue is not folded over metal, and so that stirrup edges

do not cut into the calf (peroneal nerve), posterior thigh, or low on the Achilles' tendon.

RISK OF CLEANSING

A common and dangerous error is to allow agent, particularly concentrated iodine solutions, to puddle between the buttock fold. This can lead to severe chemical burns, even requiring grafting (Fig. 10-1).

During surgery, attention to detail is mandatory. This attention must begin with the examination under anesthesia, positioning, and preparing of the patient.

CHAPTER ELEVEN

CYSTOSCOPY

JACQUELINE C. JOHNSON

Instrumentation
Indications
Operative Procedure
Complications
Advantages
Summary

Cystoscopy has many uses in gynecologic practice, and basic cystoscopy skills should be part of every gynecologic surgeon's training. Cystoscopy can be useful for preoperative evaluation before urogynecologic procedures, for the staging of gynecologic malignancies, for intraoperative guidance, and for the diagnosis and prevention of urinary tract injuries that can result from gynecologic procedures.

INSTRUMENTATION

Cystoscopes are similar to laparoscopes and hysteroscopes, instruments with which most gynecologists are familiar. The cystoscope is composed of a thin fiberoptic tube to which a light source is connected, passed through a hollow sheath. The sheath may also have channels for instruments to pass through for operative cystoscopy. A blunt obturator is placed in the sheath to facilitate its insertion, then removed. An irrigating fluid source is then attached to the sheath to provide distension of the bladder and improve visibility.

Cystoscopes vary in size. The most commonly used sizes for gynecologic procedures are 17 to 24 French. In some cases, such as those where condyloma or tumor are causing compromise of the urethral lumen, pediatric scopes (8 French) may be useful.[1] Flexible fiberoptic cystoscopes have recently come into use and are associated with less pain and postoperative morbidity than rigid cystoscopes; however, their use requires more extensive training.[2]

A variety of irrigation fluids can be used for cystoscopy.

The usual media is normal (0.9 percent) saline. For use of electrocautery, a nonconductive material such as water or glycine is required. Water is preferred in cases where bleeding is evident. The hypotonic water lyses red blood cells, improving visibility, and also has the theoretic advantage of lysing tumor cells if a malignancy is present.[3]

INDICATIONS

There are numerous indications for cystoscopy in the gynecologic patient. The procedure is standard at many institutions in the evaluation of urinary complaints, and is a requirement for some surgeons before undertaking any urogynecologic procedure.[3] Abnormalities unrecognized in the workup of stress incontinence can cause similar urinary symptoms such as urethral diverticula, bladder tumor, bladder stones, and scarring. These and permanent sutures from previous urogynecologic procedures can be identified by cystoscopy and may alter the surgical approach.[4] One case has been reported in which cystoscopy identified a stone-encrusted intrauterine device (IUD) in the bladder causing urinary symptoms 16 years after insertion, and 13 years after hysterectomy and bilateral salpingoophorectomies for pelvic abscess.[5]

Cystoscopy has long been important in the staging of cervical cancer in determining bladder involvement. It is mandatory in patients with large stage I tumors and all advanced stage disease, but has been abandoned by some in cases of small stage I tumors and microinvasive disease where bladder involvement is negligible. It is also useful in the staging of other pelvic malignancies involving the cervix or vagina, and in recurrent gynecologic malignancies. At many institutions, it remains part of the preoperative evaluation in patients being considered for pelvic exenteration for recurrent or advanced pelvic tumors. Occasionally tumors may arise in the urinary tract that appear to be gynecologic in origin. In these cases, the diagnosis can be confirmed by cystoscopy. Primary clear cell adenocarcinoma arising in a urethral diverticulum has been reported.[6]

OPERATIVE PROCEDURE

Cystoscopy can be performed in an outpatient setting with local anesthesia or under regional or general anesthesia as part of another operative procedure. The patient is placed in the dorsolithotomy position and the vulva, vagina, and periurethral area are prepared sterilely. If local anesthesia is to be used, 2 percent lidocaine jelly is drawn up into a tuberculin syringe without a needle attached. This syringe, containing about 1 ml of lidocaine gel, is easily inserted into the mid-urethra using additional gel as a lubricant. The gel is slowly injected into the urethra and 3 to 5 minutes allowed to elapse. Most patients experience a mild burning sensation during insertion of the anesthetic, but have no discomfort for the remainder of the procedure. Some authors suggest using a higher volume of gel (11 to 20 ml); however, excellent results have been achieved in the office setting with the above technique.[9] It is of interest that a randomized study of lidocaine gel versus plain lubricant did not show a significant benefit for lidocaine gel in cystoscopy.[10] However, in women, increased preprocedure anxiety was associated with

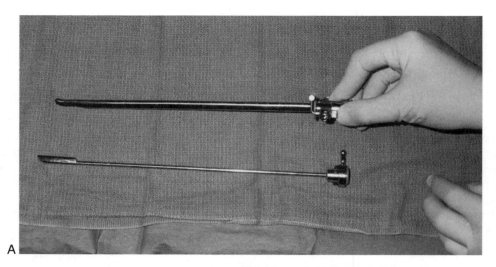

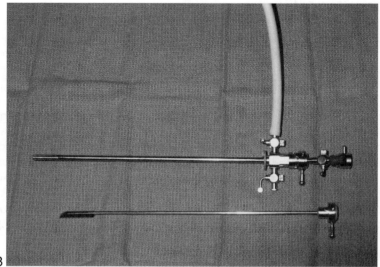

Fig. 11-1. (A) Cystoscope sleeve and blunt obturator used for insertion. (B) Cystoscope placed through sleeve; obturator removed. The obturator is removed while the sleeve is held in place in the bladder and the cystoscope is then inserted into the sleeve.

reports of more pain. Letting the patient know that local anesthesia will be used can decrease preprocedure anxiety and facilitate the procedure.

Prior to performing the procedure, the equipment should be assembled and checked. The surgeon assembles the blunt obturator into the sheath to be used (Fig. 11-1). The smallest scope that will allow adequate visualization should be used to minimize pain and urethral trauma, and to eliminate the need for urethral dilation. An 18 or 20 French cystoscope sheath should be adequate for most gynecologic uses. Cystoscopes are available with a variety of lenses: 0, 30, 70, and 120 degrees offer different fields of view. For most gynecologic procedures, a 70-degree scope will suffice. The fluid source, usually a 1- to 3-L bag suspended on an intravenous pole, is connected via tubing to the sheath (Fig. 11-2). The cystoscope is checked by attaching the light source and confirming visibility and light through the scope (Fig. 11-3).

The periurethral area is then exposed with the fingers of one hand and the lubricated cystoscope sheath and obturator are carefully inserted. The tip of the sheath is usually curved and the curve should point upward. The sheath is held nearly vertically at the urethral entrance and gently introduced, following the curve of the instrument until the upper urethral sphincter has been passed[11] (Fig. 11-4). This represents only about 2 cm in women, and with experience the surgeon can

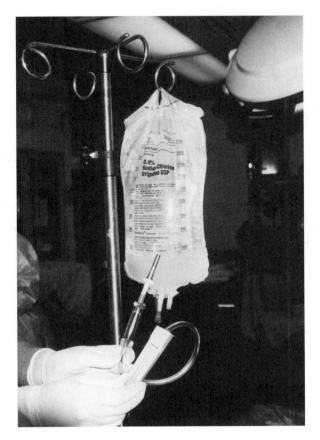

Fig. 11-2. Irrigation bag of saline to be connected to sleeve port.

feel the point at which the urethra has been cleared by the tip of the cystoscope. The obturator is then removed and sterile urine drained from the bladder. This specimen may be sent for culture or cytology. Many experienced cystoscopists insert the sheath and scope directly into the urethra without using the obturator, and with some experience this can be accomplished readily without urethral injury. This method does expose the sharper edges of the instrument to the urethral tissues and care must be taken not to cause urethral tears or bleeding.

The cystoscope, connected to the light source, is then introduced attached to a collar that provides a locking mechanism to secure the scope to the sheath. The slant of the telescope should point downward, or one will find that the tip of the sheath obscures the view. Valves are usually present on the collar or on the sheath and these should be closed before turning on the fluid source, to prevent leakage. The fluid source valve is opened and 150 to 250 ml of irrigating fluid are slowly instilled into the bladder, as the patient tolerates.

The cystoscope can be withdrawn slightly into the urethra to enable visualization of the opening of the upper urethra. The cystoscope is slowly advanced and the bladder is then visualized during filling. The trigone area directly in front of the urethra is identified by the interureteric ridge. This area is examined and the cystoscope moved slightly to each side to identify the ureteral orifices. Care is taken not to advance the scope inadvertently, as the ureteral orifices are often very close to the urethral opening, which forms one point of the trigone. The heel of the hand holding the cystoscope rests against the pubic bone, so that the scope can be rotated and moved from side to side without moving forward. This helps to reduce the risk of perforation or damage to the bladder walls.

Several minutes of observation may be needed to identify the ureteral orifices. They are often small, slit-like openings that only become apparent when opening to release a burst of urine. In cases in which the bladder is distorted by tumor or cystocele, a finger placed in the vagina and pressing upward under the bladder base may facilitate visualization of the ureteral openings. Large cervical tumors can cause a distortion of the bladder, such that the trigone sits in a valley behind the ridge made by the tumor. A bubble-like appearance to the trigone, or bullous edema may indicate tumor encroaching on the bladder, but does not document bladder invasion for staging purposes. Frond-like papillary growths or shaggy, necrotic tissue may be tumor (either primary or extending into the bladder) and should be biopsied.

After both ureteral orifices have been identified, the remainder of the bladder is inspected. The cystoscope and sheath are carefully rotated as a unit and moved slightly forward, but need not be moved far into the bladder. The dome of the bladder can often be identified by an air bubble resting there. Slight suprapubic pressure can facilitate visualization of the dome. The entire mucosa is examined 360

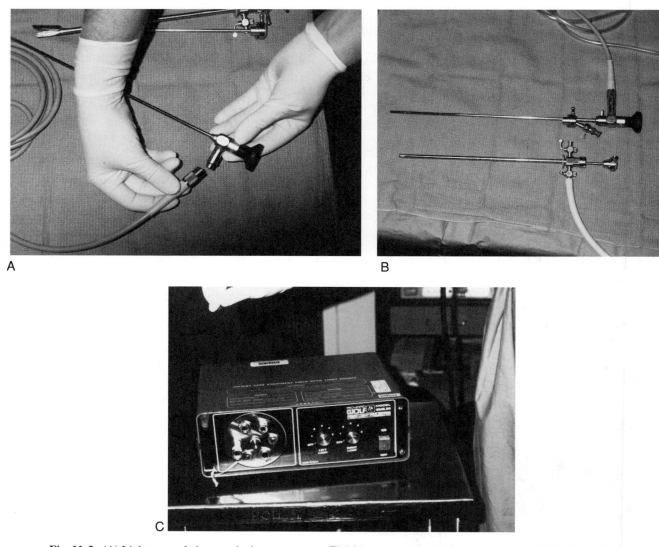

Fig. 11-3. (**A**) Light source being attached to cystoscope. (**B**) Light scource attached to cystoscope and irrigation tubing attached to sleeve with obturator in place prior to insertion. (**C**) Light source for cystoscope.

degrees for evidence of edema, stones, foreign bodies, tumor growth, erythema, or other abnormalities. Once inspection has been completed, the urethra is carefully visualized while withdrawing the scope to look for lesions (such as condyloma or erythema) and purulent exudate (which would suggest a urethral diverticulum). Some surgeons recommend inspecting the urethra at the beginning of the procedure, as movement of the cystoscope during cystoscopy may cause trauma to the urethral mucosa.

COMPLICATIONS

Complications of cystoscopy can include sepsis, hemorrhage from urethral injury or tumor, perforation of the bladder, and postprocedure dysuria. In men—whose urethra is longer, more tortuous, and often narrowed by the prostate—rectal perforation has been reported.[7] Complications can be nearly eliminated by proper technique and avoiding cystoscopy in patients suspected of having an active urinary tract infection.[8] Asymptomatic patients who have findings on cystoscopy suggestive of infection should be treated postprocedure. Those at high risk of infection, such as patients with fistulae, stents, urolithiasis, recent surgical procedures, or infected pelvic tumor, should receive preprocedure antibiotics.

ADVANTAGES

Most gynecologists will use cystoscopy to supplement their operative skills, rather than as an office diagnostic procedure for urinary complaints. Cystoscopy can be helpful in

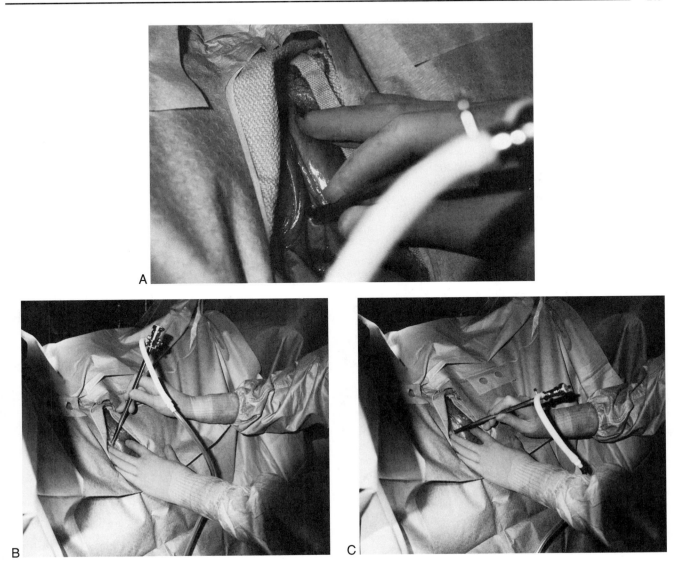

Fig. 11-4. (**A**) Cystoscope with obturator in place, being inserted into the urethra. (**B**) Cystoscope sleeve held at an upward angle to facilitate insertion. (**C**) The lubricated curved tip is inserted and the sleeve lowered as the upward curving tip passes under the pubic symphysis into the urethra.

avoiding urinary tract injuries, recognizing those that have occurred and assisting in their correction. It has now been demonstrated in a number of studies that early identification and early repair of surgical urologic injury can result in decreased morbidity to the patient and a good surgical outcome.[12,13]

Cystoscopy is very useful in identifying the two most common urinary tract injuries in gynecology: ureteral ligation or disruption, and bladder injury. Ureteral entrapment by suture with subsequent obstruction was noted clinic to occur in 0.33 percent of benign gynecologic surgeries in a large series from the Mayo Clinic.[14] Although most ureteral injury occurs in abdominal gynecologic procedures, 16 of 18 injuries in this series occurred during vaginal procedures, usually associated with a culdoplasty. This potential compli-

cation can be identified by using cystoscopy to check for ureteral patency in cases such as the following:

- Where dissection has been difficult, such as endometriosis or pelvic abscess
- When large pelvic masses have been removed
- If tumor debulking has required extensive pelvic dissection
- Where vaginal surgery has been performed, particularly with cul-de-sac obliteration

Performing cystoscopy is very simple in cases of vaginal surgery, because the periurethral area is accessible and prepared. One inserts the cystoscope, as above, while the anesthesia team injects 5 ml (20 mg) of indigo carmine intravenously. In a matter of minutes, the dye is excreted into the urine and, if both ureters are patent, flows freely from the ureteral orifices. More than 15 to 20 minutes of observation without dye excretion, or dye noted from only one ureter, is cause to explore the course of the ureters for inadvertent ligation. Blood from a ureteral orifice can also point to ureteral injury and must be investigated. Dye flow from both ureters rules out obstruction, although ureters that have been devascularized may appear intact yet develop fistulas later in the postoperative period. It has been described that using a dense irrigation medium of 10 percent glucose will cause a contrasting texture. The dye-colored urine will flow directly upward through the glucose, making visualization of each ureteral opening clear, even as dye collects at the top of the bladder.[15]

During an abdominal procedure, the ureteral orifices can be visualized either by opening the dome of the bladder, moving the patient to lithotomy position to perform transurethral cystoscopy, or by making a small incision in the dome of the bladder and inserting the cystoscope. This is held in place with a pursestring suture while the urethral catheter is occluded. Cystoscopy can be performed in this manner in the supine position, along with the dye tests described above.[3] If ureteral injury is detected, the ureter can be traced immediately throughout its pelvic course to identify the problem.

Bladder injury is often apparent to the surgeon without cystoscopy; however, cystoscopy can help ensure integrity of the bladder mucosa in cases where dissection has been difficult, and can also demonstrate sutures that have entered the bladder. Devascularization injuries, however, are not identifiable by cystoscopy, presenting later as vesicovaginal fistulas.

Cystoscopy can be useful in evaluating fistulas caused by surgical injury, pelvic irradiation, or pelvic malignancies. Enterovaginal fistulas are more accurately diagnosed by cystoscopy than by endoscopy of the gastrointestinal tract or intravenous pyelogram.[16] Ureterovaginal fistulas and vesicovaginal fistulas are most often identified by intravenous urogram, or by instilling saline and dye into the bladder or injecting indigo carmine intravenously and observing the vagina for leakage of the dye. Cystoscopy usually does not add to the initial diagnosis of ureterovaginal or vesicovaginal fistulas, but it is important for documenting the size and position of the defect before attempting repair.

Cystoscopy is a very useful adjunct in vaginal surgery, where the bladder is at risk of being entered or injured. This can include deep vaginal biopsies, excision of lesions along the anterior fornix, and vaginal hysterectomy and vault suspension in cases of prolapse where anatomy is distorted. Visualization of the interior of the bladder cystoscopically can guide the surgeon's incision depth and ensure that no sutures have been placed into the bladder, decreasing the risk of complications. Cystoscopic guidance is useful in the removal of small vaginal tumors, lesions of the vaginal cuff, and in excision of vaginal carcinoma in situ close to the

bladder and urethra. It has been suggested that cystoscopy be used routinely (and discussed with patients preoperatively) for all vaginal surgery to avoid complications involving the ureters or bladder.[17] The cystoscopy adds little to the operative time and can often facilitate the procedure by giving anatomic guidance. Probing a vaginal lesion while performing cystoscopy can show whether the lesion is actually lying over the bladder or only the vagina, and can aid in excision. In addition, in many vaginal cases, the ureters cannot be seen or palpated clearly; cystoscopy with intravenous dye injection can assure the surgeon of bilateral ureteral patency at the end of the procedure.

SUMMARY

Although operative cystoscopy such as stent placement and retrograde urography, and bladder biopsies requiring electrocautery are best left to urologists, simple cystoscopic skills can greatly benefit the gynecologic surgeon. Early diagnosis and treatment of urinary tract injury and avoidance of such injuries can be improved by the frequent use of cystoscopy, particularly during vaginal surgical procedures.

REFERENCES

1. Cervigni M, Scotto V, Panei M, Sbiroli C: Acute urethral obstruction due to condyloma acuminata. Obstet Gynecol 78:970, 1991
2. Denholm SW, Conn IG, Newsam JE, Chisolm GD: Morbidity following cystoscopy: comparison of flexible and rigid techniques. Br J Urol 66:152, 1990
3. Richardson DA: Cystourethroscopy in urogynecology. Obstet Gynecol Clin North Am 16:817, 1989
4. Ramahi AJ, Richardson DA, Ataya KM: Urethral stones in women, a case report. J Repro Med 38:743, 1993
5. Dietrick DD, Issa MM, Kabalin JN, Bassett JB: Intravesical migration of intrauterine device. J Urol 147:132, 1992
6. Wheeler JS, Flanigan RC, Young Hong H, Walloch JL: Female urethral diverticula with clear cell adenocarcinoma. J Surg Oncol 49:66, 1992
7. McDowell GC, Wise HA: Rectal perforation as a complication of urethral instrumentation: 2 case reports. J Urol 140:605, 1988
8. Bavetta S, Olsha O, Fenely J: Spreading sepsis by cystoscopy. Postgrad Med J 66:734, 1990
9. Brekkan E, Ehrnebo M, Malmstrom PU et al: A controlled study of low and high volume anesthetic jelly as a lubricant and pain reliever during cystoscopy. J Urol 146:24, 1991
10. Stein M, Lubetkin D, Taub HC et al: The effects of intraurethral lidocaine anesthetic and patient anxiety on pain perception during cystoscopy. J Urol 151:1518, 1994
11. Rosenblum D: The Practice of Cystoscopy. p. 70. Charles C Thomas, Springfield, IL, 1966
12. Blandy JP, Badenoch DF, Fowler CG et al: Early repair of

iatrogenic injury to the ureter of bladder after gynecologic surgery. J Urol 146:761, 1991

13. Tancer ML: Observations on prevention and management of vesicovaginal fistula after total hysterectomy. Surg Gynecol Obstet 175:501, 1992

14. Stanhope CR, Wilson TO, Utz WJ et al: Suture entrapment and secondary ureteral obstruction. Am J Obstet Gynecol 164:1513, 1991

15. Lin BL, Iwata Y: Modified cystoscopy to evaluate unilateral traumatic injury of the ureter during pelvic surgery (letter). Am J Obstet Gynecol 162:1343, 1990

16. Kirsch GM, Hampel N, Shuck JM, Resnick MI: Diagnosis and management of vesicoenteric fistulas. Surg Gynecol Obstet 173:91, 1991

17. Pettit PD, Petrou SP: The value of cystoscopy in major vaginal surgery. Obstet Gynecol 84:318, 1994

CHAPTER TWELVE

VAGINOSCOPY

SUSAN POKORNY

PREOPERATIVE CONSIDERATIONS

Endoscopy is the visual inspection of any cavity of the body by means of an endoscope, an instrument for the examination of the interior of a hollow viscus. Vaginoscopy has been defined as use of a special instrument to visualize the vaginal canal, usually as distinct from a speculum examination. The clinician should choose an instrument that will cause no damage to the hymen or lower genital tract of the unestrogenized child. The anatomic integrity of the child's hymenal tissue is important from a cultural and forensic point of view; families need to be assured the child will remain virginal, and anatomic disruptions of the hymenal tissues are used as forensic evidence of childhood sexual abuse. Prior to insertion of any instrument into the vaginal introitus, a recording of the anatomic features of the hymen should be made. A normal, intact hymen has a smooth contiguous rim from at least 3 o'clock clockwise around to 9 o'clock, if one is observing the child in the supine position; 12 o'clock is toward the urethra, 3 o'clock the child's left side and 6 o'clock toward the anus.[1] Comment should also be made about the amount of estrogen effect on the child's tissues,[2] since children with a high estrogen effect (newborns and peripubertal children) are able to tolerate stretch trauma to the hymen without residual effect to a higher degree than are children with a very low estrogen effect (children 3 to 8 years of age). There is no place for use of pediatric vaginal speculums in the routine examination of the prepubertal child's vagina, as there is risk of traumatizing the hymen and vaginal walls; this is true even if the child is under general anesthesia.

INSTRUMENTATION

Historically, a popular technique for examination of a child's vagina involved the Cameron-Myers vaginoscope, which has interchangeable distal tubular structures of 0.7 cm, 1.0 cm, and 1.3 cm diameters[3,4] (Fig. 12-1). This instrument was in essence a modification of a veterinary otoscope, which certain other clinicians advocate for vaginoscopy.[5,6] Still others have suggested use of the Killian nasal speculum.[7] Use of these instruments allows detection of large lesions and those that are a different color than the vaginal walls. However, if the lesion is accompanied by a large amount of mucus or debris, or is very small, its detection with these instruments is difficult.

Vaginoscopy with an irrigating endoscope is ideal for examination of the lower reproductive tract of a prepubertal female[8–10] (Fig. 12-2). The small diameter of the endoscope causes no distortion of the hymenal tissues, and the irrigation fluid will not only lavage the vagina but distend it sufficiently to allow good visualization of the cervix and vaginal canal. Lavaging the vagina of mucus and debris is important for detection of extremely small exophytic lesions that can be camouflaged by mucus. In addition, a small exophytic lesion will flap freely in the irrigating fluid, aiding in its detection.

Distension of the vaginal canal by fluid allows the cervix and the vagina to be visualized together. Use of any other instrument than an irrigating vaginoscope will not allow this panoramic view, since one can only see that which is directly adjacent to the distal portal of the Cameron-Myers vaginoscope or veterinary otoscope. This general panorama of the

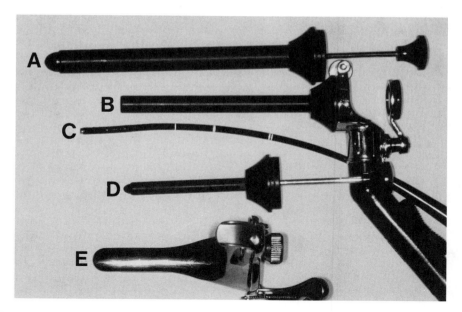

Fig. 12-1. Relative size of the Cameron-Myers vaginoscope (A, B, & D), as compared to a 3-mm hysteroscope (C) or a pediatric speculum (E).

cervix and vagina helps the examiner to appreciate any anatomic asymmetries that would be suggestive of certain congenital anomalies such as ectopic ureters (Figs. 12-3 and 12-4) and mullerian duct defects.

Any endoscope with irrigating properties can be used. Because of their shorter length, a bronchoscope or urethroscope are ideal. Nevertheless, a laparoscope, cystoscope, nephroscope, or hysteroscope can be used. (Fig. 12-5) Hysteroscopes, which have very small diameters, are necessary in certain children; but the smaller the scope used, the lower the pressure of the fluid for distension of the vaginal canal. An assistant placing pressure on the irrigating fluid bag or supplementing the pressure of the fluid with an attached large-volume syringe of fluid usually overcomes these problems. Bladder irrigating fluid or normal saline can be used as the distending fluid. High molecular weight fluids, as are used in hysteroscopy, offer no advantage and, in fact, are a deterrent to getting a good seal of the vulvar tissues around the endoscope due to their slippery consistency.

The advantages of irrigating vaginoscopy over nonirrigating vaginoscopy are as listed. Vaginoscopy with an irrigating endoscope can be performed in the office or as an examination under anesthesia. The site is determined by the child's ability to comply with instructions. The author is more comfortable using a flexible irrigating endoscope for office procedures due to concern about inadvertent patient movement that might accidentally injure her. Patient compliance can be improved when the child is informed that she too will be able to see her cervix or birth canal after completion of the examination; when a flexible scope is used, it can be bent toward the patient and she also can visualize her lower genital tract. A video attachment with a monitor will also im-

prove compliance. Topical anesthetic is applied to the vulva approximately 5 minutes before inserting the vaginoscope.[11] The author uses a 2 percent preparation of viscous lidocaine.

FINDINGS

If swabs are used to obtain cultures from the unestrogenized prepubertal vagina before vaginoscopy, one will invariably notice pink discoloration on the final swab(s) of a series. On vaginoscopy, small petechiae will be noted on the cervix or vaginal side walls. This occurs so frequently that it should be considered normal in this situation (Fig. 12-6).

Rugation of the vaginal walls is variable but usually low and minimal. Much of the prepubertal side walls are smooth and free of rugae.

Extensive papillary projections have been observed around embedded foreign objects. Lesser papillary projections have been observed at the site of other foreign objects. It seems very likely that because of the dependent position of the vaginal orifice, a foreign object could be expelled with Valsalva's maneuver before its discovery. Thus, when performing vaginoscopy for unexplained vaginal bleeding or discharge, the physician should look for and note any sites of papillary excrescences as possible evidence of an expelled foreign object.[12]

The unestrogenized vaginal walls will also frequently respond to trauma with the formation of granulation tissue. The mounds of friable tissue will look very bizarre with the magnification of vaginoscopy. Nevertheless, this granulation tissue will resolve in most cases by application of topical estrogen cream to the vulva.[13]

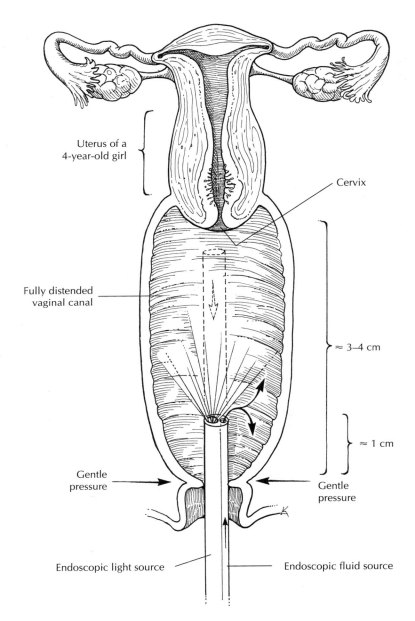

Uterus of a
4-year-old girl

Cervix

Fully distended
vaginal canal

≈ 3–4 cm

≈ 1 cm

Gentle
pressure

Gentle
pressure

Endoscopic light source

Endoscopic fluid source

Fig. 12-2. After carefully placing the irrigating endoscope into the vagina approximately 3 to 4 cm, the vulvar tissues are gently pressed against the endoscope, trapping the irrigating fluid in the vagina. At this point, the endoscope is withdrawn to approximately 1 cm from the introitus for full visualization of the vaginal canal.

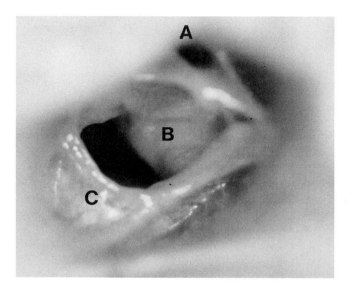

Fig. 12-3. Ectopic ureter through vaginal introitus. Urethra (A). An asymmetric ridge of tissue was observed coarsing the length of the vagina from the level of the cervix to the introitus (B). Note the smooth contiguous rim of hymenal tissue, which remained unchanged after vaginoscopy (C).

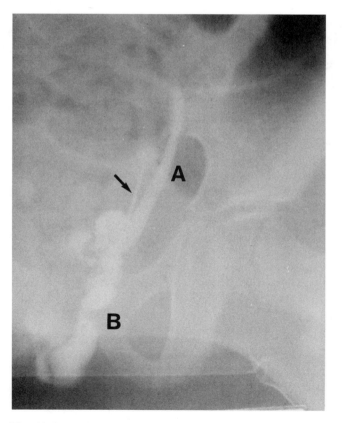

Fig. 12-4. Radiograph of patient in Fig. 12-3. Dye injected via spinal needle (arrow) placed in the suprapubic area under cystoscopic visualization, illustrating left ectopic ureter (A) and extention down the vaginal wall to introitus (B).

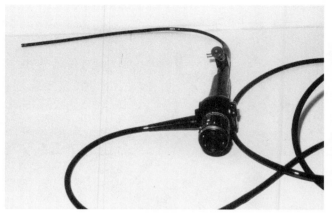

Fig. 12-5. Nephroscope.

If an irrigating vaginoscope is not used, linear lacerations noted with a pediatric speculum would have to be attributed to the trauma of the speculum examination per se. This would be very detrimental if the examination was being performed to document sexual abuse. Because abuse is always in the differential of unexplained genital bleeding in a prepubertal female, speculums should never be used for evaluation. Vaginoscopy, by contrast, will lavage the vagina and allow good definition of acute trauma. If there has been avulsion of the vaginal apex there will be no vaginal distension, since the fluid would be going into the abdominal cavity.

Advantages of Irrigating Endoscope for Vaginoscopy

- Small diameter causes no lower genital tract trauma or damage
- Mucus and debris are lavaged from the vaginal canal by the irrigating fluid
- Good visualization of the vaginal canal and cervix is provided when the irrigating fluid distends the vagina
- Superior visualization is necessary for detection of the following:
  - Very small (2 to 4 mm) exophytic, skin-colored lesions
  - Subtle asymmetry of the vaginal canal
  - Small craters/dimples of ectopic ureters
- Endoscopes are readily available

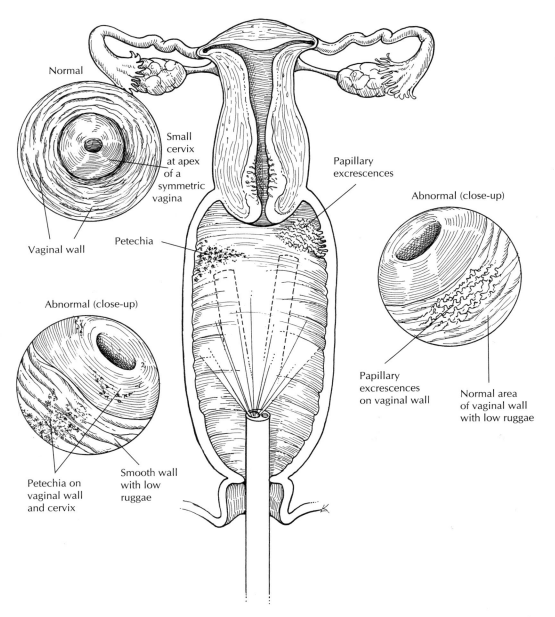

Normal

Small
cervix
at apex
of a
symmetric
vagina

Vaginal wall

Petechia

Papillary
excrescences

Abnormal (close-up)

Abnormal (close-up)

Petechia on
vaginal wall
and cervix

Smooth wall
with low
ruggae

Papillary
excrescences
on vaginal wall

Normal area
of vaginal wall
with low ruggae

Fig. 12-6. Commonly observed variations are iatrogenic petechiae (from swabs used to obtain cultures) and papillary excrescences (associated with inflammation).

Steps for Outpatient Vaginoscopy

- Patient sits semireclined with buttocks at end of gynecologic procedure table, positioned so that the irrigating fluid will collect in the drip basin
- Topical anesthetic agent is placed on vulva, approximately 5 minutes before procedure
- Fluid must be at room or slightly warmer temperature (tepid)
- Endoscope is inserted with irrigating fluid flowing
- Flexible endoscopes diminish chance of patient injury with inadvertent movement, and allow some patients the opportunity to also visualize their lower genital tract
- Patient compliance improved by promising her "a look" at the end of the procedure

---

In most cases without distinct pathology, the vaginoscopist will encounter a smooth or nodular symmetric cervix and smooth or slightly rugated symmetric vaginal canal. When asymmetry of the cervix or vagina are noted, or when there are extra craters, dimples, or folds of tissue in the upper

---

Potential Findings on Vaginoscopy of the Prepubertal Vagina

- Petechiae following serial swabs for cultures
- Papillary excrescence suggestive of inflammation such as caused by an expelled foreign object
- Lacerations or granulation tissue from trauma
- Subtle findings suggestive of genitourinary anomalies
- Small cervical polyps

---

vagina, suspicion of a urogenital anomaly must be raised. Vaginoscopy with an irrigating endoscope has led to such a superior panoramic view of the prepubertal vagina and cervix that future clinical studies are warranted to better define and outline management for cervical and vaginal variants.

REFERENCES

1. Pokorny S: Configuration of the prepubertal hymen. Am J Obstet Gynecol 157:950, 1987
2. Yordan EE, Yordan RA: The hymen and tanner staging of the breast. Adolesc Pediatr Gynecol 5:76, 1992
3. Capvaro V: Gynecologic examinations in children and adolescents. Pediatric Clin North Am 19:511, 1972
4. Droegemueller W: Pediatric gynecology. p. 251. In Droegemueller W, Herbst AL, Mishell DR Jr, Stenchever MA (eds): Comprehensive Gynecology. CV Mosby, St. Louis, 1987
5. Billmire ME, Farrell MK, Dine MS: A simplified procedure for pediatric vaginal examination: use of veterinary otoscope specula. Pediatrics 65:823, 1980
6. Brenner PF: Infancy and childhood. p. 375. In Romney SL, Gray MJ, Little AB et al (eds): Gynecology and Obstetrics: The Health Care of Women. McGraw-Hill, New York, 1981
7. Emans SJH, Goldstein DP: Office evaluation of the child and adolescent. p. 15. In Emans SJH, Goldstein DP (eds): Pediatric and Adolescent Gynecology. 3rd Ed. Little, Brown, Boston, 1990
8. Pokorny SF: The genital examination of the infant through adolescence. p. 753. In Goldfarb AA (ed): Current Opinion in Obstetrics and Gynecology. Current Science, 1993
9. Pokorny SF: Pediatric gynecology. p. 109. In Stenchever MA, (ed): Office Gynecology. Mosby–Year Book, St. Louis, 1992
10. Bascko G: Hysteroscopy for vaginoscopy in pediatric gynecology. Adolesc Pediatr Gynecol 7:221, 1994
11. Zupi E, Luciano AA, Valli E et al: The use of topical anesthesia in diagnostic hysteroscopy and endometrial biopsy. Fertil Steril 63:414, 1995
12. Pokorny SF: Long term intravaginal presence of foreign bodies in children: a preliminary study. J Repro Med 39:931, 1994
13. Pokorny SF, Pokorny WJ, Kramer W: Acute genital injuries in prepubertal females. Am J Obstet Gynecol 166:1461, 1992

CHAPTER THIRTEEN

DILATION AND CURETTAGE AND HYSTEROSCOPY

RICHARD S. GUIDO
DALE W. STOVALL

The female uterus is a dynamic organ consisting of a relatively quiescent muscular myometrium and an active endometrium. The uterus and the endometrial cavity are frequently evaluated in the presence of abnormal uterine bleeding, pelvic pain, infertility, and pregnancy complications. The practicing gynecologist has a variety of tools available for the examination of the uterus. The appropriate selection of these technologies in the evaluation of a patient presenting with complaints related to the uterus is the challenge for the practitioner. This chapter is designed to provide the practicing obstetrician/gynecologist with an understanding of the pathophysiology, evaluation, and appropriate surgical treatment of uterine diseases. Included in this chapter are the indications and techniques for office endometrial biopsy, diagnostic and therapeutic curettage, hysteroscopy, and their associated complications.

BACKGROUND

During the past 70 years there have been remarkable changes in the techniques that gynecologists use to examine the uterus for abnormalities. The dilation and curettage (D&C) procedure is one of the oldest surgical procedures, dating back to the early 1800s. Initially used for evacuation of fungal growths from the endometrial cavity, D&C became the most popular gynecologic operation performed in the United States. In 1975, over 900,000 D&Cs were performed.[1] The office endometrial biopsy, initially conceived in 1924 by Kelley[2] and championed in the 1970s, has, to a major degree, replaced the diagnostic D&C as the initial step in obtaining endometrial tissue. Both D&C and office biopsy are limited in that the procedures are performed in a blind fashion. Pantaleoni[3] in 1869 was one of the first investigators to attempt to directly view the uterine cavity. The forefathers of hysteroscopy encountered numerous technical problems, including the lack of a panoramic view, poor illumination, lack of magnification of the specimen, and inability to obtain a surgical specimen. Over the past century, developments in the technical aspects of hysteroscopic equipment have enabled the gynecologist to obtain well-illuminated, panoramic views of the uterine cavity and to perform a variety of therapeutic procedures. Finally, with the development of pelvic ultrasound, including transvaginal ultrasound, gynecologists are able to obtain detailed information about the uterus in a nonsurgical fashion.

Indications for Diagnostic Dilation and Curettage

- Abnormal uterine bleeding
- Postmenopausal bleeding
- Histologic dating of the endometrium
- Endometrial cells on Pap smear

DILATION AND CURETTAGE

Indications for Diagnostic D&C

The endometrium is evaluated in a variety of clinical settings. The most common indications for obtaining endometrial tissue include abnormal uterine bleeding, postmenopausal bleeding, and endometrial dating. The indications for the histologic assessment of the endometrial cavity are summarized in the box titled *Indications for Histologic Assessment.*

Abnormal Uterine Bleeding

Understanding the mechanisms that control normal menses is a prerequisite for the evaluation and treatment of patients with abnormal uterine bleeding. Normal menses begins, on average, at 12.5 years of age and continues until age 51. Under the control of ovarian steroids, an average woman will have approximately 500 menses during her reproductive life. The control of menses involves a complex interaction of the hypothalamic, pituitary, and ovarian hormones to produce an effect on the endometrium. Menstruation occurs in the absence of implantation of the fertilized oocyte with the withdrawal of estrogen and progesterone production from the failing corpus luteum.

The endometrium consists of two layers, the basalis and the functionalis (Fig. 13-1). The endometrium is a dynamic epithelium ranging in thickness from 2 mm during the prolif-

---

Indications for Histologic Assessment of the Endometrium

- Abnormal uterine bleeding
- Postmenopausal bleeding
- Histologic dating of endometrium
- Evaluation of abnormal glandular cells on Pap smear

---

erative phase to 6 mm during the secretory phase.[4] The functionalis layer is further subdivided into the compacta, which is a thin superficial zone that contains the straight portion of the endometrial glands, and the spongiosum, which is the deep section of the endometrium filled with tortuous glands, spiral arteries, and stroma.

A number of theories exist that explain the events leading to menstruation. In vitro studies have demonstrated that vascular constriction of spiral arteries represents one of the initiating events during menses.[5] Venous stasis, in conjunction with bleeding either directly from the vessels or into a hematoma, is responsible for menstrual blood flow. Menstrual toxins, in addition to the rupture of lysosomal enzymes, are also responsible for the tissue destruction that occurs with menstruation.

The entire functionalis layer of the endometrium is not lost during menstruation; rather, 5 percent of the endometrial cells show evidence of destruction on any given menstrual day.[6] The endometrium does regress in size during menstruation, not completely by loss of tissue, but rather by a process of autophagia (intracellular destruction of nonvital organelles), heterophagia (intracellular destruction of extracellular debris), extrusion of secretory products, and elimination of fluids through intracellular spaces. These processes, in conjunction with the presence of a protective carbohydrate coating on the endometrial cells, result in an organized loss of endometrium.

The blood loss during menstruation is difficult to quantify. However, careful analysis has shown that the mean blood loss during menstruation is approximately 30 ml.[7] In a given individual, the amount of blood loss with each menses is remarkably consistent. There is, however, a striking difference in the amount of interpersonal variation, ranging from 5 to 180 ml.

Normal menstrual cycles occur every 28 days, with a range of 7 days. Abnormalities in the duration, amount, and timing of menstrual bleeding may occur.

The gynecologist may gain a great deal of insight into the pathophysiology of a patient's bleeding abnormality by taking a good history. Goldrath and Sherman[8] studied 406 patients who presented for the evaluation of menstrual abnormality and underwent office hysteroscopy and biopsy. Table 13-1 lists the underlying pathology for each patient in relation to their presenting complaint. Patients presenting with menorrhagia were frequently found to have an underlying submucous fibroid. Endometrial polyps were found to produce a variety of symptoms ranging from intramenstrual bleeding to menorrhagia but appeared more frequently (17 percent) in patients with intramenstrual bleeding. Of the patients undergoing evaluation for postmenopausal bleeding, 12 percent were found to have a carcinoma.

The endometrium responds to the cyclic stimulation and withdrawal of estrogen and progesterone production by the ovary with proliferation, glandular secretion, and predictable menstruation. If ovulation does not occur and estrogen pro-

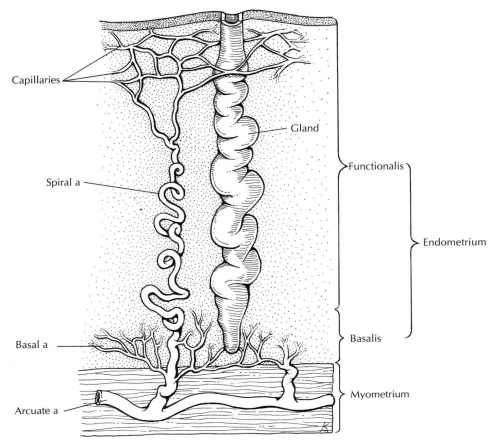

Capillaries

Spiral a

Basal a

Arcuate a

Gland

Functionalis

Endometrium

Basalis

Myometrium

Fig. 13-1. Premenstrual endometrium.

Table 13-1. Endometrial Histology As It Relates to Presenting Symptoms

Hysteroscopic and/or Pathologic Diagnosis	Intermenstrual Bleeding (n = 56)	Dysfunctional Bleeding (n = 54)	Postmenopausal Bleeding (n = 84)	Menorrhagia (n = 149)	Menometrorrhagia (n = 23)	Other (n = 40)
Normal (n = 219)	35	34	48	67	12	23
Submucous (n = 87)	5	5	7	59	8	3
Carcinoma (n = 12)	2	0	10	0	0	0
Hyperplasia (n = 14)	3	5	4	1	1	0
Endometrial polyp (n = 38)	10	5	10	11	0	2
Adenomyosis (n = 3)	0	0	0	3	0	0
Miscellaneous[a] (n = 27)	1	4	1	8	2	11
Failure to complete hysterectomy (n = 6)	0	1	4	0	0	1
Total	56	54	84	149	23	40

[a] Synechiae, 14; adenocarcinoma of the cervix, 1; T-shaped uterus in patients exposed to diethylstilbestrol, 4; septate uteri; 4; hemiuterus, 1; imbedded intrauterine device, 2; vascular anomaly, 1.
(From Goldrath and Sherman,[8] with permission.)

Definitions Commonly Used To Describe Menstrual Abnormalities

- Polymenorrhea
  - Menstrual cycle intervals less than 21 days
- Oligomenorrhea
  - Menstrual cycle intervals of more than 37 days
- Metrorrhagia
  - Bleeding that occurs between menstrual cycles
- Menorrhagia
  - Excessive or prolonged bleeding that occurs at regular intervals
- Menometrorrhagia
  - Combination of excessive or prolonged bleeding as well as bleeding that occurs between menstrual cycles
- Dysfunctional uterine bleeding
  - Excessive uterine bleeding in the absence of intrauterine or extrauterine pathology, typically a manifestation of anovulation
- Postmenopausal bleeding
  - Uterine bleeding that occurs 12 months after cessation of menses

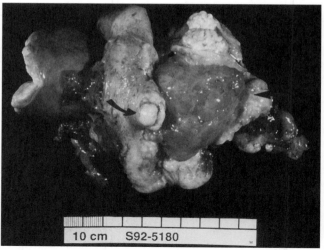

A

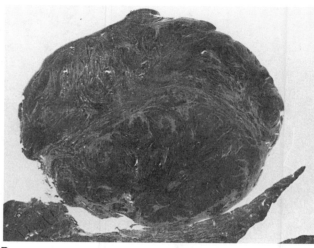

B

Fig. 13-2. Submucous leiomyoma. (**A**) Gross specimen. Curved arrow, submucous leiomyoma; straight arrow, degenerating leiomyoma. (**B**) Magnification of leiomyoma ($\times$ 2).

duction is unopposed, endometrial proliferation continues unabated. This results in irregular shedding of the endometrium and menometrorrhagia. Irregular endometrial growth, sloughing, and irregular menstrual bleeding can occur with the more subtle defects in estrogen and progesterone production that are caused by abnormalities in the follicular and luteal phases, including an inadequate synthesis and release of estrogen and/or progesterone that may be incapable of sufficient endometrial support and cause noncyclic uterine bleeding.

Leiomyoma are associated with a variety of bleeding patterns, ranging from normal menstrual flow to menorrhagia. The exact pathophysiology of menstrual abnormalities in patients with leiomyoma is unknown, although they have been postulated to increase the endometrial surface area from which bleeding may occur. Submucous fibroids in particular have been implicated as the cause of menorrhagia (Fig. 13-2). Degeneration of a submucous fibroid with subsequent hemorrhagia has been reported; however, this is an uncommon occurrence.[9] Endometrial venule ectasia has been associated with the endometrium overlying an intramural fibroid. These dilated venules may alter the normal control mechanism of menses and result in menorrhagia.

Endometrial polyps occur most frequently in the fifth dec-

ade of life and have been found in approximately 17 to 30 percent of patients undergoing a D&C.[10] The histologic diagnosis is confirmed by the presence of endometrial mucosa overlying connective tissue containing a thick-walled vessel and stromal fibrosis (Fig. 13-3). The predominant bleeding pattern in patients with endometrial polyps is metrorrhagia, although other bleeding patterns may occur. The exact pathophysiology for the bleeding is unknown. However, focal necrosis of the polyp may occur, exposing underlying vascular structures. The endometrium of the polyp may be hyperplastic, proliferative, or secretory, with the latter being the most uncommon. Endometrial polyps may arise from the basalis layer of the endometrium and therefore are less responsive to progesterone. This feature may account for the

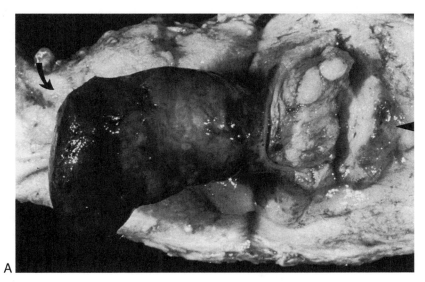

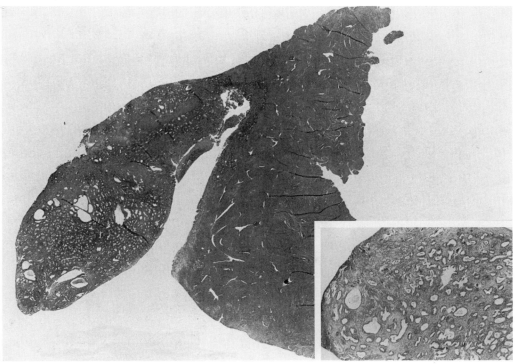

Fig. 13-3. Endometrial polyp. **(A)** Gross specimen. Curved arrow, polyp; straight arrow, submucous leiomyoma. **(B)** Magnification of polyp (× 1). (Inset, × 10.)

frequent finding of endometrium that is out of phase with the surrounding tissue and may be more susceptible to bleeding.

Endometrial hyperplasia and endometrial carcinoma frequently present with abnormal vaginal bleeding. Endometrial hyperplasia occurs most frequently in the fifth decade, whereas endometrial carcinoma is most frequent in the postmenopausal patient. The exact etiology for bleeding from endometrial hyperplasia and carcinoma is unknown; however, these tissues are extremely vascular, which may account for this symptom (Fig. 13-4).

Postmenopausal Bleeding

Postmenopausal bleeding is one of the most common indications for office endometrial biopsy or outpatient D&C. Endometrial carcinoma is a disease that presents in the postmenopausal age range, and is frequently diagnosed in an early stage due to vaginal bleeding. The detection of endometrial carcinoma is the main focus in any patient who presents with postmenopausal bleeding, and it is detected in 10 to 15 percent of patients.[11] Although the most frequent diag-

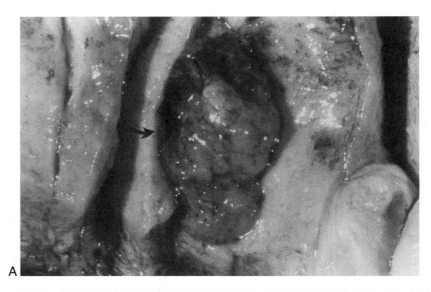

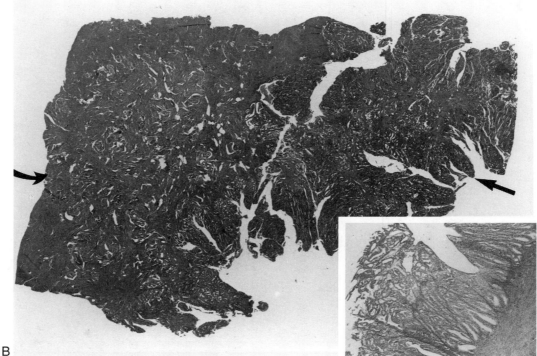

Fig. 13-4. Endometrial carcinoma. **(A)** Gross specimen. Curved arrow, carcinoma. **(B)** Magnification ($\times$ 1). Curved arrow, carcinoma; straight arrow, myometrium. (Inset, $\times$ 10.)

nosis is an atrophic endometrium, endometrial hyperplasia, endometrial polyps, and leiomyoma may also produce uterine bleeding in this age group. With the widespread use of hormone replacement therapy, a larger proportion of postmenopausal patients are susceptible to uterine bleeding. The timing of uterine bleeding in relation to the administration of cyclic progesterone has been used to predict the type of endometrial histology.[12] However, it is generally agreed that uterine bleeding that occurs beyond 6 months of initiating

hormone replacement therapy, or is irregular or excessive should be evaluated. Routine screening of the endometrium before the initiation of hormone replacement therapy has not been shown to be cost-effective in asymptomatic patients.[13]

Histologic Dating of the Endometrium

The evaluation of a couple presenting with infertility begins with a complete history and physical examination. A history of cyclic, predictable menses virtually assures the clinician that the patient is ovulating regularly. Even if additional evidence of ovulation exists (e.g., a biphasic basal body temperature curve, detection of a midcycle luteinizing hormone [LH] surge, or a serum progesterone level greater than 10 nmol/L) the endometrium may not be prepared for normal nidation in the midluteal phase. Endometrial sampling must be performed to determine whether the endometrium is responding properly to the sequential production of estrogen and progesterone. An endometrial biopsy for histologic dating should be performed in the late luteal phase. The biopsy is performed using an office biopsy technique. The timing of the biopsy is critical. The procedure should be performed 10 to 12 days after an LH surge or 4 to 5 days before an anticipated menses. The histologic menstrual date (e.g., day 21), is compared to the actual menstrual date, which can be calculated by subtracting the number of days between the day of the endometrial biopsy and the subsequent menses from 28 (the average length of a normal menstrual cycle). A luteal phase defect is defined as a delay in histologic endometrial maturation by more than 2 days in two different menstrual cycles and has been associated with infertility and recurrent pregnancy loss.

Endometrial Cells on Papanicolaou Smear

Endometrial cells may be detected during a routine Papanicolaou (Pap) smear. The desquamation of endometrial cells during the first 12 days following menses is considered normal. Endometrial cells identified during the luteal phase of the menstrual cycle or in the postmenopausal period have been associated with a variety of uterine conditions, including endometritis, endometrial polyps, and endometrial carcinoma.[14]

The cytologic characteristic of the endometrial cells is predictive of the incidence of endometrial carcinoma. Endometrial cells that are described as atypical or suspicious for malignancy are associated with endometrial carcinoma in 20 to 60 percent of postmenopausal patients.[15] All patients with atypical endometrial cells present on a Pap smear should undergo endometrial sampling. Premenopausal patients with normal-appearing endometrial cells on a Pap smear are unlikely to have associated endometrial carcinoma and could be followed with noninvasive techniques. All postmenopausal patients with any endometrial cells present on a Pap smear should undergo an endometrial sampling. The Pap smear abnormality, ''atypical glandular cells of unknown significance,'' is problematic. Endometrial biopsy, endocervical curettage, and colposcopy are probably indicated.

Prehysterectomy Endometrial Sampling

The routine use of either an office endometrial biopsy or intraoperative D&C before a hysterectomy or in conjunction with cervical conization has been a common practice in gynecology. These procedures are frequently conducted for the sole purpose of discovering unsuspected uterine carcinoma. A number of studies have demonstrated that this practice lacks scientific support. The incidence of endometrial carcinoma in patients undergoing hysterectomy for benign indications is quite rare, 0.4 percent in one study.[16] Stovall et al[17] examined the results of endometrial biopsy obtained prior to hysterectomy in 619 patients with either Vabra aspiration (10 percent), Novak curette (27.4 percent), or fractional D&C (63.1 percent). There were 30 cases of endometrial carcinoma or hyperplasia that were undetected by the prehysterectomy sampling. The results of these studies demonstrate the futility of performing a preoperative endometrial sampling in patients undergoing a hysterectomy for benign conditions.

Most patients undergoing cervical conization for the treatment of cervical dysplasia are between 20 and 40 years of age and are unlikely to be afflicted by endometrial carcinoma. The incidence of endometrial abnormalities, and specifically endometrial carcinoma, is less than 1 percent in this group. In one retrospective review of 207 cervical conizations performed for cervical dysplasia, 96 percent underwent concurrent D&C.[18] Two cases of endometrial abnormalities—one patient with cystic hyperplasia and one with mild adenomatous hyperplasia with atypia—were discovered. Three uterine perforations occurred that required hospitalization for observation. Unless a patient requires a diagnostic evaluation of the endometrium for a specific reason, the routine use of D&C is not indicated in conjunction with cervical conization.

Preoperative Evaluation

Ultrasound

Noninvasive techniques for the evaluation of the uterus, and specifically the endometrium, have improved dramatically over the past 10 years. In skilled hands, the combination of transabdominal and transvaginal ultrasound provide excellent definition and detail of the endometrium, the myometrium, and any associated pathology. The practicing gynecologist may use a pelvic ultrasound before a diagnostic D&C, or to determine the condition of an early pregnancy in a patient presenting with symptoms of a spontaneous abortion. Intraoperative transvaginal ultrasound has been used to guide surgeons in performing difficult diagnostic and therapeutic D&Cs.

Numerous studies have been conducted to evaluate the sensitivity and specificity of transvaginal ultrasound for detecting uterine pathology in patients with abnormal or postmenopausal bleeding. Goldstein et al[19] examined 30 patients with postmenopausal bleeding before the patients underwent an outpatient suction endometrial sampling. All patients with a full-thickness endometrial echo of less than 5 mm were noted to have insufficient tissue for diagnosis and were classified as having atrophic endometrium. Patients with an en-

Table 13-2. Histologic Diagnosis of Endometrium As Related to Thickness (5-mm Intervals) of Endometrium Measured by Endovaginal Scanning[a]

Histologic Diagnosis	Endometrial Thickness						Total No.
	≤5 mm	6–10 mm	11–15 mm	16–20 mm	21–25 mm	>25 mm	
Atrophy	150	6	1	—	—	—	157
Hyperplasia	—	7	6	—	—	—	13
Polyp	—	7	5	—	—	—	13
Pyometra	—	—	1	—	1	1	3
Hematometra	—	—	1	—	—	—	1
Cancer	—	1	8	4	3	2	18
Total	150	21	22	4	5	3	205

[a] Figures indicate number of women.
(From Granberg et al,[20] with permission.)

dometrial echo of greater than 6 mm were found to have a variety of histologic diagnoses, including functional endometrium, hyperplasia, and one case of endometrial carcinoma. This pilot study demonstrated the feasibility of using an endometrial thickness of less than 5 mm as a cutoff between atrophic endometrium and other histologic conditions. Granberg et al[20] preoperatively evaluated three groups of patients: 205 postmenopausal patients undergoing a D&C for vaginal bleeding, 30 postmenopausal patients without vaginal bleeding, and 30 patients with known endometrial cancer. Table 13-2 correlates the final histologic diagnoses with the endometrial thickness. The mean endometrial echo in women with endometrial cancer was 18.2 ± 6.2 mm, as compared to 3.4 mm ± 1.2 mm in those women with atrophic endometrium. No cancers were identified when the endometrial echo was less than 9 mm, and no histologic abnormalities were identified in any patients with an endometrium echo of less than 5 mm.

A pelvic ultrasound incorporating a transvaginal probe is useful in the patient who is medically unable to undergo a diagnostic D&C or office biopsy. An endometrial echo of less than 5 mm is consistent with a benign endometrium. A few reports of endometrial hyperplasia[21] and carcinoma[22] have been described in patients with an endometrial echo of less than 5 mm. Further large scale prospective studies are required using this technique before determining its role in the evaluation of patients with abnormal or postmenopausal bleeding. The lack of specificity of this technique makes it unlikely that the transvaginal pelvic ultrasound will replace the endometrial biopsy or D&C.

Sonohysterography

Sonohysterography is a relatively new technique introduced to improve the resolution of intrauterine pathology. This technique employs the instillation of saline into the uterus while performing either transabdominal or transvaginal ul-

trasound. Saline is injected for transabdominal ultrasound by using a Finkentscher and Semm cup (Wisap, Saverlach, Germany) attached to the cervix to slowly introduce 30 ml of fluid while simultaneously performing an ultrasound.[23] Transvaginal sonohysterography can be performed using either a flexible 5.5 French intrauterine insemination catheter with a 2-ml cervical balloon (HG Catheter, Co., Cranford, NJ) to instill 5 to 10 ml of saline into the uterine cavity[24] (Fig. 13-5). Internal endometrial images are obtained using either real time or cine-loop imaging. The presence of a fluid-solid interface improves the specificity of transvaginal and transabdominal ultrasound in the detection of submucous leiomyoma (Fig. 13-6) and endometrial polyps[23,25] (Fig. 13-7). Preliminary studies have shown the utility of sonohysterography in detecting intrauterine adhesions, endometrial hyperplasia,[26] and demonstrating a normal intrauterine contour in patients using Tamoxifen who otherwise were noted to have an abnormal transvaginal ultrasound.[27] Further large scale studies are required to determine the utility of this technique.

Magnetic Resonance Imaging

Magnetic resonance imaging (MRI) is a rapidly evolving technology that uses three parameters inherent to an individual tissue to develop a measurable signal and subsequently, an image of anatomic structures. The signal is a function of the T_1 relaxation time, the T_2 relaxation time, and the proton density of the tissue.[28] Since the MRI signal is derived from several parameters, it is capable of exhibiting excellent soft tissue contrast, a characteristic that is important in the imaging of pelvic structures. MRI is noninvasive, and provides a multidirectional image of the female pelvis without interference from the surrounding pelvic bones.

The T_2-weighted image of the uterus provides the greatest detail of internal uterine structures. The endometrial stripe appears as a high-intensity signal as compared to the sur-

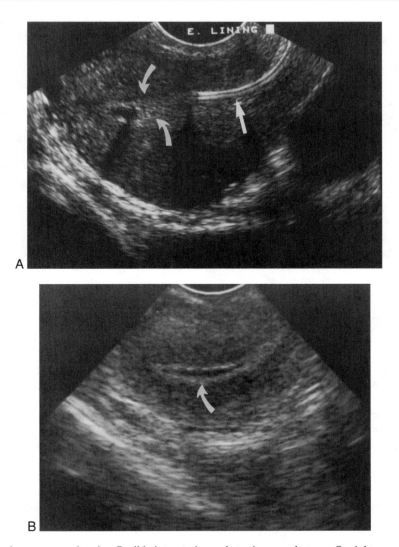

Fig. 13-5. (A) Sonohysterogram showing flexible intrauterine catheter in normal uterus. Straight arrow, catheter; curved arrows, endometrial cavity. **(B)** Sonohysterogram of normal uterine cavity. Curved arrow, endometrial cavity.

rounding myometrium (Fig. 13-8). The myometrium is further subdivided into an inner junctional zone (JZ) and an outer myometrium. The JZ represents an area of increased cellular concentration and decreased intracellular matrix per unit volume.[29] This zone is helpful in differentiating normal anatomy from pathologic conditions.

The role of the MRI in the evaluation of uterine pathology is somewhat limited by its expense and long examination time in a confined space. Ultrasound remains the most appropriate first-line noninvasive diagnostic test for uterine abnormalities. MRI of the uterus is particularly helpful in the diagnosis of adenomyosis. Ascher et al[30] used MRI of the uterus to correctly identify adenomyosis in 15 of 17 patients, as compared to 9 of 17 patients identified by transvaginal ultrasound. The soft tissue detail obtained using MRI is particularly helpful in delineating the location of uterine leiomyomas and their relationship to the endometrial canal.[31] MRI

is useful for the assessment of uterine abnormalities when an ultrasound is indeterminate, and provides outstanding detail for the evaluation of uterine anomalies. Finally, the diagnosis and staging of endometrial carcinoma has been evaluated using MRI. MRI can be used to identify endometrial carcinoma based on a thickened endometrial lining. However, tumors that only involve the endometrial canal may be frequently undetected. MRI is more helpful in identifying the depth of myometrial invasion of a carcinoma with a reported sensitivity of 66 to 82 percent.[32–35]

Office Endometrial Biopsy

The concept of an office sampling of the endometrium was first proposed in 1924; however, this idea was never adopted as routine until the 1970s. In 1970, Jensen[36] demonstrated the feasibility of performing endometrial biopsies without

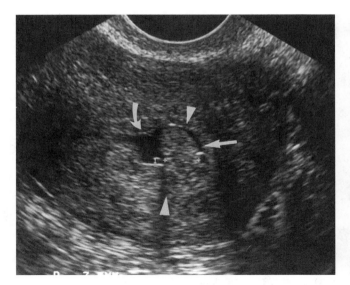

Fig. 13-6. Submucous leiomyoma by transvaginal ultrasound with saline in the endometrial cavity. Straight arrow, fibroid; curved arrow, saline; arrowheads, uterus.

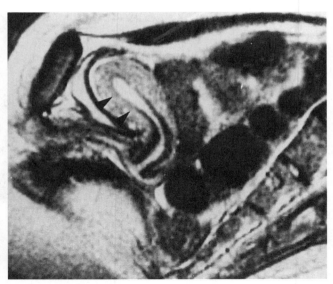

Fig. 13-8. Magnetic resonance imaging scan of normal uterus. White stripe, endometrial cavity; arrowheads, junctional zone. (From Togashi,[28] with permission.)

anesthesia in 350 patients presenting with abnormal bleeding. Adequate histologic specimens were obtained in 98.5 percent of the patients. In 1982, Grimes[37] wrote a landmark article that challenged the need for hospital-based diagnostic D&C and proposed the routine use of office Vabra aspiration. This article summarized the results of 13,598 D&Cs and 5,851 Vabra aspirations. The results (Table 13-3) demonstrated that from the standpoint of cost, convenience, and safety, the Vabra technique was as good or better than D&C. The two techniques were equally effective in detecting endometrial pathology. The author also pointed out the lack of scientific evidence for the then held belief that the D&C was superior to an office procedure.

The office endometrial biopsy offers a number of advantages to a D&C. The procedure can be conducted with minimal to no cervical dilation. Anesthesia is generally not required and the cost is approximately one-tenth of a hospital D&C. Despite some limitations, numerous studies have shown that the endometrium is adequately sampled with these techniques.[38]

The indications for office endometrial biopsy include all the indications listed for the evaluation of the endometrium: abnormal uterine bleeding in a patient older than 40, postmenopausal bleeding, dating of the endometrium, abnormal endometrial cytology on Pap smear, follow-up of patients undergoing medical therapy for endometrial hyperplasia, and an abnormal endometrium diagnosed on radiographic or ultrasonic imaging.

Recent investigations of patients being treated for breast carcinoma with the estrogen antagonist Tamoxifen have demonstrated a 6.4-fold relative risk of developing endometrial carcinoma.[39] The routine sampling of asymptomatic patients on Tamoxifen has not been adopted, but clearly, patients with abnormal uterine bleeding should undergo endometrial sampling. Cohen et al[40] recommends annual Pap smears and transvaginal ultrasound for women on Tamoxifen. Women with an endometrial thickness of 5 mm or less are followed without biopsy. Biopsy is recommended for an endometrial thickness of 8 mm or greater. Patient follow-up is individualized for those with a thickness between 5 and 8 mm.

Vabra Aspirator

A number of techniques exist for sampling the endometrium in the office. Table 13-4 lists the most frequently used techniques. The Vabra aspirator (Berkeley Medevices, Berkeley,

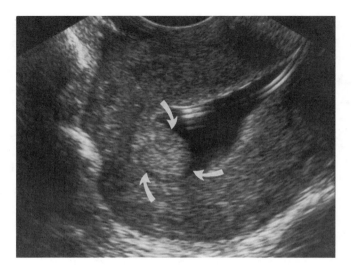

Fig. 13-7. Sonohysterogram demonstrating endometrial polyp (curved arrows).

Table 13-3. Comparison of Diagnostic D&C and Vabra Aspiration

Characteristic	D&C (n = 13,598)	VA (n = 5,851)
Safety		
Hemorrhage rate[a]	≤4	None reported
Infection rate[a]	3–5	0–4
Perforation rate[a]	6–13	0.4
Unanticipated major operation rate[a]	0.3–5	None reported
Death-to-case rate	Low	None reported
Adequacy of specimen[b]	0.77–0.94	0.85–0.99
Diagnostic accuracy[c]		
Endometrial adenocarcinoma	Unknown	0.96
Endometrial polyps	Unknown	0.80
Cost	Approximately $720	Approximately $65
Convenience:		
Patient	Inconvenient	Convenient
Physician	Inconvenient	Convenient
Discomfort	Negligible with general anesthesia	Usually minimal with no anesthesia
Examination under anesthesia	Frequent	Rare
Therapeutic effect	Limited	Limited

Abbreviations: D&C, dilation and curettage; VA, vabra aspiration.

[a] Events per 1,000 procedures.

[b] No. of procedures yielding specimens adequate for histologic interpretation per total no. of procedures.

[c] No. of cases detected by VA/total no. of cases detected by VA plus D&C or hysterectomy.

(From Grimes,[37] with permission.)

Table 13-4. Disposable Suction Devices for Endometrial Sampling

Device (Manufacturer)	Cannula Material	Suction Source	Estimated Cost (100-unit minimum)	Physician Convenience
Karman cannula and syringe (International Projects Assistance Services)	Plastic	50-ml syringe with self-locking plunger	$2.60	Convenient
Masterson endometrial biopsy system (Gyneco, Inc.)	Stainless steel	Reusable self-contained pump with handle	$12.00	Convenient
Pipelle (Unimar, Inc.)	Plastic	Internal piston	$3.19	Most convenient
Tis-U-Trap (Milex Products, Inc.)	Stainless steel, semirigid nylon, or flexible plastic	Suction pump or 50 ml self-locking syringe	$12.65	Convenient
Vabra aspirator (Berkeley Medevices, Inc.)	Stainless steel, plastic, or transparent plastic	Electric suction	$10.41 (steel) $5.00 (plastic)	Convenient
Z-Sampler (Zinnanti Surgical Instruments, Inc.)	Plastic	Internal piston	$2.99	Most convenient

(From Kaunitz,[117] with permission.)

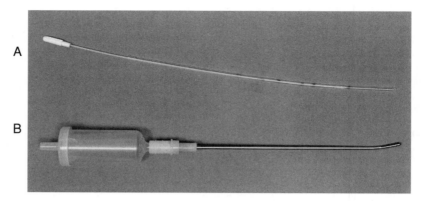

Fig. 13-9. Office endometrial biopsy instruments. (**A**) Pipelle endometrial suction curette. (**B**) Vabra aspirator.

CA) has the longest clinical experience. This stainless steel device has an outside diameter of 3 mm and is connected to a suction device that generates a vacuum of 600 mmHg. The tissue sample enters the device through a side port (Fig. 13-9B). The device incorporates both physical as well as vacuum forces to draw the endometrium into the tissue trap. The Vabra is used by first inserting the instrument through an undilated cervix to the uterine fundus, at which point the suction is initiated. In a systematic fashion, moving from the fundus to the internal os, the entire uterine cavity is sampled using gentle pressure against the uterine wall. The tissue sample is retrieved from the tissue trap and is placed in formalin.

Vuopala[41] summarized the results of over 4,000 patients who underwent a Vabra aspiration for diagnostic indications. This technique provided an adequate sample for evaluation in 93.5 percent of cases with a 10 percent failure rate secondary to a stenotic os or patient discomfort. Complications were rare, with only seven perforations and six cases of postoperative infection. The major limitation of the Vabra aspirator is that it produces uterine cramping.

Pipelle Endometrial Sampling Device

The pipelle endometrial sampling device (Unimar, Wilton, CT) has become a very popular method for sampling the endometrial lining. The device is constructed of flexible polypropylene with an outer sheath measuring 3.1 mm in diameter with a 2.4-mm distal side port, through which the endometrial sample is obtained (Fig. 13-9A). The suction to draw the sample into the device is created by withdrawing an inner piston. The device is placed in the uterus through an undilated cervix. The flexibility of the device allows the cannula to conform to the contour of the uterus. The piston is fully withdrawn and, while the device is rotated 360 degrees, the distal port is brought from the fundus to the internal os. The device is removed and the distal aspect of the instrument is severed, allowing for the expulsion of the sample into formalin.

Kaunitz et al[42] evaluated the efficacy of the endometrial pipelle as compared to the Vabra aspirator in 56 patients undergoing the procedure before a hysterectomy. The pipelle provided more tissue for evaluation in 50 percent of the cases as compared to 38 percent for the Vabra. Equal diagnostic accuracy was obtained with each instrument (89 percent). Eighty-four percent of the patients stated that the pipelle biopsy was less painful than the Vabra. Silver et al[43] compared the Pipelle to the Novak curette in 55 patients undergoing endometrial biopsy due to an increased risk of endometrial disease. This randomized study included one-half of the patients undergoing the Pipelle biopsy before the Novak curette, and one-half in the reverse order. The results demonstrated a statistically significant reduction in the patients' perception of pain with the Pipelle as compared to the Novak curette. The histologic quality and interpretation of the specimens were no different between the two techniques. Lipscomb et al[44] recently evaluated the Pipelle, Accurette, and Explora endometrial sampling devices in 248 patients in a randomized prospective fashion. The Pipelle and Explora failed to obtain tissue or had insufficient tissue for analysis in 18.8 percent and 17.3 percent of patients, respectively. The Accurette was found to be inferior to the Pipelle and Explora, with 42 percent of the cases having failed endometrial sampling or provided insufficient tissue for analysis.

Very little data is available regarding the efficacy of the Pipelle in detecting endometrial carcinoma. Stovall et al[45] studied 40 patients with known endometrial cancer, previously diagnosed by either D&C or office biopsy. The biopsies were performed preoperatively in an office setting before a staging total abdominal hysterectomy. The histologic samples were adequate for analysis in 100 percent of the cases, with a sensitivity for detecting endometrial carcinoma of 97.5 percent. The only patient who was not correctly diagnosed using the Pipelle had tumor confined to an endometrial polyp. Guido et al[46] studied the effectiveness of the Pipelle in 65 patients undergoing staging hysterectomy for endometrial carcinoma. The preoperative diagnosis of malignancy was made by D&C in 82 percent of the cases, by office biopsy in 14 percent of the cases, and by Pipelle in 4 percent of the cases. Each patient underwent a Pipelle biopsy in the operating room under general anesthesia before staging procedure. The tissue was adequate for analysis in 97 percent of the cases, with 54 of 65 cases of carcinoma correctly identified by the Pipelle biopsy (83 percent ± 5 percent). Close evaluation of the 11 patients with a false-negative Pipelle biopsy demonstrated 5 patients with tumor present only in an endometrial polyp and 3 with disease localized to less than 5 percent of the endometrial surface area.

Summary

Office endometrial biopsies are an excellent method for detecting global effects on the endometrium. These techniques are less expensive, less painful, and do not require hospitalization as compared to a D&C. Gynecologists who use these techniques must understand the limitations of these devices. Rodriguez et al,[47] in an elegant study, compared the surface area sampled by both the Pipelle and the Vabra aspirator prior to a hysterectomy. The Pipelle, on average, sampled 4.2 percent of the endometrial surface area as compared to 41 percent by the Vabra, a significant difference. The surface area sampled by the Vabra aspirator compares favorably to that of routine D&C. Stock and Kanbour[48] evaluated the surface area sampled in 50 patients undergoing prehysterectomy D&C. In 16 percent of the specimens, less than one-fourth of the cavity had been curetted; in 60 percent less than one-half of the cavity had been curetted; and in 84 percent, less than three-quarters of the cavity had been effectively curetted. Despite their limitations, D&C and office sampling techniques demonstrate adequate sensitivities for detecting endometrial pathology. Pathologic conditions of the endometrium frequently cover a large proportion of the surface area of the endometrial cavity and are therefore detectable by any of the aforementioned techniques. Focal pathologic processes may, however, go undetected by any blind procedure.

A D&C with or without a hysteroscopy should be performed on

1. Patients who are at high risk of endometrial carcinoma with a benign office biopsy
2. Patients with insufficient tissue for analysis on office biopsy
3. Patients in whom cervical stenosis prevents the completion of an office biopsy
4. Patients for whom an examination under anesthesia will contribute to the management of the patient

We prefer to perform all diagnostic D&Cs with hysteroscopy to obtain a visual image of the endometrial cavity and to rule out focal disease.

Indications for Therapeutic Dilation, Evacuation and Curettage

Dilation of the cervix with the subsequent evacuation of the contents of the uterus is used as a therapeutic modality in the following clinical settings:

Indications for Therapeutic Dilation, Evacuation, and Curettage

- Spontaneous abortions
- Molar pregnancy
- Bleeding unresponsive to medical therapy

---

1. Treatment of incomplete, inevitable, missed, septic, and induced abortions
2. Initial treatment of molar pregnancies
3. Management of patients with prolonged or excessive vaginal bleeding unresponsive to hormonal therapy

Spontaneous Abortions

Human reproduction is a relatively inefficient process. It has been estimated that as many as 70 percent of all fertilized ovum do not implant, or abort at some point during the pregnancy.[49] Fifteen to 20 percent of all clinically recognized pregnancies end in abortions, while as many as 22 percent of preclinical pregnancies are lost.[50]

Women with spontaneous abortions typically present around the 8th week of gestation (i.e., 10 weeks from the last menstrual period). Embryonic demise is most likely to have occurred weeks before the actual abortion.[51] Patients typically present with symptoms of bleeding or cramping. The following terms are useful in describing the clinical setting of an abortion. An *inevitable abortion* describes uterine bleeding from a gestation of less than 20 weeks accompanied by cervical dilation but without expulsion of any placental or fetal tissue. An *incomplete abortion* requires the passage of some but not all fetal or placental tissue through the cervix. In a *complete abortion,* all fetal and placental tissue have been expelled from the uterine cavity. Finally, an *anembryonic gestation* (blighted ovum) is used to describe an ultrasonically visualized gestational sac without a fetus in a pregnancy greater than or equal to 7.5 weeks' gestation.

The etiology of spontaneous abortions can be divided into genetic and environmental causes, with genetic abnormalities accounting for most abortions. The most frequent genetic cause of spontaneous abortion is a chromosomal aneuploidy. Autosomal trisomy is the most common abnormal karyotype and is found in approximately 50 percent of spontaneous abortions with abnormal karotype. The second most common chromosomal abnormality and the most common single chromosomal abnormality is monosomy 45,X, which is found in 15 to 20 percent of abortuses. Less frequently found chromosomal defects of abortuses include triploidy

(15 percent), tetraploidy (10 percent), and structural abnormalities (5 percent).[52]

Environmental sources of abortion include a variety of maternal factors that create an inadequate environment for fetal development. Among these factors are uterine abnormalities, endocrinologic defects, immunologic factors, infection, and environmental exposures. The actual relationship between any of these factors and the risk of abortion is hard to quantify.

Abnormalities of uterine development such as bicornuate and septate uterus are associated with abortions. The rate of abortions in this population is generally quoted to be approximately 20 percent. A unicornuate uterus is associated with the highest incidence of spontaneous abortion (50 percent).[53] Uterine abnormalities have been studied extensively for patients suffering from diethylstilbestrol (DES) exposure. The apparent risk of spontaneous abortion in DES-exposed patients is independent of the shape of the uterine cavity, with similar miscarriage rates being found in those with and without a T-shaped uterus (25.9 percent).[54]

Intrauterine pathology is associated with recurrent spontaneous abortion. Leiomyoma, especially those of the submucous type, may alter the ability of the fertilized ovum to implant in the uterus or represent a physical obstruction to growth of the developing fetus. Leiomyoma are a common finding in women in the reproductive age range, but are thought to be associated with only 2 percent of recurrent pregnancy losses.[55] Intrauterine adhesions, with the associated distortion of the uterine cavity, are also associated with a spontaneous abortion.

Endocrinologic causes of spontaneous abortion include diabetes mellitus, luteal phase deficiencies, and thyroid diseases. The spontaneous abortion rate in patients with diabetes mellitus is directly associated with glucose control. Women with poor glucose control, as demonstrated by elevated first trimester glycosylated hemoglobin, have a twofold increase in the rate of spontaneous abortion as compared to those with good control.[56] Luteal phase deficiency describes an inadequate progesterone effect on the endometrium. The diagnosis is typically made with two endometrial biopsies that are 3 days out of phase, as compared to the cycle day, as calculated by the subsequent menses. The role of luteal phase deficiency in spontaneous abortions is unknown due to a lack of well-controlled studies. Similarly, despite some data associating thyroid disorders with spontaneous abortion, no clear-cut scientific evidence exists to support a cause and effect relationship.

Pelvic ultrasound is extremely useful in assessing patients who present with signs or symptoms of a spontaneous abortion. Mansur[57] evaluated 155 patients with signs of an incomplete abortion using transvaginal ultrasound. Of these, 112 (72.3 percent) were found to have retained products of conception and subsequently required a dilation, evacuation, and curettage (DE&C). The remaining 43 patients were found to have no products of conception by ultrasound and

were followed conservatively, with only one patient subsequently requiring a DE&C. Rulin et al[58] examined the clinical reliability of pelvic ultrasound in patients with clinical findings suggestive of a complete abortion. Of 49 patients, 48 (98 percent) with an empty uterus on ultrasound had an uneventful recovery without curettage.

Molar Pregnancy

Molar pregnancies are a relatively rare occurrence affecting 1 in 1,200 pregnancies in the United States.[59] These pregnancies occur as a result of polyspermia in the case of an incomplete mole, or as the result of the fertilization of a genetically empty ovum with single sperm in the case of a complete mole. Patients typically present with uterine bleeding or passage of vesicular tissue, or are detected due to an unusually large uterus for the gestational age. The pelvic ultrasound has a characteristic "snowstorm" appearance in molar pregnancies (Fig. 13-10). The initial therapy for a molar pregnancy is a therapeutic DE&C.

Bleeding Unresponsive to Medical Therapy

Dilation and curettage is used primarily to identify a possible etiology for abnormal bleeding. However, it is frequently believed that the procedure will have a therapeutic effect as well. This effect is believed to occur as the result of the removal of the endometrium to the basalis layer with the subsequent restoration of a hormonally appropriate endometrium. There is very little data available that specifically addresses the therapeutic benefit of a curettage. Nickelsen[60] evaluated 181 consecutive patients undergoing a D&C for the diagnosis and treatment of postmenopausal bleeding, menorrhagia, and metrorrhagia. Patients were followed for a 9-month period to assess the benefit of the surgical procedure. Twenty-two percent of the patients had a histologic diagnosis established that explained their symptoms. Only 57 percent of patients were cured by the procedure at 9 months, with the lowest cure rate occurring in the menorrhagia group. This low therapeutic yield is similar to that reported by other investigators,[61] who found that only 50 percent of patients older than 40 years of age had long-term resolution of their abnormal bleeding.

Instrumentation

Vaginal Retractors

Exposure for a D&C may be accomplished with a variety of vaginal retractors. The type of vaginal retraction that is required is dependent on the patient's body habitus and the procedure being performed. The Graves speculum provides adequate exposure of the cervix and is well suited for patients undergoing a therapeutic D&C. When a hysteroscopy is being performed in conjunction with a D&C, the side-

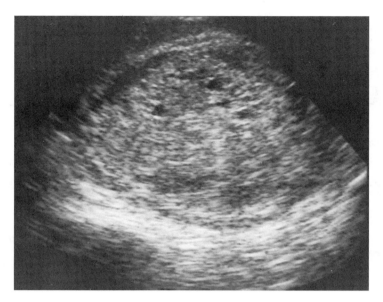

Fig. 13-10. Transvaginal ultrasound appearance of molar pregnancy.

open Graves speculum provides excellent exposure of the cervix and is easily removed, providing a maximum range of motion to the hysteroscope during the examination. Alternatively, an Auvard weighted speculum (V. Mueller, McGraw Park, IL) can be used in conjunction with Schieden vaginal side wall retractors (V. Mueller, McGraw Park, IL) (Fig. 13-11).

Dilators

There are a variety of dilators available for cervical dilation, the most common being the Pratt and Hegar dilators (V. Mueller, McGraw Park, IL) (Fig. 13-12). The Pratt dilator comes in sizes ranging from 13 to 43 French. Each French

unit is equivalent to 0.33 mm in diameter. This dilator is notable for its gradual taper at the end of the instrument. Hegar dilators have a blunt end and come in sizes ranging from 1 to 26 mm in diameter. We prefer the tapered end of the Pratt dilator to the Hegar dilator. The former has been shown to require less force for dilation and is less likely to cause a perforation of the uterus.[62]

When cervical dilation beyond 9.0 mm is required, such as in second trimester therapeutic abortions or operative hysteroscopy, osmotic dilators may be used preoperatively. There are three primary techniques for osmotic dilation: Laminaria Japonica (Milex Products, Chicago, IL), Dilapan Hygroscopic Cervical Dilator (Gynotech, Inc., Middlesex, NJ), and Lamicel Osmotic Cervical Dilator (Cabot Medical,

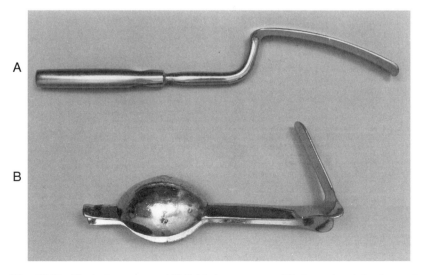

Fig. 13-11. Vaginal retractors. **(A)** Schieden retractor. **(B)** Auvard weighted speculum.

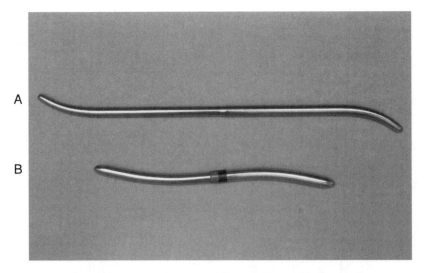

Fig. 13-12. Cervical dilators. **(A)** Pratt dilator. **(B)** Hegar dilator.

Langhorne, PA) (Fig. 13-13). Laminaria is a sea-grown plant that swells in the presence of fluid. Laminaria is available in five sizes: extra thin, thin, medium, thick, and extra thick, ranging from 2 to 6 mm in diameter. Dilapan is a synthetic hydrophilic polymer, available in 3- and 4-mm diameter sizes. Lamicel is a polyvinyl alcohol polymer sponge impregnated with 450 mg of magnesium sulfate, and is available in 3- and 5-mm diameter sizes.

Laminaria has been used extensively for dilation prior to therapeutic abortions. It reaches maximum dilation in 12 hours, with most of the dilation occurring within 4 to 6 hours. Careful attention to aseptic protocol is required for all dilators and specifically with the use of Laminaria, as it may contain spores that are resistant to the sterilization process.

Dilapan is a synthetic material that is sterile and offers the advantage of a more rapid dilation, with maximum dilation occurring within 3 to 4 hours.[63] Lamicel is a sterile product that has been shown to produce significantly less dilation than Dilapan when used before performing a second trimester abortion.[64]

The author prefers the use of Dilapan for cervical dilation before operative procedures due to its reproducible rapid dilation and sterility. Figure 13-14 demonstrates the effect of cervical preparation using Dilapan. Care must be taken in the removal of the device as it has been found to fracture more frequently than both the Laminaria and the Lamicel.[64,65] Numerous clinical studies have been conducted to evaluate these techniques for the preoperative dilation of the

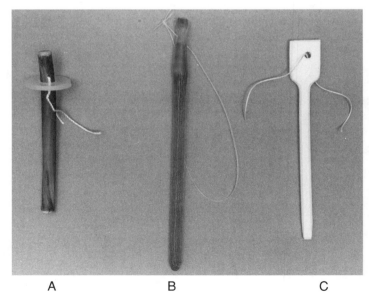

Fig. 13-13. Osmotic dilators. **(A)** Laminaria Japonica. **(B)** Dilapan. **(C)** Lamicel.

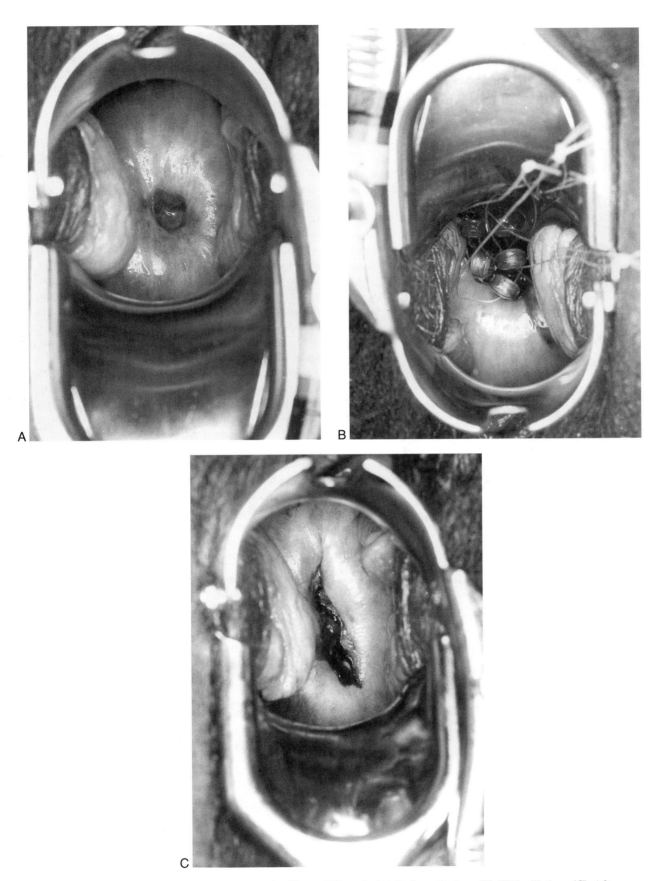

Fig. 13-14. Dilation of cervix with an osmotic dilator (Dilapan). **(A)** Before dilation. **(B)** With dilation. **(C)** After dilation.

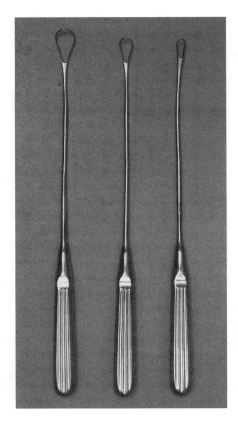

Fig. 13-15. Sharp curettes.

cervix before therapeutic abortions. A limited number of studies exist to evaluate their effectiveness prior to benign gynecologic procedures. Dilapan has been demonstrated to be an effective technique for cervical dilation in patients with inadequate colposcopy, allowing adequate examination of the distal aspect of the cervical canal.[66,67] Laminaria has been found to provide adequate cervical dilation prior to the

vaginal removal of submucous leiomyoma[68] and to significantly reduce the frequency of inadequate cervical dilation before resectoscopic surgery.[69]

Curettes

Curettes are available in blunt and sharp styles, ranging in size from #1 to 6, with 1 being the smallest curette (Fig. 13-15). The blunt curette is best suited for the removal of retained placental tissue in the postpartum uterus. The blunt edge prevents excessive removal of the basalis layer of the endometrium, which can occur in the soft postpartum uterus and result in subsequent intrauterine adhesions. The Hunter uterine curette (V. Mueller, McGraw Park, IL) is a large curette with a width of 30 mm that is especially useful in performing curettage postpartum for retained products of conception. The sharp curettes are used in all other curettage procedures. The curette is malleable, which allows the instrument to be bent slightly to conform to the ante- or retroflexed uterus.

Suction curettes exist for the removal of products of conception from the uterus in the case of spontaneous, missed, inevitable, and therapeutic abortions. The suction curette is preferred by some for a diagnostic curettage.[70] The suction curettes range in size from 6 to 16 mm in diameter. The 6-mm curette is composed of a flexible plastic while the larger curettes are rigid (Fig. 13-16). We prefer the flexible plastic 6-mm curette when performing suction curettage in a small uterus (less than 8-week size). When a larger rigid suction curette is used, the curved instrument provides better tactile sensation as compared to the straight curette.

Accessory Equipment

The cervix is generally grasped on the anterior lip with a tenaculum during the D&C. There are a variety of types, including the single tooth tenaculum and the Bierer tenacu-

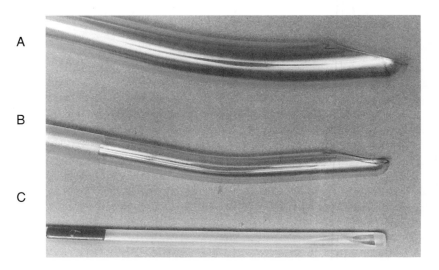

Fig. 13-16. Suction curettes. **(A)** No. 16. **(B)** No. 12. **(C)** No. 6.

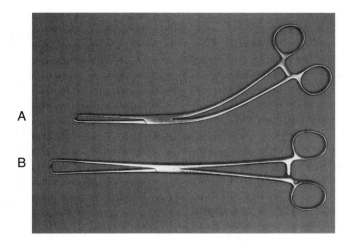

Fig. 13-17. Tenaculums. **(A)** Beirer tenaculum. **(B)** Single tooth tenaculum.

lum (V. Mueller, McGraw Park, IL) (Fig. 13-17). This author prefers the Bierer tenaculum, due to the less traumatic nature of the instrument. The single tooth tenaculum is particularly helpful in patients with a small amount of cervical tissue (i.e., the postmenopausal patient or patients who have undergone previous cone biopsy). This instrument is more likely to cause a laceration of the cervix. The ring forceps may also be used to grasp the cervix in the pregnant patient with an enlarged cervix, to reduce the risk of cervical laceration.

The endocervical curettage is generally performed using a Kevorkian-Younge (V. Mueller, McGraw Park, IL) endocervical biopsy curette. This instrument is narrow to accommodate the small endocervical canal and is slightly curved. Randall-Stone polyp forceps (V. Mueller, McGraw Park, IL) are helpful for the exploration of the fundus and removal of polyps (Fig. 13-18).

Operative Techniques

Diagnostic D&C

A D&C is best performed with the patient in the dorsal lithotomy position. This position is achieved by placing the patient in lithotomy stirrups. Care must be taken to avoid

overabduction of the hip joint, as this may be uncomfortable for the patient. The lateral aspect of the legs should not rest against the stirrups, to avoid the risk of peroneal nerve injury with subsequent foot-drop. Physicians-in-training should develop the habit of positioning the patient to their liking, a technique that is useful during all vaginal cases.

Anesthesia for D&C may be general, regional anesthesia with spinal or epidural, or paracervical. The type of anesthesia used is a function of the indication for the procedure, as well as the medical history of the patient. General anesthesia provides complete muscular relaxation, a component that is important when the examination under anesthesia is a critical element of the procedure, such as in the case of a diagnostic hysteroscopy and D&C. Regional anesthesia provides adequate muscular blockade without the known pulmonary effects of general anesthesia.

Paracervical or intracervical anesthesia with intravenous sedation is a convenient, inexpensive, and effective technique for providing anesthesia for a D&C or hysteroscopy. This technique is amenable to the outpatient setting and is particularly useful for therapeutic DE&C for spontaneous abortions. The literature on therapeutic abortions has demonstrated a decrease in the rate of perforation and infection associated with these procedures when paracervical anesthesia is used as compared to general.[71]

The examination under anesthesia is then performed. The size, shape, and position of the uterus are noted, with particular attention being paid to the axis of the cervix and the flexion of the fundus. The latter is critical to reduce the incidence of uterine perforations. The size, shape, and consistency of the adnexa are determined. The perineum, vagina, and cervix are then prepared with an aseptic solution and vaginal retractors are inserted into the vagina.

When a paracervical block is required, it is administered by placing a small amount (less than 2 ml) of 1 percent Lidocaine in the cervix at the site of the placement of the tenaculum for patient comfort. Longer-acting local anesthetics may also be used. The lateral fornices are then identified and 5 to 10 ml of local anesthetic is placed at the 3 and 9 o'clock positions below the vaginal epithelium. Before injecting the anesthetic agent, the position of the needle out-

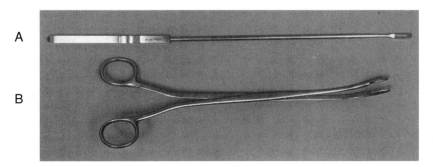

Fig. 13-18. Accessory instruments. **(A)** Kevorkian-Younge curette. **(B)** Randall-Stone polyp forceps.

side a vascular space is confirmed by withdrawing the plunger of the syringe and checking for the absence of blood. Direct intravascular injection can produce convulsions if the serum level of lidocaine is greater than the 5 μg/ml. By employing 10 ml of 1 percent lidocaine (100 mg), the peak plasma level generally is well below the toxic range and occurs 10 to 15 minutes following the injection.[72]

The anterior lip of the cervix is grasped with a tenaculum and traction is applied to align the axis of the cervix and the uterine canals. The uterus should be sounded to document the size and confirm the position. The sound should be held between the thumb and the index finger to avoid the use of excessive pressure. Dilation of the cervix may be required before sounding the uterus. The pregnant uterus should not be sounded under any circumstances, to avoid the risk of uterine perforation.

The endocervical curettage (ECC) should be performed before dilation of the cervix to avoid contamination of the histologic specimen with endometrial cells. A Kevorkian-Younge curette is introduced into the cervical canal up to the internal os. Curetting of all four quadrants of the entire canal should be conducted with the specimen placed on a Telfa pad.

The ECC is performed to detect the presence of endometrial carcinoma extending into the cervical canal or the presence of endocervical pathology. The clinical usefulness of the ECC has been questioned. The ECC is predictive of cervical involvement of endometrial carcinoma when the histology demonstrates stromal involvement. However, numerous investigators have demonstrated a false-positive rate of 80 percent when tumor alone is detected on ECC.[73] In light of the surgical staging of endometrial carcinoma, the need for an ECC is only relevant for patients who cannot undergo a full staging procedure.

Cervical dilation is then performed. The dilator is grasped in the middle of the instrument with the thumb and index finger (Fig. 13-19). The cervix is gradually dilated beginning with the 13 French Pratt dilator. The dilator should be inserted to the point where the internal os is dilated, without excessively entering the uterine cavity. This is helpful in

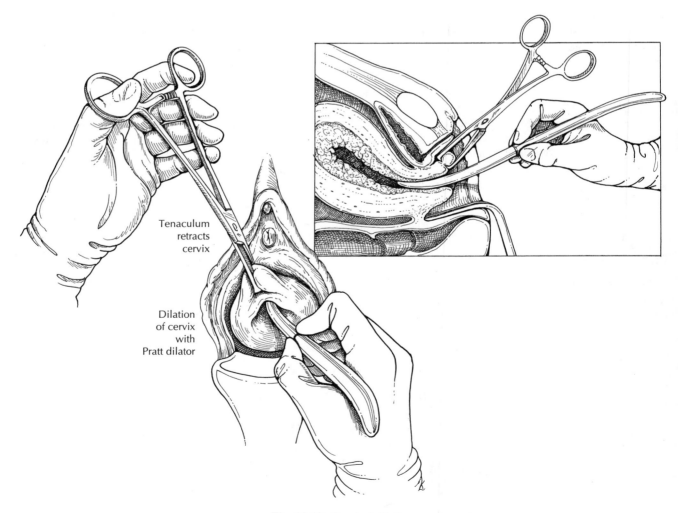

Tenaculum retracts cervix

Dilation of cervix with Pratt dilator

Fig. 13-19. Cervical dilation.

preventing uterine perforation and avoids undesirable damage to the endometrium prior to hysteroscopic examination. A stenotic cervical os may be present in as much as 10 percent of postmenopausal patients and increases the risk of cervical laceration and uterine perforation. This patient is best dilated using a series of small Hegar (1- to 4-mm) dilators. Transabdominal ultrasound is useful in guiding the gynecologist performing a difficult dilation, as in the case of cervical stenosis or in patients with a previous perforation of the uterus.[74] This technique is especially helpful in completing a DE&C if a perforation is suspected or if there is a question as to the adequacy of the evacuation.

The eventual dimension of cervical dilation is dependent on the indication for the procedure. When a diagnostic hysteroscopy and D&C are performed, the dilation is conducted to a point at which the hysteroscope may be comfortably inserted. The 17 French Pratt dilator will easily accommodate a 5-mm hysteroscope as well as a #3 sharp curette. When products of conception are to be removed, the cervix is generally dilated to a diameter in millimeters equal to the gestation age of the uterus. Dilation is easily accomplished up to 9 mm, at which time the cervix may become difficult to dilate.[75] Cervical dilation beyond 9 mm generally requires laminaria.

Curettage is performed in a systematic fashion beginning with the curette placed at the fundus and applying even pressure on the endometrial surface (Fig. 13-20). The curette is withdrawn the entire length of the uterus to the internal cervical os. The endometrial tissue is deposited on a Telfa pad placed in the vagina. Moving around the uterus in a consistent and systematic fashion, the entire surface of the endometrium is sampled. The curettage procedure is completed when the "uterine cry" (grittiness to palpation) is appreciated on all surfaces of the uterus. The size and shape of any submucous fibroids detected by tactile sensation should be noted as part of the operative note. Polyp forceps are then introduced into the uterine cavity to evaluate for the presence of uterine polyps.

Suction Curettage

Suction curettage is used for the evacuation of products of conception, as in the case of spontaneous, missed, inevitable, and therapeutic abortions, and may be used for diagnostic curettage.

Suction curettage is begun following adequate dilation of the cervix. The curette is placed at the fundus of the uterus. The instrument is then grasped with the index finger and

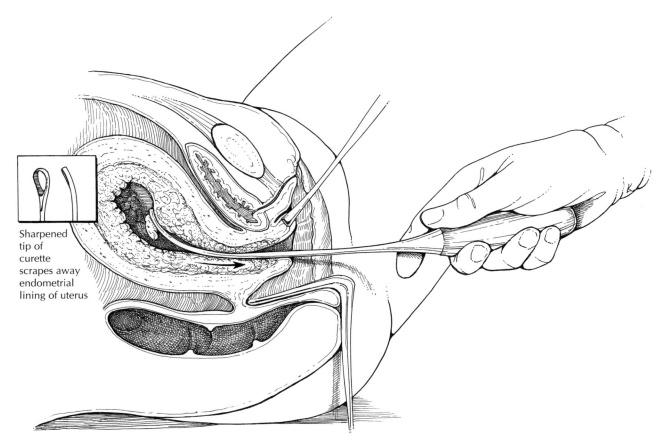

Sharpened tip of curette scrapes away endometrial lining of uterus

Fig. 13-20. Inserted sharp curette.

thumb to avoid excessive pressure. The suction tubing is applied and a vacuum of 60 mmHg is used. The cannula is slowly withdrawn while rotating the device in a clockwise or counterclockwise direction. The vacuum should be broken as the internal os is reached. This may be accomplished by disconnecting or sliding the release ring at the canula to reduce the strength of the vacuum. The cannula is subsequently withdrawn from the uterus. Two to three passes of the device are typically required to ensure adequate removal of all intrauterine contents. Suction curettage is typically completed with the entire uterine cavity being assessed for products of conception employing sharp curettage. When the "uterine cry" is appreciated, the procedure is complete.

The external cervical os is then checked for any evidence for excessive bleeding. The tenaculum is removed and the cervix is examined for any trauma. Bleeding from the tenaculum site generally responds to direct pressure or the application of Monsel's solution.

Suction Curettage for Molar Pregnancies

There are a few technical aspects of DE&C in this setting that are worth noting. Patients with molar pregnancies are at risk of hemorrhage during the procedure and therefore, blood should be available if necessary, as well as adequate venous access. The uterus should not be sounded. Pitocin is usually begun once the suction curettage is started. Unlike a suction curettage performed for the evacuation of an abortion, the suction curette is not advanced to the fundus; rather, it is placed just inside the internal os. Suction is then applied and the hydropic placental tissue is drawn into the curette. As additional tissue is evacuated, the uterus will contract and the suction curette may then be advanced to the fundus. The procedure is completed with gentle sharp curettage once the uterus has completely contracted, to assure adequate evacuation (Fig. 13-21).

Complications

Uterine Perforation

Perforation of the uterus at the time of D&C is the most common immediate complication of this procedure. The rate of perforation varies with the indication for the procedure.

Complications of Dilation and Curettage

- Uterine perforation
- Cervical injury
- Infection
- Intrauterine adhesions
- Trophoblastic embolization

Perforation is most common in the setting of the control of postpartum hemorrhage (5.1 percent).[76] Perforations occur less frequently during diagnostic curettage, with an incidence of 0.3 percent in the premenopausal patient and 2.6 percent in the postmenopausal patient. The rate of perforation occurring with therapeutic abortion ranges from a high of 1.5 percent to a generally quoted value of 0.2 percent found in a number of studies from the United States.[77]

A variety of conditions are associated with an increased risk of uterine perforation. Pregnancy is a major risk factor, due in part to the softening of the uterine wall as well as the increased size of the endometrial cavity. Surgical experience of the operator has a direct effect on the incidence of perforation, with a 5.5-fold increase in perforations occurring with inexperienced physicians, as compared to attending staff.[78] Preoperative cervical dilation with osmotic dilators has been found to decrease the risk of perforation of the uterus when used in the setting of therapeutic second-trimester abortions.

Perforation of the uterus is suspected when there is a loss of resistance during the instrumentation of the uterus, or when an instrument is found to extend into the uterine cavity for a distance that is greater than the known depth of the uterus. Severe vaginal bleeding may be a sign of a perforation, especially if the lateral aspect of the uterus is perforated and the uterine vessels are lacerated. Occult retroperitoneal hemorrhage can occur, with the first sign of a complication being hypotension. The diagnosis of perforation is occasionally made by the presence of abdominal viscera brought through a perforation.

The most frequent site of uterine perforation is the fundus, occurring in 30 to 50 percent of cases (Fig. 13-22). Less frequently, the anterior or posterior wall of the uterus is perforated. Fortunately the lateral wall of the uterus is perforated in less than 5 percent of the cases. Perforations in this region, with its proximity to the uterine vessels and decreased uterine wall thickness, can produce profound hemorrhage. The sharp curettage is the most common instrument producing a perforation; however, perforations may also occur with the suction curettage, during dilation, and when sounding the uterus (9 to 17 percent).[79]

The management of a uterine perforation is dependent on the clinical setting of the complication. Laparotomy is indicated when intraabdominal visceral injury is suspected or there is clinical evidence of severe hemorrhage. Laparotomy allows for adequate examination of the pelvis and bowel, as well as adequate exposure in the case of large vessel injury. The abdomen should be opened using a vertical incision. Midline perforations that occur during the sounding of the uterus or with dilation frequently do not produce significant hemorrhage and can be managed with observation and serial hemoglobin measurements. When a perforation occurs during the evacuation of the products of conception, the procedure may be completed with either ultrasound or laparoscopic guidance. Laparoscopy allows for the direct visualization of the perforation and an assessment of any intra-abdominal organ damage. Uterine bleeding can

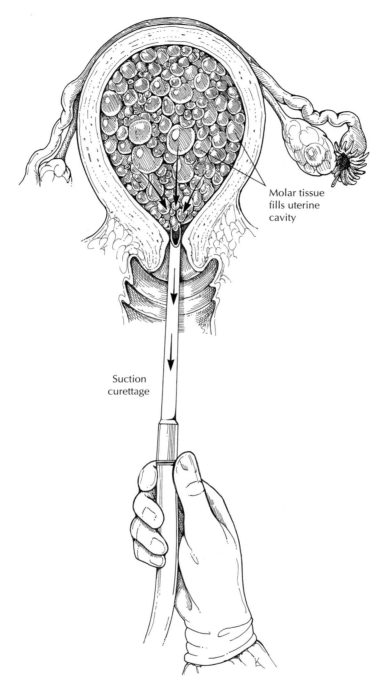

Molar tissue fills uterine cavity

Suction curettage

Fig. 13-21. Suction curettage of a molar pregnancy.

be controlled with the use of monopolar or bipolar electrocautery, or suturing. Laparotomy is clearly indicated in the setting of lateral wall perforations, and perforations that occur with either sharp or suction curettage.

Cervical Injury

Cervical injuries can arise as a direct result of dilation, or from trauma during curettage. Cervical lacerations frequently occur as excessive traction is applied to the tenacu-

lum. The single tooth tenaculum is particularly vulnerable to such injuries; therefore, the Bierer tenaculum is preferred. Lacerations that occur with the tenaculum are managed with direct pressure, with the application of Monsel's solution or, in severe cases, suture control. Lacerations that occur with dilation or with curettage that involve the cervical branch of the uterine artery may produce extensive hemorrhage. Hemorrhage in this situation may be controlled with direct suture application, or by placing hemostatic sutures at the

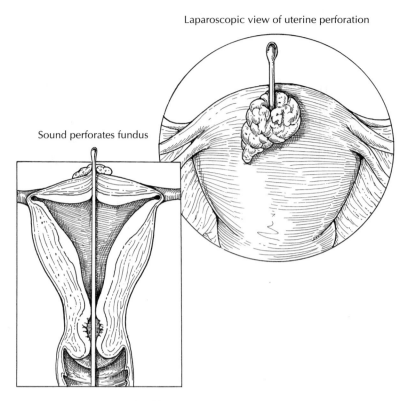

Laparoscopic view of uterine perforation

Sound perforates fundus

Fig. 13-22. Uterine perforation.

internal os. Occasionally, hysterectomy is required to control extensive bleeding.[80]

Cervical injury may be prevented by avoiding the excessive use of force for dilation. The Pratt dilators generally require less force to insert into the cervix as compared to Hegar dilators. Osmotic dilators are helpful in decreasing the force required to dilate the cervix and are useful when dilations of 9 mm or greater are anticipated.

Infection

Infection from dilation and curettage is a rare complication. The highest incidence of febrile morbidity occurs in the setting of therapeutic abortion, where the incidence is 0.34 per 100 abortions.[81]

Although bacteremia has been demonstrated in 5 percent of D&Cs, the incidence of septicemia is very low.[82] Very little is known with regard to risk factors for infection in patients undergoing D&C for diagnostic purposes. The literature regarding infection following therapeutic abortions indicates that the use of prophylactic tetracycline significantly reduced the rate of infections. The use of rigid versus flexible cannula, general versus local anesthesia, and resident versus attending physician were all associated with an increased risk of febrile morbidity.[81] Presently, no data support the routine use of prophylactic antibiotics in diagnostic D&C.

Subacute bacterial endocarditis (SBE) prophylaxis is not recommended for a routine diagnostic D&C.[83]

Intrauterine Adhesions

Intrauterine adhesions (Asherman syndrome) are one possible delayed complication of D&C. This syndrome is characterized by the presence of permanent adherence of the uterine walls, with partial or complete obliteration of the uterine cavity, in the clinical setting of a patient with menstrual abnormalities, infertility, or habitual abortion. The exact incidence of intrauterine adhesions is unknown. The rate of intrauterine adhesions in patients undergoing a hysterosalpingogram (HSG) ranges from 1.5 to 40 percent.[84]

Intrauterine adhesions appear to be directly related to endometrial damage, occurring primarily in the setting of curettage. Most, if not all, cases of Asherman syndrome arise from curettage performed on the pregnant uterus, Table 13-5 summarizes the causes of intrauterine trauma in one of the largest reported series of intrauterine adhesions.[85] Curettage of the endometrium, especially within the first 4 weeks postpartum, results in trauma to the basalis layer with subsequent granular tissue healing on opposing surfaces of the uterus, which eventually fuse to produce tissue bridges. These intrauterine adhesions range from filmy adhesions composed of endometrial tissue, to dense adhesions consisting entirely of connective tissue. Adenomyosis is reported to occur in 25

Table 13-5. Causes of Intrauterine Adhesions in 187 Patients

Antecedent Intrauterine Trauma	Patients (n)	%
Curettage	183	97.9
Incomplete abortion	92	50.3
Postpartum bleeding	44	24.0
Elective abortion	32	17.5
First trimester	14	
Second trimester	18	
Missed abortion	11	6.0
Hydatidiform mole	4	2.2
Myomectomy (hysterotomy)	2	1.1
Metroplasty (abdominal)	1	0.5
Endometritis	1	0.5

(From Valle,[85] with permission.)

percent of cases of Asherman syndrome. The resulting disruption of the normal uterine cavity accounts for the menstrual abnormalities, frequent dysmenorrhea, and habitual abortion.

Asherman syndrome is typically diagnosed by either HSG or hysteroscopy. The combination of the two techniques is helpful in that the HSG provides information as to the location and extent of the adhesions, while hysteroscopy provides information as to the character of the adhesions. Before the widespread use of hysteroscopy, careful D&C of the uterus followed by the placement of an intrauterine Foley catheter along with estrogen therapy had been the mainstay of therapy. Present day therapy for Asherman syndrome includes hysteroscopic resection of the adhesions under direct visualization. The procedure may be done in conjunction with laparoscopy to prevent inadvertent perforation of the uterus.

Trophoblastic Embolization

A rare complication of DE&C of a molar pregnancy is the embolization of trophoblastic tissue into the systemic circulation. Case reports have demonstrated the presence of trophoblastic tissue in blood retrieved from the central circulation in asymptomatic patients undergoing a DE&C for molar pregnancy.[86] Fatalities from cardiovascular collapse due to trophoblastic embolization have been described.[87]

HYSTEROSCOPY

Role of Hysteroscopy With D&C

Patients who undergo a D&C for suspected endometrial pathology should undergo a diagnostic hysteroscopy both before and after the curettage. The addition of the hysteroscopic evaluation before the curettage allows the surgeon the opportunity to directly visualize the endometrial surface and note the location of endometrial polyps or submucous fibroids, two of the most commonly missed pathologies at the time of D&C.[88] Hysteroscopy allows the surgeon to perform a directed biopsy of a focal region of the endometrium and can confirm the presence of atrophic endometrium. Hysteroscopic evaluation of the endometrium following the curettage gives the surgeon an appreciation of the percentage of the endometrial surface that has been biopsied, and allows for a directed curettage to be performed if necessary. Despite the potential slight increase in the cost associated with hysteroscopy, the additional information that is obtained is well worth the added time and expense.

Indications

D&C without hysteroscopy is a "blind" procedure and can miss focal disease. Hysteroscopy allows direct visualization of both the intrauterine cavity and the tubal ostia. There are several diagnostic indications for hysteroscopy in the gynecologic subject, including the evaluation of abnormal uterine bleeding, postmenopausal bleeding, and suspected muellerian anomalies, and the assessment of abnormal findings on HSG, such as proximal tubal occlusion and filling defects. Diagnostic hysteroscopy is useful in conjunction with a diagnostic laparoscopy performed during an infertility evaluation. Hysteroscopy has numerous therapeutic indications, including the removal of submucous myomas, endometrial polyps, and intrauterine devices. Operative hysteroscopy is also used for the excision of intrauterine adhesions, to remove uterine septa, and for the ablation of the endometrium in patients with menorrhagia unresponsive to medical therapy. The following sections review the instruments used in modern hysteroscopy and address the most commonly performed hysteroscopic procedures with regard to their indications, techniques, efficacy, and complications.

Instrumentation

Hysteroscopes

The two predominant types of hysteroscopy are contact and panoramic hysteroscopy. Contact hysteroscopy was developed as a simple mechanism for viewing the uterine cavity without the use of a distending media.[89] The instrument is 200 mm in length and outer diameters (ODs) of 4, 6, and 8 mm are available. The eyepiece has a magnification of × 1.6 and adjustable focus with a focal length of 4 mm. Only tissue that comes in direct contact with the scope can be viewed. Unless the uterine cavity is explored in a slow, systematic fashion, significant pathology can be missed. This instrument is inferior to the panoramic hysteroscope for evaluation of the endometrium.

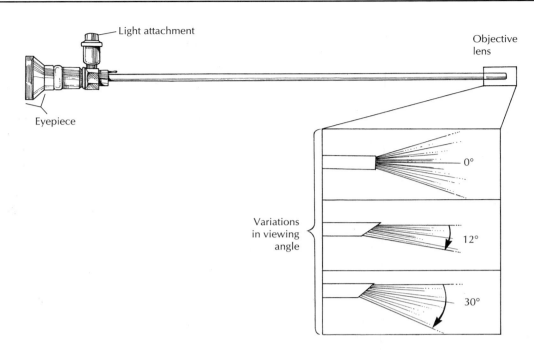

Fig. 13-23. Hysteroscope with different viewing angles.

The rigid, panoramic hysteroscope, which is derived from the cystoscope, uses distending media to obtain a wide-angle view of the uterine cavity. This hysteroscope takes advantage of a system of lenses and prisms to give the operator a well-illuminated image with excellent contrast and resolution. The most widely used panoramic hysteroscopes have an OD of 4 mm, but thinner scopes with an OD of 2.7 mm have been developed for office procedures. Most panoramic hysteroscopes are focused at infinity but some have adjustable focusing mechanisms. The overall magnification of the endoscope is the product of the magnification of the eyepiece and the objective lens. The magnification is inversely proportional to the distance of the tissue from the objective lens. A prism at the proximal end of the hysteroscope is used to form an upright image. Hysteroscopes are monocular and provide little depth perception. They are available with different viewing angles, from 0 to 70 degrees (Fig. 13-23). Zero and 15-degree scopes are most commonly used for diagnostic procedures. Larger angles of deflection are used in operative procedures.

Hysteroscope Sheaths

When performing panoramic hysteroscopy, one must instill distending media into the uterine cavity. For this purpose, the hysteroscope is inserted and securely fastened into a metallic sleeve or sheath. Removable obturators are available for easy introduction of the sheath into the uterine cavity. Obturators are especially useful when dilation is difficult or when large sheaths are being used. Diagnostic sheaths have an OD from 3.3 to 5.0 mm and operative sheaths have an OD from 7.0 to 10.0 mm. Both diagnostic and operative sheaths are fitted with stopcocks or ports for the instillation of distending media. Some operative sheaths have isolated, dual ports and provide continuous laminar flow of distending media.

Operative sheaths are designed to allow the passage of one or more operative instruments. Simple sheaths use the distending media channel for the insertion of instruments (Fig. 13-24). Although this method is easy and allows one to use a small-diameter sheath, leaks are commonly encountered. Other operative sheaths contain permanently attached operative instruments such as biopsy forceps and scissors. A right-angle hysteroscope allows for direct insertion of rigid operating instruments (Fig. 13-25). These sheaths have an OD of 8 mm. Some of the more advanced operative sheaths contain as many as four channels. Two channels are utilized for placement of the hysteroscope and the distending media, leaving two operative channels for placement of accessory instruments.

Flexible Hysteroscopes

Flexible, steerable fiberoptic hysteroscopes were patterned after the gastrointestinal endoscope[90] (Fig. 13-26) The distal tip can be deflected upward or downward from 130 to 160 degrees. Both the diagnostic and operative scopes deliver distending media through a 1-mm channel. Some diagnostic, flexible hysteroscopes have an OD as small as 3.5 mm, while flexible hysteroscopes with single operating channels have ODs starting at 5.0 mm. Each of these hysteroscopes can be inserted with little or no cervical dilation. This instrument is especially useful for evaluating the uterine cavity and tubal

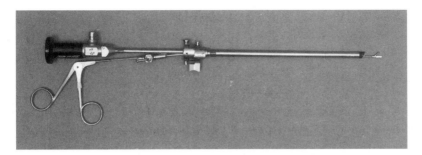

Fig. 13-24. In-line operative hysteroscope with semirigid scissors.

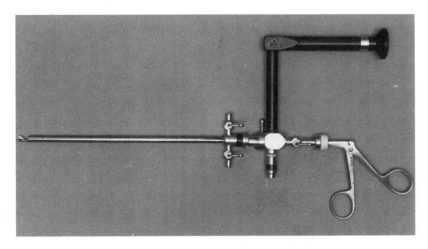

Fig. 13-25. Right-angle operative hysteroscope sheath.

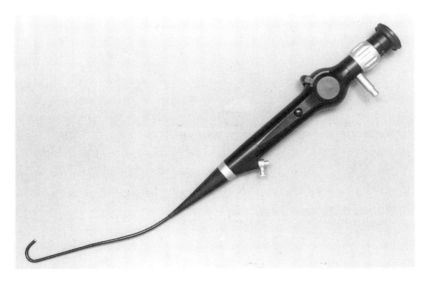

Fig. 13-26. Flexible hysteroscope. (Circon ACMI, Stamford, CT.)

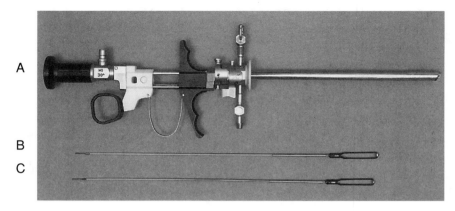

Fig. 13-27. Resectoscope. **(A)** Assembled hysteroscopic resectoscope with **(B)** roller bar and **(C)** roller ball.

ostia in patients with an irregularly shaped uterus. It can be used when performing proximal tubal cannulation and for lysis of adhesions located laterally, which are difficult to reach with the rigid hysteroscope.

Resectoscope

The hysteroscopic resectoscope is a modification of the urologic resectoscope. Its assembly requires some practice and should be mastered before surgical procedures are undertaken. The sheath has an OD of 8 mm and includes both inflow and outflow ports for distending media. The resectoscope is equipped with continuous flow and provides excellent irrigation for operative procedures. If surgical debris blocks the operative field, the resectoscope can be removed while the sheath is left in place. This allows the removal of large debris while maintaining cervical dilation.

Electrosurgical instruments can be inserted into the apparatus. The device has a spring handle that allows one to move the attached surgical instrument inward and outward (Fig. 13-27).

The resectoscope is useful in removing submucous myomas, uterine septa, endometrial polyps, and intrauterine adhesions, and for endometrial ablation. The patient must be grounded and a nonelectrolyte, nonconducting, distending media must be used. Electric shocks to the surgeon and patient from the resectoscope sheath occurred with the initial instrument design, but this problem has been resolved.

Operative Instruments

There are an assortment of rigid, semirigid, and flexible instruments that have been developed or adapted for hysteroscopic surgery. The rigid and semirigid instruments include scissors, grasping forceps, and biopsy forceps. The flexible instruments are a group of specifically adapted catheters. The rigid instruments can be categorized into two types. One type of rigid instrument is permanently fixed to the end of an operative sheath. Since these instruments must be maneuvered with the hysteroscope, it may be somewhat awkward to manipulate. Another set of rigid instruments, including

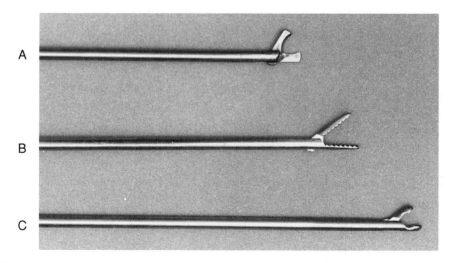

Fig. 13-28. Hysteroscopic instruments. **(A)** Scissors. **(B)** Grasping forceps. **(C)** Rigid hysteroscopic biopsy forceps.

scissors, grasping forceps, and biopsy forceps, are inserted through an offset operating hysteroscope (Fig. 13-28). By contrast, semirigid instruments and flexible catheters can be inserted through the operative port of an in-line hysteroscope. These instruments are small (7 French) and fragile. Special care should be taken when handling these instruments as the handle, shaft, and tips of these devices can he easily damaged. Catheters can be inserted through the hysteroscopic sheath for tubal cannulation and selective chromotubation. A 3-French whistle tip catheter works well for this purpose.

Both electrocautery and laser instruments are used in hysteroscopic surgery. Electrocautery instruments have been adapted for the resectoscope. Included are a loop electrode, roller ball, and punctate electrode (Fig. 13-29). Both the roller ball and the loop electrode can be used for endometrial ablation. The loop, which ranges in size from 24 to 27 French, has other applications, including the excision of submucous myomas and the resection of uterine septa. The punctate electrode can be used for pinpoint coagulation. Lasers including the neodymium-yttrium-aluminum-garnet (Nd:YAG), potassium-titanyl-phosphate (KTP), and argon are delivered by fiberoptics and, unlike the carbon dioxide,

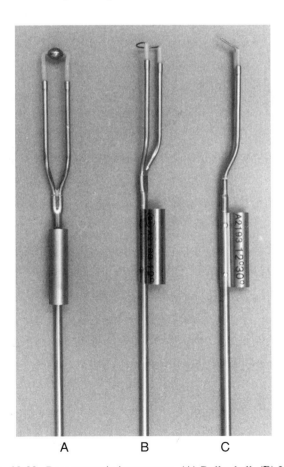

Fig. 13-29. Resectoscopic instruments. **(A)** Roller ball. **(B)** Loop electrode. **(C)** Punctate electrode.

laser, can freely pass through liquid distending media. The Nd:YAG laser is invisible with a wavelength of 1,064 nm. It penetrates tissue to a depth of 3 to 4 mm and exerts its major effects below the tissue surface. The principle effect of the Nd:YAG is photocoagulation and not vaporization. It has been used in endometrial ablation; however, in this author's experience, it offers few if any advantages over electrocoagulation and is more expensive.

Light Source

Illumination for hysteroscopy is provided by a light source that is connected to the hysteroscope by a fiberoptic cable. Fiberoptics provide the transmission of potent light from a given source to the hysteroscope without the production of significant heat. The fiberoptic system employs thousands of small glass fibers with a low refractory index cladding and a high refractory index core. In a compact light system, one can deliver sufficient illumination for both diagnostic and operative procedures. The light cable fastens directly onto the hysteroscope. Adapters are made so that one may use a single light source for several different cables or hysteroscopes. Most of the contemporary light sources contain either halogen or xenon light sources. The xenon lamps are more expensive, but both provide adequate illumination for operative procedures, photography, and videotaping.

Distending Media

The uterine cavity must be distended to perform panoramic hysteroscopy. The ideal distending media is a solution that is isotonic, no hemolytic, nonconductive, nontoxic, rapidly cleared from the body, and provides ample visualization. If a surgical procedure is planned, the distending media should minimize uterine bleeding or maintain a clear visual field, or both. The most commonly used media are carbon dioxide, low viscosity fluids, and high molecular weight dextran 70.[91] The angle of view and magnification seen varies with the refractory index of the distending media. Gaseous media allow perception of the maximal angle of view. Liquid media reduce the angle of view.[92] Table 13-6 compares the various distending media used during hysteroscopic procedures.

The use of carbon dioxide as a distending media has several advantages. It provides an excellent field of view, is widely available, has a long history of safety in tubal patency testing, is rapidly absorbed, and makes cleaning of instruments easy. Carbon dioxide is an exceptional distending media for office hysteroscopy. It is less useful in operative hysteroscopy. Intrauterine bleeding usually results in the formation of bubbles that obscure the visual field. Carbon dioxide must be insufflated with a special instrument. One such instrument uses a pressure set point, such as 100 mmHg, and gas is infused until this pressure is reached. Another

Table 13-6. Comparison of Distending Media Used in Hysteroscopy

Type	Examples	Mode of Delivery	Conductive	Advantages	Disadvantages	Special Complications
Gas	Carbon dioxide	Specialized insufflator (maximum flow 100 ml/min)	No	Clean, good for office use and taking photos	Forms bubbles with blood, requires special insufflator	Embolism with high flow (laparoscopy insufflators)
Low-viscosity distending media	Lactated Ringer's Normal saline	Gravity, pressurized system, or electrical pump	Yes	Inexpensive, readily available	Cannot be used with electrocautery, mixes with blood, large volume may be needed	Fluid overload
	5% Dextrose 1.5% Glycine 3% Sorbitol	Gravity, pressurized system, or electrical pump	No	Inexpensive, readily available, can be used with electrocautery	Large volumes may be needed, mixes with blood	Fluid overload, hyponatremia
High-viscosity distending media	Dextran 70 in 10% dextrose (Hyskon)	Manual insufflation with 50-ml syringe	No	Requires small volume, does not mix with blood	Adheres to and may damage instruments, bubble formation	Low risk of anaphylaxis and prolonged bleeding time

insufflator has an adjustable flow rate with a maximum of 100 ml/min. The laparoscopic insufflator delivers 1 L/min or more of flow and should never be used for hysteroscopy due to the potential complication of an embolism.

There are two types of low-viscosity distending media, those that contain electrolytes and those that do not. The electrolyte-containing media include normal saline and lactated Ringer's solution and cannot be used with electrocautery. The electrolyte-free solutions are 5 percent dextrose, 1.5 percent glycine, and 3 percent sorbitol. Low-viscosity media are usually delivered into the hysteroscopic sheath from 500 to 3,000 ml plastic bags. These large bags are either elevated above the patient and infused by the force of gravity or placed in a large blood pressure cuff and infused by pressurizing the cuff. Alternatively, low-viscosity fluids can be instilled into the uterine cavity by an electrically driven pump, which provides a more precise delivery of fluid at a constant pressure.

Hyskon is categorized as a high-viscosity distention media. Hyskon is a clear, viscous, sterile, nonpyogenic, electrolyte-free, nonconductive solution of dextran 70 in dextrose 10 percent. It has a tendency to crystallize if it is subjected to temperature variations or is stored for long periods of time. Hyskon has the ability to attract large volumes of water when intravasated intravascularly, which may lead to electrolyte imbalances. The extent of systemic absorption of dextran 70 by the uterine and peritoneal cavities has not been ascertained. One of the major advantages of Hyskon is its

inability to mix with blood, which maintains a clear visual field despite the presence of uterine bleeding. Electrosurgery can be performed with Hyskon because the solution is nonconductive. The major disadvantage of Hyskon is its tendency to adhere to surgical instruments. If the surgical instruments are not washed with hot water immediately after a procedure, it can damage valves and optical components. Hyskon must be poured slowly down the side of a container and then aspirated into two or more 50-ml plastic syringes for delivery, to avoid the formation of air bubbles that may distort the visual field. The delivery tubing should be filled before being attached to the inflow valve on the hysteroscopic sheath. The sheath is then filled with Hyskon before it is inserted into the uterine cavity. The amount of solution used is rarely greater than 300 ml and the infusion pressure should not exceed 150 mmHg.

Operative Procedures

Before performing any procedure, the operating surgeon must fully inform the patient regarding the realistic benefits, the cost, the chance for failure, the potential risks, and what the procedure involves. The alternatives to the procedure should be discussed in detail, and the options for anesthesia should be reviewed. All elective hysteroscopic procedures should be performed during the proliferative phase of the menstrual cycle, as this provides the most optimal view of the uterine cavity. Most hysteroscopic procedures can be

Hysteroscopy Procedures

- Resection of uterine leiomyomas
- Metroplasty
- Endometrial ablation
- Intrauterine adhesions
- Transcervical tuboplasty

performed with intravenous sedation and a paracervical block. Other options include general and regional anesthesia. When an operative hysteroscopy is scheduled, consent should be obtained for laparoscopy and in some cases laparotomy. The author does not advocate the routine use of laparoscopy with operative hysteroscopy.

The patient is positioned, antiseptically prepared, and draped in a manner that is similar to that for D&C. If the patient did not void prior to the procedure, the urinary bladder is drained and a side-opening speculum is inserted. Once adequate cervical dilation is obtained, the hysteroscope is inserted through the cervical os under direct endoscopic vision and the speculum is removed. Although a video camera is not requisite, it is strongly recommended for the benefit of the surgeon and for teaching.

One of the most important factors in performing operative hysteroscopy is the maintenance of a clear operative field. Besides using a distending media that does not mix with blood, such as Hyskon, this can be accomplished by either overdilating the cervical os and allowing the distending media to flow out around the hysteroscopic sheath, or by using a sheath that provides continuous laminar flow of media. With the former method, the assessment of media outflow can be difficult. The author prefers a dual sheath or dual port system with an outflow port that can be directly connected to a vacuum collecting system. This gives an accurate assessment of the fluid deficit as less media is lost in the drapes, towels, or on the operating room floor. Every 10 to 15 minutes the surgeon should be updated as to the fluid deficit.

The uterus is an intrinsically vascular organ and its vascularity may be enhanced by uterine myomas or other pathology. Despite this, intraoperative bleeding is usually not a significant problem. This is because the liquid distending media usually exerts an intrauterine pressure of more than 90 mmHg, which exceeds end-arterial pressure. The risk of intravasation of distending media through open, low-pressure venous channels with subsequent fluid overload exists. Corson et al[93] demonstrated that, in a prospective randomized study of patients undergoing endometrial ablation and hysteroscopic resection of fibroids, intracervical stromal in-

jection of dilute vasopressin solution statistically decreased the intravasation of distending media.

Postoperatively, both pelvic ultrasound and HSG can be used to determine whether a particular procedure was completely successful (e.g., repair of a uterine anomaly, removal of a uterine leiomyoma, or cannulation of a proximal tubal obstruction). The appropriate timing for postoperative evaluation should be individualized and is based on the recurrence of symptoms, the difficulty of the procedure, and the needs of the patient.

Uterine Leiomyomas

The American College of Obstetrician and Gynecologists (ACOG) has endorsed preoperative criteria for myomectomy.[94] Included in the ACOG criteria are the presence of either infertility or recurrent pregnancy loss when myoma(s) is believed to be the primary cause for the condition. A preoperative evaluation should be performed that will exclude other causes of these conditions. Myomas alone may be responsible for infertility in only 2 to 3 percent of cases.[95] Recurrent pregnancy loss is believed to be the result of uterine myomas and muellerian anomalies in no more than 15 percent of cases.[96] Patients with submucous leiomyomas commonly present with menorrhagia. These patients are candidates for hysteroscopic treatment.

Hysteroscopy is effective in the removal of broad-based and pedunculated, submucous myomas. Derman et al[97] reported on the long-term effectiveness of hysteroscopic treatment of menorrhagia and leiomyomas. In this study, patients underwent either myomectomy or a combination of myomectomy and endometrial ablation and were followed for up to 10 years. Of the 94 subjects included in the study, only 16 percent of patients who underwent endoscopic myomectomy required additional treatment over the next 5 to 10 years. In the group of patients who underwent endometrial ablation, only 5 of 62 (8.1 percent) required repeat surgery. Still, there are no data regarding the efficacy of hysteroscopic myomectomy in patients with recurrent pregnancy loss and very little information regarding its effectiveness in the treatment of infertility. In a group of infertile subjects with otherwise normal infertility evaluations who underwent myomectomy for a submucosal myoma of greater than 5 cm, 62 percent conceived within 1 year after surgery.[98] No control group was available for comparison.

The author and colleagues have used the resectoscope and loop electrode almost exclusively for hysteroscopic myomectomy. Hysteroscopic scissors, laser energy, or a knife electrode may be used for this purpose. The loop electrode can be used to cut directly through the base of a pedunculated myoma, or it can be used as a morcellating device to slowly "shave-away" a broad-based myoma. A combination of these two techniques is often needed. The loop should pass through the tissue with ease. A cut or blended cut and coagulation current of 100 to 120 watts is used. The resection is

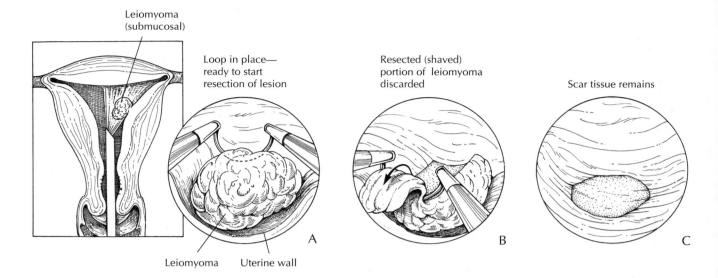

Leiomyoma
(submucosal)

Loop in place—
ready to start
resection of lesion

Resected (shaved)
portion of leiomyoma
discarded

Scar tissue remains

A

B

C

Leiomyoma   Uterine wall

Fig. 13-30. (A–C) Resection of uterine leiomyoma.

begun by placing the loop just beyond the most cephalad portion of the fibroid and gradually drawing the loop toward the operator (Fig. 13-30). This motion can be achieved by moving either the loop alone through its spring mechanism or by moving the entire resectoscope. Both techniques are acceptable and each individual surgeon should use the technique found to be most effective. As the middle of the fibroid is resected, the edges tend to fall inward, increasing the panoramic view. During the resection, small pieces of the myoma will accumulate and obstruct the operative field. When this occurs, the inner sheath of the resectoscope can be removed. This will allow for drainage of the uterine cavity and will clear the field. Polyp forceps may be needed to remove larger debris. The tissue is collected for histologic examination. The resection should not proceed past the level of the surrounding endometrial lining. Postoperatively, the surgical area will be covered with newly proliferated endometrium. Although theoretically appealing, postoperative estrogen therapy has not been proved effective in decreasing intrauterine adhesions. Concurrent laparoscopy may be helpful for the less experienced surgeon, and its use should be decided on a case-by-case basis. There are no data to suggest that concurrent laparoscopy decreases operative complications and this author has found it to be useful only with large myomas or when completing an infertility evaluation. Uterine perforation during hysteroscopic myomectomy can lead to uterine rupture during a subsequent pregnancy.[99]

With the introduction of long-acting gonadotropin-releasing hormone (GnRH) agonists (which downregulate GnRH receptors, leading to a hypogonadotropic hypoestrogenic state), there has been a resurgence of interest in the medical management of uterine myomas. In general, a 50 percent reduction in uterine volume is observed with GnRH therapy, with the greatest effect occurring after 12 weeks of treat-

ment.[100] Preoperative treatment with a GnRH agonist might be useful in decreasing the size of submucous myoma(s) making resection less difficult. When compared to oral iron therapy, GnRH agonists have not been shown to be more effective in improving the patient's preoperative hemoglobin. The author does not advocate routine preoperative medical therapy for submucous myomas and has not used size limits as a contraindication for myoma resection, as long as the cavity can be visualized and the loop electrode can be placed safely around the lesion. Until proven otherwise, the author advocates oral iron therapy for the treatment of chronically anemic patients.

Metroplasty

Lateral fusion defects of the muellerian ducts result in uterine anomalies that are associated with recurrent pregnancy loss. Once other etiologies for recurrent pregnancy loss are excluded, one may consider corrective surgery. Historically, all muellerian anomalies were repaired via laparotomy. Although this procedure is effective, it requires an incision through the uterus, which increases the risk of uterine dehiscence and necessitates a cesarean delivery. The risks of an abdominal metroplasty include excessive blood loss, pelvic adhesions, and wound infection. Although bicornuate uteri are not repairable via hysteroscopy, a septate uterus can be approached with hysteroscopy.

The author prefers the use of rigid or semirigid scissors to perform hysteroscopic metroplasty, as this avoids the risk of electrical or laser damage to the endometrium. Alternatively, one could use the resectoscope with loop electrode or laser. Concurrent laparoscopy is indicated if a definitive diagnosis of the type of anomaly has not been made. Concurrent laparoscopy is not essential and should be performed on a case-by-

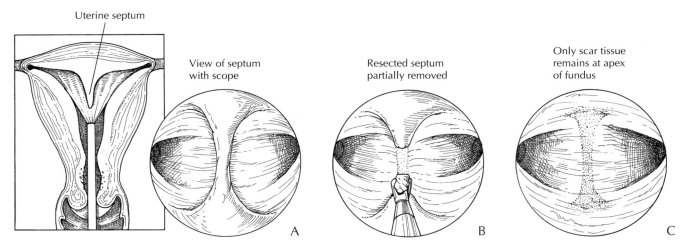

Uterine septum

View of septum with scope

Resected septum partially removed

Only scar tissue remains at apex of fundus

A   B   C

Fig. 13-31. (A–C) Resection of uterine septum.

case basis. During the procedure, a thorough inspection is made of the cervical canal, endometrial cavity, tubal recesses, and tubal ostia. The septum is approached in its midposition using sharp dissection. Uterine septa are composed of fibrous tissue and intraoperative bleeding is usually minimal. As the dissection progresses, the uterine wall will separate. Sharp dissection is continued until the fibrous tissue is even with the beginning of the tubal recesses (Fig. 13-31). In one study of 103 patients who underwent hysteroscopic metroplasty, 81 percent reported a term pregnancy.[101]

Endometrial Ablation

Abnormal uterine bleeding is commonly caused by an underlying endocrinopathy and is usually controlled with the use of progestins or estrogen, or both. If medical therapy is not successful and an underlying anatomic condition is suspected, a diagnostic hysteroscopy may shed some light on the etiology of the bleeding. In the past, hysterectomy was commonly performed when medical therapy or curettage had failed to treat patients with dysfunctional uterine bleeding. For a little more than a decade, abnormal uterine bleeding has been successfully treated by obliterating the endometrium. This process is known as endometrial ablation and was originally described using an Nd:YAG laser.[102,103] It has now been described using the roller ball[104] and loop electrode.[105] In the initial reports on endometrial ablation using the laser or roller ball, although 90 percent of all patients experienced some decrease in their uterine bleeding, only 30 to 50 percent experienced complete amenorrhea after 3 to 6 months of follow-up.[102,103] Wortman[105] has reported an 84 percent (21 of 25) amenorrhea rate after a 6-month follow-up period in patients undergoing endometrial resection with the loop electrode. In this particular study, the endometrium was not medically or surgically manipulated prior to the resection. Preoperatively, patients should be

made aware of the reported results of the procedure, as well as the fact that an intrauterine pregnancy has been reported after an endometrial ablation.[106]

Endometrial ablation with the resectoscope and roller ball or loop electrode is now much more popular then laser endometrial ablation. The resectoscope is at least as effective as the laser, is less time-consuming, and is less expensive. The resectoscope uses electrical energy to either fulgurate or resect the endometrium. Although the roller ball was originally described for use in endometrial ablations, this author prefers to use a combination of the two. The loop electrode is used with a cutting current of 100 watts to shave the endometrium to a myometrial depth of approximately 4 mm. Using this method, one can easily assess the depth of the resection, as well as obtain endomyometrial tissue for histologic review. The ablation is begun on the anterior uterine wall (Fig. 13-32). Long furrows of endometrial tissue are resected, beginning in the fundus and extending to the internal cervical os. The endometrium is resected row-by-row. The endometrium surrounding the tubal recesses is not ablated with the loop electrode. The roller ball, with a blended current from 80 to 100 watts, is used to desiccate any missed areas and to ablate around the tubal ostia. Although preoperative therapy with GnRH agonists, progestins, danazol, or endometrial curettage has been described, no randomized comparison or placebo-controlled clinical trials are available to compare the efficacy of these different therapies. Care must be taken to avoid ablation of tissue at or below the cervical os, which may result in the development of cervical stenosis. Perforations of the uterus with the loop electrode can be avoided by limiting the time of contact of the loop with the uterine tissue.

Intrauterine Adhesions

Intrauterine adhesions are most commonly caused by infection or uterine trauma such as a D&C performed after pregnancy. Adhesions are commonly diagnosed or suspected

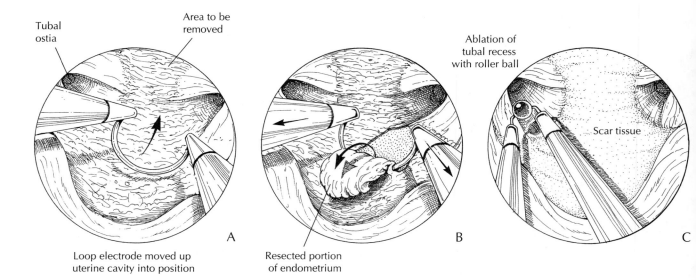

Fig. 13-32. (A–C) Resection of endometrium.

during an HSG performed for an infertility evaluation or in a patient with oligomenorrhea that is unresponsive to hormonal therapy (Fig. 13-33). Hysteroscopy provides the physician with the opportunity to diagnose and remove intrauterine adhesions using hysteroscopic scissors under direct visualization. This decreases the probability of trauma to the surrounding endometrium. Care must be taken during cervical dilation in patients with severe occlusion of the uterine cavity. The development of false passages and uterine perforation is all too common during this procedure. Concurrent ultrasonography can help define the junction between the internal os and the intrauterine cavity. The procedure is begun by placing the hysteroscope at the internal os and

carefully lysing adhesions with sharp dissection. We prefer the small rigid scissors for this procedure. Careful dissection is continued until the entire uterine cavity is free of adhesions.

When intrauterine adhesions are lysed in patients with either oligomenorrhea or amenorrhea, approximately 90 percent can expect to have normal menses restored and approximately 80 percent will achieve a term pregnancy. In a study of 187 patients, the obstetric outcome was related to the degree of occlusion of the uterine cavity.[85] Term pregnancies were realized in 81 percent of patients with mild occlusive disease, and in only 32 percent of those with severe occlusion.

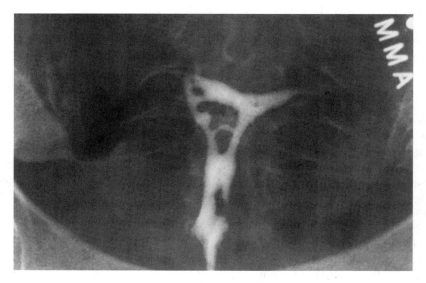

Fig. 13-33. Hysterosalpingogram of intrauterine adhesions.

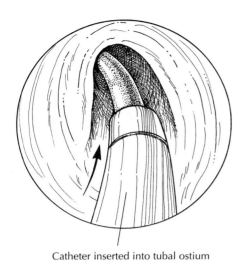

Catheter inserted into tubal ostium

Fig. 13-34. Transcervical tubal cannulation.

Transcervical Tuboplasty

The causes of proximal tubal occlusion include infection, salpingitis isthmica nodosum, intraluminal debris, tubal spasm, ectopic pregnancy, tubal ligation, and endometriosis. Proximal tubal occlusion is usually diagnosed with an HSG during an infertility evaluation. HSG may not differentiate tubocornual spasm from a mechanical obstruction and tends to overdiagnose proximal tubal occlusion.[107] Selective salpingography, using fluoroscopic guidance to selectively cannulate and inject dye into a fallopian tube, is useful and may obviate the need for surgery in some patients.[108] If proximal tubal occlusion is confirmed, hysteroscopy with concurrent laparoscopy can be used to perform transcervical tuboplasty. Laparoscopy is used to document the condition of the distal fallopian tube. Transcervical tuboplasty is more cost-effective than either transabdominal tuboplasty or in vitro fertilization.

Using a single-port operating hysteroscope, either a 3-French coaxial catheter and guidewire or a balloon catheter can be inserted under direct visualization into the tubal ostia to establish tubal patency (Fig. 13-34). Dye can be injected through the catheter to confirm patency. There are no controlled data to support the use of selective tubal cannulation for proximal tubal occlusion. In a multicenter study on balloon tuboplasty for proximal tubal occlusion, 92 percent of 77 patients had successful recanalization of at least one tube, and 23 patients subsequently conceived.[109]

Complications

Fluid Overload

Complications specifically related to distending media are rare, yet can be very serious. In one survey, complications related to distending media were reported to occur in less

than 4 percent of cases and varied according to the media used.[110] Complications related to the use of dextran 70 are twofold. The first is fluid overload and the second is an anaphylactic reaction. The introduction of dextran into the circulation can produce both pulmonary edema and disseminated intravascular coagulation. Reports of anaphylactic shock with the use of dextran 70 are sporadic and anecdotal. One report discussed using intravenous injections of small amounts of 15 percent dextran 2 minutes before the use of dextran 70 to prevent anaphylaxis.[111] Since this problem is rare, this author does not recommend prophylaxis routinely. The key to decreasing the likelihood of complications associated with dextran 70 is to restrict the volume used in any procedure to less than 500 ml, although complications can occur with lower volumes of dextran.[112]

Fluid overload and hyponatremia are complications of low-viscosity, sodium-free fluids. A fluid deficit of greater than 1,000 ml in a young, healthy patient is associated with a significant risk of fluid overload. In the older patient, or those with a history of cardiovascular compromise, a 750-ml deficit is significant. When the fluid deficit reaches these limits the procedure should be discontinued and the serum electrolytes should be assessed. A rapid decrease in serum sodium concentration can result in generalized cerebral edema, seizures, and possibly death. Diuretics and intravenous fluid restriction can be used to treat hyponatremia and fluid overload.

Electrosurgical Injury

One potential intraoperative complication of hysteroscopy is an injury sustained from either electrical or laser energy and their associated thermal effects. Although the probability for injury is low, it can be very serious. Injury can occur to both the uterine cavity and adjacent organs. Injury to adjacent organs, including the bowel, urinary bladder, and large pelvic vessels, may occur. These complication can be avoided by always moving the electrical instrument when activated. Duffy et al[113] has demonstrated in vivo that the temperature of the uterine serosal surface does not rise appreciably as long as the roller ball is not held stationary during the coagulation.

In a study on hysteroscopic coagulation of the tubal cornua

Hysteroscopy Complications

- Fluid overload
- Electrosurgical injury
- Bleeding
- Procedure failures

for sterilization, a significant risk of bowel injury was reported.[114] One must be cautious when coagulating in the tubal recesses.

Bleeding

Intraoperative bleeding is rare. The sources of intraoperative bleeding include lacerations due to cervical manipulation and uterine perforation. Bleeding from cervical lacerations may be controlled using electrocautery or sutures. Excessive bleeding can occur postoperatively. This complication can be treated by placing a Foley catheter in the uterine cavity. After insertion, the catheter is distended with 15 to 30 ml of saline solution. In one series of 216 resectoscope procedures, four patients (1.9 percent) developed postoperative uterine bleeding and were successfully treated with this procedure.[115]

Procedure Failures

Occasionally, the surgeon will be faced with a situation in which the hysteroscopic procedure failed to correct the uterine problem. There are several reasons for hysteroscopic failure. Periodically, a procedure will be progressing without difficulty, but will need to be stopped prematurely because of an excessive fluid deficit. If the uterus is perforated during cervical dilation, the uterine cavity cannot be distended and the procedure must be aborted. Other causes of failure include recurrence of the preoperative condition. Patients with uterine synechiae and recurrent pregnancy loss may experience recurrence of their adhesions after hysteroscopic adhesiolysis. Successful transcervical tuboplasty may be followed by recurrent tubal obstruction, and menorrhagia may not be satisfactorily controlled by endometrial ablation. Although the author does not advocate repeat transcervical tuboplasty for failed procedures, patients with failed endometrial ablations and less than adequate resection of submucous leiomyomas or uterine septums are candidates for repeat procedures if indicated.

Contraindications

The contraindications to hysteroscopy include pelvic infection, excessive uterine bleeding, pregnancy, and the inability to undergo anesthesia. Pelvic infections should be evaluated and treated appropriately. Upper genital tract infections increase the risk of uterine perforation. Lower genital tract infections can be spread to the upper genital tract with hysteroscopy.[116] Although patients with uterine bleeding may be candidates for hysteroscopy, heavy uterine bleeding will obscure the visual field and render the procedure ineffective. These patients are better diagnosed and treated with D&C.

REFERENCES

1. National Center for Health Statistics: Surgical operations in short-stay hospitals. United States-1975, DHEW Publication No (PHS) 78–1785, April, 1978
2. Kelly HA: Curettage without anesthesia on the office table. Am J Obstet Gynecol 9:78, 1925
3. Pantaleoni DC: On endoscopic examination of the cavity of the womb. Med Press Circ 8:26, 1869
4. Fleischer AC, Entman SS, Kalemeris GE: Sonographic depiction of normal cyclical changes of endometrium. Ultrasound Med Biol 12:271, 1986
5. Markee JE: Menstruation in intraocular endometrial transplants in the rhesus monkey. Contr Embryol Carneg Inst 28:219, 1940
6. Wilborn WH, Flowers CE: Cellular mechanisms for endometrial conservation during menstrual bleeding. Semin Reprod Endocrinol 2:307, 1984
7. Hallberg L, Nilsson L: Constancy of individual menstrual blood loss. Acta Obstet Gynecol Scand 43:352, 1962
8. Goldrath MH, Sherman MD: Office hysteroscopy and suction curettage: can we eliminate the hospital diagnostic dilation and curettage? Am J Obstet Gynecol 152:220, 1985
9. Friedman AJ: Vaginal hemorrhage associated with degenerating submucous leiomyomata during leuprolide acetate treatment. Fertil Steril 52:152, 1989
10. Van Bogaert LJ: Clinicopathologic findings in endometrial polyps. Obstet Gynecol 71:771, 1988
11. Morrow CP, Townsend DE (eds): Synopsis of Gynecologic Oncology. 3rd Ed. Churchill Livingstone, New York, 1987
12. Padwick ML, Pryse-Davies J, Whitehead MI: A simple method for determining the optimal dosage of progestin in postmenopausal women receiving estrogens. N Engl J Med 315:930, 1986
13. Archer D, McIntyre-Seltman K, Wilborn W et al: Endometrial morphology in asymptomatic postmenopausal patients. Am J Obstet Gynecol 165:317, 1991
14. Cherkis RC, Patten SF, Dickinson JC, Dekanich AS: Significance of atypical endometrial cells detected by cervical cytology. Obstet Gynecol 69:786, 1987
15. Yancey M, Magelssen D, Demaurez A, Lee RB: Classification of endometrial cells on cervical cytology. Obstet Gynecol 76:1000, 1990
16. Hofmeister FJ, Wolfgram RC, Schwartz WR: Significant tissue abnormalities found coincidental to vaginal hysterectomy and vaginal reconstructive procedures. Obstet Gynecol 21:603, 1963
17. Stovall TG, Solomon SK, Ling FW: Endometrial sampling prior to hysterectomy. Obstet Gynecol 73:405, 1989
18. Rubin SC, Battistini M: Endometrial curettage at the time of cervical conization. Obstet Gynecol 67:663, 1986
19. Goldstein SR, Nachtigall M, Snyder JR, Nachtigall L: Endometrial assessment by vaginal ultrasonography before endometrial sampling in patients with postmenopausal bleeding. Am J Obstet Gynecol 163:119, 1990

20. Granberg S, Wikland M, Karlsson B et al: Endometrial thickness as measured by endovaginal ultrasonography for identifying endometrial abnormality. Am J Obstet Gynecol 164: 47, 1991

21. Nasri MN, Shepherd JH, Setchell ME et al: The role of vaginal scan in measurement of endometrial thickness in postmenopausal women. Br J Obstet Gynaecol 98:470, 1991

22. Dorum A, Kristensen GB, Langebrekke A et al: Evaluation of endometrial thickness measured by endovaginal ultrasound in women with post menopausal bleeding. Acta Obstet Gynecol Scand 72:116, 1993

23. Cicinelli E, Romano F, Anastasio PS et al: Transabdominal sonohysterography, transvaginal sonography, and hysteroscopy in the evaluation of submucous myomas. Obstet Gynecol 85:42, 1995

24. Parsons AK, Lense JJ: Sonohysterography for endometrial abnormalities: preliminary results. J Clin Ultrasound 21:87, 1993

25. Cicinelli E, Romano F, Anastasio PS et al: Sonohysterography versus hysteroscopy in the diagnosis of endouterine polyps. Gynecol Obstet Invest 38:266, 1994

26. Romano F, Cicinelli E, Anastasio PS et al: Sonohysterography versus hysteroscopy for diagnosing endouterine abnormalities in fertile women. Int J Gynecol Obstet 45:253, 1994

27. Goldstein SR: Unusual ultrasonographic appearance of the uterus in patients receiving tamoxifen. Am J Obstet Gynecol 170:447, 1994

28. Togashi K: MRI of the Female Pelvis. Igaku-Shoin, New York; 1993

29. Scoutt LM, Flynn SD, Luthringer DJ et al: Junctional zone of the uterus: correlation of MR imaging and histologic examination of hysterectomy specimens. Radiology 179:403, 1991

30. Ascher SM, Arnold LL, Patt RH et al: Adenomyosis: prospective comparison of MR imaging and transvaginal sonography. Radiology 190:803, 1994

31. Mitchell DG: Benign disease of the uterus and ovaries. Application of magnetic resonance imaging. Radiol Clin North Am 30:777, 1992

32. Hricak H, Rubinstein LV, Gherman GM et al: MR imaging evaluation of endometrial carcinoma: results of an NCI cooperative study. Radiology 179:829, 1991

33. Hricak H, Stern JL, Fisher MR et al: Endometrial carcinoma staging by MR imaging. Radiology 162:297, 1987

34. Sironi S, Taccagni G, Garancini P et al: Myometrial invasion by endometrial carcinoma: assessment by MR imaging. AJR 158:565, 1992

35. Yamashita Y, Mizutani H, Torashima M et al: Assessment of myometrial invasion by endometrial carcinoma: transvaginal sonography vs contrast-enhanced MR imaging. AJR 161:595, 1993

36. Jensen JG: Vacuum curettage. Dan Med Bull 17:199, 1970

37. Grimes DA: Diagnostic dilation and curettage: a reappraisal. Am J Obstet Gynecol 142:1, 1982

38. Chambers JT, Chambers SK: Endometrial sampling: when? where? why? with what? Clin Obstet Gynecol 35:28, 1992

39. Fornander T, Rutquist LE, Cedermark B et al: Adjuvant tamoxifen in early breast cancer: occurrence of new primary cancers. Lancet 1:117, 1989

40. Cohen I, Altaras M, Shapiro J et al: Postmenopausal Tamoxifen treatment and endometrial pathology. Obstet Gynecol Surv 49:823, 1994

41. Vuopala S: Diagnostic accuracy and clinical applicability of cytological and histological methods for investigating endometrial carcinoma. Acta Obstet Gynecol Scand Suppl 70:1, 1977

42. Kaunitz AM, Masciello A, Ostrowski M, Rovira EZ: Comparison of endometrial biopsy with the endometrial Pipelle and Vabra aspirator. J Reprod Med 33:427, 1988

43. Silver MM, Miles P, Rosa C: Comparison of Novak and Pipelle endometrial biopsy instruments. Obstet Gynecol 78:828, 1991

44. Lipscomb OH, Lopatine SM, Stovall TG, Ling FW: A randomized comparison of the Pipelle, Accurette, and Explora endometrial sampling devices. Am J Obstet Gynecol 170: 591, 1994

45. Stovall TG, Photopulos GJ, Poston WM et al: Pipelle endometrial sampling in patients with known endometrial carcinoma. Obstet Gynecol 77:954, 1991

46. Guido RS, Kanbour-Shakir A, Rulin MC, Christopherson WA: Pipelle endometrial sampling: sensitivity in the detection of endometrial cancer. Am J Reprod Med 40:553, 1995

47. Rodriguez GC, Yaqub N, King ME: A comparison of the Pipelle device and the Vabra aspirator as measured by endometrial denudation in hysterectomy specimens: the Pipelle device samples significantly less of the endometrial surface than the Vabra aspirator. Am J Obstet Gynecol 168:55, 1993

48. Stock RJ, Kanbour A: Pre-hysterectomy curettage. Obstet Gynecol 45:537, 1975

49. Leridon H: Human Fertility. University of Chicago Press, Chicago, 1977

50. Wilcox AJ, Weinberg CR, O'Connor JF: Incidence of early pregnancy loss. N Engl J Med 319:189, 1988

51. Gabbi SG, Niebyl JR, Simpson JL (eds): Obstetrics: Normal and Problem Pregnancies. 2nd Ed. Churchill Livingstone, New York, 1991

52. Kajii T, Ferrier A: Anatomic and chromosomal anomalies in 639 spontaneous abortuses. Hum Genet 55:87, 1980

53. Heinonen PK, Saarikoski S, Pystynen P: Reproductive performance of women with uterine anomalies. Acta Obstet Gynecol Scand 61:157, 1982

54. Kaufman RH, Noller K, Adam E et al: Upper genital tract abnormalities and pregnancy outcome in diethylstilbestrol-exposed pregnancy. Am J Obstet Gynecol 148:973, 1984

55. Buttram VC Jr, Reiter RC (eds): Uterine leiomyomata: etiology, symptomatology, and management. Fertil Steril 36:433, 1981

56. Mills JL, Simpson JL, Driscoll SG et al: NICHD-DIEP study: incidence of spontaneous abortion among normal women with insulin-dependent diabetes whose pregnancies were

identified within 21 days of conception. N Engl J Med 319: 1617, 1988

57. Mansur MM: Ultrasound diagnosis of complete abortion can reduce need for curettage. Eur J Obstet Gynecol Reprod Biol 44:65, 1992

58. Rulin MC, Bornstein SG, Campbell JD: The reliability of ultrasonography in the management of spontaneous abortion, clinically thought to be complete: a prospective study. Am J Obstet Gynecol 168:12, 1993

59. Buckley JD: The epidemiology of molar pregnancy and choriocarcinoma. Clin Obstet Gynecol 27:153, 1984

60. Nickelsen C: Diagnostic and curative value of uterine curettage. Acta Obstet Gynecol Scand 65:693, 1986

61. Mikuta JJ: Surgical management of dysfunctional uterine bleeding. Clin Obstet Gynecol 13:451, 1970

62. Hulka JS, Lefler HT, Anglone A, Lachenbruch PA: A new electronic force monitor to measure factors influencing cervical dilation for vacuum curettage. Am J Obstet Gynecol 120: 166, 1974

63. Chvapil M, Droegmueller W, Meyer T et al: New synthetic Laminaria. Obstet Gynecol 60:729, 1982

64. Wells E, Hulka J: Cervical Dilation: a comparison of Lamicel and Dilapan. Am J Obstet Gynecol 161:1124, 1989

65. Hern W: Laminaria versus Dilapan osmotic cervical dilators for outpatient dilation and evauation abortion: randomized cohort comparison of 1,001 patients. Am J Obstet Gynecol 171:123, 1994

66. McCord ML, Stovall TG, Summitt RL Jr et al: Synthetic hygroscopic cervical dilator use in patients with unsatisfactory colposcopy. Obstet Gynecol 85:30, 1995

67. Stern JL, Major C, Vanle L: Preventing cervical conization by achieving satisfactory colposcopy with hygroscopic cervical dilators. Am J Obstet Gynecol 163:176, 1990

68. Goldrath MH: Vaginal removal of the pedunculated submucous myomoma: the use of Laminaria. Obstet Gynecol 70: 670, 1987

69. Ostrzenski A: Resectoscopic cervical trauma minimized by inserting Laminaria Digitata preoperatively. Int J Fertil Menopausal Stud 39:111, 1994

70. Thompson JD, Rock J: Operative Gynecology. JB Lippincott, Philadelphia, 1992

71. Grimes DA, Schulz KF, Cates W Jr et al: Local vs. general anesthesia. Which is safer for performing suction curettage abortion? Am J Obstet Gynecol 135:1030, 1979

72. Blanco LJ, Reid PR, King TM: Plasma lidocaine levels following paracervical infiltration for aspiration abortion. Obstet Gynecol 60:506, 1982

73. Chen SS, Lee L: Reappraisal of endocervical curettage in predicting cervical involvement by endometrial carcinoma. J Reprod Med 31:50, 1986

74. Hunter RE, Reuter K, Kopin E: Use of ultrasonography in the difficult postmenopausal dilation and curettage. Obstet Gynecol 73:813, 1989

75. Molin A: Risk of damage to the cervix by dilation for first-trimester-induced abortion by suction aspiration. Gynecol Obstet Invest 35:152, 1993

76. Ben-Baruch G, Menczer J, Shalev J et al: Uterine perforations during curettage: perforation rates and post-perforation management. Isr J Med Sci 16:821, 1980

77. Grimes DA, Willard C Jr: Complications from legally-induced abortions: a review. Obstet Gynecol Surv 34:177, 1979

78. Grimes DA, Schulz KF, Cates WJ: Prevention of uterine perforation during curettage abortion. JAMA 251:2108, 1984

79. Ben-Baruch G, Menczer J. Frenkel Y, Serr DM: Laparoscopy in the management of uterine perforation. J Reprod Med 27: 73, 1982

80. Lowensohn RI, Hibbard LT: Laceration of the ascending branch of the uterine artery. A complication of therapeutic abortion. Am J Obstet Gynecol 118:36, 1974

81. Park T-K, Flock M, Schulz KF, Grimes DA: Preventing febrile complications of suction curettage abortion. J Obstet Gynecol 152:252, 1985

82. Sacks PC, Tchabo J-G: Incidence of bacteremia at dilatation and curettage. J Reprod Med 37:331, 1992

83. Dejani AS, Bisno AL, Chung KJ et al: Prevention of bacterial endocarditis. Recommendations by the American Heart Association. JAMA 264:2919, 1990

84. Klein SM, Garcia CS: Asherman's syndrome: a critique and current review. Fertil Steril 24:722, 1973

85. Valle RF, Sciarra JJ: Intrauterine adhesions: hysteroscopic diagnosis, classification, treatment, and reproductive outcome. Am J Obstet Gynecol 158:1459, 1988

86. Twiggs LB, Phillips GL: Documentation of subclinical trophoblastic embolization with invasive cardiac monitoring in a woman with a molar pregnancy. J Reprod Med 31:277, 1986

87. Cohle SD, Petty CS: Sudden death caused by embolization of trophoblast from hydatidiform mole. J Forensic Sci 30: 1279, 1985

88. Loffer FD: Hysteroscopy with selected endometrial sampling compared with D&C for abnormal uterine bleeding: the value of a negative hysteroscopic view. Obstet Gynecol 73:16, 1989

89. Barbot J, Parent B, Dubuisson JB: Contact hysteroscopy: another method of endoscopic examination of the uterine cavity. Am J Obstet Gynecol 136:721, 1980

90. Brueschke EE, Wilbanks GD: A steerable fiberoptic hysteroscope. Obstet Gynecol 44:273, 1974

91. Siegler AM: A comparison of gas and liquid for hysteroscopy. J Reprod Med 15:73, 1975

92. Gardner FM: Optical physics with emphasis on endoscope. Clin Obstet Gynecol 26:213, 1983

93. Corson SL, Brooks PG, Serden SP et al: Effect of vasopressin administration during hysteroscopic surgery. J Reprod Med 39:419, 1994

94. American College of Obstetricians and Gynecologists: Quality assessment and improvement in obstetrics and gynecology. ACOG, Washington, DC, 1994

95. Buttram VC, Reiter RC: Uterine leiomyomata: etiology, symptomatology, and management. Fertil Steril 36:433, 1981

96. Salat-Baroux J: Recurrent spontaneous abortion. Reprod Nutr Dev 28:1555, 1988

97. Derman SG, Rehnstrom J, Neuwirth RS: The long-term effectiveness of hysteroscopic treatment of menorrhagia and leiomyomas. Obstet Gynecol 77:591, 1991

98. Garcia CR, Tureck RW: Submucosal leiomyomas and infertility. Fertil Steril 42:16, 1984

99. Yaron Y, Shenhav M, Jaffa AJ et al: Uterine rupture at 33 weeks' gestation subsequent to hysteroscopic uterine perforation. Am J Obstet Gynecol 170:786, 1994

100. Friedman AJ, Hoffman DI, Comite F et al: Treatment of leiomyomata uteri with leuprolide acetate depot: a double-blind, placebo-controlled, multicenter study. Obstet Gynecol 77:720, 1991

101. DeCherney AH, Russel JB, Graebe RA, Polan ML: Resectoscopic management of mullerian fusion defects. Fertil Steril 45:726, 1986

102. Goldrath MP, Fuller T, Segal S: Laser photovaporization of endometrium for the treatment of menorrhagia. Am J Obstet Gynecol 140:14, 1981

103. Lomano JM, Feste JR, Loffer FD, Goldrath MH: Ablation of the endometrium with the Nd:YAG laser: a multicenter study. Colposc Laser Surg 2:203, 1986

104. Daniell JF, Kurtz BR, Ke RW: Hysteroscopic endometrial ablation using the rollerball electrode. Obstet Gynecol 80:329, 1992

105. Wortman M, Daggett A: Hysteroscopic endomyometrial resection: a new technique for the treatment of menorrhagia. Obstet Gynecol 83:295, 1994

106. Goldberg JM: Intrauterine pregnancy following endometrial ablation. Obstet Gynecol 83:836, 1994

107. World Health Organization: Comparative trial of insufflation, hysterosalpingogram and laparoscopy with dye hydrotubation for assessment of tubal patency. Fertil Steril 46:1101, 1986

108. Thurmond AS, Novy M, Uchida BT, Rosch J: Fallopian tube obstruction: selective salpingography and recanalization. Radiology 163:511, 1987

109. Confino E, Tur-Kaspa I, DeCherney A et al: Transcervical balloon tuboplasty: a multicenter study. JAMA 264:2079, 1990

110. American Association of Gynecologic Laparoscopists: Office hysteroscopy, national statistics. 1988 AAGL membership survey. J Reprod Med 35:584, 1990

111. Renck H: Prevention of dextran-induced anaphylactic reactions. Acta Chir Scand 149:355, 1983

112. McLucas B: Hyskon complications in hysteroscopic surgery. Obstet Gynecol Surv 46:196, 1991

113. Duffy S, Reid PC, Sharp F: In-vivo studies of uterine electrosurgery. Br J Obstet Gynaec 99:579, 1992

114. Darabi K, Roy K, Richart RM: Collaborative studies on hysteroscopic sterilization procedures: final report. In Sciarra JJ, Zatuchni GI, Speidel JJ (eds): Risks, Benefits, and Controversies in Fertility Control. p. 81. Harper & Row, Hagerstown, MD, 1978

115. Serden SP, Brooks PG: Treatment of abnormal uterine bleeding with the gynecologic resectoscope. J Reprod Med 36:697, 1991

116. Siegler AM, Valle RF: Therapeutic hysteroscopic procedures. Fertil Steril 50:685, 1988

117. Kaunitz AM: Endometrial sampling in menopausal women. The tools and techniques. Menopause Management 3:7, 1990

CHAPTER FOURTEEN

CERVICAL CONIZATION

MITCHEL S. HOFFMAN

BACKGROUND AND ALTERNATIVE PROCEDURES

The Papanicolaou (Pap) smear was introduced in 1941 and screening for precancerous cervical lesions gradually came into widespread use.[1] Initially, the general management of an abnormal smear without an obvious lesion on the cervix was to paint the cervix with Lugol's iodine and take random biopsies of nonstaining areas. Alternately, the physician could go straight to cone biopsy, an operation that had previously been used for miscellaneous conditions of the cervix and was used to treat cervical cancer in 1815 by Lisfranc.[2] This management plan led to a large number of operative procedures, often for minimally abnormal Pap smears, but prevented invasive cancer from being missed.

Colposcopy

Colposcopy was first described by Hinselman in 1925, but did not come into widespread use in North America until the 1970s.[3] Colposcopy is coordinated with office or outpatient treatment of cervical cancer precursor lesions by local surface ablation. This is based on the premise that with colposcopy, the entire area of concern, the squamocolumnar transition zone—at least in younger patients—could be directly visualized and biopsied and, in experienced hands, invasive cancer could confidently be ruled out. The anticipation was that cervical conization could be replaced in most cases with the less costly and less complicated outpatient methods of treatment. The importance of colposcopic expertise in this scheme has been emphasized and numerous colposcopy educational programs are continually offered, as well as incorporated into residency training programs. The major risks of this procedure, incorrect or inadequate evaluation, are entirely dependent on the skill and expertise of the colposcopist. Failure to diagnose an invasive lesion can lead to inappropriate delay in treatment and patient morbidity, even death; while overtreatment of minimal abnormalities can also lead to patient morbidity, and excessive cost and anxiety. Extensive literature has accumulated to attest both to the accuracy of colposcopy with directed biopsy and to the efficacy of outpatient locally destructive methods of treatment.[4-14] Conization can be avoided and replaced by office management in perhaps as many as 90 percent of women with an abnormal Pap smear.

As a method of potentially eliciting the help of an expert consultant in managing patients with abnormal Pap smears, cervicography has been studied. Cervicography, originally described by Adolf Stafl in 1981, is basically the expert review of a picture taken through the colposcope. These photos must be performed uniformly, with defined camera settings. Most well-trained gynecologists believe themselves to be capable of managing these patients without consultation.

Cryosurgery

Cryosurgery, utilizing nitrous oxide as a refrigerant, can be used without anesthesia in an office setting. A double freeze technique: 3-minute freeze, thaw 3-minute freeze, with the freeze timed from the appearance of the ice ball, yields a 90 percent cure rate, for all grades of cervical intraepithelial neoplasia (CIN). The thawing causes cell disruption. Alternatively, a single 5-minute freeze may be used. Most experience is with CIN I and II, but this is largely a bias reflecting the physician's fear of treating CIN III lesions with a methodology that does not yield a histologic specimen to confirm that malignancy is absent. Many patients will experience vague lower abdominal discomfort during freezing, but this is usually not severe if treatment is done 1 week from menses. Rarely, vasovagal episodes occur, but these are easily reversed with atropine. Most patients will experience a watery discharge for 2 to 4 weeks after treatment. This relatively inexpensive and simple technique uses probe temperatures near $-60°C$. Drawbacks to cryosurgery include the lack of specimen for histologic analysis; inability to control the depth and extent of freeze beyond selecting a probe tip most likely to fit the lesion; and that the squamocolumnar junction usually resides in the endocervical canal after healing, making subsequent surveillance more difficult. Patients with large three- or four-quadrant lesions, lesions involving the endocervical canal, or with misshapen cervices are poor candidates for cryosurgery.

Triage

Despite the immense success of this triage and outpatient treatment system, several well-defined indications for cervical conization remain. These are discussed in the next section. In addition, occasional reports continue to appear describing small numbers of patients with invasive cancer following apparent failure of this triage system.[15-19] A number of factors have been cited as important in potentially reducing this problem (i.e., adequate endocervical curettage, colposcopic expertise, and so forth). More recently, the pendulum has swung back to some extent, with many individuals advocating wider application of tissue excision (over de-

structive) methods, both for treatment and histologic confirmation of intraepithelial lesions.[20-29] The clear implication (probably correct) is that conization would be much less likely to miss a diagnosis of occult invasive cancer. This has coincided with the development of simpler and less morbid methods of excision. Undoubtedly, differences will continue to exist as to when office ablation is preferable to conization, influenced by the escalating concerns over health care costs, and these procedures will find an established place in the armamentarium for management for cervical precancers, perhaps as defined ''clinical pathways.''

INDICATIONS

Cone biopsy is generally performed to excise the entire transformation zone, thus enabling the pathologist to study an intraepithelial or superficially invasive lesion in its entirety. This is based on the dogma that squamous lesions arise at the transformation zone. Certainly, conization does not always remove the entire transformation zone, and is less likely to do so in certain situations (e.g., pregnancy, large transformation zone, transformation zone high in the endocervical canal, extension onto the vaginal fornices). Broadly, cone biopsy may be categorized as diagnostic or therapeutic, although in many cases the procedure serves both purposes. It is most important to perform a diagnostic conization when, after outpatient evaluation, concern remains that invasive cervical cancer has not been completely ruled out. A diagnostic cone biopsy is also performed to evaluate the exact nature and extent of an apparently microinvasive carcinoma, diagnosed on biopsy, or when there is a two-level discrepancy between cytologic and biopsy results. Diagnostic conization may also be performed when it appears that significant disease is present in the endocervical canal beyond adequate visualization. If there is cytologic evidence of an occult high-grade intraepithelial lesion that is not identified on outpatient evaluation, including colposcopy of the vagina, vulva, anus, and urethra, then diagnostic cervical conization should be done.

A conization may also be considered therapeutic when it has been performed for diagnosis and has cleared (margins are negative) an intraepithelial lesion. The gynecologist may then be confident that the intraepithelial neoplasia has been removed, thereby virtually eliminating the likelihood of progression to invasive cancer. When margins are positive, close follow-up shows that most patients have no further problem. Only a few will require repeat colposcopic evaluation and re-treatment. When dealing with adenocarcinoma in situ of the endocervix or endocervical glandular dysplasia, however, determining adequate deep margins may be very problematic. A cone biopsy is also thought to be therapeutic for certain highly selected cases of microinvasive squamous cell carcinoma of the cervix, when uterine preservation is desired. When an adequately visualized high-grade lesion extends into the endocervical canal beyond the point where it can be confidently ablated, then a cone biopsy is performed for treatment. More controversial uses of therapeutic conization include high-grade intraepithelial neoplasia, previous failure of ablative treatment, high-grade intraepithelial neoplasia in the noncompliant patient, and large four-quadrant lesions.

In the following sections, indications for cone biopsy are discussed individually.

Microinvasion

When microinvasion is suspected after colposcopy with directed biopsy (and/or, in some cases, endocervical curettage [ECC]), then cone biopsy is necessary to study the entire lesion. Depending on the extent of invasion identified in the cone, the recommended treatment may vary widely from observation only to radical surgery or radiotherapy. The conization ensures that more deeply invasive areas were not missed, and allows vascular-lymphatic space involvement and confluency to be assessed—factors that may influence treatment decisions.

A few studies that included highly selected patients with microinvasive cervical cancer have documented good therapeutic results with cone biopsy only.[30-34] This is mainly applicable to the young patient with microinvasive cancer who is desirous of further childbearing, who is anticipated to comply with long-term close follow-up. The margins of the cone should be clear of the lesion and the microscopy should be reviewed by an experienced gynecologic pathologist and a gynecologic oncologist.

Unsatisfactory Colposcopy

In a small percentage of patients with CIN, the entire extent of the identified lesion or the transformation zone cannot be visualized colposcopically. This is more commonly the case in postmenopausal women, patients with high-grade lesions, and after certain types of prior treatment such as cryotherapy. Classically, a cone biopsy has been recommended in such instances, mainly to ensure adequate treatment of the disease extending into the endocervical canal, but to a lesser extent, to exclude occult invasion above the area of visualization. This recommendation certainly seems appropriate for higher grades of dysplasia (CIN II and III). However, cone biopsy is probably inappropriate when all evidence (colposcopy, biopsies, cytology, ECC) point to a low-grade lesion (CIN I, human papillomavirus). Such lesions may be safely followed with a high (60 percent) expectation of spontaneous regression.[35-39] In the meantime, lesser treatments may be tried at the discretion of the physician, such as trichloracetic acid.[40,41] Follow-up with cytology and possibly colposcopy on an every 6-month basis is warranted. If the lesion persists over 1 to 2 years or if there is any evidence of progression of the neoplastic process, then a repeat evaluation and probable extirpation of the lesion will be necessary.

Positive Endocervical Curettage

The role of ECC in the triage of patients with CIN is controversial.[42-54] Problems with ECC include high false-positive and false-negative rates, a large percentage of insufficient samples, interference with histologic interpretation of a subsequent cone biopsy, and the discomfort and expense associated with the procedure. A negative ECC may be defined by normal endocervical glands and stroma, a positive curettage as CIN in continuity with endocervical tissue, an equivocal curettage as isolated strips of dysplastic epithelium on the same slide as fragments of normal endocervical tissue, and an inadequate curettage as blood, mucus, and isolated cells. Endocervical curettage is done following completion of colposcopy and directed biopsies, but before hemostatic agents are applied. A standard Kevorkian curette is used, and traction on the cervix with a tenaculum may be necessary in some cases. An attempt is made to scrape the entire length and circumference of the endocervical canal, with care taken to avoid the area of the external os (doing the ECC under colposcopic guidance is helpful). The loose material freed by the curettage is collected with the aid of gently applied ring forceps.

The patient with an unsatisfactory colposcopy and a low-grade lesion on biopsy who is found to have high-grade CIN on cytology or ECC should certainly undergo cone biopsy. When the colposcopic examination is satisfactory, evaluation of the endocervical canal is aimed at uncovering a "skip" area of squamous abnormality or an endocervical glandular intraepithelial abnormality. These entities appear to be uncommon, however, and false-positive results may lead to unnecessary conization. The concern on the other hand has been that omission of the ECC may lead to inadequate treatment of dysplasia or a missed diagnosis of invasive cancer. Medicolegal considerations may be an issue here. The gynecologist who is less confident with colposcopy should probably perform an ECC as part of the evaluation of *all* patients with a significantly abnormal Pap smear (CIN II, III, or worse).

When attempting to triage the patient with a positive ECC, the gynecologist can guard against over-action by careful evaluation of the results.[55,56] It is appropriate to be less concerned over results suggesting a low-grade lesion (human papillomavirus, CIN I). Depending on the individual situation, ablative therapy may still be appropriate or the patient may be re-evaluated in 2 to 3 months with a carefully performed repeat ECC under colposcopic guidance. Conization on the sole basis of such a result is probably overzealous. An ECC that consists of strips of normal endocervical epithelium and a few fragments of dysplastic epithelium is more than likely a false-positive result as opposed to an ECC yielding strips of severely dysplastic epithelium. When the patient has a satisfactory colposcopy but the lesion does extend a short distant up the endocervical canal, the issue of a false-positive ECC is not as important, as treatment will be based on colposcopic findings and patient considerations.

A patient with an ECC demonstrating unequivocal fragmentsof invasive cancer is staged and treated appropriately. If there is any doubt about invasion or possible microinvasion then a cone biopsy should be performed. The skill, experience, and judgement of the colposcopist is the ultimate safeguard against excessive or inadequate treatment. A skilled colposcopist will know when an ECC is contaminated by ectocervical tissue, or endocervical disease is present but adequately visualized, and will differentiate this from a positive ECC that necessitates diagnostic conization.

Discrepant Cytology

When the Pap smear suggests high-grade CIN or invasive cancer and no significant abnormality has been discovered on colposcopy, biopsy, or ECC, the physician must consider the possibility of a more significant occult lesion up in the endocervical canal or deep within endocervical crypts.[57] Before resorting to cone biopsy, however, a couple of possibilities should be considered. Overreading of the Pap smear is not uncommon and, especially in postmenopausal women, it is a good idea to have the smear reviewed by an experienced cytopathologist. Additional colposcopic assessment of the vagina may disclose a vaginal neoplasm as the rare cause of such a Pap smear discrepancy. Rarely, urethral, vulvar, and anal lesions may exfoliate cells into the vagina and be detected on a Pap smear. If the Pap smear is suggestive of a significant spiglandular abnormality, then an office endometrial biopsy and careful pelvic examination should be performed in addition. This may require an examination under anesthesia and fractional dilation and curettage, which may be performed concomitantly with cone biopsy.

Cervical Intraepithelial Neoplasia III

Cone biopsy performed for CIN III as the only indication is controversial.[56,58–62] Cone biopsy has been advocated because of concern over higher failure rates for ablative methods and the increased likelihood and difficulty in discovery of an occult invasive cancer. These issues seem to be even more relevant in the presence of a large lesion. Methods recommended to overcome such difficulties include careful assessment by an experienced colposcopist, multiple directed biopsies to insure adequate sampling of the lesion, routine performance of an ECC, and use of laser vaporization in place of cryotherapy (for larger lesions out of reach of the cryotherapy probe). Several recent studies have, in fact, reported excellent results with ablative treatment of CIN III lesions. If the physician is not sufficiently confident in the colposcopic assessment of a CIN III lesion, and consultation is not readily available, then cone biopsy would seem reasonable. The use of the LLETZ (large loop excision of the transformation zone) procedure in such situations is a reasonable option. Otherwise, conization is generally not necessary in such patients.

Adenocarcinoma In Situ

When a cervical biopsy or ECC suggests adenocarcinoma in situ of the cervix, a cone biopsy must be performed to be certain the process is not invasive. There is a lack of specific colposcopic findings with glandular dysplasia and early invasive adenocarcinoma. Literature regarding the management of this entity is scarce.[63–69] When cone margins are clear and the patient desires further childbearing, informed consent with close observation, including periodic evaluation of the endocervical canal, is in order. However, the standard treatment is considered by many to be hysterectomy.

Endometrial Versus Cervical Cancer

After careful evaluation (including fractional curettage) has demonstrated adenocarcinoma, but with uncertainty remaining as to endometrial or cervical origin, cone biopsy followed by repeat endometrial curettage will usually clarify the situation. At other times, the diagnosis of endometrial cancer is clear but a question remains as to whether or to what extent the malignancy has extended to the cervix. Again, cone biopsy will clarify the situation. Whether preoperative knowledge of occult cervical involvement should alter management remains open to debate. There may be situations where proceeding to hysterectomy is appropriate.

Alternatively, the cone biopsy may be sent for frozen section if definitive surgical treatment is planned under the same anesthesia. Common sense and common courtesy would recommend that the pathologist be notified well in advance of the planned procedure; the pathologic interpretation may potentially alter planned treatment.

OPERATIVE TECHNIQUES

As stated above, cone biopsy is generally aimed at removal of the entire transformation zone. In many cases, however, the surgeon cannot be certain of the transformation zone boundary in the endocervix. The size and configuration of the cone is therefore left up to the surgeon's clinical judgment. Careful preoperative colposcopy and, in the hands of a few individuals, microcolpohysteroscopy, may help clarify the size of the cone needed. Microcolpohysteroscopy utilizes a contact hysteroscope with × 20 to 60 magnification and Waterman's blue ink. The technique requires special training and equipment, and has not come into widespread use. Several reports do indicate its potential for more thorough evaluation of the endocervical canal, better tailoring of cone biopsies, and avoidance of incomplete excision.[70,71]

The surgeon does not want to perform too small an excision with resultant inadequate removal of the lesion. By contrast, a larger cone biopsy is more likely to result in immediate and delayed complications.[72,73] The size and shape of the cone biopsy should be tailored to the individual situation.

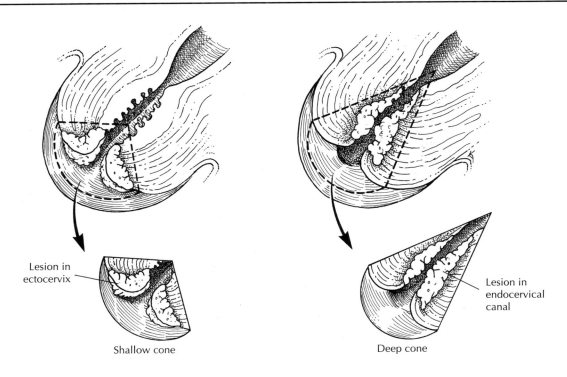

Lesion in
ectocervix

Shallow cone

Lesion in
endocervical
canal

Deep cone

Fig. 14-1. Tailoring the cone biopsy.

If the transformation zone and area of concern are in the endocervical canal and the exocervix appears normal, the cone biopsy may be made narrower to preserve the normal ectocervical tissue, but should extend well upward along the endocervical canal (Fig. 14-1). By contrast, when a lesion and transformation zone are largely confined to the ectocervix and the endocervical canal appears to be free of disease, the cone is taken wide enough to clear the transformation zone, but need excise only a minimal portion of the endocervical canal (Fig. 14-1). Many cases are not as clear-cut, but with careful preoperative colposcopy and good surgical judgement, the cone biopsy can be tailored to suit each individual patient. Colposcopy in the operating room just before cone biopsy is not always practical but may be helpful in many situations. Extending colposcopy to include evaluation of the upper vagina is worthwhile, especially in the presence of large, high grade ectocervical lesions.

Currently, three instruments for performing a cone biopsy are commonly used: a scalpel ("cold knife"), laser, or electrosurgical loop. Cone biopsy done with a scalpel is considered to be the gold standard. However, a number of reported and proposed advantages and disadvantages exist for each of these procedures. In the following sections, the techniques of each of the three methods are described, followed by a discussion of their relative merits.

Cold Knife Cone

In contradiction to the "hot knife" (cautery), the cold knife cone is done with a scalpel. In all reports to date, this procedure has been done in an operating room setting, almost always under general or regional anesthesia. The patient is positioned in the dorsal lithotomy position and the bladder is drained. A digital examination is not done, to avoid difficulty with histologic interpretation of the specimen. Likewise, only the outer vagina is prepared, to avoid trauma to the cervix. A weighted speculum of appropriate length and narrow deavers are placed to visualize the cervix. Colposcopic examination may be performed at this time, and a final decision is made as to the size and configuration of the cone. Some surgeons use Lugol's iodine solution to help demarcate the outer limits of the transformation zone. The anterior lip of the cervix is grasped with a single tooth tenaculum well outside the transformation zone, so as not to interfere with the excision. If room allows, a tenaculum placed likewise on the posterior cervical lip is also helpful. Many surgeons recommend the placement of absorbable sutures at the 3 and 9 o'clock positions just below the cervicovaginal junction to include a generous amount of cervical stroma (sutures placed too deeply may be cut during excision) (Fig. 14-2A). The intended purpose of the sutures is to ligate the cervical branches of the uterine arteries and therefore reduce blood loss resulting from the cone biopsy. The clinical effectiveness of these sutures does not appear to be substantial and is inconsistent at best.[74,75] These sutures may also be useful, however, for manipulation of the cervix and for securing hemostatic material in the cone bed. Providing there is no contraindication, a vasospastic solution may be injected into the cervix at this time. Some surgeons avoid this step, citing concerns over delayed bleeding and an increased infection rate. The evidence for this is not convincing and it

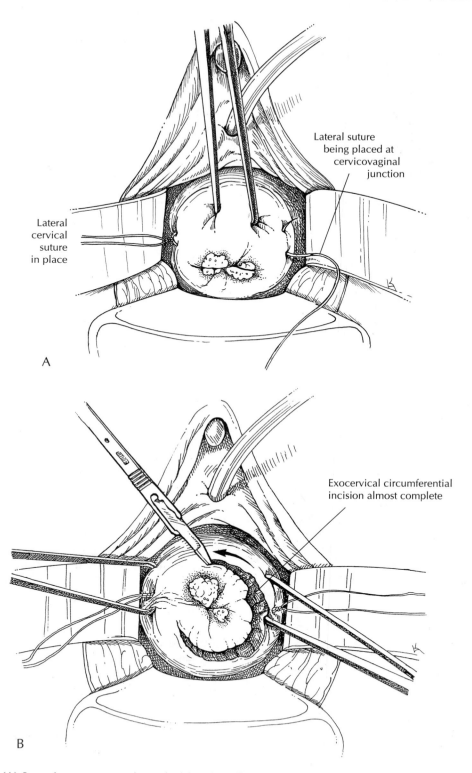

Fig. 14-2. (A) Lateral sutures at cervicovaginal junction. **(B)** Start of cone biopsy with exocervical circumferential incision. *(Figure continues.)*

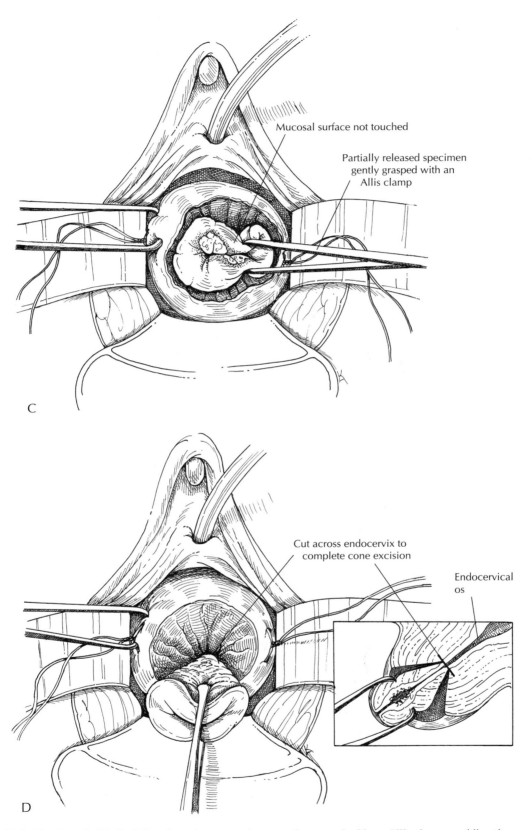

Fig. 14-2 *(Continued).* **(C)** Partially released cone specimen gently grasped with an Allis clamp, avoiding the mucosal surfaces. **(D)** Completion of cone excision by cutting across endocervix.

has not been a problem at the author's institution. Use of the solution reduces intraoperative blood loss and thereby improves operative exposure, allowing the surgeon to do a more controlled and accurate cone biopsy. It is this author's preference to inject 20 to 30 ml of pitressin (0.5 U/ml) or 1:200,000 epinephrine solution with a 1.5-in 21 gauge needle circumferentially deep into the dense cervical stroma, just lateral to the imagined line of resection. With a long-handled scalpel and a #11 blade, a circumferential incision is made just lateral to the outer limit of the transformation zone (Fig. 14-2B). Starting posteriorly, the scalpel blade is inserted to the desired depth and direction (in general, slightly toward the endocervical canal). Using a very slight sawing motion (more like pushing) in an attempt to keep the scalpel at the same depth and angle, the desired circular incision is completed. When the intention is to remove a significant portion of the endocervical canal, a uterine sound may help guide the path of the incision, with care taken not to traumatize the endocervical canal. With an Allis clamp, the partially released specimen is gently grasped, being careful to avoid the mucosal surfaces (Fig. 14-2C). The Allis clamp is only used for gentle traction and manipulation. Mayo scissors are used to complete and deepen the incision as necessary. The specimen is then removed by cutting across the remaining

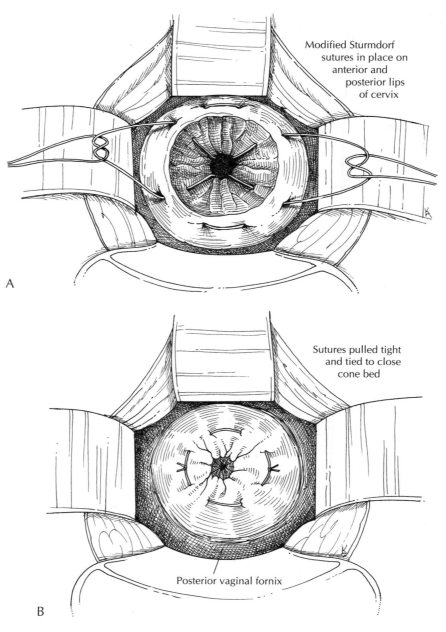

Modified Sturmdorf sutures in place on anterior and posterior lips of cervix

A

Sutures pulled tight and tied to close cone bed

Posterior vaginal fornix

B

Fig. 14-3. **(A & B)** Modified Sturmdorf sutures.

base with Jorghenson scissors (Fig. 14-2D). The remaining endocervical canal is then curetted, and if indicated, dilation and endometrial curettage is also performed at this time.

Routine dilation and endometrial curettage is unnecessary, but should be performed in peri- and postmenopausal women, those with abnormal spiglandular cytology, and women who otherwise have factors placing them at risk of endometrial pathology such as abnormal bleeding.[76,77]

Optimal management of the cone bed is not well established. A variety of suture techniques have been described, and recently good results have been reported with a modification of the Sturmdorf type sutures[78] (Fig. 14-3). The author has used these sutures when there is significant bleeding from the cone bed or when a large cone biopsy has been taken. There is some concern, however, that sutures placed into the cone bed may interfere with healing, and other studies have reported a technique that leaves the cone bed open.[74,79-81] The open cone bed technique as reported on by Trimbos et al,[81] Helmkamp et al,[80] Gilbert et al,[74] and others—and that this author has used for most cases—begins by obtaining spot hemostasis with the cautery. A piece of long narrow Surgicel is then carefully packed into the cone bed. It is secured there by tying the two lateral cervical (or similar) sutures across to each other in the midline over the surgical pack (Fig. 14-4). The patient must be warned that she will pass this pack within 1 to 2 weeks. Ideally, menstrual flow does not occur while the pack is in place. Regardless of whether the cone bed is sutured or left open, the vagina is generally not packed and the patient is sent

home the same day or the next morning. The patient is instructed to avoid intercourse, place nothing in the vagina, and not take a bath or swim for 4 weeks. She is seen in the office at 6 weeks, to be sure the cervix is healing and that the endocervical canal is patent. A Pap smear and colposcopy are performed 3 to 4 months postoperatively. These instructions also apply to the other methods of cone biopsy.

Laser Cone

The laser cone is a more demanding surgical procedure and requires a certain amount of expertise, both with cone biopsy and with laser surgery of the lower genital tract. Although most laser conizations are done in the operating room under general or regional anesthesia, there are a few reports of the procedure being done in an office setting.[28,29,82-84] This requires an experienced staff and a cooperative patient who has some degree of "pelvic relaxation," and is only appropriate when a small or shallow cone is planned.

Protective eyewear is mandatory for the operating room personnel. In addition, there must be close communication between the surgeon and the person assisting in the operation of the laser machine. Wet towels are placed externally, to protect the perineum and thighs from a misdirected laser beam. Paper drapes are avoided due to the risk of fire. The outer vagina is prepared. For office procedures, sedation is beneficial. The cervix is infiltrated as previously described with a vasospastic solution. Speculums and tenaculums

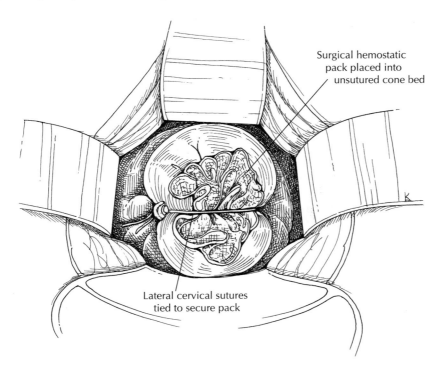

Surgical hemostatic pack placed into unsutured cone bed

Lateral cervical sutures tied to secure pack

Fig. 14-4. Surgical hemostatic pack (Surgicel) placed into unsutured cone bed, secured in place by tying across with lateral cervical sutures.

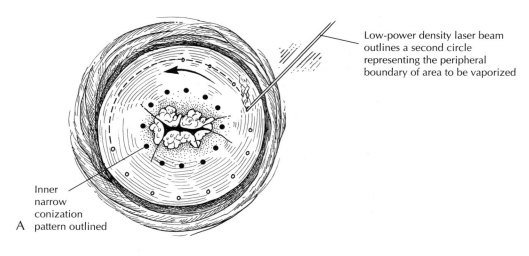

Low-power density laser beam outlines a second circle representing the peripheral boundary of area to be vaporized

Inner narrow conization
A pattern outlined

Areas planned for vaporization/conization marked out in quadrants; one quadrant vaporized at a time

B

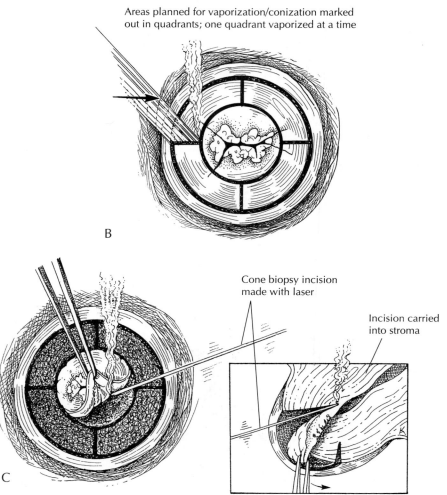

Cone biopsy incision made with laser

Incision carried into stroma

C

Fig. 14-5. (**A**) Exocervical margin of laser cone planned with a circle of dots placed with the laser. (**B**) Combined vaporization-conization. Area planned for vaporization is marked out in quadrants and one quadrant at a time is vaporized. (**C**) Cone biopsy incision being made with the laser.

should be black (these are available through several companies) to avoid reflection of the laser beam. Both weighted and Graves speculums are available with built-in hookup for suction. In the office, a Graves speculum may be used, but this author prefers a weighted speculum and deavers. Under direct vision with the colposcope, a margin around the outer limit of the transformation zone is marked. This is done by making a series of dots with the carbon dioxide laser, set on intermittent power (Fig. 14-5A). The diameter of the ectocervical portion of the cone should still be kept fairly large because of shrinkage of the specimen, which does not occur with a cold knife cone. The recommended power density used for laser conization is generally in the range of 1,000 to 1,500 watts/cm^2.

If there is extensive ectocervical disease that is clearly intraepithelial, a very large cone may be required. Alternatively, the surgeon may elect to ablate much of the ectocervical disease in concert with a smaller cervical cone biopsy.[85,86] The outer and inner margins of the planned ablation are likewise marked with the laser and divided into quadrants. Starting posteriorly, each quadrant is vaporized to a depth of 5 to 7 mm using a power density of 500 to 1,000 watts/cm^2 (Fig. 14-5B). The planned outer margin of the cone is circumferentially deepened to the extent that exposure allows. This is done with a smaller spot size (0.5 to 1 mm) and a higher power density (1,000 to 1,500 watts/cm^2). With a skin hook on the freed stromal edges of the cone specimen and simultaneous manipulation of the cervix with the tenaculum and/or lateral sutures, the laser incision is deepened along the desired depth and direction until the specimen is only attached around the endocervical canal (Fig. 14-5C). It is desirable to cut across this area with Jorghenson scissors rather than with the laser, in order to reduce thermal damage of the endocervical margin. Endocervical curettage is then performed. A "defocused" laser beam using a larger spot size (2 mm) and a lower powered density (200 watts/cm^2) is then used to obtain hemostasis at the cut endocervical margin and within the cone bed. The careful

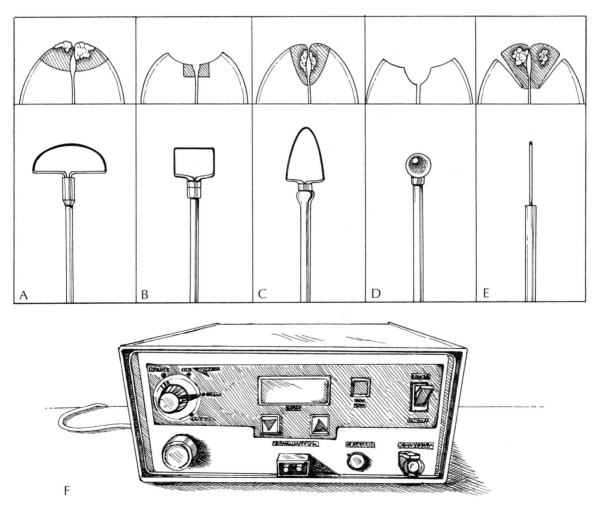

Fig. 14-6. (A–E) Loops of various sizes and **(F)** an electrosurgical generator.

application of spot cautery or the application of ferric subsulfate paste is more efficacious for this purpose, however. When bleeding is more substantial, a Surgicel pack may be tied into the cone bed as previously described.

Large Loop Excision of the Transformation Zone

The use of wire loop cautery to perform a cone biopsy dates back to 1933.[87] The technique did not come into modern use until it was modified by Cartier[88] in 1984 and then by Prendiville and Cullimore[89] in 1989. The significant modifications contributing to the currently used technique include a very thin wire, wires of larger size (often enabling excision of the entire transformation zone in one pass), and modern electrosurgical generators that allow accurate and selective blending of the current. The loops are available in a variety of sizes, allowing individualization and avoidance of excessive excision (Fig. 14-6). The loops are insulated along the shaft and crossbar to prevent injury to the patient and thermal damage to the ectocervical portion of the cone. A plastic or insulated speculum must also be used. A speculum that will connect to suction is helpful. Emphasis has been on use of the LLETZ procedure in an office setting.[20-24] As with the laser cone, however, this requires a cooperative patient and a reasonable amount of room to work.

After colposcopic assessment and selection of an appropriate loop, the cervix is thoroughly infiltrated with an anesthetic/vasoconstrictor solution. The electrosurgical generator is set at 30 to 40 watts on blend 1. A blended current mixes cutting and coagulating currents. The higher the blend, the more the coagulating current and the greater the thermal damage. Starting at one side and ending at the other, the loop is carefully passed simultaneously around and under the transformation zone, thus excising it (Fig. 14-7). The loop should be allowed to glide through the cervix, allowing the cutting current to divide the tissue. If the surgeon attempts to pull through the cervix, the loop will drag, bend, adhere to the tissue, result in a more shallow excision, and basically not perform properly. If the loop moves too slowly, however, excess thermal damage to the specimen will occur. Occasionally, it is necessary to make additional passes in order to ensure complete removal of endocervical disease. If it was determined preoperatively that disease extends well up the endocervical canal beyond the reach of the loop (i.e., 5 mm), additional tissue may be excised from this area with a smaller-diameter rectangular loop.[21,22,29,90] Additional local anesthesia should be administered to this area before proceeding. Some experts have recommended colposcopic reassessment to determine adequacy of excision.

Following completion of excision, an endocervical curettage is performed and hemostasis is obtained with a Ball electrode or regular tip cautery. It is also advisable to apply ferric subsulfate (monsel's) paste to the cone bed.

ADVANTAGES AND DISADVANTAGES OF CONIZATION METHOD

Although there are certain advantages and disadvantages of each type of conization method, it is suggested that they not be thought of as competing techniques. Rather, familiarity with all of these procedures allows the gynecologic surgeon to use the method that best suits the individual situation.

The important advantages of the cold knife cone are its technical simplicity (relatively speaking) and specimen qual-

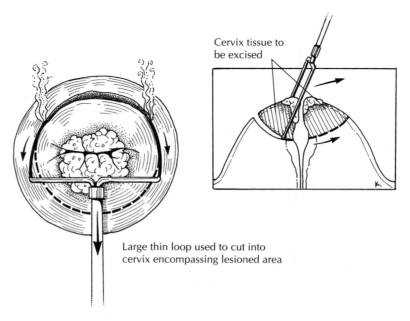

Cervix tissue to be excised

Large thin loop used to cut into cervix encompassing lesioned area

Fig. 14-7. Performing the LLETZ procedure.

ity. One disadvantage is the necessity of a general or regional anesthetic. In addition, healing and the final appearance of the cervix may not be as good, especially when sutures are used. Finally, the overall complication rate may be higher with the cold knife cone.[91–93] The main advantage with the laser cone is the simultaneous hemostasis achieved with minimal thermal damage. The specimen is therefore reasonably well preserved and interpretable and the cervix heals well. The cervix exhibits minimal distortion and follow-up colposcopy is satisfactory in most patients.[81–84,94] Cryosurgery, by contrast, usually results in the squamocolumnar juction residing in the endocervical canal. The overall complication rate of laser conization is low. In selected cases, the procedure may be carried out in an office setting. Finally, the laser allows greater flexibility in managing the ectocervical component of the disease by its ability to combine the vaporization and conization techniques.

There are several disadvantages to the laser cone, however. The procedure is technically difficult and requires a greater amount of expertise on the part of the surgeon and ancillary staff. Most hospitals and outpatient facilities require the surgeon to be credentialed in this particular type of laser surgery. To become credentialed usually requires either evidence of appropriate training during residency or taking a certifying course. Such courses include didactics and hands-on experience with tissue or animal models. Following this, a facility may require a period of supervision by an experienced peer. In addition to these factors, the laser equipment is expensive and must be maintained. Technically, it is difficult to perform a narrow, deep cone with the laser. Finally, although dependent to a large degree on technique, the laser cone specimen invariably sustains some thermal damage, which has varied among reports.[95]

The main advantage of the LLETZ procedure is that it is readily performed in an office setting. The technique is rapid and reasonably easy to master. The equipment is relatively inexpensive and its operation straightforward for the ancillary staff. Because of its ambulatory nature, lower complication rate, and the ability to produce a histologic specimen, the LLETZ procedure has been promoted by some as a method to treat patients immediately following colposcopy in one office visit.[21,23,96] The role of this approach is not well defined and pertains more to using the technique in place of ablative procedures than as a method of indicated cone biopsy. The LLETZ procedure may also have similar advantages to the laser in terms of minimizing thermal damage, better healing and colposcopic follow-up, and a lower overall complication rate. A credentialing process similar to that for the laser is common for in-facility performance of the LLETZ procedure. The main disadvantage of the LLETZ procedure is thermal damage to the specimen. As with the laser, this is dependent on technique and has varied among reports.[97–101] For larger ectocervical lesions, removal may require more than one pass with the wire loop, which further interferes with histologic interpretation. A "deep" cone biopsy for disease extending well up the endocervical canal

may be difficult to perform in an office setting, and double-excision techniques to accomplish this may also cause difficulty with histology. There is concern that the ease of the LLETZ procedure will lead to its overuse.[102,103]

COMPLICATIONS

Significant intraoperative complications are uncommon with cone biopsy. Bleeding rarely becomes severe, but when conservative measures (e.g., sutures, cautery, ferric subsulfate paste) fail, the surgeon may resort to a cerclage-type stitch, internal iliac artery ligation, or hysterectomy. Perforation also appears to be quite uncommon, but may be more likely when the uterus is acutely anteflexed and in postmenopausal women with significant atrophy. Perforation laterally may result in laceration of the uterine artery and broad ligament hematoma.[104] Laceration of the bladder and of the rectum has also been reported.[99] The likelihood of these complications probably does not vary greatly according to conization method.

Early postoperative complications include bleeding and infection. Bleeding shortly after surgery may be due to inadequate intraoperative hemostasis or wearing off of the vasoconstrictor solution. Delayed hemorrhage may occur 1 to 2 weeks after surgery, probably related to dissolving sutures or erosion of a blood vessel during the healing process. The incidence of postoperative bleeding following cold knife conization is reported to be 5 to 15 percent.[18,74,78,91,92,98,105,106] This complication may be reduced to a moderate degree with the laser (2 to 10 percent)[26–29,83,84,91,94] or LLETZ (0 to 8 percent).[20,21,23,93,96,98,107–109] Only a few comparative studies are available and possible contributing factors such as cone size (length is often mentioned) are difficult to assess from the information available. Early or delayed hemorrhage will often resolve with conservative measures in the office, such as application of silver nitrate or ferric subsulfate, suturing, or packing. Occasionally, however, a patient will need to be taken back to the operating room.

Infection occasionally occurs following cone biopsy. The reported incidence following cold knife conization is 0.2 to 6.8 percent.[58,78,91–93,105] The infection may manifest in a variety of ways, including local cervical inflammation, endometriosis, parametritis, salpingitis, and even pelvic abscess. The value of prophylactic antibiotics before cone biopsy is not known, but has been recommended by some experts. They should certainly be used in selected high-risk patients (history of gonorrhea, pelvic inflammatory disease, and so on). Infection following laser conization or the LLETZ procedure may be slightly less (0 to 2 percent).[20,21,23,28,29,82,84,86,94,98]

Late complications of cone biopsy include cervical stenosis, pregnancy complications, and infertility. Cervical stenosis is a well-known and identifiable complication of cone biopsy. By their nature, the relation of pregnancy complications and infertility to cone biopsy are less well defined.

Most studies including this complication report a low incidence of cervical stenosis (approximately 1 percent) regardless of conization method.[21,23,24,28,78,84,91,92] The condition is usually not defined, and some reports have described associated problems such as dysmenorrhea. One comparative study did show a significantly higher rate of stenosis for cold knife versus laser conization.[91] Another study reported less stenosis with open versus sutured cold knife cone techniques.[74] In order to reduce this complication, some authors have recommended periodic sounding of the cervical canal during the first few follow-up visits after cone biopsy. In practice, this is necessary only in a small percentage of patients on a selected basis.

Cervical mucous is important to the initial assent of sperm in the reproductive tract. A compromise in the cervical mucous or perhaps severe cervical stenosis may lead to infertility. However, the effect of cervical conization on fertility, if any, does not appear to be substantial.[110–113] Pregnancy complications that have been related to prior cervical conization include incompetent cervix, abortion, and premature delivery, and cervical dystocia and lacerations with labor and delivery. From the information available, there is no major increase in the incidence of any of these problems.[110,114,115] One recent study did report a smaller birth weight incidence following the LLETZ procedure, which is of concern considering the liberal attitude by some toward the use of this technique.[116] The likelihood of pregnancy complications is probably greater following larger or repeat conizations.[117,118] The role of prophylactic cerclage in these patients is unclear, but may be reasonable on a highly individualized basis.

DISPOSITION AFTER CONE BIOPSY

When the final pathologic interpretation of the cone biopsy is CIN with clear margins, a cure rate of about 95 percent can be expected.[119,120] Considering the epidemiology of cervical dysplasia and the potential role the increased prevalence of human papillomavirus may have on recurrence rates, long-term follow-up of these patients is warranted. Gynecologists must be alert to the increased incidence of vaginal and vulvar neoplasia in these patients. Follow-up consists of a Pap smear and pelvic examination every 4 months for the first 2 years, and then every 6 months thereafter. After 5 years, an annual examination is reasonable.

If dysplasia extends to the margin of the cone, the risk of persistence or recurrence is greater.[121–128] This is particularly true when CIN III extends to the endocervical margin. The risk may be further increased in postmenopausal women and when the ECC above the cone is positive. When childbearing is complete, and especially in postmenopausal women, hysterectomy is a reasonable consideration. Because most patients with positive endocervical margins will not have residual disease in a hysterectomy specimen and

the operation is becoming more controversial for CIN III, the decision to perform hysterectomy in these patients should be made on a carefully selected basis. Otherwise, close follow-up is warranted consisting of a Pap smear with attention to endocervical cytology, and a pelvic examination every 3 months for the first 2 years. Patients with persistent cervical neoplasia will generally manifest further abnormal cytology, which then prompts reinvestigation. However, the vast majority of patients with positive conization margins will remain free of disease.

Management of the patient whose cone demonstrates microinvasive squamous cell carcinoma or AIS is discussed above. If hysterectomy is not carried out, then these patients should be followed particularly closely. A Pap smear with attention to endocervical cytology and a pelvic examination every 3 months for the first 2 years is appropriate.

When hysterectomy is planned following a cone biopsy, it is probably best to proceed immediately (after a frozen section report) or wait at least 6 to 8 weeks for the inflammatory reaction in the surrounding postoperative tissues to subside.[129–136] At institutions experienced with the technique, cervical conization with frozen sections before planned hysterectomy is safe and highly accurate.[129–133] A window of 1 to 2 days following cone biopsy may be present before a significant inflammatory response has set in. This gives the pathologist time to make a final determination on the cone biopsy while still allowing the gynecologist to safely proceed with hysterectomy in a timely manner. If a radical hysterectomy is indicated following cone biopsy, the 6- to 8-week wait is not necessary or advisable, depending on the extent of disease.[137]

CONE BIOPSY IN PREGNANT WOMEN

Conization during pregnancy is associated with greater blood loss, hemorrhagic complications, and an increased risk of pregnancy loss.[138–146] To avoid injury to the pregnancy as well as increased hemorrhage, the cone is kept relatively shallow. For this reason, conization during pregnancy frequently has a specimen with a positive margin, and residual disease is left behind.[139,140,146] This limited excision may not address areas of concern higher in the endocervix of some patients. Due to all the above considerations, it is recommended that cone biopsy during pregnancy be done only when there is a strong suspicion of invasive cancer. Some investigators have recommended limiting the excision to wedge-removal of the area of concern.[13] In the latter half of pregnancy further conservatism may be warranted, by waiting until fetal maturity before proceeding. Consultation with a gynecologic oncologist may be helpful.

When performing a cone biopsy during pregnancy, a prophylactic cerclage procedure may be considered.[146,147] This may reduce pregnancy wastage and have the added benefit of aiding in hemostasis. The cerclage is placed before the conization, and tied immediately afterward. Suture of the cone bed with the modified Sturmdorf or running interlocking technique is also warranted. ECC above the cone is not performed.

REFERENCES

1. Papanicolaou GN, Traut HF: The diagnostic value of vaginal smears in carcinoma of the uterus. Am J Obstet Gynecol 42: 193, 1941

2. Lisfranc MJ: Memoire sur l'amputation du col de l'uterus. Gaza Med de Par ii:385, 1834

3. Richart RM: The patient with an abnormal Pap smear: screening techniques and management. N Engl J Med 302:332, 1980

4. Javaheri G, Balin M, Meltzer RM: Role of cryosurgery in the treatment of intraepithelial neoplasia of the uterine cervix. Obstet Gynecol 58:83, 1981

5. Stanhope CR, Phibbs GD, Stuart GCE, Reid R: Carbon dioxide laser surgery. Obstet Gynecol 61:624, 1983

6. Creasman WT, Hinshaw WM, Clarke-Pearson DL: Cryosurgery in the management of cervical intraepithelial neoplasia. Obstet Gynecol 63:145, 1984

7. Wetchler SJ: Treatment of cervical intraepithelial neoplasia with the CO_2 laser: laser versus cryotherapy. A review of effectiveness and cost. Obstet Gynecol Surg 39:469, 1984

8. Arof HM, Gerbie MV, Smeltzer J: Cryosurgical treatment of cervical intraepithelial neoplasia: four-year experience. Am J Obstet Gynecol 150:865, 1984

9. Ferenczy A: Comparison of cryo- and carbon dioxide laser therapy for cervical intraepithelial neoplasia. Obstet Gynecol 66:793, 1985

10. Bryson SCP, Lenehan P, Lickrish GM: The treatment of grade 3 cervical intraepithelial neoplasia with cryotherapy: an 11-year experience. Am J Obstet Gynecol 151:201, 1985

11. Higgins RV, van Nagell JR Jr, Donaldson ES et al: The efficacy of laser therapy in the treatment of cervical intraepithelial neoplasia. Gynecol Oncol 36:79, 1990

12. Oraeby J, Garsane M, Bruun M, Hansen K: Ten years after cryosurgical treatment of cervical intraepithelial neoplasia. Am J Obstet Gynecol 165:43, 1991

13. Anderson ES, Husth M: Cryosurgery for cervical intraepithelial neoplasia: 10 year follow-up. Gynecol Oncol 45:240, 1992

14. Benedet JL, Miller DM, Nickerson KG: Results of conservative management of cervical intraepithelial neoplasia. Obstet Gynecol 79:105, 1992

15. Cullimore JE, Rollason TP, Luesley DM et al: Invasive cervical cancer after laser vaporization for cervical intraepithelial neoplasia: a 10-year experience. J Gynecol Surg 6:103, 1990

16. Paraskevaidis E, Jandial L, Mann EMF et al: Pattern of treatment failure following laser for cervical intraepithelial neoplasia: implications for follow-up protocol. Obstet Gynecol 78:80, 1991

17. Schmidt C, Pretorius RG, Bonin M et al: Invasive cervical cancer following cryotherapy for cervical intraepithelial neoplasia or human papillomavirus infection. Obstet Gynecol 80: 797, 1992

18. Koonings PP, d'Ablaing G, Schlaerth JB, Curtin JP: A clinical-pathology review of cervical intraepithelial neoplasia following cryotherapy failure. Gynecol Oncol 44:213, 1992

19. Anderson MC: Invasive carcinoma of the cervix following local destructive treatment for cervical intraepithelial neoplasia. Br J Obstet Gynaecol 100:657, 1993

20. Mor-Yosef S, Lopes A, Pearson S, Monaghan JM: Loop diathermy cone biopsy. Obstet Gynecol 75:884, 1990

21. Keijser KGG, Kenemans P, van der Zanden PHTH et al: Diathermy loop excision in the management of cervical intraepithelial neoplasia: diagnosis and treatment in one procedure. Am J Obstet Gynecol 166:1281, 1992

22. Murdoch JB, Grimshaw RN, Morgan PR, Monaghan JM: The impact of loop diathermy on management of early invasive cervical cancer. Int J Gynecol Cancer 2:129, 1992

23. Wright TC Jr, Gagnon S, Richart RM, Ferenczy A: Treatment of cervical intraepithelial neoplasia using the loop electrosurgical excision procedure. Obstet Gynecol 79:173, 1992

24. Hallam NF, West J, Harper C et al: Large loop excision of the transformation zone (LLETZ) as an alternative to both local ablative and cone biopsy treatment: a series of 1000 patients. J Gynecol Surg 9:77, 1993

25. Burger MPM, Hollema H: The reliability of the histologic diagnosis in colposcopically directed biopsies. A plea for LLETZ. Int J Gynecol Cancer 3:385, 1993

26. Baggish MS: A comparison between laser excisional conization and laser vaporization for the treatment of cervical intraepithelial neoplasia. Am J Obstet Gynecol 155:39, 1986

27. McIndoe CAJ, Robson MS, Tidy JA et al: Laser excision rather than vaporization: the treatment of choice for cervical intraepithelial neoplasia. Obstet Gynecol 74:165, 1989

28. Partington CK, Turner MJ, Soutter WP et al: Laser vaporization versus laser excision conization in the treatment of cervical intraepithelial neoplasia. Obstet Gynecol 73:775, 1989

29. Vergote IB, Makar AP, Kjorstad KE: Laser excision of the transformation zone as treatment of cervical intraepithelial neoplasia with satisfactory colposcopy. Gynecol Oncol 44: 235, 1992

30. Creasman WT, Fetter BF, Clarke-Pearson DL et al: Management of stage IA carcinoma of the cervix. Am J Obstet Gynecol 153:164, 1985

31. Kolstad P: Follow-up study of 232 patients with stage IA1 and 411 patients with stage IA2 squamous cell carcinoma of the cervix (microinvasive carcinoma). Gynecol Oncol 33:265, 1989

32. Burghardt E, Giardi F, Lahousen M et al: Microinvasive carcinoma of the uterine cervix (International Federation of Gynecology and Obstetrics IA). Cancer 67:1037, 1991

33. Sevin B-U, Nadji M, Averette HE et al: Microinvasive carcinoma of the cervix. Cancer 70:2121, 1992

34. Morris M, Mitchell MF, Silva EG et al: Cervical conization

as definitive therapy for early invasive squamous carcinoma of the cervix. Gynecol Oncol 51:193, 1993

35. Nasiell K, Roger V, Nasiell M: Behavior of mild cervical dysplasia during long-term follow-up. Obstet Gynecol 67:665, 1986

36. Hall JE, Walton L: Dysplasia of the cervix: a prospective study of 206 cases. Am J Obstet Gynecol 100:662, 1968

37. Syrjánen K, Kataja V, Yliskoski M et al: Natural history of cervical human papillomavirus lesions does not substantiate the biologic relevance of the Bethesda system. Obstet Gynecol 79:675, 1992

38. Jones MH, Jenkins D, Cuzick J et al: Mild cervical dyskaryosis: safety of cytological surveillance. Lancet 339:1440, 1992

39. Cervical cytology: evaluation and management of abnormalities. ACOG technical bulletin #183, August 1993

40. Malviya VK, Deppe G, Pluszczynski R, Boike G: Trichloracetic acid in the treatment of human papillomavirus infection of the cervix without associated dysplasia. Obstet Gynecol 70:72, 1987

41. Benrubi GI, Shannon J, Glazer J, Nuss RC: Cervical human papilloma virus infection: is treatment possible? J Fla MA 75:799, 1988

42. Urcuyo R, Rome RM, Nelson JH Jr: Some observations on the value of endocervical curettage performed as an integral part of colposcopic examination of patients with abnormal cervical cytology. Am J Obstet Gynecol 128:787, 1977

43. Drescher CW, Peters WA III, Roberts JA: Contribution of endocervical curettage in evaluating abnormal cervical cytology. Obstet Gynecol 62:343, 1983

44. Granai CO, Jelen I, Louis F et al: The value of endocervical curretage as part of the standard colposcopic evaluation. J Reprod Med 30:373, 1985

45. Saltzman DH, Evans MI, Warsof SL, Friedman AJ: Endocervical curettage as a routine part of colposcopic examinations for abnormal cervical cytology. J Reprod Med 30:871, 1985

46. Moseley KR, Dinh TV, Hannigan EV et al: Necessity of endocervical curettage in colposcopy. Am J Obstet Gynecol 154:992, 1986

47. Spirtos NM, Schlaerth JB, d'Ablaing G III, Morrow CP: A critical evaluation of the endocervical curettage. Obstet Gynecol 70:729, 1987

48. Krebs H, Wheelock JB, Hurt WC: Positive endocervical curettage in patients with satisfactory and unsatisfactory colposcopy: clinical implications. Obstet Gynecol 69:601, 1987

49. Grainger DA, Roberts DK, Wells MM, Horbelt DV: The value of endocervical curettage in the management of the patient with abnormal cervical cytologic findings. Am J Obstet Gynecol 156:625, 1987

50. Soisson AP, Molina CY, Benson WL: Endocervical curettage in the evaluation of cervical disease in patients with adequate colposcopy. Obstet Gynecol 71:109, 1988

51. Husseinzadeh N, Carter V, Wesseler T: Significance of positive endocervical curettage in predicting endocervical canal involvement in patients with cervical intraepithelial neoplasia. Gynecol Oncol 35:358, 1989

52. El-Dabh A, Rogers RE, Davis TE, Sutton GP: The role of endocervical curettage in satisfactory colposcopy. Obstet Gynecol 74:159, 1989

53. Helmerhorst TJM: Clinical significance of endocervical curettage as part of colposcopic evaluation. A review. Int J Gynecol Cancer 2:256, 1992

54. Hoffman MS, Sterghos S Jr, Gordy LW et al: Evaluation of the cervical canal with the endocervical brush. Obstet Gynecol 82:57, 1993

55. Shingleton HM, Gore H, Austin JM: Outpatient evaluation of patients with atypical papanicolaou smears: contribution of endocervical curettage. Am J Obstet Gynecol 126:122, 1976

56. Killackey MA, Jones WB, Lewis JL Jr: Diagnostic conization of the cervix: review of 460 consecutive cases. Obstet Gynecol 67:766, 1986

57. McCord ML, Stovall TG, Summitt RL Jr, Ling FW: Discrepancy of cervical cytology and colposcopic biopsy: is cervical conization necessary? Obstet Gynecol 77:715, 1991

58. Holdt DG, Jacobs AJ, Scott JC Jr, Adam GM: Diagnostic significance and sequelae of cone biopsy. Am J Obstet Gynecol 143:312, 1982

59. Levine RU, Carillo EJ, Crum CP: Outpatient management of cervical intraepithelial neoplasia: a summary of 279 cases. J Reprod Med 30:351, 1985

60. Benedet JL, Anderson GH, Simpson ML, Shaw D: Colposcopy, conization, and hysterectomy practices: a current perspective. Obstet Gynecol 60:539, 1982

61. Matseoane S, Williams SB, Navarro C et al: Diagnostic value of conization of the uterine cervix in the management of cervical neoplasia: a review of 756 consecutive patients. Gynecol Oncol 47:287, 1992

62. Elkington KW: Cone biopsy in premenopausal women: why was outpatient management abandoned? South Med J 85:155, 1992

63. Qizilbash AH: In situ and microinvasive adenocarcinoma of the cervix. Am J Clin Pathol 64:155, 1975

64. Ostor AG, Pagano R, Davoren RAM et al: Adenocarcinoma in situ of the cervix. Int J Gynecol Path 3:179, 1984

65. Bertrand M, Lickrish GM, Colgan TJ: The anatomic distribution of cervical adenocarcinoma in situ: implications for treatment. Am J Obstet Gynecol 157:21, 1987

66. Hopkins MP, Roberts JA, Schmidt RW: Cervical adenocarcinoma in situ. Obstet Gynecol 71:842, 1988

67. Anderson ES, Arffmann E: Adenocarcinoma in situ of the uterine cervix: a clinico-pathologic study of 36 cases. Gynecol Oncol 35:1, 1989

68. Muntz HG, Bell DA, Lage JM et al: Adenocarcinoma in situ of the uterine cervix. Obstet Gynecol 80:935, 1992

69. Poynor EA, Barakat RR, Saigo PE et al: Management and follow-up of patients with adenocarcinoma in situ of the uterine cervix, abstracted. Proceedings of the 25th Annual Meet-

ing of Society of Gynecologic Oncologists, Orlando, FL, 1994

70. Hamou J: Microhysteroscopy: a new procedure and its original applications in gynecology. J Reprod Med 26:375, 1981

71. Saunders N, Anderson D, Sheridan E et al: Endoscopic localization of the squamocolumnar junction before cervical cone biopsy in 284 patients. Cancer 65:1312, 1990

72. Rubio CA, Thomassen P, Kock Y: Influence of the size of cone specimens on postoperative hemorrhage. Am J Obstet Gynecol 122:939, 1975

73. Luesley DM, McCrum A, Terry PB: Complications of cone biopsy related to the dimensions of the cone and the influence of prior colposcopic assessment. Br J Obstet Gynaecol 92:158, 1985

74. Gilbert L, Saunders NJS & G, Stringer R, Sharp F: Hemostasis and cold knife cone biopsy: a prospective randomized trial comparing a suture versus non-suture technique. Obstet Gynecol 74:640, 1989

75. Grundsell H, Larsson G, Bekassy Z: Use of an antifibrinolytic agent (tranexamic acid) and lateral sutures with laser conization of the cervix. Obstet Gynecol 64:573, 1984

76. Rubin SC, Battistini M: Endometrial curettage at the time of cervical conization. Obstet Gynecol 67:663, 1986

77. Pearl ML, Beretta S: Routine endometrial curettage is not indicated at the time of cervical cone biopsy. Surg Gynecol Obstet 176:251, 1993

78. Krebs H-B: Outpatient cervical conization. Obstet Gynecol 63:430, 1984

79. Krebs H-B, Helmkamp BF: Assuring successful cone biopsy. Contemp OB/GYN March 1991

80. Helmkamp BF, Krebs HB, Averette HE: Meeting the challenge of cervical cone biopsy. Contemp OB/GYN December 1983

81. Trimbos JB, Heintz APM, Van Hall EV: Reliability of cytological follow-up after conization of the cervix; a comparison of three surgical techniques. Br J Obstet Gynaecol 90:1141, 1983

82. Indman PD: Conization of the cervix with the CO_2 laser as an office procedure. J Reprod Med 30:388, 1985

83. Iverson T: Outpatient cervical conization with the CO_2 laser. J Reprod Med 30:607, 1985

84. Wagner AL Jr: Laser excisional conization in an office environment. J Gynecol Surg 6:47, 1990

85. Baggish MS, Dorsey JH: Carbon dioxide laser for combination excisional-vaporization conization. Am J Obstet Gynecol 151:23, 1985

86. Baggish MS, Dorsey JH, Adelson M: A ten-year experience treating cervical intraepithelial neoplasia with the CO_2 laser. Am J Obstet Gynecol 161:60, 1989

87. Hyams MN: Conization of the uterine cervix. Am J Obstet Gynecol 25:653, 1933

88. Cartier R: Practical Colposcopy. 2nd Ed. Laboratorie Cartier, Paris, 1984

89. Prendiville W, Cullimore NS: Large loop excision of the transformation zone (LLETZ): a new method of management for women with cervical intraepithelial neoplasia. Br J Obstet Gynaecol 96:1054, 1989

90. Baggish MS, Noel Y, Brooks M: Electrosurgical thin loop conization by selective double excision. J Gynecol Surg 7:83, 1991

91. Larsson G, Guilberg B, Grundsell H: A comparison of complications of laser and cold knife conization. Obstet Gynecol 62:213, 1983

92. Delmore J, Horbelt DV, Kallail KJ: Cervical conization: cold knife and laser excision in residency training. Obstet Gynecol 79:101, 1992

93. Oyesanya OA, Amerasinghe C, Manning EAD: A comparison between loop diathermy conization for management of cervical dysplasia associated with unsatisfactory colposcopy. Gynecol Oncol 50:84, 1993

94. Dorsey JH, Diggs ES: Microsurgical conization of the cervix by carbon dioxide laser. Obstet Gynecol 54:565, 1979

95. Helkjaer PE, Schultz H, Eriksen PS et al: Thermal artifacts and inter-gynecologist variation of laser cone biopsies of the cervix. Obstet Gynecol 82:435, 1993

96. Murdoch JB, Grimshaw RN, Monaghan JM: Loop diathermy excision of the abnormal cervical transformation zone. Int J Gynecol Cancer 1:105, 1991

97. Wright TC Jr, Richart RM, Ferenczy A, Koulos J: Comparison of specimens removed by CO_2 laser conization and the loop electrosurgical excision procedure. Obstet Gynecol 79:147, 1992

98. Ouesanya OA, Amerisinghe CN, Manning EAD: Outpatient excisional management of cervical intraepithelial neoplasia: a prospective, randomized comparison between loop diathermy excision and laser excisional conization. Am J Obstet Gynecol 168:485, 1993

99. Krebs H-B, Pastore L, Helmkamp F: Loop electrosurgical excision procedures for cervical dysplasia: experience in a community hospital. Am J Obstet Gynecol 169:289, 1993

100. Montz FJ, Holschneider CH, Thompson LDR: Large-loop excision of the transformation zone: effect on the pathologic interpretation of resection margins. Obstet Gynecol 81:976, 1993

101. Messing MJ, Otken L, King LA, Gallup DG: Large loop excision of the transformation zone (LLETZ): a pathologic evaluation. Gynecol Oncol 52:207, 1994

102. Jones HW III: Should conization by hot loop or laser replace cervical biopsy? Can J Gynecol Surg 7:195, 1991

103. Alvarez RD, Helm CW, Edwards RP et al: Prospective randomized trial of LLETZ versus laser ablation in patients with cervical intraepithelial neoplasia. Gynecol Oncol 52:175, 1994

104. Brown CF, Mashini IS, Turner WA, Gallup DG: Retroperitoneal hemotoma: an unusual complication of cold knife conization of the cervix. Obstet Gynecol 68:66, 1986

105. Clamen AD, Lee N: Factors that relate to complications of cone biopsy. Am J Obstet Gynecol 120:124, 1974

106. Nolan TE, Gallup DG: Managing hemorrhage associated with cold-knife conization. The Female Patient 15:57, 1990

107. Spitzer M, Chernys AE, Seltzer VL: The use of large-loop excision of the transformation zone in an inner-city population. Obstet Gynecol 82:731, 1993

108. Luesley D, Shafi M, Finn C, Buxton J: Haemorrhagic morbidity after diathermy loop excision: effect of multiple pretreatment variables including time of treatment in relation to menstruation. Br J Obstet Gynaecol 99:82, 1992

109. Gunasekera PC, Phipps JH, Lewis BV: Large loop excision of the transformation zone (LLETZ) compared to carbon dioxide laser in the treatment of CIN: a superior mode of treatment. Br J Obstet Gynaecol 97:995, 1990

110. Bjerre B, Eliasson G, Linell F et al: Conization as only treatment of carcinoma in situ of the uterine cervix. Am J Obstet Gynecol 125:143, 1976

111. Blunt VAW, Lang LP: A review of 307 cone biopsy examinations of the cervix. Med J Aust 54:64, 1967

112. Champion PK, Thompson NJ: Effect of conization of the cervix on subsequent pregnancy. Am J Obstet Gynecol 62:1321, 1951

113. Green GH: Pregnancy following cervical carcinoma in situ. A review of 60 cases. J Obstet Gynaecol Br Commonw 73:897, 1966

114. Burghardt E, Girardi F: Conization of the uterine cervix. p. 267. In Nichols DH (ed): Gynecologic and Obstetric Surgery. CV Mosby, St. Louis, MO, 1993

115. Kristensen GB: The outcome of pregnancy and preterm delivery after conization of the cervix. Arch Gynecol 236:127, 1985

116. Bloomfield PI, Buxton J, Dunn J, Luesley DM: Pregnancy outcome after large loop excision of the cervical transformation zone. Am J Obstet Gynecol 169:620, 1993

117. Leiman G, Harrison NA, Rubin A: Pregnancy following conization of the cervix: complications related to cone size. Am J Obstet Gynecol 136:14, 1980

118. Weber T, Obel E: Pregnancy complications following conization of the uterine cervix. Acta Obstet Gynecol Scand 58:259, 1979

119. DiSaia PJ, Creasman WT: Clinical Gynecologic Oncology. 4th Ed. Mosby–Year Book, St. Louis, MO, 1993

120. Kullander S, Sjoberg N-O: Treatment of carcinoma in situ of the cervix uteri by conization: a five-year follow-up. Acta Obstet Gynec Scand 50:153, 1971

121. Lubicz S, Ezekweche C, Allen A, Schiffer M: Significance of cone biopsy margins in the management of patients with cervical neoplasia. J Reprod Med 29:179, 1984

122. Buxton EJ, Luesley DM, Wade-Evans T, Jordan JA: Residual disease after cone biopsy: completeness of excision and follow-up cytology as predictive factors. Obstet Gynecol 70:529, 1987

123. White C, Cooper W, Williams R: Cervical intraepithelial neoplasia extending to the margins of resection in conization of the cervix. J Reprod Med 36:635, 1991

124. Lapaquette TK, Dinh TV, Hannigan EV et al: Management of patients with positive margins after cervical conization. Obstet Gynecol 82:440, 1993

125. Patterson-Brown S, Chappatte OA, Clark SK: The significance of cone biopsy resection margins. Gynecol Oncol 46:182, 1992

126. Vedel P, Jakobsen H: Five-year follow-up of patients with cervical intraepithelial neoplasia in the cone margins after conization. Eur J Obstet Gynecol Reprod Biol 50:71, 1993

127. Lopes A, Morgan P, Murdoch J et al: The case for conservative management of "incomplete excision" of CIN after laser conization. Gynecol Oncol 49:247, 1993

128. Murdoch JB, Morgan PR, Lopes A, Monaghan JM: Histological incomplete excision of CIN after large loop excision of the transformation zone (LLETZ) merits careful follow-up, not retreatment. Br J Obstet Gynaecol 99:990, 1992

129. DiMusto JC: Reliability of frozen sections in gynecologic surgery. Obstet Gynecol 35:235, 1970

130. Gupta RK: Frozen sections in cervical conization: a cytohistopathologic approach in the early diagnosis of carcinoma cervix. Obstet Gynecol 38:248, 1971

131. Torres JE, Moorman J, Shiu A, Gyer D: Colposcopically directed conization for frozen-section examination in the management of cervical intraepithelial neoplasia. J Reprod Med 28:123, 1983

132. Hannigan EV, Simpson JS, Dillard EA Jr, Dinh TV: Frozen section evaluation of cervical conization specimens. J Reprod Med 31:11, 1986

133. Hoffman MS, Collins E, Roberts WS et al: Cervical conization with frozen section before planned hysterectomy. Obstet Gynecol 82:394, 1993

134. Malinak LR, Jeffrey RA Jr, Dunn WJ: The conization-hysterectomy time interval: a clinical and pathologic study. Obstet Gynecol 23:317, 1964

135. Van Nagell JR, Roddick JW, Cooper RM, Triplett HB: Vaginal hysterectomy following conization in the treatment of carcinoma in situ of the cervix. Am J Obstet Gynecol 113:948, 1972

136. Elkins TE, Gallup DG, Slomka CV, Phelan JP: Postoperative morbidity in cases of cervical conization followed by vaginal hysterectomy South Med J 75:264, 1982

137. Webb MJ, Symmonds RE: Radical hysterectomy: influence of recent conization on morbidity and complications. Obstet Gynecol 53:290, 1979

138. Ferguson JH, Brown C: Cervical conization during pregnancy. Surg Gynecol Obstet 111:603, 1960

139. Hinde FC: Cervical biopsy in pregnancy. J Obstet Gynaecol Br Commonw 71:707, 1964

140. Rogers RS, Williams JH: The impact of the suspicious papanicolaou smear on pregnancy: a study of nationwide attitudes and maternal and perinatal complications. Am J Obstet Gynecol 98:488, 1967

141. Daskal JL, Pitkin RM: Cone biopsy during pregnancy. Obstet Gynecol 32:1, 1968

142. Horowitz A, Sabatelle R, Sell S: The risk of cone biopsy during pregnancy. J Reprod Med 3:9, 1969

143. Averette HE, Nasser N, Yankow SL, Little WA: Cervical

conization in pregnancy: analysis of 180 operations. Am J Obstet Gynecol 106:543, 1970

144. Hannigan EV, Whitehouse HH, Atkinson WD, Becker SN: Cone biopsy during pregnancy. Obstet Gynecol 60:450, 1982

145. Hacker NF, Berek JS, Lagasse LD et al: Carcinoma of the cervix associated with pregnancy. Obstet Gynecol 59:735, 1982

146. Roberts WS, Hoffman MS: Management of malignant and premalignant lesions of the female genital tract during pregnancy. p. 439. In Iffy L, Apuzzio JJ, Vintzileos AM (eds): Operative Obstetrics. 2nd Ed. McGraw-Hill, New York, 1992

147. Goldberg GL, Altaras MM, Bloch B: Cone cerclage in pregnancy. Obstet Gynecol 77:315, 1991

CHAPTER FIFTEEN

EXCISIONAL BIOPSY OF THE VULVA AND VAGINA

KEN HATCH

B iopsy of the vulva can be either incisional or excisional. An incisional biopsy is indicated when the lesion to be diagnosed is too large to remove with a simple outpatient procedure. Ideally, an incisional biopsy is small enough that no suturing is required for hemostasis. It should include the area of the lesion that has the most significant pathology. It is not necessary to perform a biopsy that includes the worst pathology and a normal edge of skin.

An excisional biopsy is indicated when the lesion is small enough to perform both diagnosis and treatment with the same excision (Fig. 15-1). In general, the size of lesion should be 1 cm or less, which can easily be performed under local anesthesia in the outpatient setting. An excisional biopsy is also indicated when the physician suspects an early invasive carcinoma. It is extremely important to establish the depth of invasion by examining the entire specimen and measuring the deepest penetration below the dermal papillae. To accomplish this, the entire lesion must be excised and adequately sampled. Often, these lesions are large enough to require a regional or even general anesthetic and several sutures to close. An excisional biopsy is also indicated when melanoma is suspected. Melanomas are staged according to the area of the thickest growth. To establish this the entire lesion must be removed, oriented properly, and suctioned appropriately.

INDICATIONS FOR VULVAR BIOPSY

Any ulceration of the vulva requires a biopsy. When the ulceration is large, an incisional biopsy will often establish the diagnosis. When the lesion is less than 1 cm in size, an excisional biopsy is appropriate if the ulcerated portion is small. The number of biopsies necessary depends on the size and location of lesions, the appearance of the lesions, and the age of the patient. Unifocal lesions in women over age 50 have a higher incidence of harboring a microinvasive carcinoma and excisional biopsy should be performed to rule out invasion. When a slight ulceration accompanies the lesion, then excision is mandatory. For women under age 50 with multifocal lesions and no ulcerations, two to three random incisional biopsies are sufficient to establish a diagnosis of vulvar intraepithelial neoplasia (VIN) (Fig. 15-2). An appropriate treatment can then be selected depending on the location of lesions, the desires of the patient, and the skill of the surgeon.

An incisional biopsy is indicated in patients that are suspected to have lichen sclerosis or epithelial hyperplasia (vulvar dystrophies) (Fig. 15-3). Such patients complain of vulvar itching and usually have typical clinical findings to suggest the diagnosis. The biopsy is indicated to rule out atypias. Those patients with atypia are at high risk of devel-

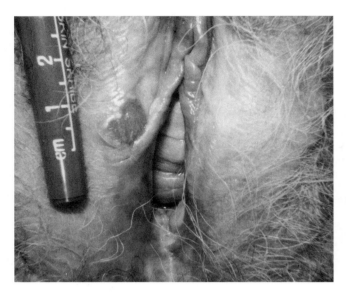

Fig. 15-1. A 58-year-old woman with a 1-cm lesion. An excisional biopsy is indicated to determine depth of suspected carcinoma.

oping invasive cancer at a later date and should be under more careful surveillance. Those without atypia can be treated in the appropriate fashion.

Incisional biopsy is also indicated in any patient in whom the vulvar condition is unclear and who has not responded to treatment. An example might be the woman who has been treated for candidiasis in an appropriate manner but has continued to have itching, erythema, and surface exudate,

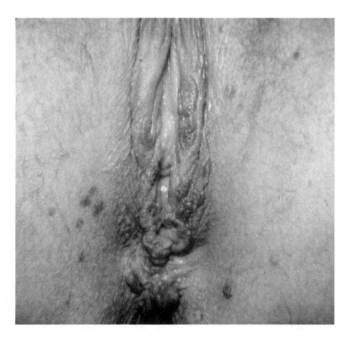

Fig. 15-2. A 28-year-old woman with multifocal pigmented vulvar intraepithelial neoplasm. Two or three incisional biopsies are sufficient to rule out invasion.

suggestive of candida. Such women may have Paget's disease. A biopsy is indicated to diagnose and direct therapy.

OPERATIVE TECHNIQUE

Incisional Biopsy

Incisional biopsies are nearly always done under local anesthesia in the outpatient setting. Those patients in whom the biopsy is to be performed on the nonhair-bearing skin can be easily biopsied with the instrument one uses for cervical biopsies. Xylocaine is injected subcuticularly so that a wheal is raised. The biopsy instrument is then used to lift off the epidermis and dermis down to the Colles' fascia layer (Fig. 15-4) Monsel's solution is then applied. A stitch is never required.

For patients whose lesion is in the hair-bearing area, the skin is often too firm to allow for a biopsy with the cervical punch instrument. Instead, the author typically uses a 15 blade knife and cuts a 3-mm square. A thumb forcep is then used to pick up the tissue and cut off under the dermis. Alternatively, the cervical biopsy instrument can be used to remove the specimen. Again, Monsel's solution will suffice for hemostasis. Healing takes place over a matter of a few days. A Keys punch biopsy can be performed; however, the author prefers the methods above because of low cost, simplicity, and excellent specimens.

Excisional Biopsy

The intent of the excisional biopsy is to diagnose and treat at the same setting. Some lesions are small enough to be done in the physician's office under local anesthesia. Lesions greater than 2 cm in size are better done in an outpatient surgical suite using a local anesthetic. Lesions of 4 cm or greater may require regional anesthetic or a short general anesthetic. The amount of local anesthetic required for local infiltration should not exceed 200 mg over a 20-minute period.

If the lesion is excised under local anesthesia, the area is given a field block by infiltration into the subcuticular level. The excision line should begin several millimeters beyond the lesion to be excised, if early invasion is suspected. If vulvar intraepithelial neoplasm is suspected, the colposcope should be used to identify the edge of the lesion and a 3 to 4 mm margin ensured. The depth of the incision is based on the type of skin being removed. The mucosal skin inside of the hair-bearing area needs only to go through the dermis to the underlying Colles' fascia level. The skin then peels off very easily in an avascular plane. The superficial excision is possible because there are no hair follicles or skin appendages that penetrate deeper than the dermis.[1,2]

On the hair-bearing tissue the incision must be deep enough to remove the skin appendages. The depth of hair

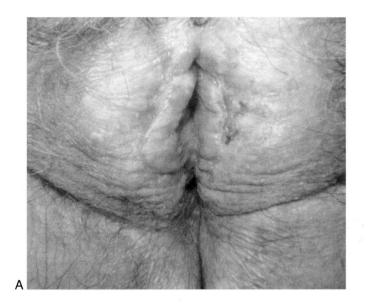

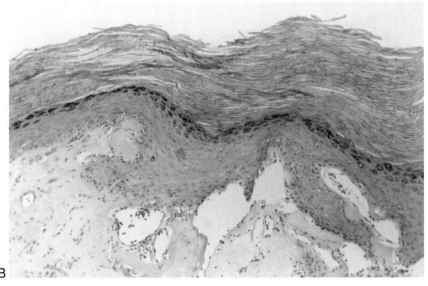

Fig. 15-3. (A) A 72-year-old woman with lichen sclerosis. Multiple excisional biopsies are necessary to rule out malignancy or atypia. **(B)** The biopsy reveals a thick Keratin layer with typical lichen sclerosis findings.

follicle involvement is up to 3.9 mm in depth. The incision should extend into the subcutaneous fat, which will ensure that the skin appendages are removed. This is necessary because carcinoma in situ (CIS) or invasive cancer can involve the skin appendages[3] (Fig. 15-5).

Closure is provided with 3–0 absorbable suture with simple interrupted stitches. Almost any defect on the labia can be closed with simple closure (Fig. 15-6). When extensive areas of the perineal skin are removed, mobilization and advancement of the lower vagina out to the perineal skin may be necessary for closure. In some instances, very large defects may require a rhomboid graft to cover the defect. Very rarely will a split-thickness skin graft be necessary to cover large defects on the vulva or perianal skin (Fig. 15-7).

INDICATIONS FOR VAGINAL BIOPSY

A biopsy of the vagina is indicated when a lesion is seen either grossly or under colposcopic vision (Fig. 15-8). Exophytic or ulcerative lesions are suspicious of vaginal cancer and usually can be seen grossly. These should be biopsied with the cervical punch biopsy instrument. If the lesion is seen on colposcopic examination (usually after an abnormal Pap smear has been noted), then the cervical punch biopsy

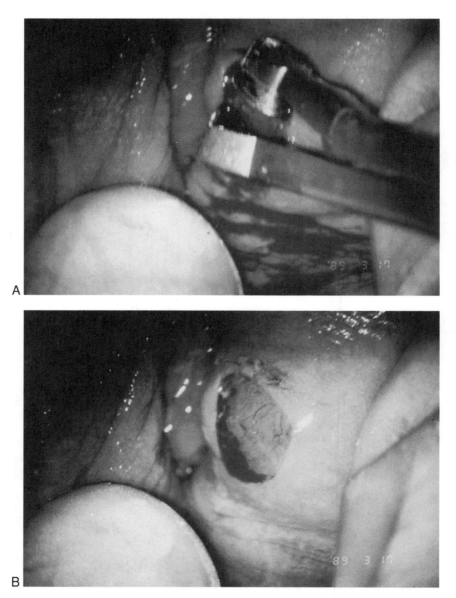

Fig. 15-4. **(A)** The cervical biopsy instrument is used to biopsy the vulvar mucosal skin. **(B)** The skin has been lifted off superficial to the Colles' fascia.

is used to biopsy the most severe site. Further treatment is then dependent on review of this biopsy.

Vaginal intraepithelial neoplasia (VAIN) III lesions require treatment. The modality selected depends on the size and location of the lesions. Most commonly, these lesions are at the apex of the vagina and follow vaginal hysterectomies for cervical intraepithelial neoplasia (CIN). They are generally under 3 cm in size and lend themselves easily to laser vaporization. If it is uncertain whether invasive cancer is present, they should not be lasered but should be excised. Patients who have had radiotherapy for cervical cancer are difficult to evaluate with the colposcope, and if the cytology or punch biopsy suggests VAIN III, these lesions should be excised to role out recurrent invasive cancer.

OPERATIVE TECHNIQUE

Laser Technique

The carbon dioxide laser should be used. For expert operators, the laser should be set to deliver 750 to 1,000 watts/mm^3. For the novice, it is better to reduce the wattage to 500 watts/mm^3. This provides a dot size of 2 mm and 20 watts of power. The procedure can be done in the outpatient setting under local anesthetic if the area is small enough to accomplish the laser vaporization with 200 mg or less of xylocaine. The lesion is identified using colposcopy and then outlined more clearly with the use of Lugol's solution. Xylocaine is injected submucosally to flatten out the vaginal epi-

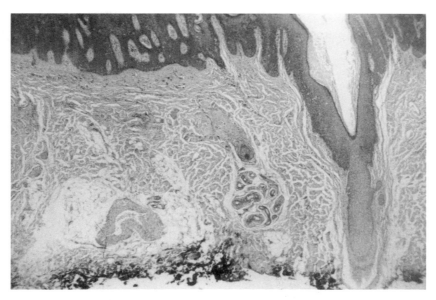

Fig. 15-5. A biopsy of carcinoma in situ (CIS) of the vulva on the hair-bearing skin shows CIS extending into the hair shaft.

thelium and to provide a liquid barrier for the laser beam. The lesion is outlined with the laser beam. The lesion is then destroyed to the papillary lamina propria below the mucosa. The mucosal layer is less than 1 mm thick, so the surface is lightly brushed. A cracking sound should be heard and the epithelium will separate from the underlying lamina propria (Fig. 15-9). There will be very little heat damage to the lamina propria. It then acts as a foundation over which the vaginal epithelium will migrate and the healing time should be rapid. The epithelium will migrate up to 2 mm/day, starting on the fifth day following the laser vaporization.

Electrosurgical Technique

There has been enthusiasm for the use of the electrosurgical unit to treat VAIN. The square loop has been advocated as the appropriate tool to use to remove VAIN. The author strongly discourages the use of the electrosurgical loop to remove strips of vaginal epithelium. The epithelial surface is less than 1-mm thick and no one is skilled enough to remove the epithelium that superficially with an electrosurgical wire. The most appropriate tool to use is the carbon dioxide laser under direct colposcopic vision, to recognize the surgical planes as the laser procedure is performed. The electrosurgical wire will remove the epithelium plus the lamina propria. If the excision extends 3 to 4 mm into the vaginal wall, the patient will experience significant scarring. This is especially true if the lesion removed is large.

If one does not have access to a carbon dioxide laser and only has an electrosurgical unit, it is much better to use a fulgeration technique with a ball electrode to destroy the surface epithelium. The electrosurgical unit is set at 50 watts of power with a 4-mm electrode ball. The vaginal epithelium is infiltrated with xylocaine so that the surface is flattened. The ball is brought into very superficial contact with the epithelium and the electrosurgical unit activated. This results in a sparking of the electrical current across to the mucosa and superficial destruction of the mucosa. It can then be moved rapidly across the surface in a manner similar to the laser beam. This will lift off the epithelium destroyed to the appropriate depth. The depth of destruction with this technique is harder to control than the depth of destruction using the carbon dioxide laser. Thus, the best instrument is the carbon dioxide laser.

Cryosurgery

The author does not recommend cryosurgery because the depth of destruction is completely uncontrolled. There may be damage to the bladder, urethra, or rectum.

Excision

When a diagnostic procedure is required, excision is the most appropriate technique. The mucosa is incised and the vaginal plane similar to that achieved with an anterior repair is achieved. This will remove the vaginal mucosa as well as the lamina propria, which is appropriate, since the reason for excision is to rule out the diagnosis of early invasion and one would need to see the lamina propria to do so. Following the excision, a closure can be accomplished by simple suturing with absorbable suture. The author has not found it necessary to apply a skin graft to an unirradiated patient when treating her for VAIN.

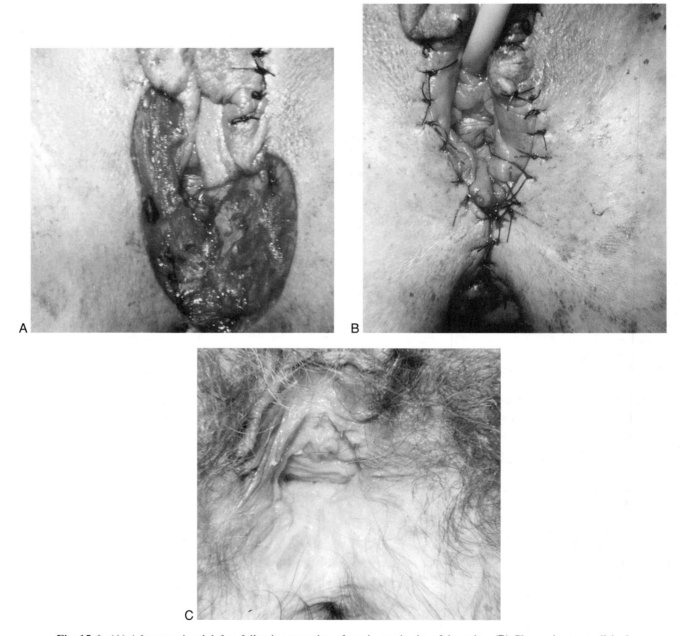

Fig. 15-6. **(A)** A large perineal defect following resection of carcinoma in situ of the vulva. **(B)** Closure is accomplished with interrupted suture. **(C)** The result of the surgery at 1 year.

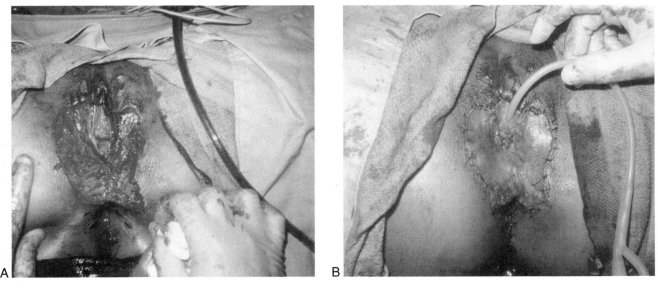

Fig. 15-7. **(A)** This skin defect is too large to cover by mobilizing skin. **(B)** A split-thickness skin graft has been placed over the defect.

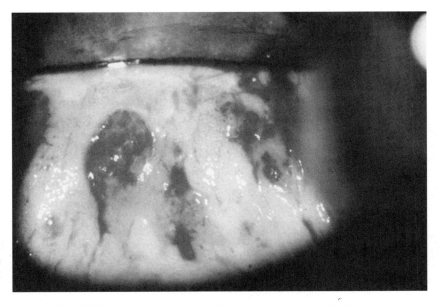

Fig. 15-8. A colposcopic photo of an early invasive vaginal cancer.

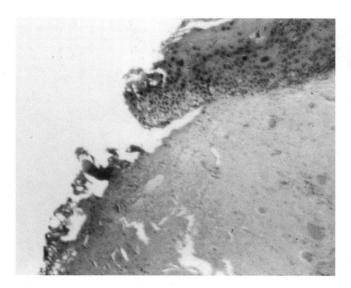

Fig. 15-9. A microscopic photo of the proper laser plane to separate the vaginal intraepithelial neoplasm from the underlying lamina propria.

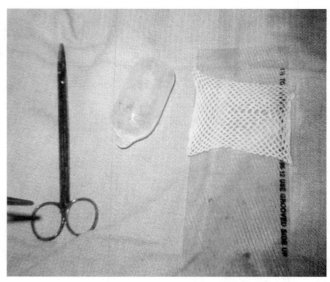

Fig. 15-11. The skin has been run through a 1 to 1.5 mesher and is ready to sew around the mold.

For patients who have had radiotherapy for cancer of the cervix or vagina, a wider excision and a skin graft is often necessary. The vagina is already shortened and stenotic due to the radiotherapy. If an area of vagina is then excised and closed, the vagina will be further shortened. If the area is less than 6 cm in depth or less than 5 cm in diameter, a skin graft is indicated. After excision of the vaginal epithelium in the radiated patient, there is generally a much larger space into which a graft can be placed and the patient's coital function will actually be improved after the excision. The graft is placed onto the base of the bladder and the surface

of the rectum. Occasionally, the peritoneal cavity will even be entered so that the graft can be placed against the intra-abdominal rectosigmoid surface or pelvic peritoneum.

The skin graft is selected from the skin of the lateral buttock. The author chooses an area that is covered by the patient's panty line, so that she can wear a two-piece bathing suit if so desired. Skin is prepared in the usual fashion and mineral oil is placed. A Browne dermitome is then used to cut a split-thickness graft of .014 in. in thickness (Fig. 15-10). This will leave the least amount of scar on the donor site, but yet give a thick enough donor skin so that excessive

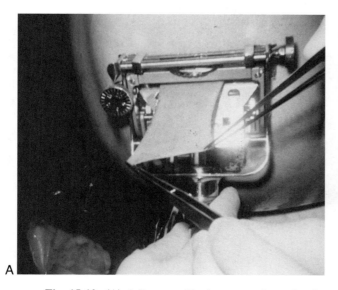

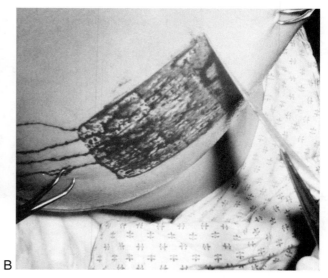

A

B

Fig. 15-10. **(A)** A Browne skin dermatome is used to harvest a split-thickness skin graft. **(B)** The donor site is from the right lateral buttock inside the panty line.

shrinkage will not take place. The skin is then placed through a 1 to 1.5 mesher, and it is sewn—with the dermal side out—onto an appropriate mold (Fig. 15-11). Many commercial molds are available. One can make one's own mold by taking a sterile condom and placing sterile foam inside it. The skin and mold is then placed into the vagina. Neovascularization will take place within 5 days. The mold is then removed at 5 days and general irrigation is carried out. A more rigid mold is then placed. The graft site has a tendency to contract over the next 2 to 6 weeks. A rigid mold is necessary so the contracture does not become severe. After the contracture period is over, the patient can then take the mold out, but must insert it several times during the day. Eventually the number of insertions per day is decreased and normal sexual relations can take place. If sexual relations are frequent enough, placement of the mold is not necessary. Fre-

quent inspection of the graft site is necessary, because patients vary, depending on healing characteristics and on whether radiotherapy has been administered.

REFERENCES

1. Benedet JL, Wilson PS, Matisic J: Epidermal thickness and skin appendage involvement in vulvar intraepithelial neoplasia. J Reprod Med 36:608, 1991
2. Mene A, Buckley CH: Involvement of the vulval skin appendages by intraepithelial neoplasia. Br J Obstet Gynaecol 92:634, 1985
3. Wright VC, Davies E: Laser surgery for vulvar intraepithelial neoplasia: principles and results. Am J Obstet Gynecol 374: 1987

CHAPTER SIXTEEN

VULVAR AND VAGINAL ANATOMY

C. WILLIAM HELM

> **Surgical Anatomy of the Vulva**
> Superficial Structures •
> Deeper Structures •
> Cutaneous Nerve Supply •
> Blood Supply • Lymph
> Drainage •
> **Surgical Anatomy of the Vagina**

SURGICAL ANATOMY OF THE VULVA

Superficial Structures

The female external genitalia are known as the vulva (Fig. 16-1). The shape of the vulva is due mainly to the mons pubis and the labia majora, which are both composed of fibrofatty tissue. The mons lies anterior and superior to the pubic symphysis and is covered by pubic hair. The labia majora form the lateral boundary of the vulva and extend from the labia minora medially to the labiocrural skin fold laterally. The overlying skin contains hair follicles together with sweat and sebaceous glands. The labia minora are smaller than the labia majora and are devoid of hair. Anteriorly, they merge to form the prepuce and frenulum of the clitoris and posteriorly, they merge into the fourchette.

The area enclosed by the labia minora is the vestibule into which the urethra and vagina open. The clitoris, the homologue of the male penis, is located anterior to the vestibule close to the symphysis and is attached to it by the suspensory ligament. The body of the clitoris is formed by the paired corpora cavernosa containing erectile tissue enclosed in a fibrous septum. These structures are each connected to the inferior pubic ramus by a crus to which the ischiocavernosus muscles are attached. The tip of the clitoris (glans clitoris) is composed of erectile tissue richly supplied with nerves.

The hymen is a thin fold of mucous membrane situated at the orifice of the vagina. The perineum is the area bordered by the fourchette anteriorly and the anus posteriorly.

Deeper Structures

The urogenital diaphragm is a fascial membrane bordered by the inferior pubic rami on each side and the transverse perineal muscles posteriorly (Fig. 16-2). It is composed of two leaves, the inferior and superior layers of fascia. These are separated by the deep perineal pouch, which contains the deep transverse perineal muscles and the sphincter urethrae. The urethra and vagina pass through the diaphragm to reach the vestibule.

The perineal muscles lie superficial to the inferior fascia of the urogenital diaphragm. The two bulbocavernosus muscles, the transverse perineal muscles and the external anal sphincter, join to form the perineal body.

The bulbocavernosus muscles are attached to the perineal body posteriorly and the corpus cavernosa of the clitoris anteriorly. They lie on the bulbs of the vestibule and pass lateral to the vaginal introitus.

The ischiocavernosus muscles arise from the inner surface of the ischial tuberosity and the ischial ramus and insert into the inferior surface of the crus of the clitoris.

Bartholin's glands lie on either side of the vagina on the inferior fascia of the urogenital diaphragm underneath the lower end of the bulbocavernosus muscles and the posterior portion of the bulb of the vestibule. Each gland drains by way of a 2-cm long duct into the vestibule immediately outside the hymenal ring at about the 4- and 8-o'clock positions.

The bulbs of the vestibule are composed of erectile tissue and lie on the inferior fascia of the urogenital diaphragm alongside the vaginal introitus. Posteriorly they are in contact with Bartholin's glands and superficially they are covered by the bulbocavernosus muscles.

Cutaneous Nerve Supply

The ilioinguinal nerve (L1) and the genital branch of the genitofemoral nerve (L1–L2) supply the anterior vulva and mons. Both nerves reach the vulva by passing through the inguinal canal and superficial inguinal ring. The ilioinguinal nerve enters the inguinal canal by piercing the internal oblique muscle, whereas the genital branch of the genitofemoral nerve passes through the deep inguinal ring.

The pudendal nerve (S2–S4) innervates the clitoris, vestibule, labia, and perineum. The nerve leaves the pelvis through the lower part of the greater sciatic foramen and

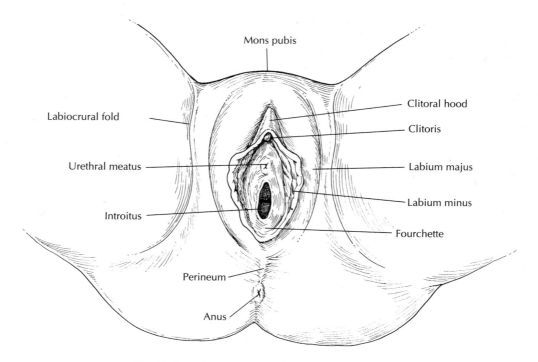

Fig. 16-1. Surface structures of the vulva and perineum.

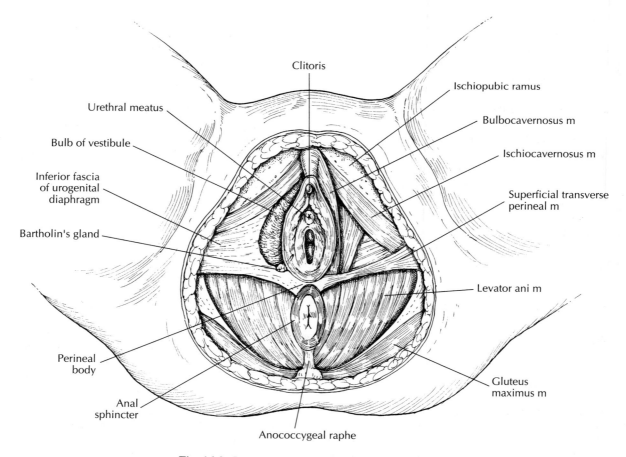

Fig. 16-2. Deeper structures of the vulva and perineum.

then passes lateral to the ischial spine before descending on the lower medial part of the ischial tuberosity in the pudendal canal to pass anteriorly across the lateral wall of the ischiorectal fossa. It divides into the dorsal nerve of clitoris and the perineal nerve.

The perineal branch of the posterior cutaneous nerve (S1–S3) supplies skin of the upper and medial thigh, the posterior vulva, and the perianal and lateral perineum. The nerve runs down the thigh posteromedial to the sciatic nerve and its perineal branch pierces the fascia lata to run toward the vulva and perineum beneath the superficial fascia.

Blood Supply

The internal pudendal artery is the main blood vessel supplying the vulva and perineum. It is one of the two terminal branches of the anterior trunk of the internal iliac (hypogastric) artery. It enters the perineum through the lesser sciatic foramen and pudendal canal, where it runs together with the pudendal nerve. It passes forward close to the medial margin of the inferior pubic ramus and splits into several branches: the perineal artery to the perineum, the posterior labial branches to the labia, the artery of the bulb to the erectile tissue of the vestibular bulb and vagina, the deep artery of the clitoris to the corpus cavernosum, and the dorsal artery of the clitoris to the dorsum, glans, and prepuce of the clitoris.

The external pudendal arteries arise from the medial side of the femoral artery and contribute further blood supply. The deep external pudendal passes medially across the pectineus muscle deep to fascia lata before piercing this muscle at the medial side of the thigh and travelling to the skin of the labium and perineum. The superficial external pudendal leaves the femoral sheath and cribriform fascia and passes medially deep to the long saphenous vein across the round ligament to supply the skin of the lower abdomen and anterior labium majus.

Lymph Drainage

The lymphatic drainage of the vulva and perineum has been described by Plentl and Friedman[1] and Parry-Jones.[2] The principal drainage is to the nodes in the groins (Fig. 16-3). Large collecting trunks pass cephalad through the labia majora receiving lymph from other parts of the vulva. Lymph channels draining the vulva do not cross the labiocrural fold.

In the groin, between 4 and 12 superficial inguinal nodes

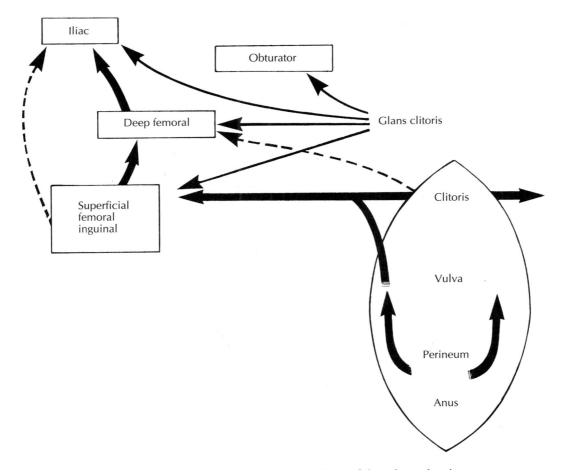

Fig. 16-3. Schematic diagram of lymphatic drainage of the vulva and perineum.

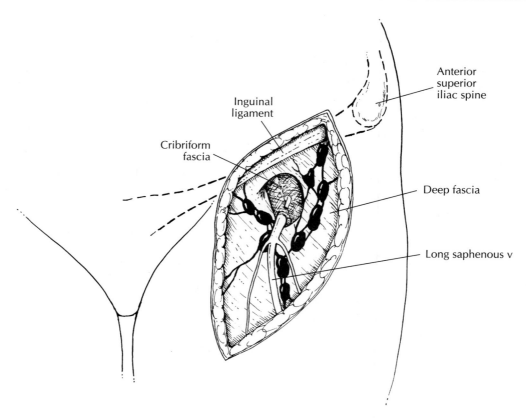

Fig. 16-4. Anatomic view of the superficial inguinal lymph nodes.

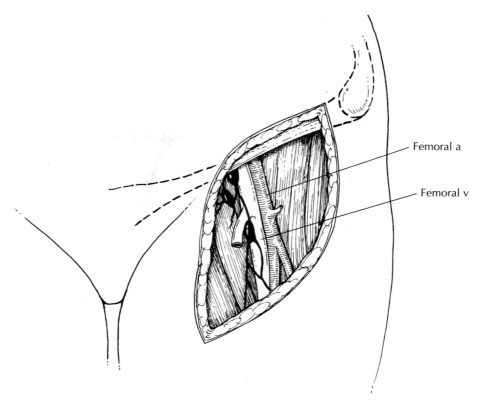

Fig. 16-5. Anatomic view of the deep femoral lymph nodes with deep fascia removed.

(Fig. 16-4) lie in the fatty layer of tissue beneath Camper's fascia anterior to the cribriform plate and fascia lata. These nodes drain mainly into the deep femoral nodes and thence to the external iliac nodes, although drainage channels from the most lateral nodes may pierce the external oblique aponeurosis or fascia lata to terminate directly in the lateral external iliac nodes.

Deep femoral nodes numbering between one and four (Fig. 16-5) are located within the femoral sheath deep to the cribriform fascia and drain to the external iliac nodes. The most constant node lies just below the saphenofemoral junction and the next most constant lies just above the junction. No nodes lie between the femoral artery and vein, lateral to the artery, or below the lower border of the fossa ovalis. The node of Cloquet, or upper deep femoral node, is absent in over 50 percent of cases.[3]

Although the lymph drainage of the prepuce of the clitoris is similar to the rest of vulva, that of the glans is distinctly different in that it may drain directly to pelvic nodes.[1] The lymph drainage from the glans passes via a presymphyseal plexus to the the superficial inguinal nodes. However, it may pass directly from here to the deep femoral nodes or under the inguinal ligament to the external iliac nodes. Alternative routes to the pelvic nodes are provided by channels that pierce the urogenital diaphragm just below the pubic symphysis then turn laterally and end in obturator or iliac nodes. Other channels run up the pubic symphysis and enter the pelvis between the insertions of the rectus muscles, turn laterally, and enter iliac nodes.

The lymph drainage of Bartholin's glands is thought to go to the groin, and possibly pelvis, directly although the exact routes have not been determined.

SURGICAL ANATOMY OF THE VAGINA

The vagina is a fibromuscular tube composed of nonkeratinizing squamous epithelium that contains no hair follicles or sebaceous glands. The upper end is contiguous with the cervix, or following hysterectomy, ends blindly at the vaginal vault. The lower end meets the body surface at the vestibule.

The submucosal layer of the vagina contains a rich network of blood vessels and lymphatic channels. This blood supply enables extensive mobilization of the vaginal tube without fear of ischemia. The arterial supply comes from the vaginal artery and branches of the uterine, middle rectal, and internal pudendal arteries. The venous plexuses drain to the internal iliac veins and to the groins. There is a network of lymphatic channels that anastomose freely throughout the mucosa and the muscularis[1] and these intercommunicating lymphatics give the potential for drainage to any pelvic nodal group from any region of the vagina. However, the upper two-thirds of the vagina drains mainly to the pelvic nodes and the lower third drains to the inguinofemoral nodes as well as the pelvic nodes.

The structures adjacent to the vagina are a major factor in the surgery of the vagina. Anteriorly, the ureters, bladder, and urethra and posteriorly, the rectum and anus limit radical excision of the vagina without the resection of these structures. However, once in the right surgical plane, dissection of the vagina away from surrounding structures is relatively straightforward. Surgery on the vagina following previous radiotherapy is hazardous due to the danger of damage to the urinary tract and rectum.

REFERENCES

1. Plentl AA, Friedman EA: Lymphatic System of the Female Genitalia. WB Saunders, Philadelphia, 1971
2. Parry-Jones E: Lymphatics of the vulva. J Obstet Gynaecol 67: 919, 1960
3. Borgno G, Micheletti L, Barbero M et al: Topographic distribution of groin lymph nodes. J Reprod Med 35:1127, 1990

CHAPTER SEVENTEEN

DIAGNOSIS AND SURGERY FOR BENIGN AND MALIGNANT DISEASE

C. WILLIAM HELM

SURGERY FOR BENIGN AND PREMALIGNANT DISEASE

Skinning Vulvectomy

Skinning vulvectomy entails removal of the vulvar skin and replacement with a split-thickness skin graft. It preserves the contours of the vulva, which are primarily a result of the underlying subcutaneous fat and fascia.

Indications

The procedure was first described in 1968 for widespread vulvar intraepithelial neoplasia[1] and later extended to the treatment of benign lichen sclerosus and vulvar atrophy.[2] It is mostly indicated for extensive vulvar intraepithelial neoplasia in younger women who wish to preserve the cosmetic appearance and function of the vulva. The procedure may be used for widespread recurrent vulvar intraepithelial neoplasia following previous treatments.

Operative Procedure

For the skinning vulvectomy procedure, general, epidural, or spinal anesthesia should be administered and the patient placed in the modified ''frog leg'' position with her legs in Allen stirrups. The excision margins are marked with a pen (Fig. 17-1) and the skin is incised down and through the dermis, but no deeper. Keeping tension on either side of the incision facilitates this procedure; the skin edges are held and elevated with forceps and the skin is dissected off the subcutaneous tissues, keeping close to the underside of the dermis (Figs. 17-2 and 17-3). The clitoris and clitoral hood may be preserved if desired. If involved with vulvar intraepithelial neoplasia, they may be treated with laser ablation at a later date.

A split-thickness skin graft is taken from the inner thigh and meshed in order to increase the area that can be covered and to prevent clot and exudate accumulating under the graft. It is important to ensure good hemostasis before the graft is applied. The undersurface of the graft is applied to the defect and the edges are secured to the wound edges by tying 3–0 polyglactin (Vicryl Ethicon, Cincinnati, OH) over dental rolls (Fig. 17-4). A paraffin gauze is laid over the graft and cotton dressings are secured over the top to maintain apposition. On each side some sutures are left long so that the dressing may be tied down. Paraffin gauze and dressings are placed over the donor site on the thigh, which is then wrapped in a crepe bandage. Excess skin is refrigerated in case the first graft does not take completely. A Foley catheter is placed per urethram at the end of the procedure.

Postoperative Management

The patient is kept either on bedrest or to chair for 7 days. The vulvar dressings are inspected daily but not taken down for 5 days, unless they show signs of infection. On or about the fifth day, the cotton dressings and paraffin gauze are removed with the dental rolls after premedication. If the graft has taken at this stage, the wound can be left open but kept clean with saline and kept dry with a hair dryer. If it has not taken, after debridement the spare stored skin may be applied in the same manner as previously. If the patient is unable to tolerate the change of dressings while awake an additional

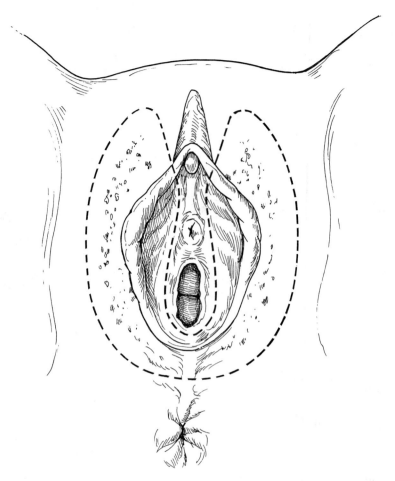

Fig. 17-1. Skinning vulvectomy: the incision.

short-term general anesthetic is sometimes necessary. The Foley catheter is left until the graft has taken.

The donor site dressing is left for 2 weeks unless it shows signs of infection.

Sequelae

Scarring around the introitus may cause dyspareunia.

Total (Simple) Vulvectomy

Total vulvectomy implies removal of the whole vulva together with perineal tissues as indicated, but usually including some of the subcutaneous tissues. It is normally performed for benign disease and therefore, wide resection margins are not necessary.

In comparison, radical vulvectomy implies removal of the whole vulva down to the level of the deep fascia of the thigh, the periosteum of the pubis, and the inferior fascia of the urogenital diaphragm. Because it is normally performed for malignant disease, the exact margins are defined by the extent of the tumor.

The desire to maintain body image and preserve sexual function has encouraged the treatment of both benign and malignant disease of the vulva with less extensive surgery. The use of partial vulvectomy has increased as a result of an effort to tailor the surgery to the disease and patient.

Indications

A total (simple) vulvectomy may be performed for benign and premalignant conditions of the vulva, including vulvar dystrophy, widespread intraepithelial neoplasia, and Paget's disease (Fig. 17-5). Total vulvectomy is a very effective treatment in older women for symptomatic vulvar dystrophy that has not responded to medical treatment.

Preoperative Preparation

In postmenopausal patients it is helpful to give estrogen replacement therapy for 6 weeks before surgery, provided there is no contraindication. This will improve the tissues of the lower genital tract, making the dissection and tissue handling easier and improving healing. Bowel preparation

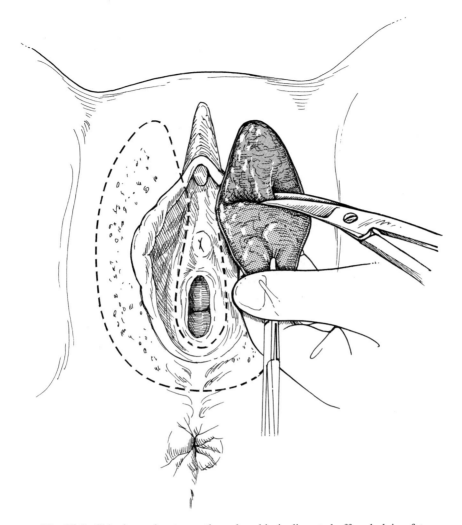

Fig. 17-2. Skinning vulvectomy: the vulva skin is dissected off underlying fat.

enables potential damage to the rectum or anus at surgery to be repaired more safely and, by delaying the return of bowel movements after surgery, allows healing of the anal sphincter if it has been repaired.

Operative Procedure

The total vulvectomy procedure requires general, epidural, or spinal anesthesia and the patient should be placed in the lithotomy position. Following skin preparation a urethral catheter is passed. The internal and external resection margins are marked (Fig. 17-6). The clitoris may be spared. In planning the incision it is best to leave as much skin of the vestibule surrounding the urethra as possible (usually 1 cm or more) to facilitate closure and avoid distortion of the meatus. The line of resection laterally depends on the extent of disease but may include all of the labia majora.

The initial dissection is in the posterior half of the vulva. The outer incision is made first through the skin across the perineum and laterally up to the level of the urethra. This incision is facilitated if the vulvar skin is stretched out.

The posterior dissection of perineal skin is performed with the aid of forceps applied to the lower edge of the specimen, which allow the operator to lift up the skin and stretch it out using two fingers placed behind the flap (Figs. 17-7 and 17-8). Dissecting scissors or scalpel are then used to carefully separate the skin from the underlying perineal tissues to a level above the intended vaginal margin. Care must be taken to avoid damaging the rectum during dissection. Mobilization of the lower vagina above the intended resection margin will help closure.

The incision is now extended upward on both sides. The lateral skin edges of the specimen are grasped with forceps and dissection is performed with curved Mayo scissors, staying within the subcutaneous fat and aiming for the internal resection margin on the vagina (Fig. 17-9). It is not necessary to resect deeply. An assistant is ready with hemostats and Bovie to deal with any blood vessels encountered.

The specimen is now detached from the vagina laterally

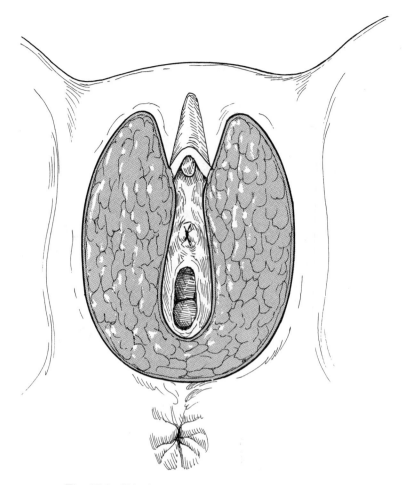

Fig. 17-3. Skinning vulvectomy: raw area to be grafted.

and posteriorly. The scissors are used to cut radially through the specimen in its posterior part to the vaginal margin. On each side, the scissors are used to divide along the vaginal margin to a point just below the level of the urethral meatus (Fig. 17-10).

The dissection is taken down toward the attachments of the clitoris, if this organ is to be excised with the specimen. The suspensory ligament is divided and ligated (Fig. 17-11). The scalpel is used to incise the skin across the vestibule above and lateral to the urethral meatus joining with the internal incision around the distal vagina. The tip of the scalpel or the Kelly forceps is then passed through the specimen in the midline to isolate the crura of the clitoris and to allow the crura to be held on each side with forceps, (Fig. 17-12) divided, and underrun with 0 polyglactin. The specimen is now detached completely and hemostasis is secured with Bovie. Venous sinuses around the urethra and vaginal margin may be difficult to control without underrunning with 2–0 polyglactin. It is helpful to orient the specimen for the pathologist and to draw a diagram on the pathology form marking the sites of disease if these are not clearly apparent.

Closure

Assessment is now made of how well the tissues will come together at all points. If it appears that there may be too much tension then the lateral and posterior vagina can be further undermined as well as the skin edges. When undermining vulvar skin, care must be taken to leave sufficient subcutaneous tissue attached to prevent devascularization. It is best to start by freeing up the lateral and posterior vaginal edges. An assessment may be made at this point as to the necessity for local skin flaps. Closure is started by inserting a stay suture to approximate the skin immediately above the urethral meatus, and continued using 3–0 polyglactin or polyglycolic acid (Dexon, Davis and Geck, Wayne, NJ) sutures (Figs. 17-13 and 17-14). The approximation of the skin immediately above the urethral meatus is made later (Fig. 17-13 inset). To reduce tension on the repair the legs may be adducted appropriately.

A suction drain is brought out on each side of the perineum and sutured to the skin. When suction is applied leakage of air may occur around the incision and extra sutures may

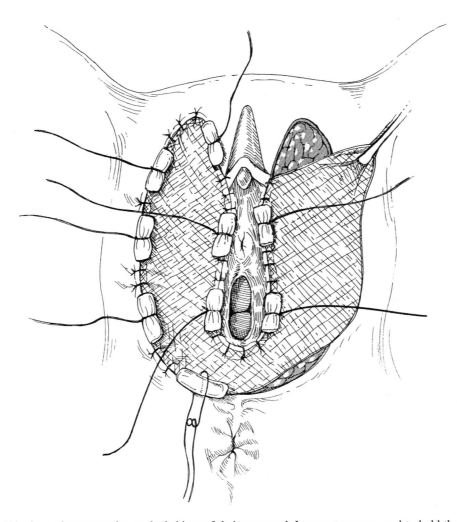

Fig. 17-4. Skinning vulvectomy: the meshed skin graft being secured. Long sutures are used to hold the dressings.

need to be inserted. Often, leakage only stops when the legs are brought together.

Postoperative Care

The catheter is left in for approximately 7 days until the wounds begin healing. The patient may be allowed out of bed to chair at an early stage but is not allowed to walk freely. Stair climbing and abduction of the legs are prohibited. The sutures may be trimmed after 7 days if they are causing irritation. Perineal hygiene with sitz baths and gentle cleansing with saline are encouraged, along with keeping the area dry using a hair dryer. Exposure to the air is helpful.

Complications

Hematoma formation is rarely a problem, provided the suction drains work well. Any infection is usually noted soon after the surgery and treated with antibiotics and continued perineal hygiene. Small separations of the wound may occur and can be left to heal spontaneously. Wide separation is unusual but can also generally be left to heal by secondary intention. Stricture of the introitus is not usually a problem following simple vulvectomy.

SURGERY FOR MALIGNANT DISEASE

By far, the most common malignant tumor of the vulva is squamous cell carcinoma. Others include malignant melanoma, basal cell carcinoma, sarcoma, and adenocarcinoma, particularly of Bartholin's and sweat glands.

Squamous cell carcinoma can remain confined to the vulva for long periods. When spread occurs, it is initially to adjacent tissues (nonvulva skin, vagina, urethra, anus, rectum, bladder, and bone) or to the inguinal lymph nodes (or both). Until recent years, the standard operation for the treatment of even a small invasive carcinoma of the vulva was a radical vulvectomy with removal of the primary tumor,

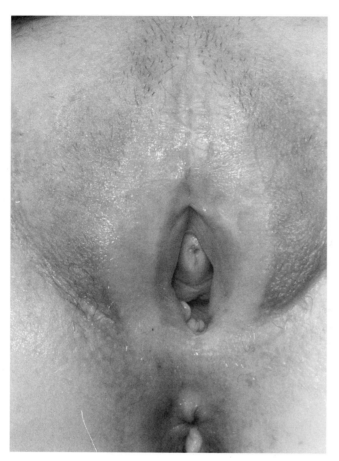

Fig. 17-5. Patient with intractable pruritus from lichen sclerosus and vulvar atrophy who will undergo total vulvectomy. The clitoris will be removed. © University of Manchester, Manchester, England.

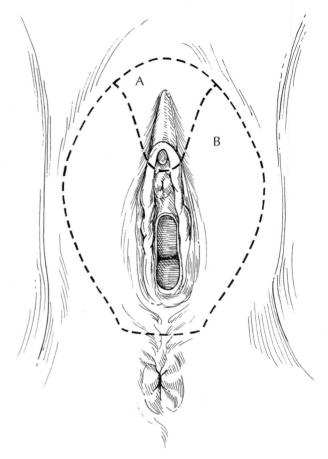

Fig. 17-6. Incisions for total vulvectomy. (A) Clitoris to be removed and (B) clitoris to be spared.

including a wide area of skin extending onto the medial thigh, groins, and lower abdomen, together with an en bloc resection of the inguinal and often the pelvic lymph nodes.[3] This operation had a high morbidity rate with approximately 50 percent of the wounds experiencing breakdown.

Surgical procedures for the treatment of carcinoma of the vulva have become more conservative and individualized to each patient. The fundamental basis of surgery for the primary tumor is now complete excision with a minimum 2-cm margin and dissection down to the deep fascia and the periosteum of the pubic symphysis. Although adenocarcinoma of the vulva is treated in much the same fashion as squamous cell carcinoma, involvement of Bartholin's gland is still thought to require radical vulvectomy. The management of malignant melanoma remains controversial.

The exact procedure used depends on the site, size, and histologic features of the tumor. In a young patient the clitoris should be left if the tumor is situated posteriorly on the vulva or lies 2 cm or more from the clitoris. When a groin node dissection is planned it is usually performed first, un-

less the patient's medical condition is uncertain, in which case it is best to excise the vulva tumor first in case the anesthetic has to be abandoned.

The extensive nature of some of the procedures, the unavoidable distortion of the appearance of the perineal area, and stoma formation can lead to major psychosexual problems for the patient. Preoperative counseling and postoperative support are vital parts of patient management.

Radical Vulvectomy

The radical vulvectomy procedure involves wide radical excision of the whole vulva together with adjacent tissues to ensure a minimum 2-cm margin around a carcinoma. It is often performed in conjunction with either a unilateral or bilateral groin node dissection. The types of incisions used are individualized depending primarily on the site and size of the tumor (Fig. 17-15).

Preoperative Preparation

All patients undergoing radical vulvar surgery require careful explanation and counseling with regard to the effects of the procedure. Good bowel preparation is also a must before

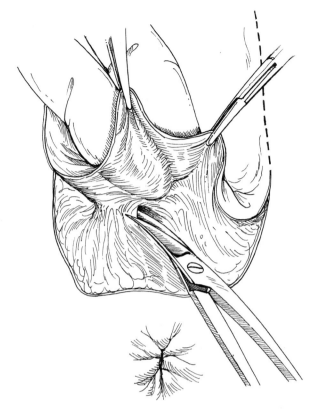

Fig. 17-7. Total vulvectomy: posterior dissection using fingers to push out posterior flap.

surgery. In view of the extensive dissection that may be necessary close to the anus, it is a good idea to document signs of anal sphincter weakness before surgery.

Operative Procedure

General, epidural, or spinal anesthesia is used for the radical vulvectomy procedure. The patient is placed in Allen stirrups with the hips abducted 45 degrees and flexed 45 degrees. It is helpful to position the patient so that the perineum protrudes over the bottom of the operating table. A pad or cushion is placed under the sacrum and the Bovie pad is kept off the thigh in case skin flaps need to be raised.

The skin is prepared to include all areas that may be required for skin flaps. The patient is examined carefully to identify the limits of spread, and the skin incisions both externally and within the vagina are marked with a pen. A catheter is inserted into the bladder per urethram. If frozen sections are required to ensure that the intended resection margins are clear of tumor, they should be taken at this time. They can be cut as small ellipses in the line of the incision.

The skin incision is begun posteriorly and extended laterally on both sides similar to the procedure for a simple vulvectomy, but the excision margins are wider and the dissection is taken down all the way through the subcutaneous fat to the deep fascia laterally using scalpel or scissors (Fig. 17-16). The tissues can be separated relatively easily off the deep fascia and pubic ramus until reaching the intended vaginal resection margin. An assistant holds forceps ready to clip vessels as they become visible so that dissection can

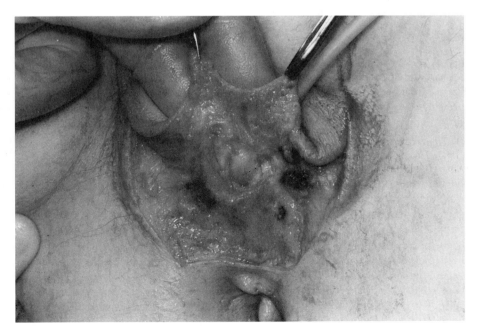

Fig. 17-8. Total vulvectomy: posterior dissection completed. The pale area in the center of the flap is the undersurface of the posterior vaginal wall. © University of Manchester, Manchester, England.

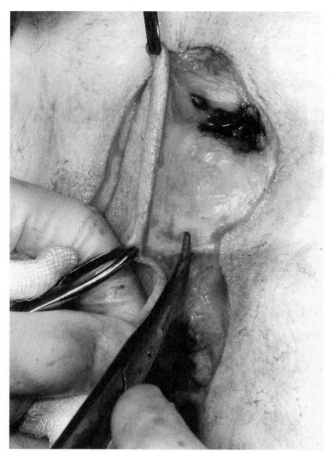

Fig. 17-9. Total vulvectomy: dissection of upper half of the vulva. The vulva specimen is elevated and stretched, and dissection proceeds in the subcutaneous fat. © University of Manchester, Manchester, England.

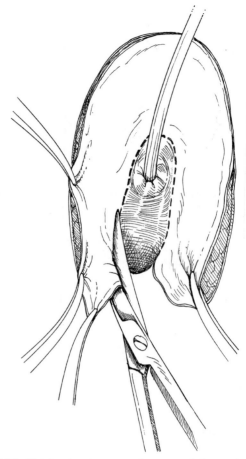

Fig. 17-10. Total vulvectomy: cutting around the vagina to the level of the urethra.

proceed rapidly. Branches of the pudendal artery will require attention as they are encountered posterolaterally.

It is important to avoid damaging the anal sphincter, while at the same time ensuring an adequate margin around a tumor placed posteriorly on the vulva or perineum. A finger in the rectum helps to guide the operator under these circumstances. As with a total vulvectomy, the posterior margin of the specimen is elevated with forceps, which can be held by the assistants while dissection proceeds (Fig. 17-7). If necessary, the anterior third of the anal sphincter can be removed with the specimen (see below).

Superolaterally, if a triple-incision procedure is being performed, the subcutaneous tissues that contain the lymphatics extending toward the groins on each side are taken with the specimen by dissecting under the skin-bridge that is left between the vulvectomy and groin dissection. Superiorly, the dissection is carried down toward the clitoral attachments by sweeping the specimen off the periosteum of the pubic bones and the deep fascia until the clitoral attachments are reached (Fig. 17-16). The suspensory ligament of the clitoris may be clamped, divided, and ligated at this point.

The vaginal incision is now made circumferentially, ensuring that the required margin around the tumor is maintained. The tip of a scalpel or Kelly forceps is passed through the specimen in the midline to isolate the crura. They are held with forceps, divided, and underrun with 0 polyglactin. The specimen is now detached completely and hemostasis is secured with Bovie. Venous sinuses around the urethra and vaginal margin may be difficult to control without underrunning with 3–0 polyglactin. The specimen is sent for histology with adequate orientation.

Closure

Closure is facilitated if the residual vagina is mobilized off the rectum and its lateral attachments. Marker sutures may be inserted to assess the way in which the edges will come together using a 2–0 polyglactin suture. In many cases the wound can be closed primarily without resorting to special techniques. A suction drain with wide holes is inserted on each side and brought out through the perineum. Paraffin gauze is placed over the wounds and covered by a gauze

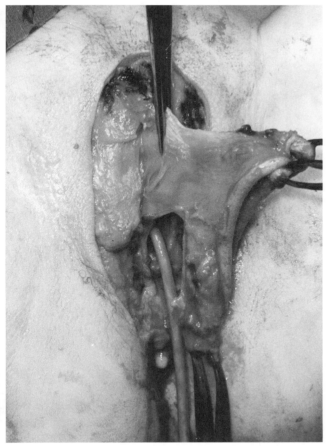

Fig. 17-11. Total vulvectomy: the suspensory ligament has been clamped ready for division. The skin above the urethra meatus has already been incised in this case. © University of Manchester, Manchester, England.

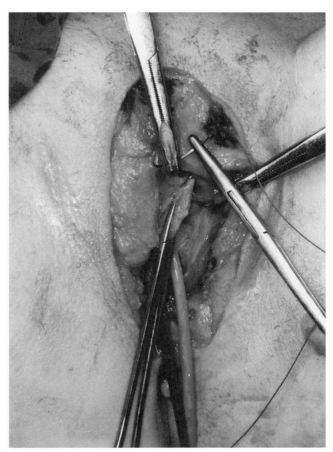

Fig. 17-12. Total vulvectomy: the crura of the clitoris have been clamped and the suspensory ligament is being ligated. © University of Manchester, Manchester, England.

dressing held in place by a diaper made out of a sterile disposable drape.

Postoperative Care

The patient is kept on bed rest for the initial postoperative period. The suction drains are left in for 3 to 4 days and the urethral catheter remains until the wounds have healed. The wound is inspected daily to ensure healing and to detect signs of infection early. The perineum is cleansed with sterile saline after the first 48 hours and dried with a hair dryer. After a few days the patient is given sitz baths.

The patient is initially fasted and given constipating agents for 3 to 4 days, particularly if the anal sphincter or rectum were repaired. Following this period a low-residue diet is prescribed together with stool softeners.

Complications

Hematoma, although unusual if adequate drains are inserted, may require evacuation. Signs of infection should prompt staff to take specimens for culture and institute antibiotics.

A small amount of wound breakdown is common but usually heals with conservative management. If the wound has been closed with skin flaps and necrosis has occurred, the dead skin should be debrided. Late sequelae include stenosis of the vaginal introitus and bladder prolapse.

Additional Procedures

Depending on the characteristics of the primary tumor, additional procedures may be required to ensure complete excision of the carcinoma (see first boxed list).

Wider Margins

Extensive areas of skin can be excised with the primary tumor. The methods available for closure of the resulting defect should be considered when planning the procedure. In the event of being unable to fashion flaps, the defect can be packed with povidone-iodine-soaked gauze and then

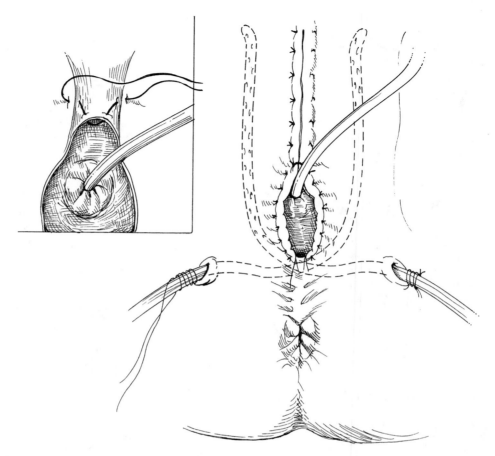

Fig. 17-13. Total vulvectomy: diagram of sutured wound. **(Inset)** Suture placed to oppose periurethral mucosa to skin edges.

allowed to granulate, with careful postoperative nursing care.

The most widely used supplementary method of closure is by skin flaps, which may be of the transposition type, such as the rhomboid flap (particularly useful for small posterior defects,[4] or myocutaneous flaps (e.g., gracilis,[5] rectus abdominis (see Fig. 17-32), and tensor fascia lata[6] (see Fig. 17-31).

Excision of Lower Uretha

If the tumor involves the urethra the distal 1 cm can be excised without affecting continence. The residual urethral mucosa is included in the closure.

Excision of Urethra and Inversion With Suprapubic Drainage

If any more than the distal 1 cm of the urethra must be excised, the patient will require an additional procedure to prevent urinary incontinence. In some patients this will be an anterior exenteration with formation of neobladder. An

alternative procedure in the palliative setting is inversion of the proximal residual urethra into the bladder. Through a suprapubic incision the cave of Retzius is entered and the upper urethra and bladder neck are exposed (Fig. 17-17). A rubber drain is passed around the urethra, which is mobilized all around with the bladder neck, and then transected and transfixed (Fig. 17-18). The anterior bladder is opened through a midline incision and the upper urethra is inverted into the bladder using forceps (Fig. 17-19). The edges of the inverted bladder neck exteriorly are approximated with 0 polyglactin sutures. The bladder incision is then closed with continuous 0 polyglactin around a suprapubic catheter (Fig. 17-20).

Vaginectomy (Partial or Total)

The extent and site of vaginal involvement will dictate the amount of surgery necessary. Involvement of the lower lateral wall can be dealt with by resection as necessary. If the tumor involves the anterior or posterior walls of the vagina, care must be taken not to damage the bladder or rectum while achieving clear margins around the tumor. Involvement of extensive amounts of the vagina will require removal of the

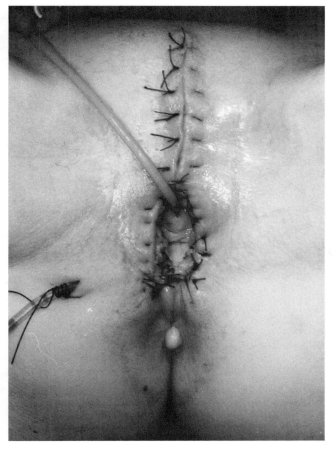

Fig. 17-14. Total vulvectomy: the operation is completed. Only a single suction drain was used in this case. © University of Manchester, Manchester, England.

Surgery for Carcinoma of the Vulva

- For lesions confined to the vulva
  Radical local excision
  Radical hemivulvectomy
  Radical vulvectomy (anterior, posterior, or total)
- For lesions that have spread beyond the vulva
  Radical vulvectomy with
    Wider skin margins
    Excision of lower uretha
    Vaginectomy (partial or total)
    Excision of anus and/or distal rectum
    Excision of pubic symphysis/pubic rami
    Exenteration (anterior, posterior, or total)

Surgical Management of Vulvar Small Cell Carcinoma

1. Well- or moderately differentiated lesions 2 cm or less in greatest dimension situated laterally on the vulva with no lymphovascular space invasion and the depth of invasion 1 mm or less
   Radical local excision without node dissection
2. Lesions 2 to 4 cm in greatest dimension with the depth of invasion greater than 1 mm or lesions 2 cm or less in greatest dimension with poor grade or lymphovascular space invasion situated laterally on the vulva
   Radical hemivulvectomy/radical local excision and ipsilateral groin node dissection
   In the case of tumors that are less than 4 cm with positive ipsilateral groin nodes, the contralateral groin should be dissected
3. Lesions greater than 4 cm placed laterally on the vulva away from the midline
   Radical hemivulvectomy with bilateral groin node dissection
4. Lesions involving midline structures
   If anterior, anterior radical vulvectomy or radical vulvectomy with bilateral groin node dissection
   If posterior, posterior radical vulvectomy or radical vulvectomy with bilateral groin node dissection
5. Locally advanced lesions involving structures other than vulva
   More extensive surgery is required depending on extent of tumor (see first boxed list)
   In cases which exenterative surgery would be necessary to effect cure, the possibility of combined chemotherapy and radiotherapy before more conservative surgery may be considered
   Disease involving the groin or groin and nodes should be excised if possible

bladder or anorectum, depending on the site of involvement (see below).

Excision of Anus and Distal Rectum

Several procedures have been described for the excision of tumor involving the anus and rectum. When the lesion just encroaches on the anus, or there is a suspicion of this en-

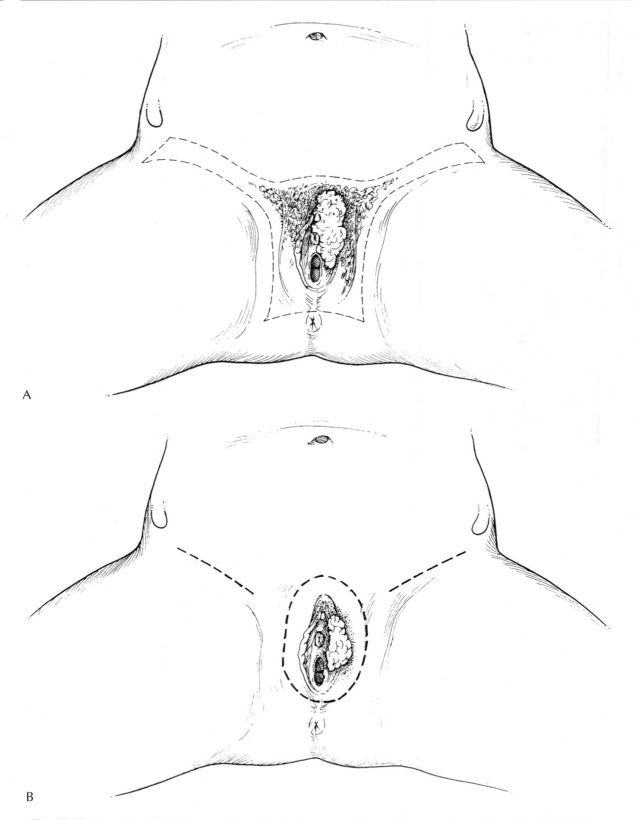

Fig. 17-15. Examples of incisions used for radical vulvectomy. **(A)** Modified butterfly incision. **(B)** Triple incision technique—a skin bridge is left between the radical vulvectomy and the groin incisions. *(Figure continues.)*

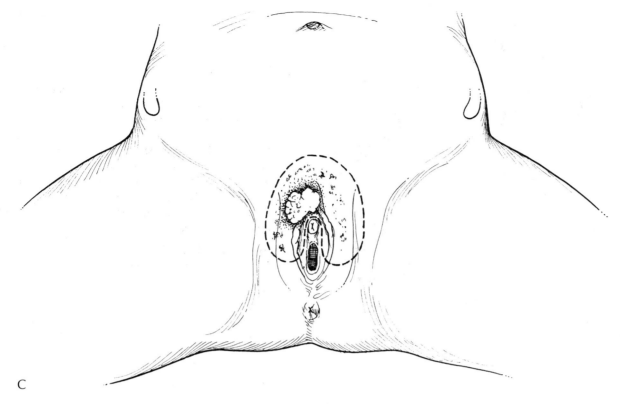

C

Fig. 17-15 *(Continued)*. **(C)** Anterior horseshoe incision.

croachment, the anterior third of the anus and sphincter can be excised without major impact on continence.[7] The external anal sphincter is repaired with 0 polyglactin sutures. For extra support of the sphincter mechanism, the distal limbs of the puborectalis may be plicated together anterior to the anus. The skin can be closed with rhomboid flaps.

In many cases partial resection of the anus would be insufficient and anovulvectomy,[8] anoproctectomy,[9] or posterior exenteration can be used. Anoproctectomy is a more extensive procedure than anovulvectomy.

Anovulvectomy With Sigmoid Colostomy

This is a most useful procedure in older women because it avoids the need for an extensive laparotomy in addition to the perineal procedure. It is well tolerated.

The operation is performed in two stages. In the first stage, a sigmoid end colostomy is raised in the left iliac fossa. Two weeks later, in the perineal phase, the tumor is excised widely including the anus and lower rectum. The rectum is transected and left opening into the perineal wound. It is usually secured to the posterior edge of the residual vagina and to the skin margins. If necessary, the two phases may be performed during the same surgery, with the lower bowel being irrigated from above to clean away fecal material.

Trephine End Sigmoid Colostomy

The patient should have undergone preoperative bowel preparation. General, epidural, or spinal anesthesia is used. The patient should be placed in the supine position. A 24 French Foley catheter is inserted into the rectum and the balloon is inflated to hold it in place. The external end is connected to the bellows used for sigmoidoscopy. A 1-in. circular incision is made in the skin of the abdomen at the site of the intended colostomy and the disc of skin is removed (Fig. 17-21). Using cutting Bovie the incision is taken down through the subcutaneous fat to the rectus sheath. Two small right-angled retractors are held by an assistant. The external oblique aponeurosis is incised obliquely in the line of the muscle fibers (Fig. 17-22). The underlying internal oblique and transversus muscles are separated (Fig. 17-23) and the retractors are inserted to expose the peritoneum. The peritoneum is picked up with hemostats and incised carefully. The intended stoma is gently stretched with the fingers to allow adequate room for the bowel.

The descending colon and sigmoid are identified. Babcock forceps are applied and used to gently elevate the bowel through the stoma site until a window of mesentery is visible (Fig. 17-24). It may be difficult to identify the nature of the bowel loop raised, although the presence of tenia will confirm large bowel. Before incising the bowel a soft bowel clamp is applied above, and the rectum and sigmoid are

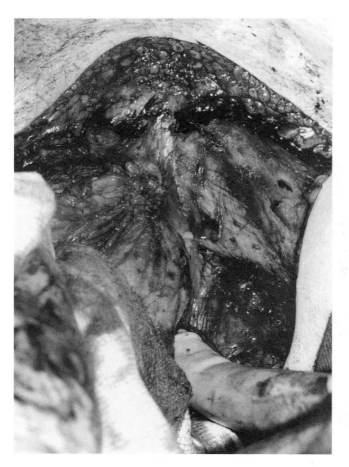

Fig. 17-16. Radical vulvectomy: dissection of fascial plane laterally (same case as in Figs. 17-27 to 17-31). The vulva is being pulled to the opposite side.

inflated with air from below to confirm the identity of the distal and proximal bowel.

A small window is made in the mesentery at the apex of the loop of bowel and widened enough to allow a GIA (gastrointestinal anastomosis) staple gun to be inserted (Fig. 17-25). The bowel is transected, and the distal end is inspected for hemostasis and placed back within the abdomen.

The proximal part is prepared for the stoma. The staple line is excised and discarded. The bowel is opened out and sutured to the skin with interrupted 3–0 polyglactin polyglactin or catgut mucocutaneous sutures (Fig. 17-26).

Anovulvectomy

The anesthesia used is either general, epidural, or spinal. The patient is placed in Allen stirrups in the modified ski position with the thighs abducted 45 degrees and flexed 45 degrees. It is important to position the patient well over the end of the table to allow access behind the anus.

The incision margins are marked with a pen. The exact extent of resection depends on the size of the tumor but encompasses the anus (Fig. 17-27). A 1 polyglactin suture

is inserted circumferentially around the anal margin, pulled tight, and tied in order to stop secretions and to provide for traction on the anal canal and rectum. The dissection differs from a radical vulvectomy only in the posterior part. Mayo scissors allow dissection in the ischiorectal fossa. In the midline posteriorly the fascia of the anococcygeal raphe may be palpated and divided. The levator muscles are incised on both sides and the anus and lower rectum are freed laterally and posteriorly (Fig. 17-28). The rectum is transected above the tumor together with the posterior vagina usually after the rest of the surgical specimen has been mobilized (Fig. 17-29). Skin flaps may be required to close the defect (Figs. 17-30 to 17-32). During closure of the wound the rectal mucosa can be secured to the posterior vaginal edge and the perineal skin closure.

Postoperative Care. The postoperative care is similar to that for patients who have undergone a radical vulvectomy.

Sequelae. The patient will intermittently discharge a small amount of mucus from the rectum into the perineum. This is not usually a problem. Occasionally the mucus may be retained in the residual rectum and requires release either digitally or by dilation of the perineal opening.

Partial Excision of Pubic Symphysis and Ischial Rami

Involvement of bone by tumor is a poor risk factor, but small areas of bone can be excised if necessary. Excision of the central part of the pubic symphysis or parts of the ischial pubic rami can be performed with the Gigli saw. The opinion of an orthopaedist should be sought if this is contemplated, because of potential problems with pelvic stability.

Groin Node Dissection

Indication

A groin node dissection is performed in certain cases of malignancy of the vulva, first, to assess the nodes for evidence of metastasis, which may indicate the need for further therapy and second, to help cure the patient of the disease or reduce the chance of recurrence.

The groin nodes have been shown to be the most significant prognostic indicator in squamous cell carcinoma of the vulva.[10] It has also been shown that if cancer recurs in a previously undissected groin, the outlook is grim.[11]

The practice of groin node dissection is controversial in the management of malignant melanoma but is probably not indicated for primary disease.

Superficial Versus Deep

It has been proposed that since lymph drainage from the vulva rarely bypasses the superficial nodes, a superficial node dissection is all that is required for small carcinomas,

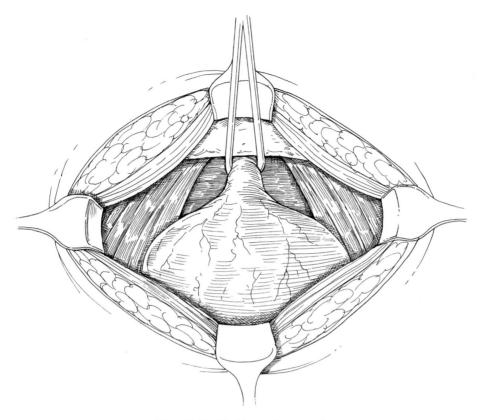

Fig. 17-17. Bladder neck exposed.

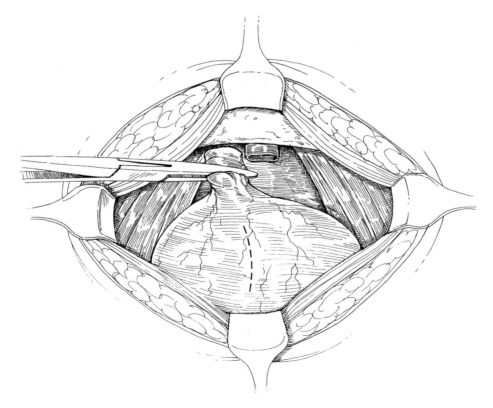

Fig. 17-18. Upper urethra transected. Line of cystotomy incision.

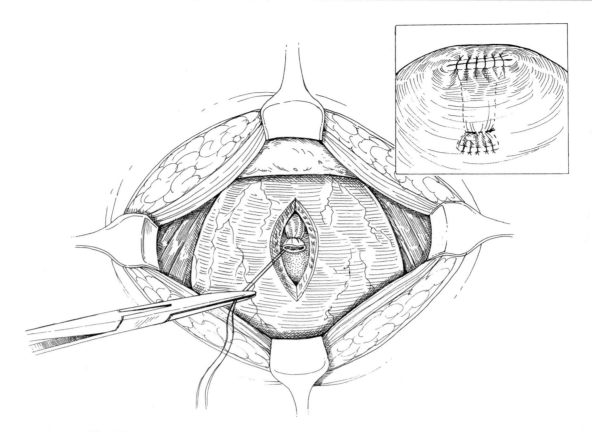

Fig. 17-19. Inverted urethra transfixed and lying in bladder. **(Inset)** Inverted urethra.

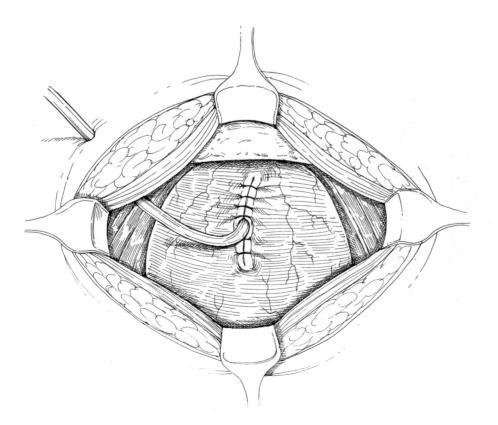

Fig. 17-20. Closed bladder incision with suprapubic catheter.

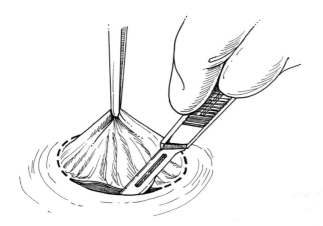

Fig. 17-21. Trephine sigmoid colostomy: cutting disc of skin for colostomy.

provided these nodes are negative.[12] However, no studies have compared the use of superficial versus superficial plus deep groin node dissection. Since it has been shown that the deep lymph nodes can be removed relatively easily without extensively disrupting the deep fascia[13] and with minimal additional morbidity, they should probably be removed.

Sampling Versus Dissection

Since the actual site of the first "sentinel" node involved in the groin varies widely, all nodes in the groin should be removed.

Operative Procedure

General, epidural, or spinal anesthesia is used. If the groin node dissection alone is to be performed, the patient is placed supine with the legs abducted 30 degrees and externally rotated. If the vulva is also to be removed, the patient is placed in Allen stirrups in the same position. After the groin node dissection the legs can be repositioned so that the hips and knees are flexed.

Provided the groin nodes are clinically negative, the groin incision runs 2 cm below and parallel to the inguinal ligament starting 3 cm distal and medial to the anterior superior iliac spine and ending below the superficial inguinal ring (Fig. 17-33). If there is concern for groin node metastases, an elliptical skin incision can be made in the same line so that this overlying segment of skin can be excised with the nodes.

The incision is taken through the full thickness of the skin and 2 to 3 mm into the fat. Allis forceps are applied to the dermal surface of the upper skin incision to provide traction while Mayo scissors or scalpel are used to dissect down through the subcutaneous fat to expose the glistening fascia of the aponeurosis of the external oblique muscle 3 cm above the inguinal ligament (Figs. 17-34 and 17-35). Care must be taken not to dissect too close to the skin of the flaps because this will jeopardize the blood supply and may lead to flap necrosis. Scarpa's (superficial) fascia, when prominent, can occasionally be mistaken for the external oblique aponeurosis but does not have the glistening silver color. Once the

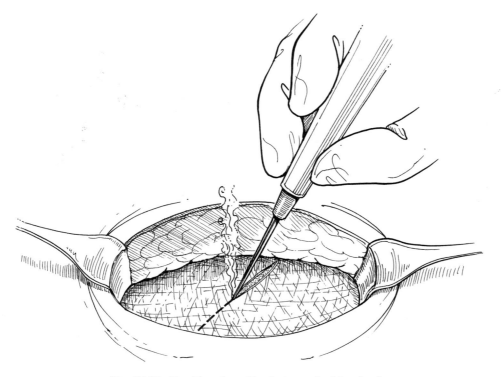

Fig. 17-22. Trephine sigmoid colostomy: incising fascia.

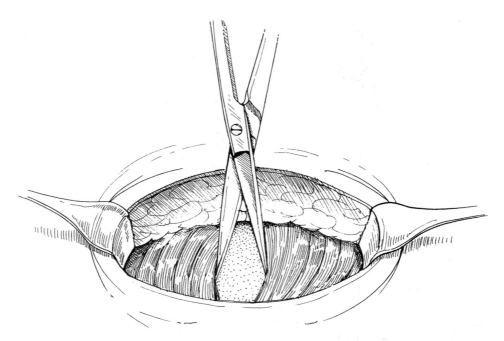

Fig. 17-23. Trephine sigmoid colostomy: separating muscle.

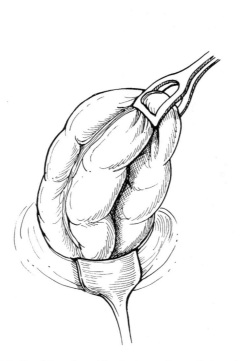

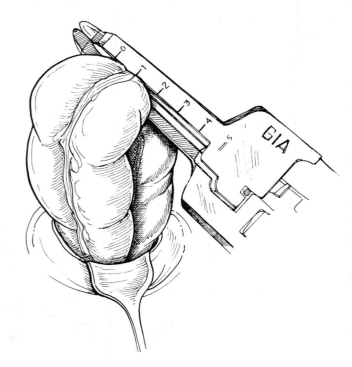

Fig. 17-24. Trephine sigmoid colostomy: loop of sigmoid pulled through incision.

Fig. 17-25. Trephine sigmoid colostomy: after confirming the proximal and distal segments the bowel is divided with GIA (gastrointestinal anastomosis) stapler.

external oblique aponeurosis is identified, the fatty tissue containing the inguinal nodes can be dissected off easily so that the lower margin of the inguinal ligament is exposed (Figs. 17-36 and 17-37).

The posterior skin flap is now raised and dissection is taken down through the subcutaneous fat to the deep fascia of the thigh approximately 6 cm from the inguinal ligament. Although the initial incision and dissection should span the entire length of the posterior flap, it is easier to identify the deep fascia at the lateral end. Once the deep fascia has been reached dissection of the fatty bundle containing the groin nodes off the deep fascia is performed heading from lateral to medial. Laterally, the circumflex iliac vessels need to be electrocauterized but throughout the dissection a sharp eye should be kept for venous and arterial vessels. A finger is passed beneath the round ligament as it exits from the superficial inguinal ring. Traction on the proximal end of the round ligament and the medial end of the groin node bundle facilitates the dissection of tissues containing lymphatic vessels leaving the vulva (Fig. 17-38).

The fatty nodal bundle is grasped with forceps and elevated by the operator or assistant. Anteromedially the long saphenous vein (LSV) is identified ascending into the thigh from the medial side. The vein can be left in situ but it is generally easier to ligate and divide with 1 polyglactin at the distal margin of the dissection.

Following ligation of the LSV the tissues on the medial and caudal side are dissected from the deep fascia. The cranial end of the ligated LSV is followed down to the saphenofemoral junction (Fig. 17-39). Although the pulsation of the

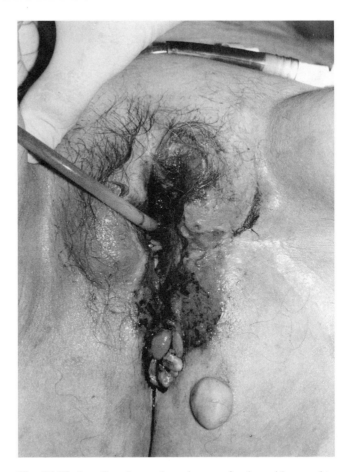

Fig. 17-27. Locally advanced carcinoma of vulva with spread to anus, urethra, and vagina.

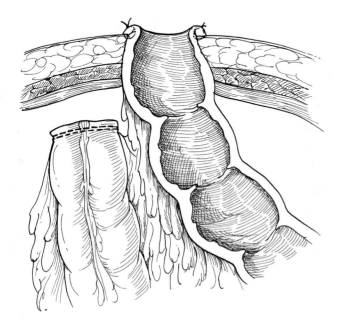

Fig. 17-26. Trephine sigmoid colostomy: cross-sectional representation of end result.

femoral artery is a good landmark for identifying the position of the femoral vein it is best approached by following down the medial side of the cranial end of the LSV. This end of the LSV is dissected free on all sides and the LSV is now ligated with a 1 polyglactin suture and divided approximately 0.5 to 1 cm from the saphenofemoral junction, taking care not to narrow the femoral vein. Traditionally, the vessel has been transfixed and ligated. The specimen is removed, leaving the saphenofemoral junction and floor of the femoral triangle exposed (Fig. 17-40).

The deep femoral nodes may have been removed with the specimen but if not, residual tissue is dissected from the anterior and medial surfaces of the femoral vein above the lower limit of the fossa ovalis. Any fatty tissue in the femoral canal is excised.

If the deep fascia has been extensively removed to expose much of the femoral artery and vein in the floor of the femoral triangle, and especially following preoperative radiation, a sartorius muscle flap can be swung across to protect the femoral vessels. The muscle forms the lateral boundary of

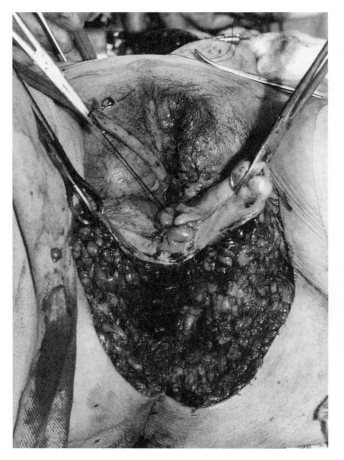

Fig. 17-28. Anovulvectomy: posterior dissection. The anus has been closed with a pursestring suture.

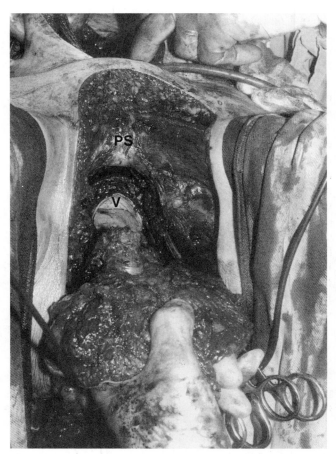

Fig. 17-29. Anovulvectomy: only the posterior vagina and rectum need to be transected to free the specimen. PS, pubic symphysis; V, vagina.

the femoral triangle running from the medial condyle of the tibia to the anterior superior iliac spine. A finger is passed underneath the belly of the upper part of the muscle and, using cutting Bovie, the muscle is divided close to the anterior superior iliac spine (Fig. 17-41). It is then swung across and sutured with 3–0 polyglactin to the inguinal ligament just above the femoral vessels (Fig. 17-42).

Before closure the skin flaps are checked to ensure that they are viable. If not they may need to be trimmed back to viable skin. The skin is closed with staples or interrupted 3–0 polyglactin vertical mattress sutures, ensuring that the skin edges are neatly apposed and everted (Fig. 17-43). A suction drain is brought out laterally above the groin and secured. If a large defect is left, such as after a more radical resection of disease in the groin, the defect can be closed with a skin flap.

Postoperative Management

Suction drainage is applied for up to 14 days to allow time for the incision to heal and the underlying space to be obliterated. Once the wound has healed the drain can be removed,

even if significant volumes of lymph are still draining. The wound is kept dry but inspected for signs of necrosis or infection. The staples can be removed at 14 days if the wound has healed cleanly.

Sequelae

Immediate complications of groin node dissection are unusual, provided that care is taken with the dissection. A small tear in the femoral vein should be repaired with 5–0 prolene while a larger tear may require a patch from the residual LSV. Damage to the femoral artery will necessitate repair with 5–0 prolene. A divided inguinal ligament can be repaired with 0 polyglactin or prolene.

It is not unusual for large volumes of lymph to collect in the drains. The staples are not removed until the wounds have healed at 2 to 3 weeks. At this time the drains can be removed even if lymph is still draining. Infection can occur early or chronically and is usually responsive to antibiotics. Persistent lymphocele is uncommon and usually the wound becomes adherent to the underlying tissues, obliterating the cavity that allows the fluid to collect.

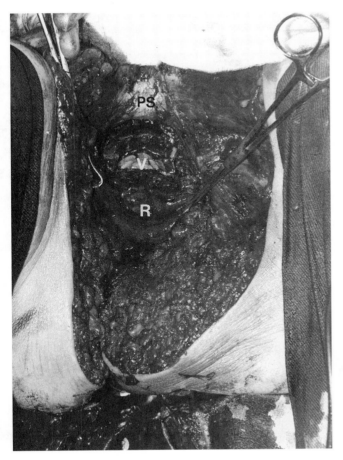

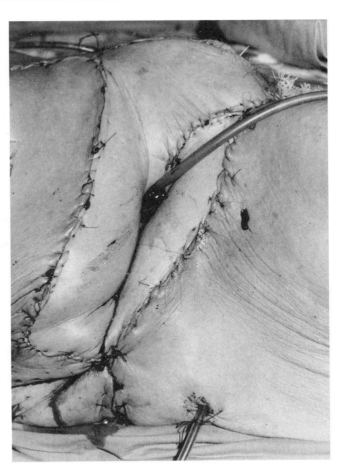

Fig. 17-30. Anovulvectomy: following tumor resection an assessment is made of the method of closure. PS, pubic symphysis; V, vagina; R, rectum.

Fig. 17-32. Anovulvectomy: a larger defect closed with a single rectus abdominis myocutaneous flap. (Courtesy of Mrs. A. Brain, FRCS.)

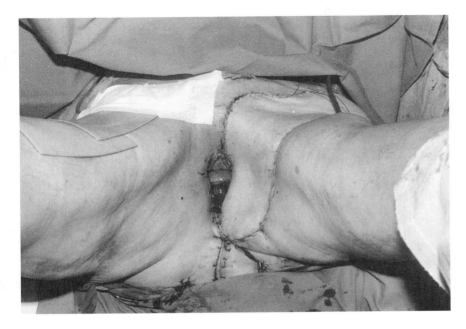

Fig. 17-31. Anovulvectomy: closure using a tensor fascia lata flap on the left side. (Courtesy of Mrs. A. Brain, FRCS.)

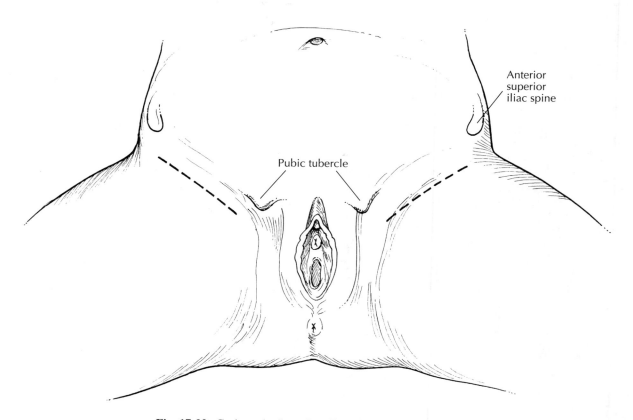

Fig. 17-33. Groin node dissection: line of incision and landmarks.

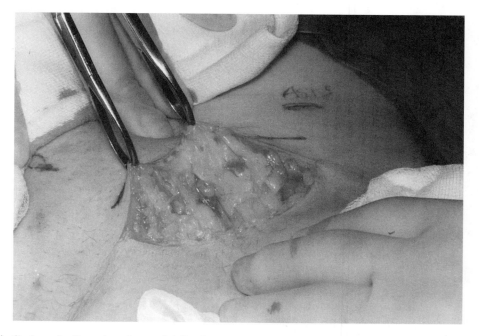

Fig. 17-34. Groin node dissection: the cranial flap is elevated with forceps. © University of Manchester, Manchester, England.

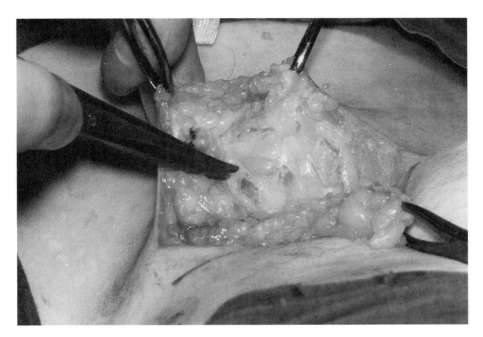

Fig. 17-35. Groin node dissection: dissection in subcutaneous fat toward the external oblique aponeurosis. © University of Manchester, Manchester, England.

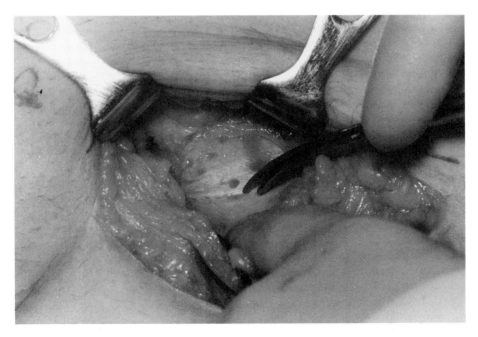

Fig. 17-36. Groin node dissection: the inguinofemoral fat pad is dissected off the external oblique aponeurosis. © University of Manchester, Manchester, England.

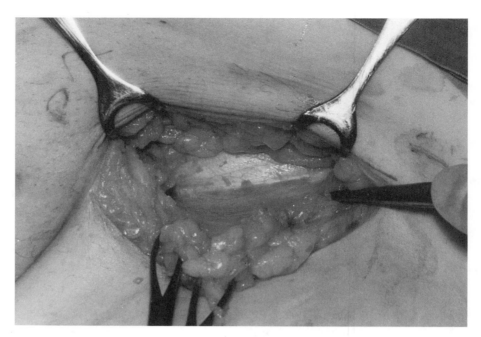

Fig. 17-37. Groin node dissection: lower edge of inguinal ligament exposed. © University of Manchester, Manchester, England.

The skin flaps may necrose partially or completely, particularly after radiation treatment. Dead tissue should be excised and the wound should be allowed to granulate.

Chronic swelling of the leg may occur as a consequence of the dissection, particularly if performed in association with radiation therapy, and this may be associated with recurrent bouts of infection. Infections can be treated with elevation and antibiotics but the swelling may be less responsive to therapy. The patient can try compression stockings and elevation.

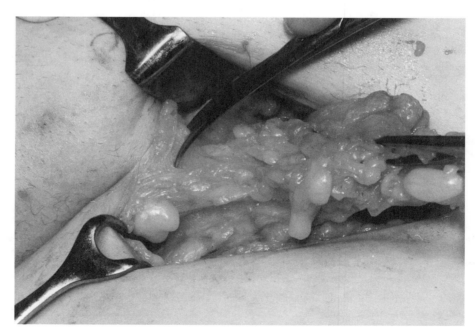

Fig. 17-38. Groin node dissection: with the inguinofemoral fat pad pulled laterally, the fatty tissue containing efferent lymphatics from the vulva is dissected off the skin and deep fascia. © University of Manchester, Manchester, England.

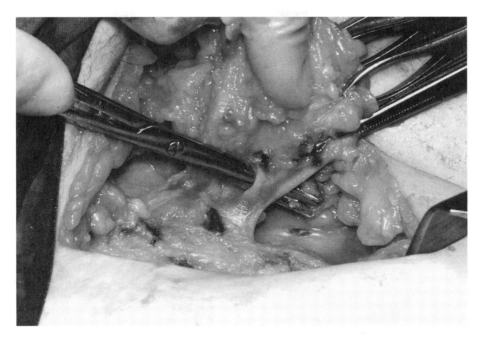

Fig. 17-39. Groin node dissection: the saphenofemoral junction has been isolated ready for ligation. © University of Manchester, Manchester, England.

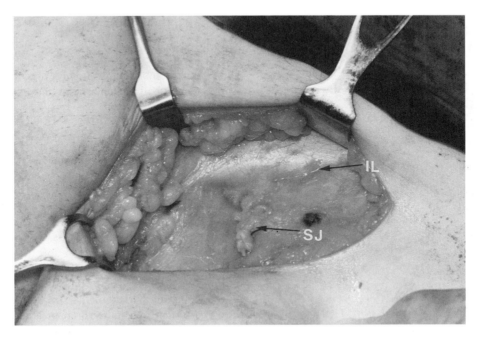

Fig. 17-40. Groin node dissection: the field after superficial node dissection. IL, inguinal ligament; SJ, saphenofemoral junction. © University of Manchester, Manchester, England.

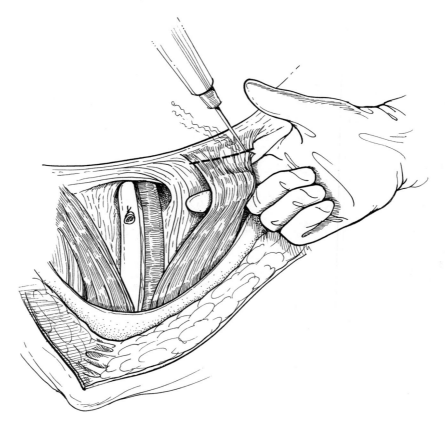

Fig. 17-41. Groin node dissection: sartorius muscle divided close to origin.

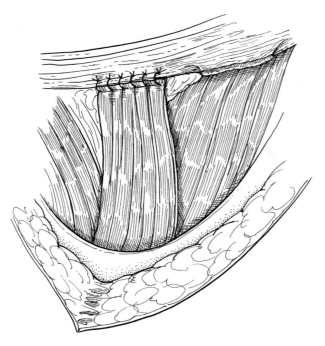

Fig. 17-42. Groin node dissection: sartorius muscle sutured to the inguinal ligament over the femoral vessels.

Excisional Biopsy of the Vagina

Indications

The most common indication for biopsy is to diagnose vaginal intraepithelial neoplasia and invasive carcinoma.

Operative Procedure

Punch biopsies of the vagina may be performed under local anesthetic but larger or multiple biopsies should be performed under general, epidural, or spinal anesthetic. This allows for optimal visualization of all parts of the vagina as well as ensuring patient comfort. The patient should be placed in the lithotomy position.

The technical difficulties of operating in the vagina make it easy for specimens to be less than adequate if due care is not given. Good visualization is provided by lateral wall retractors appropriate to the size of the vagina. The traditional Auvard speculum is rarely satisfactory. Initial examination and insertion of retractors should be performed gently to avoid trauma to the vaginal skin, which may interfere with interpretation of abnormalities.

Once the lesion to be excised has been examined, the area to be excised may be infiltrated with 1 in 100,000 epinephrine in 1-percent lidocaine solution to elevate the skin and

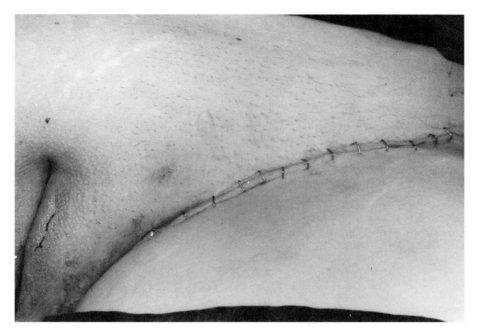

Fig. 17-43. Groin node dissection: incision closed with staples. © University of Manchester, Manchester, England.

reduce bleeding. Traction on small forceps applied to adjacent vagina will help to bring the area closer to the operator.

Although the exact incision will depend on the size and position of the lesion, an ellipse will give the best chance of closure. After the incision is made through the full thickness of the vagina the lower edge of the specimen is held with forceps while Metzenbaum scissors are used to dissect the tissue away. Bleeding points can be electrocauterized or, in the case of a punch biopsy, with silver nitrate sticks. Whether bleeding or not, it is usually a good idea to close vaginal biopsies with interrupted sutures to reduce the chance of postoperative hemorrhage. Care should be taken to ensure that the skin edges are everted so that residual disease, if present, is not buried. If closure is difficult or impossible, wounds can be left open to heal primarily.

Vaginectomy (Partial or Total)

Indication

Partial or total vaginectomy implies removal of the vaginal skin only without concern for tissues in the paracolpium, particularly at the upper end. The most common indication is for the treatment of vaginal intraepithelial neoplasia. Rarely, chronic benign conditions such as lichen planus may be severe enough to warrant vaginectomy.

Preoperative Preparation

Careful explanation to the patient is necessary before all vaginal procedures, particularly with regard to complications. Depending on the amount of vagina to be removed, the question of vaginal reconstruction should be raised. A thorough bowel preparation is mandatory in case of damage to the rectum or anus.

Operative Procedure

The anesthesia is either general, epidural, or spinal. If the approach is to be only via the perineum, and vaginal reconstruction is not planned, the patient may be placed in lithotomy. For all other procedures the patient is placed in a modified frog leg position in Allen stirrups.

For patients with an intact uterus who require total vaginectomy or upper partial vaginectomy, a total abdominal hysterectomy is usually performed at the same time. If two surgeons are available a combined abdominoperineal approach facilitates and speeds up the surgery. For patients who have previously undergone hysterectomy it is possible to perform total vaginectomy entirely from below. Great care must be taken to include all vaginal skin in the angles and vault of the vagina.

The vagina is initially inspected and the lower limit of resection identified. Since the vaginal part of the procedure is usually quicker than the abdominal, the vaginal operator may delay this dissection. The lower incision is made with a scalpel circumferentially around the vagina. Forceps are applied to the upper edge and gentle traction allows the operator to dissect the vaginal skin off underlying structures with scissors. Care must be taken anteriorly over the urethra because the tough underlying connective tissue makes dissection less easy. Buttonholes and tears of the vagina should be avoided. Dissection is continued as far up the vagina as can be reached easily. Bleeding from venous sinuses often requires underrunning.

The abdominal surgeon performs the first stages of a total abdominal hysterectomy (see Ch. 24). Broad ligaments are taken, uterine arteries are divided and ligated in the normal fashion, and the uterovesical fold of peritoneum is divided and the bladder dissected off the vagina. The bladder dissection is aided by traction on Kelly forceps applied to the peritoneal edge over the bladder and simultaneous traction on the uterus, which stretches up the vagina. Sharp dissection should be used to reduce bleeding and preserve tissue planes. The dissection should be continued laterally underneath the path of the distal ureters on each side. The peritoneum in the cul-de-sac is incised close to its attachment to the cervix and vagina, and the rectum is dissected gently away. With the assistance of the perineal surgeon this dissection can be completed readily.

Straight Zeppelin forceps are placed on the paravaginal tissues along the line of the vagina medial to the uterine artery pedicles. A scalpel is used to divide the tissues on the vaginal side and the pedicle is transfixed and ligated. It is important to ensure that the ureters are not caught in the forceps or resulting pedicle. If there is concern for the ureters, they should be dissected off the parametrium after deroofing the ureteric tunnel similar to the fashion discribed for radical hysterectomy (see Ch. 27). Further pedicles are taken until the lower limit of resection is reached. At a convenient moment the vagina is opened anteriorly from above, with the perineal surgeon guiding the point of entry.

Following removal of the specimen hemostasis is secured using electrocauterization and sutures. The procedure now depends on the extent of the vaginectomy and the need for vaginal reconstruction.

After a total vaginectomy, if no vaginal reconstruction is to be performed, the vaginal defect can be allowed to close off. A suction drain may be brought out through the abdomen or perineum. If there is persistent oozing a povidone-iodine-soaked pack can be inserted for 24 to 48 hours with its tail brought out through the perineum.

If an upper vaginectomy has been undertaken and vaginal reconstruction is not planned, the edges of the residual vagina may be run from above with continuous 0 polyglactin suture for hemostasis and left open. If there is only residual vaginal skin at the lower end, no special closure is necessary, although it is sometimes possible to mobilize the residual skin and sew the anterior and posterior edges together to prevent burial of possible intraepithelial neoplasia. Vaginal reconstruction is discussed below and in Chapter 18.

Following the extensive dissection close to bladder and ureters the competence of the ureters and bladder may be tested by injecting 5 ml of indigo carmine intravenously before closure. The dye will turn the urine blue. With the catheter temporarily occluded the bladder will distend and allow better examination of the bladder.

If the patient has had a previous hysterectomy, total or partial vaginectomy can be performed separately from above or below. There are proponents of both routes but the abdominal approach has the advantage of allowing better visualiza-

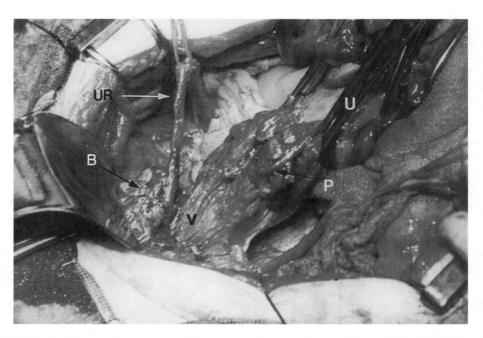

Fig. 17-44. Radical vaginectomy/hysterectomy. The uterus and upper vagina are being pulled cephalad. The right ureter has been dissected clear. UR, ureter; B, bladder, V, vagina; P, parametrium; U, uterus.

tion and dissection of the ureters, and a more complete excision of the vault and the corners of the vaginal vault where intraepithelial neoplasia can be hidden. Bowel adherent to the vault can also be dissected free.

In the abdominal approach the vault of the vagina is identified with a gauze roll on a sponge-holder placed in the vagina. The peritoneum over the vault is incised and the bladder is dissected off the vagina with dissecting scissors. The cul-de-sac peritoneum is incised and the rectum is separated from the vagina and uterosacral ligaments. The course of the ureters may have been somewhat distorted as a result of the previous hysterectomy. Great care must therefore be taken to identify them, and they may require dissecting out as per a radical hysterectomy in order to clear the area of

the upper vagina. Once the bladder, ureters, and rectum are clear the dissection continues as previously described.

Radical Vaginectomy

Indication

Usually performed at the time of pelvic exenteration for pelvic malignancy involving or encroaching on the vagina, a radical vaginectomy is rarely indicated for a highly select group of patients with early invasive carcinoma involving the upper vagina. If the uterus is present, radical hysterectomy is performed as part of the procedure.

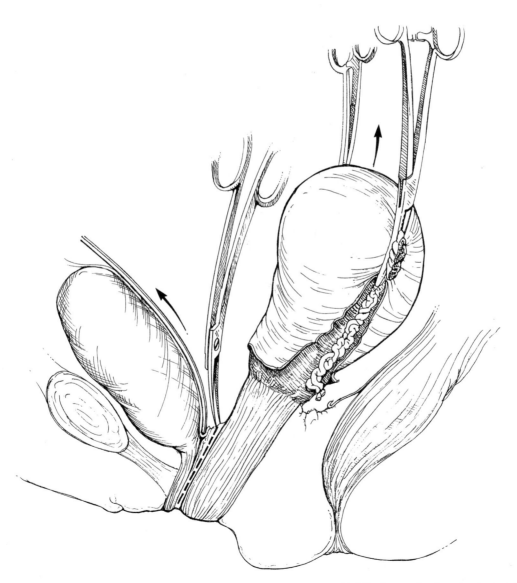

Fig. 17-45. Radical vaginectomy: the distal ureters and bladder are retracted while the proximal vagina is stretched up to facilitate further dissection.

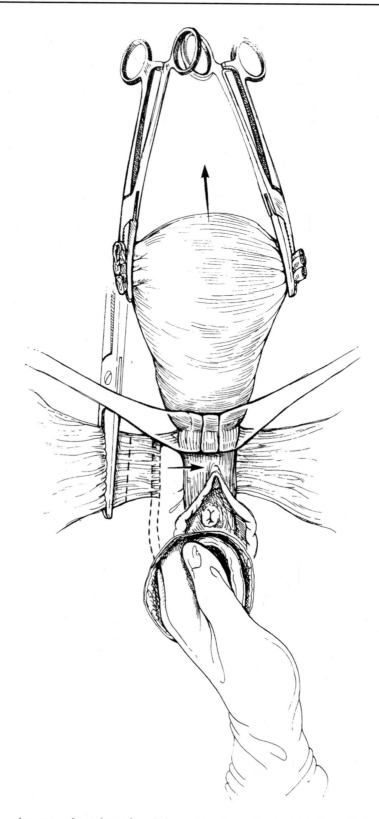

Fig. 17-46. Radical vaginectomy: the assistant from below guides the application of the Zeppelin forceps to the paravaginal tissues, protecting the vagina.

Operative Procedure

The principal difference between radical and nonradical vaginectomy is the extent of resection of tissues lateral to the upper half of the vagina.

When performed together with radical hysterectomy but not as part of an exenteration procedure, the distal ureters and bladder are dissected from the upper vagina, paracolpium, and parametrium; the rectum is separated from the vagina and uterosacral ligaments; and the uterosacral ligaments are divided as part of the radical hysterectomy (see Ch. 27). The parametrial tissues are clamped and ligated (Fig. 17-44). Following this, the bladder and ureters are gently elevated by retractors and while the uterus and vagina are stretched cephalad, the surgeon dissects the bladder distally off the vagina (Fig. 17-45). The perineal surgeon incises the vagina circumferentially and dissects the distal vagina off the rectum and urethra/bladder. With the index and middle fingers placed anterior and posterior to the tissues lateral to the vagina, the perineal surgeon (Fig. 17-46) pushes the vagina medially and guides the placement of the Zeppelin forceps onto these tissues by the abdominal surgeon. The upper lateral tissues of the paracolpium are clamped, divided, and ligated until the vagina is freed on both sides.

Hemostasis is then secured and vaginal reconstruction is performed if planned. A suction drain may be left in the pelvis.

Postoperative Management

If the bladder has been left in situ a 16 French Foley catheter is inserted suprapubically at the time of surgery. This allows bladder function to be assessed postoperatively before catheter removal. If a perineal pack has been placed it is removed after 24 to 48 hours. The patient is encouraged to resume a normal diet after return of flatus.

Sequelae

The major specific problems with regard to vaginectomy are urinary and rectal fistula and chronic bladder and rectal dysfunction. These complications are more common after radical vaginectomy. Radical vaginal surgery may alter body image perception and cause severe psychosexual problems.

Vaginal Reconstruction

Vaginal reconstruction (see Ch. 18) is best performed at primary surgery because the cavity is "ready" and does not require further dissection.

If a vaginectomy only has been performed without removal of the bladder or rectum, a number of techniques are available. A split-thickness skin graft may be applied to the residual tissues, if sufficient, or to an omental tube. A full-thickness skin graft, a transposition skin flap (e.g., pudendal thigh flap[14]), or a sigmoid colon neovagina are alternatives. Myocutaneous flaps are too bulky after nonradical surgery.

Following vaginectomy in combination with exenteration, reconstruction of a neovagina with skin flaps is inadequate. Myocutaneous flaps bring bulky vascularized tissue into the pelvis, which reduces the chance of the empty pelvis syndrome developing. Possibilities include gracilis[15] and the more reliable rectus abdominis flaps.[16] Recently, the use of a rectus abdominis flap with a paddle including transversus abdominis muscle and underlying peritoneum has been described.[17]

REFERENCES

1. Rutledge F, Sinclair M: Treatment of intraepithelial carcinoma of the vulva by skin excision and graft. Am J Obstet Gynecol 102:806, 1968
2. Rettenmaier MA, Braly PS, Roberts WS et al: Treatment of cutaneous vulvar lesions with skinning vulvectomy. J Reprod Med 30:478, 1985
3. Way S: The anatomy of the lymphatic drainage of the vulva and its influence on the radical operation for carcinoma. Ann R Coll Surg Engl 3:187, 1948
4. Helm CW, Hatch KD, Partridge EE, Shingleton HM: The rhomboid transposition flap for repair of the perineal defect after radical vulvar surgery. Gynecol Oncol 50:164, 1993
5. Wheeless CR, McGibbon B, Dorsey JH, Maxwell GP: Gracilis myocutaneous flap in reconstruction of the vulva and female perineum. Obstet Gynecol 54:97, 1979
6. Chafe W, Fowler WC, Walton LA, Currie JL: Radical vulvectomy with use of tensor fascia lata myocutaneous flap. Am J Obstet Gynecol 145:207, 1983
7. Hoffman MS, LaPolla JP, Roberts WS et al: Use of local flaps for primary anal reconstruction following perianal resection for neoplasia. Gynecol Oncol 36:348, 1990
8. Grimshaw RN, Ghazal Aswad S, Monaghan JM: The role of ano-vulvectomy in locally advanced carcinoma of the vulva. Int J Gynecol Cancer 1:15, 1991
9. Adams J, Daly JW: Proctectomy combined with vulvectomy for carcinoma of the vulva. Obstet Gynecol 54:643, 1979
10. Homesley HD, Bundy BN, Sedlis A et al: Assessment of current International Federation of Gynecology and Obstetrics staging of vulvar carcinoma relative to prognostic factors for survival. Am J Obstet Gynecol 164:997, 1991
11. Hacker NF: Current treatment of small vulvar cancers. Oncology 4:21, 1990
12. DiSaia PJ, Creasman WT, Rich WM: An alternative approach to early cancer of the vulva. Am J Obstet Gynecol 133:825, 1979
13. Borgno G, Micheletti L, Barbero M et al: Deep femoral lymph-

adenectomy with preservation of the fascia lata. J Reprod Med 35:1130, 1990

14. Wee JTK, Joseph VT: A new technique of vaginal reconstruction using neurovascular pudendal-thigh flaps: a preliminary report. Plast Reconst Surg 83:701, 1989

15. Copeland LJ, Hancock KC, Gershenson DM et al: Gracilis myocutaneous vaginal reconstruction concurrent with total pelvic exenteration. Am J Obstet Gynecol 160:1095, 1989

16. Tobin GR, Pursell SH, Day TG: Refinements in vaginal reconstruction using rectus abdominis flaps. Clin Plast Surg 17:705, 1990

17. Hockel M, Shumsky A, Konerding M et al: Myoperitoneal composite flaps—a new surgical principle for partial vulvovaginal reconstruction following anterior and posterior exenteration, abstracted. Society of Gynecologic Oncologists, San Francisco, 1995

CHAPTER EIGHTEEN

CREATION OF A NEOVAGINA

LISA JANE JACOBSEN
ALAN H. DECHERNEY

V aginal reconstructive surgery is used in a variety of clinical situations. Patients with congenital absence of the vagina are in need of a neovagina, as are patients with androgen insensitivity syndrome or extensive scarring from trauma, infection, or radiation. Replacement of the vagina may also be considered after extirpative surgery for urologic or gynecologic malignancies or cloacal malformations.

Throughout the world, there are a number of operative approaches to the construction of a neovagina. Certain procedures have fallen in and out of favor over the last 60 years and some have found greater popularity in Europe than in the United States. There are at least 15 different techniques used today and the choice of a specific technique depends on the needs and motivation of the patient as well as the skill and experience of the surgeon. The primary goal of this type of reconstructive surgery is to form a vagina that will enables the patient to have a sexual relationship that includes sexual intercourse.

CONGENITAL ABSENCE OF THE UTERUS AND VAGINA

The most common indication for vaginal reconstructive surgery seen by the gynecologic surgeon is congenital absence of the uterus and vagina. The incidence is quite low and cannot be stated with any precision, as evidenced by the variation in incidence rates given by different authors (1 in 4,000 to 80,000 female births).[1–5] The most frequently sited incidence is 1 in 4,000. Evans et al[6] estimated that vaginal agenesis occurred once in 10,588 female births in Michigan from 1953 to 1957.

Background

Matteo Realdo Columbo is generally credited with the first description of congenital absence of both the vagina and the uterus in 1572.[7] In 1829, Mayer described congenital absence of the vagina as one of the abnormalities found in stillborn infants with multiple birth defects. Rokitansky (1838) and Kuster (1910) described an entity in which the vagina was absent, a small bipartite uterus was present, the ovaries were normal, and anomalies of other organ systems (renal and skeletal) were frequently observed. Hauser (1961) emphasized the associated anomalies.[8] Over the years, the disorder became known as the Mayer-Rokitansky-Kuster-Hauser syndrome (Fig. 18-1).

Presentation

These patients usually present to the gynecologist's office between the ages of 15 and 18 years with primary amenorrhea or inability to accomplish intercourse. On examination,

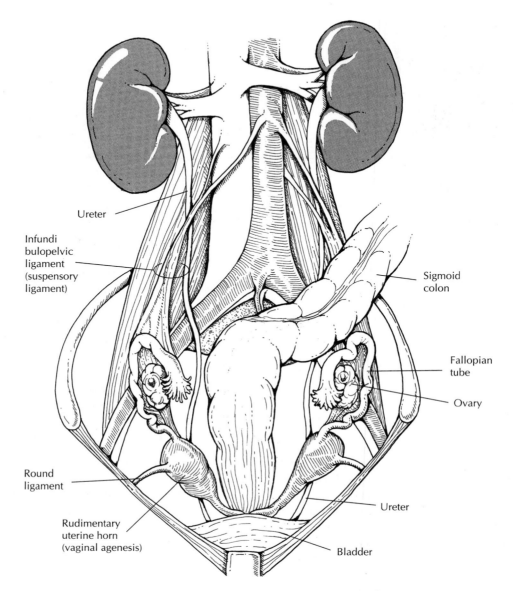

Ureter

Infundi
bulopelvic
ligament
(suspensory
ligament)

Sigmoid
colon

Fallopian
tube

Ovary

Round
ligament

Rudimentary
uterine horn
(vaginal agenesis)

Ureter

Bladder

Fig. 18-1. Internal anatomy of a patient with Mayer-Rokitansky-Kuster-Hauser syndrome.

they have normal secondary sexual characteristics and normal appearing external genitalia. In place of a vagina they have a dimple or a small pouch. The internal anatomy usually consists of two small, rudimentary uterine anlagens connected only by peritoneum. The uterine anlagens lack endometrial tissue and each is attached to a fallopian tube. The ovaries are normal.

Approximately 30 to 40 percent of patients with vaginal agenesis will also have a concomitant urologic abnormality.[2,9] Fore et al[5] reports that 47 percent of patients in whom an evaluation of the urinary tract was performed had associated urologic abnormalities, such as unilateral renal agenesis, unilateral or bilateral pelvic kidney, horseshoe kidney, hydronephrosis, hydroureter, and ureteral duplication.

Five to 28 percent of patients will have skeletal anoma-

lies.[2,9] Griffin[3] reviewed 574 cases and found 12 percent had skeletal abnormalities. Two-thirds involved the spine (wedge vertebrae, fusions, rudimentary vertebral bodies, supernumerary vertebrae) and the rest involved the limbs and ribs (malformed arms or legs, syndactyly, rib deformity, or extra ribs). The incidence of these anomalies was probably underestimated, as most patients did not get a full radiologic evaluation.

Embryology

True vaginal agenesis is thought to result from dysgenesis of the müllerian ducts, which also leads to agenesis of the uterus. Occasionally, a patient with a long transverse septum that extends through almost the entire vagina will be diagnosed as having a true vaginal agenesis, but these patients differ in that they have a functioning uterus and, usually, cervix. Both complete and ''partial'' vaginal agenesis fall into class IA of the American Fertility Society's classification of müllerian anomalies (segmental müllerian agenesis/hypoplasia—vaginal)[10] but their embryologic origins are different. Complete vaginal agenesis is thought to be due to dysgenesis of the inferior portion of the müllerian ducts. Partial vaginal agenesis (or transverse septae) represents a problem with vertical fusion—a disorder in the junction between the down-growing müllerian ducts (müllerian tubercle) and the up-growing derivative of the urogenital sinus.[9]

All embryos develop a wolffian (mesonephric) duct system. In females, the müllerian (paramesonephric) duct system is stimulated to develop over the wolffian system, which regresses in early fetal life (Fig. 18-2A). The cranial parts of the wolffian ducts may persist as the epoophoron—cystic structures in the mesosalpinx. The caudal parts may persist as Gartner's duct cysts in the vagina The two lateral müllerian ducts grow in a medial and caudal direction. They eventually meet in the midline and become fused together. The septum between the two müllerian ducts gradually disappears, leaving a single uterovaginal canal that will form the uterus and part of the vagina (Fig. 18-2B). Persistence of this septum between the two lumina can result in a septate uterus (arcuate, bicornuate, or uterine didelphis). The most cranial portions of the müllerian ducts remain separate and form the fallopian tubes.

The vagina is formed from the lower end of the fused müllerian ducts and the urogenital sinus. A solid vaginal cord grows from a proliferation of cells at the caudal tip of the fused müllerian ducts. The cord elongates in a caudal direction toward the urogenital sinus. Sinovaginal bulbs begin to grow cranially from the urogenital sinus toward the solid vaginal cord (Fig. 18-2C). They finally fuse with the vaginal cord to form the vaginal plate. The proliferation continues at the cranial end of the plate, thus increasing the distance between the uterus and the urogenital sinus. Canalization of the vaginal cord then occurs and is complete by the fifth month (Fig. 18-2D).

There is controversy regarding whether the vaginal plate is derived from the müllerian and wolffian ducts or from the urogenital sinus. Since it is believed that this plate gives rise to most of the vagina, the embryologic origin of the vagina is uncertain. Some report that the top two-thirds of the vagina comes from the paramesonephric ducts,[11] while others report that it is only the top one-third, with the urogenital sinus contributing the rest.[8,12] It has been reported that the vaginal plate and vagina may develop under the influence of the müllerian ducts and estrogenic stimulation.[13]

The close developmental relationship of the müllerian ducts and the wolffian ducts can explain why anomalies of the female genital system and urinary tract are often associated. The wolffian ducts give rise to the ureteric bud from which the bladder, ureters, and the collecting system of the kidney are derived. They are also essential in the development of the müllerian ducts and serve as a template for their growth. Dysplasia of the wolffian ducts can lead to abnormal development of both systems. Given their close proximity, any insult that affects müllerian duct development could potentially lead to agenesis of the renal system by inhibiting growth of the ureteric bud from the wolffian duct.

Etiology

The etiology of Mayer-Rokitansky-Kuster-Hauser syndrome is unclear. No teratogen likely to cause a lesion between the sixth and eighth week of embryonic life has been identified. A genetic etiology has been suggested, although a discordance of vaginal agnesis in three sets of monozygotic

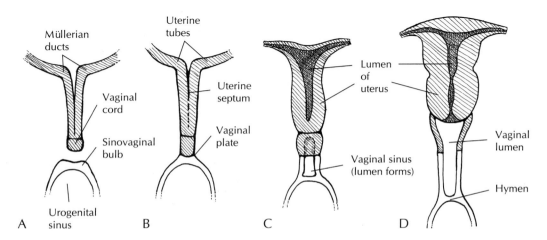

Fig. 18-2. **(A)** Embryologic development of the vagina and uterus. **(B)** Note disappearance of the uterine septum. **(C)** The tissue of the sinovaginal bulbs. **(D)** Complete canalization of the vaginal chord.

twins is evidence against an exclusively genetic etiology.[14] Griffen[3] hypothesizes that the finding of occasional familial occurrence is consistent with several different interpretations. First, some cases may be due to a hereditary abnormality and the remainder to some other type of developmental defect. Second, all cases may result from a mutant gene, but due to natural selection against the transmission of the gene, familial cases are unusual. Finally, if congenital absence of the vagina can represent only one manifestation of a variably expressed genetic defect, ascertainment may not be adequate in most instances, so that the real frequency of familial involvement has been underestimated.

DIAGNOSTIC EVALUATION

The patient who presents with primary amenorrhea and has an abnormal vagina needs a workup to determine the underlying cause so that the appropriate surgical intervention can be made. One needs to be able to differentiate between an imperforate hymen, transverse septum, and vaginal agenesis, because each condition is treated differently. The patient with androgen insensitivity needs to be identified because she must also undergo surgery for removal of the testes because of the risk of malignant transformation. A proper diagnosis is important. The most common indication for a second operation is a missed diagnosis where there has been an unplanned exploration of the space between the rectum and bladder in search of a vagina through what was expected to be an imperforate hymen.[9]

An imperforate hymen is the most frequent obstructing müllerian malformation. The incidence is reportedly 1 in 1,000 women.[15] Patients with imperforate hymens usually present with not only the complaint of primary amenorrhea, but also have a pelvic mass and pain from the menstrual blood that has accumulated behind the obstruction. The hymen usually bulges from the force of the fluid or with bearing down. These patients will occasionally present in infancy with a mucocolpos from accumulated mucous secretions. The hymen is often somewhat transparent. To rule out an absent vagina in unclear cases, a metal instrument can be placed in the urethra and a rectal examination performed. If this object is easily palpated through the anterior rectal wall, the vagina may be absent. An intervening mass may be a hematocolpos.

A transverse vaginal septum is one of the least common müllerian abnormalities, occurring in 1 of every 80,000 women.[4] These patients also present with primary amenorrhea, cyclic pelvic pain, and a pelvic-abdominal mass. Most have a central microperforation that helps to make the diagnosis. A rectal examination can help to differentiate a transverse septum from vaginal agenesis. In cases in which the transverse septum is quite thick, the diagnosis may be hard to make. These patients should all have a uterus and cervix, and ultrasound can help to identify these structures if they are not easily palpated on rectal examinations. Some centers are using magnetic resonance imaging to identify the uterus and to better determine the thickness of the septum.

An absent vagina can be diagnosed in a patient who presents with a vaginal dimple or a small pouch at the introitus, no palpable structures between the rectum and urethra, and no uterus on rectal examination or ultrasound. Before identifying the abnormality as Mayer-Rokitansky-Kuster-Hauser syndrome, androgen insensitivity must be ruled out.

Patients with androgen insensitivity are usually tall, have large breasts, and have normal appearing external genitalia except that they may have sparse or no pubic hair. The vagina can vary from a simple dimple to a pouch that is 2 cm deep. A testosterone level and a karyotype will help make the diagnosis. Patients with androgen insensitivity are candidates for the same vaginal reconstructive procedures available to the girl with vaginal agenesis. It is imperative that they undergo gonadectomy after puberty is complete but before age 20, when the risk of malignant transformation becomes significant. They will also require lifelong hormone replacement.

If congenital vaginal agenesis is diagnosed, an intravenous pyelogram should be obtained to look for urologic abnormalities. Occasionally a patient with vaginal agenesis will present with cyclic pelvic pain from endometrial tissue within the uterine anlagens. Attempts have been made to use these rudimentary uterine bulbs to reconstruct a midline uterus, which is then connected to a newly constructed vagina.[16,17] Many of these patients developed cyclical bleeding, but recurrent stenosis and obstruction of the horns was the most common outcome. Four pregnancies have been reported after metroplasty and attachment to a neovagina.[17-20] Much more frequently, however, repeated surgical procedures, sepsis, and ultimately, hysterectomy have resulted.[21,22] Removal of the uterine remnants is generally advocated in cases in which cyclical pelvic pain is a problem.[8,10,22] Laparoscopic removal has recently been reported.[23]

PREOPERATIVE CONSIDERATIONS AND APPROPRIATE TIMING

Deciding on which procedure to perform depends on the special circumstances of the patient. Gynecologic oncologists tend to use myocutaneous flaps and bowel to create neovaginas at the time of exenteration. A gynecologic surgeon treating a patient with vaginal agenesis or androgen insensitivity may choose a nonsurgical pressure technique or an Abbe-Wharton-McIndoe procedure. Williams' vulvovaginoplasty and full-thickness skin grafts are preferred by others. The Vechietti procedure is popular in Europe. The gynecologist should be familiar with a few different techniques and be able to choose the one that will be of greatest benefit given the patient's situation.

The most frequent indication for a neovagina that the

gynecologic surgeon comes across is vaginal agenesis and occasionally, androgen insensitivity. These patients present in adolescence and the appropriate time to create the neovagina appears to be when the patient has shown the emotional maturity necessary to be able to reliably participate in the procedure. The patient must be cooperative for the operation to be successful. She must have strong motivation and personal commitment. Her understanding of the necessary aftercare and its critical importance in determining the success of the procedure are essential.[1] If emotional maturity is lacking, the surgery should be postponed.

The single most important factor in determining the success of vaginoplasty is the psychosocial adjustment of the patient to her congenital vaginal anomaly. Some never adjust and, despite a successful surgical result, are emotionally unable to use the vagina for sexual relations.

The diagnosis of vaginal agenesis usually occurs when adolescents are extremely sensitive about the appearance of their bodies. Patients often exhibit varying degrees of depression[24] and may develop feelings of defectiveness and inadequacy.[25] A patient's sexual identity may be compromised and she may have concerns about her ability to ever become a wife and mother. The diagnosis of congenital absence of the vagina is an indication for a psychiatric referral. Therapy should include the parents as well, because their adjustment to the disorder will greatly affect the patient's acceptance of it. Kaplan,[25] in a study of 17 patients with vaginal agenesis, found that parents often react with feelings of guilt, anxiety, disappointment, depression, and pity. From this reaction, a young girl can get the message of defectiveness, with a lasting imprint on self-image. He advised early diagnosis of the disorder so that there would be time to deal with the irrational reactions of the parents and patient and facilitate "a conscious acceptance of the defect in a realistic light."

The psychiatrist can help make the decision as to when the patient is ready for the procedure. It should be early enough that the patient has time to form a positive body image and develop self-confidence so that she can eventually have romantic relationships. She must, however, be emotionally mature enough to think of herself as a woman capable of sexual intercourse. If the patient is not motivated enough to have a functional vagina for coitus, she may find the vaginal procedure, as well as the necessary postoperative manipulation of the dilators or mold, intolerable.

Most patients are ready for the procedure around the age of 16. This also is the time when medical insurance coverage under a parent's plan is close to running out, another incentive to perform the procedure before age 18. The beginning of summer vacation can be an ideal time.

NONSURGICAL METHODS

In 1938, Robert Frank[26] described a method of forming a neovagina without an operation. His method involves a system of progressive dilation by applying pressure to an introital dimple to stretch it through the fibroareolar tissue between the bladder and rectum.[27] A dilator (1.5 cm by 1.5 cm) is introduced into the center of the hymenal region and pressure is applied in a caudad direction away from the urethra (Fig. 18-3). This is performed for 20 minutes, once a day. This stretches the mucosa so that further dilation does not dilate or distort the urethral meatus. After the first week, a caudal pouch 2 to 3 cm in depth is created and the direction of the pressure is changes to cephalad. The patient continues to apply pressure like this for 20 to 30 minutes every day. In 2 to 4 weeks, the depression is sufficient to permit one-half of the tube to be retained and within 6 to 8 weeks, a 7.5-cm vagina should be created. The patient then starts to use a wider dilator (2 cm) to increase the vaginal width. An adequate vagina is formed in approximately 4 to 6 months[28] but it is important to continue dilating the vagina several times a week or have regular intercourse in order to keep the opening sufficiently dilated. Frank[29] found, in his follow-up of eight patients, that the vagina remained permanent in depth and caliber, even in patients who neglected dilation for more than 1 year.

Ingram,[30] in 1975, altered Frank's approach by building a bicycle seat stool on which patients could sit with a dilator in place (Fig. 18-4). Ingram believed that the Frank method had not been accepted with enthusiasm by gynecologists or patients because the technique was too time-consuming and uncomfortable for the patient. It was not a lack of motivation on the part of the patient but rather three factors: (1) sheer fatigue of hands and fingers, (2) necessity for use of awkward lithotomy, squatting, or Sims' position, and (3) inability to perform other productive activities during the hours of required pressure. The bicycle seat enables the weight of the trunk of the body to be substituted for manual and digital exertion. The patient sits upright and a Lucite dilator held in place by a girdle under the clothes, presses against the bicycle seat. Activities such as homework, that can be performed in a sitting position, can be carried out during this time.

The first objective in this technique is to establish a narrow canal 1.5 cm wide and about 6 cm long. This can be created in 4 to 6 weeks and does not dilate the urethral meatus as it is so narrow. By increasing the length but not the width of the mold, a vaginal depth of 10 cm can be achieved within another 4 weeks. The neovagina can then be enlarged to a diameter of 3.5 cm by the use of progressively wider dilators. The patient needs to use the dilator for at least 2 hours per day. A prime component of the technique is using previous patients who had successful outcomes to volunteer as role models for the girls, to encourage them in their efforts.

Ingram used this technique on patients with vaginal agenesis, androgen insensitivity, stenosis from contracture after a MacIndoe or Wharton procedure, and partial transverse vaginal septa. Of the 26 he performed between 1975 and 1980, 20 were successful and 6 failed (coitus was impossible). He believed that having a vaginal dimple or an introital

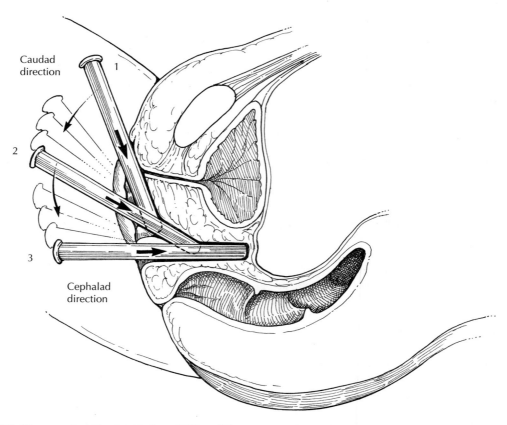

Fig. 18-3. Nonoperative: Frank technique. With a dilator, pressure is applied to the center of the hymenal region in a caudad direction. After a 2 to 3 cm pouch is created, the direction of the pressure changes to cephalad. Within 6 to 8 weeks, a 7.5-cm vagina is created.

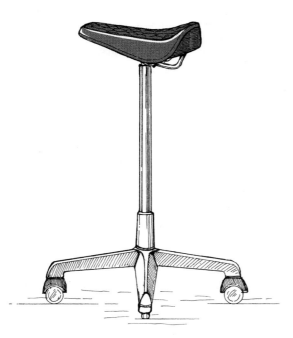

Fig. 18-4. Ingram bicycle seat stool.

pouch was not a requirement for proceeding with a nonsurgical technique. The technique took 4 to 6 months to achieve an adequate vagina and there were no complications.

Few complications are associated with this procedure, although prolapse of the neovagina and enterocele have been reported.[31] Contraction of the cavity can result if the neovagina is not dilated regularly or the patient is not having regular intercourse.

SURGICAL METHODS

Background

Over the last 180 years, many different methods of creating a neovagina have been used. Certain techniques have fallen out of favor, while others have been improved on over the years and are frequently used today. Pediatric surgeons, general surgeons, gynecologic oncologists, and operative gynecologists tend to have particular techniques that have become popular within their specialties. It is important for all surgeons doing this type of surgery to be familiar with several different techniques so that the operation most appropriate for the patient's particular situation will be chosen.

Dupuytren is credited with the first attempt at surgical correction of an absent vagina in 1817.[7] His attempt was unsuccessful, resulting in death from septicemia. Amussat, in 1832, described using his finger to dissect between the bladder and rectum of a patient with vaginal agenesis and then packing the cavity with sponge tampons. In 1898, Abbe modified the procedure by placing into the cavity a split-thickness skin graft from the thigh, wrapped around a rubber pouch stuffed with iodoform gauze.[7] In 1938, Wharton[32] combined adequate dissection of the vaginal space with continuous dilation by a balsa form covered with a thin rubber sheath. This was based on the principle that vaginal epithelium would proliferate and, in a short time, would cover the raw surface. Occasionally, however, the epithelium does not cover the entire vault and coital bleeding and leukorrhea result from persistent granulation tissue. This leads to scarring of the vagina in the upper portion.[8]

In 1938, Sir Archibald McIndoe[33] at Queen Victoria Hospital in England popularized a method that combined many of the principles developed before him. He emphasized, first, the dissection of an adequate space between the rectum and bladder. Second, an inlay split-thickness skin graft was placed so that the newly formed cavity would have an epithelial lining. Third, he recognized the most important principal of continuous and prolonged dilation during the contractile phase of healing of the skin graft. He advised wearing a mold continuously for 6 months following surgery. Counsellor and Flor[34] modified this technique in 1958, by using a foam rubber mold covered by a condom instead of the acrylic shells used by McIndoe. Human amnion has since been used successfully in place of the split-thickness skin graft.[35–37]

While this technique was being developed, some vastly different operations were being performed. Surgeons were using bowel to create neovaginas in the early part of the 20th century. Others used skin flaps from the labia and inner thighs. Myocutaneous flaps using the gracilis rectus abdominis muscle or gained popularity. Vechietti's technique was used frequently in Western Europe and Asia and involved traction from within the abdomen to stretch the introital pouch into a full length vagina. The Williams vulvovaginaplasty to create a pouch out of vulvar skin was also popular because of its relative simplicity. Each of these procedures has its useful application; but most have significant drawbacks as well.

Abbe-Wharton-McIndoe Procedure

This procedure is the most popular one among gynecologists. Patients should be given a full bowel preparation because of the risk of bowel-lumen entry during the initial dissection of the vaginal space. Prophylactic antibiotics should be given before surgery and for 1 week following.

The first step involves harvesting the split-thickness skin graft. The skin graft should be taken from the buttocks, if possible, as the scar is more cosmetically desirable than one taken from the hip or thigh. Patients can be asked to sunbathe in a bathing suit prior to surgery so that tan lines can be used to guide the best location. A Padgett or Reese electric dermatome is used to obtain a graft that is 0.016 to 0.020 in. thick and 8 to 9 cm wide. The total graft length should be 20 to 25 cm. If it is not possible to take the graft from one buttock, two separate grafts measuring 10 to 13 cm long from each buttock can be used.

The skin is prepared by scrubbing it with an antiseptic solution that is washed away thoroughly. The skin is stretched and the graft is obtained, taking care not to create any breaks in the continuity of the graft. The graft is placed between two layers of saline-moistened gauze and the donor sites are dressed. A dilute solution of epinephrine for hemostasis is placed over the donor site and a sterile pressure dressing is applied. This dressing stays in place until the postoperative day 7.

Passing the graft through a meshing device has been advocated by some.[28] This makes the graft more expandable, and the fenestrations prevent serous drainage buildup behind the graft, so that there is a higher percentage of graft-take. The disadvantage lies in the increased risk of formation of granulation tissue in areas not completely covered by graft tissue. For this reason, it is not advocated.

The patient is then placed in a dorsal lithotomy position in preparation for the creation of the neovaginal space. A transverse incision is made through the mucosa of the vaginal vestibule. A space between the urethra and bladder anteriorly and rectum posteriorly is bluntly dissected with fingers (Fig. 18-5A). The dissection is continued superiorly and laterally, creating a channel on each side of a median raphe, until the peritoneum is reached (Fig. 18-5B). A catheter should be placed in the urethra and a finger in the rectum in order to guide the dissection in the proper plane. Hegar dilators or Kelly clamps may also be helpful in the dissection. The median raphe is then divided so that one continuous cavity results (Fig. 18-5C). The puborectalis muscles may need to be incised bilaterally along the midportion of the median vagina to avoid a subsequent narrowing of the vagina at the level of the pelvic diaphragm. The cavity should be continued as high as possible without entering the peritoneal cavity and without cleaning away all tissue beneath the peritoneum (Fig. 18-5D). The split-thickness skin graft will not take well when applied against a base of thin peritoneum. It is also thought to increase the chances of future prolapse and enterocele formation if the dissection is too close to the peritoneum.

It is important to ligate all bleeders along the way. If no specific bleeding vessel can be identified, microfibrillar collagen (Avitene) can be used. It is essential to have a vaginal cavity that is dry, to prevent bleeding beneath the graft. Bleeding will cause the graft to separate from its base, prevent it from implanting in that area, and part of the graft may necrose.

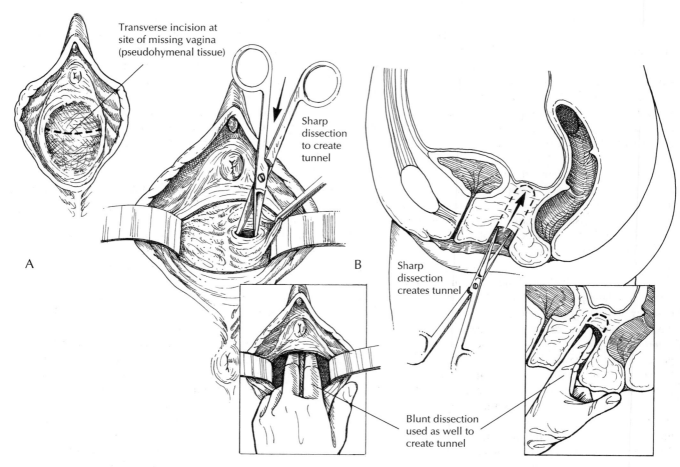

Fig. 18-5. McIndoe technique. **(A)** A space is made between the urethra and bladder anteriorly and rectum posteriorly. **(B)** The dissection is continued until a median raphe is created. (*Figure continues.*)

If the rectum is entered during the dissection, it must be repaired and the procedure terminated to allow it to fully heal. If the bladder is entered, it can be repaired and the procedure can continue. If the peritoneum is entered, it can be primarily closed with a pursestring suture before proceeding.

With the assistance of another surgeon, the skin graft can be sewn over the vaginal form at the same time the neovaginal space is being dissected. A commercially available vaginal stent, consisting of a watertight silicone elastomer shell filled with polyurethane foam, can be used (Mentor mold). This stent has a drainage tube through the center and can be inflated with normal saline to adjust the size. If this is not available, one can be made using the technique described by Counsellor and Flor.[34] The mold can be cut from a foam rubber block. It should be cut approximately twice the desired size and compressed by covering it with a condom. The form is placed into the vagina and left in place to allow the foam rubber to expand and conform to the space. The condom is then closed and the form is withdrawn. The external end is tied with 2–0 silk, and an additional condom is placed over the form and tied securely.

The skin graft is placed over the form with its raw surface exteriorized (Fig. 18-6). It is then sewn over the form with interrupted stitches using a 5–0 nonreactive suture. The suture line should be along the longitudinal axis of the mold. Care should be taken not to have a seam at the apex of the form, as this will impede the chances of the graft taking. Granulation tissue can grow any place where the form is not covered with skin.

The form can then be placed into the neovaginal space and the edges of the graft are sutured to the skin edge with 5–0 nonreactive absorbable suture, allowing space between sutures for drainage to occur. The form should not be so large as to cause pressure on the urethra or rectum. A suprapubic catheter is placed in the bladder to avoid pressure necrosis of the urethra, caused when a large form presses against a Foley catheter. The labia can be sutured together with a few nonreactive sutures, to hold the form in place. The patient should be placed on a low-residue diet, prescribed a stool softener, and kept supine in bed for 7 to 10 days. She may benefit from physical therapy during this time.

After 7 to 10 days, the form is removed and the cavity is irrigated with saline and inspected. This should be done in

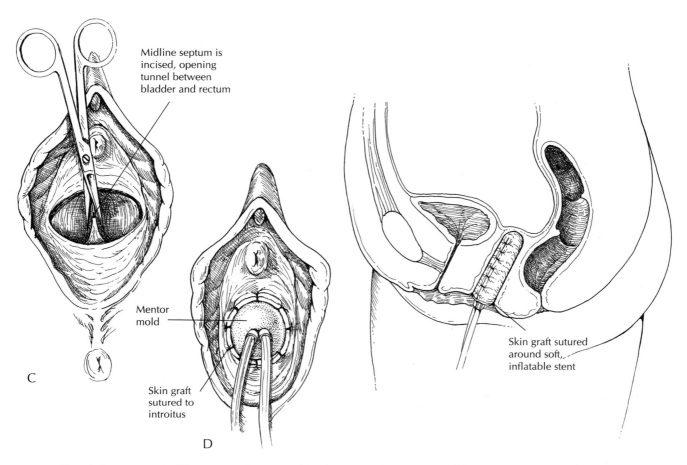

Midline septum is
incised, opening
tunnel between
bladder and rectum

Mentor
mold

Skin graft
sutured to
introitus

Skin graft sutured
around soft,
inflatable stent

C

D

Fig. 18-5 (*Continued*). **(C)** The raphe is cut, resulting in one continuous cavity. **(D)** The depth and axis of the tunnel of the neovagina is shown.

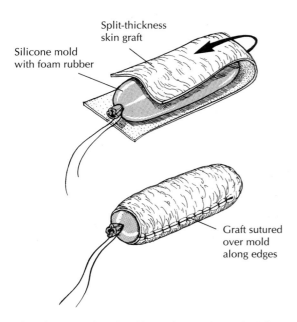

Split-thickness
skin graft

Silicone mold
with foam rubber

Graft sutured
over mold
along edges

Fig. 18-6. Suturing the skin graft over the vaginal form.

the operating room with mild sedation. The form is replaced with a firm dilator (many brands are available). The dilator can be held in place by wearing a girdle and a sanitary napkin. The patient is instructed to remove it daily and reinsert it after washing the cavity with a low-pressure, warm water douche. It is to be removed only for urination and defecation, but otherwise should be worn for 2 weeks continuously. The patient continues to wear it for 6 months, but may remove it for intercourse. The contractile phase of the graft, when constriction is most likely to occur, lasts 6 months. She then decreases usage to 3 nights per week until she is sexually active on a regular basis. If there is ever any difficulty in inserting the mold, the patient should be advised to wear it continuously again.

McIndoe[33] reported on 63 cases that he performed over a 12-year period. Of the cases, 61 were for congenital atresia and 2 were for acquired strictures. Of the patients, 89 percent had "excellent" results, meaning that the vagina measured 12 cm by 3 cm, and normal intercourse was possible. In Counseller's series of 70 patients using the same technique, 78 percent had excellent results and 7 percent failed.[38] Thompson et al[11] reported an 81 percent success rate with their series of 29 patients. Evans[39] had good results with 75 percent of 110 patients, fairly satisfactory results with 13 percent, and a very poor outcome with 13 percent. Most of these failures were due to improper or inadequate use of the obturator. Cali and Pratt[40] followed 71 patients for 10 to 37 years after surgery (mean of 19 years) and found that 93 percent reported satisfactory coitus, despite some contraction in one-half of the patients.

The mucosa created by this procedure appears like normal vaginal mucosa and responds normally to hormones.[24] Masters and Johnson[41] showed that it even has the ability to emulate the native vagina throughout the phases of sexual excitement. Evans et al[6] reports that more than 90 percent of his patients are orgasmic after the McEndoe procedure.

The procedure is, however, associated with a few troublesome complications. Graft failure can occur, although Rock[8] reported that 83 percent of 94 patients who had McEndoe procedures done at John Hopkins Hospital had 100 percent take of the graft: In areas not covered by the graft, troublesome granulation tissue can grow. The canal can become infected, which inhibits healing and promotes scarring. Contracture can be a big problem in patients who have difficulty using the dilator and who are not sexually active on a regular basis. The rectum, bladder, and urethra can be injured during surgery. Rectovaginal and urethrovaginal fistulas have been described. Intraoperative and postoperative hemmorhage can occur.

Prolapse of the neovagina with enterocele has been reported. It is thought that the weakness of the support structures of the neovagina can be made greater if the underside of too much peritoneal cul-de-sac is exposed during creation of the tunnel.[1] Nichols and Randall[1] suggest transabdominal sacral colpopexy or transvaginal sarospinous ligament fixations in such patients.

Despite the wide variety of possible complications, their occurrence is infrequent and, in general, this is a reasonably safe procedure that usually brings good results.

Vaginoplasty Using Human Amnion

Human amnion has been used in place of a split-thickness skin graft in creating neovaginas with the McIndoe technique.[35–37] Amnion is an inexpensive allograph with low antigenicity, high antimicrobial activity, and the ability to enhance epithelialization.[36] Membranes are taken immediately postpartum from a patient who has been afebrile and who has been ruptured for less than 12 hours. A woman undergoing an elective cesarean section is ideal. The amnion is separated from the chorion, leaving a small portion of chorion adherent in order to distinguish each side of amnion. The amnion is then rinsed in sterile saline until free of contaminants such as blood, vernix, or meconium and stored at 4°C in saline containing 50,000 U/100 ml of crystalline penicillin. It should be harvested close to the time it will be used for the neovaginal surgery, but it has been shown to last for days.

Once a cavity has been dissected, the amnion is draped over a mold with its chorion side outwards and inserted into the cavity. After 7 days, the mold is removed and a clean mold covered with a new piece of amnion is inserted. After 7 more days, the mold is removed and the patient is instructed to use a vaginal dilator at least three times daily for 15 minutes to keep the cavity open.

Morton and Dewhurst[35] showed that by the time of the second mold change, epithelialization was complete in 24 of 27 patients undergoing this procedure. By 4 weeks after the operation, healthy pink vaginal epithelium was visible. Dhall[37] showed that vaginal biopsies taken 4 to 6 weeks after operation showed early epithelialization, which was replaced by mature epithelium by the end of 8 to 10 weeks. The ultimate results, however, depend on the motivation of the patient. Postoperative dilation is essential to prevent vaginal contraction, which has a tendency to occur in this procedure, as it does when the split-thickness skin graft technique is used. The degree of contraction does not seem to be greater, and possibly is less than when a skin graft is employed.

Dhall[31] reported that the entire procedure took 15 minutes. Other advantages to the use of amnion are that there is no painful buttock wound and no scar. The major disadvantage, which has limited the use of the procedure, is the concern about the transmission of the human immunodeficiency virus.

Williams Vulvovaginoplasty

The Williams vulvovaginoplasty is a relatively simple way of creating a pouch-like vagina by sewing together vulvar skin incisions overlying the labia majora.[42]

A U-shaped incision is made along the inner surface of the labia majora, as close to the hairline as possible, about 4 cm lateral to the urethra (Fig. 18-7A). The patient must have sufficient skin available to form a pouch. The skin is then undermined and, after it is well mobilized, the inner skin margins are sutured together with knots tied inside the vaginal lumen (Fig. 18-7B). A second layer of interrupted sutures reapproximates the subcutaneous fat and perineal muscles for support (Fig. 18-7C). The external skin margins are then approximated with interrupted sutures (Fig. 18-7D). The pouch should be at least 3 cm deep and wide enough to insert two fingers. These patients are placed on bed rest for 1 week to avoid tension on the suture line. Williams[43] reported in 1976 that 51 of 52 patients on whom he performed this procedure had successful results. The simplicity of this surgery makes this option attractive. Postoperative care is simple.

The major drawback to this procedure is that the resultant canal is at a vertical angle, but it is reported to straighten

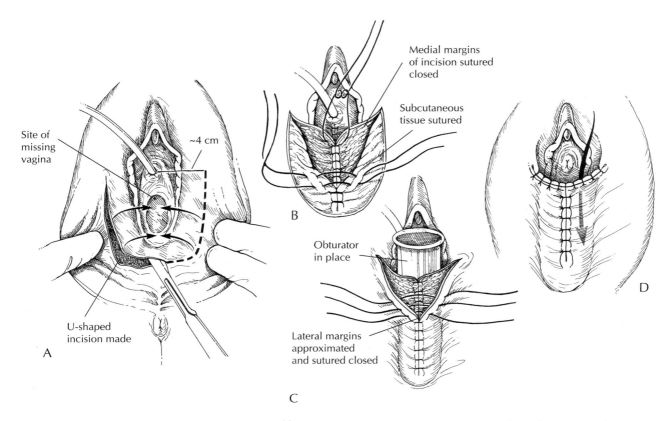

Fig. 18-7. Williams vulvovaginoplasty. **(A)** A U-shaped incision is made along the inner surface of the labia majora, as close as possible to the hairline, and the skin is then undermined (broken line). **(B)** The inner skin margins are sutured together. **(C)** A second layer of sutures approximates the subcutaneous tissue. **(D)** The external skin margins are formed with interrupted sutures.

out as it is gradually pressed posteriorly by the penis during intercourse.[44] This same result can be achieved if patients use dilators in what, in essence, is the Frank pressure technique. Three case reports describe a satisfactory outcome of a variant of the Williams procedure combined with cavitation and subsequent dilation.[45]

Other drawbacks include a problem with urine collecting in the pouch. Some patients complain of a dry pouch and excessive stimulation against the clitoris. This procedure should not be done in patients with a patulous urethral meatus due to concern that the urethra might be stretched farther by coitus.

Vechietti Procedure

The Vechietti procedure is used frequently in Western Europe and Asia. A cavity is created using continuous progressive pressure to the vaginal dimple.

Two threads are attached to a 2-cm acrylic olive and then passed through the pseudohymenal tissue at the introitus, up through the potential neovaginal space and out through the abdominal wall. The threads are then connected to a traction device on the abdomen that draws the olive upward. The

elastic skin stretches as the olive moves upward over the course of several days, creating a vaginal cavity of desired depth. Within 7 to 8 days in the hospital, a vagina of sexually usable depth is created, but regular sexual intercourse or the use of vaginal molds is necessary to maintain vaginal depth and patency. Fedele[46] described a laparoscopic version of this procedure.

Use of Bowel In Vaginoplasty

In 1904, Baldwin[47] described the use of a double loop of ileum to line the space between the bladder and rectum, leaving the mesentery connected to the bowel. The continuity of the intestinal tract was re-established by an end-to-end anastamosis. In 1910, Popoff constructed an artificial vagina using a portion of the rectum that was moved anteriorly.[33] This operation was modified in 1911 by Schubert, who severed the rectum above the anal sphincter and moved it anteriorly to serve as the vagina.[33] The sigmoid was then sutured to the anus (Fig. 18-8). The use of sigmoid has since been advocated,[48] but the colocecal reconstruction appears to be the most reliable and functional.[49] The caliber is appropriate and it is easy to mobilize.

Vaginal reconstruction using section of sigmoid colon

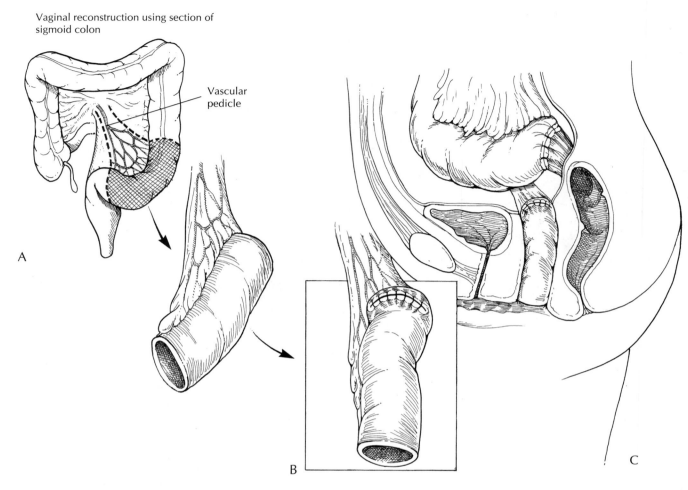

Vascular pedicle

A

B

C

Fig. 18-8. Sigmoid vaginoplasty. (**A**) Distal sigmoid is identified and (**B**) the distal end of the bowel segment is divided and pulled through to perineum and sewn in place. The bowel must come down with adequate slack and no tension on its mesentery. The upper end of the bowel segment is divided while preserving adjacent blood supply. (**C**) The upper end is closed and the colon anastomosed and the bowel vagina is complete.

The colocecal interposition is performed by isolating the colocecum with its mesentery. An appendectomy is performed and the colonic segment is inverted and sutured to the vaginal introitus. An ileoascending enterocolostomy and closure of the mesenteric defect restores intestinal continuity (Fig. 18-9).

Turner-Warwick and Kirby[49] achieved good results with no complications in the three patients in whom they performed this procedure. In Freundt et al's group of patients, who received sigmoid transplants, 25 of 32 patients who were examined 6 weeks postoperatively were found to have a vagina suitable for intercourse.[50] The advantages to these techniques are that shortening does not seem to occur and stenting is not required. The major disadvantage is that these procedures involve a laparotomy and bowel surgery, with all the associated risks. In addition, the bowel tends to secrete a malodorous mucoid discharge and regular douching is required. Some patients develop introital stenosis[51] that re-

quires surgical intervention, and prolapse of bowel out of the introitus[51,52] has been reported. Adenocarcinoma[53] and ulcerative colitis[54] can also develop in the transplanted colon.

Flaps for Vaginal Reconstruction

In the second half of the 19th century, C. L. Heppner described a new procedure in which he used an H-shaped incision of the rectovaginal septum and lined the cavity with flaps from the labia majora and thighs.[7] The use of flaps from the perineum and thigh have not gained much popularity over the years. Some of the reported complications with the procedure include vulvar pain, chronic vaginal discharge, hair growth in the neovagina, and protrusion of the flaps.[55] These vulvovaginal symptoms discourage patients and their partners from genital contact. Gleeson et al[55] described ne-

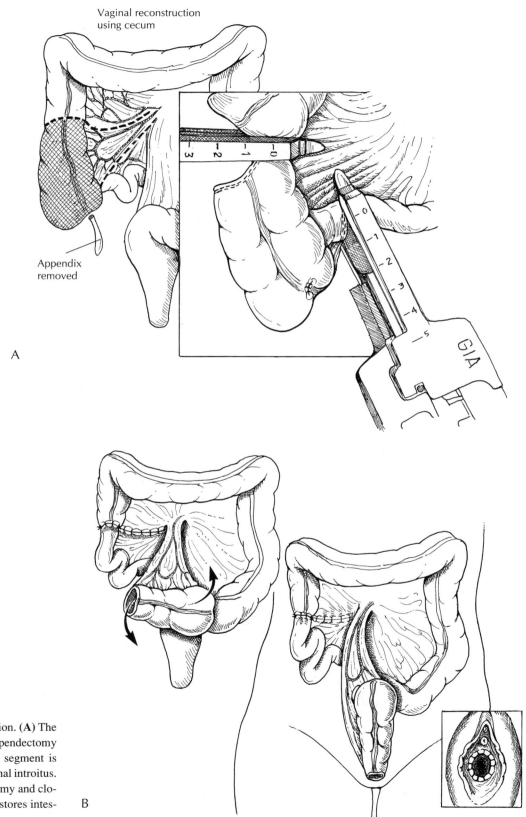

Vaginal reconstruction
using cecum

Appendix
removed

A

B

Fig. 18-9. Colocecal interposition. **(A)** The colocecum is isolated and an appendectomy is performed. **(B)** The colonic segment is inverted and sutured to the vaginal introitus. An ileoascending enterocolostomy and closure of the mesenteric defect restores intestinal continuity.

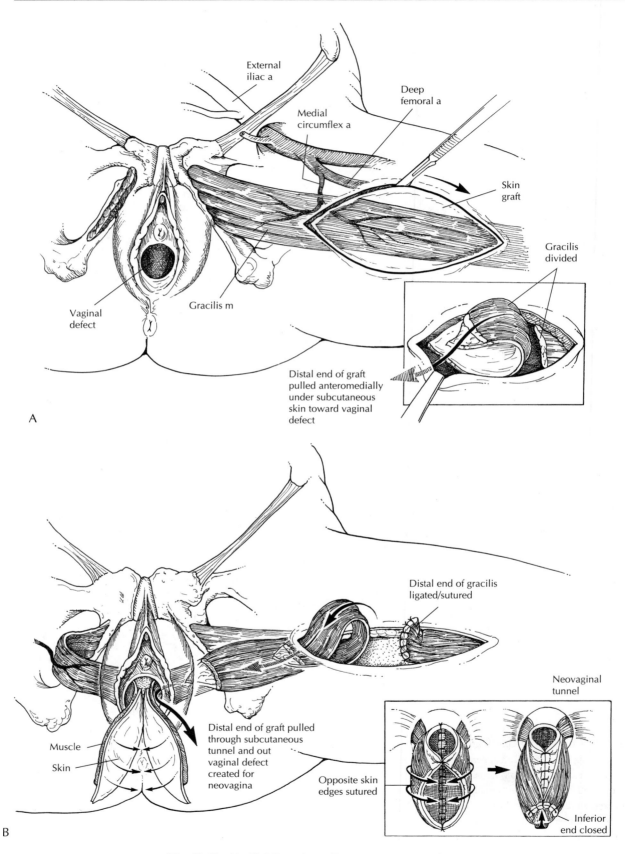

Fig. 18-10. (A–C) Bilateral gracilis myocutaneous graft.

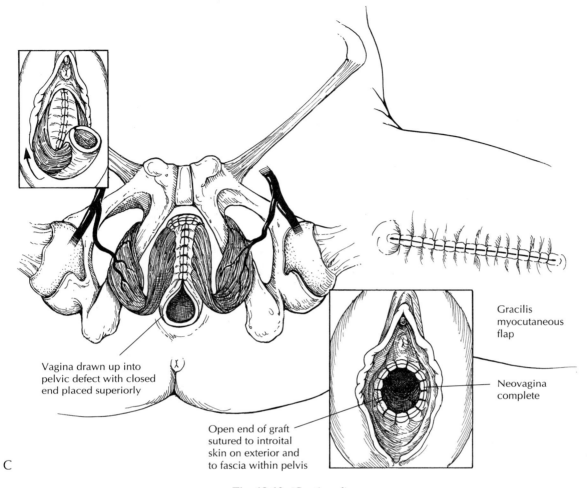

Gracilis myocutaneous flap

Neovagina complete

Vagina drawn up into pelvic defect with closed end placed superiorly

Open end of graft sutured to introital skin on exterior and to fascia within pelvis

C

Fig. 18-10 *(Continued).*

crosis in 62 percent of the pudendal thigh fasciocutaneous flaps in their series. Although the procedure was technically easy to perform, the functional results were disappointing. Free flap vaginal reconstruction with a full-thickness graft from the scapular region has been described,[56] but is a major surgical undertaking with microvascular anastomosis to vessels in the groin.

Myocutaneous flaps, using the gracilis, vulvobulbocavernosus, and rectus muscles have become the most popular technique for neovaginal construction in gynecologic oncology. The bilateral gracilis myocutaneous graft is used best after a pelvic exenteration that removes the perineal body and the anus.[57] It fills the empty pelvic space and brings a new blood supply, which decreases the postoperative morbidity from the exenteration itself. The neovagina is surrounded by the subcutaneous fat and muscle, which leads to a softness and pliability that is not achieved with split-thickness skin graft techniques (Fig. 18-10). Patients in whom the vaginal introitus perineal body and anus are preserved are not candidates for this procedure as the graft is too large to place into the vagina without compromising the

vascular pedicle. These patients are candidates for either a vulvobulbocavernosus graft or the rectus abdominis graft. Copeland et al[57] showed that there was no increase in operating room time, blood loss, or length of hospital stay when this procedure was done after radical surgery. Complications, however, include a 10 to 20 percent incidence of flap loss due to vascular compromise and the potential for prolapse. The frequency of prolapse was decreased from 65 to 6 percent in the study by Copeland et al by using smaller flaps and by anchoring the neovagina to the levator and retropubic fascia.

The vulvobulbocavernosus graft uses the skin, fat, and underlying muscle to form part of a vaginal cylinder.[58] The grafts, one from each side, are sewn together to form the posterior and lateral walls. The omental pedicle is used to form the anterior wall of the vagina. A split-thickness skin graft is reportedly not required over the omental tissue, as long as a vaginal mold can be left in place while normal epithelialization occurs. The omental pedicle forms a protective coital cushion. Satisfactory results have been found in patients who are able to maintain the vaginal volume by having an active sexual partner. The cosmetic results are reportedly superior to those of the gracilis flaps as there are no thigh scars, which can be painful and disfiguring. The sexual response is more normal because the tissue is innervated by the pudendal nerve. The disadvantage of this graft is the presence of vulvar hair in the vagina, which leads to a vaginal discharge and, at times, a strong odor.

The rectus abdominis myocutaneous graft is a reliable technique for vaginal reconstruction at the time of pelvic exenteration.[59] The flap is raised from the upper abdomen and is based on the inferior epigastric vessels. Disruption to these vessels during the pelvic lymphadenectomy poses a potential threat to flap viability. This type of flap enables the surgeon to create a neovagina of varied size and bulk (Fig. 18-11). The major disadvantage is repair of the donor site, which is closed under tension.

Choosing the Appropriate Procedure

Choosing the appropriate technique to create a neovagina is based on the clinical situation of the patient as well as the skills of the surgeon performing the procedure. Being able to perform several different operations is important so that the patient and surgeon have several options available from which they can choose.

In most circumstances, the patient with congenital absence of the vagina or androgen insensitivity would benefit most from the Ingram modification of the Frank pressure technique or from a McIndoe procedure. The nonoperative technique is ideal for a mature, highly motivated patient who can reliably devote a few hours each day toward this process. The advantages include the avoidance of surgery and low risk of complications. The disadvantages include the length of time it takes to get a result. The McIndoe procedure also

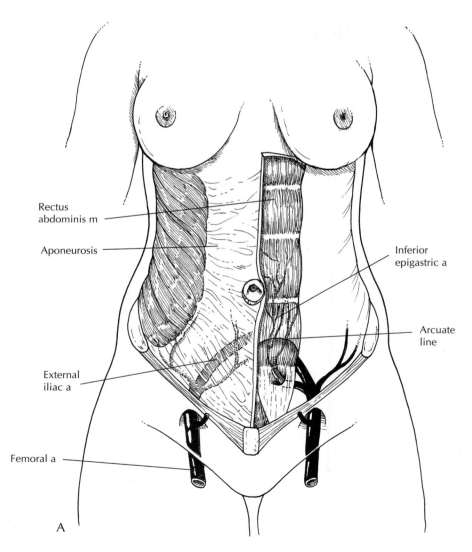

Rectus
abdominis m

Aponeurosis

Inferior
epigastric a

Arcuate
line

External
iliac a

Femoral a

A

Fig. 18-11. Rectus myocutaneous graft. **(A)** The rectus abdominis is based on an inferior pedicle with the vascular supply from the inferior epigastric vessels off the external iliacs. *(Figure continues.)*

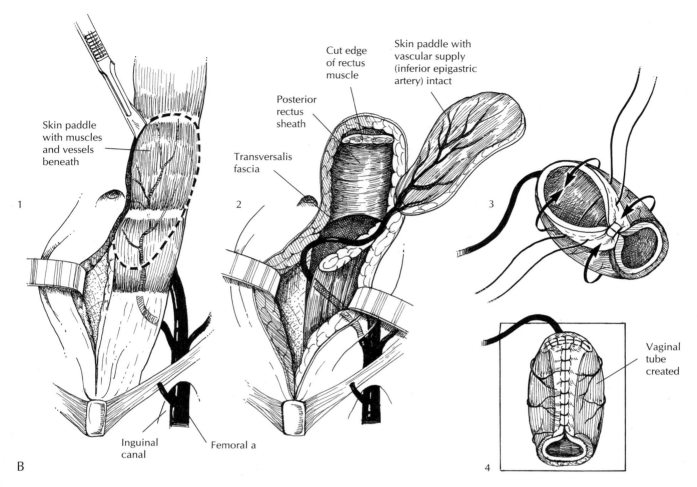

Fig. 18-11 *(Continued).* **(B)** The paddle is 10 to 14 cm wide and 14 to 20 cm long. The rectus abdominis muscle is transected superiorly and dissected free from its fascial bed. The vaginal tube is formed by inverting the lateral and inner margins. *(Figure continues.)*

requires a good deal of cooperation from the patient, who has to use the mold reliably in order to keep the vagina from contracting. This procedure avoids a laparotomy but does expose the patient to the general risks of surgery. The uncomfortable skin graft and subsequent scar is another disadvantage, although this can be avoided if amnion is available. Both of these procedures leave a nice cosmetic result with a normal-appearing perineum.

The patient who is not motivated to participate in the creation of her neovagina may be better suited for a bowel interposition or flap procedure. The Vechietti technique is also an option, although there has been little experience with this procedure in the United States. The patient with secondary atresia from infection, trauma, or failed colporrhaphy may be a candidate for a McIndoe procedure if the scarred tissue can be excised and a suitable rectovesicle space is available. The patient who has failed the nonoperative pressure technique would also be a good candidate for the procedure. In the case of a failed McIndoe procedure from contraction,

the nonoperative pressure technique or vaginal reconstruction with bowel are possibilities. The patient with an obliterated vagina after radiation is not a candidate for the pressure technique or the McIndoe procedure and would benefit most from a bowel interposition or a flap procedure.

The oncology patient who has recently undergone exterpative surgery has a number of options available. The McIndoe procedure is not particularly suited to postexenteration patients because of the large pelvic cavity created after surgery and the need for cushioning around the canal. Omentum, however, can be used to create a cylinder, which provides anterior, posterior, and lateral walls for the vagina.[60] The cylinder is sutured to the introitus and a foam rubber vaginal form covered with a split-thickness skin graft is placed within. Often times, however, cancer patients are too preoccupied and overwhelmed to devote the time required for stent management.

The bowel procedures can be a good choice in these patients. This can be done at the time of the radical cancer

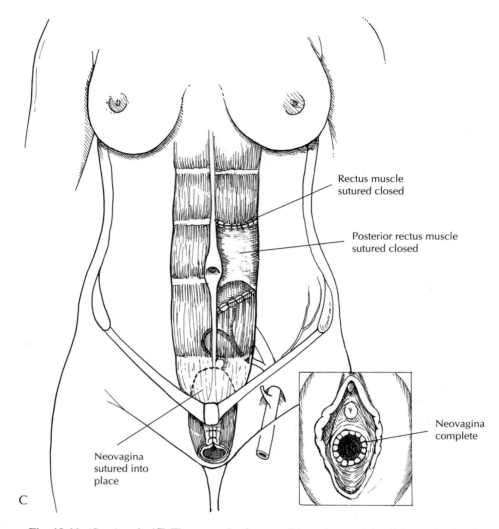

Rectus muscle
sutured closed

Posterior rectus muscle
sutured closed

Neovagina
complete

Neovagina
sutured into
place

C

Fig. 18-11 *(Continued).* **(C)** The neovagina is sutured into place and the abdomen is closed.

surgery, when a laparotomy is already required. These patients can have their normal functional anatomy restored at the same time as the extirpative surgery, and this may allow them to begin the psychological recovery phase and return to a normal lifestyle sooner. Much less maintenance is required, except for a regular douching of the vagina to try to clear the mucous-like secretions. Prolapse can be a troublesome complication.

The myocutaneous flap procedures are also frequently used in oncology patients. These are also done at the time of the radical surgery. The subcutaneous fat and muscle provides a soft, pliable encasing for the neovagina, which is not achieved with the McIndoe procedure. The cosmetic results, however, are not as pleasing as with the vagina created using the McIndoe technique.

Whichever technique is chosen, it should be one that is most likely to approximate the normal female anatomy, enable the patient to have sexual intercourse, and, it is hoped, improve her quality of life.

REFERENCES

1. Nichols DH, Randall CL: Creation of a neovagina. p. 413. In Vaginal Surgery. 3rd Ed. Williams & Wilkins, Baltimore, 1989
2. Gould SF, Evans TN: Diagnosis and management of total vaginal agenesis. Clin Consult Obstet Gynecol 6:210, 1994
3. Griffen JE: Congenital absence of the vagina: the Mayer-Rokitansky-Kuster-Hauser syndrome. Ann Intern Med 85:224, 1976
4. Farber M, Noumoff J, Freedman M: Understanding and correcting genital anomalies. Contemp Ob Gyn 113, December 1984
5. Fore SR, Hammond CB, Parker RT et al: Urologic and genital anomalies in patients with congenital absence vagina. Obstet Gynecol 46:410, 1975
6. Evans TN, Poland ML, Boving RL: Vaginal malformations. Am J Obstet Gynecol 141:910, 1981
7. Goldwyn RM: History of attempts to form a vagina. Plast Reconstr Surg 59:319, 1977

8. Rock JA: Surgery for anomalies of the müllerian ducts. p. 603. Int Thompson JD, Rock JA (eds): TeLinde's Operative Gynecology. JB Lippincott, Philadelphia, 1992

9. Jones HW: Reconstruction of congenital uterovaginal anomalies. p. 246. In Rock JA (ed): Female Reproductive Surgery. Williams & Wilkins, Baltimore, 1992

10. American Fertility Society: Classification of müllerian anomalies. Fertil Steril 49:952, 1988

11. Thompson JD, Wharton LR, TeLinde RW: Congenital absence of the vagina: an analysis of 32 cases corrected by the McIndoe operation. Am J Obstet Gynecol 74:397, 1957

12. Sadler TW: Langman's Medical Embryology. Williams & Wilkins, Baltimore, 1990

13. Boving RL, Pelusa JJ, Boving BG: Estrogen binding sites in genital tracts of human female fetuses. Anat Rec 190:344, 1978

14. Lischke JH: Discordance of vaginal agenesis in monozygotic twins. Obstet Gynecol 41:920, 1973

15. Farber M, Noumoff J, Freedman M, Oberkotter L: Understanding and correcting genital anomalies. Contemp Ob Gyn 113, December 1984

16. Chakravarty BN: Congenital absence of the vagina and uterus—simultaneous vaginoplasty and hysteroplasty. J Obstet Gynecol (India). 27:627, 1977

17. Singh J, Devi YL: Pregnancy following surgical correction of nonfused müllerian bulbs and absent vagina. Obstet Gynecol 101:267, 1983

18. Zarou GS, Esposito JM, Zarou DM: Pregnancy following the surgical correction of congenital vaginal atresia of the cervix. Int J Gynaecol Obstet 11:143, 1973

19. Fraser IS: Successful pregnancy in a patient with congenital partial cervical atresia. Obstet Gynecol, suppl. 74:443, 1989

20. Hampton HL, Meeks GR, Bates W, Wiser W: Pregnancy after successful vaginoplasty and cervical stenting for partial atresia of the cervix. Obstet Gynecol 76:900, 1990

21. Valdes C, Malini S, Malinak LR: Sonography in the surgical management of vaginal and cervical atresia. Fertil Steril 40: 263, 1983

22. Maciulla GJ, Heine MW, Christian CK: Functional endometrial tissue with vaginal agenesis. J Reprod Med 21:373, 1978

23. Yeko TR, Parsons AK, Marshall R, Maroulis G: Laparoscopic removal of müllerian remnants in a woman with congenital absence of the vagina. Fertil Steril 57:218, 1992

24. Addison WA, Hammond CB: Successful management of vaginal agenesis—a team effort. Contemp Ob Gyn 17:61, 1981

25. Kaplan EH: Congenital absence of vagina: psychiatric aspects of diagnosis and management. NY State J Med July 15:1937, 1968

26. Frank RT: The formation of an artificial vagina without operation. Am J Obstet Gynecol 35:1053, 1938

27. Wabrek AJ, Millard PR, Wilson WB, Pion RJ: Creation of a neovgina by the Frank nonoperative method. Obstet Gynecol 37:408, 1971

28. Copeland LJ: Reconstructive surgery in gynecologic oncology. p. 607. In Gershenson, DeCherney, Curry (eds): Gynecologic Oncology. WB Saunders, Philadelphia, 1993

29. Frank RT: The formation of an artificial vagina without operation. NY State J Med 40:1669, 1940

30. Ingram JM: The bicycle seat stool in the treatment of vaginal agenesis and stenosis: a preliminary report. Am J Obstet Gynecol 140:867,

31. Peters WA: Prolapse of a neovagina created by self-dilatation. Obstet Gynecol 76:904, 1990

32. Wharton LR: A simple method of constructing a vagina. Ann Surg 107:842, 1938

33. McIndoe AH: The treatment of congenital absence and obliterative conditions of the vagina. Br J Plast Surg 2:254, 1950

34. Counsellor VS, Flor FS: Congenital absence of the vagina: further results of treatment and a new technique. Surg Clin North Am 37:1107, 1957

35. Morton KE, Dewhurst CJ: Human amnion in the treatment of vaginal malformations Br J Obstet Gynaecol 93:56, 1986

36. Tancer ML, Katz M, Veridiano NP: Vaginal epithelialization with human amnion. Obstet Gynecol 54:345, 1979

37. Dhall K: Amnion graft for treatment of congenital absence of the vagina. Br J Obstet Gynecol 91:279, 1984

38. Counsellor VS: Congenital absence of the vagina. JAMA 136: 861, 1948

39. Evans TN: The artificial vagina. Am J Obstet Gynecol 99:44, 1967

40. Cali RW, Pratt JH: Congenital absence of the vagina. Am J Obstet Gynecol 100:752, 1968

41. Masters WH, Johnson VE: The artificial vagina: anatomic, physiologic, psychosexual function. West J Surg Obstet Gynecol 63:192, 1961

42. Williams EA: Congenital absence of the vagina: a simple operation for its relief. J Obstet Gynecol Brit Common 21:511, 1964

43. Williams EA: Uterovaginal agenesis. Ann R Coll Surg Engl 58:266, 1976

44. Feroze RM, Dewhurst CJ, Welply G: Vaginoplasty at the Chelsea hospital for women: a comparison of two techniques Br J Obstet Gynecol 82:536, 1975

45. O'Brien BM, Mellow CG, MacIsaac IA: Treatment of vaginal agenesis with a new vulvoplasty. Plastie Reconstr Surg 85: 942, 1990

46. Fedele L: Laparoscopic creation of a neovagina in Mayer-Rokitansky-Kuster Hauser syndrome by modification of Vecchietti's operation. Am J Obstet Gynecol 171:268,

47. Baldwin JF: The formation of an artificial vagina by intestinal transplantation. Ann Surg 40:398, 1904

48. Pratt JH: Vaginal reconstruction with a sigmoid loop. Am J Obstet Gynecol 96:31, 1966

49. Turner-Warwick R, Kirby RS: The construction and reconstruction of the vagina with the colocecum. Surg Gynecol Obstet 170:132, 1990

50. Freundt I, Toolenaar TA, Huikeshoven FJ: A modified technique to create a neovagina with an isolated segment of sigmoid colon. Surg Gynecol Obstet 174:11, 1992

51. Hendren WH: Use of bowel for vaginal reconstruction. J Urol 152:752, 1994

52. Freundt I, Toolenaar TA, Jeekel H: Prolapse of the sigmoid neovagina: report of three cases. Obstet Gynecol 83:876,

53. Munkarah A, Malone JM, Budev HD: Mucinous adenocarcinoma arising in a neovagina. Gynecol Oncol 52:272, 1994

54. Froese DP, Haggitt RC, Friend WG: Ulcerative colitis in the autotransplanted neovagina. Gastroenterology 100:1749, 1991

55. Gleeson NC, Roberts WS, Hoffman MS: Pudendal thigh fasciocutaneous flaps for vaginal reconstruction in gynecologic oncology. Gynecol Oncol 54:269, 1994

56. Johnson N, Lilford RJ, Batchelor A: The free-flap vaginoplasty: a new surgical procedure for the treatment of vaginal agenesis. Br J Obstet Gynecol 98:184, 1991

57. Copeland LJ, Hancock KC, Gershenson DM: Gracilis myocutaneous vaginal reconstruction concurrent with total pelvic exenteration. Am J Obstet Gynecol 160:1095, 1989

58. Hatch KD: Construction of a neovagina after exenteration using the vulvobulbocavernosus myocutaneous graft. Obstet Gynecol 63:110, 1984

59. Benson C, Soisson AP, Culbertson G: Neovaginal reconstruction with a rectus abdominis myocutaneous flap. Obstet Gynecol 51:871, 1993

60. Wheeless CR: Recent advances in surgical reconstruction of the gynecologic cancer patient. p. 1. In Thompson JD, Rock JA (eds): TeLinde's Operative Gynecology Updates, Vol. 1. JB Lippincott, Philadelphia, 1992

CHAPTER NINETEEN

USE OF THE VAGINAL PESSARY

DENISE M. ELSER

For a patient with pelvic organ prolapse, an alternative to surgical procedures, such as colporrhaphy or sacrospinous ligament fixation, is to fit the patient for a vaginal pessary.

The physician who has not had much hands-on experience managing pelvic organ prolapse with a pessary should not be discouraged. After reading this chapter, any clinician should feel confident enough to counsel a woman regarding nonsurgical treatment of prolapse, choose and insert the appropriate pessary, and provide continuing care for that patient.

INDICATIONS

Pelvic Organ Prolapse

In 1951, Colmer[1] reported that uterine displacement was the most frequent indication for the pessary. Although we may think of a prolapsed uterus as being displaced, in this case, he was referring to a retroverted organ, which was thought to be the cause of many gynecologic and obstetric ailments, including backache, dysmenorrhea, pelvic pain, infertility, abnormal uterine bleeding, and miscarriage. Colmer added that the general consensus was that uterine prolapse is best treated by surgery. He believed there were four situations in which use or continuation of the pessary may be advisable:

1. Patients having only slight or moderate prolapse and who are kept perfectly comfortable by the pessary

2. Patients with marked prolapse who are poor operative risks and who can be made fairly comfortable with pessary support
3. Patients with marked prolapse who prefer to get by with the inconvenience and limited relief of pessary treatment rather than undergo surgery
4. Younger women with prolapse who desire additional children. The beneficial effects of extensive vaginal repairs in such patients may be nullified by subsequent childbirth

In general, the four situations hold true today. Although the contemporary consensus remains that pelvic organ prolapse is best treated with surgery, a pessary is indicated for any woman with symptomatic prolapse, for as long as she is comfortable using the device and wishes to postpone or forego surgery. A recent study by Sulak et al[2] found that approximately 50 percent of women fitted with a pessary to treat pelvic organ prolapse were still satisfied with this treatment an average of 16 months later.

In fact, there are women with certain conditions for which pessary use should not only be suggested but strongly encouraged. In cases of severe prolapse, when the vaginal mucosa has been exposed, resulting in ulcerations, or in a postmenopausal woman who is not taking hormone replacement therapy, the use of a pessary for 2 to 4 weeks while estrogen is administered will allow the vaginal mucosa to become as healthy as possible before the actual day of surgery. Women who desire surgical repair of prolapse but are unable to schedule surgery until the distant future, may gain symptomatic relief by using a pessary in the meantime. Patients who are at high risk of suffering recurrent prolapse after a surgical repair, such as those with morbid obesity or chronic obstructive pulmonary disease (COPD), should be encouraged to use a pessary indefinitely in lieu of surgery, provided that the pessary provides relief.

Urinary Incontinence

Although pelvic organ prolapse is the predominant reason to recommend a pessary, its use is also indicated in the treatment of urinary incontinence and the diagnosis of occult urinary incontinence. Several pessaries have been designed with the intent of providing differential support to the urethrovesical junction for treatment of stress urinary incontinence. These include the Milex incontinence ring (Milex Products, Inc., Chicago, IL), the Cook Continence Ring (VPI, A Cook Group Company, Spencer, IN), and the Bladder Neck Support Prosthesis (BNSP) (Johnson & Johnson, Arlington, TX).

The Milex Incontinence Ring is a flexible ring pessary with a ball incorporated onto the ring. This ball is placed posterior to the pubic bone to provide support to the bladder base (Fig. 19-1). The Cook Continence Ring is also a flexible ring pessary with an inflatable balloon that lies under the urethrovesical junction. The balloon obstructs the flow of urine during rest and episodes of physical stress. When an urge to urinate is experienced or when a specified time interval on a voiding schedule has passed, the balloon is deflated to allow voiding. The Bladder Neck Support Prosthesis is a ring-shaped device with two prongs located at one end. When properly positioned, the prongs provide retropubic support to the urethrovesical junction.

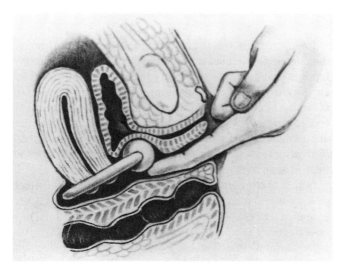

Fig. 19-1. Milex incontinence ring. The ball portion of the pessary lies below the urethrovesical junction. (Courtesy of Milex Products, Inc., Chicago, IL.)

The risk of occult urinary incontinence surfacing after the correction of severe pelvic organ prolapse is recognized by pelvic surgeons. The only continence mechanism in women with extreme relaxation of the anterior vaginal wall may be a "kinking" of the urethra.[3] If normal anatomic relations are restored, whether by placement of a pessary or by surgical correction, then the lack of urethral sphincter function may become apparent, resulting in stress urinary incontinence. A woman who experiences urinary incontinence with a pessary in place may simply choose to abandon the pessary. The consequences are more extreme in a woman who has undergone operative repair of her prolapse. No matter how perfect her post operative anatomy, she is likely to be displeased with the results if she has traded in a bulge for continuous wetness. The best way to detect occult urinary incontinence is to employ barrier studies[4] or a pessary test during preoperative urodynamics. If urodynamic measurements made with the prolapse placed reveal occult incontinence (which may be defined as a significant decrease in maximum urethral closure pressure or lowered pressure transmission during stress), then the patient requires additional support to the urethrovesical junction at the time of prolapse surgery.

A vaginal pessary can also be used to help predict successful outcome of surgical therapy in a woman with genuine stress incontinence and a correctable anatomic defect. Bhatia et al[5] found that a Smith-Hodge pessary provides support to the urethrovesical junction, resulting in increased functional urethral length, maximum urethral closure pressure, and improved pressure transmission to the urethra during physical stress without obstructing the urethra. These are the same physiologic changes effected by successful incontinence surgery. In the study by Bhatia and Bergman,[6] 80 percent of the patients tested became continent with the pessary in place.

Retrodisplacement of the Uterus

Previously blamed for any number of gynecologic maladies, currently, the finding of retroversion of the uterus may be attributed as the cause of lower back pain. Since most women with a retroverted uterus are asymptomatic, other disease processes must be ruled out before making this diagnosis. Pessaries themselves are not used to antevert the uterus, but rather the lever pessaries are used to maintain the uterus in anteflexion once it has been manually returned to the normal position.[7]

PESSARY CHOICE

Most gynecologists will never see, let alone use every type of pessary that is available; however, it is wise to become familiar with several pessaries (Fig. 19-2), as different types are best suited to correct different types of support defects.

Finding the proper pessary size is basically a matter of

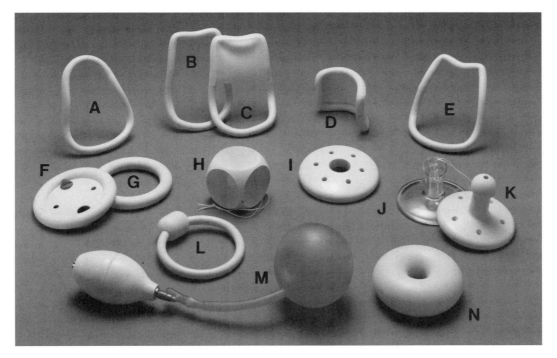

Fig. 19-2. Commonly used pessaries: A, Smith; B, Hodge; C, Hodge with support; D, Gehrung; E, Risser; F, Ring with diaphragm; G, Ring; H, Cube; I, Shaatz; J, Rigid Gellhorn; K, flexible Gellhorn; L. incontinence Ring; M, Inflatoball; N, Donut. (Courtesy of Milex Products, Inc., Chicago, IL.)

Pessary Choices by Pelvic Floor Defect

- Uterine prolapse
  - Ring
  - Donut
  - Gellhorn
  - Cube
- Anterior vaginal defect
  - Ring with Support
  - Donut
  - Gelhorn
  - Smith-Hodge
- Posterior vaginal defect
  - Gehrung
- Uterine displacement
  - Smith-Hodge
  - Risser
- Urinary incontinence
  - Milex incontinence ring
  - Cook continence ring
  - Bladder Neck Support Prosthesis

trial and error. In general, the best size to use is the largest pessary that the patient can comfortably wear. Some postmenopausal women have a stenotic introitus that does not allow introduction of a sufficiently large pessary. A few weeks of estrogen therapy may make insertion much easier. More commonly, the introitus is widened from chronic protrusion of the pelvic organs. After the pessary has been worn for several weeks, the width of the introitus should decrease, and the pessary then ought to be changed for one of smaller diameter to allow for easier removal and insertion.

To initially fit a woman for a pessary, the clinician should perform a bimanual examination after the "bulge" has been manually replaced (Fig. 19-3). Depending on the length of the vagina, the index or middle finger should be placed at the vaginal apex or in the posterior vault if the cervix is present. The examiner should note where the posterior edge of the pubic symphysis rests on the vaginal hand. When the hand is removed, the index finger of the other hand can be immediately placed on the spot where the pubic bone was felt. The assistant can then hold up different sized pessaries to the clinician's hand to approximate the diameter of pessary that will best match the size of this particular patient's pelvis.

Ring Pessary

The Ring pessary (Fig. 19-2F & G) is one of the most commonly used pessaries. This pessary will provide support

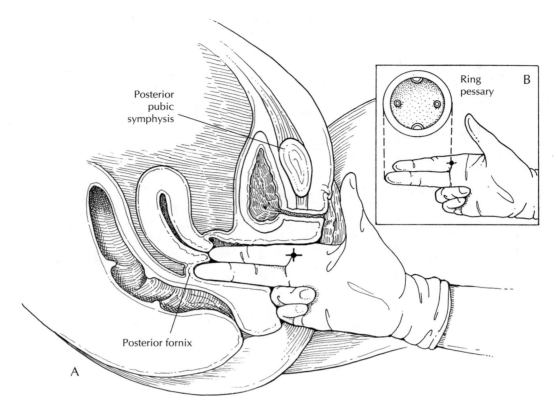

Posterior
pubic
symphysis

Ring
pessary

B

Posterior fornix

A

Fig. 19-3. (A) A bimanual examination is performed to judge the distance from the posterior fornix to the posterior pubic symphysis. **(B)** The spot where the pubic symphysis rests on the examining hand is mentally marked. Sample pessaries are then held up to the examining hand to estimate the proper pessary size.

for uterine or apical prolapse. A modification, the Ring with support, is useful for uterine prolapse with accompanying cystocele. Most gynecologists are familiar with fitting a diaphragm and therefore, with fitting a patient with a Ring pessary. The outer Ring folds, allowing easy insertion and removal, even by older patients with moderately decreased manual dexterity. Another advantage of the Ring pessary is that coitus is possible with the device in place.

To insert the Ring pessary, the outer ring is squeezed using the thumb and middle finger at the arrows, until the Ring resembles a crescent shape (Fig. 19-4). A finger on the nondominant hand applies pressure to the perineal body. Most authors recommend inserting the folded Ring into the vagina with the concave surface up to avoid painful pressure on the urethra. The author prefers to insert the Ring with the concave surface downward (Fig. 19-5). This way, the pessary arcs nicely over the perineal body during insertion. The folded Ring pessary is narrow enough that undue pressure on the external urethra is easily avoidable. Gentle pressure should be applied until the edge of the Ring reaches the apex of the vagina or the posterior fornix. The Ring is then allowed to open to its circular shape. The lower rim of the pessary should rest behind the pubic symphysis. The Ring should be turned one-quarter turn, so that it will not easily fold on itself and be expelled.

The Ring pessary is available in sizes 0 to 13. The diameter of the pessary increases with the larger number size. Most patients will be accommodated with sizes 5, 6, or 7.

Gellhorn Pessary

The Gellhorn pessary provides excellent support for women with more pronounced uterine vault prolapse or cystocele, or both. The Gellhorn pessary resembles a tripod, consisting of a broad base with a stem protruding from the center (Fig. 19-2J & K). The broad base provides support to a relatively large prolapse. Because of the concavity of the base, suction forms, helping to hold the organs and pessary in place (Fig. 19-6). Disadvantages are that this pessary requires a vaginal canal wide enough to allow the base to rest above the levators, and a perineal body of adequate substance to support the knob. The wide base and presence of suction make this pessary more difficult to remove, especially for older patients. The presence of a Gellhorn pessary makes coitus virtually impossible. Recently, the Gellhorn has become available in flexible silastic to make placement easier. A string is attached to the stem to aid in removal. One should attempt to tuck this string into the vagina to avoid soiling with urine and feces.

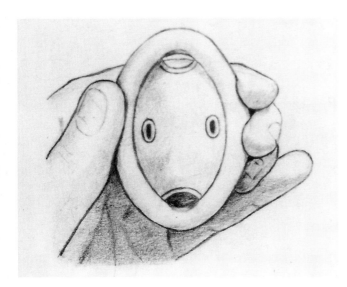

Fig. 19-4. The Ring pessary is folded into a crescent shape by squeezing at the arrows. (Courtesy of Milex Products Inc., Chicago, IL.)

The Gellhorn pessary is inserted by first holding the stem so that the base of the pessary is vertical and at a 90-degree angle to the introitus. A finger from the opposite hand is used to help depress the perineal body. A leading edge of the base is then placed into the vagina until it reaches the posterior fornix and rotated into place until the remainder of the base can be tucked under the pubic symphysis. The base of the flexible Gellhorn pessary can be folded partially during insertion. When properly in position, the base will be underlying the apex and bladder, with the stem or knob resting on the inner surface of the perineal body.

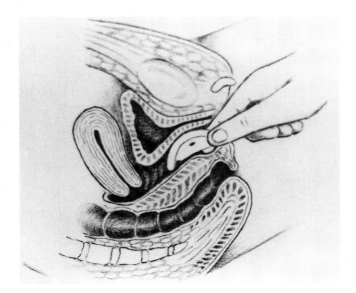

Fig. 19-5. Insertion of the Ring pessary, (Courtesy of Milex Products Inc., Chicago, IL.)

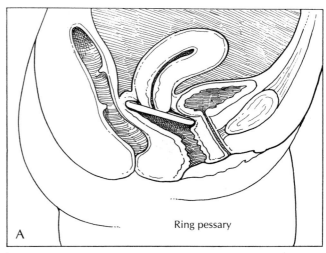

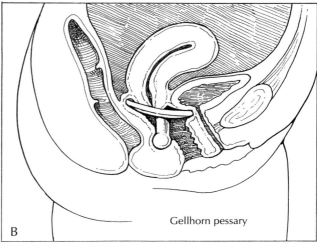

Fig. 19-6. Diagram showing (**A**) Ring pessary and (**B**) Gellhorn pessary in position.

The Gellhorn sizes reflect the diameter of the base and are available in $1\frac{1}{2}$- to $3\frac{1}{2}$-in. sizes in one-quarter-inch increments.

Donut Pessary

The Donut pessary consists of a large hollow rubber ring (Fig. 19-2M). The Donut pessary basically occludes the upper vagina and is quite effective in reducing a pronounced uterine or apical prolapse. This pessary is more likely to be successful in women with poor perineal support than the previous pessary designs. The size and shape of the Donut make removal by the patient herself almost impossible.

The Donut compresses only slightly and a pair of sponge forceps are very useful in compressing the pessary as much as possible during insertion (Fig. 19-7). Lubrication should be used sparingly during insertion or it will be impossible to grasp the donut with the required force. One should begin

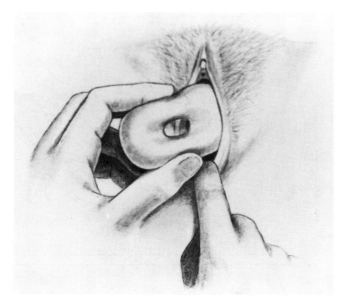

Fig. 19-7. Insertion of the Donut pessary. (Courtesy of Milex Products, Inc., Chicago, IL.)

by holding the pessary vertically and then rotating it to a horizontal position during placement. Sponge forceps or a single-tooth tenaculum may be required for pessary removal.

The Donut pessary is available in diameter sizes similar to the Gellhorn, ranging from 1½- to 3½-in. sizes in one-quarter-inch increments.

Inflatoball Pessary

The Inflatoball Pessary (Fig. 19-2M) is similar to the Donut pessary, except the design was altered to facilitate removal and insertion. The hollow rubber ring has a port with an inflating site that protrudes from the vagina (Fig. 19-8). A bulb may be attached to inflate or deflate the pessary. The port that protrudes from the vagina may cause unacceptable discomfort. Some women, however, find this more comfortable than the prolapse.

The Inflatoball is placed in a similar manner to the Donut pessary, except that it is inflated after insertion. The inflating bulb is then removed.

The Inflatoball pessary is available in diameters of 2 to 2¾ in. in one-quarter-inch increments.

Cube Pessary

The Cube pessary is a six-sided device (Fig. 19-2H). All the sides are concave. This allows the Cube to hold the vaginal walls together by suction, preventing the organs above it from descending (Fig. 19-9). Many consider this to be a last choice of pessary. The Cube is very effective in reducing massive prolapse in women who have little or no perineal

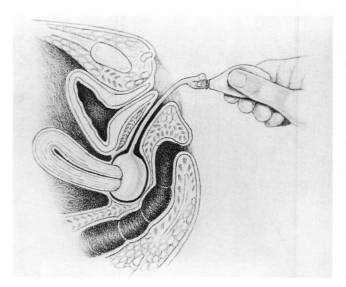

Fig. 19-8. The Inflatoball pessary in position. (Courtesy of Milex Products, Inc., Chicago, IL.)

support. Unfortunately, even short-term use of the Cube pessary is associated with a profound malodorous discharge. The author has used this pessary in demented women who themselves did not mind the odor, but the choice can be very unpopular with the patient's family or nursing home attendants. Because of the discharge, it is recommended that the Cube pessary be removed nightly and left out until morning.

To insert the Cube pessary, the flexible rubber is squeezed together and the device is placed at the vaginal apex.

The Cube pessary is available in sizes 1 to 7, with diameters ranging from ³⁄₁₆ to 2¼ in.

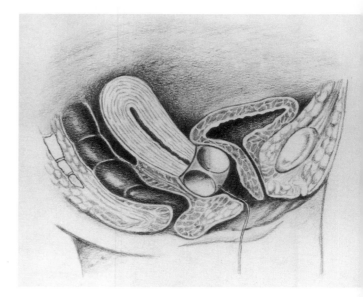

Fig. 19-9. The Cube pessary in position. (Courtesy of Milex Products, Inc., Chicago, IL.)

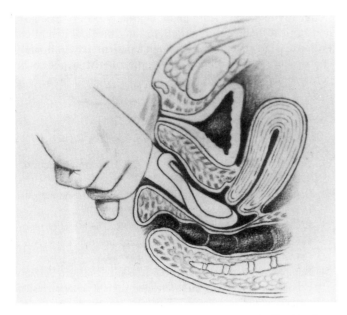

Fig. 19-10. Insertion of lever pessary. (Courtesy of Milex Products Inc., Chicago, IL.)

Smith, Hodge, and Risser Pessaries

The Smith (Fig. 19-2B), Hodge (Fig. 19-2C), and Risser (Fig. 19-2E) pessaries are collectively referred to as lever pessaries. These devices were originally intended to treat uterine retroversion. Indications for employing lever pessaries now include incompetent cervix, relief of uterine prolapse and cystocele, and diagnosis of occult urinary incontinence associated with correction of severe prolapse.

When inserting a lever pessary, the uterus is manually anteverted if it has been retrodisplaced. The pessary is then folded and inserted into the vagina. The index finger is placed against the posterior bar until it rests posterior to the cervix (Fig. 19-10). The anterior bar should rest posteriorly to the pubic symphysis.

The Smith, Hodge, and Risser pessaries are available in sizes 0 to 9.

AFTER PESSARY PLACEMENT

Choosing the best pessary size is often not accomplished on the first try. Still, it is necesary to make sure that a reasonably good fit has been accomplished before the patient leaves the office. While she is still on the examination table, the woman should be asked to bear down. A well-placed pessary will just be visible at the introitus but will not descend past the hymenal ring. The pessary should return to its prior position when the patient relaxes. Afterwards, the patient should be left alone in the room for a few minutes. The patient is asked to walk back and forth several times, to squat, and to sit on the toilet and bear down as if she were attempting to have a bowel movement. If she is comfortable during these maneuvers and the pessary has not been expelled, one can be assured for a reasonably good fit. Each patient should be informed that it is not an emergency if the pessary is expelled when she gets home, she should be counseled to bring the pessary with her to the office, and reassured that other pessaries can be tried for a better fit.

The author generally does not teach a patient how to remove, replace, or care for her pessary until the follow-up visit. This education can be time-consuming, especially with an elderly patient. If the pessary design needs to be changed after a few days, the information will be confusing for her as well. Thus, one wants to be sure that the pessary chosen is the right size, shape, and design, before the patient is taught how to care for it.

The patient should be asked to return to the office for a "pessary check" 2 to 3 days after initial placement. At this time, the patient should be asked about comfort, urinary incontinence, and the ability to have a bowel movement, as well as any vaginal bleeding or discharge. The pessary is then removed and cleaned with soap and water. A speculum examination is performed to ensure no mucosal erosions have developed. If the patient is able to remove and replace her own pessary, she is taught to do so at this visit. If all is well, the pessary is then replaced. The author has all patients return at 3 months. Follow-up thereafter is determined based on the patient's manual dexterity, mental status, and the type of pessary chosen. If a patient is managing her own pessary, the author allows her to decide the frequency at which she removes and cleans her pessary, but encourages her to do so at least weekly. The pessary is cleaned simply with soap and water. Douching is not specifically recommended, but is not discouraged if the patient brings it up. The author suggests leaving the pessary out overnight, but finds that most women are more comfortable leaving the device in place. Women who are sexually active and wearing a Ring or lever pessary are counseled that they may engage in coitus with or without the pessary, whichever way she and her partner are more comfortable. Patients who lack the mobility, dexterity, or mental functioning to manage their pessaries are seen in the office at least every 3 months and occasionally monthly.

Postmenopausal women ought to be placed on estrogen before initiating pessary use, and remain on hormone replacement during the entire time that they use a pessary in order to decrease the chance of the device eroding through thin atrophic vaginal mucosa. The best route of estrogen administration (oral, transvaginal or transdermal) has not been established in clinical studies. Thus, the route of administration should be left up to patient or physician preference. If a woman has an absolute contraindication to the use of estrogen, this does not preclude her from using a vaginal pessary. She will, however, require more frequent vaginal examinations to detect any early mucosal erosions.

COMPLICATIONS

Complications arising from the use of a vaginal pessary, such as erosion into the bladder and rectum, incarceration, embedment into the mucosa, renal failure secondary to hydronephrosis, colonic obstruction, and an association with vaginal cancers, have all been reported.[8-10] All were associated with the ''neglected'' pessary, usually in an elderly, demented patient who is unable to inform health care workers that she has a vaginal device in place. All of the above situations are avoidable with routine care and follow-up of the patient who uses a pessary. In the elderly patient, this requires communication with her family or caretakers to ensure that follow-up will be accomplished.

More commonly, a woman will develop side effects that are less serious but nonetheless sufficiently annoying to cause her to cease using the pessary. Typical complaints are new onset of urinary incontinence, recurrent urinary tract infections, interference with coitus, inability to have a bowel movement, vaginal bleeding due to mucosal erosions, irritative symptoms from ulcers and granulation tissue, and development of a foul vaginal discharge.

SUMMARY

Pelvic reconstructive surgery remains the ultimate cure for pelvic organ prolapse. Improved technology allows gynecologists to operate on older and sicker patients than was possible in years past. Along with the growing enthusiasm for pelvic reconstruction, the art of using the vaginal pessary has for the most part been lost. Modern women continue to become more educated consumers of medical treatment and frequently request to learn about alternative, and especially, nonsurgical therapeutic options for any medical condition. Prolapse is no exception. Although a patient may ultimately choose surgical correction, her gynecologist ought to be comfortable enough with the use of the vaginal pessary to be able to offer her this option.

REFERENCES

1. Colmer WM: Use of the pessary. Am J Obstet Gynecol 65: 170, 1953
2. Sulak PJ, Kuehl TJ, Shull BL: Vaginal pessaries and their use in pelvic relaxation. J Reprod Med 38:919, 1993
3. Richardson DA, Bent AE, Ostergard DR: The effect of uterovaginal prolapse on urethrovesical pressure dynamics. Am J Obstet Gynecol 146:901, 1983
4. Bump RC, Fantl JA, Hurt WG: The mechanism of urinary continence in women with severe uterovaginal prolapse: results of barrier studies. Obstet Gynecol 72:291, 1988
5. Bhatia NN, Bergman A, Gunning JE: Urodynamic effects of a vaginal pessary in women with stress urinary incontinence. Am J Obstet Gynecol 147:   , 1983
6. Bhatia NN, Bergman A: Pessary test in women with urinary incontinence. Obstet Gynecol 65:220, 1985
7. Deger RB, Menzin AW, Mikuta JJ: The vaginal pessary: past and present. Postgrad Obstet Gynecol 13:1, 1993
8. Poma P: Management of incarcerated vaginal pessaries. J Am Geriatr Soc 24:325, 1981
9. Meinhardt W, Schuitemaker NWE, Smeets MJGH, Venema PL: Bilateral hydronephrosis with urosepsis due to neglected pessary. Scand J Urol Nephrol 27:419, 1993
10. Zeitlin MP, Lebherz TB: Pessaries in the geriatric patient. J Am Geriatr Soc 40:635, 1992

CHAPTER TWENTY

SURGICAL REPAIR OF PELVIC RELAXATION

STEPHEN H. CRUIKSHANK

Preventing vaginal vault prolapse by supporting the vaginal cuff is an essential part of a hysterectomy—whether abdominal or vaginal. The incidence of vaginal prolapse varies from 0.2 to 43 percent.[1,2] Most American medical literature gives an incidence of 1 to 2 percent, but in the world literature and with the advent of increasing longevity, more women are presenting with posthysterectomy vaginal prolapse. Therefore, the incidence has been estimated to be much higher. Preventing complications is a sine quo non in surgery. In either transvaginal or transabdominal hysterectomy, it is necessary to use the most obvious pelvic supporting structures (uterosacral and cardinal ligaments) to support the vaginal cuff. Any successful repair will restore normal anatomy and a functioning vagina.

This chapter discusses various principles of vaginal fixation during hysterectomy. These include attaching the vagina to the pelvic supporting structures, correcting or preventing an obvious or potential enterocele, and vaginal and abdominal colpopexy.

ANATOMY

The normal vaginal axis lies almost horizontal, superior to the levator plate.[3] The levator plate is the area where the levator ani muscle has fused posterior to the rectum, points caudally, and attaches to the coccyx. The vagina lies parallel to the levator ani and not directly over the genital hiatus, the separation in the levator ani muscles through which pass the urethra, vagina, and rectum. With increased intra-abdominal pressure, the levator plate and the endopelvic fascia (especially the cardinal–uterosacral complex) hold the cervix and upper vagina in position. The endopelvic fascia includes the cardinal and uterosacral ligaments and the fascia on the superior surface of the levator ani; it attaches to the arcus tendineus fascia pelvis, a line of fascial condensation between the levator muscle and the obturator internus muscle.

Stretching and laceration of the above supportive structures can result in uterine or vaginal prolapse, or both. Etiologic factors include trauma, menopausal atrophy and attenuation, and possibly pudendal neuropathy, with loss of levator and endopelvic fascia integrity. The uterus and vagina then overlie the genital hiatus, leading to prolapse.

The rest of this chapter discusses and pictorially represents methods to help prevent posthysterectomy prolapse. These steps are performed both routinely and adjunctly. They call strict attention to attaching the uterosacral and cardinal ligaments to the vaginal membrane. Also discussed are techniques to close the cul-de-sac of Douglas to prevent enterocele formation.

PREVENTING VAGINAL PROLAPSE AT HYSTERECTOMY

During transvaginal hysterectomy, it is vital to attach the uterosacral–cardinal ligament complex to the vagina. The following steps can be performed at the beginning or end of the case. The author's preferred method is to perform these steps in the beginning of a transvaginal hysterectomy so that the sutures are not cut by mistake later in the case, and so that these steps are not forgotten should the case become difficult or complicated.

After the anterior and posterior cul-de-sacs are entered, the uterosacral and cardinal ligaments are cut and ligated. If these supporting structures are not frail or attenuated, the pedicles are immediately sutured to the vaginal membrane (Fig. 20-1). The vaginal membrane includes the vaginal epithelium, as well as the fascia layers (sheath) that surround the vagina. By securing these to the lateral angles of the vagina, the vault is supported and the lateral angles of the vaginal cuff are readily sutured, preventing a common source of postoperative bleeding. These steps are completed during any transvaginal hysterectomy. If the indication for hysterectomy includes uterovaginal prolapse, laxity in these ligaments will require shortening. This can be done at the beginning of the case, as long as the anterior cul-de-sac has been entered and the bladder retracted. This step elevates the bladder and ureters out of harm's way. Should the uterosacral and cardinal ligaments need shortening but the hysterectomy is performed without being in the anterior cul-de-sac, the shortening steps can be done after the uterus is extirpated and the bladder and ureters then elevated. A recent study shows that in all patients, except those with severe uterovaginal prolapse or procidentia (or both), the ureters are actually protected by the cutting of the cardinal ligaments at the start of the case.[4] This step allows the ureters to fall laterally and be retracted toward the lateral pelvic side wall.

The McCall culdoplasty or its modification is another means of supporting the vaginal cuff during transvaginal hysterectomy.[5,6] This type of culdoplasty aids in supporting the posterior vagina by attaching the uterosacral and cardinal ligaments to the posterior peritoneal surface. The sutures are attached in such a method that, when tied, the uterosacral and cardinal ligaments are drawn toward the midline, helping to close off the cul-de-sac. In addition, when the suture is tied,

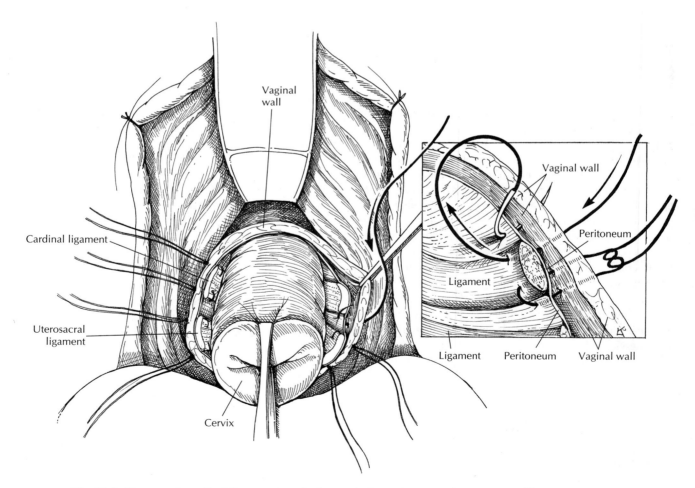

Fig. 20-1. Uterosacral–cardinal ligaments attached to vaginal membrane. (From Cruikshank,[24] with permission.)

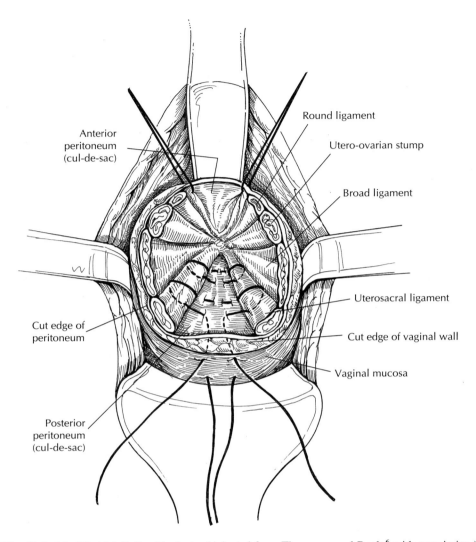

Fig. 20-2. Modified McCall culdoplasty. (Adapted from Thompson and Rock,[6] with permission.)

it draws the posterior vaginal apex up to the supporting structures, elevating it to a normal position. This can be performed with one or several sutures (Fig. 20-2). The only drawback to this type of culdoplasty is a theoretically increased incidence of kinking or ligating of the ureter, since it is close to the uterosacral ligament. No specific type of hysterectomy requires using the McCall culdoplasty. It is one way to close the deep cul-de-sac and support the vaginal cuff at the time of hysterectomy. Other methods are discussed below.

Any modification of the two above mentioned procedures that attach the supporting structures to the vagina work. It is important to remember these steps during the transvaginal hysterectomy. During abdominal hysterectomy, the cardinal and uterosacral ligaments should also be attached to the vaginal cuff. As soon as the uterus and cervix are removed, the cardinal and uterosacral pedicles are sewn to the lateral angles of the vagina. This does not have to be any type of

elaborate angle suture as long as the endopelvic fascia (specifically, the uterosacral–cardinal complex) are sutured to the vaginal fascia at either angle, taking care not to incorporate the ureter. The ureter at this point is crossing the vagina at approximately a 45-degree angle into the base of the bladder. It is not necessary to incorporate the round ligaments to the cuff, as these do not aid in cuff suspension and in fact may draw the ovaries to a position overlying the vaginal apex, predisposing to dyspareunia.

Emphasis should be on preventing posthysterectomy vault prolapse. Prolapse of the vagina is due to loss of normal pelvic supports or to omitting the steps using these pelvic support tissues during a hysterectomy. This complication occurs after either transvaginal or transabdominal hysterectomy, and surgeons must realize that hysterectomy by itself will not cure uterovaginal prolapse. Hysterectomy permits the pelvic surgeon to visualize the supportive ligaments and attach them to the vaginal membrane.

PREVENTING ENTEROCELE

An enterocele, much like any other type of hernia, is a peritoneal lining filled with bowel. In this chapter, an enterocele that divides the rectovaginal septum (or the fascia of Denonvillier) is discussed. When this happens, the peritoneal sac can elongate and become deepened, dissecting the rectovaginal septum. Often, this will present as a bulge in the superior segment of the vagina along the posterior wall. This can be present with the cervix or it can be present when the cervix is absent. Many times, this is misinterpreted as a rectocele or vaginal vault prolapse. It is readily diagnosed by having the patient examined in the standing position. With the examiner's first finger in the rectum and the thumb in the vagina, the patient is asked to bear down. Should there be a bowel in this area, it will fall into the peritoneal sac and can be palpated. At other times, no bowel falls in the sac, but there is a large peritoneal sac dissecting the rectovaginal septum and this could be called a culdocele. Any time there is a superior vaginal bulge, an enterocele should be suspected. Another step that aids in preventing complications following transvaginal or transabdominal hysterectomy is closure of the cul-de-sac of Douglas.

Peritoneal Closure

Peritoneal closure should be performed during vaginal hysterectomy to prevent enterocele formation. It is now known that closure of peritoneum itself is unnecessary for proper healing. However. if a deep cul-de-sac or obvious enterocele is not repaired, this will lend itself to future enterocele formation and possible vaginal vault prolapse. At the time of transvaginal hysterectomy the author prefers to close the cul-de-sac as follows:

1. Beginning at the 12-o'clock position, a full-length, long-acting, absorbable or permanent suture is placed through the anterior peritoneum (Fig. 20-3)
2. In a clockwise fashion, a running pursestring suture is placed in the peritoneum (may be counterclockwise if lefthanded)
3. At the level of the uterosacral and cardinal ligaments, a bite is taken through each of these, proximal to the ligature connecting the pedicle to the vagina
4. The suture is then passed through the rectal serosa and muscularis about 3 to 4 cm above the level of the peritoneal reflection; it is carried around to meet the free end of the tie and is drawn and tied to ensure adequate and high abdominal peritoneal closure (Fig. 20-4)
5. The suture is then held and sewn to the vagina at the level of the cardinal ligaments as the vaginal cuff is closed

Several other methods have been described to close the posterior cul-de-sac of Douglas in both transvaginal and

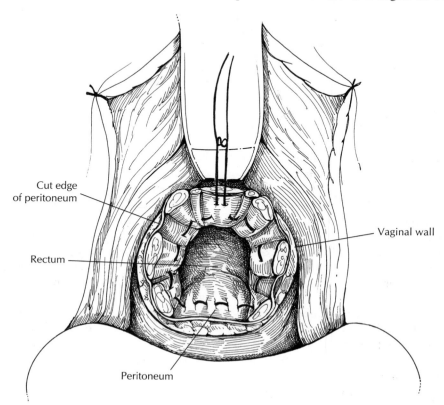

Fig. 20-3. Closing the cul-de-sac and peritoneal cavity during vaginal hysterectomy. (From Cruikshank,[24] with permission.)

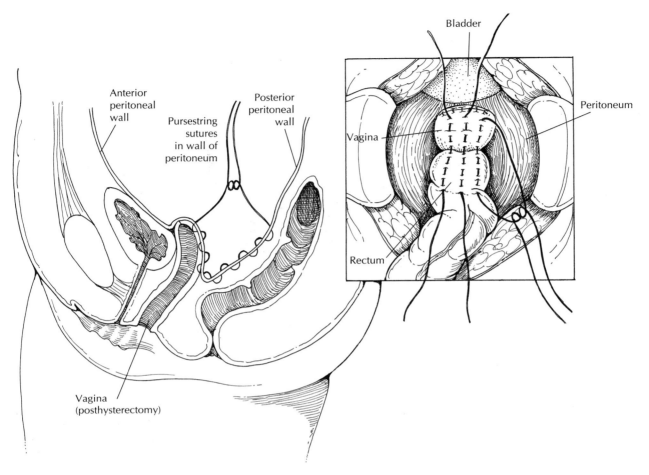

Fig. 20-4. Peritoneal closure complete. (From Nichols,[25] with permission.)

transabdominal hysterectomy.[5–9] These vary only slightly in technique, while the goal remains the same—to prevent or repair an enterocele.

Halban cul-de-sac Closure

The Halban cul-de-sac closure is a vertical-type closure of the peritoneum that was first described for abdominal procedures (Figs. 20-5 and 20-6). Ureteral damage is averted in this type of closure because the stitches close the peritoneum in a vertical manner and do not encompass the lateral peritoneal walls, where the ureters are in close proximity to the cardinal and uterosacral ligaments. This procedure is good for transvaginal surgery as well (Fig. 20-7). It will repair the cul-de-sac, but at the same time, places no sutures near the ureters. It also accomplishes high peritoneal ligation, an important step in closing a deep cul-de-sac.

Moschcowitz Procedure

The Moschcowitz procedure was first described as a method to close off a deep cul-de-sac in conjunction with prolapse

of the rectum. It has since been modified and heralded as a technique to close the cul-de-sac during the course of different kinds of abdominal procedures (i.e., hysterectomy, abdominal sacral colpopexy, abdominal procedures for genuine stress incontinence). It is a circumferential suture (Fig. 20-8) that closes the cul-de-sac. The anterior portion of this ligature is attached to the posterior side of the lower uterine segment, if the uterus is left in situ, or the posterior vaginal wall peritoneum after hysterectomy. The author's method of cul-de-sac closure described above for transvaginal hysterectomy is in essence a modification of the abdominal Moschcowitz suture. Whether performed abdominally or vaginally, care must be taken to avoid the ureter as it proximates the uterosacral ligaments. This can be done by direct palpation and identification of these structures while placing the cul-de-sac plicating ligatures.[11]

Summary

Enterocele formation is more common than is often recognized. Ranny[7] reported an incidence of 18.1 percent in patients undergoing major gynecologic operations. Failure to

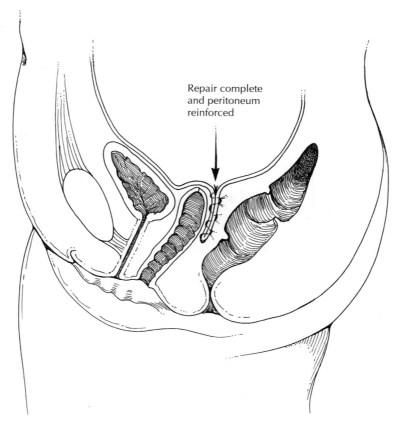

Fig. 20-5. Halban cul-de-sac closure (abdominal, uterus extirpated). (Adapted from Nichols,[25] with permission.)

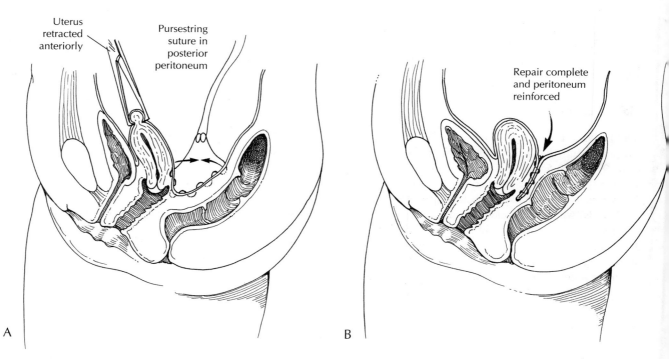

Fig. 20-6. (A & B) Halban type cul-de-sac closure (abdominal, uterus in-situ). (From Nichols,[25] with permission.)

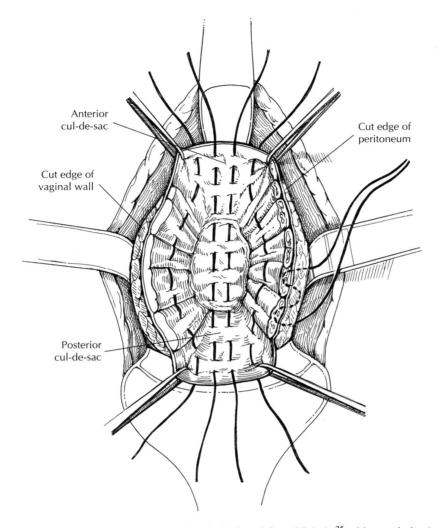

Anterior
cul-de-sac

Cut edge of
vaginal wall

Cut edge of
peritoneum

Posterior
cul-de-sac

Fig. 20-7. Halban-type closure (vaginal). (Adapted from Nichols,[25] with permission.)

close a deep cul-de-sac at the time of hysterectomy or other procedure can result in hernia formation. Whether repairing or preventing an obvious or potential enterocele, the objectives are the same:

1. To restore function and anatomy
2. To prevent recurrences
3. To use an appropriate procedure

As stated at the beginning of this section, it is important to do a preoperative, as well as intraoperative, evaluation of the cul-de-sac. Some authors advocate laparoscopic obliteration of the cul-de-sac, but this not been proved effective by any randomized controlled prospective study. It is truly a difficult operative laparoscopic procedure that should not be taken lightly.

The time to evaluate the cul-de-sac and to prevent an anterocele is intraoperatively during the transvaginal hysterectomy or transperitoneal abdominal procedure. High peritoneal ligation using the anterior rectal wall will help prevent

enterocele. Either a circumferential or vertical obliterative technique of the cul-de-sac may be used.

ADJUNCT SUPPORT TO THE VAGINAL CUFF

Pelvic Support Evaluation

Most women who undergo a transvaginal hysterectomy have some degree of uterovaginal descensus. At times, the primary indication for the hysterectomy is symptomatic pelvic relaxation. In cases in which moderate or severe uterovaginal prolapse exists, adjunct vaginal apex support may be necessary. Moderate uterovaginal prolapse is defined as the presentation of the cervix past the midportion of the vagina or to the introitus as a result of Valsalva's maneuver. This is grade I and II by the International Continence Society's Classification. Severe uterovaginal prolapse is defined as the presentation of the cervix past the introitus with or without Valsalva's maneuver[12] (Fig. 20-9 and 10). This is

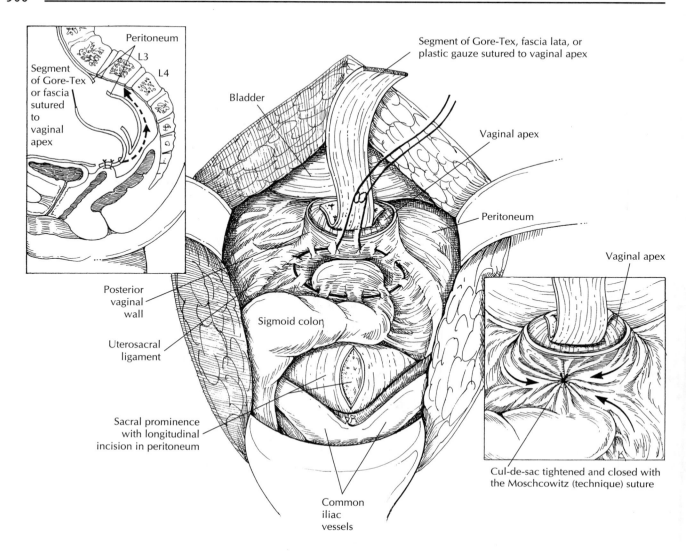

Peritoneum

L3

L4

Segment of Gore-Tex or fascia sutured to vaginal apex

Segment of Gore-Tex, fascia lata, or plastic gauze sutured to vaginal apex

Bladder

Vaginal apex

Peritoneum

Vaginal apex

Posterior vaginal wall

Sigmoid colon

Uterosacral ligament

Sacral prominence with longitudinal incision in peritoneum

Cul-de-sac tightened and closed with the Moschcowitz (technique) suture

Common iliac vessels

Fig. 20-8. Moschcowitz procedure to close deep cul-de-sac during an abdominal colposacropexy. (Adapted from Thompson and Rock,[6] with permission.)

grade III or IV by the International Continence Society's definition. If either degree of relaxation is present, the patient may be a candidate for more than uterosacral–cardinal ligament complex attachment to the vaginal membrane. Moreover, there will be patients who do not present like this preoperatively but for whom, after vault support and plastic vaginal repairs, the vaginal vault may still be pulled to or past the introitus. This is an intraoperative diagnosis, and needs to be repaired. Thus, both preoperative and intraoperative evaluation of pelvic support is needed to repair all defects present. There are several ways in which to define uterine or uterovaginal prolapse. Many societies, including the International Incontinence Society, have been working on this but, to date, none has been accepted. The important thing to remember is individual consistency. If one has a particular way of grading or defining uterovaginal prolapse, this should be used consistently. At all times one should

have some bony landmark that acts as a point of reference for normal.[11] Once a personal system has been defined, office evaluation of the pelvic support proceeds as follows. The patient should be examined in the supine, as well as the standing position, and in these positions she should be asked to perform the Valsalva maneuver to perform Kegel's exercise, and then to relax. The Valsalva maneuver will show the extent of the pelvic support defect. The Kegel support will show what compensatory support the patient has left, and the relaxation will demonstrate, once the Kegel is released, how far past normal the pelvic support allows the uterovaginal prolapse to fall in the absence of a Valsalva maneuver. At all times during the examination, it is paramount to visualize the patient's pelvic organs and their supportive structures and to palpate them as well.

Traditionally, sacrospinous fixation of the vagina and abdominal sacral colpopexy have been regarded as therapeutic

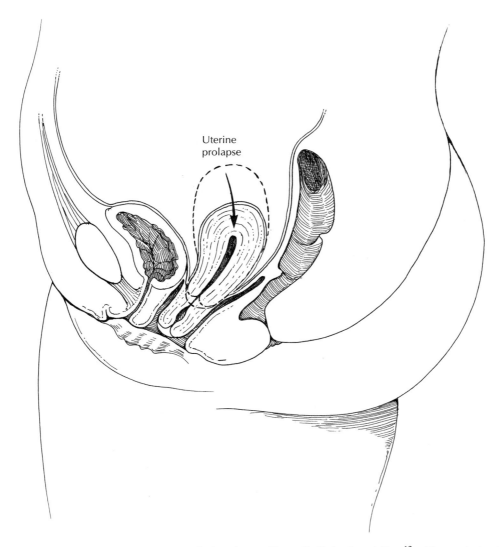

Uterine
prolapse

Fig. 20-9. Moderate (grade I) uterovaginal prolapse. (From Cruikshank and Cox,[12] with permission.)

tools to be used only for the repair of vaginal vault prolapse and certain types of enteroceles.[13,14] However, these procedures may also be used as an adjunct to prevent posthysterectomy vault prolapse. Not every hysterectomy patient is a candidate. If there is a loss of the pelvic supportive structures (uterosacral–cardinal ligament complex) noted at the time of hysterectomy, an attempt to use their remnants should be made. However, sacrospinous fixation as an adjunct will prevent further vault prolapse. If for some reason an abdominal hysterectomy is indicated in a woman with uterovaginal prolapse, the abdominal sacral colpopexy can be performed as an adjunct.

Sacrospinous Colpopexy

If the preoperative or intraoperative evaluation during transvaginal hysterectomy reveals the need for adjunct vaginal support, a sacrospinous colpopexy is easy to perform

after the hysterectomy. The sacrospinous ligament fixation is an excellent procedure for replacing the vagina to its normal anatomic position, by attaching the posterior vaginal epithelium to the sacrospinous–coccygeus complex. The sacrospinous ligament is embedded in the upper one-half of the coccygeus muscle. Once the suture has been placed through the sacrospinous ligament and the coccygeus muscle, it is attached to the posterior vaginal epithelium at the apex of the vagina. When this is pulled into the ligament, it is well attached in its almost horizontal position in the pelvis.

Preoperative Evaluation

The preoperative evaluation for a patient undergoing sacrospinous ligament fixation is much the same as for any patient undergoing any major gynecologic procedure. If she has not yet been prescribed estrogen, conjugated estrogen or estrogen cream (or both) should be given for approximately 1 to 2

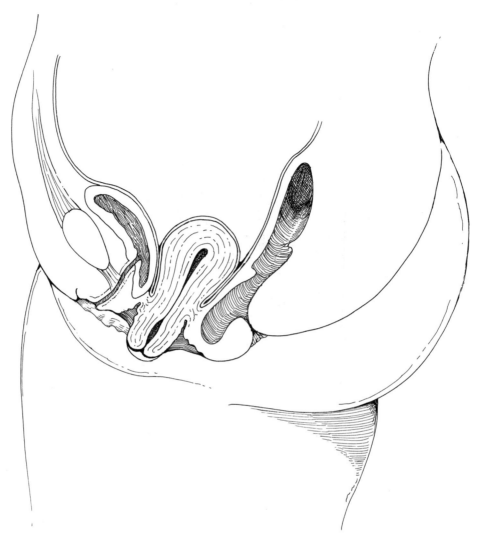

Fig. 20-10. Severe (grade III) uterovaginal prolapse. (From Cruikshank and Cox,[12] with permission.)

months before the operation. This will help increase the tone and elasticity in the vagina. This will also provide more epithelium with which to place the sutures when attaching the sacrospinous ligament and the top of the vagina together. In addition, should a patient have procidentia or vaginal vault prolapse that is long standing prior to evaluation, an intravenous pyelogram is warranted to ensure that the patient does not have ureteropelvic obstruction or silent dead kidney (or both) on one or both sides. This will advert any problems that might show up postoperatively and be blamed on the surgeon.

Sacrospinous Ligament Fixation Procedure

The sacrospinous ligament fixation procedure is performed as follows:

1. The posterior vaginal wall is opened to the apex and the rectovaginal space entered

2. This space is dissected with the operator's finger to the level of the ischial spines
3. At that time, the descending rectal septum (pillar) is perforated, opening the pararectal space (Fig. 20-11)
4. With additional blunt dissection, the ischial spine and coccygeus muscle–sacrospinous ligament complex are palpated and identified visually
5. Long-acting, absorbable sutures or monofilament, permanent sutures are placed through the ligament
6. These are held and left untied until any additional reconstructive procedures are finished
7. Finally, the ligament fixation is carried out using both safety and pulley stitches (Fig. 20-12)

If for some reason an abdominal hysterectomy was indicated in spite of the presence of uterovaginal prolapse, an abdominal sacral colpopexy can be performed.

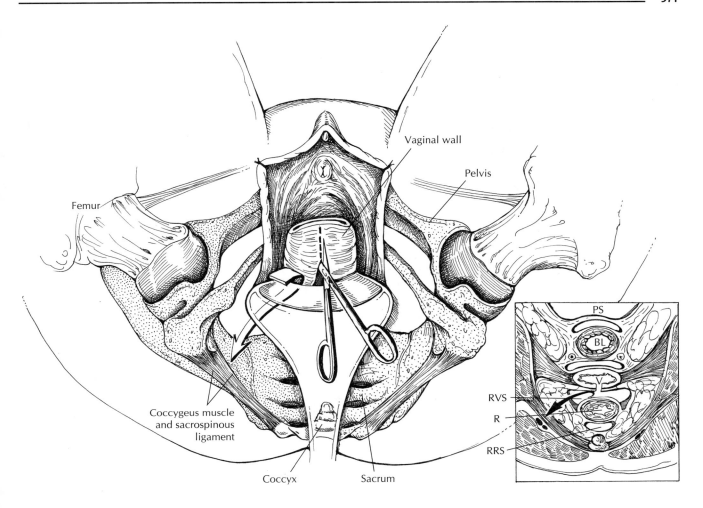

Fig. 20-11. Dissecting rectovaginal and pararectal spaces. PS, pararectal space; BL, bladder; V, vagina; RVS, rectovaginal space; R, rectum; RRS, (From Cruikshank and Cox,[12] with permission.)

Complications

The sacrospinous ligament fixation procedure is not to be undertaken lightly, although it can be a relatively short and efficacious procedure. There have been cases of death resulting from the procedure (hemorrhage) and of neuropathy from tying off branches of the sciatic nerve, Also pudendal nerve and vessel damage have occurred.

Postoperative Considerations

Postoperatively in these patients, it is important to emphasize that heavy lifting (greater than 20 pounds) or anything that increases intra-abdominal pressure on a chronic basis, such as smoking should be avoided. At the 3-month postoperative evaluation, the patient should again be evaluated in the standing and supine position and asked to perform the Valsalva maneuver to ensure that the procedure has worked and that there are no recurrent or new vaginal defects identifiable. These same examinations should be done again at 6 and 12 months, and annually thereafter. Estrogen replacement should be continued postoperatively to help the patient maintain adequate vaginal tone and elasticity.

Abdominal Sacral Colpopexy

There are several modifications relating to the type of graft material used in performing abdominal sacral colpopexy, but this discussion is limited to a modification of two of those.[15,16]

1. An incision is made in the peritoneum in the hollow of the sacrum from the sacral promontory downward as far posteriorly as possible
2. The cul-de-sac is obliterated by the Moschcowitz operation
3. Three to five permanent sutures are placed in the periosteum approximately 1 cm apart; these sutures are used to hold one end of the graft (Teflon, Mersilene, Gore-tex, or homologous fascia) to the sacrum

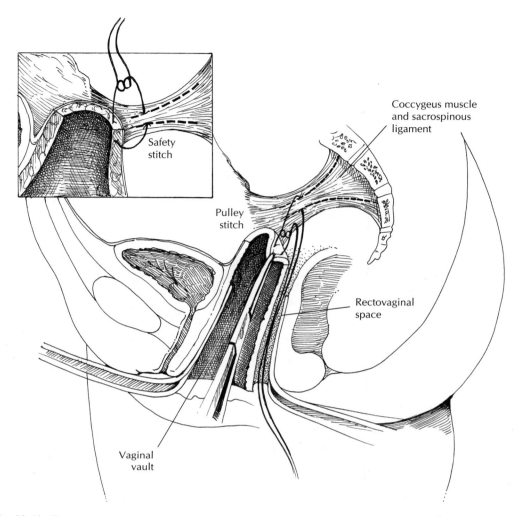

Fig. 20-12. Fixation demonstrating pulley and safety stitches. (From Cruikshank and Cox,[12] with permission).

4. The other end of the graft is sewn to the vaginal vault and sacral promontory periosteum and the graft is secured to the underlying serosa of the sigmoid with two or three 2–0 nonabsorbable sutures (Fig. 20-13)

The author's preference for this type of a graft is homologous fascia or Gore-Tex.

Summary

The literature is replete with attempted nonsurgical and surgical management of genital prolapse. Over 1,500 articles exist on the management of prolapse. Before the 20th century, most therapies were only partial or had serious drawbacks. This chapter discusses only a few anatomically correct operations for supporting the vaginal vault. Others exist and it is not meant to slight any of these. Various principles of vaginal fixation during hysterectomy are recognized

today. It is paramount that the surgeon note the laxity of the supporting structures and attempt to repair this at the initial operation. Hysterectomy offers a good opportunity to evaluate all anatomic aspects of pelvic support and to prevent future vaginal prolapse. Attaching the pelvic supportive structures to the vagina, repairing an obvious or potential enterocele, and using adjunct procedures when needed are all part of the surgical armamentaria to support the vaginal cuff.

VAGINAL VAULT PROLAPSE

Vaginal vault prolapse poses quite a challenge to the gynecologic surgeon. This is evidenced by the numerous historical attempts to surgically repair it. Although there have been over 40 proposed procedures, few have reconstructed the vagina in its normal anatomic position. This is of utmost importance so that the anatomy is not distorted and does

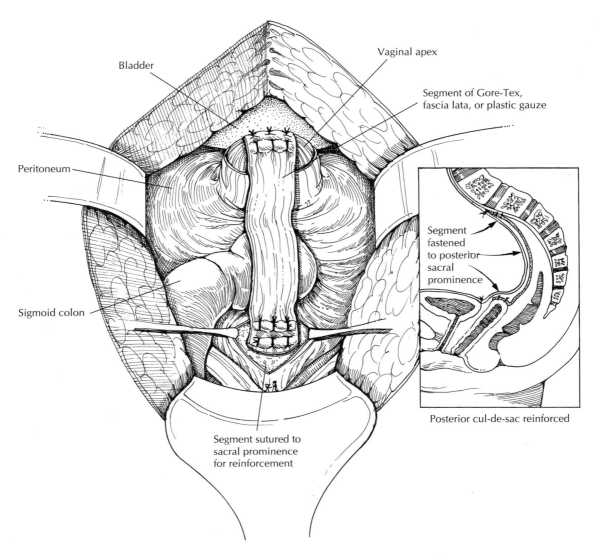

Fig. 20-13. Abdominal sacral colpopexy. (Adapted from Thompson and Rock,[6] with permission.)

not predispose to enterocele formation, and so the vagina functions normally. With any reconstructive procedure, there will be some incidence of operative failure. Advanced age, poor tissue, scar tissue, increased abdominal pressure, and neuropathies optimal reconstruction and lead to less than perfect results. The previous described methods of attaching the vagina (via an abdominal sacral colpopexy or through the vaginal sacrospinous fixation) represent two methods of good anatomic restoration.

Procedure Selection

Each patient must be treated individually. If good support and good function of the vagina are to be the result of an operative repair of posthysterectomy prolapse, there may be considerable variation in the techniques from patient to pa-

tient. However, the end result will be replacing the vagina to its normal anatomic position. Preventing recurrence is one of the goals in reconstructive surgery for vaginal vault prolapse. Recurrences are frequently caused by one or more of the following:

1. An enterocele sac had been ignored
2. The vaginal vault had been suspended in a much too anterior position—possibly to the anterior rectus abdominal wall, thereby predisposing to a rapid recurrence of an enterocele
3. Both above factors may be present
4. The procedure was performed incorrectly

One of the most important factors in selecting the procedure of choice is whether the patient will remain sexually active. Currently women are maintaining their sexual function longer and longer, and it is of paramount importance to ensure that a woman is positive that she will not be sexually active if an obliterative technique is being considered. Recent studies on the Neugebauer-LeFort operation[17] for vaginal prolapse have demonstrated good results. However, every effort should be made to preserve vaginal function, length, and axis.

Of the 40-plus procedures described over the past century for vaginal vault prolapse, three major categories have evolved:

1. Complete obliteration (colpocleisis)
2. Abdominal sacral colpopexy or vaginal sacrospinous fixation (or a modification thereof)
3. Anterior abdominal wall/ventral fixation, which is rarely used because of the lack of restoration of normal anatomy

What remain as anatomically correct procedures for vaginal vault prolapse are those described above—the transvaginal sacrospinous fixation and the transabdominal sacral colpopexy, with either the use of an artificial type of graft or an analogous fascial-type graft.

It is not intended to discuss every type of repair that has been described for this tragic complication of hysterectomy. However, a partial review of the different types of abdominal repairs and vaginal repairs can be found in the reference section.[12–22] The most important aspect is that normal anatomy is restored and that the specific site or sites of damage are properly reconstructed.

Posthysterectomy Vault Prolapse

It has been demonstrated both clinically and anatomically, that the site of damage that results in vaginal vault prolapse is that of suspensory fibers that attach to the vaginal vault.[23] These include the fibers that make up the endopelvic fascia of the cardinal–uterosacral ligament complex. When these are destroyed, surgically lax, or not used for prevention of posthysterectomy prolapse at the time of hysterectomy, vaginal vault prolapse can result. Therefore, every effort should be made to to reattach them to the vaginal vault during the hysterectomy to prevent posthysterectomy prolapse.[24] Theoretically, this should work in almost every case to prevent prolapse. However, a diminution in the suspensory fibers, menopausal atrophy, or a loss of the neural supply to this area may still result in vaginal vault prolapse, and one of the anatomic repairs for vault prolapse will have to be used.

Traditionally, transvaginal sacrospinous fixation has been regarded as a therapeutic tool to be used only for vaginal vault prolapse. However, the procedure can also be used as an adjunct against posthysterectomy vault prolapse. Not every vaginal hysterectomy patient will be a candidate. However, if there is a loss of the pelvic supportive structures (uterosacral–cardinal ligament complex) noted at the time of hysterectomy, an attempt should be made to use their remnants. In addition, sacrospinous fixation as an adjunct will prevent further vault prolapse and restore normal anatomy. If the abdominal approach is used, an abdominal sacral colpopexy should be performed when vaginal apex's suspensory fibers are surgically lax.

Summary

It is obvious from the numerous attempts reported in the literature of a vault prolapse repair, that this is a significant problem to the gynecologic surgeon. However, careful reconstruction of anatomy at the time of hysterectomy will prevent a most of the incidences of posthysterectomy prolapse. However, should prolapse occur, restoration of the normal anatomic relationships should be attempted either transvaginally or transabdominally. In addition, each and every other defect should be corrected at that time. Treatment only of the vaginal vault prolapse without taking care of a cystocele, an enterocele, a rectocele, or a paravaginal defect can result in recurrence of other anatomic hernias and failure of the initial repair. An anatomic vaginal or abdominal repair can be accomplished in this group of patients without any reduction in the vaginal depth, diameter, or function.

REFERENCES

1. Symmonds RE, Williams TJ, Lee RA, Webb MJ: Post-hysterectomy enterocele and vaginal vault prolapse. Am J Obstet Gynecol 140:852, 1981
2. Kaser O, Ikg FA, Kirsch HA: Atlas of Gynecologic Surgery. 2nd ed. Thieme-Stratton, New York, 1985
3. Nichols DH, Milley PS, Randall CL: Significance of restoration of normal vaginal depth and axis. Obstet Gynecol 36:251, 1970
4. Cruikshank SH, Kovac SR: Role of the uterosacral-cardinal ligament in protecting the ureter during transvaginal hysterectomy. Int J Gynecol Obstet 40:141, 1993
5. McCall ML: Posterior culdoplasty. Obstet Gynecol 10:595, 1957
6. Thompson JD, Rock JA (eds): TeLinde's Operative Gynecology, JB Lippincott, Philadelphia, 1992
7. Ranny B: Enterocele, vaginal prolapse, pelvic hernia: recognition and treatment. Am J Obstet Gynecol 140:852, 1981
8. Torpin R: Excision of the cul-de-sac of Douglas—for surgical care of hernias through the female caudal wall, including prolapse of uterus. J Int Coll Surg 24:322, 1955
9. Moschcowitz AV: The pathogenesis, anatomy, and cure of prolapse of the rectum. Surg Gynecol Obstet 15:7, 1912

10. Halban J: Gynakologische Operations. Urgan and Schwarzenberg, Berlin-Vienna, 1932
11. Cruikshank SH, Pixley RL: Surgical method of identifying the ureters during total vaginal hysterectomy. Obstet Gynecol 67:277, 1986
12. Cruikshank SH, Cox DW: Sacrospinous fixation at the time of transvaginal hysterectomy. Am J Obstet Gynecol 162:1611, 1990
13. Randall CL, Nichols DH: Surgical treatment of vaginal invasion. Obstet Gynecol 38:327, 1971
14. Morley GW, DeLancey JOL: Sacrospinous ligament fixation for eversion of the vagina. Am J Obstet Gynecol 158:872, 1988
15. Lansman HA: Post-hysterectomy vault prolapse: sacral colpopexy with dura matter graft. Obstet Gynecol 63:577, 1984
16. Feldman GB, Birnbaum SJ: Sacral colpopexy for vaginal vault prolapse. Obstet Gynecol 53:399, 1979
17. Ahranjani M, Nora E, Rezai P, Bujewski S: Neugebauer-LeFort operation for vaginal prolapse. J Reprod Med 37:959, 1992
18. Ridley JH: A composite vaginal vault suspension using fascia lata. Am J Obstet Gynecol 126:590, 1976
19. Stanton SL, Cardozo CA: Results of the colposuspension operation for incontinence and prolapse. Br J Obstet Gynaecol 86:693, 1979
20. Lee RA, Symmonds RE: Surgical repair at post-hysterectomy vault prolapse. Am J Obstet Gynecol 112:953, 1972
21. Langmade CF, Oliver JA, White JS: Cooper ligament repair of vaginal vault prolapse twenty-eight years later. Am J Obstet Gynecol 131:134, 1978
22. Palma PCR, Pinotti JA: Endoscopic suspension of vaginal prolapse. Int J Gynaecol Obstet 27:451, 1988
23. Delancey JOL: Anatomic aspects of vaginal eversion after hysterectomy. Am J Obstet Gynecol 166:1717, 1992
24. Cruikshank SH: Preventing post-hysterectomy vaginal vault prolapse and enterocele during vaginal hysterectomy. Am J Obstet Gynecol 156:1433, 1987
25. Nichols DH: Vaginal Surgery. Williams & Wilkins, Baltimore, 1989

CHAPTER TWENTY-ONE

COLPOCLEISIS

DENISE M. ELSER

It has been advocated that gynecologic surgeons identify and correct all pelvic support defects when performing pelvic reconstructive surgery. However, what is advisable when one is presented with an elderly patient who is clearly not interested in maintaining sexual function and who desires only symptomatic cure? Should she be submitted to several hours of surgery in order to meticulously reconstruct a functional vagina defect by defect? In selected patients, colpectomy and colpocleisis provide permanent relief of symptoms, require minimal surgery, and result in an excellent long-term cure.

Colpectomy involves removing the vaginal mucosa, and allowing the raw surfaces to granulate together without suturing the surfaces to one another. Excision of the vaginal epithelium to the hymenal ring is performed at the beginning of a colpocleisis procedure. A partial colpocleisis closes any portion of the upper vagina down to within 2 cm of the hymenal ring. A partial rather than a total colpocleisis may be done in an attempt to prevent stress urinary incontinence during prolapse repair by avoiding distortion of the urethrovesical junction. The Latzko procedure, or partial colpocleisis of only the most proximal portion of the vagina, is frequently used to repair a vesicovaginal fistula located at the apex. The LeFort procedure is a method of treating procidentia by closing the vagina yet leaving the uterus in situ. During a LeFort procedure, narrow tunnels of vaginal mucosa are created at the lateral aspects of the vaginal mucosa to allow drainage of blood and mucus.

INDICATIONS

The obvious advantages of colpocleisis are that the procedure is relatively easy to perform, is accomplished within a short period and can be done under general, regional, or even local anesthesia. Postoperative recovery and convalescence are short, as there is no abdominal incision and thus less associated atelectasis, ileus, and incisional pain. Colpocleisis, therefore, is an ideal operation for the treatment of severe pelvic organ prolapse in elderly women who are considered poor surgical risks because of multiple coexisting medical problems.

It is imperative before performing a colpocleisis that the patient fully understands that her vagina will be closed and she will be unable to engage in sexual intercourse. One must never assume that a woman is not sexually active or not interested in future sexual activity no matter what her age, physical condition, or marital status. Regardless of her current interest in sexual intercourse, we must respect the wishes of a patient who is reluctant to undergo colpocleisis. It is perfectly understandable why some women are hesitant to give up an organ that has been identified with female sexuality, even if she has not been active sexually for many years. However, we should not assume that an older woman with a youthful appearance is interested in preserving vaginal function. Colpocleisis should be considered as an alternative therapy for severe pelvic organ prolapse repair in selected patients.

OPERATIVE PROCEDURE

A balloon catheter should be placed to aid in identification of the urethrovesical junction. If indicated, a vaginal hysterectomy is performed at the beginning of the procedure.

Removing the Vaginal Mucosa

The vaginal cuff is grasped at each corner of the apex with two clamps. The vaginal mucosa is then infiltrated with a dilute vasoconstrictive solution. A marking pen is used to divide the mucosa into two halves, separated in the midline anteriorly and posteriorly. The vaginal mucosa is removed with sharp dissection, starting at the midline and working laterally. Large vessels that require clamping and suturing may be encountered laterally, at the location of the bladder pillars and cardinal ligament attachments. Dissection is completed to within 1 to 2 cm of the hymenal ring, Leaving some vaginal mucosa will result in a cosmetically more acceptable introitus. This technique also avoids excessive distortion of the urethrovesical junction (Fig. 21-1).

Resecting an Enterocele

An enterocele is usually encountered in women with large prolapse. Recurrence of many prolapse operations is blamed on failure to recognize and repair an enterocele. An enterocele, if present, should be resected. If the peritoneal cavity is entered, a high obliteration of the cul-de-sac should be performed using permanent suture (Fig. 21-2).

Urethrovesical Junction Support

Particular attention is paid to providing differential support to the urethrovesical junction. Using permanent suture, the endopelvic fascia is plicated in the midline under the urethrovesical junction. A second layer of two sutures is placed beneath the first. A third layer of three serial plicating

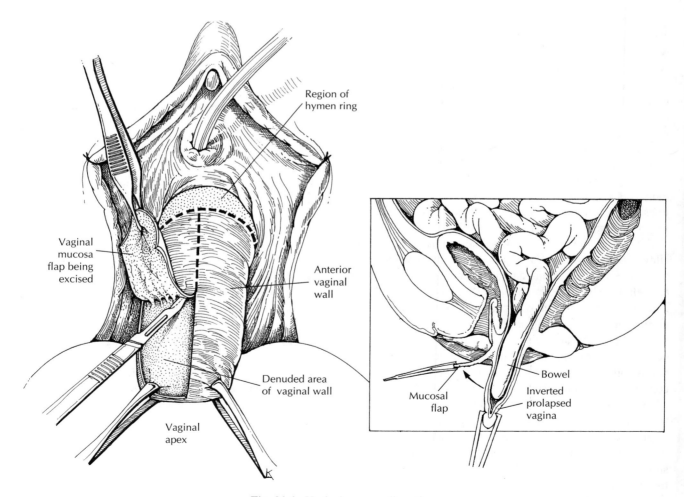

Fig. 21-1. Vaginal mucosa dissection.

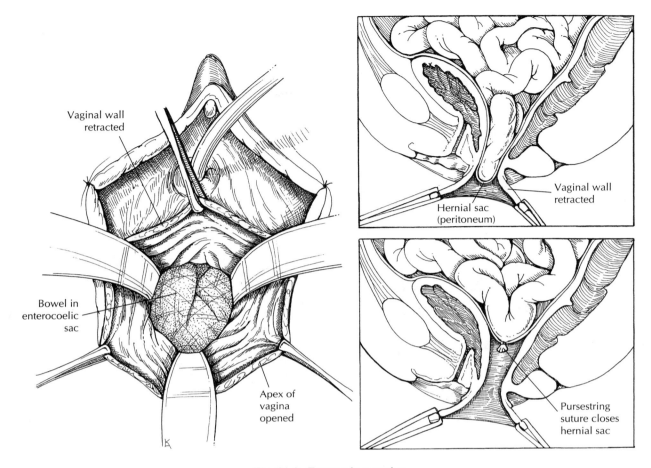

Vaginal wall retracted

Bowel in enterocoelic sac

Apex of vagina opened

Vaginal wall retracted

Hernial sac (peritoneum)

Pursestring suture closes hernial sac

Fig. 21-2. Enterocele resection.

sutures completes the differential wedge of support intended to prevent postoperative stress urinary incontinence (Fig. 21-3).

Vaginal Closure

The bladder is closed to the rectum in running imbricating layers using a delayed absorbable suture, beginning at the apex. As each layer is completed, the vagina will begin to fold in on itself; with the protruding organs becoming smaller and smaller (Fig. 21-4).

The levator ani muscles are then approximated in the midline using interrupted stitches of number 0 permanent suture. These sutures are inverted to bury the knot. Finally, the edges of the vaginal mucosa are closed to within 2 cm of the hymen using interrupted 2–0 delayed absorbable suture. The bladder is drained the first day postoperatively. No drains are placed. The usual inpatient stay is 2 to 3 days (Fig. 21-5).

COMPLICATIONS

Long-term complications of colpocleisis include recurrent prolapse, stress urinary incontinence, and the loss of sexual function. Since colpocleisis is traditionally reserved for

women who are elderly and in poor health, the evaluation of long-term success and complications is limited by the generally short-term survival of the patients.

Recurrent Prolapse

The surgical literature contains many articles that describe variations of technique, but little information on recurrence and complication rates. Many authors concur with Adams,[1] who believed that colpocleisis fills the need for a procedure that relieves the incapacitating symptoms of prolapse completely and provides permanent support without fear of recurrence. In Adam's series of 30 patients, none developed recurrent prolapse. Ridley[2] performed colpocleisis on 58 women for prolapse. Three women with recurrent prolapse were considered complete failures. Symmonds et al[3] provided data regarding recurrence in the Mayo experience, where there were 3 cases of recurrent prolapse out of a total of 16 vaginectomies. Nearly 5 percent of 288 women who underwent a LeFort operation for prolapse developed a recurrence, according to Hanson and Keettel.[4] None of the above reports are specific regarding the length of follow-up. In a somewhat larger, better documented series, Langmade

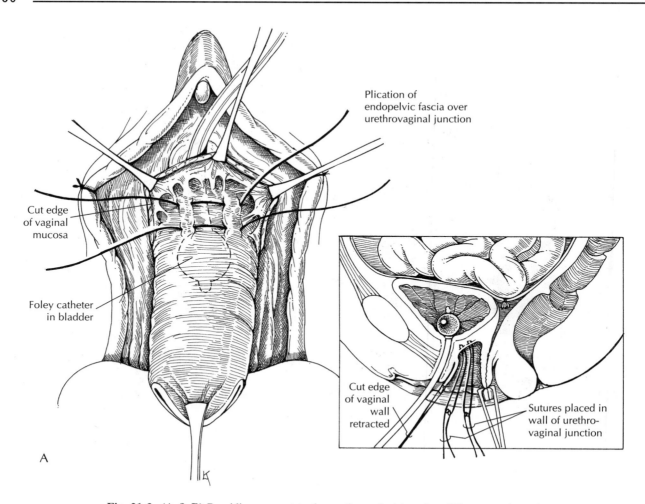

Plication of endopelvic fascia over urethrovaginal junction

Cut edge of vaginal mucosa

Foley catheter in bladder

Cut edge of vaginal wall retracted

Sutures placed in wall of urethro-vaginal junction

A

Fig. 21-3. (A & B) Providing support to the urethrovesical junction. *(Figure continues.)*

and Oliver[5] followed 102 women after colpocleisis for an average of 3 years. None of these women developed a recurrence of prolapse.

Urinary Incontinence

The undesirable development of de novo stress urinary incontinence after a colpocleisis is frequently mentioned in descriptions of complications of colpocleisis. The incontinence theoretically develops because the anterior segment of the vagina is pulled downward when the bladder is sewn to the rectum.[3] Although many authors mention that there is a risk of stress incontinence after the surgery, Ridley[3] is one of the few to report the incidence of incontinence after colpocleisis. In his series, 4 of 11 patients who reported incontinence preoperatively continued to suffer incontinence postoperatively and 4 patients developed new urinary incontinence after the procedure. Thus, 8 of 58 patients were incontinent of urine after the procedure. As a result of the experience of incontinence after a colpocleisis, some sur-

geons have altered their technique so that the vagina is closed only to within 2 cm of the introitus, thus avoiding distortion of the urethrovesical junction.[5] Another alternative is to support the urethrovesical junction by plicating the endopelvic fascia.

Loss of Sexual Function

Colpocleisis, by definition, results in a loss of coital function. Before counseling a patient regarding surgical choices that preserve vaginal function versus colpocleisis, we need to be realistic about the sexual function of women who undergo more extensive pelvic reconstructive surgery. Richter and Albrich[6] reported that 8 of 38 patients undergoing anterior and posterior colporrhaphy with sacrospinous ligament fixation were afraid to resume sexual relations because of a narrowing of the vagina. Similarly, Morley and DeLancey[7] found that 9 of 71 patients undergoing colporrhaphy and sacrospinous ligament fixation developed vaginal stenosis. In a series reported by Jeffcoate,[8] 30 percent of women

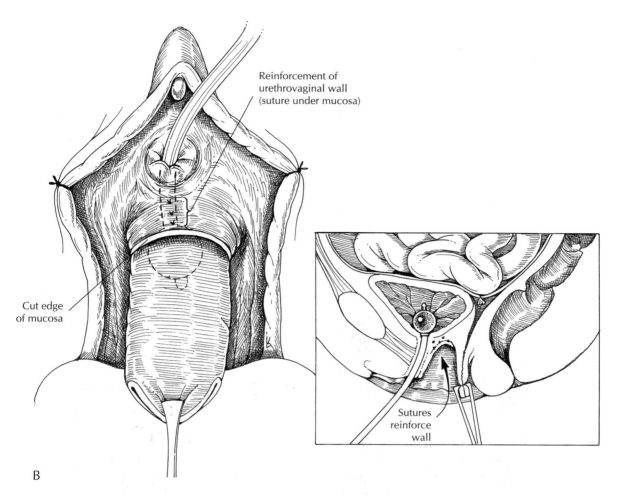

Reinforcement of
urethrovaginal wall
(suture under mucosa)

Cut edge
of mucosa

Sutures
reinforce
wall

B

Fig. 21-3 *(Continued).*

undergoing colporrhaphy experienced permanent apareunia or dyspareunia postoperatively. This last figure does not include the widows who were noted on postoperative examination to have extremely stenotic vaginas. Thus, any prolapse surgery may have a significantly negative effect on coital function.

Other Complications

The most significant acute complication of colpocleisis is injury to the ureters during the repair. For this reason, injection of intravenous indigo carmine, followed by cystoscopy to confirm ureteral function after the procedure is recommended.

Women with procidentia or significant vault prolapse are inevitably found to have an enterocele as a component of their prolapse. Thus, it is imperative to give attention to enterocele repair at the time of any pelvic reconstructive surgery, including colpocleisis.

If possible, a vaginal hysterectomy should be performed prior to colpocleisis. Removing the uterus prevents the postoperative problems of hematocolpos or mucocolpos, and the dilemma of how to evaluate postmenopausal bleeding in a uterus that lies behind a closed vagina. However, hysterectomy will increase operative time, bleeding, and risk of injury to intraabdominal contents. In very elderly or frail patients, hysterectomy can be omitted to decrease perioperative complications.

SUMMARY

Colpocleisis is a simple, effective procedure for treating severe pelvic organ prolapse in carefully selected patients. It allows patients who are otherwise too ill for major surgery to experience permanent relief from their prolapse symptoms. The procedure remains a viable alternative in those women for whom more conservative surgery may not realistically be expected to result in preservation of vaginal function.

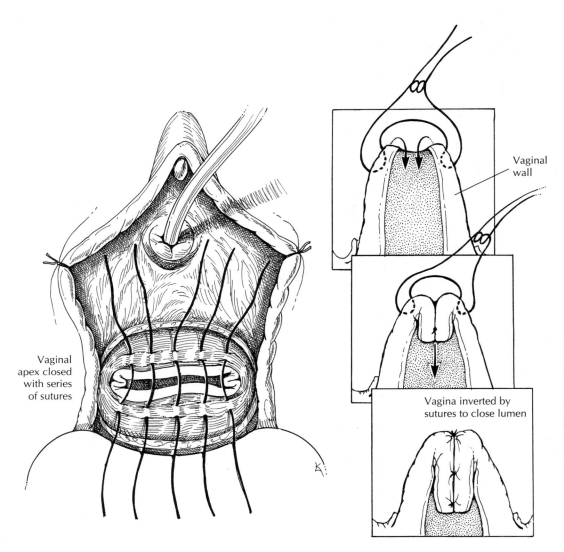

Vaginal apex closed with series of sutures

Vaginal wall

Vagina inverted by sutures to close lumen

Fig. 21-4. The bladder is closed to the rectum.

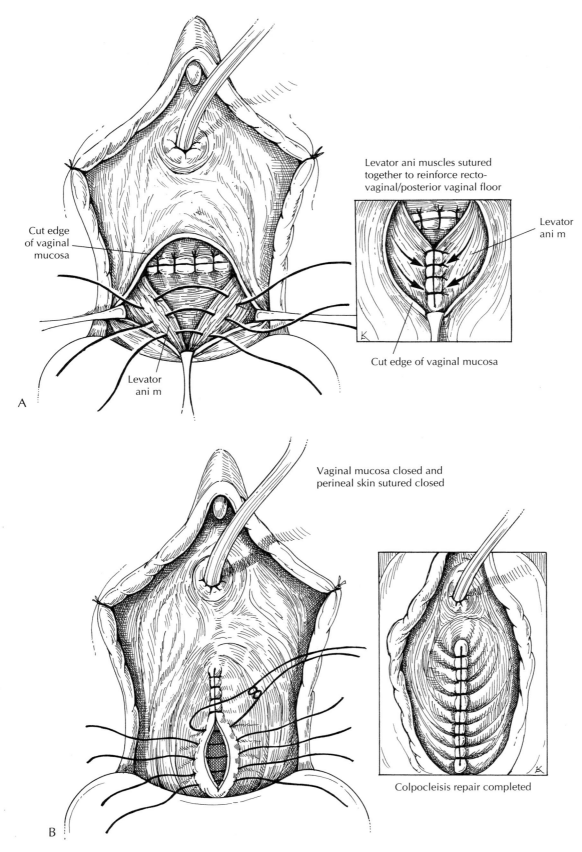

Cut edge
of vaginal
mucosa

Levator
ani m

Levator ani muscles sutured
together to reinforce recto-
vaginal/posterior vaginal floor

Levator
ani m

Cut edge of vaginal mucosa

A

Vaginal mucosa closed and
perineal skin sutured closed

Colpocleisis repair completed

B

Fig. 21-5. (A & B) Suture and closure.

REFERENCES

1. Adams HD: Total colpocleisis for pelvic eventration. Surg Gynecol Obstet 92:321, 1951
2. Ridley JH: Evaluation of the colpocleisis operation: a report of fifty-eight cases. Am J Obstet Gynecol 113:1114, 1972
3. Symmonds RE, Williams TJ, Lee RA, Webb MJ: Posthysterectomy enterocele and vaginal vault prolapse. Am J Obstet Gynecol 140:852, 1981
4. Hanson GE, Keettel WC: The Neugebauer-LeFort operation. Obstet Gynecol 34:352, 1969
5. Langmade CF, Oliver JA Jr: Partial colpocleisis. Am J Obstet Gynecol 154:1200, 1986
6. Richter K, Albrich W: Long-term results following fixation of the vagina on the sacrospinal ligament by the vaginal route (vaginaefixation sacrospinalis vaginalis). Am Obstet Gynecol 141:811, 1981
7. Morley GW, DeLancey JOL: Sacrospinous ligament fixation for eversion of the vagina. Am J Obstet Gynecol 158:872, 1988
8. Jeffcoate TNA: Posterior colpoperineorrhaphy. Am J Obstet Gynecol 77:490, 1959

CHAPTER TWENTY-TWO

CONGENITAL ANOMALIES OF THE UTERUS

RONALD E. IVERSON, JR.
ALAN H. DECHERNEY

Congenital anomalies of the uterus are often asymptomatic and therefore unrecognized. They may affect a woman's obstetric as well as her gynecologic health. Although the diagnosis of these anomalies is not difficult, the appropriate treatment requires much consideration. Therefore, in order to better serve patients and to contribute to the understanding of these problems, the physician should be alert to the possibility of a congenital mullerian anomaly.

INCIDENCE

Since many women with mullerian anomalies are not diagnosed, it is difficult to know how often such conditions occur. Many authors have stated that the rate of anomalies is 0.1 to 1.0 percent. Simon et al, studied 679 women with normal reproductive outcomes who had evaluations with laparoscopy or laparotomy for tubal ligation with a follow-up hysterosalpingogram (HSG) at 5 months. The uterine congenital anomaly rate was 3.2 percent, with 90 percent being septate uteri, 5 percent bicornuate, and 5 percent didelphic. Cooper[2] found a 6 percent incidence of uterine structural abnormalities (septate or bicornuate uteri) in women who had normal reproductive performance and were undergoing hysteroscopic sterilization.

UTERINE DEVELOPMENT

In order to understand these defects and their repair, it is important to study their embryologic basis. Normally, by the fifth week of gestation, the urogenital ridges develop from the mesoderm on the dorsal wall of the coelomic cavity. Germ cells migrate from the yolk sac to the genital ridge and initiate gonadal development by the sixth week of gestation. Two pairs of genital ducts begin to develop along the coelomic cavity: the mesonephric, or wolfian and the paramesonephric, or mullerian ducts.

The mullerian duct is initially a longitudinal invagination of the coelomic epithelium on the anterolateral surface of the urogenital ridge. It opens cranially into the coelomic cavity. The caudal portion begins by coursing laterally to the mesonephric duct, but soon crosses it ventrally to grow in a caudal and medial direction. The apposing ducts soon abut and eventually fuse. The intervening septum disappears at approximately 10 weeks, with the remaining uterine canal lined by cuboidal epithelium. The caudal tip of the uterine canal ends at the posterior wall of the urogenital sinus, forming the paramesonephric, or mullerian tubercle.

In the absence of mullerian-inhibiting substance, the paramesonephric system continues to develop, while without induction from the Y chromosome and androgens, the mesonephric duct system regresses. The unfused cranial portions of the ducts continue to connect with the coelomic cavity as the fallopian tubes. The fused portion eventually becomes the uterine corpus down to the upper third of the vagina. As the mullerian ducts fuse, a transverse pelvic fold is created; with further development, this becomes the broad ligament. The renal system develops concomitantly from the mesonephric duct (collecting system) and surrounding metanephric tissue (kidney).

There are three common developmental defects of the mullerian system to consider: agenesis, vertical fusion defects, and lateral fusion defects. The Mayer-Rokitansky-Kuster-Hauser syndrome is the result of mullerian agenesis. The vertical fusion defects relate to either defective fusion of the caudal end of the mullerian duct and the urogenital sinus or problems with vaginal canalization. The resulting vaginal septum or cervical agenesis or dysgenesis may either be obstructed or nonobstructed. The amount of obstruction will determine symptomatology, including obstetric outcomes. The lateral fusion defects are the most common and are evident as uterine malformations. The resulting organs are either symmetric or asymmetric, and obstructed or nonobstructed. These fusion defects result from the failure of formation of one mullerian duct, migration of a duct, fusion of the mullerian ducts, or absorption of the intervening septum.

The unicornuate uterus is an example of an asymmetric lateral fusion defect. One cavity is usually normal, with a fallopian tube and cervix, while the failed mullerian duct is varied. The affected mullerian duct may not develop at all, or it may develop only partially as either a horn on the uterus or an anlager. This horn or anlager may develop endometrial tissue, and may communicate with the uterus. It may or may not, therefore, be able to pass menstrual flow out through the uterus.

Abnormal mullerian duct fusion results in symmetric uterine defects. These are often called ''double uteri.'' In the extreme case, uterus didelphys, with two uteri and two cervices, may occur. There is an increased incidence of longitudinal vaginal septa associated with all uterine fusion defects, especially uterus didelphys. More common than didelphys is the bicornuate uterus, with two cornua and one cervix. Finally, the arcuate uterus is noted to simply have an indentation at the center of the fundus.

Defective resorption of the septum between the fused mullerian ducts results in a uterine septum, which may extend either partially down the uterus or the full length to the cervix. This is the most common of the uterine defects.

Women who were exposed to diethystilbestrol (DES) in utero classically have a T-shaped or hypoplastic uterus.

It is important to note whether an obstruction is present, not only for symptomatology, but as it relates to the renal system. Ipsilateral renal agenesis is invariably noted with obstructive defects. Obstruction may occur in a unicornuate uterus with a functioning, noncommunicating horn, an obstructed cavity in one of the double uteri, or if there is a vaginal septum leading to obstruction. Obstructions have only been observed unilaterally; most likely, if there is bilateral obstruction, there was bilateral renal agenesis as well, which is incompatible with fetal life.

Other congenital renal anomalies are often found in conjunction with mullerian defects. Upper urinary tract anomalies such as horseshoe kidney, duplication of the collecting system, pelvic kidney, and ectopically located ureteral orifices have all been noted. Thompson and Lynn[3] found that 37 percent of women with a solitary kidney have genital abnormalities. Therefore, all women with mullerian defects should undergo a radiologic renal investigation, such as an intravenous pyelogram or renal ultrasound.

CLASSIFICATION OF ABNORMAL DEVELOPMENT

A classification system is an attempt to group by symptomatology, treatment, and prognosis. Classification of uterine defects varied widely until recently, making it difficult to compare research statistics and to counsel patients appropriately. The American Fertility Society in 1988 produced a standard form for classification of mullerian defects.[4] This descriptive form focuses largely on vertical fusion defects and, therefore, on uterine dysgenesis. The associated anomalies in the vagina, cervix, fallopian tubes, and renal system are to be noted as well. It is through use of these standardized forms that physicians can more accurately codify the symptomatology, treatment, and outcome of these patients.

ETIOLOGY

The underlying etiology of the congenital defects is not well understood. The karyotype of most women with these anomalies is 46,XX. Rubella virus may cause defects of the genital tract, heart, eye, and ear. Teratogens such as DES, which causes serious genital tract defects, are also known. Most likely, these defects are polygenic and multifactorial.

PRESENTATION AND COMPLICATIONS

Congenital anomalies of the uterus are often diagnosed incidentally during the workup of common gynecologic and obstetric problems. The symptoms of mullerian anomalies vary greatly, depending on the defect involved. Adolescents may have increased pelvic pain (either cyclic or noncyclic), dysmenorrhea, abnormal vaginal bleeding, or vaginal pain. Hypomenorrhea may occur if there is minimal endometrium; amenorrhea may be a sign of Mayer-Rokitansky-Kuster-Hauser syndrome or of a vertical fusion defect. Longitudinal vaginal septum may occur alone, but is usually seen with didelphic or other forms of double uterus; this may lead to dysparaunia, leukorrhea, and dystocia at delivery. If one side of the vagina is obstructed, complications such a hydrocolpos and hematocolpos may occur. Finally, the patient may present with endometriosis and its associated symptoms if a noncommunicating functioning horn seeds the peritoneum through retromenstruation.

Many women present with obstetric complications. Most authors believe that infertility is not a result of uterine abnormalities, but that carrying the pregnancy is compromised by the defect. Ben-Rafael et al,[5] found that 21 percent of the 67 women with uterine anomalies in their study presented for HSG complaining of primary infertility. By contrast, Heinonen and Pystynen[6] found that of 228 women with uterine anomalies, only 9.1 percent had primary infertility, and that most of these cases could be explained by other defects. In addition, Daly[7] has reported that metroplasty is not a worthwhile treatment for unexplained infertility. Although other reports have suggested an association between the problems, most authorities agree that primary infertility in the presence of uterine anomalies is not an indication for metroplasty. After all other diagnostic and therapeutic attempts have been made, metroplasty may be considered.

There is a high rate of recurrent first and second trimester abortion in women with mullerian dysgenesis. Harger et al[8] reported mullerian anomalies in 12 percent of women from a prospective evaluation of 155 couples with two or more consecutive pregnancy losses. Many women, however, have normal reproductive histories in spite of mullerian anomalies. The only abnormality that is consistently noted on routine gynecologic examination is the uterus didelphys, which also has two hemicervices and likely a longitudinal sagittal vaginal septum. Because there have been no good prospective studies on patients with various uterine anomalies and their reproductive outcome, it is difficult to know what are the true spontaneous abortion risks for these women. The estimated spontaneous abortion rate is 33.8 percent for bicornuate uterus, 22.2 percent for septate uterus, and 34.6 percent for unicornuate uteri according to Jewelewicz and colleagues.[9]

The didelphic uterus is thought to have the best reproductive performance after the arcuate uterus. Heinonen et al[6] found a fetal survival rate of 64 percent without repair, while Musich and Behrman[10] found a 57 percent chance of successful pregnancy. The didelphic uterus may not, however, have better outcomes than the unicornuate uterus according to Moutos et al.[11] They compared 25 women with 28 pregnancies in didelphic uteri to 29 women with 40 pregnancies in unicornuate uteri, and found no statistical difference in the percentage ending in living children (61 percent versus 53 percent, respectively).

The most common uterine anomaly found during evaluation for recurrent abortion is the septate uterus. Again, it is difficult to know what is the risk of miscarriage with this anomaly, as it is so commonly found in women with normal reproductive histories. The uterine septum is thought to be

unable to support a gestation because of its poor vascularity. Candiani et al[12] showed an absence of organized vasculature in the septum's intermediate myometrium and scanty differentiation of the endometrial basal stratum. Burchell et al[13] have shown that myometrial vascular inadequacies have an important impact on pregnancy outcomes. It seems that the longer the septum, the worse the prognosis; Buttram and Gibbons[14] noted fetal loss in 88 percent of pregnancies with a complete septum and 70 percent with an incomplete septum. Although the septate uterus is generally considered to have the worst outcome of the uterine anomalies, Heinonen et al[15] found in a review of the reproductive histories of 182 women that the fetal survival was 86 percent with septate uterus, 50 percent with bicornuate uterus, and 40 percent with the unicornuate uterus.

As noted above, 53 percent of 40 pregnancies resulted in living children in one study of unicornuate uteri. In another study of 13 women with 29 pregnancies, there was a 59 percent spontaneous abortion rate and 38 percent living children.[16] Pregnancy in an obstructed horn is of great concern; a study of 328 pregnancies showed that only 1 percent of such pregnancies were alive at term and that 89 percent of the horns ruptured.[17]

DES is associated with increased fetal loss as well. In a study of 120 conservatively managed pregnancies in 50 women with and without gross anomalies, Levine and Berkowitz[18] reported that 59 percent of these pregnancies resulted in liveborn children with a significantly higher spontaneous abortion and preterm birth in the anomalous group (25.8 and 12.4 percent, versus 12.9 and 0 percent respectively).

Other obstetric complications also occur more commonly with uterine anomalies. There are increased risks of prematurity, intrauterine growth retardation,[19] antepartum bleeding, cervical incompetence, abnormal fetal presentation, cesarean section, and retained placenta associated with uterine abnormalities.

Premature births may be explained by the decreased size of the uterine cavity, especially in the unicornuate uteri. Growth retardation may be secondary to a small uterine cavity or abnormal vascularization of the uterus, with resultant uteroplacental insufficiency. Antepartum bleeding may be secondary to threatened abortions or bleeding from a decidualized horn that is not bearing a pregnancy. At present, it is not believed necessary to perform routine cerclage in all women with uterine anomalies; standard indications for cerclage placement are followed. The increased risk of malpresentation[20] and occasional occurrence of other anomalies in the vagina are the main reasons for the increased risk of cesarean section. Postpartum hemorrhage may also occur in these pregnancies, as the placenta may be partially trapped in an accessory or opposite horn.

Ben-Rafael et al[5] studied the outcomes of 67 women with uterine malformations—86.5 percent bicornuate uterus, 7.5 percent unicornuate, and 6 percent didelphys, with septate and arcuate uteri excluded. In comparison with 130 women with normal HSG, they found a significantly higher rate of the following: prematurity, intrauterine fetal death, and premature rupture of the membranes in women who had earlier presented with infertility; decreased birth weight in preterm infants; antepartum bleeding; breech presentation; and cesarean section.

Ludmir et al[21] studied 42 women with 101 pregnancies. There were 5 unicornuate, 61 bicornuate, 25 septate, and 10 didelphic uterine anomalies. All of these women were managed at high-risk clinics. The authors found that 60 percent of the pregnancies of the unicornuate and didelphys group reached term, 39 percent in the bicornuate group, and 48 percent in the septate group. Twenty-one percent of bicornuate and 15 percent of the septate group had preterm labor, requiring tocolysis. Five percent of the bicornuate uteri required cerclage. The fetal survival before their care was 52 and 53 percent with bicornuate and septate uteri respectively, and 58 and 65 percent under their care; these differences were not significant. Therefore, the cure for these poor obstetric outcomes does not seem to lie in more intensive pregnancy management.

DES exposure leads to a 50 to 70 percent risk of vaginal adenosis, and a 20 to 50 percent risk of various cervical structural abnormalities. Spontaneous abortion, premature labor, increased perinatal mortality, and ectopic pregnancy are more common.

DIAGNOSIS

Uterine anomalies are often first diagnosed on HSG during the workup for infertility. When an abnormal endometrial cavity is shown with this study, the external contour of the uterus requires further workup. Description of the external uterus has traditionally been performed with diagnostic laparoscopy.

Radiologic diagnosis of uterine anomalies has become very effective. Imaging studies should be performed during the luteal phase, when the endometrium is thickest and cavities can be better identified. While abdominal ultrasound is not effective, endovaginal sonography (EVS) has been shown to be very good. Pellerito et al[22] showed that in 12 cases of uterine anomaly, EVS was 100 percent sensitive and 80 percent specific for septate uterus, but 100 percent specific for anomalies not requiring surgery. Reuter et al[23] found that 90 percent of women with HSG and then ultrasound-suspected septate uteri had confirmation of this finding on laparoscopic examination. Ultrasound is also able to diagnose obstructive anomalies, such as hematometria or hematosalpinx. Magnetic resonance imaging (MRI) was shown to be 100 percent sensitive and 100 percent specific in 24 cases studied by Pellerito[22] and 29 patients by Carrington.[24]

Fedele et al[25] has suggested specific radiologic criteria for the diagnosis of septate uterus. The diagnosis relies on three points identified on a longitudinal scan of the uterus—the two ostia and the midpoint of the fundal perimetrium. If the midpoint was at least 5 mm above the straight line drawn between the ostia, he treated the uterus as septate. In a study of 29 women with abnormal uterine cavities, he defined 23 of these as septate uteri. Using this radiologic diagnosis, he performed hysteroscopic metroplasty safely on all 23 women, including 4 who at the time of laparoscopy were thought to have a fusion defect (bicornuate or didelphic uterus).

SURGICAL REPAIR

Indications

The most common indication for repair of congenital anomalies is repetitive pregnancy loss. Fetal wastage is greatly decreased in women who undergo metroplasty for this indication. Few authors suggest its use for primary infertility. A noncommunicating rudimentary horn in a unicornuate uterus, regardless of the presence of functioning endometrium, may be an indication because of the increased risk of ectopic pregnancy or endometriosis. Finally, some gynecologists advocate hysteroscopy for dysmenorrhea in the presence of a uterine anomaly.

Prior to surgical intervention, other causes for recurrent miscarriage must be ruled out. This workup should begin with a full history, including information on family reproductive problems, medical illness, and infectious and toxic etiologies, including DES exposure. An HSG to evaluate the uterine cavity and tubal patency is necessary. Basal body temperature, progesterone levels, and a timed luteal phase endometrial biopsy will evaluate luteal phase defects. Blood tests include a thyroid screen, antinuclear antibody, anticardiolipin antibody, lupus anticoagulant, and prolactin levels. Finally, chromosomal studies on both parents should be done.

Background

Prior to hysteroscopy, some physicians used blind transcervical approaches to uterine anomaly repair. In 1884, Ruge[26] performed a blind transcervical division of a septum for a patient with pregnancy wastage. In 1919, Hirsh[27] incised a septum for habitual abortion by placing his fingers through the cervix and cutting the palpated septum. In 1936, Luikart[28] performed a transcervical metroplasty by dilating the cervix, clamping the septum anteriorly and posteriorly, then cutting the intervening septum. The clamps were removed 24 hours later. Like Hirsh's patient, Luikart's later delivered vaginally at term.

Abdominal procedures are not new either. In 1907, Paul Strassman developed and then his son Erwin Strassman promoted a unification procedure for the bicornuate uterus.

Jones and Jones in 1953, and then Thompkins in 1962 presented valuable abdominal approaches for the repair of the septate uterus.

Hysteroscopic Repair

Hysteroscopic metroplasty has become the method of choice for repair of most uterine septa. Edstrom[29] first proposed the hysteroscopic technique in 1974; but improvements in instruments, distension media, and illumination were required before this procedure became widely used.

The procedure may be performed in an outpatient setting, usually under general anesthesia. It can be done with laparoscopic assistance, both to evaluate the external uterus and to observe for perforation. Some operators use progestational agents preoperatively to further atrophy the lining, but this is not necessary.

Various techniques and instruments are used either to incise the septum or actually remove it. Two of the most common instruments are the semirigid or rigid scissors (7 French) or the 8-mm wire loop urologic resectoscope used through the 21 French sheath. One may also use lasers: potassium-titan–phosphate (KTP/532), neodynamic:yttrium aluminum garnet (Nd:YAG), and argon lasers have all been used. In comparison studies, similar results have been shown for the many techniques.[30,31]

After evaluation with the laparoscope, the uterus is dilated with dextran or another appropriate medium. If two cervices are noted, a Foley balloon may be inserted into one os to prevent leakage of the distension media (Fig. 22-1).

Sometimes, the septum might only need incision, such as for partial septa or in the case of arcuate uterus. In the case of a complete septum, a zigzag approach may be used to remove tissue. In deciding which technique to use, the surgeon should remember that the goal of this procedure is to reduce the septal surface area. It can be difficult to recognize when the base of the septum has been reached. Remembering that the septum often has poor blood supply, the surgeon may continue until increased bleeding is noted. This will not work if a coagulative instrument is used. On completion, the surgeon should be able to visualize the fundus and sweep easily between the ostia in a normal appearing cavity.

No further treatment is required postoperatively. Intrauterine devices, Foley balloons, high-dose estrogen, and antibiotics are not necessary.[32] Formation of intrauterine synechiae is rare, as are postoperative infections, and the body's own estrogen is sufficient to promote new endometrium. Candiani et al[33] demonstrated microscopically the repair of the uterine fundus within 2 months after hysteroscopic metroplasty. Therefore, attempts at pregnancy may begin after two menstrual cycles. An HSG should be performed 2 months after surgery to assess success. Typically, over 90 percent of the septum is removed during the procedure. Occasionally, further repairs of the septum are required, again

in an ambulatory setting. Vericellini et al[32] reported that 4 of 12 septi treated with the resectoscope, and 2 of 11 repaired with microscissors required a second procedure to complete removal of the septum. Fedele et al[34] reported that of 102 metroplasties using the microscissors (n = 80), argon laser (n = 10), or electroresectoscope (n = 12), 35 required repair of a residual fundal notch of greater than 1 cm noted on follow-up hysteroscopy; 32 of these were done in the office and 5 required general anesthesia.

There has been some study of the use of ultrasound to guide a transcervical metroplasty using microscissors, with results similar to those of hysteroscopic procedures.[35] This procedure is still being evaluated, however and cannot yet be recommended.

Abdominal Procedures

Until hysteroscopy, uterine septum repair was performed with either the Jones or Thompkins metroplasty. If the septum cannot be safely removed hysteroscopically, then the abdominal approach may still be used. In addition, these repairs have be used on the DES-exposed uterus. The Strassman procedure, traditionally reserved for the bicornuate uterine repair, has not been sufficiently shown to be effective and therefore is not recommended.

The Jones procedure is in fact a wedge resection of the uterine fundus (Fig. 22-2). The operator first draws a triangular incision line forming a wedge in the anterior-posterior plane. Some surgeons will inject vasopressin (Pitressin) into the myometrium (10 U in 30 ml of saline) at this juncture to reduce bleeding. Alternatively, a system of tourniquets may be placed. A 0.5 Penrose drain may be placed through an avascular space in the broad ligament just lateral to the uterine vessels and tied at the junction of the lower uterine segment and the cervix. Using the same holes in the broad ligament, tourniquets should also be secured on the infundibulopelvic ligaments bilaterally. It is important that arterial flow is stopped, as uterine congestion and increased bleeding will occur if only the venous flow is staid.

Sutures should be placed bilaterally for traction. The wedge resection is then performed until the common uterine cavity is found and the septum totally removed. The reconstruction of the uterus begins at the lower portion of the uterine cavity. The anterior and then the posterior walls are closed in either a continuous or interrupted fashion. Some operators inject methylene blue into the uterine cavity prior to the incision, so that the endometrium is easily identified. The first layer should include the endometrium and a small amount of myometrium. The knot should be tied so that it remains in the uterine cavity. The second closure layer of interrupted sutures includes the remainder of the myometrium, beginning inferiorly. The final layer, using light suture in a continuous or interrupted fashion, includes the remainder of the myometrium and the serosa, attempting to imbricate the rough serosal edges.

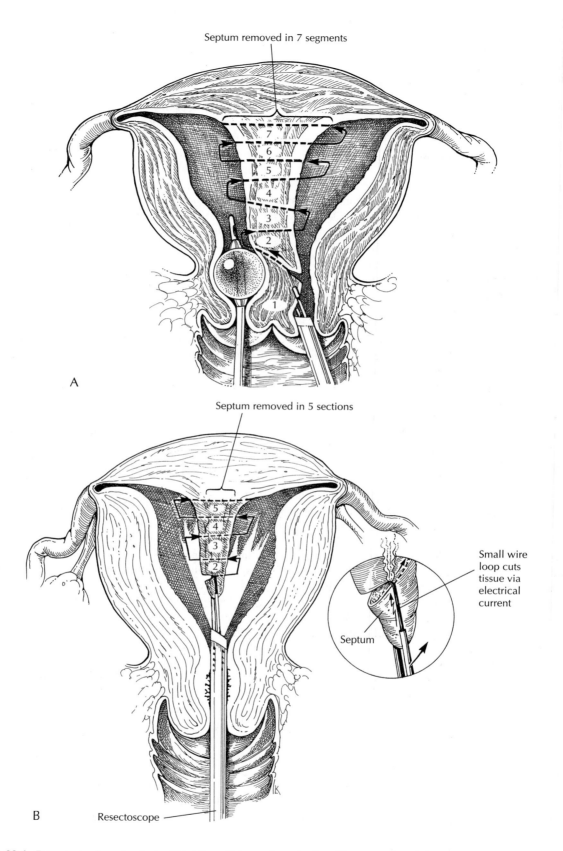

Septum removed in 7 segments

7
6
5
4
3
2
1

A

Septum removed in 5 sections

5
4
3
2

Small wire
loop cuts
tissue via
electrical
current

Septum

B   Resectoscope

Fig. 22-1. Resectoscopic metroplasty. **(A)** After a Foley catheter is placed in one cavity of the complete septate uterus, the resectoscope is inserted into the opposite cavity. The septum is then incised with the resectoscope until the Foley catheter is visualized. The septum is removed in small portions until both internal oses are visible. **(B)** In a similar fashion, the septate uterus may be repaired with stepwise resectoscopic excision of the septum.

390

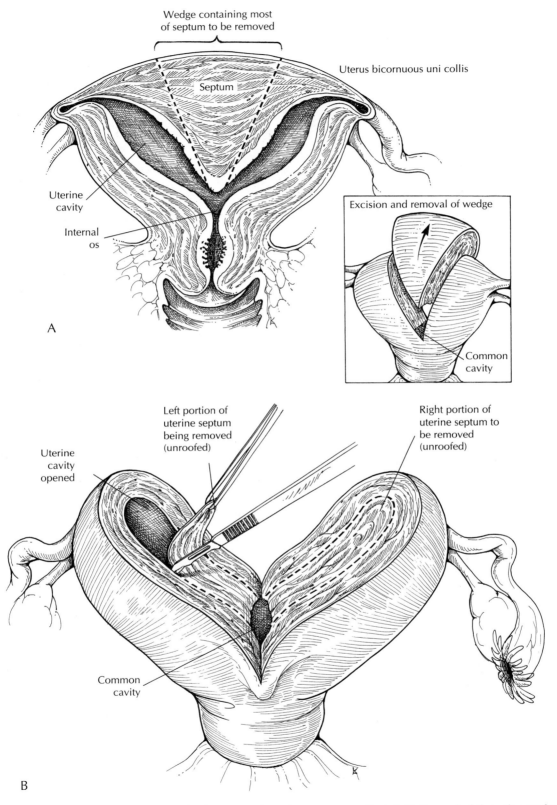

Fig. 22-2. The Jones procedure. **(A)** In the Jones procedure, the common cavity is initially reached through a wedge resection of the septum. **(B)** The septum is totally removed as the two cavities are unroofed. *(Figure continues.)*

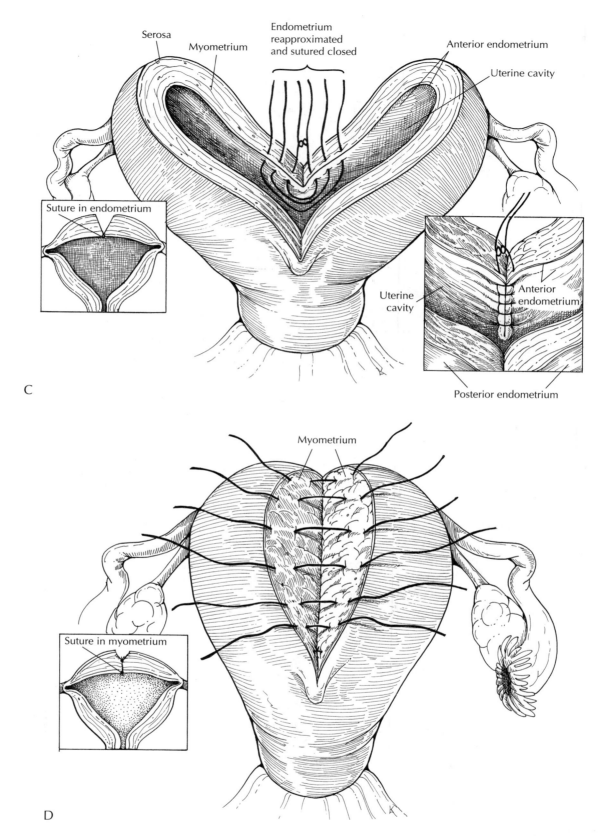

Fig. 22-2 *(Continued).* **(C)** Uterine closure is begun in the lower portion of the cavity. The anterior and then the posterior walls are closed, including the endometrium and a small portion of myometrium. The suture may be continuous or interrupted. **(D)** Beginning inferiorly, a row of interrupted sutures is then placed in the remaining thickness of the uterine wall. *(Figure continues.)*

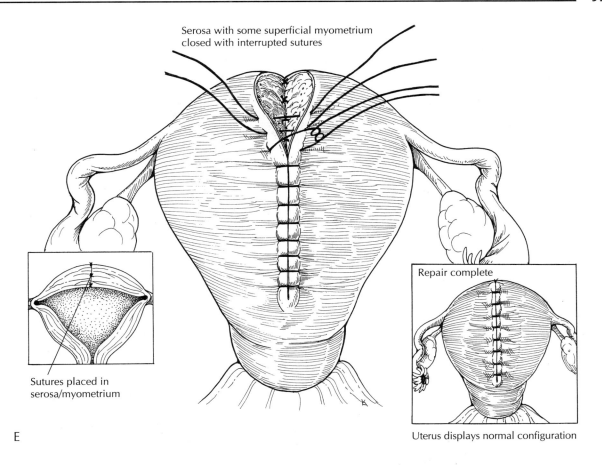

Serosa with some superficial myometrium
closed with interrupted sutures

Sutures placed in
serosa/myometrium

E

Repair complete

Uterus displays normal configuration

Fig. 22-2 *(Continued)*. **(E)** Using the lightest possible suture, the third layer approximates the superficial myometrium and serosa. The rough edges should be imbricated as much as possible to prevent adhesions along the suture line.

The Thompkins procedure is very similar to the Jones procedure, except that no tissue is removed (Fig. 22-3). The uterus is incised in the midline anterior-posterior plane until the uterine cavity is reached. The bilateral cavities are then unroofed, using sharp dissection, and the uterus is closed as in the Jones procedure. The benefit of this procedure is a resultant larger uterine cavity.

Outcome

Improved fetal survival has been demonstrated for all of the above described procedures. Although some early studies reported lower rates, the successful pregnancy rate after hysteroscopic metroplasty is 85 to 90 percent, which was much improved compared to the patients' preoperative fetal salvage rates.[36–39] Hysteroscopic metroplasty was also found to be of benefit in DES-associated anomalies.[40]

Rock and Jones[41] reported that of 58 pregnancies after Jones metroplasty in 43 women, 70 percent resulted in living children. Prior to surgery, these women had 140 pregnancies with 3 percent resulting in living children.[41] Khalifa and colleagues[42] performed abdominal metroplasties (Jones or Strassman) on 15 women with bicornuate uteri (n = 2), T-shaped uteri (n = 3), or septate uteri (n = 13) in women with concomitant intra-abdominal lesions such as endometriosis, adhesions, or myoma, or because of a wide arcuate septum. They reported that the fetal wastage rate dropped from 87.9 to 9.1 percent, and 13 of 16 patients attempting pregnancy conceived and delivered postoperatively. Candiani et al[43] reported on 70 women with septate uteri and 73 women with bicornuate uteri who underwent abdominal metroplasty, primarily with the Tompkins (n = 62 for septate uteri, and n = 55 for bicornuate uteri), Jones (n = 7 for septate uteri, and n = 6 for bicornuate uteri), and Strassman procedures (n = 4 for septate uteri, and n = 5 for bicornuate uteri), for sterility or recurrent miscarriage. They reported delivery rates of 70 and 73 percent in women with septate and bicornuate uteri, respectively, after surgery. Although the pregnancy outcomes are improved, either the uterine anomaly diagnoses or the types of repair are incorrect. In a comparison of abdominal and hysteroscopic metroplasty, Fayez[42] found that of the 14 women who underwent Thompkins procedure for septate uteri, 70 percent of pregnancies resulted in liveborn infants. In a study on 40 women with bicornuate uteri and 49 women with septate uteri who underwent either

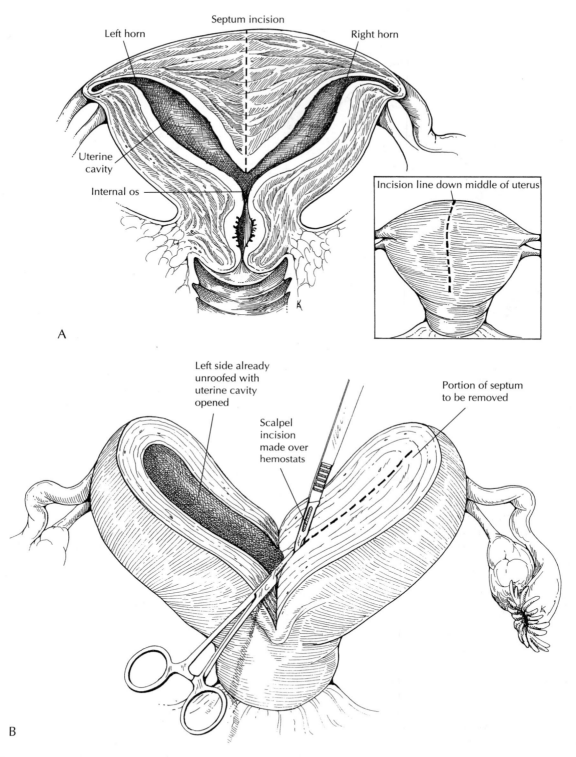

Fig. 22-3. The Tompkins procedure. **(A)** In the Tompkins procedure, the septum is incised but not removed. An initial incision is made down the middle of the septum until the common cavity is reached. **(B)** The septal tissue is incised bilaterally to unroof the two cavities. *(Figure continues.)*

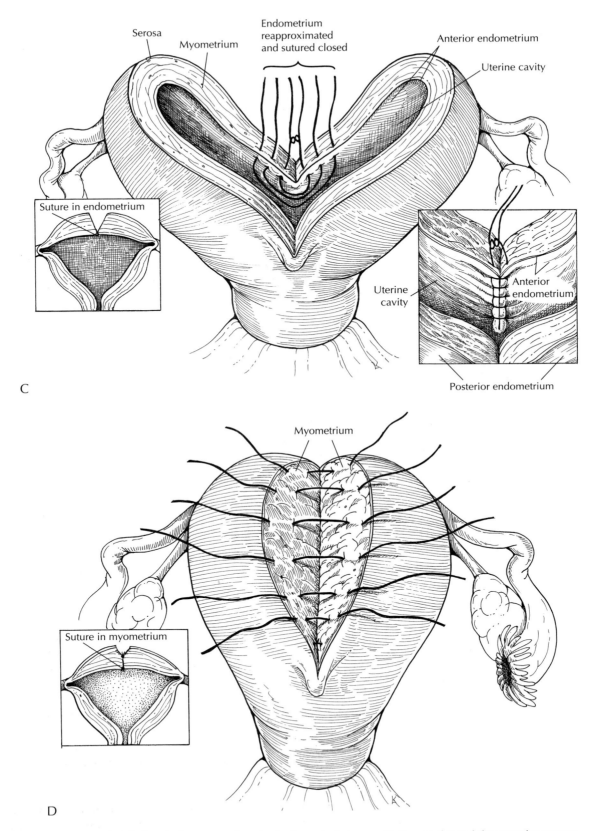

Fig. 22-3 *(Continued).* **(C)** Repair then proceeds as in the Jones technique, with the anterior and the posterior aspects being approximated with continuous or interrupted sutures. **(D)** The deep myometrium is repaired. *(Figure continues.)*

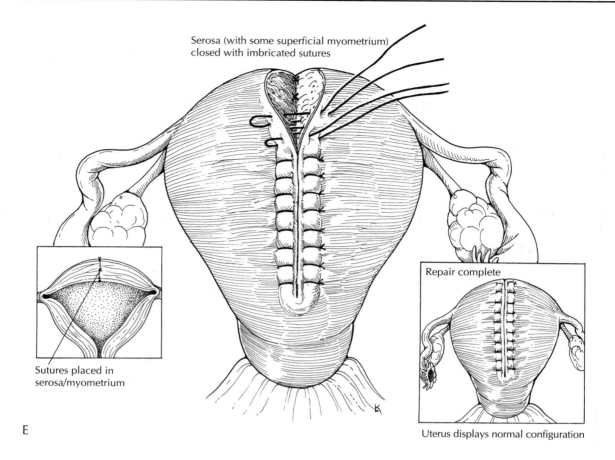

Serosa (with some superficial myometrium) closed with imbricated sutures

Sutures placed in serosa/myometrium

Repair complete

Uterus displays normal configuration

E

Fig. 22-3 *(Continued).* **(E)** After which the superficial myometrium and serosa are closed with an imbricating suture.

Jones, Tompkins, or Strassman procedures, Ayhan et al[44] found fetal survival increased from 3 to 83.3 percent and 4 to 65.2 percent respectively. Much improved fetal outcomes were also noted by Capraro et al[45] using the abdominal unification procedures.

Kirk et al[46] have questioned whether metroplasty truly improves outcome for repetitive abortions. In a study of 146 women with bicornuate, septate, or didelphic uterus, 30 of whom were matched, no increase in the number of living children was found after metroplasty in the matched group. Some believe that consecutive pregnancies in abnormal uteri will carry longer and that these women will eventually deliver at term.

In summary, the repairs for septate uteri are believed to be useful, while use of the abdominal repair of the bicornuate uterus is not believed by the authors to be sufficiently supported by the existing data.

Fedele and colleagues[47] have presented a prospective study on dysmenorhea reported by women who underwent Tompkins (n = 28) or hysteroscopic (n = 62) metroplasty for septate uteri. They found that the frequency of dysmenorhea fell from 50 to 32.1 percent after the Tompkins procedure (0.1< P >0.05) and from 54.8 to 17.7 percent hysteros-

copic treatment (P <0.001). Strassman was a proponent of metroplasty for dysmenorrhea as well. Therefore, dysmenorrhea in women with septate uteri may be considered by some an indication for hysteroscopic metroplasty.

Obstetrically, one would expect that the incidence of malpresentation, bleeding, and other risks associated with mullerian abnormalities would return to that of the general population after repair. There is an increased risk, however, of uterine rupture with abdominal procedures. Most authors recommend cesarean delivery for these patients. Uterine rupture has been reported after hysteroscopic procedures as well. One case involved use of the microscissors complicated by perforation.[48] In another, metroplasty was performed with a KTP laser without known perforation.[49] Still, vaginal delivery is generally pursued after hysteroscopic repair.

In addition to equivalent or better pregnancy outcomes, there are many other benefits to the transcervical approach. There is much less morbidity, no abdominal incision, and patients are able to return to normal activity quickly. As there is no abdominal incision, possible infections and intra-abdominal adhesions that may cause future infertility problems or pain are avoided. Patients are able to become pregnant again in 2 months instead of 3 to 6 months, and are able to attempt vaginal delivery. Additionally, this is an outpatient procedure, so it is much more cost-effective.

SUMMARY

Thus, the physician must remember that congenital uterine anomalies are not infrequent, and recognize signs and symptoms of their presence. A relatively simple workup has been defined, but the presence of anomalies without significant symptoms is not an indication for their repair.

REFERENCES

1. Simon C, Martinez L, Pardo F et al: Mullerian defects in women with normal reproductive outcome. Fertil Steril 56: 1192, 1991
2. Cooper J, Houck RM, Rigeberg HS: The incidence of intrauterine abnormalities found at hysteroscopy in patients undergoing elective hysteroscopic sterilization. J Reprod Med 8:659, 1983
3. Thompson DP, Lynn HB: Genital anomalies associated with solitary kidney. Mayo Clin Proc 41:538, 1966
4. The American Fertility Society: The American Fertility Society classifications of adnexal adhesions, distal tubal occlusion, tubal occlusion secondary to tubal ligations, tubal pregnancies, mullerian anomalies, and intrauterine adhesions. Fertil Steril 49:952, 1988
5. Ben-Rafael Z, Seidman DS, Recabi K et al: Uterine anomalies: a retrospective, matched-control study. J Reprod Med 36:723, 1991
6. Heinonen PK, Pystynen PP: Primary infertility and uterine anomalies. Fertil Steril 40:311, 1988
7. Daly DC, Maier D, Soto-Albors CS: Hysteroscopic metroplasty: six years' experience. Obstet Gynecol 73:201, 1989
8. Harger JH, Archer DP, Marchese SG: Etiology of recurrent pregnancy losses and outcome of subsequent pregnancies. Obstet Gynecol 62:574, 1983
9. Jewelewicz R, Husarni N, Wallach EE: When uterine factors cause infertility. Contemp Obstet Gynecol 16:95, 1980
10. Musich JR, Behrman SJ: Obstetric outcome before and after metroplasty in women with uterine anomalies. Obstet Gynecol 52:63, 1978
11. Moutos DM, Damewood MD, Schlaff WD et al: A comparison of the reproductive outcome between women with a unicornuate uterus and women with a didelphic uterus. Fertil Steril 58:88, 1992
12. Candiani GB, Fedele L, Zamberletti D et al: Endometrial patterns in malformed uteri. Acta Eur Fertil 14:311, 1983
13. Burchell RC, Creed F, Rasoulpour M et al: Vascular anatomy of human uterus and pregnancy wastage. Br J Obstet Gynaecol 85:698, 1978
14. Buttram V, Gibbons W: Mullerian anomalies: a proposed classification. Fertil Steril 32:40, 1979
15. Heinonen P, Saarikoski S, Pystynen P: Reproductive performance of women with uterine anomalies: an evaluation of 182 cases. Acta Obstet Gynecol Scand 61:157, 1982
16. Fedele L, Zamberletti D, Vercellini P et al: Reproductive performance of women with a unicornuate uterus. Fertil Steril 47:416, 1987
17. O'Leary JL, O'leary JA: Rudimentary horn pregnancy. Obstet Gynecol 22:371, 1963
18. Levine RU, Berkowitz KM: Consevative management and pregnancy outcome in diethylstilbestrol-expose women with and without gross genital tract abnormalities. Am J Obstet Gynecol 169:1125, 1993
19. Andrews MC, Jones HW Jr: Impaired reproductive performance of the unicornuate uterus: intrauterine growth retardation; infertility and recurrent abortion in five cases. Am J Obstet Gynecol 144:173, 1982
20. Green LK, Harris RE: Uterine anomalies: frequency of diagnosis and associated obstetric complications. Obstet Gynecol 47:427, 1976
21. Ludmir J, Samuels P, Brooks S, et al: Pregnancy outcome of patients with uncorrected uterine anomalies managed in a high-risk obstetric setting. Obstet Gynecol 75:906, 1990
22. Pellerito JS, Diagnosis of uterine anomalies: relative accuracy of MR imaging, endovaginal sonography, and hysterosalpingography. Radiology 183:795, 1992
23. Reuter KL, Daly DC, Cohen SM: Septate versus bicornuate uteri: errors in imaging diagnosis. Radiology 172:749, 1989
24. Carrington BM, Hricak H, Nuruddin RN et al: Mullerian duct anomalies: MR limaging evaluation. Radiology 176:715, 1990
25. Fedele L, Dorta M, Brioschi D et al: Re-examination of the anatomic indications for hysteroscopic metroplasty. Eur J Obstet Gynecol Repro Biol 39:127, 1991
26. Ruge P: Einen fall von schwangerschaft bei uterus suptus. Z Geburtshife Gynakol 10:141, 1884
27. Hirsh BC: The operative treatment of uterus subseptus or semipartus with a case report. Trans Obstet Soc Phila 791:1919
28. Luikart R: Technique of successful removal of the septum uterine septus and subsequent deliveries at term. Am J Obstet Gynecol 31:797, 1936
29. Edstrom KGB: Intrauterine surgical procedures during hysteroscopy. Endoscopy 6:175, 1974
30. Candiani GB, Vercellini P, Fedele L et al: Argon laser versus microscissors for hysteroscopic incision of uterine septa. Am J Obstet Gynecol 164:87, 1991
31. Vercellini P, Vendola N, Colombo A et al: Hysteroscopic metroplasty with resectoscope or microscissors for the correction of septate uterus. Surg Gynecol Obstet 176:439, 1993
32. Vercellini P, Fedele L, Arcaini L et al: Value of intrauterine device insertion and estrogen administration after hysteroscopic metroplasty. J Reprod Med 34:447, 1989
33. Candiani GB, Vercellini P, Fedele L et al: Repair of the uterine cavity after hysteroscopic septal incision. Fertil Steril 54:991, 1990
34. Fedele L, Arcaini L, Parazzini F et al: Reproductive prognosis

after hysteroscopic metroplasty in 102 women: life table analysis. Fertil Steril 59:768, 1993

35. Querleu D, Brasme TL, Parmentier D: Ultrasound-guided transcervical metroplasty. Fertil Steril 54:995, 1990

36. March CM, Israel R: Hysteroscopic management of recurrent abortion caused by septate uterus. Am J Obstet Gynecol 156:834, 1987

37. Valle RF, Sciarra JJ: Hysteroscopic treatment of the septate uterus. Obstet Gynecol 67:253, 1986

38. Fayez JA: Comparison between abdominal and hysteroscopic metroplasty. Obstet Gynecol 68:399, 1986

39. Choe JK, Baggish MS: Hysteroscopic treatment of septate uterus with neodymium-YAG laser. Fertil Steril 57:81, 1992

40. Nabel TC, Malo JW: Hysteroscopic metroplasty in the diethylstilbestrol-exposed uterus and similar nonfusion anomalies: effects on subsequent reproductive performance; a preliminary report. Fertil Steril 59:502, 1993

41. Rock J, Jones H Jr: The clinical management of the double uterus. Fertil Steril 28:798, 1977

42. Khalifa E, Toner JP, Jones HW: The role of abdominal metroplasty in the era of operative hysteroscopy. Surg Gynecol Obstet 176:208, 1993

43. Candiani GB, Fedele L, Parazzini F et al: Reproductive prognosis after abdominal metroplasty in bicornuate or septate uterus: a life table analysis. Br J Obstet Gynecol 97:613, 1990

44. Ayhan A, Yucel I, Tuncer ZS et al: Reproductive performance after conventional metroplasty: an evaluation of 102 cases. Fertil Steril 57:1194, 1992

45. Capraro VJ, Chuang JT, Randall CL: Improved fetal salvage after metroplasty. Obstet Gynecol 31:97, 1968

46. Kirk EP, Chuong CJ, Coulam CB et al: Pregnancy after metroplasty for uterine anomalies. Fertil Steril 59:1164, 1993

47. Fedele L, Bianchi S, Bocciolone L: Relief of dysmenorrhea associated with septate uteri after abdominal or hysteroscopic metroplasty. Acta Obstet Gynecol Scand 73:56, 1994

48. Halvorson LM, Aserkoff RD, Oskowitz SP: Spontaneous uterine rupture after hysteroscopic metroplasty with uterine perforation: a case report. J Reprod Med 38:236, 1993

49. Lobaugh ML, Bammel BM, Duke D et al: Uterine rupture during pregnancy in a patient with a histrory of hysteroscopic metroplasty. Obstet Gynecol 83:838, 1994

CHAPTER TWENTY-THREE

UTERINE ANATOMY

WILLIAM J. MANN, Jr.

> **Uterus**
> **Bladder**
> **Ligaments**
> **Pelvic Vasculature**

UTERUS

The uterus is a pear-shaped, muscular, hollow organ located in the midpelvis, with a cervical portion extending approximately 2 cm into the vagina and a body, or corpus, extending 5 to 6 cm into the abdomen. At the point where the cervix and corpus meet, there is a surface constriction referred to as the isthmus. The portion of the corpus extending above the entrance of the fallopian tubes is known as the fundus. The normal uterus may weigh 40 to 80 g, depending on a patient's parity and menstrual status.

BLADDER

The bladder lies over the upper vagina and cervix, and the rectum lies against the posterior upper vagina. Both organs are covered by pelvic peritoneum, with the depth of the posterior space between the uterus and rectum quite variable. If this posterior pelvic peritoneum is incised, a potential space exists between the posterior vagina and anterior rectum, which at the midline is avascular. The anterior peritoneum may be elevated and incised, and then sharp and blunt dissection can develop an anterior space between the bladder and cervix, which is also avascular at the midline (Fig. 23-1).

LIGAMENTS

The lateral attachments of the uterus consist of the paired round, broad, and uterosacral ligaments. The round ligaments run anterolaterally from the ventral surface of the uter-

ine fundus just below the attachment of the tube, to cross the external iliac vessels and enter the deep inguinal ring. The ring is usually 2 to 4 ml in diameter, and contains a small artery and vein. The broad ligaments are covered with peritoneum anteriorally and posteriorally, and run from the lateral aspects of the uterus to the pelvic sidewall. The uterine vasculature, lymph nodes, fat, and connective tissues lie within this ligament. The ureter passes through it in its pelvic course. The lower part of the broad ligament, where the connective tissue is condensed and thicker, is often referred to as the cardinal ligament. The cardinal ligament attaches to the cervix and upper vagina laterally. The uterosacral ligaments run posterolateral from the cervix to the sacrum, and are a continuation of the posterior cardinal ligament. In elderly women, the round and uterosacral ligaments may be extremely tenuous.

PELVIC VASCULATURE

The pelvic vasculature arise from branches of the external and internal iliac arteries, and the middle sacral artery. The uterine artery courses medially from the internal iliac to the uterine isthmus, where it divides into an ascending and descending branch. These vessels give off subserosal arteries, which then give off radial arteries that course into the myometrium (Fig. 23-2).

The branches of the internal iliac artery are of great varia-

399

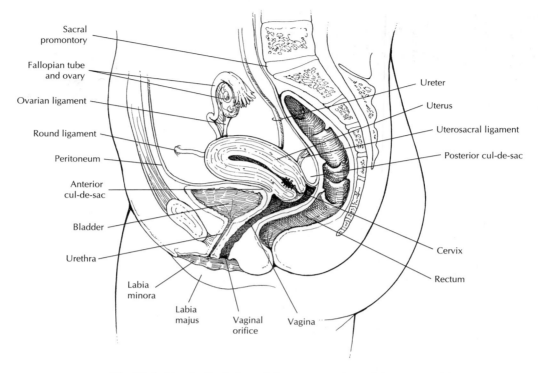

Fig. 23-1. Longitudinal view of the anatomy of an adult woman.

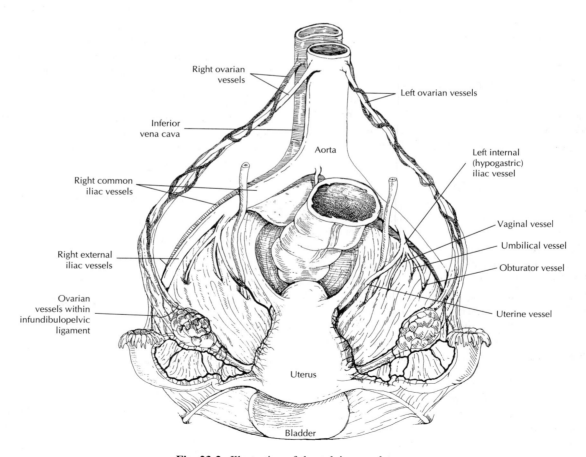

Fig. 23-2. Illustration of the pelvic vasculature.

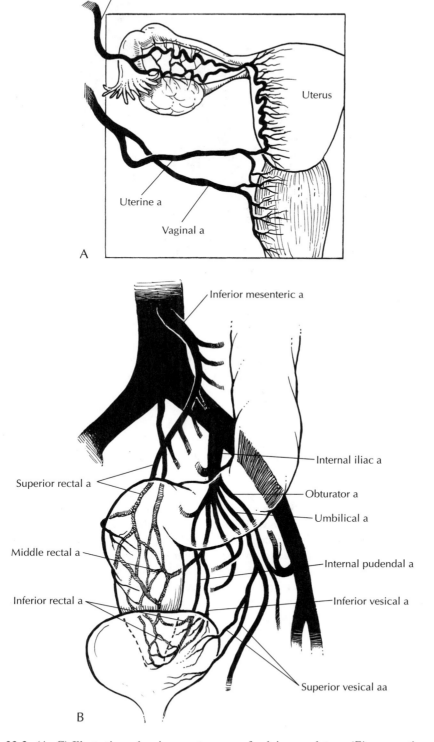

Fig. 23-3. (**A–C**) Illustrations showing anastomoses of pelvic vasculature. *(Figure continues.)*

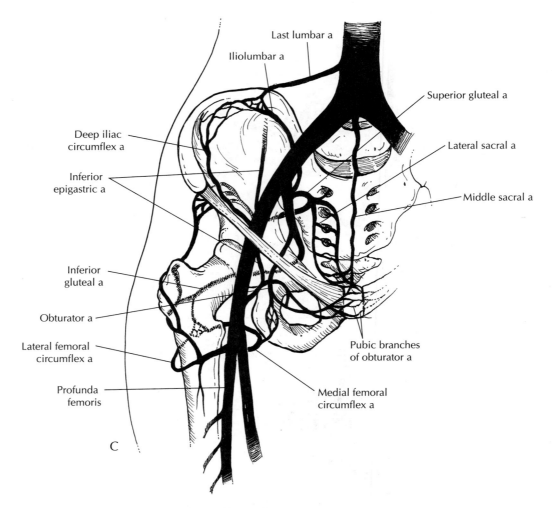

Last lumbar a

Iliolumbar a

Superior gluteal a

Deep iliac
circumflex a

Lateral sacral a

Inferior
epigastric a

Middle sacral a

Inferior
gluteal a

Obturator a

Pubic branches
of obturator a

Lateral femoral
circumflex a

Medial femoral
circumflex a

Profunda
femoris

C

Fig. 23-3 *(Continued).*

tion. In addition, generous collateral circulation in the pelvis allows for adequate blood flow to the pelvic viscera despite ligation of multiple vessels. The uterine, vaginal, and ovarian arteries anastomose with their contralateral equivalent, and with each other on each side (Fig. 23-3A). In addition, the vesical arteries on each side, as well as the rectal branches of the internal iliac and inferior mesenteric arteries also anastomose (Fig. 23-3B). The obturators anastomose with each other via a pubic branch, and with the inferior epigastric and medial femoral vessels on each side. Anastomoses also occur between the profunda femoris and inferior gluteal; the superior gluteal and the lateral sacral; the iliolumbar and the last lumbar; the lateral sacral and the middle sacral; and the iliac circumflex and the iliolumbar and superior gluteal (Fig. 23-3C). It is almost impossible to devascularize the female pelvis because of this rich anastomotic bed.

CHAPTER TWENTY-FOUR

VAGINAL, ABDOMINAL, AND LAPAROSCOPIC-ASSISTED HYSTERECTOMY

THOMAS G. STOVALL

For the gynecologic surgeon, hysterectomy represents the cornerstone of surgery, and is one of the most common and controversial surgical procedures performed by gynecologists. In an effort to best serve their patients, every gynecologist should be familiar with the issues surrounding the performance of hysterectomy and the variety of surgical techniques to accomplish the procedure.

BACKGROUND

Benrubi[1] has written a comprehensive review of the history of hysterectomy. In 1507, Berengarius of Bologna described the removal of the uterus through the vagina, al-though some credit Andreas of Cruce for performance of the first vaginal hysterectomy in 1560. Still others credit Ambrose Pare for removal of an inverted uterus as early as 1575. Although many procedures may have involved only partial uterine removal, Palletta did a transvaginal hysterectomy with complete uterine removal in 1812. This case was done inadvertently, however, as he was trying to remove only the cervix.

Ephraim McDowell is credited for performing the first abdominal gynecologic surgical procedure and first ovariectomy. Heath, in 1842, inadvertently performed a supracervical hysterectomy during an attempted oophorectomy. The first total abdominal hysterectomy with bilateral salpingo-oophorectomy was performed by Clay in 1844, although the patient subsequently died. Thus, Burnham in 1853 is credited with performance of the first successful abdominal hysterectomy.

INCIDENCE

The number of hysterectomies performed in the United States peaked in 1975 when 724,000 procedures were performed. Hysterectomy was the second most frequently performed major surgical procedure in the United States during 1995. In 1975, the average length of stay for hysterectomy was 9.4 days, which decreased to only 4.5 days in 1991. This length of stay is expected to decrease still further as a greater number of patients are enrolled in managed care organizations, and the safety of shorter hospital stay is determined. The most recent data available indicates that approximately 75 percent of hysterectomies are performed abdominally, with only 25 percent performed through the vagina.[2,3]

The rate of hysterectomy per 1,000 women has varied between 6.1/1,000 and 8.6/1,000 women in all age groups, with the average age of women undergoing hysterectomy remaining relatively constant over the past 20 years at 42.7 years (median age 40.9 years). Approximately 75 percent of all hysterectomies are performed in women between the ages of 20 and 49 years. The rate of hysterectomies varies by region of the country, with the South having the highest overall rate, and the northeast portion of the United States having the lowest rate. Hysterectomy is also more commonly performed in blacks than whites, and tends to be done more frequently by male gynecologists than female gynecologists.[4–7]

As the population ages, it is estimated that the number of hysterectomies will increase. Using 1987 age-specific hysterectomy rates and the population projections supplied by the Census Bureau, it is projected that approximately 824,000 hysterectomies will be done in 2005.[8,9]

INDICATIONS

The indications for hysterectomy vary somewhat between surgeons and also vary depending on the patient's age. Except for gynecologic and nongynecologic pelvic malignancy, medical therapy should always be considered before performing hysterectomy. In many instances, the decision to proceed with a hysterectomy is based on the patient's perception that the procedure will better the patient's overall life quality. For example, observational therapy or conservative surgical treatment can certainly be used for virtually all benign gynecologic conditions. However, some patients simply prefer hysterectomy. At present, little data is available to guide the patient's decision-making process in this regard. The decision to proceed with hysterectomy is a decision that should be mutually made by the patient and her physician.

Commonly Cited Indications for Hysterectomy

- Leiomyomata uteri
- Dysfunctional uterine bleeding
- Intractable dysmenorrhea
- Pelvic pain
- Cervical dysplasia
- Genital prolapse
- Obstetric injury
- Sterilization
- Pelvic inflammatory disease
- Endometriosis
- Gynecologic cancer
- Nongynecologic pelvic cancer

Increasingly, other parties such as third-party payers and professional standards review oganizations are having input on which patients are allowed to undergo hysterectomy.

Leiomyomata Uteri

Leiomyomata uteri is the most common indication for hysterectomy and should only be considered for the patient who does not desire future fertility. Hysterectomy can be used for management of symptoms commonly associated with myomas, including abnormal uterine bleeding, pelvic pressure, and pain. Other indications for hysterectomy in the patient with myomas include rapid uterine enlargement, ureteral compression, or growth following menopause. Rapid uterine enlargement (more than 6 weeks increase in gestational size in less than 12 months) has been thought in the past to be associated with a higher incidence of sarcomatous change. A recent study did not confirm this, and patients with rapid uterine enlargement did not have an increased incidence of leiomyosarcomas.[10,11] Some gynecologists suggest that the uterus should be removed even if asymptomatic when it reaches 12 gestational weeks in size. Reasons given for this view include the possibility of malignancy, inability to palpate the ovaries on bimanual examination, and the suggestion that, as the uterus enlarges, the morbidity for hysterectomy increases. However, it must be remembered, that the incidence of leiomyosarcomas is rare, adnexal palpation is not possible in up to 20 percent of patients, and even if palpable, this practice has not been shown to decrease the morbidity of ovarian cancer or lead to earlier detection. Studies also suggest that there is no difference in surgical morbidity in patients with a 12-week size uterus when compared to those with a 20-week size uterus if both procedures are done abdominally. However, most uteri that are 12 weeks in size can best be removed through the vagina.[12,13] Thus, when all of this is considered hysterectomy should probably only be considered in the symptomatic patient who does not desire future fertility.

Dysfunctional Uterine Bleeding

Dysfunctional uterine bleeding as an indication for hysterectomy accounts for approximately 20 percent of all hysterectomies performed. Hysterectomy for this indication should only be done after other etiologies for abnormal bleeding have been excluded and the patient has not responded to medical treatment. Although dilation and curettage has been commonly performed as a diagnostic and therapeutic procedure prior to hysterectomy, it is not successful in controlling the bleeding and is not necessary before considering hysterectomy.[14] Alternatives to hysterectomy such as endometrial ablation or resection may be considered and have been found to be cost-effective when compared to abdominal hysterectomy.[15,16] This study must be questioned, since most of these patients can undergo vaginal hysterectomy and no studies have yet compared ablation to outpatient vaginal hysterectomy. Nor have studies been done to address the long-term implications of ablation. For example, endometrial carcinomas and pregnancy have been reported after endometrial ablation.[17-19]

As with dysfunctional uterine bleeding, hysterectomy for dysmenorrhea should only be done in the patient who does not respond to medical treatment. Certainly, most patients can be controlled using nonsteroidal anti-inflammatory drugs alone or in combination with oral contraceptives.[20-22] Patients with secondary dysmenorrhea may have associated myomas, endometriosis, or adenomyosis.

Chronic Pelvic Pain

For the patient with chronic pelvic pain that has not responded to medical or conservative surgical therapy, hysterectomy may be considered. Before the hysterectomy, a multidisciplinary team approach, including physical therapy, has been shown to be beneficial.[23-25] Following hysterectomy, Carlson et al[26] found a significant reduction in symptoms which was associated with an improvement in the patient's life quality. Stovall and colleagues[27] reviewed 104 patients who underwent hysterectomy for chronic pelvic pain that was thought to be of uterine etiology. Patients were followed for a mean of 21.6 months, with 78 percent of patients showing significant improvement in their pain. However, 22 percent of patients had no improvement or an exacerbation of their pain. These findings suggest that hysterectomy should only be done in those patients who have pain that does not

respond to nonsurgical treatment modalities and in those patients where the pain is of uterine origin.

Cervical Intraepithelial Neoplasia

In the past, hysterectomy was done as primary treatment of cervical intraepithelial neoplasia. Conservative treatment modalities such as cryotherapy, laser ablation/conization, or loop excision are far less expensive and associated with less morbidity. These modalities can provide successful treatment in most patients and thus can minimize the use of hysterectomy as treatment for cervical dysplasia. Hysterectomy can probably be considered for the patient who develops recurrent cervical dysplasia and does not desire future fertility. This is especially true if the patient has had a previous conization or loop procedure. Rarely, hysterectomy is indicated in patients with biopsy-proven dysplasia who, for technical reasons related to markedly distorted anatomy, cannot undergo conization.

Pelvic Relaxation

Hysterectomy for pelvic relaxation accounts for approximately 15 percent of all hysterectomies performed in the United States. This indication for hysterectomy is more common in the older patient and is generally associated with other pelvic support defects that require correction during the same procedure in order to decrease the incidence of future recurrence. For the patient who desires future fertility, correction of the support defects can be corrected and uterine suspension can be accomplished while leaving the uterus in place. Regardless of the patient's age, nonsurgical treatment alternatives should be offered. This is an example of a surgical indication that is done primarily for improvement of the patient's life quality rather than because of a medical necessity.

Obstetric Complication

Hysterectomy for treatment of postpartum hemorrhage should only be considered after failure of uterotonic agents, as these medications are generally quite successful. Other obstetric indications include uterine rupture that cannot be repaired or when the patient develops a postcesarean or postpartum pelvic abscess that is not responsive to intravenous antibiotic therapy. In addition, patients with placenta accreta or increta will occasionally require hysterectomy. Cesarean hysterectomy is discussed in Chapter 26.

Pelvic Inflammatory Disease

Hysterectomy, with or without adnexal removal, in the patient with pelvic inflammatory disease should not be done unless the patient has not responded to broad-spectrum intravenous antibiotic therapy. Other treatment methods include abscess drainage alone by colpotomy or radiographically, laparoscopic drainage, or removal of a single adnexum. These treatment modalities should be considered for the patient who desires future fertility. The long-term implications in terms of development of chronic pain or future pelvic infections are uncertain. Laparotomy is also indicated if the patient has acute abdominal findings associated with peritonitis or sepsis in the presence of a ruptured tubo-ovarian abscess. In patients who desire future fertility, consideration should be given to leaving the uterus in place even if bilateral adnexectomy is necessary, so that the possibility of ovum donation and in vitro fertilization is maintained.

Endometriosis

Although a common etiology for infertility, endometriosis is an uncommon reason for hysterectomy as it can generally be treated with medical or conservative surgical approaches. Most patients with endometriosis who require hysterectomy do so because of pelvic pain or dysmenorrhea. Less common reasons include endometriosis involving other organ systems such as the urinary or gastrointestinal tract.

Gynecologic and Nongynecologic Malignancy

Primary gynecologic malignancy or metastases from nongynecologic sites may require that a patient undergo hysterectomy (i.e., colorectal cancer). Generally, hysterectomy with bilateral salpingo-oophorectomy should be considered for the patient with colorectal carcinoma, since these patients are at risk of either synchronous pelvic cancers or occult metastases.[28,29] Occasionally, symptomatic patients with breast cancer metastatic to adnexae or uterus will also benefit from hysterectomy.

Persistent Adnexal Mass

Hysterectomy is often done concurrently when a patient requires surgical intervention for a benign but persistent ovarian tumor. As with other benign conditions, the uterus should not be removed if the patient desires future fertility. Gambone et al[30] reviewed the records of 100 patients who underwent adnexectomy plus incidental hysterectomy for benign adnexal disease and compared these to a group of risk-matched women who underwent adnexectomy without hysterectomy for similar conditions. These authors found a significant increase in operative and perioperative morbidity, estimated blood loss, and longer hospital stay in patients who underwent an incidental hysterectomy at the time of adnexectomy. The long-term effects of this practice are not known.

Sterilization

In the past, hysterectomy was performed as a method to achieve sterilization. This is no longer considered an appropriate indication for hysterectomy because tubal occlusion is safer and more cost-effective. Vaginal and abdominal hysterectomy, when compared with tubal sterilization, are associated with greater morbidity, longer postoperative and convalescence periods, a higher risk of transfusion, and greater cost.[31,32] Vasectomy is also a cost-effective alternative.

ROUTE OF HYSTERECTOMY

Once the decision has been made to proceed with hysterectomy, the physician must then decide whether the procedure will be performed abdominally, vaginally, or with laparoscopic assistance. The route chosen should be the one that best accomplishes the procedure in a particular patient in question. The surgeon must also give consideration to surgical experience and expertise, as well as the patient's disease process. How the gynecologist chooses the route of hysterectomy varies between surgeons. Absolute and relative contraindications for vaginal hysterectomy have been proposed. Although there is no general agreement regarding these contraindications, most authors agree that contraindications to the vaginal approach include

1. Lack of uterine mobility
2. Presence of an adnexal mass requiring removal
3. Contracted bony pelvis
4. Need to explore the upper abdomen
5. Lack of surgical expertise

One must remember that many of these contraindications are relative. For example, how is uterine mobility determined and how should the bony pelvis be evaluated? Although some authors have suggested that obesity and previous pelvic surgery represent contraindications to a vaginal approach, studies have been done that actually indicate that previous pelvic surgery is not a contraindication to vaginal hysterectomy and that a vaginal approach is the procedure of choice for the obese woman requiring hysterectomy.[33–35]

Several studies have compared vaginal and abdominal hysterectomy. The most often quoted and complete study is a large multicenter retrospective study that was conducted by the Centers for Disease Control between 1978 and 1981, in which the risks and outcome of abdominal and vaginal hysterectomy were compared.[5] The study included 1,851 patients (568 vaginal and 1,283 abdominal hysterectomies), performed in women aged 15 to 44 years for benign gynecologic disorders. The overall complication rate was 24.5 per 100 women who had a vaginal hysterectomy, compared with 42.8 per 100 women who underwent abdominal hysterectomy. The risk of having one or more complications was 1.7

times more likely if the patient underwent an abdominal hysterectomy. The risk of infection was 2.1 times higher and the risk of transfusion was 1.9 times higher for the abdominal hysterectomy group. This data must be interpreted with a word of caution, since the patients undergoing abdominal hysterectomy may have had more severe disease and the guidelines for transfusion have changed in the last decade.[5] These authors also suggested that as many as 50 percent of patients in this study who underwent abdominal hysterectomy could have potentially undergone vaginal hysterectomy. This may indeed be the case, as two studies done recently have suggested that most hysterectomies can be completed vaginally without laparoscopic assistance.[36,37]

The role of laparoscopic assistance remains controversial, but may be used as either a diagnostic or operative instrument. Diagnostic laparoscopy before hysterectomy has been reported as a method to assess whether vaginal hysterectomy is possible and was thought to increase the utilization of the vaginal approach. However, patients in these studies had relative contraindications to a vaginal approach and could have undergone a vaginal approach without prehysterectomy laparoscopy.[38,39] If this approach is adopted, the cost and complication rate of hysterectomy will be higher. If selective laparoscopy is used only in patients with risk factors for endometriosis and adhesive disease, many patients will undergo laparoscopy who do not require the procedure. Clinical experience and expertise would likely allow selection of patients for vaginal surgery more efficiently through utilizing diagnostic laparoscopy. However, laparoscopy may contribute to developing these skills. Studies have been done demonstrating that the presence or absence of pelvic adhesions cannot be predicted based on either history or physical examination.[40] In addition, skilled and experienced vaginal surgeons may place less weight on relative contraindications than novices.

Numerous studies have reported case series of laparoscopic-assisted vaginal hysterectomies (LAVHs). Most of these studies lack randomization and most do not define the patient population such that conclusions can be drawn from the data presented. Many of these studies have suggested that patients included had contraindications to a vaginal approach, but the reasons for this decision are unclear. Nezhat et al[41] excluded patients from their study with a uterine size of 14 weeks or larger gestational size. Patients with leiomyomata who have a uterine size in this range can undergo vaginal hysterectomy. Daniell et al[42] reported a series of 68 patients who were said to require an abdominal approach for hysterectomy. Of these 68 patients, 13 were operated on for uterovaginal relaxation. Again, one must wonder why these patients require an abdominal approach. These two studies are representative of much of the current literature.[43–46]

It has been suggested that LAVH offers advantages over vaginal hysterectomy. Summitt et al[47] randomized patients who were candidates for vaginal hysterectomy to either LAVH or standard vaginal hysterectomy. All procedures were performed on an outpatient basis, with patients included who had a uterine size up to 16 weeks gestational size. No differences were found between the groups in terms of uterine weight, febrile morbidity, or the need for transfusion. Patients undergoing LAVH had a lower hematocrit value on postoperative days 1 and 2 and required more pain medication on postoperative day 2. This study suggests that LAVH does not reduce perioperative morbidity when compared to a vaginal approach. Charges for LAVH were significantly higher than for vaginal hysterectomy, with the largest component of this difference being secondary to the use of disposable equipment. Virtually all gynecologic surgeons now agree that if vaginal hysterectomy is possible, it is the procedure of choice.[47]

Davis et al[48] reported a group of patients with stage III and stage IV endometriosis in whom LAVH was attempted. These patients normally require an abdominal approach, even by experienced gynecologists. These authors were successful in performing the procedure in 40 of 46 patients. In this group of patients, the rate of surgical complications seemed high. However, because no comparison group was included in this study, no definite conclusions can be made. Also, the number of gynecologic surgeons who have the expertise to perform a procedure such as this is unknown.

LAVH has been proposed to increase the use of the vaginal approach for patients with uterine immobility or a narrow vaginal outlet. No studies have been done such that conclusions can be made regarding this indication. The classic teaching is that the major supporting structures of the uterus are the uterosacral ligaments and lower cardinal complex.[49] These structures are generally not transected through the laparoscope. Thus, one must question whether laparoscopic assistance is of real benefit in this group of patients.

As discussed later in this chapter, when desired, most oophorectomies can be completed at the time of vaginal hysterectomy. Thus, the use of either the laparoscopic or abdominal approach is not warranted solely for ovarian removal. Laparoscopic assistance is also not required for patients with mild pelvic adhesions or when the surgical indication is chronic pain. Even in this situation, a vaginal approach can generally be used successfully.

OPERATIVE PROCEDURES

The surgical technique of any individual surgeon varies between cases, evolves with experience, and is dependent on the pathologic conditions or anatomic variations encountered. Therefore, what is presented below is a step-by-step approach that works well for most cases encountered.

Vaginal Hysterectomy

Vaginal hysterectomy is performed with the patient in the dorsal lithotomy position. Patient positioning is critical to obtain optimal exposure. Once adequate anesthesia is obtained, a bimanual pelvic examination is performed to confirm the findings of the office examination, to assess uterine mobility and descent, and to confirm that no unsuspected adnexal pathology is found. Once completed, the final decision is made to proceed with a vaginal or abdominal approach to hysterectomy. Vaginal hysterectomy is most commonly performed using regional or general anesthesia, although the use of local anesthesia has been described.[50] The patient is then prepared and draped, and the bladder drained. Some surgeons prefer not to drain the bladder and believe that if urine is left in the bladder, it aids with recognition of a bladder injury should it occur. Still other surgeons prefer to place a Foley catheter in the bladder, empty the bladder, and then clamp the catheter.

A posterior weighted speculum is placed into the vagina, and a Dever retractor is placed anterior to the cervix. The anterior and posterior lips of the cervix are grasped with a single- or double-toothed tenaculum. For the surgeon operating alone, the use of a self-retaining vaginal retractor may be of benefit.[51] If vasopressin is to be used, it is injected into the cervical, paracervical, and submucosal tissues (Fig. 24-1). A solution composed of 10 to 20 U of vasopressin in a 50-ml solution is most commonly used. Other surgeons prefer to use a solution of 0.5 percent Xylocaine. Surgeons who prefer to use these vasoconstrictive agents believe that they aid with identification of tissue planes and reduce blood loss.[52] Still others use normal saline without a vasoconstric-

tive agent. This is preferable if the patient has heart disease or severe hypertension.[53,54] Finally, there are surgeons who do not use any vasoconstrictive agents, but rely on traction and prompt ligation alone for reducing blood loss.

Traction is placed on the cervix to expose the posterior vaginal mucosa, which is placed on traction. Using Mayo scissors, the posterior cul-de-sac is entered sharply, and the peritoneum identified (Fig. 24-2). A common error is to make exceedingly small cuts into the tented-up posterior peritoneum, as opposed to a generous bite. Once identified, a figure-of-eight suture is placed to attach the peritoneum to the posterior vaginal mucosa. If difficulty is encountered isolating the posterior peritoneum, the vaginal mucosa may be incised vertically to the point at which the cul-de-sac becomes more apparent. If vaginal mucosal dissection has occurred in the wrong plane, the hysterectomy may be begun in an extraperitoneal fashion by clamping and cutting the uterosacral and cardinal ligaments close to the cervix. If these steps fail, the anterior peritoneum can be entered and the posterior peritoneum identified by placing a finger or instrument behind the uterus. Other conditions such as endometriosis or extensive adhesive disease resulting from previous surgery or pelvic inflammatory disease may cause posterior cul-de-sac obliteration. In such circumstances, entry into the cul-de-sac may not be possible as an initial step. In such cases, one can continue clamping/ligation of the uterosacral

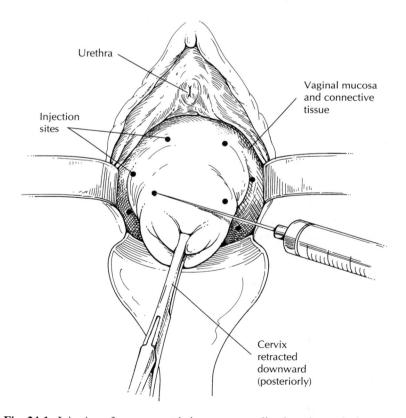

Fig. 24-1. Injection of a vasoconstrictive agent or saline into the vaginal mucosa.

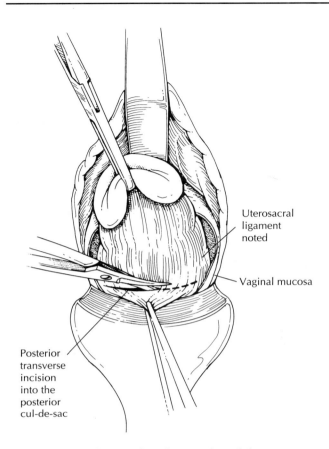

Fig. 24-2. Entry into the posterior cul-de-sac.

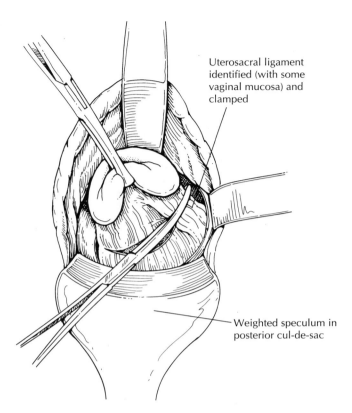

Fig. 24-3. Clamping and suture ligation of the uterosacral ligaments.

and cardinal ligaments until such time that posterior cul-de-sac entry becomes possible.

Rather than direct entry into the posterior cul-de-sac, some surgeons prefer to make a circumferential incision in the vaginal epithelium at the junction of the cervix just below the bladder reflection. The vaginal epithelium may be dissected sharply for the underlying tissue or may be pushed bluntly with an open sponge. If the initial incision is made too close to the external cervical os, there is a greater amount of dissection required and associated bleeding.

A Steiner-Anvard weighted speculum is placed into the posterior cul-de-sac. The uterosacral ligaments are clamped, with the tip of the clamp placed to incorporate the lower portion of the cardinal ligaments (Fig. 24-3). The clamp is placed perpendicular to the uterine axis, and the pedicle cut so that there is approximately 0.5 cm of tissue distal to the clamp. When learning this technique, it is helpful for the young surgeon to exaggerate rotating the elbow of the operating hand upward and toward the patient's buttocks. More tissue than this may become necrotic and provide a culture medium for microorganisms. A transfixion suture is placed at the tip of the clamp. Once ligated, the uterosacral ligaments are transfixed to the posterior lateral vaginal mucosa in an effort to further support the vagina and provide hemostasis (Fig. 24-4). This suture is held with a hemostat to facili-

tate location of any bleeding at the completion of the procedure and to aid vaginal mucosal closure. An alternative approach is to suture the uterosacrals to the internal vagina and then tie and cut the suture without holding it in place. Still another approach is to suture ligate the uterosacral pedicles and then use one end of the suture to run along the posterior vaginal cuff. The two suture ends are then tied in the midline. These various methods are mentioned for completeness and to illustrate that there are various techniques that can be used to accomplish the same objective.

Downward traction is placed on the cervix to provide countertraction for the vaginal mucosa. The anterior vaginal mucosa is incised at the level of the cervicovaginal junction (Fig. 24-5). Using an open moistened 4 × 8 gauze sponge, the bladder is advanced upward. Alternatively, sharp dissection can be performed using Metzenbaum scissors with the tips directed toward the uterus (Fig. 24-6). At this point, the vesicovaginal peritoneal reflection is usually identified and can be entered sharply using scissors (Figs. 24-7 and 24-8). If this reflection is not easily seen, there is no danger in delaying this step, as long as the operator has ascertained that the bladder has been advanced. To further protect the bladder, a Deaver or Heaney retractor is placed in the midline to keep the bladder out of the operative field. Blunt or sharp advancement of the bladder should precede each clamp placement until the vesicovaginal space is entered. If abla-

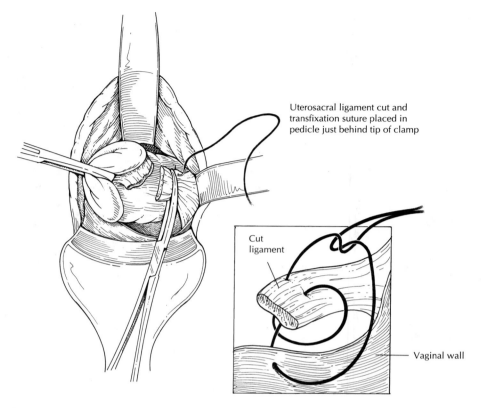

Uterosacral ligament cut and
transfixation suture placed in
pedicle just behind tip of clamp

Cut
ligament

Vaginal wall

Fig. 24-4. Suture transfixion of the uterosacral ligaments with attachment to the posterior vaginal mucosa.

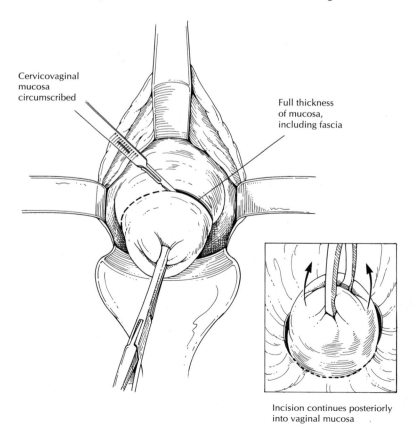

Cervicovaginal
mucosa
circumscribed

Full thickness
of mucosa,
including fascia

Incision continues posteriorly
into vaginal mucosa

Fig. 24-5. Incision into the anterior vaginal mucosa at the level of the cervicovaginal mucosa.

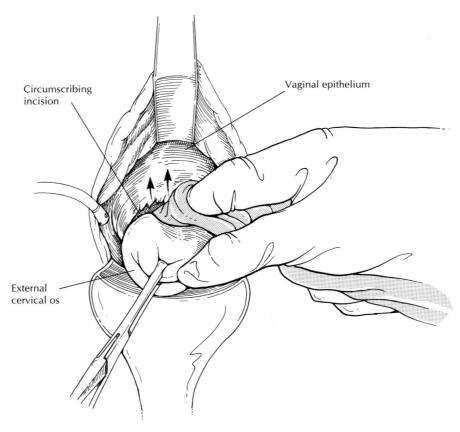

Fig. 24-6. Advancement of the anterior portion of the vaginal mucosa.

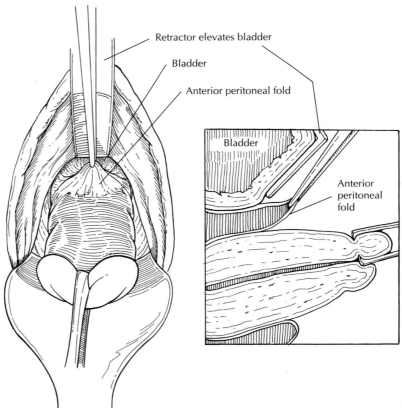

Fig. 24-7. Identification of the anterior peritoneal reflection.

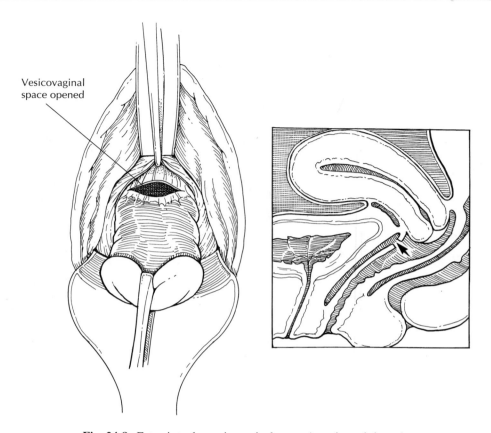

Vesicovaginal
space opened

Fig. 24-8. Entry into the vesicovaginal space (anterior cul-de-sac).

tion laceration occurs, the cystotomy may be repaired before completion of the hysterectomy, or some surgeons prefer to complete the procedure and then repair the cystotomy.

The cardinal ligaments are identified, clamped, cut, and suture ligated in a manner similar to that used for the uterosacral ligaments. Continued traction on the cervix aids with the identification of these structures and with hemostasis (Fig. 24-9). Again the bladder is advanced out of the operative field using either a blunt or sharp dissection technique. Sharp dissection is generally preferred in those patients whose bladder is adhered to the lower uterine segment from previous surgery.

Constant traction is maintained on the cervix, and at this point, the traction is directed to the contralateral side from the operative site. That is, if the left uterine artery is to be ligated, the uterus is directed downward and to the right. This simple step aids visualization of the operative site. The uterine vessels are clamped in such a manner as to incorporate the anterior and posterior leaves of the visceral peritoneum (Fig. 24-10). Although a double-clamp technique has been described, a single-clamp technique is adequate and decreases the potential risk of ureteral injury. In the patient with a large uterus, a second pedicle may be necessary to make certain that all branches of the uterine vasculature have been ligated (Fig. 24-11).

The anterior peritoneal fold is now usually easily visual-

ized and the anterior cul-de-sac can be entered. The anterior peritoneal fold appears as a crescent-shaped line. The peritoneal reflection is grasped with smooth forceps, tented, and opened with scissors with the tips pointed toward the uterus. A Heaney or Deaver retractor is placed into this space, to protect the bladder and to aid visualization of the abdominal contents. If the anterior cul-de-sac cannot be identified, a bent uterine sound can be placed through the posterior cul-de-sac to assist with visualization of the anterior peritoneal fold.[55]

For the patient with an enlarged uterus, uterine morcellation can begin after ligation of the uterine vasculature. If this is not necessary, the uterine fundus is delivered posteriorly. This is done by placing a tenaculum on the uterine fundus in a successive fashion. The surgeon's index finger is used to identify the utero-ovarian ligament and aid in clamp placement (Fig. 24-12). The remainder of the utero-ovarian ligaments are clamped and cut (Fig. 24-13). Again a double-clamp technique has been described, but is not necessary. However, this pedicle is double-ligated first with a suture tie and followed by a suture ligature medial to the first tie. A hemostat is placed on the second suture to aid in the identification of any bleeding and to assist with peritoneal closure if this is to be done. A hemostat is not placed on the first tie, as traction on a tied suture risks loosening the tie.

If the adnexa are to be removed, traction is placed on the

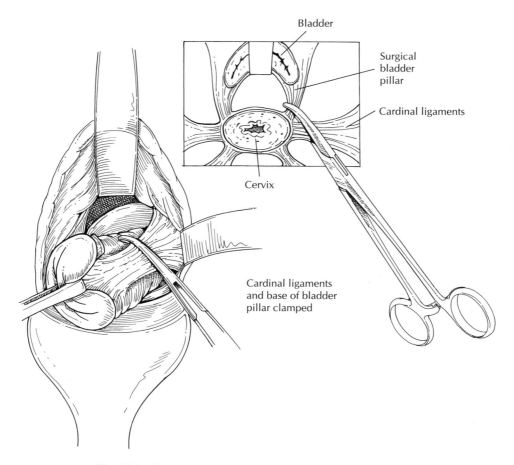

Bladder

Surgical
bladder
pillar

Cardinal ligaments

Cervix

Cardinal ligaments
and base of bladder
pillar clamped

Fig. 24-9. Clamping and suture ligation of the cardinal ligaments.

ovary by grasping it with a Babcock clamp. If the infundibulopelvic ligament is mobile and elongated, a Heaney clamp is placed across the infundibulopelvic ligament and the ovary and tube are excised. Both a suture tie and transfixion suture ligature are placed on this pedicle (Fig. 24-14). If the tissue pedicle is too large, the fallopian tube can be taken as a separate pedicle. Most adnexa can be removed transvaginally in this manner.[56–58] If the ovaries are not readily accessible, a pre-tied surgical loop can be used for ligation of this pedicle. When this technique is used, it is preferable to removal the round ligament as a separate pedicle, to reduce the size of the pedicle that is ligated using the surgical loop.[59] Yet another author has described using laparoscopy equipment placed through the vagina to accomplish ovarian removal.[60] However, this is rarely if ever necessary.

To ensure that hemostasis has been obtained, a lap-strip is placed into the peritoneal cavity and each of the pedicles is visualized and inspected. If any bleeding points are identified, a suture is used to ligate the bleeding vessel under direct vision. The pelvic peritoneum can be closed or left open. When left open, the peritoneum reforms in 24 to 48 hours. Although this is preferable, some surgeons believe that re-

peritonealization is important. If it is to be closed, the anterior peritoneal edge is identified and grasped using smooth tissue forceps. A continuous absorbable zero suture is begun at the 12-o'clock position. The suture is continued in a pursestring fashion and incorporates the distal portion of the left upper pedicle and the left uterosacral ligament. The posterior peritoneum is sutured as high as is practical; some surgeons believe that this helps to prevent the formation of an enterocoele in the future. The right uterosacral ligament and the distal portion of the right upper pedicle are incorporated, and this continuous suture ends at the point on the anterior peritoneum where it was begun. Before tieing the peritoneal suture, the lap strip is removed and again the pedicles are checked for hemostasis. As the suture is tied, the surgeon must make certain that no viscera has prolapsed beyond the suture or that no viscera is ligated as the suture is secured (Fig. 24-15).

The vaginal mucosa is reapproximated in either a vertical or horizontal manner using either a continuous suture or a series of interrupted sutures (Fig. 24-16). The sutures are placed through the entire thickness of the vaginal mucosa, making certain that the bladder is not entered. If one desires,

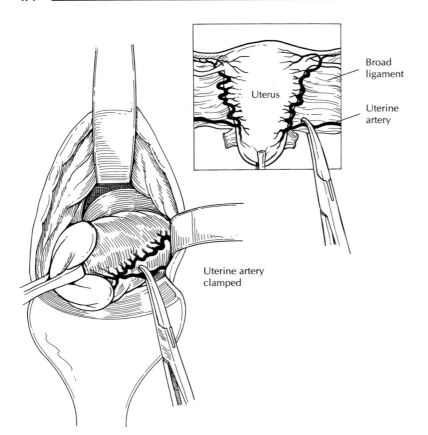

Fig. 24-10. Clamping and suture ligation of the uterine vasculature.

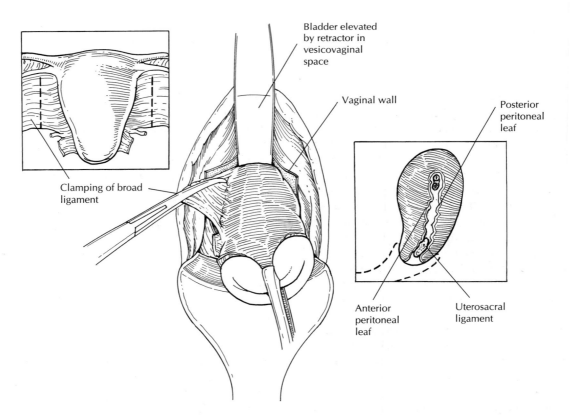

Fig. 24-11. Clamping of the remaining portion of the broad ligament.

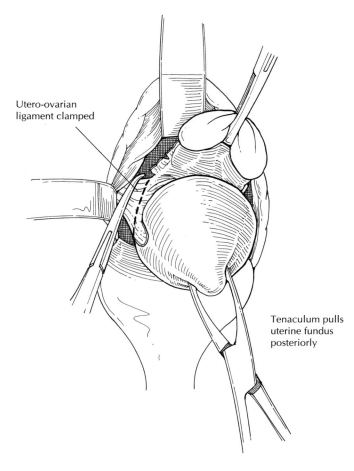

Utero-ovarian
ligament clamped

Tenaculum pulls
uterine fundus
posteriorly

Fig. 24-12. The posterior uterine fundus is delivered posteriorly.

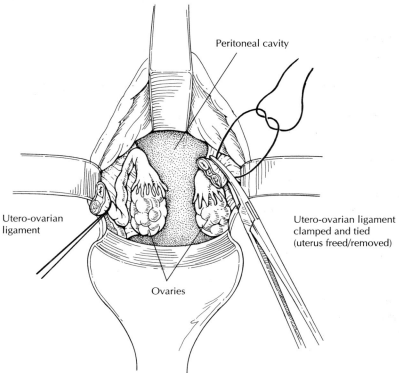

Peritoneal cavity

Utero-ovarian
ligament

Utero-ovarian ligament
clamped and tied
(uterus freed/removed)

Ovaries

Fig. 24-13. Clamping of the utero-ovarian ligament.

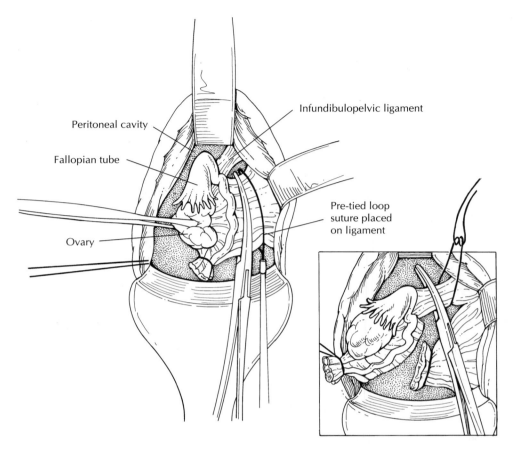

Fig. 24-14. Cutting and suture ligature and suture tie ligation of the utero-ovarian pedicle.

the peritoneum can be incorporated into these sutures. Whether the cuff is closed vertically or horizontally does not affect postoperative morbidity or vaginal depth.[61] A culdoplasty is recommended by some gynecologic surgeons. It is their opinion that the placement of this type of suture decreases the subsequent risk of enterocoele formation and the potential for development of vaginal vault prolapse. If this is done, an absorbable suture is placed through the full thickness of the posterior vaginal wall at a point where the highest portion of the vaginal vault will be. The suture is then passed through the left uterosacral ligament pedicle, the posterior peritoneum, and then the right uterosacral ligament. This stitch is completed by passing the suture from the inside to the outside at the same point that it was begun. The suture is then tied, which approximates the uterosacral ligaments and posterior peritoneum. Although recommended by many vaginal surgeons, there is no randomized or prospective follow-up data that demonstrates that this technique reduces the subsequent formation of vaginal vault prolapse or enterocoele formation.[62]

If the case has been prolonged, the bladder can be drained. However, little urine may have collected during a normal procedure. Unless a vaginal repair has been performed, it is

not necessary to use any type of vaginal pack. In these patients, suture placed into the levator muscles may cause sufficient discomfort and prevent spontaneous voiding. It is also not necessary to leave a bladder catheter in place, and in fact, doing so may increase the risk of a postoperative infection and increases the cost incurred by the patient.

Yet another method for vaginal hysterectomy is the Doderlein vaginal hysterectomy.[63–65] Using this method, an incision is made in the vaginal mucosa at the junction of the bladder and anterior cervix. The pubovesicocervical fascia is dissected from the lower uterine segment and the anterior cul-de-sac is entered. The cervix is pushed posteriorly and the uterine fundus is delivered through the anterior cul-de-sac. The hysterectomy is then begun much in the same manner that one would proceed with an abdominal procedure.

A wise (or wizened) vaginal surgeon will have multiple approaches in his armamentarium to deal with unusual or expected intraoperative findings.

Uterine Morcellation

Uterine morcellation, or removal of the uterus piecemeal, is a procedure most often used for the large myomatous uterus. Several methods have been described for uterine morcella-

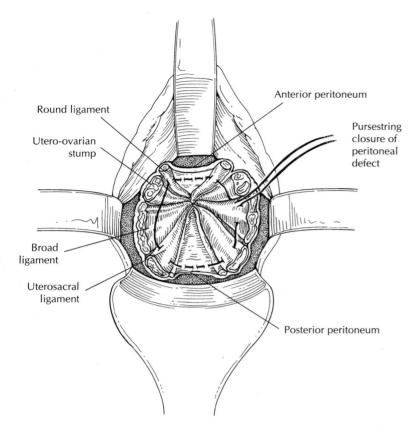

Round ligament

Utero-ovarian stump

Broad ligament

Uterosacral ligament

Anterior peritoneum

Pursestring closure of peritoneal defect

Posterior peritoneum

Fig. 24-15. Peritoneal closure using a continuous synthetic absorbable suture.

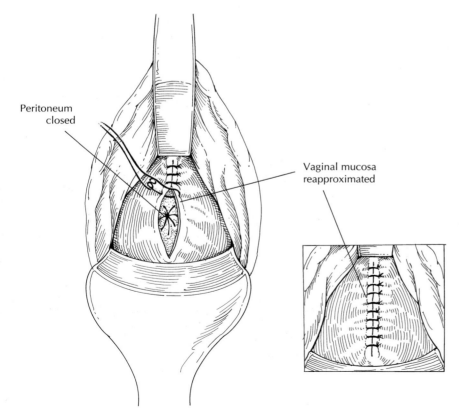

Peritoneum closed

Vaginal mucosa reapproximated

Fig. 24-16. Closure of the vaginal mucosa.

Surgical Tips for Uterine Morcellation

- Patient positioning: the patient's buttock should be positioned at the edge of the table to provide maximum exposure
- Lighting: the use of a headlight can be invaluable
- Experienced surgical assistant
- Retractors: malleable ribbon, Deaver, Steiner-Anvard weighted speculum with elongated tip
- Heaney needle holder
- No excess vaginal mucosa should be removed
- Traction should be maintained throughout the procedure to decrease blood loss
- The peritoneal cavity should be entered before beginning morcellation
- The uterine arteries must be clamped before beginning morcellation
- Beaver knife blade facilitates morcellation
- Preoperative consent to proceed with an abdominal hysterectomy, if necessary, should always be obtained

tion, including hemisection or bivalving, wedge/V-type incision or intramyometrial coring/Lash procedure. The latter two methods are most commonly used, generally in combination. Before beginning any type of morcellation, the uterine vasculature must be ligated and the peritoneal cavity entered either posteriorly or anteriorly.

Uterine hemisection or bivalving is rarely used. The uterus is split in the midline beginning at the cervix. One side of the uterus is then removed, followed by removal of the opposite side. If the uterus is still too large to remove after it has been bisected, the uterine half can be further morcellated (Fig. 24-17). This method seems best suited in the patient with a fundal, midline myoma.

Wedge morcellation is accomplished by removal of V-shaped tissue pieces, and is most commonly used for removal of anterior or posterior myomas or when a broad ligament myoma is encountered. Using a tenaculum, the posterior fundus is grasped and a knife is used to make a V-type incision. A second tenaculum is attached to the piece of tissue that is to be removed and the incision is completed (Fig. 24-18). It is important not to extend the incision into the broad ligament or through the anterior portion of the uterine fundus. At times, it is often possible to perform a myomectomy for removal of a myoma intact. This will greatly reduce the overall size of the uterus.

Intramyometrial coring is best suited for the diffusely enlarged uterine fundus. Coring generally begins with a circumferential incision into the lower uterine segment just above the cervix. The incision is continued circumferentially and cephalad in a slightly enlarging diameter. Constant traction should be maintained on the cervix as the uterus begins to elongate, to aid exposure of the incisional plane and to decrease blood loss. Care should be taken not to remove a small core of tissue, but to remove a significant volume of the central portion of the uterus. The overall result is an elongation of the uterus[66,67] (Fig. 24-19).

The use of uterine morcellation to remove the enlarged uterus transvaginally is a safe and effective procedure. Studies suggest that the associated morbidity is less than that encountered at the time of abdominal hysterectomy.[68] Other research suggests that there are no significant differences in the mean uterine weight, estimated blood loss, and complication rate in unsuccessful versus successful vaginal hysterectomies. Thus, uterine size alone is not an absolute contraindication to vaginal hysterectomy, and large uteri weighing more than 300 g was not related to a significant increase in failed vaginal hysterectomy.[69]

A rare problem in excision of a myoma with loss of the specimen into the peritoneal cavity is due to clamp slippage. If this occurs, retrieval of the specimen can be difficult. After finishing removal of the remainder of the specimen, the patient's head can be elevated and lavage of the peritoneal cavity will bring the errant fibroid into the pelvis.

Lack of Uterine Descensus

At times, the examination under anesthesia does not reveal the degree of uterine mobility that was anticipated following the examination in the office. At other times, the procedure is begun and the uterus does not descend as much as one anticipated. The surgeon must decide whether to proceed with a vaginal approach or whether to stop and make an abdominal incision. If the problem relates to introital narrowing on access, a midline or mesiolateral episiotomy can be performed or a Schuchardt type incision, in which the perineal and levator muscles are incised, can be used. If the problem stems from an enlarged uterus, morcellation can be begun after the uterine arteries have been ligated. If, by contrast, the problem results from extensive adhesive disease, an abdominal incision may be considered or packing the vagina and accessing the pelvis by means of laparoscopy.

Abdominal Hysterectomy

The patient is placed in the dorsal supine position. After obtaining adequate anesthesia, the patient's legs are placed in the frog-leg position and an examination under anesthesia is preformed to validate the operative indication and verify the pelvic anatomy. A Foley catheter is placed in the bladder and the vagina is cleansed with an antiseptic solution. The patient's legs are then replaced in the dorsal supine position, and a bovie pad is placed on the lower extremity.

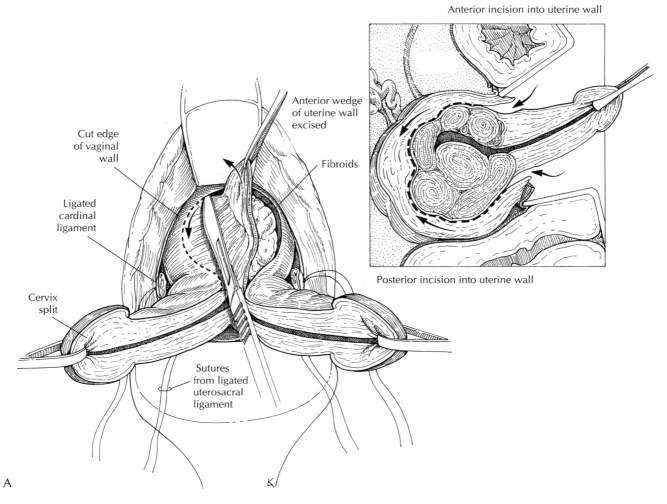

Anterior incision into uterine wall

Anterior wedge of uterine wall excised

Fibroids

Cut edge of vaginal wall

Ligated cardinal ligament

Cervix split

Sutures from ligated uterosacral ligament

Posterior incision into uterine wall

A

Fig. 24-17. **(A–C)** Uterine hemisection technique for uterine morcellation. *(Figure continues.)*

A variety of skin preparation have been advocated, including a betadine scrub followed by application of a betadine solution, or a betadine scrub followed by alcohol with application of an iodine-impregnated occlusive drape. However, the simplest and equally effective preparation is the application of a betadine solution followed by placement of the surgical drapes.

The choice of incisions is determined by a variety of conditions, which are discussed in Chapter 8. Once the peritoneal cavity is entered, the upper abdomen and then the pelvis are explored in a systematic fashion to make certain that the examination is complete. If cytologic sampling is needed, this should be obtained before abdominal exploration.

A variety of retractors have been designed for pelvic surgery, including the Balfour retractor, the O'Connor-O'Sullivan retractor, and others. The Bookwalter retractor is excellent for the obese patient, as it has a variety of adjustable blades. It is advisable to protect the wound edges with moist laps before placing the retractor blades.

The first step of any hysterectomy is to normalize the pelvic anatomy by separating any omental or intestinal adhesions as well as any abdominal wall adhesions. It is virtually always possible to locate the uterine fundus or round ligaments. This is a good landmark to remember and a good place to begin any hysterectomy.

The uterus is elevated by placing a large Kelly clamp at each uterine cornu so that the tip of the clamp incorporates the round ligament. This placement serves to ensure uterine elevation as well as to prevent back bleeding when the round ligament is ligated and cut (Fig. 24-20).

The uterus is deviated to the patient's left, which places the round ligament on stretch. The lateral portion of the round ligament is ligated with suture ligature or clamped using an Oshsner clamp (Fig. 24-21). The round ligament is then cut, which facilitates separating the anterior and posterior leaves of the broad ligament. The anterior leaf of the broad ligament is incised with Metzenbaum scissors along the vesicouterine fold and separates the peritoneal reflection of the bladder from the lower uterine segment (Fig. 24-22). The retroperitoneum is entered by extending cephalad the

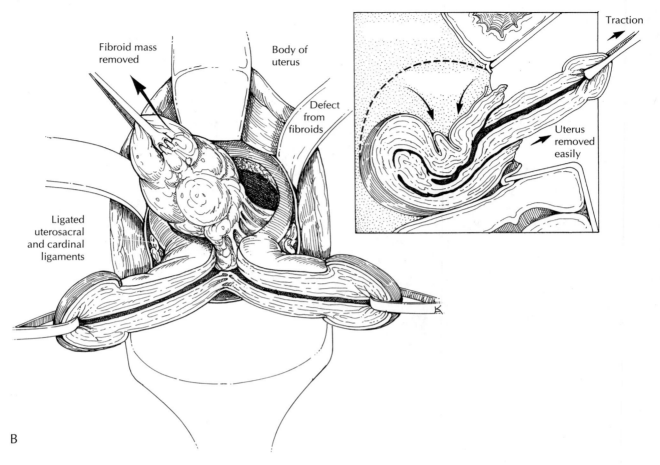

Fibroid mass removed

Body of uterus

Defect from fibroids

Ligated uterosacral and cardinal ligaments

Traction

Uterus removed easily

B

Fig. 24-17 *(Continued). (Figure continues.)*

incision on the posterior leaf of the broad ligament, making certain to remain lateral to both the infundibulopelvic ligament and iliac vessels. Blunt or sharp dissection is used to separate the loose connective tissue overlying the external iliac artery. By following the artery cephalad to its bifurcation, the ureter is identified crossing the common iliac artery. The ureter is left attached to the medial leaf of the broad ligament so as not to disrupt its blood supply (Fig. 24-23). The same procedure is completed on the opposite side. The left ureter is usually more medial than the right ureter. If the patient has extensive pelvic disease, the ureter may be dissected down toward the bladder as far as necessary. The position of the ureter should never be assumed and should always be kept under direct visualization. Palpation is not an adequate alternative to direct visualization.

If the ovaries are to be preserved, the uterus is retracted toward the pubic symphysis and deviated to one side, placing the contralateral infundibulopelvic ligament, tube, and ovary on tension. With the ureter under direct vision, an opening is created in the posterior leaf of the broad ligament under the utero-ovarian ligament and fallopian tube. The utero-ovarian ligament on each side is clamped with a curved

Heaney or Ballentine clamp, cut, and ligated with both a free tie and suture ligature (Fig. 24-24). The medical clamp at the uterine cornu will control back bleeding. By contrast, if the ovaries are to be removed, the peritoneal opening is enlarged and extended cephalad to the infundibulopelvic ligament and caudad to the uterine artery. This allows for proper exposure of both the uterine artery and infundibulopelvic ligament. In addition, the ureter is released from its close proximity to the uterine vessels and the infundibulopelvic ligament. A curved Heaney or Ballentine clamp is placed lateral to the ovary, making certain that the entire ovary is included in the surgical specimen (Fig. 24-25). The infundibulopelvic ligament on each side is cut and ligated with a suture tie followed by a suture ligature (Fig. 24-26). Tieing the pedicle before suturing it prevents creating an expanding hematoma by inadvertently puncturing the ovarian vessels.

Using Metzenbaum scissors with the tips pointed toward the uterus, the bladder is sharply dissected off the lower uterine segment and cervix (Fig. 24-27). An avascular plane exists between the lower uterine segment and bladder, which allows for its mobilization. Vanderbilt clamps may be placed on the bladder edge to provide countertraction and easier

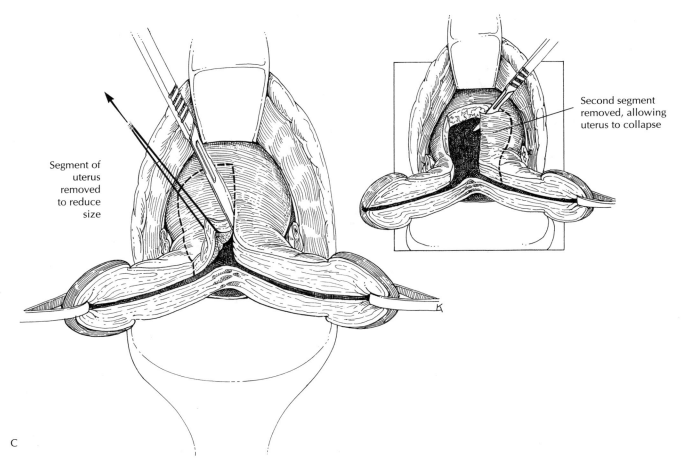

Segment of uterus removed to reduce size

Second segment removed, allowing uterus to collapse

C

Fig. 24-17 *(Continued).*

dissection. After this dissection is completed, a lap sponge can be placed beneath the bladder retractor to tamponade any small bleeding vessels.

The uterus is then retracted cephalad and deviated to one side on the pelvis, placing the lower uterine ligaments on stretch. Any loose connective tissue overlying the uterine vessels is sharply removed, skeletonizing the vessels, and a curved Heaney clamp is placed perpendicular to the uterine artery at the junction of the cervix and body of the uterus. Care is taken to place the tip of the clamp adjacent to the uterus at this site of anatomic narrowing (Fig. 24-28). The opposite side is managed in a similar fashion, and then the uterine artery pedicles are cut and suture ligated.

If the rectum requires mobilization from the posterior cervix, the posterior peritoneum between the uterosacral ligaments just beneath the cervix and rectum is incised. A relatively avascular tissue plane exists in this area, which allows mobilization of the rectum inferiorly out of the operative field (Fig. 24-29). The cardinal ligament and any remaining broad ligament is divided by placing a straight Heaney clamp medial to the uterine vascular pedicle for a distance of 2 to 3 cm parallel to the uterus. The pedicle is cut and ligated with a suture ligature (Fig. 24-30). The procedure is completed on

the contralateral side. A series of pedicles may be required depending on the size of the uterus.

The uterus is placed on traction cephalad and the tip of the cervix is palpated. A curved Heaney clamp is placed bilaterally to incorporate the uterosacral ligament and upper vagina just below the cervix (Fig. 24-31). Care should be taken to avoid foreshortening the vagina. The uterus is then removed using heavy curved scissors. At this point, an intrafascial hysterectomy can be preformed. To do this, a transverse incision is made on the anterior and posterior surfaces of the cervix below the level of the uterine vasculature. The cardinal and uterosacral ligaments are clamped inside the vaginal cuff.[70]

Numerous techniques have been described for vaginal cuff closure. One effective method is to place a figure-of-eight suture of a 0 or 2–0 gauge synthetic absorbable suture material between the tips of the two clamps. This suture is used for both traction and hemostasis. Sutures are then placed at the tip of each clamp and then the pedicle is transfixed with the suture ligature. This suture incorporates the uterosacral and cardinal ligament at the angle of the vagina (Fig. 24-32). Some surgeons prefer to leave the cuff open and allow it to heal secondarily. If this method is used, a

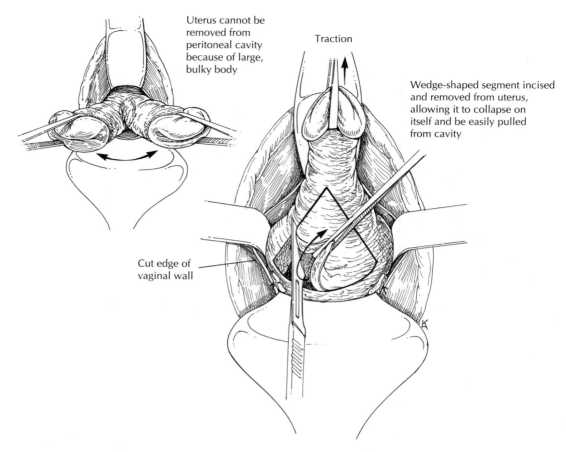

Uterus cannot be removed from peritoneal cavity because of large, bulky body

Traction

Wedge-shaped segment incised and removed from uterus, allowing it to collapse on itself and be easily pulled from cavity

Cut edge of vaginal wall

Fig. 24-18. Uterine morcellation using a wedge resection technique.

running locking suture is used for hemostasis along the cuff edge (Fig. 24-33). There appears to be no difference in postoperative febrile morbidity whether the vaginal cuff is closed or remains open.[71]

The pelvis is thoroughly irrigated with saline or Ringer's lactate solution. Meticulous care is taken to ensure hemostasis throughout the pelvis. Ureteral position and integrity are checked to ensure they are intact and do not appear entrapped by a suture.

It is not necessary to reapproximate the visceral or parietal peritoneum. The fascia and skin are reapproximated as described above.

Every practitioner has developed a system for postoperative care. However, it must be remembered that many of our postoperative regimens are based in the past, when patients were allowed to remain hospitalized for several days. In an effort to reduce hospital stay, many postoperative regimens have been modified and will be modified further. For example, it is not generally necessary to leave a bladder catheter in place postoperatively. However, if a catheter is used, it should be removed on the morning following surgery. An intravenous line is generally used for the first 24 hours to ensure that the patient remains well hydrated, especially if the patient experiences any nausea or vomiting. A clear liq-

uid diet is begun on the evening of surgery or the morning following surgery. The patient's diet is advanced as quickly as she tolerates it. Some surgeons are now beginning a regular diet immediately postoperatively. The patient is encouraged to use a regimen of deep breathing and coughing in an effort to prevent atelectasis, and ambulation is encouraged as soon as feasible. Adequate control of postoperative pain is necessary. Patient-controlled analgesia can be utilized, or a narcotic pain medication can be given as an intravenous or intramuscular injection. Yet another method that can be used is a morphine or meperidine drip. This infusion is prepared using 100 mg of meperidine or 10 mg of morphine in 250 ml of 5 percent dextrose water or saline and infused at 25 ml/hr. At this rate and concentration the patient receives 1 mg of morphine or 10 mg of meperidine per hour. Intravenous narcotic analgesia is generally not required after the first postoperative day and more stoic patients may use only oral agents.

Laparoscopic-Assisted Vaginal Hysterectomy

A variety of methods have been described to accomplish an LAVH, such as endoscopic staples, electrosurgery, and suture ligatures. At present, no single method has been

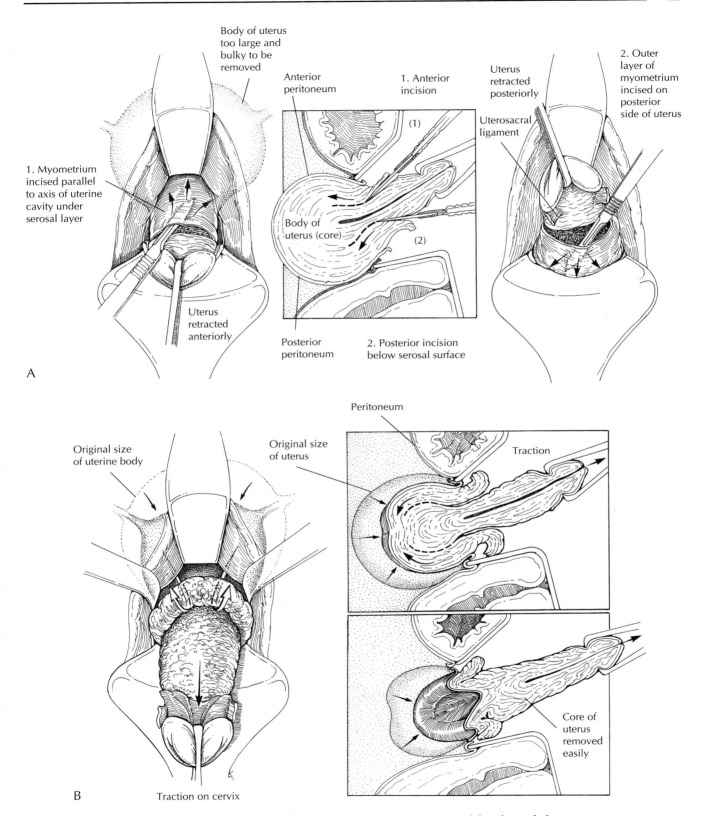

Fig. 24-19. (A & B) Uterine morcellation using an intramyometrial coring technique.

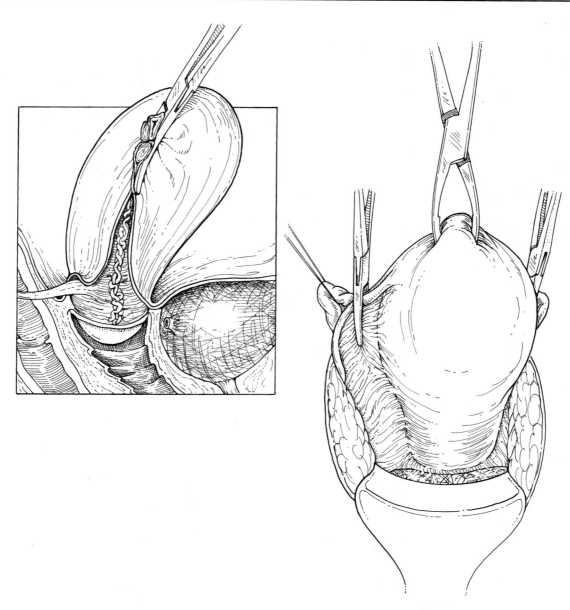

Fig. 24-20. Elevation of the uterus using broad ligament clamps incorporating the utero-ovarian and round ligaments.

proved to be better than another. No laparoscopic instruments are unique to laparoscopic hysterectomy, and these instruments can be used for a variety of operative laparoscopic procedures.

Following an examination under anesthesia, the perineum, vagina, and lower abdomen are prepared with dilute povidone-iodine solution. A uterine manipulator is attached to the cervix through a side-opening Graves speculum, making certain to antevert the uterus. A Foley catheter is inserted and the patient is draped using standard laparoscopy drapes. A trocar is inserted periumbilically. Following correct placement and gas insufflation of the abdomen, either two 12-mm trocars (if endoscopic staples are used), or two 5-mm

trocars are placed in the right and left lower quadrants, 6 to 8 cm above the pubic rami and lateral to the inferior epigastric vessels (Fig. 24-34). If endoscopic staples are to be used, the insertion of three 12-mm trocars allows for maximum flexibility of insertion and direction of the endoscopic stapling device. Once the trocars are in place, an intra-abdominal survey should be performed and should include examination of the uterus, tubes, ovaries, and cul-de-sac.

Once the abdominal and pelvic surveys are complete, the round ligaments are desiccated or ligated, and incised. Beginning at the left round ligament, the peritoneum of the vesicouterine fold is incised with the hook scissors. Attachment of unipolar cautery to the scissors allows for dissection

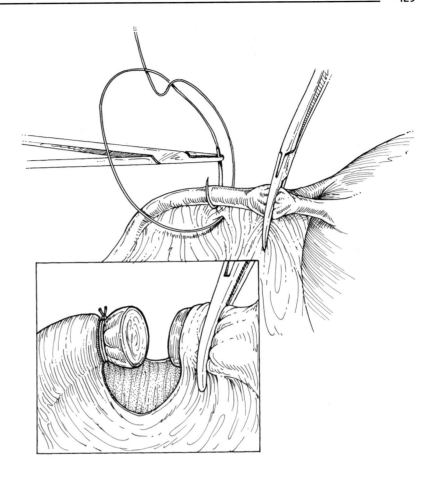

Fig. 24-21. Suture ligation of the round ligament.

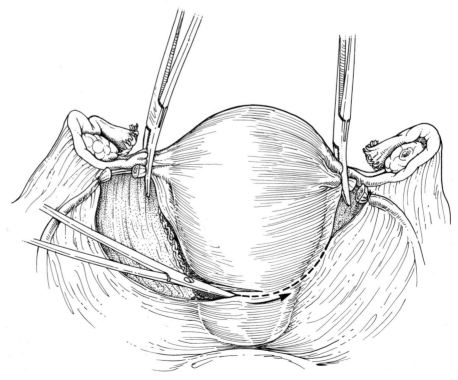

Fig. 24-22. Creation of the vesicouterine fold.

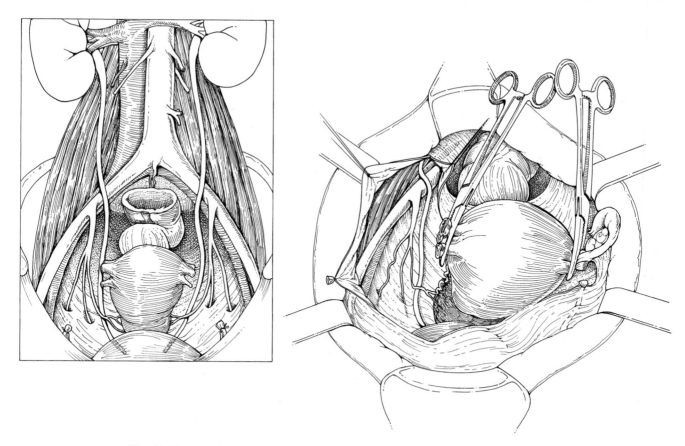

Fig. 24-23. Identification of the ureter located on the medial leaf of the broad ligament.

and desiccation of peritoneal vessels and maximizes visualization. The incision is continued across the lower uterine segment to the opposite round ligament (Fig. 24-35). On completing the incision, the bladder is sharply dissected off the lower uterine segment and cervix. This is best accomplished by lifting the lower peritoneal edge with graspers, and using curved scissors to incise and dissect the loose areolar tissue and bladder from the uterus. To maintain good hemostasis, the electrocautery is activated prior to cutting. Some surgeons prefer to use a contact-tip neodynium:yttrium-aluminum-garnet laser for dissection. This extremely expensive instrument has not been shown to be superior to cautery. Once the bladder flap has been developed, the ureters are identified by incision of medial leaf of the broad ligament and dissection of the retroperitoneal space in a manner similar to that of performing an abdominal hysterectomy.

If staples are to be used, the proper staple size is chosen and inserted through one of the lower abdominal ports on the same side of the uterus that is to be stapled. If electrosurgery is to be used, the bipolar coagulation instrument is inserted. If the ovaries are to be removed, the infundibulopelvic ligament is ligated or desiccated lateral to the ovary. If the ovary is not removed, the same procedure is completed medial to the ovary. The tip of the stapler should be past

the cut edge of the anterior peritoneum (Fig. 24-36). Once positioned, the stapling unit is closed and locked in place. The closed position is inspected, paying particular attention that no bowel is enclosed and that the ureter is visualized and is free. The safety is released and the stapling unit is activated. After removing the stapling unit, the cut and stapled edges are inspected for hemostasis and proper staple alignment (Fig. 24-37). If satisfactory, the same procedure is performed on the opposite side. Some surgeons stop the laparoscopic portion of the procedure at this point while others proceed with ligation or desiccation of the uterine vasculature.

With the ureter under direct vision, the uterine vasculature is desiccated and cut. If staple-ligation is used, the uterus is again pushed upward and to the opposite side from the one being stapled. The endoscopic staples are opened and aligned along the uterus, incorporating the uterine artery. The open stapling device is pushed down to the apex of the previously cut pedicle, the stapler is closed, and again the position of the ureter is inspected (Fig. 24-38). If satisfactory, the stapler is fired and removed slowly, checking for hemostasis. The procedure is repeated on the opposite side. Again, some surgeons stop the laparoscopic portion of the procedure at this point while others proceed with ligation of the cardinal liga-

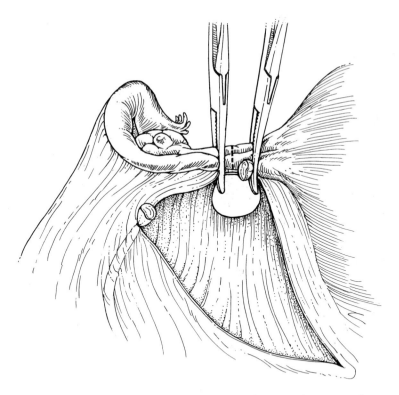

Fig. 24-24. Clamp placement when the ovaries are to be preserved.

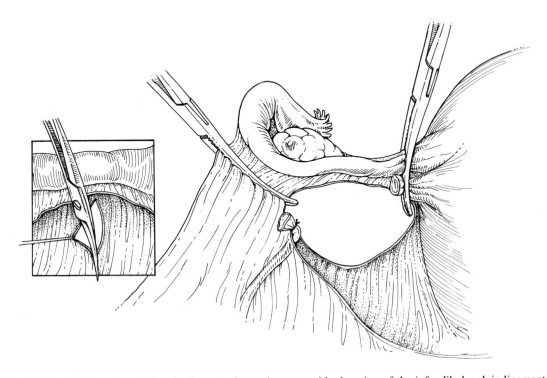

Fig. 24-25. Creation of a window in the posterior peritoneum with clamping of the infundibulopelvic ligament.

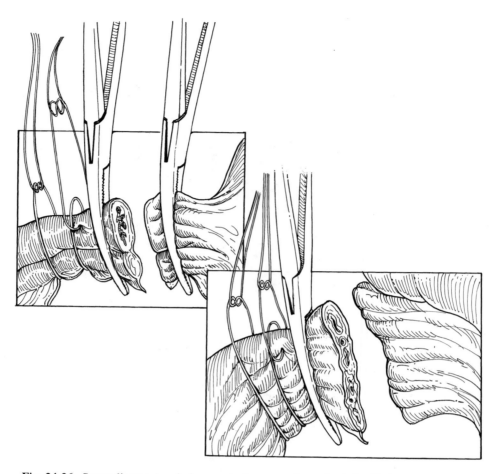

Fig. 24-26. Suture ligament and placement of a suture tie on the infundibulopelvic ligament.

ments with or without opening of the anterior or posterior cul-de-sac.

Before any further surgery, the level of the bladder must be well mobilized. The cardinal ligaments can either be staple-ligated or desiccated with electrocautery. It is extremely important to visualize and avoid the ureter during this step. Once completed, the vagina can be entered through an anterior colpotomy incision. A posterior colpotomy incision can also be made, although it is not necessary and can be made much more easily during the vaginal portion of the surgical procedure.

Once the endoscopic dissection is complete, the vaginal approach is begun. Adequate exposure is obtained and the uterine manipulator is removed. A tenaculum is applied to the cervix and the vaginal hysterectomy is begun in standard fashion through a posterior cul-de-sac incision as described above. Following uterine removal and closure of the vagina, it is suggested that a pneumoperitoneum be re-established for inspection of the surgical pedicles, irrigation of the pelvis, and to confirm hemostasis. The trocars are removed and the skin incisions closed in standard fashion. The patient

is then taken to the recovery room and most patients are discharged on the afternoon of surgery.

DISCHARGE INSTRUCTIONS

At the time of discharge, the patient is encouraged to resume her normal daily activities as quickly as is comfortable. As a general rule, patients who have undergone a vaginal hysterectomy can generally return to their normal activities more quickly than patients who have undergone an abdominal hysterectomy. However, this is just a general rule, as patients differ widely depending on their preoperative expectations and their ability to tolerate the postoperative discomfort. Patients should avoid lifting over approximately 20 lb of weight for 4 to 6 weeks after surgery to minimize stress on the healing fascia. Sexual intercourse is not recommended until after 4 to 6 weeks to allow the vaginal cuff to heal completely. In addition, patients are instructed to avoid driving until full mobility returns and until they are no longer requiring narcotic analgesia. In the past, patients were not

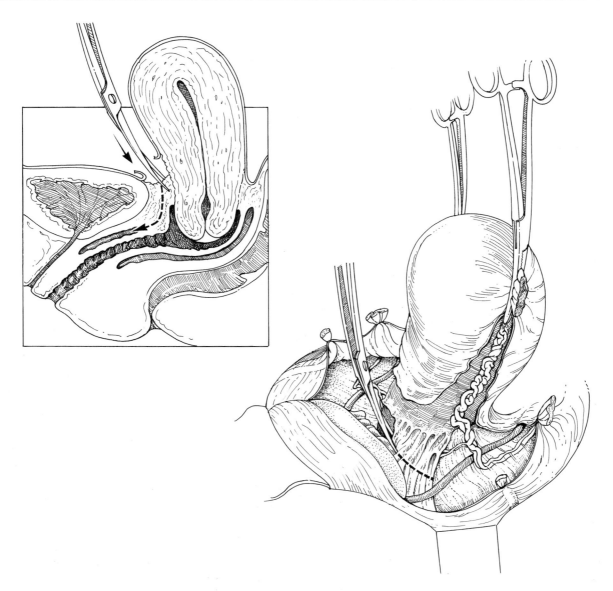

Fig. 24-27. Sharp dissection of the bladder from the lower uterine segment.

allowed to return to work for 6 to 8 weeks. However, this is not necessary and patients are now allowed to return to work as soon as they have regained sufficient strength. Walking and stair climbing are encouraged. Tub baths or showers are permissible. At the time of discharge, the patient is given these instructions as well as educated about any medications that she will be given. She is also told to make contact with her surgeon if she experiences an increase in pain, persistent nausea or vomiting, bleeding heavier than a menstrual period, or any signs or symptoms of infection.

OUTPATIENT VAGINAL HYSTERECTOMY

Over the past decade, there have been vast improvements in the types and numbers of patients on whom operations are performed on an outpatient basis. In this same period,

an era of health care reform, pressure has been exerted to decrease surgical cost by decreasing postoperative hospital stay. There is no question that by decreasing the need for hospitalization, one can substantially decrease the cost associated with any surgical procedure. However, safety must precede cost issues and thus, studies must be done to demonstrate that early discharge is safe before it is put into practice.

Over the past two decades, the length of hospital stay after vaginal hysterectomy has been reduced. Moolgaoker et al[72] reported that the average hospital stay after vaginal hysterectomy in their institution was 12.7 days prior to 1992. At the end of the next 2 years, the average postoperative stay was reduced to 7.2 days. During a similar time period in the United States, the average stay following vaginal and abdominal hysterectomy was 10.3 days.[73] In 1980, the mean

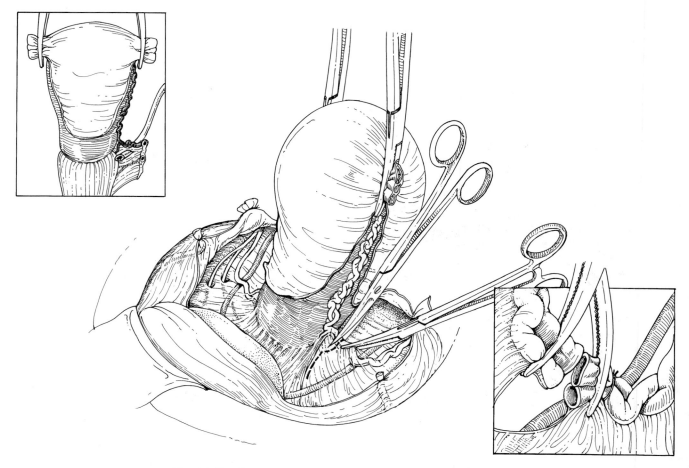

Fig. 24-28. Clamp placement perpendicular to the uterine vasculature.

postoperative stay after vaginal hysterectomy was 5.0 days, and 7.0 days for abdominal hysterectomy.[5]

Moore[7] reported a protocol used at an ambulatory surgery center in which patients were discharged accompanied by a private duty nurse who stayed with the patient in her home for approximately 30 hours. Reiner[75] in 1988 reported 41 patients who were candidates for same-day discharge following vaginal hysterectomy. However, patients remained in the hospital, with all but one patient being discharged the following morning.

With this background, a clinical trial was begun in January 1991 in which selected patients were offered the option of early discharge following vaginal hysterectomy. Since beginning this protocol, it has been modified to increase patient eligibility.

Counseling during the preoperative visit is one of the most important means of ensuring patients' acceptance and compliance during the immediate postoperative period. Patients are provided with positive statements both preoperatively and postoperatively, along with a standard surgical informed consent.

The vaginal hysterectomy is scheduled as early in the workday as possible, and all patients are given a single dose of a preoperative antibiotic. Synthetic absorbable sutures are used for all pedicles and for vaginal cuff closure. No vaginal packs or postoperative bladder drainage is used, as this increases patient discomfort and is unnecessary.

Patients receive traditional care in the recovery room for about 1.5 to 2.0 hours. Intravenous access is maintained at a rate of 25 to 50 ml/hr until the patient is discharged. This rate is used to minimize any hemodilutional effect on the patient's hematocrit level. The patient is then transferred to the ambulatory surgery unit, which provides an environment that encourages early ambulation; the nursing personnel are familiar with the care of this patient population. Patients are offered a clear liquid diet and ambulate with assistance as early as possible. Only rarely are intravenous or intramuscular narcotics required once the patient leaves the recovery room.

Patients are discharged only after the postoperative hematocrits have been obtained and are stable, the patient has ambulated, and is able to tolerate clear liquids. Patients are

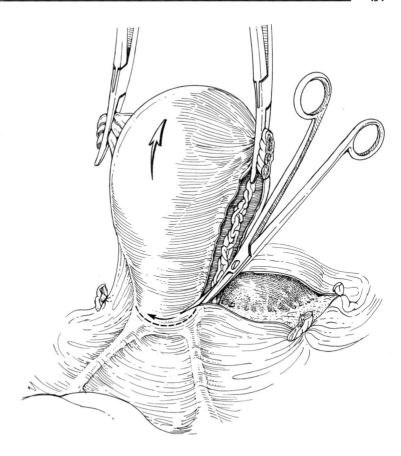

Fig. 24-29. Mobilization of the rectum and detachment for the posterior uterus.

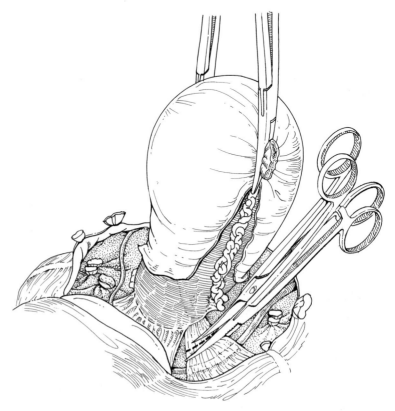

Fig. 24-30. Clamp placement across broad ligament and cardinal ligaments.

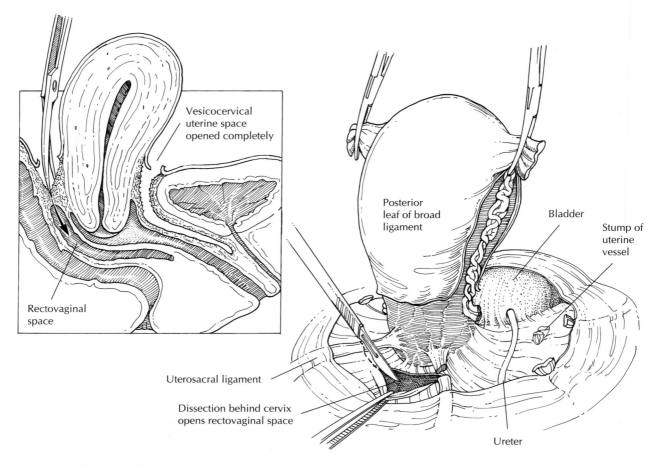

Vesicocervical
uterine space
opened completely

Rectovaginal
space

Posterior
leaf of broad
ligament

Bladder

Stump of
uterine
vessel

Uterosacral ligament

Dissection behind cervix
opens rectovaginal space

Ureter

Fig. 24-31. Two clamps are placed just beneath uterine cervix and incorporate the uterosacral ligaments.

not required to void prior to discharge, and no patients have been readmitted or required emergency care because of urinary retention. Discharge medications include

1. Promethazine suppository 25 mg every 4 hours as need for nausea
2. Oxycodone-acetaminophen tablet (one or two) every 4 hours as needed for pain
3. Docusate sodium 100-mg tablet twice daily for 2 weeks
4. Iron sulfate 325 mg one tablet twice daily for 1 month if the discharge hematocrit level is less than 35 percent

Estrogen replacement therapy is also begun at the time of discharge if the patient underwent oophorectomy. Before discharge, a home health care visit is arranged and the patient must have an understanding of the discharge instructions.

Stovall et al[76] and Summitt et al[77] reported on a series of patients who underwent vaginal hysterectomy with or without salpingo-oophorectomy on an outpatient basis. To date, well in excess of 250 cases have been completed. Approximately 9 percent of patients are not discharged from the

hospital on the day of surgery for a variety of reasons. Approximately 5 percent of patients require readmission, all but one of whom was readmitted secondary to a postoperative infection. Given these favorable results, outpatient vaginal hysterectomy or LAVH can be safely accomplished, with an acceptably low hospital readmission rate, and is well accepted by most patients.

INTRAOPERATIVE COMPLICATIONS

Intraoperative complications can be minimized using good lighting, a good surgical assistant, proceeding without undue haste, and by normalizing any abnormal pelvic anatomy before proceeding with the intended surgical procedure. However, even with careful attention to detail and use of proper surgical technique, there will be an irreducible number of operative injuries and postoperative complications. The most common injuries that occur at hysterectomy are ureteral, bowel, and bladder injuries along with intraoperative and postoperative hemorrhage.

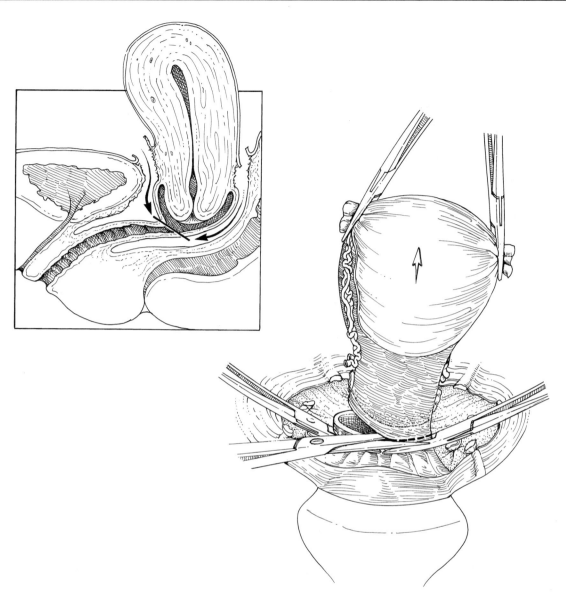

Fig. 24-32. Suture closure of the vaginal cuff.

Ureteral Injury

Injury to the ureter remains one of the most feared complications of gynecologic surgery. Attention should always be paid to the relationship of the ureter to the other pelvic structures. Most ureteral injuries can be avoided by opening the retroperitoneum and visualizing the ureter during abdominal hysterectomy. Palpation alone is inadequate, as the internal iliac artery, ovarian vessels, and vessels of the broad ligament are easily confused for the ureter. During vaginal hysterectomy, the ureter can sometimes be visualized and/or palpated. However, the best way to avoid ureteral injury is to place all clamps close to the uterus and keep the bladder out of the operative field, which displaces the ureters out of the operative field. With abdominal hysterectomy, the blad-

der flaps should be well displaced inferiorly to allow a lateral displacement of the ureters. The use of ureteral catheters is of little help in patients with extensive fibrosis or scarring due to endometriosis, pelvic inflammatory disease, or ovarian cancer. In fact, their use may lead to additional ureteral injury. If a ureteral injury is suspected, confirmation may be obtained by intravenous injection of indigo carmine, opening the dome of the bladder, and observing the presence or absence of bilateral spill of colored urine. This does not rule out ureteral ''nicks,'' partial transection, or kinking of the ureter. Seeing dye in the Foley catheter is inadequate, as this only indicates one ureter is patent. Alternatively, ureteral patency may be established by opening the dome of the bladder and passing retrograde ureteral stents. Cystoscopic evaluation may replace opening the bladder and is especially

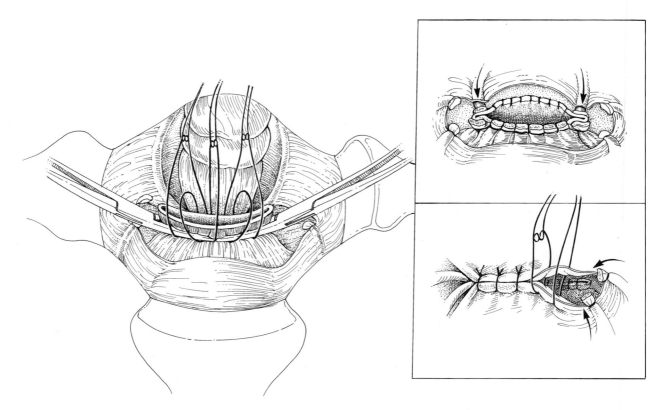

Fig. 24-33. Open technique to obtain hemostasis of the vaginal mucosa.

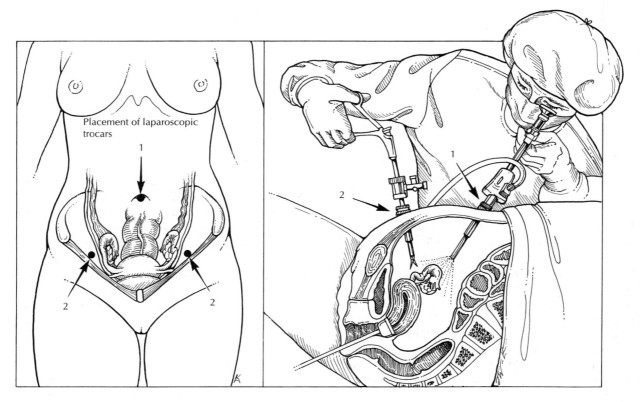

Placement of laparoscopic trocars

Fig. 24-34. Trocar placement for laparoscopic-assisted vaginal hysterectomy.

Instruments Commonly Used to Perform Laparoscopic-Assisted Vaginal Hysterectomy

- Pelviscopic surgical equipment
- A 10-mm, 0-degree telescope
- A 45-degree-angled-lens telescope
- Three 12-mm trocars and sleeves if endoscopic staples are used
- One 10-mm trocar and sleeve, and two 5-mm trocars and sleeves if electrosurgery or sutures are used
- 5-mm grasping forceps (atraumatic/traumatic)
- Two 5.5-mm operating port converters and one 10.5-mm converter if 12-mm trocars are used
- Hook scissors with electrocautery capability
- Unipolar or bipolar cautery
- Suction/irrigation system
- Hulka tenaculum or other type of uterine manipulator
- Endoscopic surgical stapler, if used
- Vaginal hysterectomy equipment
- ''Candy-cane'' stirrups

helpful during vaginal hysterectomy. Operative cystoscopy can be used to place ureteral stents retrograde. Dissection of the entire ureter is occasionally necessary to assure its integrity.

Bladder Injury

At abdominal hysterectomy, bladder injury may occur on opening the peritoneum or, more frequently, during dissection of the bladder off the lower uterine segment, cervix, and upper vagina. Unless there is involvement of the bladder trigone, a bladder laceration is easily repaired. During vaginal hysterectomy, the bladder is most commonly injured during entry into the anterior cul-de-sac. As long as the bladder has not been irradiated, a one- or two-layer closure with a small caliber absorbable suture such as 3–0 is adequate. The length of time the bladder should be drained postoperatively is controversial, but at a minimum, the catheter should be left until any gross hematuria has cleared. A more conservative approach is to continue drainage for 3 to 4 days.

Small Bowel Injury

Small bowel injury is the most common intestinal injury that occurs during hysterectomy, and generally occurs during abdominal hysterectomy. Small defects of the serosal or muscularis may be repaired using a single layer of continuous or interrupted 3–0 silk or synthetic absorbable suture material. Single layer closure of small bowel is adequate in most cases. If a large area has been injured, resection with reanastomosis may be necessary. Small bowel injury is rarely encountered during vaginal hysterectomy.

Colonic Injury

The ascending colon can be repaired in a similar manner to small bowel, and the transverse colon is rarely injured in normal gynecologic procedures, as it is well out of the operative field. However, the descending colon and rectum can be injured during either abdominal or vaginal hysterectomy. If the bowel has not been cleansed prosperatively, and the injury is larger than 5.0 cm, a diverting colostomy may be necessary, especially if there is gross spillage of bowel content.

Hemorrhage

When significant arterial bleeding occurs, it is usually from the uterine arteries or the ovarian vessels near the insertion of the infundibulopelvic ligaments. Binding clamping or mass ligature placement in bleeding areas should always be avoided, as one risks unnecessary ureteral or bowel injury. It is best to apply a pressure pack to tamponade the bleeding and then slowly remove the pack in an effort to visualize, isolate, and individually clamp the bleeding vessels. The use of surgical clips may be helpful. Venous bleeding is often more bothersome than arterial bleeding. This type of bleeding can usually be controlled with pressure and/or suture ligation. Bleeding from peritoneal edges or denuded surfaces may be controlled using cautery or by applying topical hemostatic agents. If a vascular pedicle is lost during a vaginal hysterectomy and efforts at visualization from below are unsuccessful, blind clamping or suturing is ill advised. Laparoscopy can be used to identify and control the bleeding site, with laparotomy reserved for bleeding inaccessible to laparoscopic techniques or beyond the skill of the surgeon.

Early postoperative hemorrhage after vaginal hysterectomy may present in one of two ways. First, bleeding from the vagina may be noted, or secondly and less commonly, the patient may be noted to have little bleeding from the vagina, but have deteriorating vital signs, falling hematocrit level, and flank or abdominal pain. The first presentation usually represents bleeding from the vaginal cuff or one of the pedicles, while the second presentation may represent retroperitoneal hemorrhage. These two situations are approached differently in evaluation and treatment, but both involve prompt stabilization of vital signs, fluid and blood product replacement, and constant surveillance of the patient's condition. The patient should be taken promptly to the examining room where the operative site is viewed and

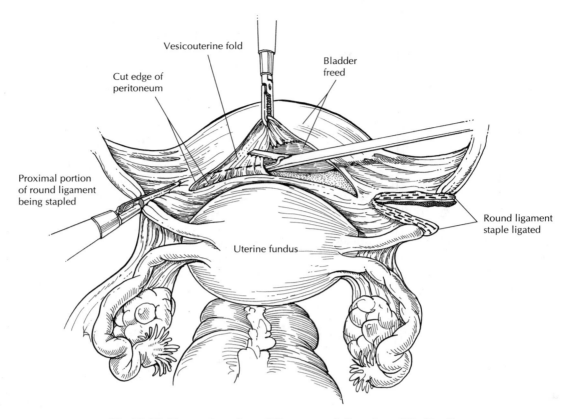

Fig. 24-35. Transection of round ligament and dissection of bladder flap.

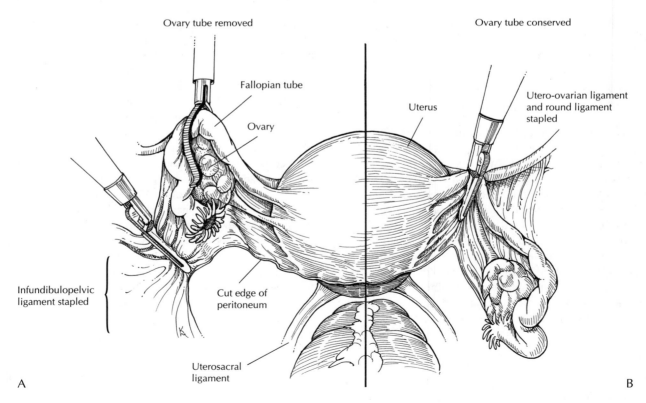

Fig. 24-36. (A & B) Placement of stapling device for ligation of utero-ovarian or infundibulopelvic ligaments.

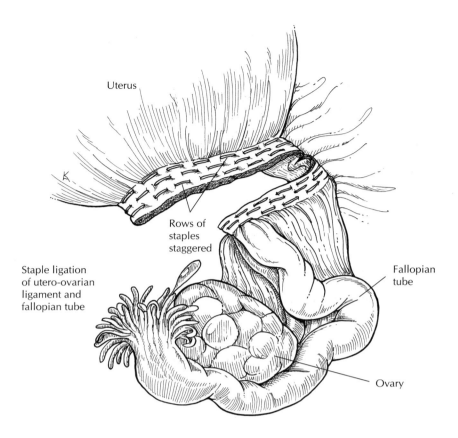

Uterus

Rows of
staples
staggered

Staple ligation
of utero-ovarian
ligament and
fallopian tube

Fallopian
tube

Ovary

Fig. 24-37. Appearance of staple line following tissue transection.

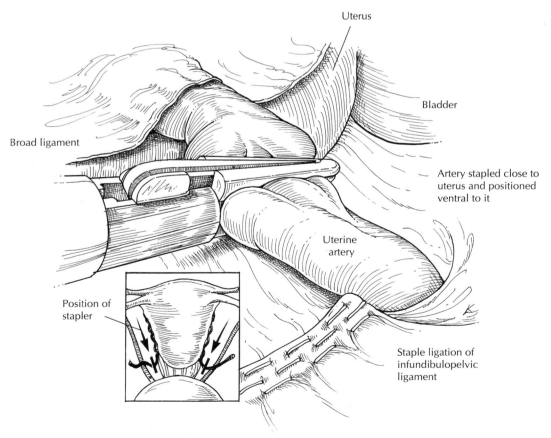

Uterus

Bladder

Broad ligament

Artery stapled close to
uterus and positioned
ventral to it

Uterine
artery

Position of
stapler

Staple ligation of
infundibulopelvic
ligament

Fig. 24-38. Placement of the stapling device for ligation of uterine arteries.

Criteria Used for Selecting Patients for Outpatient Vaginal Hysterectomy

- No medical condition requiring special postoperative care, such as uncontrolled diabetes mellitus, class II or IV heart disease
- No condition that limits ambulation such as severe arthritis
- Working telephone in the home
- Support person available for the first postoperative night
- No anterior or posterior colporrhaphy required
- Postoperative criteria
  - Does not sustain an intraoperative complication requiring hospital admission (gastrointestinal or urinary tract injury)
  - Less than 3 volume percent change in two hematocrits separated by 3 to 4 hours, with the first being at least 1 hour postoperative
  - Understands postoperative instructions
  - Tolerating clear liquids
  - Ambulates with assistance
  - Temperature less than 100.4°F

Patient Discharge Instructions for Outpatient Hysterectomy

- Record your temperature every 4 hours for 2 days
- If your temperature is greater than 100°F, notify your surgeon
- Drink at least six glasses of liquid during the first 24 hours after surgery
- Begin a regular diet after 24 hours
- Have a support person to assist and stay with you for the first 24 hours after surgery
- Refrain from heavy lifting or strenuous exercise for 1 week
- Do not drive for at least 48 hours and until you can turn quickly and do not require sedative pain medication
- No douching or vaginal intercourse for 4 weeks
- Notify your surgeon if you develop vaginal bleeding heavier than a menstrual period, persistent nausea, vomiting, or pain not relieved by your pain medication
- You may contact your surgeon at [insert phone number]
- A nurse will visit you at your home in the morning about 9:00 AM
- You may return to work as soon as you are capable, usually 1 to 2 weeks
- An appointment for an office visit is scheduled for you on [insert date] at [insert time]

the vaginal cuff inspected. Bleeding from the vaginal cuff can usually be sutured in the examination room. If bleeding is coming from above the cuff, the patient should be taken to the operating room. General anesthesia should be administered and the vaginal operative site explored. If the patient is stable, a laparoscopy may be useful. However, an exploratory laparotomy will be necessary to ligate most bleeding vessels. In some patients, radiographic ligation of the hypogastric vessels may be used in an effort to avoid surgery.

If the patient has little vaginal bleeding and vital signs have deteriorated, retroperitoneal hemorrhage should be suspected. A hematocrit should be ordered immediately, along with crossmatching of blood. Physical examination reveals tenderness and dullness in the flank and abdominal distension may be present. If the patient's condition stabilizes rapidly with intravenous fluids, the patient can be transfused and followed with serial hematocrits and vital signs. In many instances, the bleeding will tamponade and stop, forming a hematoma that will eventually reabsorb. The risk of this approach is that the hematoma will later also become infected, necessitating surgery if antibiotic therapy is not successful. The other option is to perform an abdominal exploration while the patient is stable and in good condition. This approach brings the added morbidity of a second anesthesia and an abdominal incision, but avoids the possibility of the patient's condition deteriorating with continued delay or the

possibility of a pelvic abscess later. Very infrequently, an otherwise stable patient will demonstrate an unexpected and confirmed significant drop in hematocrit during the postoperative period, usually days 2 to 4. Ultrasound may demonstrate free intraperitoneal fluid. The patient may ultimately drain a large amount of watery brown fluid from the vagina. Antibiotics are not necessary.

Postoperative Infection

Infection after vaginal hysterectomy can be classified as vaginal cuff cellulitis, pelvic cellutis, pelvic abscess, and infected pelvic hematoma. Although some degree of cuff cellulitis probably occurs after every hysterectomy, antibiotics are not required unless the fever persists. Pelvic cellulitis usually begins about the third day after surgery. It is an infection of the soft tissue of the surrounding pelvic structures. Regardless of the type of infection, the initial treatment consist of broad-spectrum intravenous antibiotic therapy. The antibiotics should be continued for 24 to 48 hours after the resolution of fever and symptoms. Oral antibiotics are not necessary once the patient is discharged from the hospital. An ultrasound may be helpful if the pelvic examination findings are uncertain or if the patient does not respond to parenteral antibiotic therapy. In addition, if the patient does not respond to antibiotic therapy, the vaginal cuff should be opened using a Kelly clamp or uterine dressing forceps. Rarely is the infection of such a degree that a repeat surgical procedure is needed.

Postoperatively, most patients will have an increase in cul-de-sac fluid following hysterectomy. The importance of these fluid collections is uncertain, as some authors have found that women who develop posthysterectomy fluid collections are at increased risk of the development of febrile morbidity, while other authors found no significant association between the presence of a postoperative fluid collection and the development of febrile morbidity.[78,79]

Postoperative Urinary Retention

Urinary retention is the only postoperative complication that is higher in patients undergoing vaginal hysterectomy when compared to patients undergoing abdominal hysterectomy.[80] Urinary retention usually results from either pain or bladder atony and is most common after vaginal repair. Bladder drainage is not necessary following either vaginal or abdominal hysterectomy but is used by many surgeons. The use of catheter drainage may be associated with increased febrile morbidity and increased cost. When not used, it also preserves the possibility of earlier ambulation and outpatient vaginal hysterectomy.[81]

Fallopian Tube Prolapse

Posthysterectomy prolapse of the fallopian tube is an uncommon postoperative complication and is often confused with granulation tissue at the vaginal apex. Predisposing factors for the development of fallopian tube prolapse include development of a hematoma or abscess formation at the vaginal apex. If the tissue at the top of the vaginal cuff does not respond to conservative treatment, such as silver nitrate application or cryotherapy, a biopsy of the area is warranted to make certain that the tissue is tubal epithelium. Once diagnosed, the patient should be taken to the operating room and the surrounding vaginal mucosa opened, undermined widely, and the tube resected.

Vaginal Cuff Evisceration

Evisceration of the small intestine into the vagina is extremely rare, but when it does occur, it most often occurs in the immediate postoperative period. It may be associated with the Valsalva maneuver or severe vomiting or coughing. Treatment for evisceration is immediate laparotomy with replacement and inspection of the mesentery and small bowel. Any necrotic vaginal mucosa should be resected and the cuff closed. Postoperatively, broad-spectrum antibiotic coverage is usually used.

Mortality

The mortality for any surgical procedure is somewhat dependent on the patient's age, surgical indication, health status, and surgical route. The mortality rate for hysterectomy for a 40-year-old woman is approximately 5 per 10,000 cases, but increases to about 75 per 10,000 for a 50 year old woman.[82] If all women 15 to 44 years of age are included, the mortality rate is about 20 per 10,000 cases.[80] Given these mortality rates, about 350 deaths will occur annually as a result of women undergoing hysterectomy. Patients undergoing hysterectomy avoid certain long-term health risks such as the development of cervical or endometrial cancer. It is estimated that women who undergo hysterectomy have an increased life expectancy of 14 to 73 days.[81,83]

CONCURRENT SURGICAL PROCEDURES

Appendectomy

Appendectomy is performed at hysterectomy to prevent the development of appendicitis later in life, and for the possibility that unsuspected appendicial pathology will be removed. The incidence of appendectomy peaks in the second and third decades of life, and the peak age for hysterectomy is some 10 to 20 years later.[84] The incidence of histologic abnormalities was found in 32 or 45 appendices in one study and in 22 percent of patients in another study.[85,86]

When appendectomy is performed with hysterectomy, the operative time is increased by approximately 10 minutes and thus is associated with slightly higher cost.[87] However, it does not seem to be associated with increased intraoperative or postoperative morbidity.[88,89] Although not commonly done, prophylactic appendectomy can be done at the time of vaginal hysterectomy and like appendectomy at abdominal hysterectomy, does not seem to be associated with increased operative or postoperative morbidity.[90–93] The technique is the same as when the procedure is performed at the time of abdominal hysterectomy. That is, the appendix is grasped with a Babcock clamp, the mesoappendix clamped and divided, and the base of the appendix is ligated and removed.

Cholecystectomy

Gallbladder disease is about four times more common in women than men and has its highest incidence in the fifth and sixth decades of life. This is obviously the time when hysterectomy is most common. When cholecystectomy is done in conjunction with hysterectomy, there does not seem to be a significant increase in febrile morbidity or hospital stay.[94,95] Laparoscopic cholecystectomy can be combined with operative laparoscopic gynecologic procedures.

Abdominoplasty/Liposuction

Abdominoplasty can be combined with abdominal hysterectomy. Studies indicate that there is shorter hospital stay, shorter operating time, and lower intraoperative blood loss when the procedures are combined rather than being done separately.[96,97] Liposuction has been reported with vaginal hysterectomy and like abdominoplasty, appears to be safe.[98]

Prophylactic Oophorectomy

Prophylactic oophorectomy is the most common concurrent surgical procedure performed at the time of hysterectomy. The procedure is done to decrease the incidence of ovarian cancer and to prevent the potential need for reoperation. The major reason for leaving the ovaries is to delay the need for estrogen replacement therapy and because the long-term implications of hormone replacement are not understood, nor are the potential functions of the ovary in postmenopausal women. Although standard teaching suggests that oophorectomy should be offered to women undergoing hysterectomy beginning at about age 40 years, the decision to proceed with oophorectomy should be individualized after the patient has been informed of the risks and benefits of ovarian removal.[99–101]

PSYCHOSOCIAL ASPECTS OF HYSTERECTOMY

The patient faces many issues and risks once she has decided to proceed with hysterectomy. Many women wonder whether the procedure will cause a loss of femininity or sexual satisfaction, or interpersonal problems with her spouse. The emotional response to the patient may be greater because the uterus is being removed as compared to removal of another intra-abdominal organ.[102] Because of the many issues surrounding hysterectomy and the potential for misconceptions, the importance of preoperative counseling and preparation cannot be overemphasized.

Drellich and Bieber[103] studied 23 women following hysterectomy, most of whom regretted the loss of menstruation. This was true even for women who had experienced dysmenorrhea. Several of these women viewed the menstrual cycle as a way for the body to rid itself of waste and many of these women said they had felt refreshed following menstruation.

Whether psychological changes result from hysterectomy or whether there is an increased incidence of psychiatric symptoms or depression remains controversial. Some investigators have reported an increased incidence of these symptoms, while other investigators have not found an association with hysterectomy.[104–107] In fact, some studies actually report a decrease in the incidence of psychiatric symptoms following hysterectomy.[108–110] Given the conflicting results of these studies it is probable that there is a wide variation of patient responses and this variation probably depends on the patient's preoperative condition and cultural background.

Before hysterectomy most patients experience some degree of anxiety. Patients who experience a moderate amount of preoperative anxiety tend to do better postoperatively than patients with little or no anxiety or patients who have an exaggerated preoperative response. It has also been shown that long delays prior to surgery increase anxiety, as does a very short preoperative period. Therefore, women should be scheduled for surgery a couple of weeks in advance, if possible, to minimize this problem.[111] Other preoperative factors noted to increase a patient's emotional response following hysterectomy include a desire to maintain fertility, a great deal of investment in motherhood, and the patient who has not dealt well with a previous loss.[112]

The changes in sexual functioning (if any) following hysterectomy are also uncertain. The reported incidence of sexual dysfunction after hysterectomy ranges from 10 to 40 percent. Studies addressing this issue vary greatly in their collection methods, cultural variations, and definitions of sexual dysfunction. Some studies indicate that libido is decreased following hysterectomy while other studies actually suggest that it is increased, because patients no longer have to fear conception.[113] Humphreis[114] found that most patients do not have a change in their sexual practices following hysterectomy, while other studies report a deterioration of sexual relations.[115] It also appears that preoperative anxiety about deterioration of sexual function is often associated with an overall deterioration of sexual relations.[116]

The role of the cervix in sexual satisfaction is also controversial. Kikku et al[117–120] reported a group of 212 patients who underwent hysterectomy, 105 of whom had a total abdominal hysterectomy and 105 of whom who had a supracervical hysterectomy. These authors found an increase in psychiatric symptoms in both groups, while sexual desire and functioning was unchanged in either group. Both groups had a significant decrease in dyspareunia following hysterectomy. Following supracervical hysterectomy, patients reported an increased orgasmic frequency when compared to patients in which the cervix was removed.

In summary, patients do not appear to have psychiatric sequelae or diminished sexual functioning following hysterectomy. It appears that the best predictor of postoperative sexual function is the patient's sexual satisfaction preoperatively. Before hysterectomy, these issues should be discussed with the patient, and her questions and concerns addressed. Just this simple discussion will help alleviate the patient's fears and anxieties.

SUPRACERVICAL/SUBTOTAL HYSTERECTOMY

In certain intraoperative situations, removal of the cervix might place the patient at undue risk, although these clinical situations are very unusual. Among these potential indications are endometriosis with obliteration of the anterior and posterior cul-de-sac at cesarean hysterectomy, when the cervix is fully dilated and effaced, making cervical identification difficult. In some cultures, the woman's femininity is tied directly to her ability to menstruate; in these instances, menstruation will continue if the cervix and a portion of the lower uterine segment is left in place. There are also patients who desire to retain the cervix, given the information presented above regarding sexual satisfaction after hysterectomy. With cul-de-sac obliteration, an alternative approach would be to proceed with an intrafascial hysterectomy. The minority of gynecologic surgeons believe that removal of the cervix leads to increased operative and postoperative morbidity, vaginal shortening, subsequent vault prolapse, abnormal cuff granulations, and the potential for fallopian tube prolapse. These gynecologists believe that the cervix should not be removed unless there is a specific reason, such as the patient who is undergoing hysterectomy for treatment of cervical dysplasia.[121,122] If the cervix is left, the patient remains at risk of the development of cervical dysplasia and cervical cancer, and many patients will continue to experience menstruation. Therefore, the patient is also at risk of development of endometrial cancer and should probably be given progestins as a component of her estrogen replacement therapy. If the cervix is to be left on an elective basis, the patient should have a negative cervical cytology and preoperative informed consent regarding the risks and benefits of leaving the cervix.

REFERENCES

1. Benrubi GI: History of hysterectomy. J Fla Med Assoc 75: 533, 1988
2. National Hospital Discharge Survey, Annual Summary. U.S. Department of Health and Human Services, Public Health Services, Centers for Disease Control (Vital and Health Statistics. Series 13, data from the National Health Survey), 1985–1991. Hyattsville, MD, 1993
3. Pokras R: Hysterectomy: past, present and future. Stat Bull Metrop Insur Co 70:12, 1989
4. Ross NP: Hysterectomy: variations in rates across small areas and across physicians' practices. Am J Public Health 74:327, 1984
5. Dicker RC, Scally MJ, Greenspan JR et al: Hysterectomy among women of reproductive age: trends in the United States, 1970–1978. JAMA 248:323, 1982
6. Domenighetti G, Luraschi P, Marazzi A: Hysterectomy and sex of the gynecologist. N Engl J Med 313:1482, 1985
7. Kjerulff KH, Guzinski GM, Langenberg PW et al: Hysterectomy and race. Obstet Gynecol 82:757, 1993
8. Spencer G: Projections of the population of the United States, by age, sex, and race, 1983 to 2080 (Current Population Reports. Population estimates and projections. Series P-25; no. 952.) U.S. Department of Commerce, Bureau of the Census, Washington, DC, 1984
9. Pokras R, Hufnagel VG: Hysterectomy in the United States, 1965–84. Am J Public Health 78:852, 1988
10. Leibsohn S, d'Ablaing F, Mishell DR, Schlaerth JB: Leiomyosarcoma in a series of hysterectomies performed for presumed uterine leiomyomas. Am J Obstet Gynecol 162:968, 1990
11. Parker WH, Fu YS, Berek JS: Uterine sarcoma in patients operated on for presumed leiomyoma and rapidly growing leiomyoma. Obstet Gynecol 83:414, 1994
12. Peiter RC, Wagner PL, Gambone JC: Routine hysterectomy for large asymptomatic uterine leiomyomata: a reappraisal. Obstet Gynecol 79:481, 1992
13. Friedman AJ, Haas ST: Should uterine size be an indication for surgical intervention in women with myomas? Am J Obstet Gynecol 168:751, 1993
14. Nilsson L, Rybo G: Treatment of menorrhagia. Am J Obstet Gynecol 110:713, 1971
15. Gannon MJ, Holt EM, Fairbank J et al: A randomised trial comparing endometrial resection and abdominal hysterectomy for the treatment of menorrhagia. BMJ 303:1362, 1991
16. Brooks PG, Clouse J, Morris LS: Hysterectomy vs. resectoscopic endometrial ablation for the control of abnormal uterine bleeding: a cost-comparative study. J Reprod Med 39:755, 1994
17. Copperman AB, DeCherney AH, Olive DL: A case of endometrial cancer following endometrial ablation for dysfunctional uterine bleeding. Obstet Gynecol 82:640, 1993
18. Goldberg JM: Intrauterine pregnancy following endometrial ablation. Obstet Gynecol 83:578, 1994
19. Mongelli JM, Evans AJ: Pregnancy after transcervical endometrial resection. Lancet 338:578, 1991
20. Dawood MY: Current concepts in the etiology and treatment of primary dysmenorrhea. Acta Obstet Gynecol Scand Suppl 138:7, 1986
21. Halbert DR, Demers LM, Fontana J, Jones DE: Prostaglandin levels in endometrial jet wash specimens in patients with dysmenorrhea before and after indomethacin therapy. Prostaglandins 10:1047, 1975
22. Chan WY, Dawood MY, Fuchs F: Prostaglandins in primary dysmenorrhea: comparison of prophylactic and nonprophylactic treatment with ibuprofen and use of oral contraceptives. Am J Med 70:535, 1981
23. Gambone JC, Reiter RC: Nonsurgical management of chronic pelvic pain: a multidisciplinary approach. Clin Obstet Gynecol 33:205, 1990
24. Reiter RC, Gambone JC: Demographic and historic variables in women with idiopathic chronic pelvic pain. Obstet Gynecol 75:428, 1990

25. Rapkin AJ, Kames LD: The pain management approach to chronic pelvic pain. J Reprod Med 32:323, 1987

26. Carlson KJ, Miller BA, Foweler FJ: The Maine women's health study. I. Outcomes of hysterectomy. Obstet Gynecol 83:556, 1994

27. Stovall TG, Ling FW, Crawford DA: Hysterectomy for chronic pelvic pain of presumed uterine etiology. Obstet Gynecol 75:676, 1990

28. Enblad P, Adami HO, Glimelius B et al: The risk of subsequent primary malignant disease after cancers of the colon and rectum: a nationwide cohort study. Cancer 65:2091, 1990

29. Stearns MW Jr: Benign and malignant neoplasms of colon and rectum: diagnosis and management. Surg Clin North Am 58:605, 1978

30. Gambone JC, Reiter RC, Lench JB: Short-term outcome of incidental hysterectomy at the time of adnexectomy for benign disease. J Womens Health 1:197, 1992

31. Deane RT, Ulene A: Hysterectomy or tubal ligation for sterilization: a cost-effective analysis. Inquiry 14:73, 1977

32. Laros RK, Work BA: Female sterilization. III. Vaginal hysterectomy. Am J Obstet Gynecol 122:693, 1975

33. Pratt JH, Daikoku NH: Obesity and vaginal hysterectomy. J Reprod Med 35:945, 1990

34. Pitkin RM: Vaginal hysterectomy in obese women. Obstet Gynecol 49:567, 1977

35. Coulam CB, Pratt JH: Vaginal hysterectomy: is previous pelvic operation a contraindication. Am J Obstet Gynecol 116:252, 1973

36. Kovac SR: Guidelines to determine the route of hysterectomy. Obstet Gynecol 85:18, 1995

37. Richardson RE, Bournas N, Magos AL: Is laparoscopic hysterectomy a waste of time? Lancet 345:36, 1995

38. Kovac SR, Cruikshank SH, Retto HF: Laparoscopy-assisted vaginal hysterectomy. J Gynecol Surg 6:185, 1990

39. Cartwright DS: Diagnostic laparoscopy immediately preceding elective hysterectomy. Proceedings of the 18th Annual Meeting of American Association of Gynecologic Laparoscopists, p. 88, 1992

40. Stovall TG, Elder RE, Ling FW: Predictors of pelvic adhesions. J Reprod Med 34:345, 1989

41. Nezhat F, Nezhat C, Gordon S, Wilkins E: Laparoscopic versus abdominal hysterectomy. J Reprod Med 37:247, 1992

42. Daniell JF, Kurtz BR, McTavish G et al: Laparoscopically assisted vaginal hysterectomy: the initial Nashville, Tennessee, experience. J Reprod Med 38:537, 1993

43. Jones RA: Laparoscopic hysterectomy: a series of 100 cases. Med J Aust 159:447, 1993

44. Kaye WB, Espy GB III, Bishop MR et al: Laparoscopic Doderlein hysterectomy: a rational alternative to traditional abdominal hysterectomy. Surg Laparosc Endosc 3:88, 1993

45. Liu CY: Laparoscopic hysterectomy. Report of 215 cases. Gynaecol Endos 1:73, 1992

46. Raju KS, Auld BJ: A randomized prospective study of laparoscopic vaginal hysterectomy versus abdominal hysterectomy each with bilateral salpingo-oophorectomy. Br J Obstet Gynaecol 101:1068, 1994

47. Summitt RL Jr, Stovall TG, Lipscomb GH, Ling FW: Randomized comparison of laparoscopic-assisted vaginal hysterectomy with standard vaginal hysterectomy in an outpatient setting. Obstet Gynecol 80:895, 1992

48. Davis GD, Wolgamott G, Moon J: Laparoscopically assisted vaginal hysterectomy as definitive therapy for stage III or IV endometriosis. J Reprod Med 38:577, 1993

49. Mengert WF: Mechanisms of uterine support and position. I. Factors influencing uterine support (an experimental study). Am J Obstet Gynecol 31:775, 1936

50. Sheth SS, Malpani A: Vaginal hysterectomy for high-risk patients under local anesthesia. J Gynecol Surg 8:65, 1992

51. Magrina JF: Self-retaining retractor for vaginal operations. J Gynecol Surg 7:33, 1991

52. Lazar MR, Krieger HA: Blood loss in vaginal surgery: a comparative study. Obstet Gynecol 13:707, 1959

53. England GT, Randall HW, Graves WL: Impairment of tissue defenses by vasoconstrictors in vaginal hysterectomies. Obstet Gynecol 61:271, 1983

54. Evans DG, Miles AA, Niven JSF: The enhancement of bacterial infections by adrenaline. Br J Exp Pathol 29:20, 1948

55. Hoffman MS, Jaeger M: A new method for gaining entry into the scarred anterior cul-de-sac during transvaginal hysterectomy. Am J Obstet Gynecol 162:1269, 1990

56. Sheth SS: The place of oophorectomy at vaginal hysterectomy. Br J Obstet Gynaecol 98:662, 1991

57. Sheth SS, Malpani A: Routine prophylactic oophorectomy at the time of vaginal hysterectomy in postmenopausal women. Arch Gynecol Obstet 251:87, 1992

58. Capen CV, Irwin H, Magrina J, Masterson BJ: Vaginal removal of the ovaries in association with vaginal hysterectomy. J Reprod Med 28:589, 1993

59. Hoffman MS: Transvaginal removal of ovaries with endoloop sutures at the time of transvaginal hysterectomy. Am J Obstet Gynecol 165:407, 1991

60. Magos AL, Bournas N, Sinha R et al: Transvaginal endoscopic oophorectomy. Am J Obstet Gynecol 172:123, 1995

61. Cruikshank SH: Methods of vaginal cuff closure during vaginal hysterectomy. South Med J 81:1375, 1988

62. Symmonds R, Williams TJ, Lee RA, Webb MJ: Posthysterectomy enterocele and vaginal vault prolapse. Am J Obstet Gynecol 140:852, 1981

63. Doderlein A, Kronig S: Die Technik Der Vaginalen Bauchhohlen-Operationen. Verlag Von S Hirzel, Leipzig, 1906

64. Bohm JW, Lee FYL: Vaginal hysterectomy by anterior delivery of the uterine corpus. South Med J 69:1543, 1976

65. Kaminski PF, Podczaski ES, Pees RC et al: The Doderlein vaginal hysterectomy: a useful approach for the neophyte vaginal surgeon. J Gynecol Surg 6:123, 1990

66. Kovac SR: Intramyometrial coring as an adjunct to vaginal hysterectomy. Obstet Gynecol 67:131, 1986

67. Lash AF: A method for reducing the size of the uterus in vaginal hysterectomy. Am J Obstet Gynecol 42:452, 1941

68. Grody MH: Vaginal hysterectomy: the large uterus. J Gynecol Surg 5:301, 1989

69. Mazdisnian F, Kurzel RB, Coe S et al: Vaginal hysterectomy by uterine morcellation: an efficient, non-morbid procedure. Obstet Gynecol 86:60, 1995

70. Jaszczak SE, Evans TN: Intrafascial abdominal and vaginal hysterectomy: a reappraisal. Obstet Gynecol 59:435, 1982

71. Neuman M, Beller U, Chetrit AB et al: Prophylactic effect of the open vaginal vault method in reducing febrile morbidity in abdominal hysterectomy. Surg Gynecol Obstet 176:591, 1993

72. Moolgaoker AS, Rizvi JH, Payne PR: Reducing the hospital stay following vaginal hysterectomy. Obstet Gynecol 49:570, 1977

73. Ledger WJ, Child MA: The hospital care of patients undergoing hysterectomy: an analysis of 12,062 patients from the Professional Activity Study. Am J Obstet Gynecol 117:423, 1973

74. Moore J: Vaginal hysterectomy: its success as an outpatient procedure. AORN J 48:1114, 1988

75. Reiner IJ: Early discharge after vaginal hysterectomy. Obstet Gynecol 71:416, 1988

76. Stovall TG, Summit RL Jr, Bran DF, Ling FW: Outpatient vaginal hysterectomy: a pilot study. Obstet Gynecol 80:143, 1992

77. Summitt RL Jr, Stovall TG, Lipscomb GH et al: Outpatient hysterectomy: determinants of discharge and hospitalization in 133 patients. Am J Obstet Gynecol 171:1480, 1974

78. Slavotinek J, Berman L, Burch D, Keefe B: The incidence and significance of acute post-hysterectomy pelvic collections. Clin Radiol 50:322, 1995

79. Toglia MR, Pearlman MD: Pelvic fluid collections following hysterectomy and their relation to febrile morbidity. Obstet Gynecol 83:766, 1994

80. Dicker RC, Greenspan JR, Strauss LT et al: Complications of abdominal and vaginal hysterectomy among women of reproductive age in the United States: the collaborative review of sterilization. Am J Obstet Gynecol 144:841, 1982

81. Summitt RL Jr, Stovall TG, Bran DF: Prospective comparison of in dwelling bladder catheter drainage with no catheter after vaginal hysterectomy. Am J Obstet Gynecol 170:1815, 1994

82. Bunker JP, McPherson K, Hennenman PL: Elective hysterectomy. In Bunker JP, Baines BA, Mosteller F (eds): Costs Risks and Benefits of Surgery. Oxford University Press, New York, 1977

83. Cole P, Berlin J: Elective hysterectomy. Am J Obstet Gynecol 129:117, 1977

84. Storer EH: Appendix. p. 1257. In Schwartz SI (ed): Principles of Surgery. 3rd Ed. McGraw Hill, New York, 1979

85. Melcher DH: Appendectomy with abdominal hysterectomy. Lancet 1:810, 1971

86. Waters EG: Elective appendectomy with abdominal and pelvic surgery. Obstet Gynecol 50:511, 1977

87. Voitk AJ, Lowry JB: Is incidental appendectomy a safe practice? Can J Surg 31:448, 1988

88. Waters EG: Elective appendectomy with abdominal and pelvic surgery. Obstet Gynecol 50:511, 1977

89. Loeffler F, Stearn R: Abdominal hysterectomy with appendectomy. Acta Obstet Gynecol Scand 46:435, 1967

90. Massoudnia N: Incidental appendectomy in vaginal surgery. Int Surg 60:89, 1975

91. Reiner IJ: Incidental appendectomy at the time of vaginal surgery. Tex Med 76:46, 1980

92. McGowan L: Incidental appendectomy during vaginal surgery. Am J Obstet Gynecol 95:588, 1966

93. Kovac SR, Cruikshank SH: Incidental appendectomy during vaginal hysterectomy. Int J Gynecol Obstet 43:62, 1993

94. Pratt JH, O'Leary JA, Symmonds RE: Combined cholecystectomy and hysterectomy: a study of 95 cases. Mayo Clin Proc 42:529, 1967

95. Murray JM, Gilstrap LC, Massey FM: Cholecystectomy and abdominal hysterectomy. JAMA 244:2305, 1980

96. Hester TR, Baird W, Bostwick J et al: Abdominoplasty combined with other major surgical procedures: safe or sorry? Plast Reconstr Surg 83:997, 1989

97. Voss SC, Sharp HC, Scott JR: Abdominoplasty combined with gynecologic surgical procedures: Obstet Gynecol 67:181, 1986

98. Kovac SR: Vaginal hysterectomy combined with liposuction. Mo Med 86:165, 1989

99. Averette HE, Nguyen HN: The role of prophylactic oophorectomy in cancer prevention. Gynecol Oncol 55:S38, 1994

100. Speroff T, Dawson NV, Speroff L, Haber RJ: A risk-benefit analysis of elective bilateral oophorectomy: effect of changes in compliance with estrogen therapy on outcome. Am J Obstet Gynecol 164:165, 1991

101. Boike G, Averette HE, Hoskins W et al: National survey of ovarian carcinoma. I. A patient care evaluation study of the American College of Surgeons. Cancer 71:1629, 1993

102. Massler DJ, Devanesan MM: Sexual consequences of gynecologic operatings. p. 153. In Comfort A (ed): Sexual Consequences of Disability. George F. Stickley, Philadelphia 1978

103. Drellich MG, Bieber I: The psychological importance of the uterus and its function. J Nerv Ment Dis 126:322, 1958

104. Lindemann E: Observations on psychiatric sequelae to surgical operations in women. Am J Psychiatry 98:132, 1941

105. Richards DH: Depression after hysterectomy. Lancet 2:430, 1973

106. Hollender MH: A study of patients admitted to a psychiatric hospital after pelvic operations. Am J Obstet Gynecol 79:498, 1960

107. Bragg RL: Risk of admission to mental hospital following hysterectomy or cholecystectomy. Am J Public Health 55:1403, 1965

108. Martin RL, Roberts WV, Clayton PJ: Psychiatric status after hysterectomy. A one year prospective follow-up. JAMA 244:350, 1980

109. Moore JT, Tolley DH: Depression following hysterectomy. Psychosomatics 17:86, 1976

110. Hamptom PT, Tarnasky WG: Hysterectomy and tubal liga-

tion: a comparison of the psychological aftermath. Am J Obstet Gynecol 119:949, 1974

111. Janis IL: Psychological stress; psychoanalytical behavioral studies of surgical patients. John Wiley & Sons, New York; 1958

112. Menzer D, Morris T, Gates P et al: Patterns of emotional recovery from hysterectomy. Psychosom Med 9:379, 1957

113. Huffman JW: The effect of gynecologic surgery on sexual relations. Am J Obstet Gynecol 59:915, 1950

114. Humphries PT: Sexual adjustment after a hysterectomy. Issues Health Care Women 2:1, 1980

115. Dennerstein L, Wood C, Burrows GD: Sexual response following hysterectomy and oophorectomy. Obstet Gynecol 49: 92, 1977

116. Lindgren HC: Personality as a Social Phenomenon. 2nd Ed. John Wiley & Sons, New York 1973

117. Kikku P, Lehtinen V, Hirvonen T, Gronroos M: Abdominal hysterectomy versus supravaginal uterine amputation: psychic factors. Ann Chir Gynaecol Suppl 76:62, 1987

118. Kilkku P, Hirvonen T, Gronroos M: Supravaginal uterine amputation vs. abdominal hysterectomy: the effects on urinary symptoms with special reference to nocturia and dysuria. Maturitas 6:197, 1981

119. Kikku P, Gronroos M, Hirvonen T, Rauramo L: Supravaginal uterine amputation vs. hysterectomy. Acta Obstet Gynecol Scand 62:141, 1983

120. Kikku P: Supravaginal uterine amputation vs. hysterectomy. Acta Obstet Gyneeol Scand 62:141, 1983

121. Hasson HM: Cervical removal at hysterectomy for benign disease: risks and benefits. J Reprod Med 38:781, 1993

122. Drife J: Conserving the cervix at hysterectomy. Br J Obstet Gynaecol 101:563, 1994

MYOMECTOMY

THOMAS G. STOVALL

U terine myomas are the most common tumors in women of reproductive age, occurring in up to 50 percent of women. They are more common in black women than whites[1] and are the most common indication for hysterectomy in the United States. These tumors are also referred to as leiomyomas, fibroids, myomas, fibromyoma, fibroleiomyoma, and leiomyofibroma.[1]

Although myomas can be found in any organ that has a smooth muscle component, this discussion deals only with those that are uterine. They may be single or multiple, and vary in size from microscopic to exceedingly very large. Fibroids weighing in excess of 100 lb have been reported.[2,3] Clinically, these tumors are categorized by location within the uterus (Fig. 25-1). The subserous and intramural fibroids are the most common and are located entirely within the myometrium. Pedunculated myomas arise from below the serosal surface or from the submucosal myometrium, develop on a stalk, and are located external to the body of the uterus. The pedicle may be broad-based or narrow. Submucosal fibroids can prolapse through the cervix and are then called prolapsed myoma. Fibroids can also arise directly from the cervix or be intraligamentous in location. The parametrial or perisalpingeal type are the least common form of fibroids. Finally, fibroids can become parasitic. Fibroids of this type arise from a pedunculated subserosal myoma that undergoes torsion, with the fibroid then deriving its blood supply from a source other than the uterus. Parasitic fibroids are most commonly found within the omentum.

The etiology of leiomyomas is unknown, although they are known to be estrogen dependent. This assumption is supported by the fact that they occur during the reproductive years, are rarely seen before menarche, decrease in size following menopause, and can be induced by giving large doses of estrogen.[4] Estrogen and progesterone receptors have been isolated in the fibroids and it has been shown that estrogen receptors are more concentrated in the myomas than in the myometrium surrounding them.[5–8] Cytogenetic studies support the theory that myomas arise from a single smooth muscle cell. Because there are many different cytogenetic abnormalities described, it is thought that multiple genetic loci are responsible for fibroid development.[9,10]

Only 20 to 40 percent of patients report symptoms, with the severity dependent on fibroid size, location, and whether there is any associated degeneration. The most common symptoms are abnormal uterine bleeding, abdominal/pelvic pain, and lower abdominal pressure. Abnormal bleeding is more common when the fibroids are submucosal. Uterine enlargement may also compress adjacent organs, causing urinary retention or constipation. Although described, ureteral compression or obstruction is uncommon. Pedunculated fibroids may undergo torsion and lead to the onset of acute lower abdominal pain. Submucosal pedunculated fibroids are most frequently associated with heavy and prolonged vaginal bleeding. They may prolapse through the cervix and undergo necrosis, leading to marked hemorrhage. Infertility or recurrent pregnancy loss associated with fibroids may result from blockage of the tubal ostia or endometrial compression.

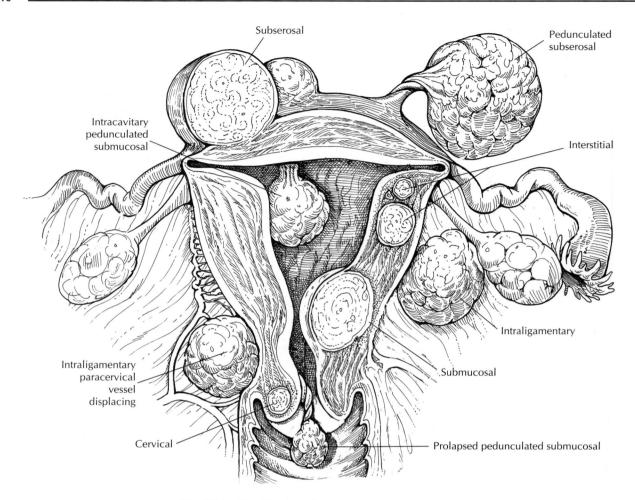

Fig. 25-1. Classification of uterine myomas by location.

INDICATIONS

The various indications that have been proposed for surgical removal of are given in the boxed list. Abdominal or pelvic pain most often results from torsion of a pedunculated fibroid or when the myoma outgrows its blood supply. This most commonly occurs during pregnancy or with rapid growth of a uterine myoma. Pain may also be secondary to cervical dilation from a prolapsed submucous myoma. More commonly, patients experience lower abdominal or pelvic pressure that results from the weight of the uterus and compression on surrounding organs. Pressure on the urinary bladder may produce dysuria or frequency. When the myoma compresses the ureterovesical angle, acute urinary retention may occur. Chronic compression of the ureters may produce renal parenchymal changes. Once the compression is relieved, these changes are generally reversible, unless it has been a long-standing process. Constipation, rectal pressure, or tenesmus are uncommon symptoms but may be associated with a large posterior leiomyomata.

Most fibroids grow slowly over several years or maintain a constant size. If rapid uterine growth is documented, or if uterine enlargement occurs following menopause, surgical intervention is indicated to make certain that no malignant change (sarcomatous degeneration) has occurred. This is exceedingly rare.

Size alone as an indication for surgical removal of asymptomatic fibroids is controversial. A uterine size of 12 weeks gestation has generally been the discriminatory zone between nonsurgical and surgical intervention.[11] However, there is no objective data to suggest that a particular uterine size is an absolute indication for intervention. Size alone as a surgical indication has been suggested because of difficulty in palpating the adnexa and because of the possibility of a leiomyosarcoma. This reasoning is flawed in that uterine sarcoma is rare, not all adnexa can be palpated even when the uterus is absent, and adnexal palpation has never been shown to decrease the morbidity or mortality of ovarian carcinoma.[10,11] The perimenopausal patient may desire more conservative therapy than patients of younger age, as they can be assured that their symptoms will diminish following menopause.

Proposed Indications for Surgical Removal of Leiomyomata Uteri

- Uterine size greater than 12 weeks' gestation
- Abnormal uterine bleeding
- Abdominal/pelvic pain or pressure
- Rapid growth
- Growth after menopause
- Infertility
- Recurrent pregnancy loss
- Ureteral/bladder compression or obstruction

Myomas, unless multiple or large, are rarely associated with recurrent pregnancy loss or infertility. In the infertile patient with leiomyomata, every effort should be made to exclude other etiologies of infertility or fetal loss before the patient undergoes myomectomy for this indication.

THERAPEUTIC CONSIDERATIONS

There is no known preventive strategy for the prevention of uterine myomas. Once the decision has been made between the patient and her gynecologist to proceed with treatment, surgical treatment is usually the best approach. Medical therapy with gonadotropin-releasing hormone (GnRH) agonist has been shown in multiple trials to reduce uterine size. This size reduction is temporary unless the agonist is continued and combined with estrogen replacement therapy.

This approach is generally not chosen because of its associated expense. The therapeutic approach selected is also based on the patient's desire for future pregnancy. If the patient desires preservation of her reproductive potential, myomectomy should be chosen. If the patient does not desire future fertility, then hysterectomy becomes a treatment alternative and the treatment approach must be based on the patient's desire and an understanding of the risks and benefits of surgical treatment. Uterine size in an of itself should not dictate whether myomectomy or hysterectomy is chosen, as even patients with very large myomas can often undergo successful myomectomy (Fig. 25-2).

Some authors have suggested that the uterus never be removed if myomectomy is possible. A reason cited for this belief is that the loss of the uterus is associated with diminished sexual feelings and decreased orgasmic intensity. They also cite data that indicates that uterine removal is associated with early onset of menopause.[12-14] Whether the uterus should be preserved in the patient who does not desire future fertility remains controversial. Clearly it is prudent to discuss these issues with the patient and allow her to make an informed decision.

PREOPERATIVE EVALUATION

The preoperative evaluation should begin with a complete history and physical examination. Cervical cytology should be within normal limits before myomectomy is considered. For the patient with intermenstrual bleeding or abnormal bleeding who is over 35 years of age, endometrial sampling should be performed to eliminate the possibility of endometrial carcinoma. The role of preoperative hysterosalpingography is controversial; some gynecologists suggest that it

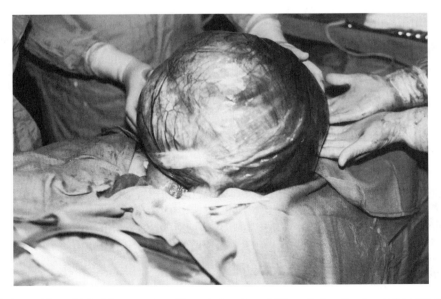

Fig. 25-2. Patient with multiple leiomyomata with a uterine size of 40 cm in length who underwent myomectomy.

should be done in all patients, while others suggest that it be done only if there is a question regarding tubal patency. Even if hysterosalpingography shows tubal occlusion, the tubes may become patent following myomectomy.[15] Hysteroscopy may be helpful in selected patients with heavy or prolonged menses to eliminate the possibility of a submucosal myoma. Ultrasound or computed tomography (CT) scan may be needed if there is a question as to whether the pelvic mass is uterine or adnexal in origin. However, from a practical standpoint, this is not necessary if the radiographic results will not alter the need for surgery. Laparoscopy is rarely indicated unless the information gained would alter the approach to the patient. For example, if the patient was found to have endometriosis or adhesive disease, she might opt for hysterectomy rather than myomectomy.

If the patient has an associated anemia, this should be corrected preoperatively. This is best accomplished using a combination of oral iron therapy combined with a GnRH agonist. Not only will vaginal bleeding be diminished, but uterine size will also be decreased. The preoperative storage of autologous and directed donor blood donation can be discussed with the patient. Generally, the patient can store up to 2 U of blood within a relatively short period. Whether this is cost-effective is uncertain at present, and thus the decision to proceed along this line should be based on the individual patient and her needs.

Whether a preoperative semen analysis is obtained is also controversial. For the nulliparous patient in a stable relationship who is undergoing the procedure because of infertility, a semen analysis should probably be done to make certain that the etiology of the infertility is not male factor. By contrast, for the patient undergoing myomectomy because of symptomatic fibroids, whether there is an associated male factor is of less importance.

The American College of Obstetricians and Gynecologists (ACOG) Quality Assessment and Improvement in Obstetrics and Gynecology[16] states that myomectomy should be done in those patients with leiomyomata who desire to retain their uterus. The indication should be confirmed by asymptomatic leiomyomata of such size that they are palpable abdominally and are a concern to the patient, or ovulatory patients with leiomyomata as probable cause of excessive uterine bleeding evidenced by either profuse bleeding with flooding or clots, repetitive periods lasting for more than 8 day, or anemia due to acute or chronic blood loss.

PREOPERATIVE USE OF GnRH AGONIST

GnRH agonist treatment induces a reversible hypoestrogenism that can lead to a temporary reduction in myoma volume. Although the reduction in individual patients may vary, most patients will have a 50 to 80 percent reduction in myoma volume after 6 months of treatment.[17–23] The maximum rate of reduction in uterine or myoma size occurs

---

Before Performing a Myomectomy

1. An absence of cervical malignancy should be documented by negative cervical cytology
2. Anovulation and other causes of abnormal bleeding should be eliminated
3. When abnormal bleeding is present with ovulatory cycles, the possible presence of submucous fibroid should be assessed by dilation and curettage, hysteroscopy, or imaging technique
4. Surgical risk from anemia and need for treatment should be determined
5. Advantages and disadvantages of myomectomy versus hysterectomy should be discussed with the patient and documented in the patient's record

In addition, the physician should

1. Evaluate other causes of male and female infertility or recurrent pregnancy loss
2. Evaluate the endometrial cavity and fallopian tubes (e.g., hysterosalpingogram)
3. Document discussion that complexity of disease process may require a hysterectomy

Note: In patients undergoing myectomy because of infertility, there should not be a more likely explanation for failure to conceive or recurrent pregnancy loss

---

during the first 12 weeks of treatment, after which point little further reduction occurs. However, once treatment is discontinued, a rapid increase in uterine/myoma size occurs in virtually all patients. Because these agents induce a relative amenorrhea, they are beneficial in the anemic patient to increase the hemoglobin and hematocrit before surgical intervention.[24,25] Their use before hysterectomy has also been shown to be cost effective. Side effects do occur, and can be serious, as in the case of degeneration of a submucous myoma leading to hemorrhage.[27] The development of ascites, although rare, has also been reported.[28] GnRH agonist pretreatment has also been shown to reduce intraoperative blood loss in patients undergoing myomectomy.[21,30] This reduced blood loss is probably a result of decreased uterine artery and myoma blood flow induced by use of these agents.[31,32] Some surgeons have suggested that GnRH agonist treatment induces fibrous changes within the myoma capsule, making it difficult to remove. No studies have been done to assess this, although the histology of myomas has been reported and did not show a difference in histopathologic appearance of the myomas. In addition, there was no increase in fibrosis among these patients.[33,34]

The use of GnRH agonist prior to hysteroscopic surgery was assessed in a prospective comparative trial reported by Perino et al.[35] In patients pretreated prior to hysteroscopic myomectomy, there was a significant reduction in operating time, intraoperative bleeding, infusion volume, and failure rate.[35–37]

The use of GnRH agonist prior to myomectomy has not been shown to increase the subsequent pregnancy rate or decrease adhesion formation.[36,37] Whether preoperative treatment with the resulting smaller uterine size allows more patients to undergo myomectomy rather than hysterectomy remains uncertain.

Friedman et al[38] followed 18 women for 27 to 38 months following myomectomy, in which they were pretreated with GnRH agonist. These authors found no difference in the recurrence rate among women who were pretreated with GnRH agonist and those women treated with progesterone. Women who had at least four myomas removed had a greater incidence of recurrent.[38] Other investigators found an increase in recurrence following agonist pretreatment (63 percent versus 13 percent) when transvaginal ultrasound was used to document recurrence of myomas of more than 1.5 cm.[39]

OPERATIVE PROCEDURES

Once the decision has been made to proceed with surgical management of her leiomyomata, the next decision point is for the patient to determine whether she desires to maintain the potential for future childbearing. If she does, and surgical intervention is required, myomectomy is the operative procedure of choice at present. The surgical approach to the patient undergoing myomectomy is somewhat dependent on the location of the myomas. Myomectomy can be performed by

---

Surgical Goals of Myomectomy

1. Total excision of the myoma
2. Restoration of the myometrial integrity
3. Closure of the uterine serosal surface in an attempt to minimize adhesion formation
4. Minimization of the number of uterine incisions
5. Avoidance of posterior uterine and cornual incisions if possible
6. Minimization of blood loss

---

laparotomy, via the vagina, laparoscopically, or using hysteroscopy. For the patient with intramural myomas, the abdominal approach is the gold standard to which other methods must be compared. For the patient with prolapsed myomas, vaginal myomectomy is the most appropriate approach, while hysteroscopic resection is most appropriate for submucosal leiomyomatas.

Abdominal Myomectomy

Although recommended by some authors, the use of prophylactic antibiotics before myomectomy has not been shown to be beneficial. Most abdominal myomectomies can be performed using a Pfannenstiel or transverse-type incision. The advantages, disadvantages, and techniques for these incisions are described in Chapter 8. Surgical principles used for myomectomy are similar to those used for other gynecologic surgical and infertility procedures. These techniques include meticulous hemostasis and avoidance of adhesiogenic materials. Hemostatic aids include myometrial injection of vasoconstrictors such as epinephrine or vasopressin (Pitressin). A vasopressin solution is made by diluting 10 to 20 U in 40 to 50 ml normal saline. In a randomized placebo-controlled trial, the use of vasopressin significantly reduced operative blood loss.[40] Tourniquet techniques using a Penrose drain or catheter to compress the uterine vasculature can be used. The tourniquet should be placed to compress the infundibulopelvic ligaments as well as the cervical blood supply.[41] Yet another method described is to use a long vascular-type clamp with rubbershods applied over the clamp's jaws.[42] Ginsburg et al[43] compared vasopressin with the use of an occlusive tourniquet. These authors found no differences in blood loss morbidity or transfusion between the use of pharmacologic vasoconstriction and mechanical vascular occlusion techniques. In their study, blood loss during myomectomy was correlated with preoperative uterine size, total weight of fibroids removed, and operating time.[43] Other methods that are thought to reduce blood loss include use of electrosurgery or laser to make the uterine incision(s).[44–48] Methods to reduce adhesion formation include using moistened laparotomy pads only. Placing these packs inside plastic bags will reduce lint deposition. Whether this is necessary is uncertain. Copious irrigation using a solution of heparinized Ringer's lactate should be used throughout the case. As much as possible, one should avoid the use of a posterior uterine incision as it is more likely to lead to postoperative adhesions. Use of adhesion prevention solutions or application of adhesive barriers should be considered, but is controversial.

The initial uterine incision should be made to allow removal of the maximum number of myomas so that the number of incisions can be minimized. When possible, the incision should be made on the anterior uterine surface in a vertical direction in an effort to avoid the more vascular

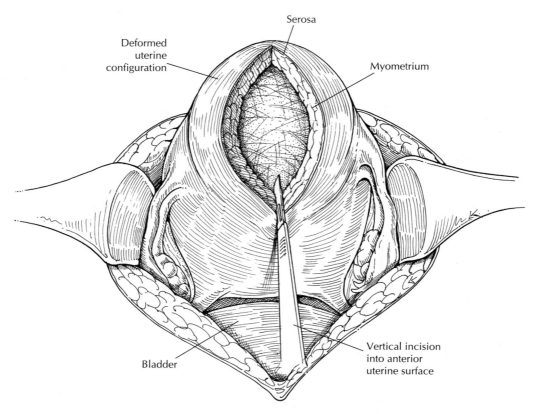

Deformed
uterine
configuration

Serosa

Myometrium

Bladder

Vertical incision
into anterior
uterine surface

Fig. 25-3. Abdominal myomectomy. Initial vertical incision into the anterior uterine surface.

areas of the uterus (Fig. 25-3). The serosa is incised and the incision is carried down so that the myoma itself is incised. This allows for identification of the plane between the myoma capsule and the myometrium (Fig. 25-4). An Allis clamp or towel clip is applied to the myoma and traction is applied (Fig. 25-5). As traction is applied, the plane between the myoma capsule and myometrium is developed using blunt and sharp dissection (Fig. 25-4). To minimize blood loss, any loose connective tissue or vascular tissue between the capsule and myometrium is desiccated as the dissection progresses (Fig. 25-6). The base of the myoma is identified and the remaining connective tissue and blood supply is clamped and ligated (Fig. 25-7). Hemostasis is then achieved using electrosurgery to desiccate any bleeding vessels. The myometrial defect is then closed using interrupted sutures in several layers (Figs. 25-8 and 25-9). Another approach is to use a continuous suture in concentric circles to close this dead space. The serosa can be reapproximated using a base-ball-type suture or using a subserosal suture (Fig. 25-10). The potential advantage of this technique is that no suture material is exposed and it might reduce adhesion formation. A delayed absorbable suture material is preferable.

At the time of myomectomy, every effort should be made to remove all of the myomas identified.[49] If myomas remain, there is a potential for these to grow and become symptomatic. Myomas can be identified by digital palpation and also

all myomas identified with preoperative ultrasound should be removed. A review of abdominal myomectomy in 128 women was reported by LaMorte.[50] The average intraoperative estimated blood loss was 342 ml, with five patients having a blood loss greater than 1,000 ml. Twenty percent of patients required blood transfusions, with 70 percent of patients receiving autologous blood. Hysterectomy was required in only one patient. Febrile morbidity occurred in 12 percent of patients.[50] Although generally not fraught with life-threatening complications, Sacks[51] reported the removal of 52 uterine fibroids in a patient with a uterine mass extending 36 cm above the pubic symphysis. This case was complicated by the development of disseminated intravascular coagulation, hemolytic anemia, and acute renal failure.

Although not always possible, every effort should be made to avoid endometrial cavity entry as this could lead to adhesion formation and the development of Asherman syndrome. For cornual myomas, special care must be taken to avoid injury to the fallopian tubes.

Weinstein and colleagues[52] performed hysterography following myomectomy in 12 patients. In 11 cases, the uterine cavity was of normal shape and size after surgery, regardless of the degree of distortion prior to surgery. In one patient, the hysterosalpingogram showed several myomas that were missed at the time of the initial surgery. Beyth et al[53] followed patients using ultrasound after myomectomy. These

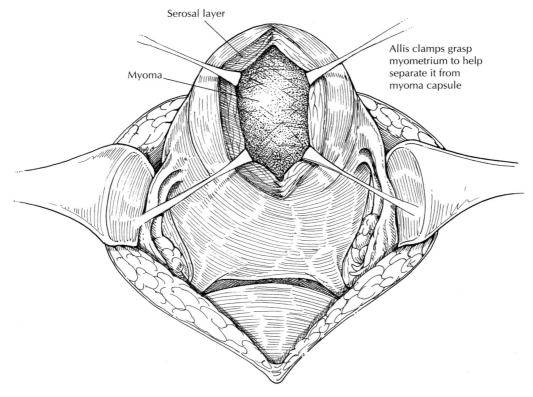

Fig. 25-4. Placement of Allis clamps for traction on the myometrium.

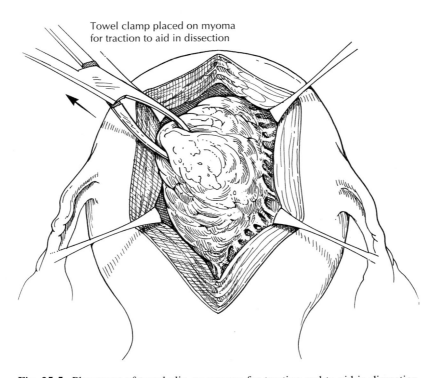

Fig. 25-5. Placement of towel clip on myoma for traction and to aid in dissection.

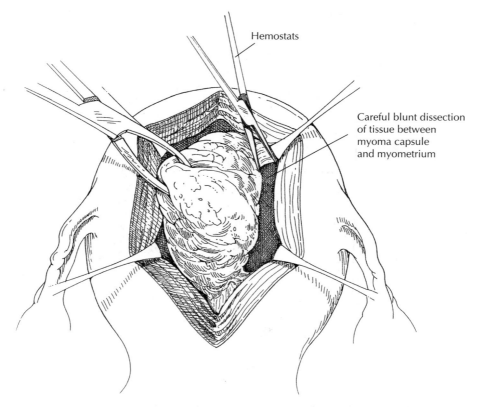

Hemostats

Careful blunt dissection
of tissue between
myoma capsule
and myometrium

Fig. 25-6. Identification and dissection of the tissue between the myoma capsule and overlying myometrium.

authors noted a gradual decrease in uterine volume in all patients during the 6 months following removal of intramural and submucosal leiomyomata. The greatest decrease occurred during the initial 2 to 3 months. These authors raised the question as to whether patients should avoid pregnancy during this interval.

Vaginal Myomectomy

Prolapse of a submucous myoma dictates a vaginal approach through an already dilated cervix.[54] As with abdominal myomectomy, the use of prophylactic antibiotics is generally recommended, although no data is available on its use. Most often, the procedure is straightforward and rapid (Fig. 25-11). The pedicle can be clamped, cut, and sutured ligated using a delayed absorbable suture material. For large myomas, it is not always possible to identify the base and place a clamp. In such cases, the myoma must be morcellated to a point that this can be done. Alternatively, a pretied surgical loop may be passed over the myoma and the base ligated. For patients with submucous myomas that are not prolapsed, the cervix can be dilated with laminaria tents and the myomas removed by grasping the fibroids with uterine polyp forceps or uterine dressing forceps.[55] Once the initial procedure is completed, it seems prudent to preform a diagnostic hysteroscopy to determine whether other submucous myo-

mas are present. If they are, the surgeon must then decide whether to proceed with hysteroscopic resection as a primary procedure or wait until the patient can be more fully evaluated and then perform the procedure as a second procedure. Often, these patients are anemic as a result of acute bleeding, and this must be taken into consideration before proceeding with additional surgery. A very uncommon situation has been reported in which the prolapsed uterine myoma leads to complete uterine inversion.[56–58] If this occurs, great care should be taken to identify the bladder and ureters as these will be extraperitoneal. Morbidity following vaginal myomectomy is lower than with an abdominal approach.[59] If bleeding becomes excessive a Foley catheter can be placed into the endometrial cavity and inflated to tamponade the bleeding.

Success with vaginal myomectomy is in excess of 90 percent.[60] The risk of recurrent vaginal myomectomy is approximately 9 percent with a 5-year follow-up; approximately 6 percent of patients requiring hysterectomy.

Uterine leiomyomas occur in approximately 2 percent of pregnant women and most often do not interfere with the course of pregnancy.[61,62] The need for myomectomy during pregnancy is uncommon, and should be avoided if at all possible. On occasion, a myoma may begin to degenerate and the patient becomes symptomatic and does not respond to hydration and antibiotic therapy. In these cases, myomec-

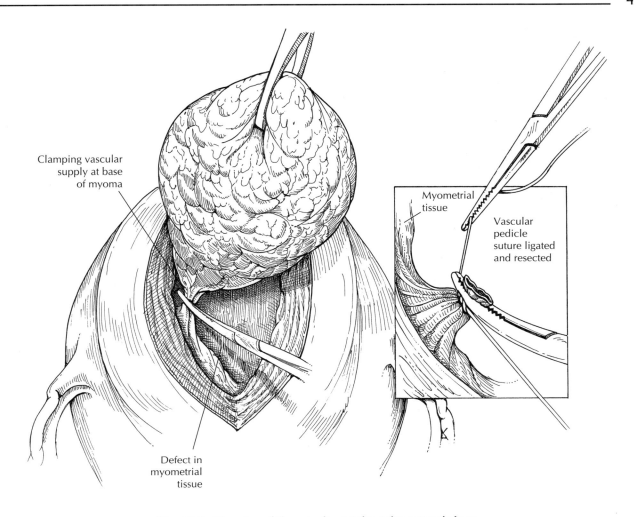

Fig. 25-7. Clamping of the vascular supply at the myoma's base.

tomy must be considered.[63] Criteria for myoma removal during pregnancy are not solid and must be based on the individual patient's symptoms. Generally pedunculated myomas can be removed without great difficulty.[64] Removal of intramural myomas has been associated with intraoperative hemorrhage and subsequent pregnancy loss.[65,68]

Laparoscopic Myomectomy

The ability to perform a myomectomy laparoscopically should not be the sole determinant for performing the procedure. Selection of cases for laparoscopic therapy should be based on the equivalent indications to those that would be performed at laparotomy.

Dubuisson et al[69,70] reported a group of 70 patients undergoing laparoscopic myomectomy. Of the 70, 46 (65.7 percent) were pretreated with GnRH agonist. Techniques used included (1) coagulation when the implantation surface was 1 cm^2 or less, and (2) uterine incision with enucleation and one- or two-layer uterine closure with 3–0 delayed ab-

sorbable suture. No complications were observed and no patient required laparotomy. Second-look laparoscopy was done in seven patients, six had no adhesions, and one had severe bowel–uterine adhesions. These authors recommend that laparotomy be used in myoma greater than 10 cm in size or if more than four myomas were present.

Daniell and Gurley[71] reported a series of 17 patients who underwent laparoscopic myomectomy following pretreatment with GnRH agonist. Techniques used included electrosurgery, cautery, potassium-titanyl-phosphate (KTP) laser, morcellation, and colpotomy for myoma removal. The uterine serosa was not closed, but was covered with an adhesive barrier. The mean blood loss was 78 ml, with an average operating time of 100 minutes. There were no postoperative hemorrhages infections or long-term complications reported. Hasson et al[72] reported 56 patients in which 144 myomas were removed through the laparoscope. These myomas ranged in size from 3 to 16 cm. The mean operative time was 157 minutes, with a range of 45 to 443. None of the patients required laparotomy or transfusion. A second-look laparoscopy was performed in 24 patients. Of these, 8 (33

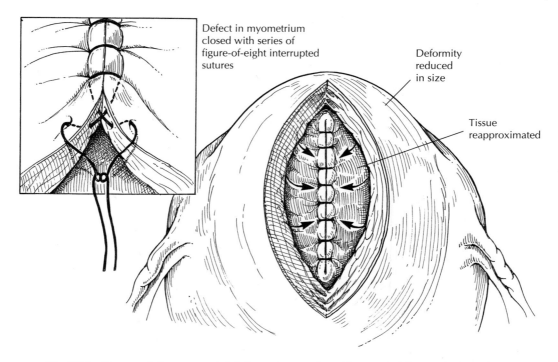

Fig. 25-8. Closure of the myometrial defect using a series of interrupted figure-of-eight sutures.

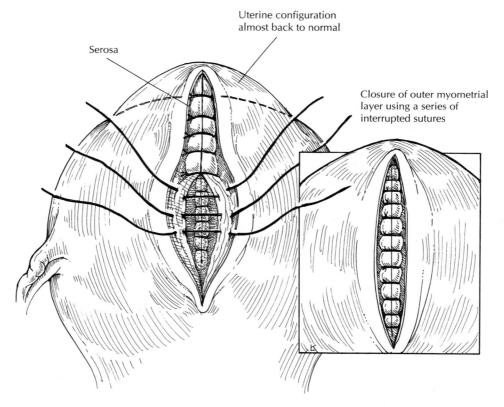

Fig. 25-9. Closure of the outer myometrial layer using a series of interrupted sutures.

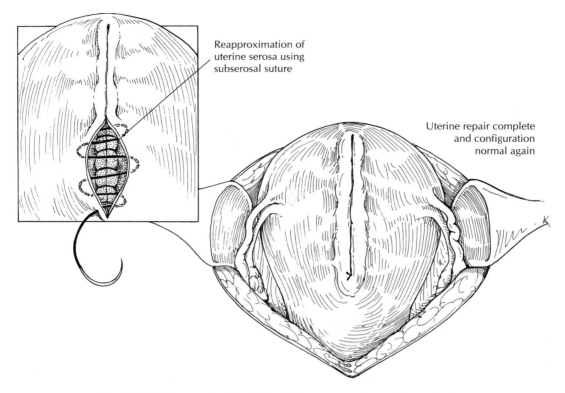

Reapproximation of
uterine serosa using
subserosal suture

Uterine repair complete
and configuration
normal again

Fig. 25-10. Reapproximation of the uterine serosa using a subserosal suture.

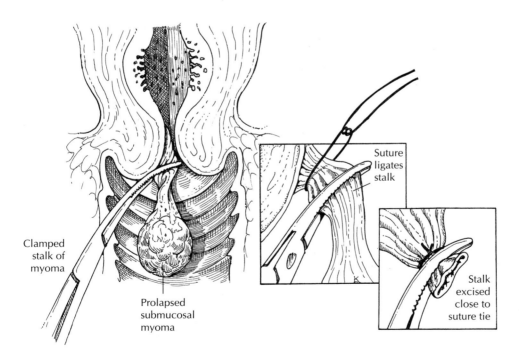

Clamped
stalk of
myoma

Prolapsed
submucosal
myoma

Suture
ligates
stalk

Stalk
excised
close to
suture tie

Fig. 25-11. Transvaginal removal of a prolapsed submucosal myoma.

percent) had no adhesives, 5 (21 percent) had minimal adhesions, and 11 (46 percent) had moderate or extensive adhesion formation. Nezhat et al[73] performed laparoscopic myomectomy on 154 women, removing 347 leiomyomata ranging in size from 2 to 15 cm. One patient required a laparotomy incision for removal of a calcified myoma. The mean operative time was 116 minutes with a range of 50 to 190. Two patients required a transfusion, and the mean duration of hospitalization was 19.6 hours, with a range of 7 to 48. Six of 24 (25 percent) of the subjects who underwent intramural myomectomy developed a uteroperitoneal fistula.

To date, no prospective randomized trials have been reported comparing conventional myomectomy by laparotomy with laparoscopic myomectomy. Thus, laparoscopic myomectomy should be seen as an alternative procedure, which cannot be recommended on a routine basis. Several issues remain regarding the use of laparoscopic myomectomy, including the following:

1. Uteroperitoneal fistula formation as a result of difficulty in closure of the uterine incision
2. The possibility of uterine rupture with a subsequent pregnancy,[76]
3. Techniques of uterine incision closure
4. Incidence of adhesion formation
5. Subsequent fertility following the procedure

Laparoscopic Myolysis

A relatively new procedure has been described in which the neodymium:yttrium aluminum garnet (Nd:YAG) laser is used to coagulate and devascularize myomas through the laparoscope. This method involves pretreatment of patients with GnRH agonist for a 2 to 6-month period. A 10 percent vasopressin solution is injected directly into the serosa of the myomas. The Nd:YAG laser is set at 50 watts of power using a 600-μm fiber. The bare fiber is used to pierce the myoma in multiple places at 5-mm intervals. Thus, for a myoma measuring 5 cm, 75 to 100 punctures are used. Following this procedure, myomas regress over a period of 3 to 6 months by 50 to 90 percent of their original volume. During 14 months of follow-up there were no recurrences.[75] Nisolle et al[78] reported similar results in a group of 48 women. In this study, 7 patients underwent a second look laparoscopy, and in all cases, dense and fibrous adhesions were found. Thus, until additional data are collected, this procedure is only recommended for patients who do not wish to have further childbearing but wish to retain their uterus. Patients should be counseled about this adhesion formation and its future implications.

Hysteroscopic Resection

Often, hysteroscopic diagnosis is the only method that allows for detection of submucous myomas. The ideal myoma for hysteroscopic removal is a pedunculated submucous myoma. For myoma located in the uterine musculature, hysteroscopic resection becomes very difficult. In 1976, Neuwirth and Amin[77] were the first to describe excision of submucous myomas using hysteroscopic surgery. Advances in technique allowed investigators to use a resectoscope to remove the myomas using a "shaving" technique.[78,79] This technique is the one that is most commonly used for hysteroscopic myoma removal (Fig. 25-12).

To accomplish the procedure, the uterine cavity is distended with a high-viscosity fluid such as Hyskon or a low-viscosity fluid media such as 1.5 percent glycine or 4 percent sorbitol. The fluid is delivered under pressure by using an electronic pump or, more commonly, gravity. A continuous flow hysteroscope is used so that an bleeding can be easily cleared. Laparoscopy is used routinely by some authors, but is a must if there is any significant degree of intramural extension. Energy sources include the Nd:YAG laser or, more commonly, electrosurgical generators.

For pedunculated myomas, the pedicle is cut near its base. This is accomplished by positioning the wire loop behind the myoma, and cutting the stalk. A pure cutting current is used to avoid tissue sticking on the loop itself. The myoma must then be removed, which can be done using polyp forceps or by morcellation of the myoma and removing it piecemeal. If not all of the pieces can be removed, they can be left inside the uterus and will undergo degeneration over a 2- to 3-week period. The base of the pedicle is then resected with special care being taken to remove minimal endometrium and surrounding myometrium.

Removal of sessile myomas that are embedded within the myometrium generally requires the use of hysteroscopy and laparoscopy. The intramural portion is removed ming the resectoscope loop and shaving the myoma, while the intramural portion is resected in a similar fashion, making certain that the uterus is not perforated and the serosal surface injured. It is generally suggested that if there is more than 50 percent intramural extension of the myoma, hysteroscopic resection should not be attempted.

Outcomes of patients following hysteroscopic resection have been reported in several series. Brooks et al[80] published the follow-up of 52 patients, of whom 91 percent had resumption of normal menses, with 33 percent of 15 infertile patients achieving pregnancy.[81] Loffer[82] reported 53 patients undergoing this procedure, with 45 patients followed for more than 12 months. Although 93 percent had resumption of normal menses, 9 percent required hysterectomy and 2 patients required a repeat hysteroscopic resection. Derman et al[33] reported on 94 patients followed for 9 years. In these patients, 15.9 percent required further surgery. Similar results have been reported by Valle,[86] who reported on 59 patients and Baggish et al[85] who reported 23 women undergoing myoma resection.

The most serious complication with this procedure is fluid overload, which can result in pulmonary edema, electrolyte disturbances, and death. Thus, as with all hysteroscopic sur-

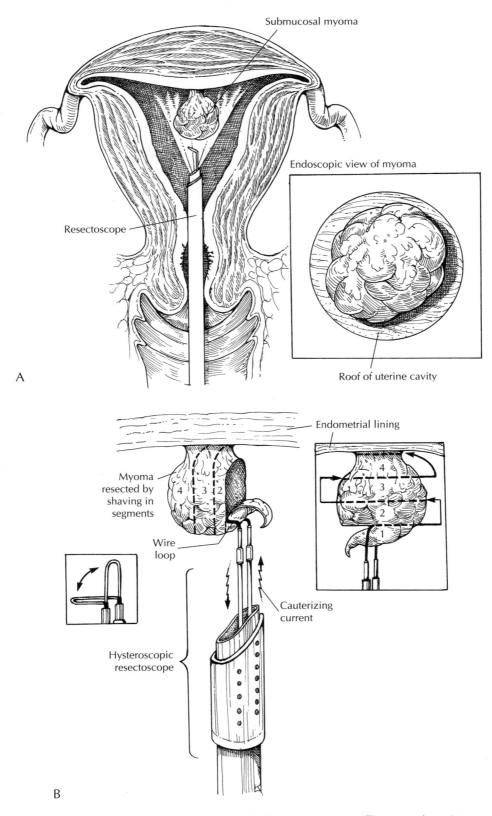

Submucosal myoma

Endoscopic view of myoma

Resectoscope

Roof of uterine cavity

A

Endometrial lining

Myoma resected by shaving in segments

Wire loop

Cauterizing current

Hysteroscopic resectoscope

B

Fig. 25-12. **(A–C)** Hysteroscopic resection of submucous myomas. *(Figure continues.)*

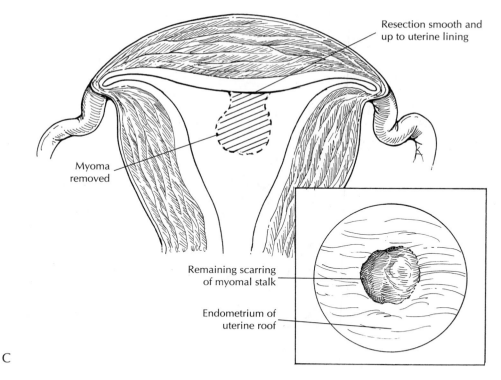

Resection smooth and
up to uterine lining

Myoma
removed

Remaining scarring
of myomal stalk

Endometrium of
uterine roof

C

Fig. 25-12 *(Continued).*

gery, fluid absorption should be calculated closely. Other potential complications can include bleeding and uterine perforation; if this occurs, there is potential for damage to the bowel.[86]

REPRODUCTIVE OUTCOME

In one of the largest series reported, Candiani et al[82] reviewed 622 patients who underwent myomectomy over a 14-year period. The cumulative 10-year recurrence rate was 27 percent, increasing with length of follow-up. There were no differences observed in recurrence rates by age at diagnosis or site of the myomas, although patients with more than one myoma tended to recur more frequently. Interestingly, women who gave birth to a child after myomectomy had a 10-year recurrence rate of 15 percent, compared to 30 percent for those women who did not become pregnant. The recurrence rates reported vary widely, raging from 5 to 10 percent to 35 percent.[88-92]

Myomectomy has long been considered a risk factor for obstetric-related uterine rupture. It has been thought that if the uterine cavity was entered at the time of myomectomy, this potentially increased this risk. In one study, the incidence of uterine rupture was increased with entry into the endometrial cavity.[93] In other studies, however, no increase was noted.[94,95]

The rate of pregnancy following myomectomy for infertil-

ity or fetal loss has been assessed by several authors.[96-100] Generally, one can expect a 50 to 65 percent pregnancy rate following myomectomy for infertility or recurrent pregnancy loss. Adhesion formation is a significant cause of infertility following myomectomy. Tulandi et al[101] found that a myomectomy incision on the posterior wall of the uterus was associated with more adnexal adhesions than that on the fundus or anterior uterine wall.

REFERENCES

1. Buttram VC Jr, Reiter RC: Uterine leiomyomata: etiology, symptomatology and management. Fertil Steril 36:433, 1981
2. Jonas HS, Masterson BJ: Giant uterine tumor: case report and review of the literature. Obstet Gynecol 50:2S, 1977
3. Singhabhandhu B, Akin JT Jr, Ridley JH et al: Giant leiomyoma of the uterus: report of a case and review of the literature. Am J Surg 39:391, 1973
4. Nelson WO: Endometrial and myometrial changes, including fibromyomatous nodules, induced in the uterus of the guinea pig by the prolonged administration of oestrogenic hormone. Anat Rec 68:99, 1937
5. Puukka M, Kontula KK, Kauppila AJI et al: Oestrogen receptors in human myoma tissue. Mol Cell Endocrinol 6:35, 1976
6. Soules KMR, McCarty KS Jr: Leiomyomas: steroid receptor content: variation within normal menstrual cycles. Am J Obstet Gynecol 143:6, 1982

7. Tamaya T, Fujimoto J, Okada H: Comparison of cellular levels in steroid receptors in uterine leiomyoma and myometrium. Acta Obstet Gynecol Scand 64:307, 1985

8. Wilson EA, Yang F, Rees ED: Estradiol and progesterone binding in uterine leiomyomata and in normal uterine tissues. Obstet Gynecol 55:20, 1980

9. Mark J, Havel G, Grepp C et al: Cytogenetical observations in human benign leiomyomas. Anticancer Res 8:621, 1988

10. Rein MT, Friedman AJ, Barbieri RL et al: Cytogenetic abnormalities in uterine leiomyomata. Obstet Gynecol 77:923, 1991

11. Reiter RC, Wagner PL, Gambore JC: Routine hysterectomy for large asymptomatic uterine leiomyomata: a reappraisal. Obstet Gynecol 79:481, 1992

12. Beavis EL, Brown JB, Smith MA: Ovarian functions after hysterectomy with conservation of the ovaries in premenopausal women. J Obstet Gynecol Br Commonwealth 76:969, 1969

13. Centerwall BS: Premenopausal hysterectomy and cardiovascular disease. Am J Obstet Gynecol 139:58, 1981

14. Sidle N, Sarrel P, Whitehead M: The effect of hysterectomy on the age of ovarian failure. Fertil Steril 47:94, 1987

15. Lev-Toaff AS, Karasick S, Toaff ME: Hysterosalpingography before and after myomectomy: clinical value and imaging findings. Am J Radiol 160:803, 1993

16. Quality Assessment and Improvement in Obstetrics and Gynecology. American College of Obstetricians and Gynecologists, Washington, DC, 1995

17. Friedman AJ, Barbieri RL, Benacerraf BR, Schiff I: Treatment of leiomyomata with intranasal or subcutaneous leuprolide, a gonadotropin-releasing hormone agonist. Fertil Steril 48:560, 1987

18. Andreyko JL, Blumfel DZ, Marshall LA et al: Use of an agonistic analog of gonadotrophin-releasing hormone (Nafarelin) to treat leiomyomas: assessment of magnetic resonance imaging. Obstet Gynecol 158:903, 1988

19. West CP, Lumsden MA, Lawson S et al: Shrinkage of uterine fibroids during therapy with goserelin (Zoladex): a luteinizing hormone-releasing hormone agonist administered as a monthly subcutaneous depot. Fertil Steril 48:45, 1987

20. Coddington CC, Collins RL, Shawker TH et al: Long-acting gonadotropin hormone-releasing hormone analog used to treat uteri. Fertil Steril 48:383, 1987

21. Kessel B, Liu J, Mortola J et al: Treatment of uterine fibroids with agonist analogs of gonadotrophin-releasing hormone. Fertil Steril 49:538, 1988

22. Friedman AJ, Hoffman DI, Comite F et al: Leuprolide Study Group. Treatment of leiomyomata uteri with leuprolide acetate depot: a double-blind, placebo-controlled, multicenter study. Obstet Gynecol 77:720, 1991

23. Schlaff WD, Zerhouni EA, Huth JAM et al: A placebo-controlled trial of depot gonadotropin-releasing hormone analogue (Leuprolide) in the treatment of uterine leiomyomata. Obstet Gynecol 74:856, 1989

24. Stovall TG, Ling FW, Henr LC, Woodruff MR: A randomized trial evaluating leuprolide acetate before hysterectomy as treatment for leiomyomas. Am J Obstet Gynecol 77:406, 1991

25. Stovall TG, Summitt RL Jr, Washburn SA, Ling FW: Gonadotropin releasing hormone use prior to hysterectomy. Am J Obstet Gynecol 170:1744, 1994

26. Bradham DD, Stovall TG, Thompson CD: Use of GnRH agonist before hysterectomy. A cost simulation. Obstet Gynecol (in press)

27. Friedman AJ: Vaginal hemorrhage associated with degenerating submucous leiomyomata during leuprolide acetate treatment. Fertil Steril 52:152, 1989

28. Harding SG, Pesce A, McMillan L: Symptomatic ascites complicating GnRH analogue use for myoma shrinkage. Br J Obstet Gynecol 100:1054, 1993

29. Friedman AJ, Rein MS, Harrison-Atlas D et al: A randomized, placebo-controlled, double-blind study evaluating leuprolide acetate depot treatment before myomectomy. Fertil Steril 52:728, 1989

30. Smith S, Levi C: On the utility of preoperative leuprolide acetate depot therapy prior to abdominal myomectomy. Am J Gynecol Health 5:121, 1991

31. Reinsch RC, Murphy AA, Morales AJ, Yen SSC: The effects of RU 486 and leuprolide acetate on uterine artery blood flow in the fibroid uterus: a prospective randomized trial. Am J Obstet Gynecol 170:1623, 1994

32. Matta WH, Stabile I, Shaw RW, Campbell S: Doppler assessment of uterine blood flow changes in patients with fibroids receiving the gonadotropin-releasing hormone agonist buserelin. Fertil Steril 49:1083, 1988

33. Gutmann JN, Thornton KL, Diamond M, Carcangiu ML: Evaluation of leuprolide acetate treatment on histopathology of uterine myomata. Fertil Steril 61:622, 1994

34. Upadhyaya NB, Doody MC, Googe PB: Histopathological changes in leiomyomata treated with leuprolide acetate. Fertil Steril 54:811, 1990

35. Perino A, Chianchiano N, Petronio M, Cittadini E: Role of leuprolide acetate depot in hysteroscopic surgery: a controlled study. Fertil Steril 59:507, 1993

36. Hutcins FL Jr: Myomectomy after selective preoperative treatment with a gonadotropin releasing hormone analog. J Reprod Med 37:699, 1992

37. Coddington CC, Brzyski R, Hansen KA et al: Short term treatment with leuprolide acetate is a successful adjunct to surgical therapy of leiomyomas of the uterus. Surg Gynecol Obstet 175:57, 1992

38. Friedman AJ, Daly M, Juneau-Norcross M et al: Recurrence of myomas after myomectomy in women pretreated with leuprolide acetate depot or placebo. Fertil Steril 58:205, 1992

39. Fedele L, Vercellini P, Bianchi S et al: Treatment with GnRH agonists before myomectomy and the risk of short-term myoma recurrence. Br J Obstet Gynaecol 97:393, 1990

40. Frederick J, Fletcher H, Simeon D et al: Intramyometrial vasopressin as a haemostatic agent during myomectomy. Br J Obstet Gynaecol 101:435, 1994

41. Rubin IC: Progress in myomectomy. Surgical measures and diagnostic aids favoring lower morbidity and mortality. Am J Obstet Gynecol 44:196, 1942

42. DeLancey JOL: A modified technique for hemostasis during myomectomy. Surg Gynecol Obstet 174:153, 1992

43. Ginsburg ES, Bensen CB, Garfield JM et al: The effect of operative technique and uterine size on blood loss during myomectomy: a prospective randomized study. Fertil Steril 60:956, 1993

44. McLaughlin DS: Metroplasty and myomectomy with the CO_2 laser for maximizing the preservation of normal tissue and minimizing blood loss. J Reprod Med 30:1, 1985

45. Reyniak JV, Corenthal L: Microsurgical laser technique for abdominal myomectomy. Microsurgery 8:92, 1987

46. McLaughlin D: Micro-laser myomectomy technique to enhance reproductive potential: a preliminary report. Lasers Surg Med 2:109, 1982

47. Weather L: Carbon dioxide laser myomectomy. J Natl Med Assoc 78:933, 1986

48. Starks GC: CO_2 laser myomectomy in an infertile population. J Reprod Med 33:184, 1988

49. Lock FR: Multiple myomectomy. Am J Obstet Gynecol 104:642, 1969

50. LaMorte AI, Lalwani S, Diamond MP: Morbidity associated with abdominal myomectomy. Obstet Gynecol 82:897, 1993

51. Sacks PC, Hoyne PM: Disseminated intravascular coagulation, hemolytic anemia, and acute renal failure associated with extensive multiple myomectomy. Obstet Gynecol 79:835, 1992

52. Weinstein D, Aviad Y, Polishuk WZ: Hysterography before and after myomectomy. AJR 129:899, 1977

53. Beyth Y, Jaffe R, Goldberger S: Uterine remodelling following conservative myomectomy: ultrasonographic evaluation. Acta Obstet Gynecol Scand 71:632, 1992

54. Brooks GG, Stage AH: The surgical management of prolapsed pedunculated submucous leiomyomas. Surg Gynecol Obstet 141:397, 1975

55. Goldrath MH: Vaginal removal of the pedunculated submucous myoma: the use of laminaria. Obstet Gynecol 70:670, 1987

56. Henderson PR: A large submucous fibroid polyp causing inversion of the uterus. Aust NZ J Obstet Gynecol 20:251, 1980

57. Riley P: Treatment of prolapsed submucous fibroids. S Afr Med J 62:22, 1982

58. Dicker D, Feldberg D, Dekel A et al: The management of prolapsed submucous fibroids. Aust NZ J Obstet Gynaecol 26:308, 1986

59. Ben-Baruch G, Schiff E, Menashe Y, Menczer J: Immediate and late outcome of vaginal myomectomy for prolapsed pedunculated submucous myoma. Obstet Gynecol 72:858, 1988

60. Goldrath MH: Vaginal removal of the pedunculated submucous myoma: historical observation and development of a new procedure. J Reprod Med 35:921, 1990

61. Katz VL, Dotters DJ, Droegemueller W: Complications of uterine leiomyomas in pregnancy. Obstet Gynecol 73:593, 1989

62. Rice JP, Kay HH, Mahony BS: The clinical significance of uterine leiomyomas in pregnancy. Am J Obstet Gynecol 160:1212, 1989

63. Makar AP, Schatteman EA, Vergote IB, Desmedt E: Myomectomy during pregnancy: uncommon case report. Acta Chir Belg 89:212, 1989

64. Burton CA, Grimes DA, March CM: Surgical management of leiomyomata during pregnancy. Obstet Gynecol 74:707, 1989

65. Gemmell AA: Abdominal myomectomy. J Obstet Gynaecol Br Commonwealth 43:715, 1936

66. Barter RH, Parks J: Myoma uteri associated with pregnancy. Clin Obstet Gynecol 19581:519, 1958

67. Campbell RE: Pregnancy and labor complicated by myomatous tumors of the uterus. Am J Obstet Gynecol 26:1, 1933

68. Buckell EWC: Fibroids in pregnancy. J Obstet Gynaecol Br Commonwealth 54:70, 1947

69. Dubuisson JB, Lecuru F, Foulot H et al: Gonadotropin-releasing hormone agonist and laparoscopic myomectomy. Clin Ther 14:51, 1992

70. Dubuison JB, Lecurur F, Foulot H et al: Myomectomy by laparoscopy: a preliminary report of 43 cases. Fertil Steril 56:827, 1991

71. Daniell JF, Gurley LD: Laparoscopic treatment of clinically significant symptomatic uterine fibroid. J Gynecol Surg 7:37, 1991

72. Hasson HM, Rotman C, Rana N et al: Laparoscopic myomectomy. Obstet Gynecol 80:884, 1992

73. Nezhat C, Nezhat F, Silfen SL et al: Laparoscopic myomectomy. Int J Fertil 36:275, 1991

74. Harris W: Uterine dehiscence following laparoscopic myomectomy. Obstet Gynecol 80:545, 1992

75. Goldfarb HA: Nd:YAG laser laparoscopic coagulation of symptomatic myomas. J Reprod Med 37:636, 1992

76. Nisolle M, Smets M, Malvaux V et al: Laparoscopic myolysis with the Nd:YAG laser. J Gynecol Surg 9:95, 1993

77. Neuwirth RS, Amin HK: Excision of submucous fibroids with hysteroscopic control. Am J Obstet Gynecol 126:95, 1976

78. Neuwirth RS: A new technique for an additional experience with hysteroscope resection of submucous fibroids. Am J Obstet Gynecol 131:91, 1978

79. Hallez JP, Netter A, Cartier R: Methodical intrauterine resection. Am J Obstet Gynecol 156:1080, 1987

80. Brooks PG, Lofer FD, Serden SP: Resectoscopic removal of symptomatic intrauterine lesions. J Reprod Med 34:435, 1989

81. Neuwirth RS, Amin HK: Excision of submucous fibroids with hysteroscopic control. Am J Obstet Gynecol 126:96, 1976

82. Loffer FD: Removal of large symptomatic intrauterine growth by the hysteroscopic resectoscope. Obstet Gynecol 76:836, 1990

83. Derman SG, Rehnstrom J, Neuwirth RS: The long-term effectiveness of hysteroscopic treatment of menorrhagia and leiomyomas. Obstet Gynecol 77:591, 1991

84. Valle RF: Hysteroscopic removal of submucous leiomyomas. J Gynecol Surg 6:89, 1990

85. Baggish MS, Sze EHM, Morgan G: Hysteroscopic treatment of symptomatic submucous myomata uteri with the Nd:YAG laser. J Gynecol Surg 5:27, 1989

86. Sullivan B, Kenney P, Seibel M: Hysteroscopic resection of fibroid with thermal injury to sigmoid. Obstet Gynecol 80: 546, 1992

87. Candiani GB, Fedele L, Parazzini F, Villa L: Risk of recurrence after myomectomy. Br J Obstet Gynaecol 98:385, 1991

88. Berkeley AS, DeCherney AH, Polan ML: Abdominal myomectomy and subsequent fertility. Surg Gynecol Obstet 156: 319, 1983

89. Bonney V: The technique and result of myomectomy. Lancet 1:171, 1931

90. Finn WF, Muller PF: Abdominal myomectomy: special reference to subsequent pregnancy and to reappearance of fibromyomas of the uterus. Am J Obstet Gynecol 60:109, 1950

91. Loeffler FE, Noble AD: Myomectomy at the Chelsa Hospital for Women. J Obstet Gynecol Br Commonwealth 77:167, 1970

92. Malone LJ: Myomectomy: recurrence after removal of solitary and multiple myomas. Obstet Gynecol 34:200, 1969

93. Roopnarinesingh S, Suratsingh J, Roopnarinesingh A: The obstetric outcome of patients with previous myomectomy or hysterotomy. West Indian Med J 34:59, 1985

94. Davids AM: Myomectomy. Surgical techniques and results in a series of 1150 cases. Am J Obstet Gynecol 63:592, 1952

95. Brown JM, Malkasian GD, Symmonds RE: Abdominal myomectomy. Am J Obstet Gynecol 99:126, 1967

96. Babatinia A, Rock JA, Jones HW Jr: Pregnancy success following abdominal myomectomy for infertility. Fertil Steril 30:644, 1978

97. Rosenfeld DL: Abdominal myomectomy for otherwise unexplained infertility. Fertil Steril 546:328, 1986

98. Omu AE, Ehigiegba A: Myomectomy: a repraisal and postoperative reproductive performance. Asia Oceania J Obstet Gynaecol 9:43, 1983

99. Verhauf BS: Myomectomy for infertility enhancement and preservation. Fertil Steril 58:1, 1992

100. Berkeley AS, DeCherney AH, Polan ML: Abdominal myomectomy and subsequent fertility. Surg Gynecol Obstet 156: 319, 1983

101. Tulandi T, Murray C, Guralnick M: Adhesion formation and reproductive outcome after myomectomy and second-look laparoscopy. Obstet Gynecol 82:213, 1993

CHAPTER TWENTY-SIX

PERIPARTUM HYSTERECTOMY

ALBERT DIKET

Hysterectomy following a cesarean section or a vaginal delivery is an operation that is most commonly performed when the mother's life is in danger. In these situations, the mother is often in shock, has unstable vital signs, and is often receiving blood and blood products through transfusion. The anatomy is obscured by massive hemorrhage, and vessels that are tiny in the nonpregnant state are massive. The surgeon must act quickly to control the bleeding; however, if a large blood vessel slips from a clamp or from a poorly thrown knot, the resulting hemorrhage may cause death. In addition, this operation is one with which most surgeons have limited experience, as the indication is rarely seen, thereby heightening the surgeon's anxiety level.

It is easy to understand why many obstetricians are reluctant to perform peripartum hysterectomies. The intent of this chapter is to describe the indications for and techniques of the operation, while highlighting the differences between this procedure and a nonpregnant hysterectomy. This operation can be safely performed and, when all conservative measures fail, the surgeon should not hesitate to perform this life-saving procedure. Finally, this author argues that elective cesarean hysterectomy is an operation that can be safely performed with acceptable morbidity rates, and that in ap-

propriate circumstances, it is the best method for teaching residents this procedure.

EMERGENCY INDICATIONS

The most common indications for cesarean hysterectomy are given in the boxed lists. The least controversial are those performed for emergency indications.

Placenta Accreta, Percreta, and Increta

Abnormal placentation has been shown to be the most common indication for emergency peripartum hysterectomy.[1-4] If the placenta fails to separate properly, as in placenta accreta, percreta, and increta, the uterus will continue to bleed from the placental bed. If the bleeding is massive and does not respond to uterine contraction stimulants, uterine curettage, or bilateral hypogastric artery ligation, cesarean hysterectomy is the only procedure that will successfully stop the bleeding. It is important to note that placenta accreta is becoming more common due to increasing numbers of

463

Emergency Indications for Peripartum Hysterectomy

- Abnormal placentation
  - Placenta accreta, percreta, and increta
  - Placenta previa
  - Abruptio placentae
- Ruptured uterus
  - Rupture of a previous uterine scar
  - Spontaneous rupture of an intact uterus
  - Traumatic rupture of the uterus
- Uterine atony
- Cesarean incision extension
- Cervical lacertion with extension

cesarean sections; placental implantation over the scarred portion of the lower uterine segment can lack Nitabauch's layer, which leads to placenta accreta.

In the fundus of the uterus there is a much greater ratio of smooth muscle to connective tissue. In the lower uterine segment and the cervix, the amount of smooth muscle diminishes. If the placenta implants over this region, a placenta previa will occur. After the delivery of the placenta, the uterus will contract less efficiently, and this can lead to a massive postpartum hemorrhage. This bleeding is frequently unresponsive to measures taken to cause the uterus to contract. One of the most important things to remember is that even at the time of cesarean section, this bleeding can go unrecognized, because most will pass through the vagina, not upward toward the cesarean incision. The placental implantation site should be examined carefully, and someone

Nonemergency Indications for Casarean Hysterectomy

- Uterine leiomyomata
- Cervical intraepithelial neoplasia
- Severe dysmenorrhea and/or menorrhagia unresponsive to medical management
- Adnexal pathology
  - Tumors
  - Endometriosis
  - Residual pathology from pelvic inflammatory disease
- Sterilization (not recommended by the author)

should look under the drapes as well, to see if hemorrhage is occurring.

Conservative treatments for this condition include all those appropriate for uterine atony (see the section, *Uterine Atony*). Frequently, these attempts are unsuccessful and hysterectomy is required. The surgeon will not have the luxury of performing a subtotal hysterectomy; the cervical area will be bleeding, and it has to be removed to stop the bleeding.

Uterine Rupture

Figure 26-1 shows a uterus removed because of uterine rupture. Rupture of an unscarred uterus is most commonly seen in grand multiparous patients.[5] Obstructed labor with oxytocin stimulation is a common cause and, as such, oxytocin should only be given to women of high parity with careful continuous evaluation.[6] When this type of rupture occurs, bleeding is usually massive, and the defect is so large that repair is impossible and hysterectomy is the only appropriate treatment.

Rupture of a scarred uterus is much more common. In recent years, several studies have shown that a trial of labor following a previous low transverse cesarean section can be safely undertaken and will be successful in most cases.[7–9] However, catastrophic rupture even of a low transverse scar can occasionally occur. Farmer et al[10] reported their experience at the University of Southern California. During a 7-year period, they experienced 77 uterine ruptures. These were associated with one maternal and one perinatal death, and 14 required hysterectomy. Scott[11] reported 12 catastrophic uterine ruptures in one community during the 1980s. In spite of this, the author recently has noticed an almost cavalier attitude toward previous cesarean section patients who were given trials of labor. Although it is a relatively

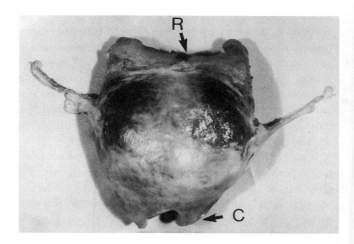

Fig. 26-1. Gross specimen of the first recorded ceasarean hysterectomy case on the Louisiana State University Service at Charity Hospital in New Orleans, LA (1938). Note the rupture (R) in the fundus of the uterus. C, cervix. (Courtesy of Dr. Abe Mickal, MD.)

rare occurrence, the possibility of uterine rupture always exists, requiring appropriate diagnosis and treatment. Often, a simple scar revision with preservation of the uterus can be performed. However, a ruptured low transverse scar sometimes extends into the broad ligament, making repair not only impossible but dangerous. The surgeon should be ready to abandon the conservative approach and proceed with hysterectomy.

Uterine Atony

Uterine atony is one of the most common indications for emergency hysterectomy.[12] With the better understanding of uterine contraction mechanisms, there are now more treatments available to alleviate this condition than in the past. When uterine atony is suspected, a dilute solution of 20 U of oxytocin in 1 L of a balanced salt solution should be begun. High intravenous doses of oxytocin should not be given, because of the danger of precipitating hypotension. The vagina and uterus should be explored immediately for lacerations, rupture of the uterus, and retained placental fragments. The uterus is massaged to stimulate contraction. When bleeding is massive, a second large-bore intravenous transfusion should be started, and the patient typed and matched for packed red blood cells. Two units of blood should be ready in the blood bank in case transfusion is necessary. Urine output is monitored with an indwelling urinary catheter. If the bleeding continues, 0.2 mg of methylergonovine should be given intramuscularly, if the patient is not hypertensive. (Some practitioners give this medication intravenously, but the author has witnessed dangerous hypertension resulting from this method.) If this fails, 0.25 mg of a 15 methyl derivative of prostaglandin $F_{2\alpha}$ should be injected into the uterine musculature. Finally, if these measures fail, laparotomy is indicated. Often, an undiagnosed uterine or cervical laceration is discovered, thereby providing an explanation for the inability to stop the hemorrhaging medically. At this point, bilateral hypogastric artery ligation is recommended, as it will lower arterial pressure in the pelvic vessels to venous levels, while extensive collateral circulation will only modestly decrease blood flow. Therefore, packing the pelvis, which usually is only appropriate posthysterectomy, is more likely to control bleeding. With the uterine in situ, the rationale for hypogastric artery ligation is weak. Bilateral uterine artery ligation, rather than ovarian artery ligation, would be more logical. Of course, none of these procedures is without risk in a blood-filled pelvis with large dilated veins. In addition, there is concern that if uterine and ovarian vessels are ligated, subsequent pregnancies may have inadequate perfusion.

However, with true uterine atony, it is difficult to see how decreasing the pulse pressure can stop the bleeding if the uterus refuses to contract. At this point, most patients are unstable. Careful isolation of the arteries takes time and may

not be completely effective; it is best to proceed directly to performing a hysterectomy. If the patient's vital signs are stable, bilateral hypogastric artery ligation can be attempted, after checking, under the drapes for vaginal or uterine bleeding. If the bleeding continues, one should proceed with a hysterectomy.

Uterine and Pelvic Infections

In older literature, peripartum hysterectomy was frequently performed for postpartum endometritis that was unresponsive to antibiotics of the day.[1,13] Because of improvements in antibiotics, this indication is now rarely seen. However, in rare cases, infections will not respond to modern antibiotics. Hysterectomy is the last resort and is usually curative, if total sepsis has not intervened. Postpartum pelvic sepsis is so rare that diagnosis is often delayed, with ominous results.

NONEMERGENCY INDICATIONS

The indications for hysterectomy at the time of cesarean section vary little from those for the procedure in nonpregnant patients. On the Louisiana State University Charity Hospital obstetric service, the author and colleges have been more liberal with our indications for nonemergency situations than many institutions. The reasons for this policy include that, between 1873 and 1973, Charity Hospital was administered within the strict rules governing a Catholic institution. During this time, tubal sterilization was forbidden and many cesarean hysterectomies were performed for this purpose.[13] Furthermore, it is our belief that if a patient has an indication for cesarean section and a hysterectomy, it is better to perform both during one operation. Two operations require twice the anesthesia and increase the chance for infectious morbidity and excessive blood loss. With every repeat cesarean section, scarring of the bladder to the anterior surface of the uterus worsens, making a hysterectomy in the future that much more difficult to perform. Additionally, with two procedures, the patient is away from her family twice, and undergoes two recovery periods, with attendant loss of work time. Finally, the author and colleges believe performing nonemergency cesarean hysterectomies are important for resident education. The controlled environment of elective cases is an easier way to teach and learn the procedure. The staff can go over the details of performing the operation before the case. The resident will have the opportunity to study the procedure from a textbook well in advance and thus, should be less apprehensive and more confident when performing the procedure. An emergency situation, when a patient is suffering from massive hemorrhage, is not the time to teach a resident this procedure, or worse, to have a private practitioner perform the operation for the first time. When a true emergency arises later, and the patient's life is in the balance, the physician will be able to perform the operation more efficiently and with greater expertise having performed several elective cases.

For the uterine and adnexal pathologic conditions listed in the second box, if the patient was symptomatic before pregnancy, then cesarean hysterectomy is a reasonable treatment option. Some physicians argue that in patients with significant medical problems, where future pregnancy is a threat to the life of the mother, cesarean hysterectomy is a better choice of sterilization because of the risk of failure from tubal sterilization. They also believe that cesarean hysterectomy may be offered in the case of a failed tubal sterilization that is ready to be delivered. An alternative is to perform a tubal sterilization procedure that has been proved to have very low failure rates, such as the Uchida bilateral tubal ligation.

Some would argue that the morbidity from cesarean hysterectomy far outweighs any benefit obtained from the single procedure or educational considerations. However, many physicians have only seen emergency cases, and elective cases are far less difficult. The reasons for this are, first, that these patients are hemodynamically stable and actually have extra blood volume because of the physiologic changes in pregnancy.[14] They can easily tolerate the extra 500 ml of blood loss without difficulty; the need for blood transfusions on the author's service was not different from that associated with elective cesarean section cases.[15] Staff members who are experienced in performing the procedure are present for all cases. When disaster strikes at 3 o'clock in the morning, a surgeon experienced with this procedure may or may not be immediately available. Another difference is that, since the procedure is performed before the onset of labor, the cervix is more readily identified and can be removed with much less difficulty. Once the cervix has dilated and effaced, its identification is much more difficult. There is no question that a cesarean section hysterectomy involves much more blood loss than an uncomplicated cesarean section, and thus the need for surgical expertise is greater. For these reasons, an elective cesarean hysterectomy should only be done when there are clear indications for both the cesarean section and the hysterectomy.

PREOPERATIVE EVALUATION

Cesarean hysterectomy is a major procedure, and requires careful planning to ensure success. Obviously, in emergency cases, very little time is available, but a thorough history and physical examination is necessary in both elective and emergency case. Since blood loss is a major concern in elective cases, the patient should be in good health and without major medical problems such as chronic heart or lung diseases. The patient should be thoroughly counseled about the risks and benefits of the procedure and understand that

sterilization will be permanent. If there is the slightest doubt about the patient's desire for future pregnancies, and the patient does not have a condition that contraindicates pregnancy, a hysterectomy should be strongly discouraged. The need for both the cesarean section and the hysterectomy should be carefully examined, and the operation performed only if both procedures are indicated.

In elective cases on women without medical problems, the only laboratory data required are a complete blood count; and a blood type and screen for antibodies. Electrolytes, clotting studies, and chest radiographs are not mandatory and are a waste of money. For an elective cesarean hysterectomy, the patient's hematocrit level should be above 28 to 30 percent. If it is below this amount, the risks and benefits of blood transfusion should be discussed; this author has given blood to raise the preoperative hematocrit level in selected cases. For emergency cases, hematocrit level can be maintained above 30 percent with packed red blood cell transfusions. Clotting studies become more important in emergencies. With severe postpartum hemorrhage, it is easy to lose enough blood to deplete the patient's clotting factors. Likewise, abruptio placentae, hemorrhage, and disseminated intravascular coagulation are common. In these cases, serum fibrinogen and platelet levels should be monitored. If the fibrinogen value falls below 150 mg/ml, it can be replenished with cryoprecipitate or fresh frozen plasma, or if the platelet count falls below 50,000/ml, platelets can be transfused to restore the count. If possible, these transfusions should be given before the incision is made. Some authors follow the prothrombin, partial thromboplastin, and bleeding times to assess clotting function, but this author has found these measures to be of little value.

ANESTHESIA

The choice of either regional vs general anesthesia depends on the indication for the procedure. Most emergency cases involve patients with large blood losses, in whom the intravascular volume is depleted. Because of the sympathetic blockade from epidural or spinal anesthesia, dangerous, uncontrollable hypotension can be precipitated. Thus, continued heavy bleeding with signs of shock contraindicates regional anesthesia and general anesthesia is preferred.[16]

For elective, nonemergent cases, epidural anesthesia seems ideal. Delayed gastric emptying is a well-known problem in pregnancy and this makes aspiration pneumonitis a concern any time a pregnant woman is administered general inhalation anesthesia.[17] Epidural anesthesia has the advantage of having the patient awake and able to protect her own airway. Other advantages of epidural anesthesia are that the mother will be able to immediately see the baby, and, if the case is extended, the anesthetic can be given for an extended period through the epidural catheter. Uncomplicated elective cases performed by the author and colleagues usually take about 90 minutes to complete. However, occasionally unexpected problems (e.g., adhesions of the bladder or bowel to the uterus) extend the time required to perform the procedure. In these cases, spinal anesthesia wears off and general anesthesia is required. If the patient has a contraindication to regional anesthesia, general anesthesia is acceptable, as long as the airway is carefully protected during the induction of anesthesia.

OPERATIVE TECHNIQUE

Incision

Many times, at the beginning of emergency cases, the exact etiology of the bleeding is uncertain. Possible etiologies are uterine atony, a cervical laceration that has extended into the broad ligament, or a ruptured uterus. For this reason, the author prefers a midline vertical incision. Initially the incision extends from the pubic symphysis to just below the umbilicus. This type of incision can be extended around and above the umbilicus if needed for proper exposure.

Many elective cases will be performed on patients who have a previous low transverse skin incision, and most would prefer not to have two scars. The Pfannenstiel or Maylard incision is used if the uterus is not enlarged with leiomyoma, and if the patient is not obese. When the hysterectomy is planned, the author prefers the Maylard incision because of the greater exposure given. This incision can be performed even when the Pfannenstiel incision has been performed in the past. If the indication for hysterectomy is enlarged leiomyoma, a midline vertical incision is preferred.

Obese patients make a potentially difficult cesarean hysterectomy that much more difficult. Exposure is not easily obtained, especially deep in the pelvis, and extra-long instruments should be available. Wound healing can be delayed and infection is more common. Because of the problem with infection under the panniculus, some authors discourage low transverse incisions, and recommend an upper vertical midline incision that goes around the umbilicus.[18] Because of these difficulties, an elective cesarean hysterectomy on morbidly obese patients is seldom scheduled.

Cesarean Section

The delivery is similar to nonhysterectomy cesarean sections. One difference is that, when the bladder flap is created, the dissection should be extended more laterally to the round ligament, then the bladder should be dissected inferiorly off the lower uterine segment (somewhat more inferiorly than usual). This can be performed more easily when the uterus is fully distended before the delivery. Care must be taken when performing this dissection, especially in patients with prior cesarean deliveries. In pregnancy, tissues are soft and more easily disrupted. This author has witnessed the floor

of a bladder being ripped open by blunt dissection. For this reason, sharp dissection should be used, until the dissection is below the scarring from the previous surgery. Once the correct plane is obtained, gentle blunt dissection can be performed. The author prefers wrapping a lap sheet around the index finger and pushing inferiorly between the bladder and uterus instead of using a sponge stick.

The next decision is what type of uterine incision to perform to deliver the baby. The author prefers a low vertical incision when it is known that hysterectomy will follow. Since the uterus will be removed, the problems associated with its poor healing and rupture in future pregnancies are nonexistent. Transverse incisions can extend into the broad ligament, making identification of where to place the clamps during the hysterectomy more difficult. Another advantage is that it is easier to clamp the vertical incision following delivery with towel clamps for hemostasis, and the top of the incision can be used by the assistant's index finger to lift the uterus. At this point, the baby and placenta are delivered and the uterus is lifted into the incision. If time permits, a self-retaining retractor is placed, and the bowel packed. If the patient is in deep shock, or if massive hemorrhage is encountered from a uterine rupture, the self-retaining retractor and bowel packs are placed after the blood supply to the uterus is secured.

Next, one must decide whether to close the uterine incision. At times, reasonable hemostasis can be achieved by reapproximating the incision with two or three towel clamps. At other times, the uterus contains large sinuses that bleed profusely. In these cases, the incision is closed with a single running and locking layer with a large suture. If the upper part of the incision is not bleeding, it can be left open to aid in traction.

Hysterectomy

The initial step in the hysterectomy is to divide the round ligaments (Fig. 26-2). The ligament is clamped approximately 2 to 3 cm lateral to the uterus. The ligament is then divided between the clamps and the lateral stump is secured with large absorbable sutures on a swagged needle. The needle is placed just under the round ligament and just lateral to the clamp. At all phases of the operation, extra care must be taken to ensure that the knots are correctly thrown and secured squarely. In pregnancy, vessels are dilated and more friable, tissues are edematous, and sutures seem to slip off their pedicles more easily. The round ligament is a good example. In nonpregnant hysterectomies, if the round ligament is divided, it will bleed very little. In pregnancy, Sampson's artery is much larger and if severed, it will bleed a surprising amount. At this point, the anterior leaf of the broad ligament from the round ligament is divided inferiorly until the incision of the bladder flap is met. The peritoneum can be incised superiorly to open the broad ligament and allow ureteral identification on the posterior sheaf of peritoneum.

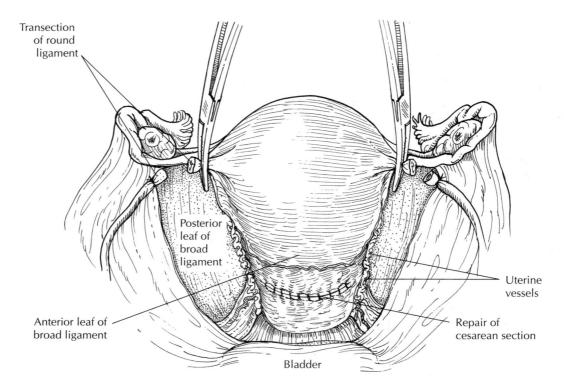

Fig. 26-2. Completion of cesarean section and transection of round ligaments.

The next step is to divide the fallopian tube and utero-ovarian ligament (Fig. 26-3). The clear space of the broad ligament under the fallopian tube is identified, and either an index finger or clamp is used to bluntly open the posterior leaf of the broad ligament. The fallopian tube and utero-ovarian ligament are then clamped. In pregnancy, the ovary can be smaller than expected and the utero-ovarian ligament relatively short. It is easy to clamp on or behind the ovary. The clamp on the medial stump of the round ligament is then repositioned to incorporate the round ligament, fallopian tube, and utero-ovarian ligament just medial to the opposing clamp. A knife or scissors is used to cut between the two clamps. The distal stump is secured with a freehand tie of absorbable suture. The clamp is opened slightly and quickly closed ("flashed") while this suture is tied down, to allow the tissue to be crushed and the vessels secured. Next, a suture with a swagged needle is placed in the middle of the stump between the freehand tie and the clamp. The needle is removed, the free ends of the suture are brought around the tips of the clamp, and a square knot is thrown around the stump facing the finger-holds of the clamp. The two free ends are then swung around again, and a square knot is placed around the pedicle closest to the tips. The clamp is then removed. The author likes to place square knots in front and back because sometimes these two sutures slip off the pedicle and cause a large amount of bleeding. This is the largest pedicle that must be secured and the author believes that the suture slips when the pedicle shrinks as

edema resolves. Since the author has employed the above technique, slippage of the suture ligature has not been a problem.

The uterine vessels are then dissected free from the soft tissue of the broad ligament, and doubly clamped just lateral to the uterus with two curved Heaney clamps (Fig. 26-4), where the incision would be made for a low transverse cesarean section. Care must be taken in placing these clamps. In a nonpregnant hysterectomy, it is easy to distinguish the uterine substance from the broad ligament, since the uterus is firm. The clamp over the uterus is opened and rolled off the uterine substance laterally until the edge of the uterus is felt, and then the clamp is closed. This is done to ensure that the clamp is placed as medially as possible to prevent ureteral injury. The pregnant uterus is much softer. If one tries to roll off the uterus in this manner, one can actually clamp into the uterine substance, or worse, lacerate the surface of the uterus with the clamp, causing significant bleeding. The author prefers to place two fingers around the uterine vessels, feel exactly where the lateral margin of the uterus is, and then place the clamps directly on it. Another important point is that the second clamp should always be placed medial to the first to avoid ureteral injury. There are surgeons who use a single-clamp technique, believing that it gives a smaller pedicle, but the author prefers two clamps. A straight clamp is placed medial to the curved clamps to control back bleeding from the uterus, which can be significant. Mayo scissors are used to divide the uterine vessels between the

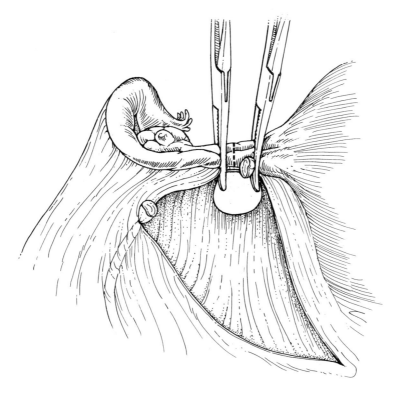

Fig. 26-3. Dividing the fallopian tubes and utero-ovarian ligaments.

clamps. As before, a suture with a swagged needle is placed just inferior to the tip of the lateral-most clamp, through the broad ligament, and then secured. As the knot is tightened, the lateral clamp is removed and the medial clamp flashed. A second swagged needle suture is placed just inferior to the tip of the remaining clamp through the broad ligament, as before. The same needle and suture is placed through the lateralmost portion of the pedicle just lateral to the clamp. The suture is tied and the clamp is removed, thus forming a transfixion ligation. This is done to prevent slipping. The author prefers not to transfix the first clamp because of the fear of passing the second throw through a uterine vessel. The ligature securing the second clamp's pedicle has the ligature of the first clamp to act as a safety in case the needle is placed through a large vessel. In the same order and manner, the opposite side's round ligament, fallopian tube, utero-ovarian ligament, and uterine vessels are divided and suture ligated. When this is completed, the major blood supply to the uterus from the uterine and ovarian vessels are secured.

There are variations of the above technique that are purported to decrease the time required to interrupt the blood supply to the uterus. Dyer and collegues[18] describe a delayed ligation technique in which the above ligaments are clamped and divided, and then placed aside to be ligated later when the entire blood supply to the uterus has been interrupted. Dr. Leon Gallard taught a technique in which, just after the uterine incision is closed following cesarean section, the clear space in the broad ligament is opened bluntly with a clamp bilaterally. The free ends of a rubber tourniquet are passed front to back through the opened broad ligaments and then brought together in the midline behind the uterus. The tourniquet is pulled tight and then clamped with a hemostat. The tourniquet can be pulled even tighter by pulling on the hemostat, stretching the tourniquet even further, and then applying a second clamp closer to the uterus. This tamponades the blood supply to the uterus via the uterine arteries, reducing blood loss that normally takes place before the ovarian and uterine arteries are ligated.

The author prefers this technique for the following reasons. With delayed ligation, all the instruments that are left in place tend to fall into the surgical field and get in the way of the dissection. When these clamps are being retracted out of the way, a pedicle could be pulled too hard and the tissue could slip or tear from the clamp, causing hemorrhage. The tourniquet is surprisingly effective in diminishing the blood supply to the uterus. Frequently, following the placement of the tourniquet, the uterine fundus blanches, and bleeding from the uterus greatly diminishes. The author does not routinely perform this technique because it takes some time to open the broad ligaments, properly apply the tourniquet, and then tighten and clamp it. For experienced surgeons, the time required to ligate the uterine blood supply by the technique described is surprisingly short, and that time is better spent ligating these vessels than applying the tourniquet. However, the tourniquet technique is excellent for teaching purposes, in that more time can be taken to secure the blood supply

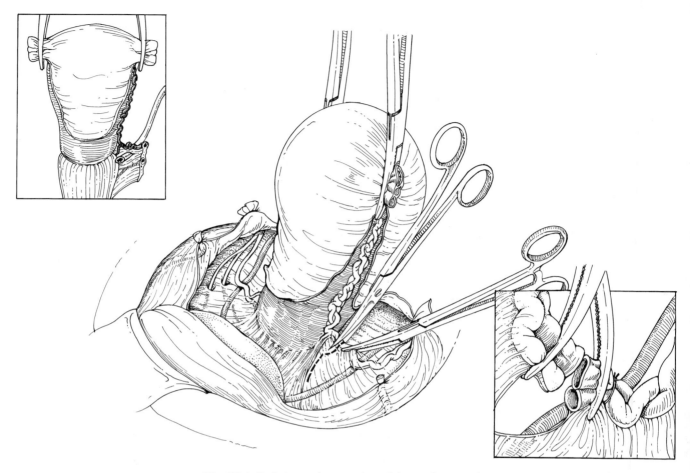

Fig. 26-4. Isolation and transection of the uterine vessels.

to the uterus without as much fear of excessive blood loss in the process.

In emergency cases, this is a good time to stop, take a deep breath, and assess the damage. This gives the anesthesiologist time to catch up with fluid and blood replacement. The surgeon should check for retroperitoneal bleeding from a lacerated and retracted vessel. The upper abdomen can be explored, and a self-retaining retractor placed and the bowel packed, if this was not done initially. If the patient's vital signs are stable and no other bleeding is found, removal of the cervix should be performed. However, if the patient has lost a large amount of blood and is unstable, and all vaginal bleeding has stopped, rarely a supracervical hysterectomy is in the patient's best interest. There are times when the cervix must be removed, such as in cases of bleeding from a placenta previa or a cervical laceration. Sometimes a high cervical laceration is very difficult to identify from vaginal inspection and can be misinterpreted as simply uterine atony hemorrhage. If a supracervical hysterectomy is contemplated, it must be carefully determined that all vaginal bleeding has stopped, even if that involves breaking scrub and looking under the drapes. All the old blood must be cleared

away from the perineum and vagina. Remember, if the patient's blood pressure is down, what appears to be only a small amount of bleeding can later become a hemorrhage when the blood pressure rises. For these reasons, the author almost always removes the cervix.

Subtotal Hysterectomy

For a subtotal hysterectomy, one must first ensure that the bladder has been dissected from the cervix to allow ligation of the cardinal ligaments. The author prefers sharp and careful blunt dissection in the midline to be carried down just as far as necessary to place the next cardinal ligament clamp. An Ochsner clamp is placed about 2 cm down the cardinal ligament medial to the previous uterine artery ties and flush with the lateral margin of the uterus (Fig. 26-5). Uterine bleeding is usually not a problem here, so back clamping is not normally necessary. The cardinal ligament is divided with the knife and a swagged needle with attached suture is placed just below the tip of the clamp. If one takes larger bites down the cardinal ligament with each clamping (although not recommended), it is a good idea to doubly clamp

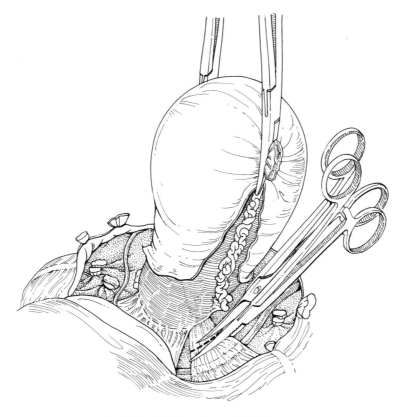

Fig. 26-5. Dividing the cardinal ligaments.

and tie the pedicle, with the second tie being a transfixion suture. Only one or two bites are required because the cervix is not removed. The uterine corpus is then excised above the level of the last suture with a knife and removed. Bleeding from the bare surface of the remaining cervix is easily controlled with series of figure-of-eight sutures or a continuous running and locking suture through the cervix.

Total Hysterectomy

For a total hysterectomy, the bladder is dissected as before, in the midline and inferiorly off the cervix. One or two cardinal ligament bites are taken successively on each side, divided, and ligated as described for a subtotal hysterectomy (Fig. 26-5). Each successive bite should be medial to the last to prevent ureteral injury, and the dissection should remain symmetrical on both sides. The bladder must be dissected low enough to allow for the next cardinal ligament clamping. This is continued until the uterosacral ligaments are reached.

Identification of the cervix must now be accomplished, which is probably the most difficult part of a cesarean hysterectomy, especially if the cervix had previously effaced and dilated. The easiest way the author has found to identify the position of the cervix is to extend the vertical cesarean section incision inferiorly in the midline just above the last

lateral suture level. If a transverse uterine incision was made, the author creates a vertical incision with the knife in the midline into the uterine cavity (again, above the last lateral suture ligation). The index finger is placed through this incision into the cervical canal and downward into the vagina. The cervix can usually be hooked with the inside index finger and its position confirmed. The bladder is dissected approximately 1 cm below the junction of the vagina and cervix. A curved Heaney clamp is opened wide and placed around the uterosacral ligaments (Fig. 26-6). The still-opened clamp is aimed medially and closed just below the junction of the cervix and vagina, incorporating the lateral aspect of the anterior and posterior vaginal cuffs. The temptation of taking too large of a bite, and having tissue extend more than halfway into the clamp from the tip should be resisted. If the distance between the uterosacral ligament and cervicovaginal junction is too far, the uterosacral ligaments are divided and ligated separately. The lateral vaginal cuff is clamped, divided, and suture ligated. Curved Mayo scissors are used to cut the tissue medial to the clamp. The incision is extended just past the tip of the clamp and the vagina entered. A nonswagged needle and suture are passed at the tip of the clamp and then a second pass is done through the lateralmost aspect of the pedicle to transfix the pedicle. This pedicle should be secured with great care, because the

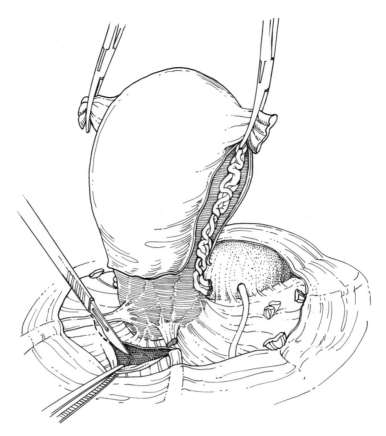

Fig. 26-6. Isolation and transection of the uterosacral ligament.

tissue can easily slip through the clamp, especially if too much tissue was taken by the clamp. Bleeding at this location is difficult to control because it can be brisk and because of the close proximity of the ureters. The needle from the suture will be used later and should not be removed. The free end is tagged with a hemostat, and the procedure is repeated on the opposite side.

A circumferential incision is then made by placing one blade of the Mayo scissors into the opening of the vagina and incising the vaginal cuff 360 degrees at the cervicovaginal junction by direct visualization (Fig. 26-7). Care must be taken not to remove too much vagina, and not to leave behind a portion of the cervix. The uterus and attached cervix are then removed. The vaginal cuff is elevated with the uncut uterosacral ligatures. Clamps are employed to elevate the medial portions of the anterior and posterior cuffs. The sutures that were used to ligate the uterosacral ligaments are now used to control the bleeding of the cuff and to suspend the cuff to the uterosacral ligaments. The operator on the right side takes the uterosacral ligament suture with the needle still attached and runs the anterior vaginal cuff away from himself. The surgeon on the left sutures away from himself and runs the posterior cuff; this way the needle is always aimed away from the bladder and rectum. These sutures are tied to the short end of the opposite uterosacral

ligature. The vaginal mucosa (especially the lateral vaginal mucosa) should be carefully incorporated when placing these running sutures, since the vaginal epithelium can retract deep into the vagina and bleed significantly.

The next question is whether to close the vaginal cuff. If there are no signs of infection, hemostasis is good, and there is no injury to bowel or bladder, the author will close the cuff by placing a series of interrupted sutures between the anterior and posterior cuffs. If collection of fluids in the pelvis is likely or if infection is suspected, the author prefers to leave the cuff open to allow drainage through the vagina. This includes most emergency cases. If the opening into the vagina appears to be gaping, a single suture is placed between the anterior and posterior cuffs in the midline to prevent prolapse of the abdominal contents. For most cases, reperitonealizing the broad ligament and vaginal cuff prolongs the case without any proven benefit, and increases anesthesia time. The length of an operation directly relates to infectious morbidity[19] and critically ill patients need to be off the operating table as soon as possible. Reperitonealization may also increase adhesion formation, and occasionally kink a ureter.

All pedicles are now thoroughly inspected for bleeding, the ureters are checked for dilation and peristalsis, and the bladder is inspected for injury. If in doubt, the bladder is

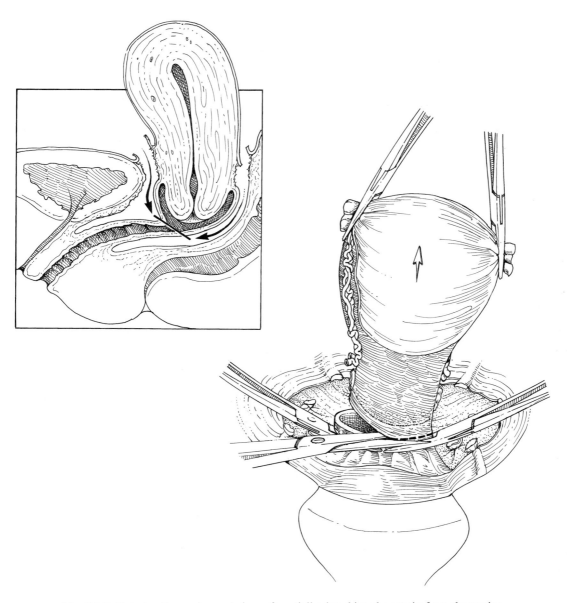

Fig. 26-7. Entering the vagina and circumferentially detaching the cervix from the vagina.

filled with 200 to 300 ml of fluid and checked for leakage. Sterile milk is used to check the integrity of the bladder.[20] The advantages of formula milk are that it is premixed, presterilized, easily obtained from any hospital nursery, easily seen when extravasation occurs through a defect in the bladder, and does not stain tissues. Sterile water dyed with methylene blue or indigo carmine stains the tissues. When a bladder injury is found, if the surrounding tissues are stained with dye, it can be difficult to see whether a small defect remains when the bladder is again filled following the repair.

All sponges and instruments are removed. The sponge and needle counts are checked. Many emergency cases are begun before a careful sponge and needle count can be made. This requires the surgeon to carefully explore the abdomen to ensure that all were removed. If in doubt, a flat abdominal radiologic film is ordered. The abdomen is then closed identical to any other abdominal operation. Before transferring the patient to the recovery room, it is a good idea to wipe the blood and lochia from the vagina. If this is not done and the recovery room staff call about vaginal bleeding, one will not know whether this is old blood oozing from the vagina or active bleeding.

POSTOPERATIVE CARE

Elective cases require no different postoperative care than other major abdominal cases. Signs of concealed intra-abdominal bleeding should be watched for during the immediate postoperative period by monitoring urine output, pulse, and blood pressure. If significant bleeding occurs from the vagina, the most likely source is from the cuff, but other higher sites of bleeding are possible. The author places a sterile speculum in the vagina and, if active bleeding is seen, takes the patient back to the operating room and, with adequate anesthesia (usually general anesthesia is required), attempts to identify and ligate the bleeding source, first from vaginal inspection and then via repeat laparotomy if necessary. The recommendations for early ambulation, deep coughing, and breathing exercises are the same as for cesarean section. The patient should have no problems breast feeding. Essentially all lactation suppressants have problems and the Food and Drug Administration has removed breast engorgement as an indication for the use of bromocriptine and sex hormones.[21]

In emergency or complicated elective cases, there is a greater need to monitor the fluid status of the patient, and many patients require admission to the intensive care unit. If the patient is critically ill and large amounts of blood and fluid are being quickly infused, central monitoring of central venous pressure or pulmonary artery wedge pressure may be appropriate. These central monitoring methods are not without risk and are not always needed. Urine output, pulse, and blood pressure assessments (the so-called poor man's Swanz-Ganz catheter) aid in the management of fluids. The author give fluids to maintain the urine output above 30 ml/hr. Blood is transfused to maintain the hematocrit level above 28 to 30 percent, until the patient is asymptomatic. Clotting dysfunction can be corrected with fresh frozen plasma or cryoprecipitate. If the patient has hypofibrinogen-emia and continues to bleed, cryoprecipitate has the advantage of having a higher concentration of fibrinogen than fresh frozen plasma, and more fibrinogen can be transfused with less volume and in a shorter time period.

If the patient develops a fever, careful evaluation is necessary to determine the cause. Early fever could originate from pulmonary atelectasis, but group B, β-hemolytic streptococcus vaginal cuff infections can cause fever within the first 24 hours postoperatively.[22] If vaginal cuff cellulitis is suspected, a broad-spectrum penicillin or second- or third-generation cephalosporin is the usual first-line antibiotic while the culture results are pending. If this fails, the results of blood cultures should help decide the next course of treatment.

The author begins the patient on a clear liquid diet in uncomplicated cases the day following the operation, and advances the patient to a regular diet as tolerated. The dietary plan is altered if gastrointestinal manipulation or injury occurred. These cases require more caution, since ileus is more likely. Often, nasogastric suctioning is needed to prevent vomiting and possible dehiscence of the abdominal incision. When bowel sounds and flatus return, a trial of liquids is appropriate.

COMPLICATIONS

Perioperative Complications

Peripartum hysterectomy is a formidable operation with significant maternal morbidity and mortality. Data was collected by the Commission on Professional and Hospital Activities between 1979 and 1980.[23] The commission reviewed 317,389 abdominal hysterectomy procedures and found 477 deaths, for an overall mortality rate of 12 per 10,000 procedures. When radical hysterectomies and pregnant cases were excluded, the mortality rate was 6 per 10,000. The number of hysterectomies performed on women who were pregnant was 5,435 and the mortality rate was 29.2 per 10,000 cases. This would indicate a nearly five times greater risk of death from peripartum hysterectomy than from nonpregnant hysterectomy. However, emergency and elective cases were not distinguished, making comparison of the two groups difficult.

In a series of 943 peripartum hysterectomy cases, Plauche' et al[12] reported the experience of the Louisiana State University at Charity Hospital between 1951 and 1984. A total of 6 deaths occurred for a mortality rate of 70 per 10,000. Three cases involved very complex management problems in which the performance of the hysterectomy played little role in the demise of the patients. The other three deaths were thought to be directly related to the procedure. Between 1975 and 1981 there was only one death, which occurred secondary to anesthetic and infectious complications. Chestnut and colleagues[24] reported their experience with 117 peripartum hysterectomies between 1963 and 1983, and no deaths were reported.

Cesarean hysterectomy is often performed as a life-saving operation in which patients are moribund when the procedure begins. Elective cases are less complicated, but since these are rarely done, most series combine emergency and elective cases and are collected over many years. Advances in treating critically ill patients have occurred over the past decade, and most series show a decreasing maternal mortality from cesarean hysterectomy. Five recent articles in the literature shown no maternal deaths in 457 elective and emergency procedures[3,15,24–26] (Table 26-1).

Intraoperative Complications

Blood Loss

The average blood loss from cesarean hysterectomy is significantly higher than for cesarean section alone. This is probably the reason that many obstetricians are reluctant to perform this procedure electively. While performing this procedure one must be extra careful in handling the tissues because of the increased friability during pregnancy. Clamps slip from or can avulse pedicles with surprising ease. The need for proper suturing techniques is crucial, since knots can slip when edema resolves and needles can puncture large vessels.

Blood loss for emergency procedures, by their nature, will be high. In the study by Zelop et al.[3] 50 percent of emergency cases had an estimated blood loss of greater than 3,000 ml, and 102 of 117 cases required blood transfusions (Table 26-1). Chestnut et al[24] reported a 100-percent transfusion rate in emergency procedures.

Are elective cases less morbid? Three recent studies in the literature by Gonsolin et al[25] (Table 26-2), Strickland et al,[27] and Chestnut et al[24] compared elective and emergency cases. The average blood loss and the need for blood transfusions were significantly greater for emergency procedures. However, in the study by Chestnut et al,[24] 65 percent of elective cesarean hysterectomy patients received blood transfusions. Two other studies showed a significant increase in blood loss and transfusion rates when elective cesarean

Table 26-1. Perioperative Complications for Emergency Cesarean Hysterectomy[a]

Complications	N
Infection (n = 58)	
Febrile morbidity	39
Wound infection	4
Pneumonia	1
Sepsis	4
Urinary tract infection	7
Hepatitis B	1
Infected hematomas	1
Septic thrombophlebitis	1
Respiratory (n = 25)	
Adult respiratory distress syndrome	4
Prolonged intubation	12
Pulmonary edema	5
Atelectasis	2
Chest tube placement	2
Urologic (n = 10)	
Cystotomy	9
Ureteral injury	3
Neurologic (n = 3)	
Coma	1
Seizure	1
Stroke	1
Gastrointestinal (n = 3)	
Ileus	3
Hemorrhagic (n = 102)	
Disseminated intravascular coagulation	32
Loss of adnexa because of bleeding	20
Transfusion requirement	102
Re-exploration because of bleeding	3
Other (n = 2)	
Compartment syndrome	1
Transfusion reaction	1

[a] Complications from 117 cases of emergency peripartum hysterectomies between 1983–1991.[3]

Table 26-2. Comparison of Perioperative Complications from Elective Cesarean Hysterectomy With Emergency Cesarean Hysterectomy

Morbidity	Elective C/Hyst (n = 109)	Emergency C/Hyst (n = 22)
Operative time (min)	83 ± 27	105 ± 38[a]
Estimated blood loss (ml)	875 ± 396	1495 ± 772[a]
Hospital stay (days)	4.2 ± 1.8	5.5 ± 2.3[a]
Wound complications (# of pts)	2	0
Ileus (# of pts)	1	1
Vesicovaginal fistula (# of pts)	0	0
Febrile morbidity (# of pts)	12	4
Pelvic abscess (# of pts)	0	0
Pelvic cellulitis (# of pts)	8	5
Pelvic hematoma (# of pts)	1	0
Cystotomy (# of pts)	1	0
Pneumonia (# of pts)	1	0
Ureteral injury (# of pts)	0	0
Urinary infections (# of pts)	2	1
Blood transfusions (# of pts)	16	15
Re-exploration (# of pts)	1	0

Abbreviations: C/Hyst, cesarean hysterectomy; # of pts, number of patients with given complication.
[a] $P < .05$
(Data from Gonsolin et al.[25])

hysterectomies were compared with cesarean section. Bukovsky et al[28] compared 86 cesarean hysterectomy cases with 86 bilateral tubal ligation cases; 64 percent of the cesarean hysterectomy cases required blood transfusions compared with only a 12-percent transfusion rate for cesarean bilateral tubal ligation patients. Yancey et al[26] compared elective cesarean hysterectomy to cesarean section, and again, a significantly higher number of cesarean hysterectomy patients required blood transfusions (Table 26-3). One study by Bey et al[15] compared cesarean section hysterectomy with cesarean section bilateral tubal ligation procedures and found no difference in the blood transfusion rates, even though the average blood loss from cesarean hysterectomy cases was significantly higher (Table 26-4).

Transfusion practices have changed dramatically in recent years. We now know that pregnant women can tolerate higher blood losses without transfusion because of the increased blood volume now seen as a normal physiologic change of pregnancy. We also tolerate much lower hematocrits and find that patients do very well without transfusions. One of the problems this author has seen is that blood loss can be easily overestimated. It is important to remember that amniotic fluid will be mixed in with blood when suctioning the abdominal cavity. This should be kept in mind when the suction canister appears to be full of only blood, because

Table 26-3. Comparison of Perioperative Complications from Elective Cesarean Hysterectomy With Cesarean Section and Subsequent Hysterectomy

Morbidity	C/Hyst (n = 43)	C/S (n = 86)	Hysterectomy (n = 86)
Operative time (min)	123.4 ± 36	54.9 ± 21.2[a]	118 ± 45
Estimated blood loss (ml)	1435 ± 624[a]	900 ± 283	508 ± 358
Hematocrit change (vol %)	5.0 ± 5.0	5.5 ± 4.6	8.4 ± 4.9
Hospital stay (days)	6.0 ± 1.5	6.1 ± 3.1	7.4 ± 3.7
Wound complication (# of pts)	1	3	2
Ileus (# of pts)	0	2	0
Vesicovaginal fistula (# of pts)	0	1	0
Pelvic abscess (# of pts)	0	2	1
Pelvic cellulitis (# of pts)	4	10	13
Pelvic hematoma (# of pts)	2	0	4
Cystotomy (# of pts)	1	0	7
Penumonia (# of pts)	0	0	1
Ureteral injury (# of pts)	0	0	1
Urinary infections (# of pts)	NA	NA	NA
Blood transfusions (# of pts)	17[a]	3	12

Abbreviations: C/hyst, cesarean hysterectomy; C/S, cesarean section; # of pts, number of patients with given complications; NA, not available.

[a] $P < .05$

(Data from Yancey et al.[26])

Table 26-4. Comparison of Perioperative Complications from Elective Cesarean Hysterectomy with Cesarean Section and Bilateral Tubal Ligation

Morbidity	C/Hyst (n = 82)	C-BTL (n = 103)
Operative time (min)	114.5 ± 36.9	73.5 ± 26.4[a]
Estimated blood loss (ml)	1201 ± 472	718 ± 364[a]
Hematocrit change (vol %)	6.0 ± 4.4	4.5 ± 3.4[a]
Hospital stay (days)	5.1 ± 2.4	5.0 ± 1.5
Wound complications (# of pts)	7	9
Ileus (# of pts)	0	0
Vesicovaginal fistula (# of pts)	0	0
Febrile morbidity (# of pts)	41	70[a]
Pelvic abscess (# of pts)	0	0
Pelvic cellulitis (# of pts)	21	43
Pelvic hematoma (# of pts)	1	0
Cystotomy (# of pts)	2	1
Pneumonia (# of pts)	0	2
Ureteral injury (# of pts)	0	0
Urinary infections (# of pts)	11	14
Blood transfusions (# of pts)	19	22

Abbreviations: C/hyst, cesarean hysterectomy; C-BTL, cesarean section with bilateral tubal ligation; # of pts, number of patients with given complication.

[a] $P < .05$

(Data from Bey et al.[15])

much of its contents may in fact be amniotic fluid. The amount of lap sponges used will also be increased because of spillage of amniotic fluid into the peritoneal cavity. Blood loss can also be overestimated because, even after ligation of the ovarian and uterine vessels, the uterus can still appear to be actively bleeding from the blood contained within its cavity and substance oozing out. For all these reasons, if the vital signs are stable, the urine output is good, and the true estimate of blood loss is not excessive, the patient should not be transfused (our anesthesiology colleagues often will need the most reassurance). Postoperatively, if the patient is asymptomatic, she should not be automatically transfused because of some arbitrary hematocrit cutoff level. If the patient needs blood, she will usually exhibit dizziness, orthostatic hypotension, or other signs of hypovolemia. In the past, some have advocated transfusing patients to aid in volume expansion or to enhance wound healing, especially in patients with fever. This has never been proved to be of any benefit, and this practice has been discouraged by the U.S. Department of Health and Human Services, the Public Health Service, and the National Institutes of Health.[29] The study by Chestnut et al[24] appears to illustrate how these patients can be overtransfused. They report a 65-percent transfusion rate for elective procedures. However, the average hematocrit level of these patients at the time of discharge was almost 34 percent, with the highest being 43 percent. Clearly, it is not necessary to replace every milliliter of blood that is lost, and one can speculate that many of these patients could have done well without transfusion. Since these guidelines have been followed, the rate of transfusion for this operation has been greatly reduced at the author's institution, and it is very similar to the transfusion rate of the institution's cesarean section patients.[15]

It has now been shown that it is safe for pregnant women to have blood donated for autologous blood transfusion.[30–33] During the donation process, maternal vital signs are unchanged, and the fetal heart tones measured during and after the transfusion show no sign of fetal distress. This blood can be stored for up to 6 weeks, so a second unit can be drawn 4 to 7 days after the first. If performed starting at 34 weeks' gestation there will be enough time for the patient to replace her own blood, and the two donated units will be available if needed during or after the surgery. Elective cesarean hysterectomy patients are perfect candidates for autologous blood donation, as are any other patients at risk of postpartum hemorrhage.

Urinary Tract Injuries

A frequent complication from cesarean hysterectomy is inadvertent cystotomy. This occurs most often in patients with multiple prior cesarean sections and occurs while dissecting the bladder from the cervix. If adherent, it is strongly recommended to employ sharp instead of blunt dissection, and when in doubt about bladder injury, to fill the bladder with sterile milk to find a defect. Cystotomy is usually not a serious complication if recognized and can be easily repaired. However, if the diagnosis is not made at the time of surgery, intra-abdominal leakage of urine and vesicovaginal fistula can be a consequence.

Plauche' and colleagues[12] reported a 3-percent inadvertent cystotomy rate in 100 cesarean hysterectomy cases. In the survey by Zelop et al,[3] cystotomy occurred in 9 of 117 cases of emergency hysterectomy. Only one occurred in 129 elective cesarean section hysterectomy cases in the series reported by Gonsolin et al.[25] It is interesting to note that in the study by Yancey et al,[26] there was only one cystotomy in 43 cesarean hysterectomy cases, compared with seven in 86 cesarean section patients when those patients subsequently received hysterectomies. One can speculate that this occurs because in pregnancy, tissue planes are more easily dissected and patients having hysterectomies at a later date would have more scarring of the bladder and cervix from the additional cesarean section. Finally, Bey et al[15] reported two inadvertent cystotomies in 82 (2.4 percent) cesarean hysterectomy procedures. This was not statistically different from the cesarean section bilateral tubal ligation group, which had one cystotomy in 103 (0.97 percent) procedures.

Ureteral injuries most often occur when the anatomy is distorted by hematomas or when uterine incisions or ruptures extend into the broad ligament and retroperitoneal space. The location of the ureters should always be kept in mind. If its location is obscured by excessive bleeding, bleeding can be controlled by hypogastric artery ligation, or by the assistant placing a fist over the aorta just above its bifurca-

tion. This will allow time to evacuate hematomas, and to find the ureter and the specific bleeding source. This is much preferred over blindly clamping in hopes of controlling a major hemorrhage. This technique not only places the ureter in jeopardy, but is usually unsuccessful and causes even more bleeding. In pregnancy, the ureters are dilated and located closer to the uterus. For this reason, when clamping and dividing the uterine vessels and cardinal ligaments, clamps should always be placed medial to the previous pedicle, and as close to the uterus as possible. When removing the adnexa, the ureters should be visualized always before clamping the infundibulopelvic ligament. If a ureteral injury is suspected, passage of ureteral stents with cystoscopy or via a cystotomy incision through the dome of the bladder or intravenous injection of dye is diagnostic.

Ureteral injuries are a rare occurrence in elective and emergency cases. In a review of 5,185 cesarean hysterectomy cases, Plauche'[34] reported only 23 cases (0.44 percent) of ureteral injuries. No ureteral injuries occurred in the previously mentioned studies by Bey et al,[15] Gonsolin et al,[25] and Chestnut et al.[24] In the study by Yancey et al,[26] no ureteral injuries occurred in cesarean hysterectomy cases, but one occurred in a patient receiving a hysterectomy at a later time. Zelop et al[3] reported the highest rate in emergency cases (nine ureteral injuries in 117 emergency peripartum hysterectomies).

Postoperative Complications

Hemorrhage

Postoperative bleeding can occur from a variety of sources. Vaginal cuff bleeding can occur when a portion of vaginal cuff retracts into the vagina and is not properly ligated. Bleeding at the angles of the vaginal cuff can be particularly heavy. For this reason the author prefers to run the anterior and posterior vaginal cuffs separately to ensure that all vaginal cuff epithelium is included in the line of suture. The next most likely source is from a pedicle whose ligature has loosened or slipped completely off when the edema resolved. When this occurs, bleeding can spill into the abdomen and will usually be seen escaping the vagina if the vagina is left open. Occasionally a loop of bowel or large clot will obstruct an open cuff and conceal intra-abdominal bleeding. However, the ovarian and uterine vessels very often retract into the retroperitoneal space, leading to massive retroperitoneal bleeding and hematoma formation. When this occurs the bleeding is very often concealed. Pulse and blood pressures are monitored carefully in the immediate postoperative period. The author has found that the earliest indication of hemorrhage is a fall in the urine output, and orders hourly urine output determinations for the first 8 hours postoperatively.

If it is suspected that the patient is bleeding, reoperation is almost always necessary. Even vaginal cuff bleeding is difficult to control vaginally and usually requires suture placement from above. Before any hematoma is drained the patient should be properly fluid resuscitated, which is indicated by a stable blood pressure pulse and urine output. Very often the hematoma has tamponaded much of the bleeding and once the hematoma is drained, bleeding will begin again. An unstable patient will probably not be able to withstand any further significant bleeding. If the hematoma is expanding, holding firm pressure over the bleeding site, hypogastric artery ligation, or compression of the aorta allow time to infuse blood and intravenous fluids.

Infectious Morbidity

Fever is one of the most common complications to occur from peripartum hysterectomy. In recent surveys, Bey et al[15] reported a 50-percent febrile morbidity rate, Gonsolin et al[25] reported 12.2 percent, and Yancey et al[26] reported an 11.6-percent incidence of significant infectious morbidity. Differences among patient populations probably explain this wide range of infectious morbidity. Inner-city training hospitals have historically had higher infection rates. Interestingly, most studies find the incidence of febrile morbidity for cesarean hysterectomy to be significantly lower than for cesarean section alone.[15,26] This is thought to be due to removal of the uterus, which is the source of infection following cesarean section.

When patients develop a fever, a diligent search for the cause should be undertaken. An abscess should be suspected when antibiotics fail, and can be diagnosed with ultrasound or computed tomography. If an abscess is found, surgical drainage is indicated. Vaginal cuff abscesses occur as a complication of hematoma formation, and can usually be managed by opening the vaginal cuff and allowing drainage from the vagina. Subfascial or intra-abdominal abscesses require drainage in the operating room with general anesthesia. If no abscess is found and the patient continues to spike fevers despite broad-spectrum antibiotics, septic pelvic thrombophlebitis should be considered. A trial of heparinization should promptly lyse the fever. If this continues for 24 to 48 hours, antibiotics and heparin can be discontinued.

Wound complications are another common problem following cesarean hysterectomy. At Charity hospital, wound infection or separation occurred in 5.3 percent of cases.[15] Wound complications were not higher in cesarean hysterectomy cases compared to cesarean sections with subsequent hysterectomies.[26] This complication is avoided by employing strict sterile technique during the procedure, and by careful ligation of all bleeding sites in the subcutaneous layer and skin edges before closure.

Overall Morbidity

Many institutions will not perform elective cesarean hysterectomies because of increased morbidity. All studies indicate increased blood loss from this procedure compared to cesar-

ean section, and most show increased rates of blood transfusion. However, at Louisiana State University, the rate of transfusion is not significantly increased over cesarean tubal ligation cases,[15] and for the two most recent surveys from three different hospitals, the overall rate of transfusion was 18 percent.[15,25] The author and colleagues believe this is to be acceptable rate of transfusion. In the only study of its kind, Yancey et al[26] compared patients receiving elective cesarean hysterectomies with patients who delivered a child by cesarean section and then required a hysterectomy within 1 year. The overall morbidity rate was significantly higher in those patients having their hysterectomy performed later (Table 26-3). Bukovsky et al[28] compared cesarean hysterectomy and cesarean tubal ligation and found the number of patients experiencing morbidity was higher in the cesarean bilateral ligation group. Bey et al[15] found no difference in overall morbidity between cesarean hysterectomy and cesarean bilateral tubal ligation.

SUMMARY

Cesarean hysterectomy is a formidable operation that should not be performed by inexperienced operators or for trivial indications such as for sterilization alone. It was first devised to control life-threatening hemorrhage, and today this is the most common and least controversial indication. As illustrated, performance of cesarean hysterectomy is similar to nonpregnant hysterectomies, but important differences exist.

Whether a cesarean hysterectomy should be performed electively remains a controversial issue depending on how one views the risks of the procedure. The author and colleagues believe that when the operation is performed or supervised by experienced operators, and if the patient's symptoms warrant both a cesarean delivery and hysterectomy, elective cesarean hysterectomy carries only a slightly increased risk to the mother. Recent literature appears to support this view, except for an increased risk of blood loss and possibly blood transfusion rates. However, with the use of autologous blood donation, and by not overtransfusing, the number of patients receiving donor transfusions should be lessened to an acceptable rate. Our patients are given informed consent and, if they accept the risk, the operation is offered. Having learned to perform this operation from elective cases, the author considers this to be a far superior way to teach residents the performance of cesarean hysterectomies. This experience will enable them to perform this operation more rapidly, with more skill, and with less apprehension when the true emergency arises.

REFERENCES

1. Barkley DL: Cesarean hysterectomy at Charity Hospital—1000 consecutive operations. Clin Obstet Gynecol 12: 635, 1969

2. Stanco LM, Schrimmer DB, Paul RH, Mishell DR: Emergency peripartum hysterectomy and associated risk factors. Am J Obstet Gynecol 168:879, 1993

3. Zelop CM, Harlow BL, Frigoletto FD et al: Emergency peripartum hysterectomy. Am J Obstet Gynecol 168:1443, 1993

4. Sturdee DW, Rushton DJ: Caesarean and post-partum hysterectomy 1968–1983. Br J Obstet Gynaecol 93:270, 1986

5. Fuchs K, Peretz BA, Marcovici R et al: The "grand multipara"—is it a problem? A review of 5785 cases. Int J Gynaecol Obstet 23:321, 1985

6. Cunningham GF, MacDonald PC, Gant NF et al (eds): Williams, Obstetrics. 19th Ed. Appleton & Lange, East Norwalk, CT, 1983

7. Flam BL, Newman LA, Thomas SJ et al: Vaginal birth after cesarean delivery: results of a 5-year multicenter collaborative study. Obstet Gynecol 76:750, 1990

8. Flam BL, Lim OW, Jones C et al: Vaginal birth after cesarean delivery: results of a multicenter study. Am J Obstet Gynecol 158:1079, 1988

9. Rosen MG, Dickerson JC, Westhoff CL: Vaginal birth after cesarean: a meta-analysis of morbidity and mortality. Obstet Gynecol 77:465, 1991

10. Farmer RM, Kirschbaum T, Potter D et al: Uterine rupture during trial of labor after previous cesarean section. Am J Obstet Gynecol 165:996, 1991

11. Scott JR: Mandatory trial of labor after cesarean delivery: an alternative viewpoint. Obstet Gynecol 77:811, 1991

12. Plauche' WC, Wycheck JG, Tannessa MJF et al: Cesarean hysterectomy on the LSU Service of Charity Hospital, 1975–1981. South Med J 76:1261, 1983

13. Mickel A, Plauche WC: Cesarean hysterectomy. In Ledger WJ (ed): Mediguide to Ob/Gyn. Vol. 4. 1985

14. Pritchard JA: Changes in the blood volume during pregnancy and delivery. Anesthesiology 26:393, 1965

15. Bey MA, Pastorek JG II, Lu P et al: Comparison of morbidity in cesarean section hysteretomy vs. cesarean section tubal ligation. Obstet Gynecol Surv 177:357, 1993

16. Datta S: Anesthetic and Obstetric Management of High-risk Pregnancy. Mosby–Year Book, St. Louis, 1991

17. Gallop DG, Nolan TE, Smith RP: Primary mass closure of midline incisions with a continuous polyglyconate monofilament. Obstet Gynecol 76:872, 1990

18. Dyer I, Nix GF, Weed JC et al: Total hysterectomy at cesarean section and the immediate puerperal period. Am J Obstet Gynecol 65:517, 1953

19. Hemsell DL. p. 143. In Pastorek JG (ed): Obstetric and Gynecologic Infectious Diseases. Raven Press, New York, 1994

20. Plauche' WC, Morrison JC, O'Sullivan MJ (eds): Surgical Obstectrics. WB Saunders, Philadelphia 1992

21. American College of Obstetricians and Gynecologists: Newsletter, April 1990

22. Faro S. p. 429. In Pastorek JG (ed): Obstetric and Gynecologic Infectious Diseases. Raven Press, New York, 1994

23. Wings PA, Huezo CM, Rubin GL et al: The mortality risk associated with hysterectomy. Am J Obstet Gynecol 152:803, 1985

24. Chestnut DH, Eden RD, Gall SA, Parker RT: Peripartum hysterectomy: a review of cesarean and postpartum hysterectomy. Obstet Gynecol 65:365, 1985

25. Gonsolin W, Kennedy RT, Guidry KH: Elective versus emergency cesarean hysterectomy in a residency program: a review of 129 cases from 1984 to 1988. Am J Obstet Gynecol 165:91, 1991

26. Yancey MK, Harlass FE, Benson W, Brady K: The perioperative morbidity of scheduled cesarean hysterectomy. Obstet Gynecol 81:206, 1993

27. Strickland JL, Griffin WT, Lorens AS, Sowash JJ: Cesarean hysterectomy: a procedure for modern obstetrics? South Med J 82:1245, 1989

28. Bukovsky I, Schneider D, Weinraub Z et al: Sterilization at the time of cesarean hysterectomy: tubal ligation or hysterectomy? Contraception 28:349, 1983

29. U.S. Department of Health and Human Services Transfusion Alert: indications for the use of red blood cells, platelets, and fresh frozen plasma. Public Health Service, National Institutes of Health, 1989

30. Sander SG, Beyth Y, Laufer N et al: Autologous blood transfusions and pregnancy. Obstet Gynecol 53:62S, 1979

31. Kruskall MS, Leonard S, Klapholtz H: Autologous blood donation during pregnancy: analysis of safety and blood use. Obstet Gynecol 70:938, 1987

32. Widmann FK (ed): Technical Manual of the American Association of Blood Banks. JB Lippincott, Philadelphia, 1981

33. Herbert WNP, Owen HG, Collins ML: Autologous blood storage in obstetrics. Obstet Gynecol 70:938, 1987

34. Plauche' WC: Cesarean hysterectomy. In Schiarra J (ed): Gynecology and Obstetrics. Vol. 2. 1988

CHAPTER TWENTY-SEVEN

RADICAL HYSTERECTOMY

WILLIAM J. MANN, JR.

The radical hysterectomy is one of the most difficult, elegant, and aesthetically pleasing operations in the gynecologist's armamentarium. It requires a thorough knowledge of pelvic anatomy, meticulous attention to sharp dissection, and careful technique to allow dissection of the ureters and mobilization of both bladder and rectum from the vagina. Particular care must be taken with the vasculature of the pelvic side walls, and the venous plexuses at the lateral corners of the bladder, to avoid excessive blood loss. When completed, the resulting pelvic dissection provides a superb display of practical, clinically significant anatomy for teaching young gynecologic surgeons and medical students.

Radical hysterectomy offers high cure rates when used as primary therapy for early stage cancer of the cervix, as well as selected patients with cancer of the endometrium and other infrequent gynecologic oncology events. Controversy exists over which patients, if any, benefit from the addition of adjuvant pelvic irradiation to primary radical hysterectomy.

In a few previously irradiated patients with small central pelvic recurrences, radical hysterectomy may offer curative salvage treatment, as an alternative to exenterative surgery.

Complications of this procedure are uncommon, but may be devastating. Proper identification continues to evolve, as does perioperative management, to minimize patient disability, improve patient selection, and lessen associated expense.

RATIONALE AND DEVELOPMENT OF RADICAL HYSTERECTOMY

Radical resection of a cancer implies excision of the primary organ in which the malignancy arose, the contiguous soft tissue into which the growth would first spread by direct extension, and frequently is combined with removal of the first set of regional lymph nodes. A radical hysterectomy, then, involves excising the uterus en bloc with the parametrium (i.e., the bilateral round, broad [including the cardinal], and uterosacral ligaments) and the upper vagina. Usually, the surgeon also performs a bilateral pelvic lymph node dissection. In a simplified overview, the operation is designed to cure the patient by removing "all" of the cancer—by removing, in entirety, the sites in which the cancer might reside or first spread.

An appreciation for the concept of removing cervical cancer with a radical approach is best developed by thoughtfully reading the landmark papers in the late 1800s and early 1900s in which early pioneers in pelvic surgery exchanged their differing experiences. With no blood transfusions, minimal anesthetic support, no antibiotics, and unsophisticated patient selection, these early surgeons tried varying degrees of extended surgery, reported their results, and sought to improve them. It is interesting to note that even early in the development of the radical hysterectomy, these surgeons were questioning the therapeutic value of node resection, the causes of bladder and ureteral fistula, and the best closures of the vagina and peritoneum—issues not yet resolved.

In the late 1800s and early 1900s, cervical cancer was treated with cautery and varying degrees of excision. Central persistent disease was common and cure seldom. Attempts to treat cervical cancer with vaginal or abdominal hysterectomy were excessively morbid. Freund the first surgeon to attempt the abdominal approach, in 1878 reported a 30 percent mortality for abdominal hysterectomy. In addition, 50 percent of patients undergoing vaginal hysterectomy had recurrence of their cervical malignancy within 1 year, and only 10 to 17 percent were disease free for 2 years.[1]

Mackenrodt in 1894 described a combined abdominal and vaginal approach that removed part of the vagina, the uterus, and parametrium. Clark,[2] working under Kelly at Johns Hopkins in 1895, developed the concept of radical resection of cervical cancer and carefully described his initial cases, in which he resected the uterine arteries at their origin, dissected out the ureters from their soft tissue attachments, and attempted to remove part of the vagina. He emphasized that in abdominal hysterectomy, the broad ligament was divided too close to the uterus, and insufficient vagina was removed. He did not attempt lymphadenectomy, but did remove enlarged or clinically suspicious pelvic lymph nodes, although he questioned the value of doing this.[3] Werder,[4] in Pittsburgh in March 1898, and Wertheim[5] of Germany, in the Autumn of the same year, independently developed an extended operation resecting the parametrium at the point where the ureter was crossed by the uterine artery. Wertheim believed enlarged lymph nodes should be removed. Based on careful observation of patients with recurrent and terminal disease, Clark, Rumpf, and Ries independently developed an extended hysterectomy, removing the uterus, parametrium, and part of the vagina with all three, particularly Ries, also advocating resection of the pelvic lymph nodes.[3,6] These authors were also aware of the work of Halstead and others in using radical mastectomy for breast cancer, and saw a parallel in their efforts at treating cervical cancer. They dissected the ureter out of the soft tissues of the broad ligament and attempted to resect the parametrium as far laterally as possible. Ureteral injury was often reported in these early studies and was treated by intraoperative repair or reimplantation, with successful outcomes.

Criteria for patient selection were rudimentary. Frequently, ureters were dissected out of gross cancer, and occasionally portions of involved bladder and ureter were resected. Parametrial induration was attributed to infection, and if found to be due to malignancy, the parametrium was resected. Operability was essentially defined as being physically possible to do the planned procedure. Gross extrauterine disease was not necessarily considered a contraindication to radical surgery. In 1912, Wertheim[7] reported that he had 30 deaths in his first 100 cases, 22 in the second 100, 17 in the third, and a total of 93 (18.6 percent) in his first 500 cases. Of these deaths, 39 were from peritonitis, and 22 from "feeble heart and cachexia." Of the patients who survived surgery and were followed for at least 5 years, 57.6 percent had no evidence of cancer. The majority of recurrences were in the pelvic lymph nodes. Wertheim removed only enlarged nodes that he believed were the only nodes at risk of metastasis, while Sampson[7,8] and many others accumulated data showing that small, apparently normal nodes could contain metastasis. In the early 1900s, radiotherapy was developed, with overall cure rates similar to reported surgical series, but with less apparent complications and patient deaths. This led to a general acceptance of radiotherapy for cancer of the cervix, although several pelvic surgeons continued to press ahead with radical surgery.

Taussig[10,11] argued for the therapeutic value of pelvic lymphadenectomy, suggesting it be combined with pelvic irradiation. He believed cancer in lymph nodes was resistant to radiation, and reported long-term survivors in patients with removal of lymph nodes containing metastatic disease. Wertheim and Taussig carefully studied removed nodal tissue, and ultimately recognized the size or clinical assessment was inadequate for determining the presence of metastasis—a point modern surgeons occasionally forget. It was recognized that parametrial involvement did not necessarily mean nodal spread, and that nodal spread could occur with small cervical lesions. Taussig argued that perhaps as many as 20 percent of patients with positive lymph nodes could be cured with resection of those nodes. He also argued for a "step-wise" spread through the lymph nodes.

In 1921, Okabayaski[14] reported that his teacher, Takayama, was able to do 200 Wertheim hysterectomies each year, and in over a decade had extended the operation to be more radical. Okabayaski described his operation, which was essentially a modern radical hysterectomy with complete resection of the parametrium and dissection out of both ureters. He originally favored resecting enlarged lymph nodes, which then evolved to a complete lymphadenectomy. Interestingly, he favored preserving an ovary in premenopausal women. Overall cure rates of 62.5 percent were obtained, with 90 percent cure of early cases, but all patients received postoperative radiation.[13] Operative mortality was 7.2 percent.

Bonney[14] aggressively continued to use radical hysterectomy combined with pelvic lymphadenectomy for cervical cancer, reporting in 1935 a 14 percent operative mortality, which was constantly being improved.[14] Of 70 operative deaths, 43 were due to vascular or toxic shock. He reported a 43 percent 5-year cure rate, and believed that 23 percent of patients with nodal disease could be cured.[15] This survival data compares favorably with contemporary series of irradiated patients, but operative mortality was excessive. Bonney[16] continued to champion this operation, and in reviewing the procedure's development, refers to an operative mortality of 3 percent by 1949.[12]

By the 1940s, attention focused on better patient selection, lessening morbidity, and improving postoperative care and rehabilitation. Meigs[17,18] believed in combining the radical hysterectomy with pelvic node dissection, and was able to reduce the operative mortality to nearly zero. Ureteral fistula occurred in 8 to 10 percent of the initial patients, but ultimately, greater care in preserving the ureteral blood supply markedly lowered the incidence of this complication. More importantly, Meigs emphasized that patient selection was the key to operative safety, "patients selected . . . should be young, preferably below 50 . . . in good physical condition . . . thin," and their cancer should "involve the cervix in part or entirely . . . advance upon the vaginal walls to not over 1 cm." Most patients received preoperative radiation as the operation was developed, but Meigs[19] ultimately concluded that surgery alone was preferable to surgery and radiation. Overall, 5-year survival was 82.1 percent. When he presented his initial data in 1944, his audience pointed out that his success with treating and curing early stage disease justified their nascent efforts at cancer screening (i.e., annual gynecologic examination, and the then newly developed Papanicolaou smears). By 1955, Liu and Meigs were able to report 473 patients with an operative mortality of 1.7 percent, and a 9 percent incidence of urinary tract fistulas.

All of this occurred due to thoughtful clinicians with a strong surgical orientation, looking closely at their patients, watching the natural history of a disease, and then meticulously assessing their interventions. Surgical skills were developed in the autopsy suite and operating room. Surgeons traveled to learn new operations and to observe their colleagues in the operating suite. Individuals with an interest in treating unfortunate women with cervical cancer developed knowledge of the disease's natural history, recognized the inadequacies of prior treatment, and developed a specific operation aimed at meeting their understanding of how this disease could be cured. The literature of 1895 to 1944 serves to emphasize the effect that clinically active surgeons and their associates can have on progressively improving medical care. This is a heritage occasionally forgotten in modern medicine, but hopefully remembered by young gynecologic surgeons.

TERMINOLOGY

Although the author prefers the term *radical hysterectomy*, this operation has been referred to as a *Wertheim hysterectomy*, *Wertheim-Meigs hysterectomy*, *extended hyster-* *ectomy*, and by multiple other locally preferred names. Clearly, Wertheim's original descriptions were less radical than those now used, with less parametrium resected. *Extended hysterectomy*, as a term, fails from imprecision. Also, at least as primary treatment, pelvic lymphadenectomy, although a completely separate procedure, is now considered a standard accompaniment of radical hysterectomy (although a few diehards still argue whether node resection is of prognostic or therapeutic value).

Piver, Rutledge, and Smith,[26] three acknowledged experts in gynecologic oncology, recognized that *radical hysterectomy* was a phrase applied to a wide and divergent range of surgical procedures. One surgeon's radical hysterectomy might differ radically from another surgeon's definition. To try to bring order to this chaos, they offered five carefully defined operations, differing on extent of resection, to classify this procedure. Their class I is essentially a nonradical, extrafascial hysterectomy, while class II removes the parametrium medial to the ureter. A close reading of this paper reveals that the procedure is dictated by the surgeon's assessment of the underlying diagnosis leading to surgery, and the risk of recurrence. Their class III hysterectomy corresponds to a radical hysterectomy, with attention being paid to leaving a lateral attachment of the most distal ureter to theoretically preserve better blood supply. This fits the definition most clinicians use for a radical hysterectomy, although many, including the author, would complete the entire ureteral dissection to the bladder. Their class IV hysterectomy completes the ureteral dissection, sacrifices more of the internal iliac vessels, and attempts to resect three-fourths of the vagina. Their class V hysterectomy includes partial resection of the ureter or vagina, or both. Although not universally accepted, this thoughtful paper helps gynecologic oncologists define the scope of the procedure they consider to be radical surgery for cervical cancer.

In this chapter, radical hysterectomy refers to removal of the uterus and upper one-half of the vagina, complete dissection of the pelvic ureters, and removal of the parametrium as completely as possible. Referring to operations as radical hysterectomies, when they resect less of the parametrium or vagina or leave portions of the pelvic ureter undissected, will compromise assessing results of primary surgical treatment for invasive cancers. There is no place for radical surgery in noninvasive cervical disease. When reporting results of clinical series of radical hysterectomy, it is reasonable to expect the authors to briefly define the scope of their procedure. Wertheim[7] emphasized the need to be consistent in surgical technique, and disagreed with those who believed "that this operation should be carried out according to the idea of the individual operator."

Since 1969, the recognition of gynecologic oncology as a subspecialty in obstetrics and gynecology has led to concentrating radical pelvic surgery among a smaller number of gynecologic surgeons. Although he hoped they led to better results in management, it has decreased the number of surgeons willing to undertake radical hysterectomy, and this operation has essentially become the domain of gynecologic oncologists.

INDICATIONS

Cervical Cancer

The most common indication for radical hysterectomy and pelvic lymphadenectomy is early stage invasive cancer of the cervix (i.e., International Federation of Gynecology and Obstetrics [FIGO]) stages IB and IIA (see Appendices 27-1 and 27-2). The cure rates for a primary surgical approach equal those of irradiation therapy. A review of survival before and after 1970 suggests that improved anesthesia, patient selection, blood replacement, and surgical technique raised patient survival from 50 to 70 percent to as high as 92.5 percent.[22] At the same time, operative death rates fell from 3 to 4 percent to less than 1 percent, with many series noting no patient deaths in large numbers of cases.[22-26] When radical hysterectomy with pelvic node dissection is used for treating cervical cancer, survival is related to clinical stage and nodal status. With stage IB cervical cancer, survival is reported to range from 82.9 to 90 percent, while with stage IIA, survival approximates 68 to 75 percent.[23,26,27] Lymph nodes contain metastatic cancer in 4 to 17 percent of patients with stage IB disease, with the usual frequency quoted being approximately 15 percent.[23,24,26-28] In stage IIA, these same authors report positive nodes in 25 to 28.5 percent of patients. Regardless of stage, the presence of metastatic disease in lymph nodes decreases survival.[26] It is not prove that administering postoperative radiation to patients with positive lymph nodes improves survival, and personal prejudices of the physician decides which patients receive radiation and which do not.[29,30] This author only recommends radiation when more than three nodes are positive on one side, there are bilateral positive nodes, or the common iliac or aortic chains contain metastases—but recognizes that few of these women are cured.

In the United States, stage IIB cervical cancer is infrequently treated surgically. However, survival for these patients, when treated with radical hysterectomy and pelvic node dissection, had been reported to be 60.1 percent, with radiation given to patients with positive nodes (35.2 percent) or positive margins.[26]

Infrequently, after primary pelvic irradiation, cervical cancer will persist or recur as a small central lesion. Radical hysterectomy may offer an alternative to exenterative surgery in this uncommon event.[31,32] In this situation, ovarian preservation is not a consideration, since radiation would have already terminated hormonal function. Pelvic lymphadenectomy may or may not be performed, depending on intraoperative findings and the surgeon's assessment of the value of resecting previously irradiated nodes. Although an uncommon indication for radical hysterectomy, small central recurrences thus treated spare the patient the morbidity of exenterative surgery. In this situation, operative and postoperative complications such as fistula and bowel obstruction are significantly higher than when radical hysterectomy is used as primary treatment.

Endometrial Cancer

Infrequently, selected patients with stage II endometrial cancer (i.e., endometrial cancer extending to the endocervix) may also be treated with radical hysterectomy and bilateral pelvic lymphadenectomy.[27,33,34] The adnexae are removed. Many of these patients with stage II endometrial cancer will be obese, and have severe intercurrent medical problems that may not allow radical surgery. Furthermore, the current surgical staging of endometrial cancer has almost eliminated this indication. However, when cervical extension of endometrial cancer is found on curettage or conization, this is a consideration. True endocervical involvement needs to be confirmed and clearly distinguished from contamination of endocervical curettings by endometrial tissue. Treatment of endometrial cancer continues to evolve, with less use of postoperative radiotherapy, and the future role of radical hysterectomy in this disease will likely be minimal.

Vaginal Carcinomas

Very small vaginal carcinomas arising in the upper vagina may also lend themselves to radical hysterectomy and pelvic lymphadenopathy, although the overwhelming number of patients with cancer of the vagina are treated with pelvic irradiation. Other rare indications include unusual cervical malignancies, such as sarcomas or melanomas, adenocarcinomas in which the primary site cannot be determined to be endocervical versus endometrial, and low-grade uterine sarcomas that have spread in a worm-like manner into the parametrium (endolymphatic stromal myosis).

If the patient has access to both surgical and radiotherapy, radical hysterectomy offers the potential for ovarian preservation, provides pathologic material to assess actual extent of disease, and gives to the anxious patient the knowledge the cancer is "out." The sexual function of the shortened vagina after radical hysterectomy is superior to the contracted radiated vagina. Major surgical complications are infrequent, usually acute, and correctable, while major complications of irradiation, equally infrequent, tend to occur 18 to 24 months or longer after surgery and may not be correctable.

PATIENT SELECTION

Initially, the feasibility of tumor resection determined operability. However, it is now clear that advanced cervical cancer is better treated with irradiation. In fact, in early cervical cancer, irradiation offers an equal cure rate when compared with radical surgery. This had led to a shift toward selecting patients for radical hysterectomy who have early stage cancers and thus, are least likely to have surgical complications. This would suggest that the ideal candidates would be young, thin, have no intercurrent medical problems, and be highly motivated toward a rapid return to normal function. However, improvements in pre- and postoperative care, the philosophical bent of the gynecologic surgeon, and the uniqueness of the individual patient add considerable complexity to this most basic treatment decision. Elderly patients, properly selected, do very well with radical surgery. There is a greater incidence of concurrent medical conditions (particularly hypertension and cardiac disease) in older women, but postoperative morbidity and mortality is similar to that in the younger patients.[34–36] It has been suggested that, although markedly uncommon, pulmonary embolism and bowel obstruction occur more often in the elderly,[37] but this has not been a uniform finding. Furthermore, some have suggested that blood loss and febrile morbidity is less in elderly women after radical surgery,[38] although this is not found in all studies.[34,39] Hospital stays were often longer in older women undergoing radical hysterectomy than in younger women, but this cannot be shown to be associated with any specific morbidity, suggesting possible physician bias.[40] It must be recognized that sexual function is important to elderly women, and, as previously noted, the surgical patient may have a more functional vagina than the irradiated patient. As the American population ages, elderly women will increasingly be considered for radical hysterectomy, and biologic age, not chronologic age, must be carefully weighed. Many elderly women have excellent cardiac and respiratory function, with no underlying medical diseases, and are fine operative candidates.

Obesity, which is not uniformly defined, is thought by some surgeons to be a relative contraindication to radical hysterectomy. Habitus may be more important than simply considering weight. Very large women may not have excessive abdominal fat. Similarly, one needs to consider width of pelvic girdle, height, and distribution of fat, not just weight. Obesity is a relative term, and some surgeons do not find it as difficult a problem to deal with as other. However, it is foolhardy to attempt radical surgery in an obese female without having access to long instruments, including retractor blades, and adequate surgical assistants. Patients who are obese—whether this is defined by exceeding ideal weight by a given percentage or by exceeding a given arbitrary weights—make radical hysterectomy more difficult.[41,42] Meticulous attention must be paid to both pre- and postoperative preparation. This author will selectively perform a panniculectomy before opening the abdomen and starting the radical hysterectomy, based on the experience that this often simplifies placement of fixed and movable retractors, and enhances visualization of the pelvis. However, blood loss in the tissue removed may exceed that of the radical hysterectomy, and wound healing can be prolonged.

There are also some medical conditions, such as Crohn's disease, connective tissue disorders, past history of peritonitis, or extensive pelvic adhesions, which prohibit radiotherapy, and push the clinician toward surgery. Prior radiation to the pelvis is also a contraindication to radiotherapy and may greatly complicate surgical intervention.

Finally, for whatever reason, there are women who flatly refuse nonsurgical therapy.

ENSURING INFORMED CONSENT

To ensure that the patient and her family understand the nature of the procedure, not only is it appropriate to outline the proposed preoperative testing and preparation, the procedure itself, its risks, and the postoperative stay, but it is also necessary to allow her to consider the alternative of radiation treatment. At a minimum, the following points need to be raised with each patient.

If cure is the only consideration, both radical surgery and pelvic irradiation offer the same survival. However, because of the rare operative or postoperative death, this equality of survival is only apparent with continued patient follow-up.

Radiotherapy clearly has the advantage of avoiding operative complications, such as hemorrhage, visceral injury, dehiscence, wound infection, postoperative pain, and anesthetic misadventures. It is almost unheard of for someone to be too ill from intercurrent medical disease to tolerate radiotherapy. But radiation does damage bladder and bowel with a progressive and occasionally clinically significant endarteritis, often causes acute enteritis and cystitis, rarely depresses bone marrow, and nearly always induces short-term malaise. Bowel obstruction, bladder and bowel fistula, and rarely, ureteral obstruction may be encountered in less that 5 percent of patients treated. The vagina may undergo apical stenosis and lose pliability, although hormone replacement therapy and vaginal rehabilitation with dilators may minimize this. If the patient has a significant connective tissue disease that has compromised tissue vascularity, active enterocolitis, extensive prior pelvic or abdominal surgery, or prior radiation to the pelvis, radiotherapy is contraindicated. Ovarian function will be lost, unless the ovaries are surgically moved out of the radiation field. If fistula or obstruction occurs, surgical repair is fraught with difficulty, and diversion of the urinary or gastrointestinal tract is often needed. Radiation damage to tissue never heals and is progressive.

With radical hysterectomy, the patient must undergo a major operative procedure requiring anesthesia, extensive pelvic dissection, and all the risks associated with any major abdominal operation (i.e., dehiscence, infection, hemorrhage, ileus or small bowel obstruction, injury to the bladder, ureters or rectum, atelectasis, pneumonia, and pulmonary embolus).[42] All these complications can be minimized by a well-trained and thoughtful gynecologic surgeon, but not eliminated.

Visceral injury presents intraoperatively or within the immediate postoperative period and can usually be managed with preservation of organ function. Return to normal daily activities can be as rapid as a few weeks, but bladder dysfunction may persist for months, even permanently. The operation provides maximum tissue for histologic analysis, which may aid in planning adjunctive therapy or offering a prognosis. Once the patient has recovered from her surgery, onset of delayed complications is exceedingly rare.

Finally, the surgeon's preoperative perception of whether postoperative radiation will be recommended ought to be explained to the patient. Otherwise, she may be very unhappy and shocked to find that when her surgery is over, yet another series of treatments must be endured.

CHARACTERISTICS OF THE CANCER

Most radical hysterectomies are performed for squamous cell cancer of the cervix, with a smaller number done for mixed adenosquamous and adenocarcinoma of the cervix. Cell type, degree of differentiation, depth of invasion, area of tumor, and vascular space involvement are controversial prognostic entities.[43] There is no evidence that the squamous lesions do better or worse than the glandular lesions, and here, cell type is of no significance in patient selection. There is a strong clinical impression that small cell neuroendocrine cancers of the cervix do not do well if treated with radical surgery alone. There is also no convincing evidence that the degree of differentiation or mitotic indices influence outcome. Vascular-lymphatic space involvement or extension

of cervical lesions to the endometrial cavity are also not significant in selecting patients for surgical therapy. A surgeon planning radical surgery for cervical cancer needs a thorough understanding of the biology of cervical cancer, a topic extensively discussed in other, more specialized texts.[44,45]

Clinical stage is an important factor, and radical hysterectomy is usually believed to be appropriate and indicated for invasive disease confined to the cervix and upper vagina. Parametrial extension of cancer by contiguous growth, or metastasis to extrapelvic sites is considered by most a contraindication to radical surgery. However, infrequently, after advancing well into the procedure, parametrial disease that was clinically inapparent preoperatively will be encountered. In this circumstance, the operation is usually completed, occasionally requiring partial ureteral resection with reimplantation. These cases are particularly interesting, as not infrequently, all the pelvic nodes and margins of resection will be clear. Although some believe no other treatment is needed, others suggest pelvic irradiation.

Lesion size may influence some in determining the appropriateness of radical surgery. There are those who believe that large, bulky, cervical lesions are best treated with irradiation, or with irradiation and extrafascial hysterectomy. When combined therapy is planned, the total dose of radiation is usually decreased from what would be used if only pelvic irradiation was planned.[46] Presumably, the nonradical hysterectomy removes the primary cancer organ, preventing central recurrence and eliminating a reservoir of potentially metastatic cancer cells.

There are occasional squamous cell carcinomas that expand the entire cervix, so-called barrel-shaped lesions, in which the cervix actually becomes larger than the fundus.

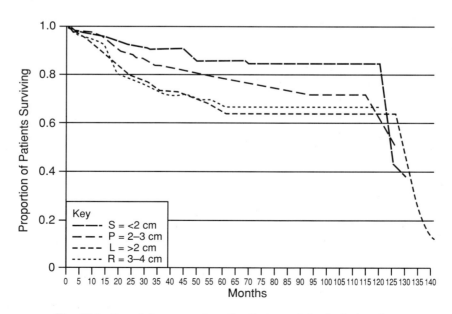

Fig. 27-1. Cumulative proportion of patients surviving by lesion size.

These lesions actually represent parametrial extension and are best treated with irradiation, or combined therapy. Similarly, large endophytic lesions may erode the vaginal cervices, and again, these are best treated as bulky stage IIB disease, using pelvic irradiation at curative doses.

However, large exophytic cancers, in which the examining finger can pass around the cancer on all sides, revealing an intact vagina, can be treated with radical hysterectomy and bilateral pelvic lymphadenectomy.[47] The problem is trying to define a cancer size above which the incidence of lymph node metastasis is thought to be so high as to make surgical therapy inadequate. Since nodal metastasis reflects an embolic phenomenon, there will be patients with distant metastases and negative nodes, and patients extensive nodal disease without dissemination.[48] In addition, there is disagreement as to whether adjunctive radiation is needed for a single positive node, multiple nodes, or bilateral posisitive nodes. A review of 172 radical hysterectomies with pelvic lymphadenectomy, done by the author and associates at Stony Brook, showed that lesion size influenced survival, but not operative complications (Fig. 27-1). Even the largest lesions were associated with negative lymph nodes and parametrium in half of the cases. Regardless of lesion size, the patients with bilateral positive lymph nodes all died, despite postoperative pelvic irradiation. This suggests that radical hysterectomy with pelvic lymph node dissection will select out patients with negative nodes and margins who can be followed, and high-risk patients with positive lymph nodes in whom adjunctive radiation is inadequate salvage therapy. Lesion size alone does not independently influence the author's decision to offer radical surgical treatment, but enters into the overall evaluation of the given patient.

PREOPERATIVE PATIENT ASSESSMENT

Prior to contemplating radical surgery, the appropriate medical assessment must confirm the diagnosis of cancer, determine the apparent extent of disease, and assess the patient for known medical problems, as well as ensuring no unknown problems exist. This topic is covered in detail in Chapter 1. Specific to radical hysterectomy and pelvic lymphadenectomy, there are certain areas of the history and examination that need be emphasized.

Any history of cardiac or pulmonary disease, or symptoms suggestive of such, must be evaluated in detail, since one is proposing a major surgical intervention. Personal contact with the physicians managing the patient's problem is requisite. Simply reviewing medical records is inadequate. All current medications need to be reviewed, to assess whether the current regimen is optimal, or whether any drugs can be deleted. Colleagues in anesthesia will rely on this history to direct them toward potential problems such as drug interactions, and the data must be as accurate and complete as possible. If nurse practitioners or physician assistants are used in preoperative assessment, the physician still remains responsible for the accuracy of their evaluation and for following up on problems these mid-level health care providers identify.

Asthmatics and patients with chronic pulmonary disease deserve preoperative pulmonary function studies to ensure their health is optimized for surgery. Clinical assessment alone is not adequate. Occasionally, patients will be encountered who are taking large doses of steroids. This author believes there are no problems related to wound healing as a result of this, but they will need adequate replacement corticosteroids in the pre-, intra- and postoperative period.

Patients with diabetes must be under good control, and the plan for immediate perioperative management should include the patient's primary care physician. This, after all, is the physician who best knows the total patient. This author tends to admit the patient on the morning of surgery, begin an intravenous line, and measure a blood glucose level. In insulin-requiring diabetic patients, low doses of regular insulin are used for control in the immediate pre- and postoperative period. Postoperatively, glucose levels are kept within the normal range.

Management of hypertension is complicated, particularly with many patients being on long-acting agents. This requires that operative management be planned well in advance. Postoperatively, antihypertensive medications are started only when the patient demonstrates elevated blood pressures.

Other more chronic conditions, such as hypothyroidism, can usually be minimized in the management plan. Although rarely found, every patient should be asked about symptoms of sciatica, (i.e., unilateral flank pain radiating to the anterior thigh or lateral thigh). This is very suggestive of common iliac/external iliac metastatic disease, and probably warrants abdominal and pelvic computed tomography (CT) scan.

With elderly patients, ambulation must be assessed. Will this otherwise healthy elderly woman require physical therapy postoperatively? Will she need nursing assistance on a one-to-one basis?

Along with the usual complete and thorough history, a detailed urologic history is mandatory. Failure to recognize patients with voiding disorder preoperatively will lead to considerable anguish postoperatively. Urodynamic testing should be ordered if there is any suggestion of voiding difficulty. Some would argue that urodynamic testing should be done on all women prior to radical hysterectomy. There is no obvious flaw in this logic, but in this author's experience, the yield in women who report normal voiding is nil.

A complete physical examination is performed on every patient. Every gynecologist can determine whether a cardiac and respiratory examination is normal. If abnormal, then either further evaluation or consultation can be done. Special emphasis is placed on the breast, abdominal, and pelvic examinations, and the lymph node survey, particularly of the inguinal and scalene area. Second primaries in the breast must be excluded. Disease metastasis to the groin or supraclavicular area contraindicates radical surgery. The abdomen must be addressed as the chosen portal to the procedure. Where are the previous scars? Where does the panniculus lie. Are there hernias that need attention? Obviously, ankle edema is a pertinent physical finding. Just as important is unilateral edema attributed to past injury or disease. These patients need to have occult pelvic side wall disease ruled out by examination and probably CT scan.

Usually, as a result of staging, the patient has had a chest radiograph and an intravenous pyelogram (IVP). If a rectal examination is negative for occult blood, this author does not order a barium enema in patients under the age of 40, or do a sigmoidoscopy. Both studies are done on women over the age of 40, or who have occult blood on rectal examination. Use of colonoscopy in these high-risk patients may be appropriate. Mammograms are ordered on all patients over the age of 40, and any abnormalities detected are resolved prior to radical hysterectomy. There is no need, in patients with clinical stage IB or IIA cancer of the cervix, to order liver/spleen scans or CT scans. Similarly, in the absence of hematuria, cystoscopy is of extraordinarily low yield, and best omitted. With neuroendocrine cancers of the cervix, cervical sarcoma, or other bizarre cancer, all of the above studies are done. With stage II endometrial cancer, the same routine is followed. For patients with recurrent cancer after previous radiation, barium enema, CT scan of abdomen and pelvis, cystoscopy, and sigmoidoscopy are always done to assess the extent of recurrence and to help decide whether exenterative surgery would better serve the patient.

Deciding to recommend a radical hysterectomy to a patient is a complex and difficult decision, involving a thoughtful weighing of risks and benefits. It must never be done without confirmation of cancer. A written pathology report from elsewhere is not adequate. The surgeon in charge must confirm the cancer diagnosis. Ideally, this is done by review of the actual pathology slides at a multidisciplinary conference that includes the primary care physician, a gynecologic oncologist, radiation oncologist, and other physicians and health care providers in the community who are recognized as being involved in cancer care. Often, input from a multidisciplinary team identifies potential problems in the pre- or postoperative period that can be addressed, and family problems may be identified. It cannot be emphasized too much that social services and home nursing services are vital components of preoperative planning. This author requests an evaluation for discharge planning from these services as part of the admitting orders.

PATIENT PREPARATION

Patients are admitted on the morning of surgery, unless other medical problems require admission earlier to optimize patient status. The patient is placed on a nothing-by-mouth diet (NPO) after midnight; it is emphasized she must eat or drink nothing. She may brush her teeth. This is an anesthesia concern and should be addressed with one's colleagues. For the day before surgery, at home, is suggested to the patient that she take clear fluids only. This author does not routinely use an osmotic bowel preparation prior to radical surgery, unless there is a history of extensive prior surgery. If the patient is elderly or taking diuretics or cardiac medications, bowel preparations are not give on an outpatient basis. The patient is told to remain active, get a good night's rest, and to spend a quiet evening. It is assumed the surgeon will do the same.

On admission on the morning of surgery, the patient is identified, all preoperative radiographs and laboratory tests are placed on the chart (especially the pathology report), and the consent is confirmed prior to the administration of any medication. A housestaff officer or the surgeon does a limited examination to ensure there have been no acute changes in the patient's condition. Obviously, if there are known medical problems, a more thorough assessment is carried out to ensure the patient is ready for surgery.

The patient is instructed in incentive spirometry, and this is documented. A shower with antimicrobial soap is given, and *no shaving* of body hair is allowed. Patients who are heavy or have hygienic problems or a large panniculus receive a Phisohex shower, and usually are requested to take these showers for 1 week at home before admission. The procedure of transfer to the operating room and the preoperative holding area are reviewed with the patient and her family. A hematocrit and type and cross for 2 U of blood is performed. In the author's institution, this will allow preparation of up to 6 U of blood or more, should they be needed in the operating room. Other laboratory tests are based on the patient's known medical problems.

Prophylactic antibiotics probably decrease complications postoperatively.[42] Therefore, an inexpensive generic penicillin or comparable drug is given on call to the operating suite. The family is encouraged to stay with the patient until she leaves for the operating room. Arrangements are made for the family to be readily available during and after surgery. Throughout the entire preoperative stay, all staff members who encounter the patient are trained to display a caring, positive attitude toward the patient and her family. This includes those who draw blood and the transport personnel.

In the preoperative holding area, the record is reviewed for completeness and the anesthesiologist greets the patient. Epidural anesthesia is started, if the patient is agreeable. She is then transferred to the operating theater, where the anesthesiologist readies the patient. The temperature is kept at 70 to 72°F to aid in preventing patient heat loss; it is not kept chilly for the staff's comfort. Additional thermal retention sheets are placed by the anesthesiologist prior to preparing and draping the patient.

Although the operation can be performed with the patient in the dorsal recumbent position, the use of a modified dorsal lithotomy position allows for vaginal examination if there is any question near the time of specimen removal of adequacy of margins. It also allows a vaginal pack to be placed to elevate the pelvic viscera to facilitate parametrial dissection in the obese patient or the patient with an excessively deep pelvis. This pack will need to be removed after completing ureteral dissection to facilitate parametrial resection. An assistant placed between the legs is in a good position for retracting during the dissection of the most inferior parts of the lymphadenectomy procedures and the bladder dissection. When positioning the patient, it is important to ensure that the patient's fingers are not near movable table parts, and that there is no excessive pressure on bony protuberances or excessive tension or weight on joints. One light needs to be placed above the patient's head for pelvic work, and another over the incision for deep dissection. A headlamp is an excellent aid. Intermittent pneumatic compression booties are applied while the patient is being positioned, in an attempt to prevent venous thrombosis and pulmonary embolism.[49] Although not proved, this author believes low-dose heparin increases blood loss.[42] In addition, this author finds that patients tolerate the intermittent compression devices well and dislike subcutaneous heparin injections. If low-dose heparin is used for pulmonary embolis prophylaxis, the dosage must be adjusted in obese patients, and platelet counts followed to identify the uncommon heparin-associated thrombocytopenia.[50]

OPERATIVE TECHNIQUE

Preliminary Preparation

Radical hysterectomy with pelvic lymphadenectomy may be performed through either a transverse or vertical incision. The transverse muscle-splitting incision provides superb access to the pelvic side walls, although care must be taken not to place the incision too high above the symphysis. The skin incision can be tailored to be within the area covered by a bathing suit bottom, and the fascial incision moved up or down to ensure it is 2 fingerbreadths above the pubic bone. Rarely, in particularly slender women, a Pfannenstiel incision will be adequate. For heavy women and patients with a narrow pelvis or a previous vertical scar, this author prefers a vertical incision. The transverse incisions offer beautiful exposure to the pelvic side wall and lymph nodes, but occasionally present difficulties with exposure for the para-aortic lymph node biopsies, if done. The vertical incision offers excellent exposure at all sites.

On opening the abdomen, any adhesions encountered are lysed to allow complete and thorough abdominal exploration. This includes palpation and, if possible, visualization of the undersurface of the diaphragm, the liver and gallbladder, the stomach and omentum, the entire large and small bowel, both kidneys, and the para-aortic area. If metastatic

disease, a second primary, or other abnormalities are detected, a decision can be made as to how to deal with this unexpected problem, and the procedure terminated, if appropriate. Radical hysterectomy would be inappropriate if metastasis were detected outside of the pelvis (i.e., in the omentum or bowel) or if tumor has broken through into the peritoneal cavity.

If gall stones are found, it is reasonable to perform a cholecystectomy at the same sitting. This author has operated on over 120 patients in whom concurrent cholecystectomy was performed during major gynecologic oncology procedures, with no significant extension of operating time and only one cholecystectomy-related complication. Postoperative cholangitis is an uncommon but severe complication of gall stones left in situ.

Washings are next taken of the pelvis, for academic interest. A self-retaining retractor is then placed. This author prefers a Balfour retractor, with a C-arm upper extension to which one may attach a malleable blade to hold back the bowel. Rarely, it may be necessary to attach more than one malleable blade. The Balfour gives excellent lateral exposure, but care must be taken to ensure that the lateral blades retract only the abdominal wall, and do not put direct pressure on the soft tissues of the side wall. Deep blades are available for larger patients. Wet laparotomy pads are then placed in each paracolic gutter and at the midline beneath the malleable blade, which is then tightened. It should not be necessary to adjust this retractor during the rest of the procedure.

Standing on the patient's left, the surgeon has two assistants opposite, or one assistant opposite and another between the patient's legs. The table is adjusted to be at the level of the surgeon's waist, and stools are provided for assistants as needed. Cautery and suction systems are checked and fastened to the drapes.

The pelvis is inspected carefully, and the parametrium palpated. The finding of cancer that has broken through into the peritoneal cavity, bladder, or rectum, indicates that radical hysterectomy will be inadequate therapy. This is also true if there is obvious adnexal metastasis. These findings must be confirmed pathologically. Prognosis for these patients is very poor.

Both the side wall and para-aortic areas are inspected for obviously enlarged or matted lymph nodes. There are surgeons who believe that finding a lymph node in the pelvis that contains metastatic disease is a reason for terminating the procedure. Others may elect to resect obviously enlarged nodes containing cancer, and then stop, while still others may elect to proceed as long as the nodes are resectable. This diversity of approaches reflects the lack of agreement on which patients benefit from postoperative radiotherapy, and the effect of prior radical hysterectomy and node dissection on morbidity of subsequent radiation.

Similarly, although many surgeons will stop if a para-aortic lymph node is positive for metastasis, others will persist, or persist if able to resect a higher para-aortic node that is negative for metastasis.

Determining metastasis intraoperatively must depend on frozen section analysis. There is the obvious risk of both false-negative and false-positive readings, depending on sampling error, the skill of the pathologist, and the "luck" of the surgeon in selecting the appropriate node for study. Clinical assessment of lymph nodes is notoriously inaccurate.

Para-aortic Node Sampling

The area above the bifurcation of the aorta may be approached transperitoneally by elevating and directly incising the peritoneum; from a lateral approach by dividing the peritoneum over the paracolic gutter and mobilizing the colon toward and across the midline; or, from an inferior approach by dividing the peritoneum lateral to the iliac vessels and dissecting upward toward the duodenum. Regardless of the approach, the key to success is adequate exposure, good lighting, and meticulous dissection. Struggling through too small an incision is foolish, frustrating, and dangerous.

On approaching the para-aortic area, small but troublesome little bleeders may be encountered. These should be cauterized, clipped, or ligated, lest their small volume of blood loss nonetheless be sufficient to obscure the anatomy. Often simple pressure with a wet sponge will suffice. The aorta should be visualized at or near its bifurcation, and the overlying peritoneum retracted laterally either by holding it with clamps or placing a Harrington or similar retractor. The closer the dissection is to the aorta, the safer it will be. By identifying the aorta, particularly in patients with extensive retroperitoneal fat, the inferior vena cava is more safely dissected. Care must be taken to ensure that the ureters are identified and displaced laterally from the operative field. This author knows of two cases in which portions of the ureter were resected and not recognized until the pathologic specimens returned (with both patients seemingly doing well postoperatively). A right angle or tonsil clamp can be used to elevate the soft tissues anterior to the great vessels, and the afferent and efferent trunks ligated or clipped. Alternately, the cautery can be used to dissect and cauterize simultaneously. Care must be taken to avoid the inferior mesenteric vessels. Occasionally, it will be necessary to mobilize the duodenum slightly to allow the para-aortic sampling. Placing clips at the extremes of the sampling area allows identification if subsequent irradiation if appropriate. No attempt is made to dissect out nodes posterior to the vessels. In slender women, the nodes may actually be easily visualized and removed. Gentle pressure to the operative site usually suffices for hemostasis, with hemoclips or cautery reserved for small vessels. The finished dissection will extend from lateral to the inferior vena cava on the right, to lateral to the aorta on the left.

If a rent in either vessel occurs, digital pressure must be rapidly applied. The operative site should be checked to ensure adequate exposure and appropriate assistants. Gentle pressure above and below the defect with wet sponge sticks allows visualization. Before attempting to suture a bleeder, it is prudent to first apply pressure for a few minutes. Often nothing else will be required. Small defects can be closed with a single interrupted suture (4–0 prolene), while larger holes may be closed with a running suture. As with any hemorrhage, if excessive blood loss occurs, it is best to control bleeding with pressure while anesthesia personnel stabilize the patient, and seek help if necessary. Mindless persistence may lead to major morbidity, even death.

There is no need to close the retroperitoneum over the biopsy site. This wastes time, and theoretically could entrap serum or lymph.

This procedure is usually accomplished in approximately 20 minutes or less, and has not been shown to be associated with significant postoperative complications independent from the primary surgery. Nonetheless, a surgeon undertaking this procedure should be familiar with the anatomy of the area and be able to handle the complications that may arise.

Pelvic Lymphadenectomy

It is possible to first perform the radical hysterectomy and to then do the node dissection. Advocates of this approach argue that in the event of an untoward intraoperative medical complication necessitating termination of the operation, at least the primary tumor will have been removed. This argument has always seemed specious to this author. If the anatomy is "set up" for the lymphadenectomy, the vascular supply to the pelvis and the anatomy of the ureter are clear, allowing complete control of any problems that may occur during the hysterectomy. The author prefers performing the lymphadenectomy first on each side, except when operating on a pregnant uterus, 16 to 18 cm or larger. In this situation, the floppy nature of the fundus makes visualization difficult, and it is easier to proceed with the radical hysterectomy first. When the patient has first undergone a caesarean section, performing the hysterectomy immediately after closing the high vertical uterine incision also minimizes blood loss from continued oozing. Transverse lower uterine segment incisions are unwise in this situation, as extension into the parametrium can occur and is problematic. If the fetus is nonviable, hysterotomy is not wise, as it significantly increases blood loss. It is better to operate on the intact uterus.

Throughout the surgery it will be necessary to manipulate the uterus to provide traction and countertraction. This is easily done by placing oversized, large Kelly clamps along each side of the uterus, incorporating the utero-ovarian ligaments, fallopian tubes, and down below each round ligament. These clamps provide an excellent handle for the uterus, and also control all back bleeding from the lateral aspects of the uterus.

The surgeon, standing on the patient's left, begins by suture ligating and dividing the right round ligament at its point of entry into the pelvis. Back bleeding is controlled by placing a hemoclip. This opens up the peritoneum of the broad ligament. While the assistant keeps the round ligament stump under traction laterally and the uterus medially and superiorly, the surgeon extends the peritoneal incision superiorly, staying well lateral to the external iliac artery, up to the beginning of the peritoneum of the right paracolic gutter. The peritoneal incision is then continued slightly inferiorly and medially, while the assistant now elevates the bladder serosa, allowing the surgeon to cut to the anterior midline of the pelvic peritoneum. Using nontraumatic forceps, the surgeon frees the peritoneum laterally from its soft tissue attachments, then sharply develops the right perivesical (Latzko's fossa) space, bounded by the iliac vessels laterally, the corner of the bladder medially, and the bony pelvis inferiorly. The posterior medial broad ligament peritoneum is retracted towards the midline with the ureter on it, and the perirectal space, bounded by the bifurcation of the iliac vessels laterally and the ureter medially, is opened. All of this should be accomplished smoothly, without repetitive grasping and releasing of instruments or excessive soft tissue palpation. Unnecessary putting down and picking up of scissors and pickups wastes considerable time and reflects indecision on the surgeon's part.

If the ovaries are to be removed, at this time, the infundibulopelvic ligament containing the ovarian artery and vein is lifted free of the ureter and the iliac vessels, and is ligated, suture ligated, and divided 2 cm or more above the iliacs. If the ovaries are to be preserved, the fallopian tube and utero-ovarian ligament may be divided, suture ligated, and the ovary placed under the laporotomy pad in the paracolic gutter, out of the surgeon's way. The left round ligament is now elevated, the uterus retracted superiorly and to the right, and the same procedure is carried out on the left.

After the left side of the bladder peritoneum is incised, upward traction is placed on the bladder by the assistant, and sharp dissection is used to free the bladder from the anterior uterine surface, and the bladder is displaced inferiorly. Cancer invasion through the cervix to the base of the bladder is infrequently found. This is, after all, the closest margin in a radical hysterectomy to a cervical malignancy, and cancer beneath the bladder or into its base would contraindicate radical hysterectomy unless partial cystectomy were considered.

The surgeon may then introduce an index finger, or preferably, the tip of the sucker, into the spaces just created, gently widening them with circular motion. Palpation now, by placing the index finger into the perivesical space and the middle finger into the perirectal space, will allow assessment of the parametrium, which lies between the two fingers. The superior vesical artery can be identified and mobilized medi-

ally. The ureter can be seen crossing the iliac vessels at or near their bifurcation, and elevated off of them. Usually, the ureter is freed from its soft tissue attachments, including the medial broad ligament peritoneum, approximately 2 cm above the vessels, and the posterior sheaf of the broad ligament is retracted medially. A Penrose drain, umbilical tape, or Babcock clamp may now be used to manipulate the ureter.

The pelvic lymph nodes lie medially, laterally, superior, and inferior to the iliac vessels. They may appear as discrete, easily visualized nodes, or as a band of soft tissue running along the vessels. Using ring pickups, the lymphatic tissue is lifted off the external iliac artery and sharply dissected free of the artery. As with the para-aortic dissection, it is advantageous to be as close as possible to the artery. Individual small vessels are clipped or cauterized. The dissection begins above the bifurcation of the iliac vessels (or where the para-aortic dissection has stopped) and frees the lymphatics down toward the inguinal ligament, until the external vein crossing from medial to lateral is identified. The lymphatic bundle is divided inferior to this vessel, and the external chain is then dissected off of the psoas muscle, moving superiorly toward the common iliacs. A vein retractor, the sucker tip, or a clamp, can be used to retract the artery lateral while the nodal tissue overlying the muscle and vessel are freed, and then the vessel can be manipulated while the attachments to the vessel are freed. This author prefers to use Metzenbaum scissor with the tips slightly open as a dissecting tool, but fine-tipped clamps will also work, as will the sucker tip.

The genitofemoral nerve runs lateral to the external iliac artery on the psoas. It may be sacrificed, causing numbness over the anterior thigh and upper labia, if it prevents adequate lymph node resection. At the bifurcation of the common iliac artery, small arterioles are often encountered lateral to the vessels and can be annoying if cut. The dissection of the iliac lymphatics may then be carried sharply superior to the point where the ureter crosses the vessels, and then further to the bifurcation of the aorta. This author prefers to use hemoclips to manage vessels and lymphatics that need to be divided. A moist laparotomy pad is occasionally used to blot the side wall, to minimize unnecessary attempts at ligating or clipping tiny vessels. The lymphatics overlying the external iliac vein are dissected from lateral to medial, and allowed to drop into the pelvis. Sharply, from the bifurcation of the common iliac to where the external circumflex vein crosses, the external iliac artery can be freed from its lateral attachments. This will provide access into the lateral aspect of the obturator fossa, by retracting the vessels medially, and lymph tissue can be sharply freed from the side wall and the obturator nerve identified. The vessels can then be placed under traction with a vein retractor and displaced laterally. The bundle of lymphatics in the obturator fossa are then freed from the undersurface of the external iliac vessels. Care is taken to clean the area of the bifurcation of the common iliac, where relatively constant lymph nodes, "the node at the notch," are found. Some believe this is the node most commonly involved in metastasis.

The dissection is carried 1 to 2 cm down the internal iliac artery, and the obturator nerve then again identified in the obturator fossa by gently spreading the tips of Metzenbaum scissors parallel to the vessels. A right-angle clamp can then be used to free the lymphatics above the obturator nerve and this bundle traced inferiorly to the pelvic muscles and divided. The vein retractor and sharp dissection can now be used to separate the external iliac artery and vein, and re-move the lymphatics between them. Nodes adjacent or be-neath the obturator nerve may be seen and removed, taking care to avoid injury to the obturator artery or vein, either or both of which may be sacrificed. Troublesome veins run lateral to the side wall into the internal iliac vein, and deserve respect. Injury to the obturator nerve, the motor nerve to the adductors, should be avoided. However, on occasion, resection of cancer-replaced obturator nodes has led to its intentional resection. Morbidity from unilateral obturator nerve is minimal; bilateral injury interferes with ambulation.

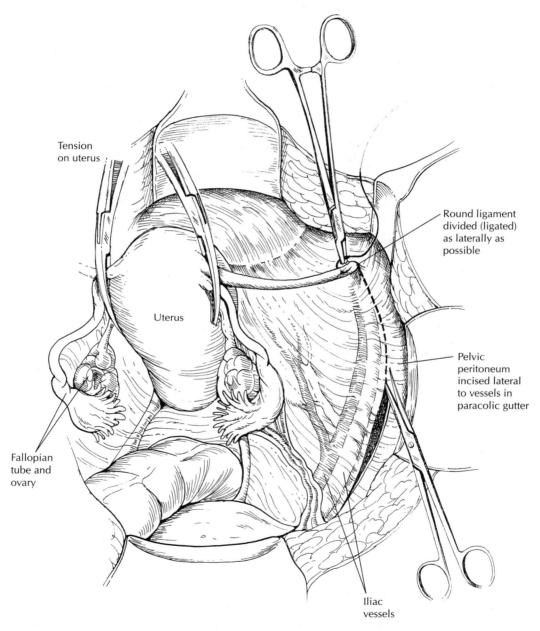

Fig. 27-2. Uterus put under tension and round ligament divided as far laterally as possible. The pelvic peritoneum is then incised lateral to the external iliac artery and vein, and the incision carried cephalad to the corresponding paracolic gutter.

At the conclusion of the node dissection, the external, common, and internal chains are inspected to be sure no nodes have been missed and to insure hemostasis. This author places a moist sponge in the obturator fossa during the remainder of the case, to quell venous-lymphatic oozing. The external artery and vein are separated through their length to be sure no lymphatic tissue lies between them. In dissecting the obturator fossa, medial tension on the superior vesical artery enhances exposure, as does placing a retractor into the perivesicale space.

The same procedure is now carried out on the left side, after the surgeon changes sides of the table, or the assistant now becomes the surgeon. The rectosigmoid lies on the left, and will need to be retracted medially and superiorly to do the left side. The ureter crosses the iliac vessels more medially on the left than on the right, and this should be borne in mind. Despite meticulous attention to sharp dissection, a complete resection of the pelvic lymph nodes is essentially impossible.[51]

Radical Hysterectomy

Figures 27-2 to 27-10 illustrate the description that follows. The assistant retracts the uterus inferiorly and to the left, while gently elevating the ureter. Beginning at the pelvic brim, the ureter is sharply dissected free of its soft tissue attachments. There is a relatively constant arterial branch to the ureter 3 to 5 mm below the common iliac bifurcation that should be identified and divided. The ureteral dissection is easiest if the initial dissection is sufficiently close to the ureter itself to allow easy visualization of the vascular web, which runs along the surface of the ureter. It is poor technique to leave chunks of fat or peritoneum on the ureter,

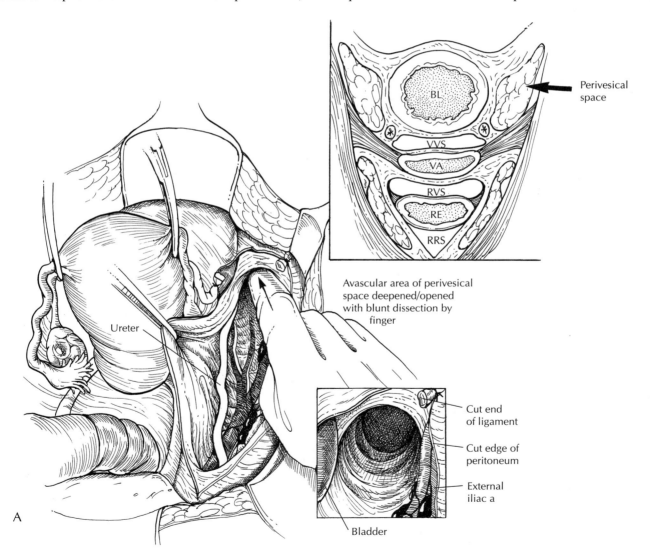

Fig. 27-3. (A) The perivesical and perirectal spaces are then developed with sharp and blunt dissection. *(Figure continues.)*

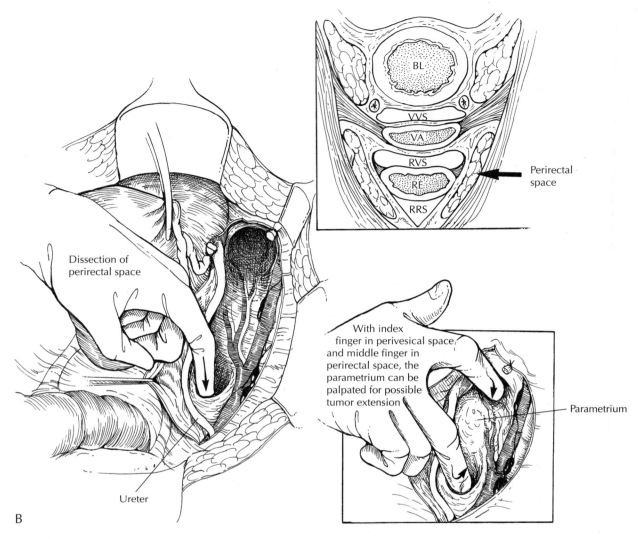

Fig. 27-3 *(Continued).* **(B)** Placing the index finger in the perivesical space and the middle finger in the perirectal space allows the tissue in between (parametrium) to be palpated to assess for tumor extension. BL, bladder; VVS, vesicovaginal space; VA, vagina; RVS, rectovaginal space; RE, rectum; RRS, retrorectal space.

and this is usually attributable to the surgeon not dissecting close enough to the ureter.

As the dissection proceeds down into the pelvis, tension can be placed on the previously identified superior vesical artery; this will cause the medial pelvic branches of the internal iliac vessels to become taught, facilitating identification of the uterine artery. The uterine artery is then dissected free and divided and ligated at its origin. A tonsil clamp or slightly opened Metzenbaum scissors make excellent dissecting tools. Blunt dissection is hazardous. The uterine vein(s) will be identified as the artery is skeletonized, and should be individually divided and ligated next. If the artery and vein are resected into a single pedicle, freeing the ureter medially is more difficult. The entire internal iliac artery can be resected, but the author only does this when intraoperative findings suggest that an en bloc resection of the parametrium

will be more easily accomplished in this manner (i.e., unexpected tumor infiltration along the uterine artery, endometriosis). Although it has been suggested that resecting the entire anterior branch of the internal iliac artery increases the risk of fistula, the data are not convincing.[52] Although identifying and dividing the artery is usually quite simple, there may occasionally be problems dealing with the uterine vein. If injured, bleeding can be difficult to quell. Applying pressure with a laparotomy pad, placing the uterus under tension, and positioning retractors will facilitate control. Bulk suturing or blind clip placement should be discouraged. Taking the uterine artery in a large bulky pedicle is also bad technique, since this pulls the tissues together, making subsequent ureteral dissection more difficult.

Tonsil or right-angle clamps are used to free the ureter down to the uterine artery pedicle, which is gently retracted

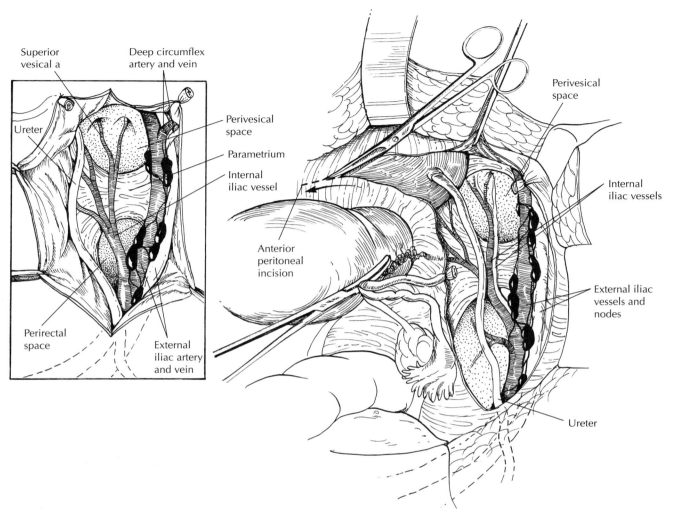

Fig. 27-4. The peritoneal reflection anterior to the uterus is incised and the bladder reflected inferiorly with sharp dissection. The ureter is identified on the medial aspect of the broad ligament during the development of the perivesical and perirectal spaces, as is the superior vesical artery.

medially; freeing the ureter sharply will allow it to be rolled laterally. The dissection of the ureter inferior to the uterine artery can be done by applying upward traction to the bladder (a right-angle clamp may be briefly applied to the bladder peritoneum, or a Harrington retractor placed at the bladder-vagina junction), using the Penrose to place lateral tension on the ureter, and introducing a right-angle clamp along the superior surface of the ureter. When the tip of the clamp is visible through the web of tissue at the corner of the bladder, the clamp may be gently opened and closed to widen the space, and one side of a second right-angle clamp may then be placed into the tunnel, rolled toward the bladder, and closed. This freeing of the distal ureter may be done in more than one step. There are aggravating veins at the corner of the bladder that can bleed copiously. Consequently, clamping the pedicle is preferable to sharply trying to dissect free the last 1 to 2 cm of the ureter. The same dissection is then

carried out on the opposite side. There are surgeons who believe this last part of the ureteric dissection should be avoided to lessen fistula risk, but this author does not concur. The worst complication of radical hysterectomy is failure to cure the patient when curative resection is possible.

The uterus is then reflected over the symphysis, the rectum retracted upward and posteriorly, and the cul-de-sac sharply incised. The posterior vagina and anterior rectum are separated with sharp and minimal blunt dissection, taking care to appreciate the curve of the posterior pelvis. Failure to recognize this curve can cause one to enter the anterior rectum. The index finger is then placed into the space posterior to the uterus and the middle finger just lateral to the uterosacral ligament, and the soft tissues are stroked first toward the cervix, then toward the rectum, consolidating the pedicle. The posterior peritoneum is incised, and the uterosacral pedicle is clamped as close to the rectum as possible with a

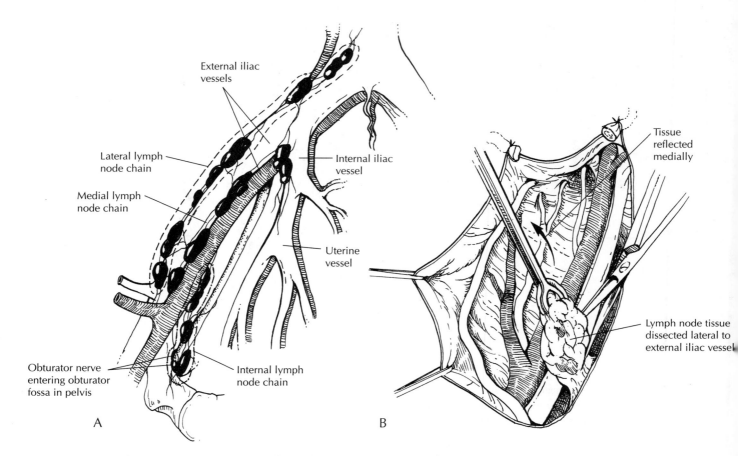

Labels in figure A:
External iliac vessels
Lateral lymph node chain
Medial lymph node chain
Internal iliac vessel
Uterine vessel
Obturator nerve entering obturator fossa in pelvis
Internal lymph node chain

A

Labels in figure B:
Tissue reflected medially
Lymph node tissue dissected lateral to external iliac vessel

B

Fig. 27-5. (A–D) Lymph node dissection is begun by sharply and bluntly mobilizing the tissue lateral to the external iliac artery and vein, and moving this tissue immediately until the external iliac artery can be identified. The closer the dissection is carried to the external iliac artery, the more readily the dissection can be accomplished. Using Metzenbaum scissors and single node pickups, the lymphatic tissue is then sharply dissected off of the surface of the external iliac artery and the common iliac artery, and reflected medially. In doing this, the external iliac vein can be identified, and with lateral traction, the obturator fossa also identified. *(Figure continues.)*

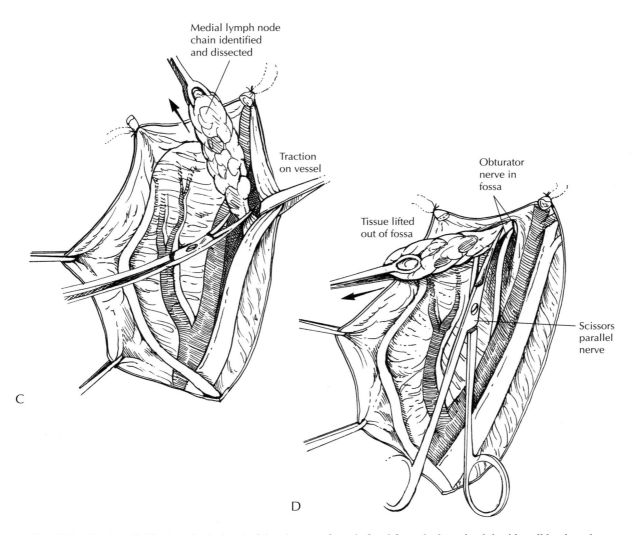

Fig. 27-5 *(Continued).* The lymphatic tissue of the obturator fossa is freed from the lateral pelvic sidewall by dropping down bluntly lateral to the external iliac artery and vein and sharply from the undersurface of the external iliac artery and vein. The obturator nerve is then identified coursing through the obturator fossa and freed for the lymphatic tissue by running the Metzenbaum scissors parallel to the nerve. The lymphatic tissue is then lifted out of the obturator fossa, care being taken to identify the internal iliac artery and vein. A similar procedure is then performed on the left.

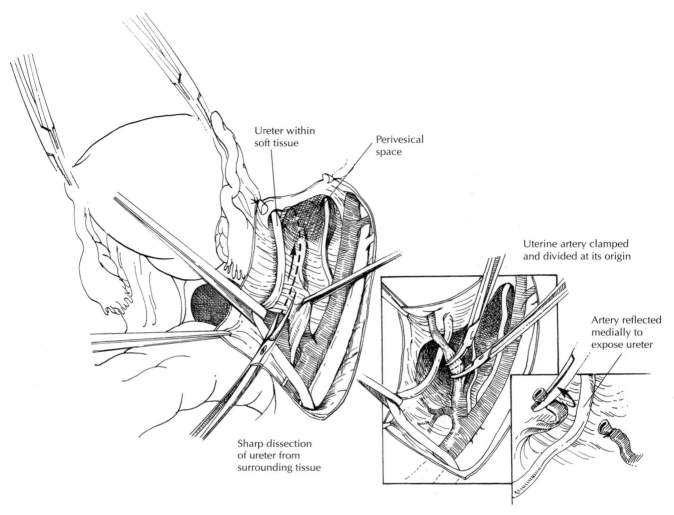

Fig. 27-6. With sharp dissection, the ureter is then dissected free of its soft tissue attachments from its point of entry into the pelvis until its insertion into the bladder. In doing this, the uterine artery is identified, divided at its origin, and reflected medially. Identification of the uterine artery can be facilitated by placing downward tension on the superior vesical artery on the ipsolateral side. This causes all of the branches of the internal ileac artery to be tensed and makes them more readily identified.

Wertheim clamp. The ureters are retracted laterally during this part of the operation. The pedicle is then divided and suture ligated bilaterally. More than one bite is usually required on each side, with the second bite adjusting to the curve of the rectum anteriorly. As these pedicles are taken, the uterus can be felt to rise while retracted. The sponges are removed from the obturator fossae. The surgeon uses one hand to retract the parametrium medially, while the assistant retracts the ureter laterally. The surgeon sharply isolates the parametrium and places a Wertheim clamp down across it. The parametrium is divided and suture ligated. The bladder is inspected, and sharply dissected free until half the vagina is free. With the subsequent parametrial bites, the anterior blade of the Wertheim clamp is placed as close as possible to the bladder corner, while the posterior blade approximates

the uterosacral pedicle. The ureteral insertion into the bladder and the vertical fibers of the rectal musculature should both be visible at this point. When placing the parametrial clamps, it may be helpful to place a long Kelly clamp on the specimen side, and to apply traction medially to help define the tissue in the pedicle clamped with the Wertheim clamp.

The vaginal tube is then sharply divided. Clamps may be placed across the vagina, and then excision carried out distal to the clamps to prevent spillage or contamination. As the vagina is cut across, long Kocher clamps are placed on the vaginal edge, taking care to exclude the bladder. If the clamps block the surgeon's view, the vagina can be cut across, the specimen removed, and the vaginal edges then clamped. Occasionally, in the very deep pelvis, finding the

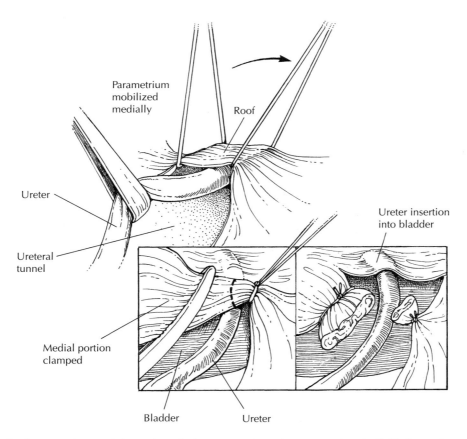

Fig. 27-7. As the ureter is traced down through the parametrium, the parametrium is divided superior and lateral to the ureter and mobilized medially, until the actual insertion of the ureter into the bladder can be seen.

vaginal edge is difficult. An assistant can introduce a gloved hand or lubricated sponge into the vagina and push the vaginal edges towards the surgeon, facilitating identification. The vagina is carefully inspected to ensure an adequate margin. If any question exists, a section of the distal vagina (not the specimen side) can be removed and sent for frozen section to assure a satisfactory margin. The vagina is then closed; the author prefers interrupted sutures. Copious irrigation of the pelvis is carried out with warm saline, and the ureters and all pedicles inspected. The pelvic vessels are examined to ensure completeness of the lymphadenectomy. Indigo carmine may be injected intravenously to test for integrity of the ureters and bladder; alternately, the bladder can be filled through the Foley catheter with methylene blue or sterile milk.

Because of the extensive bladder dissection and resection of the uterosacral ligaments, bladder dysfunction is expected postoperatively. In the past, this was handled by long-term transurethral or suprapubic catheter drainage. Catheters were either removed or clamped at an arbitrary time and postvoid residual urine volumes measured, or known volumes of sterile saline instilled and voiding volumes measured. Alternately, urodynamic testing could be performed at fixed intervals postoperatively. Many patients are now being taught intermittent self-catheterization, and being managed by following self-recorded postvoid residual urine volumes. Prejudice suggests that use of oral antibiotics may prevent urinary tract infections if given until normal voiding resumes.

Although in the past it was customary to place closed suction drains in the pelvis, there is now a movement away from this.[53] If used, soft, pliable drains are placed, one in each obturator fossa, and brought out through separate stab wounds. It has been argued that these drains prevent collections of blood, serum, and lymph, and thus would prevent pelvic abscesses or reduce the number of lymphocysts. Yet, there are a number of physicians, including the author, who no longer drain the pelvis after radical hysterectomy with pelvic lymphadenectomy.[54]

No attempt is made to close the pelvic peritoneum. There is no evidence that this if of any value, and it is time consuming. If the pelvic peritoneum is closed and defects are left in this peritoneal closure, herniation of loops of bowel is possible, and sutures placed in the lateral peritoneum may kink the ureters when tied. The ureters are not suspended in the pelvis, but left lying on the side walls. If the ovaries are being preserved, it is prudent to suspend them out of the pelvis, so that they do not attach to the vaginal apex and cause deep dyspareunia, and so that if postoperative radia-

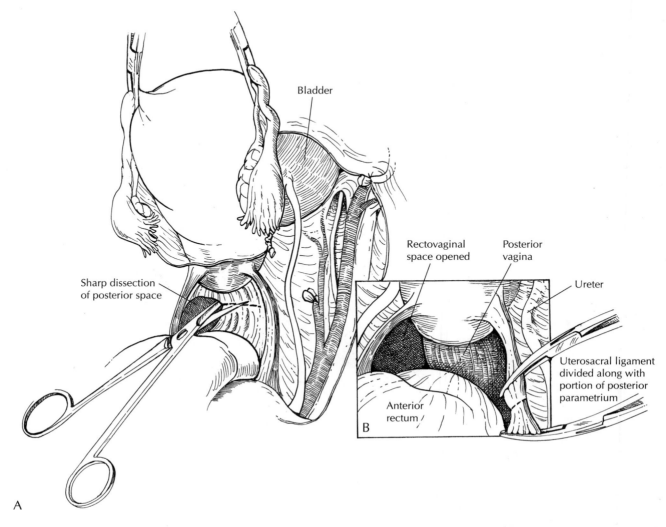

Fig. 27-8. (A & B) Sharp dissection is then used to incise the peritoneum between two uterosacral ligaments, and to develop the potential space between the posterior vagina and the anterior rectum. The uterosacral ligaments are then clamped far lateral at their origin and divided, as is the posterior aspect of the parametrium.

tion is required, they will be out of the field. The ovaries can be marked with hemoclips to facilitate identification for radiation field planning. Ovarian preservation is reasonable in patients with squamous cell carcinoma of the cervix, but not in patients with adenocarcinoma of the cervix. Squamous lesions seldom metastasize to the ovaries, while adenocarcinomas may.[55] However, transposed ovaries do not always function normally and may have a shorter life span than expected. If postoperative pelvic radiation is given, many ovaries will fail. Therefore, the prudent surgeon will follow patients with preserved ovaries closely to detect menopausal symptoms when they occur.

The abdomen is closed with a bulk closure, preferably using permanent suture material. No subcutaneous sutures are used, and the skin is closed with clips or a subcuticular suture. The author prefers a spray dressing to the wound. If

drains are used, it is wise to sew them in at the skin to prevent accidental removal.

POSTOPERATIVE CARE

Patient-controlled epidural or intravenous analgesia is used for all patients. It is emphasized to patients that being stoic and suffering is not conducive to rapid recovery; rather, if they keep themselves comfortable they are more likely to be able to hasten their recovery. By 72 hours, oral analgesics are usually sufficient.

Early ambulation is encouraged by physicians and nursing staff. When in bed, intermittent pneumatic compression devices are used until discharge. Heparin is not used. Physical therapy consultations are used frequently. Incentive spirom-

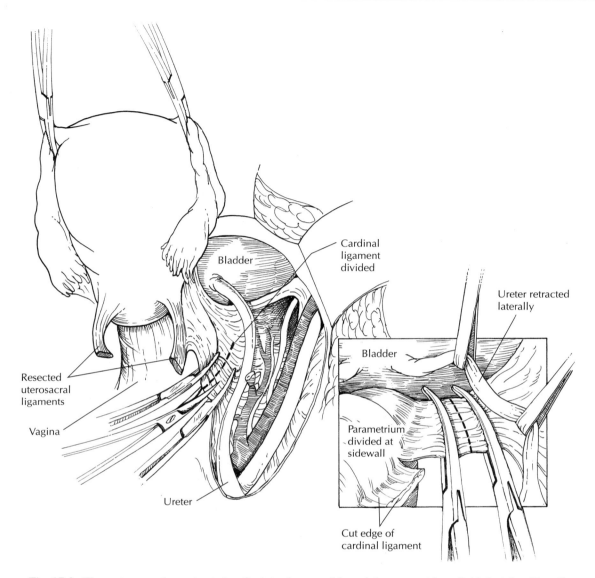

Fig. 27-9. The ureters are then retracted as far lateral as possible and the parametrium divided at the sidewall.

etry is continued until the patient is at least 72 hours out of surgery, with the primary goal prevention of atelectasis in the first 48 hours.

A hematocrit is checked postoperatively, and if acceptable, again at 72 hours. Transfusions in stable, asymptomatic patients are not given for hematocrits above 26. Transfusion does not affect survival, but is prudent to avoid in asymptomatic patients in this age when acquired immunodeficiency syndrome (AIDS) is a constant risk.[56,57] Other laboratory tests are individualized to each patient, based on her concurrent medical problems.

Nasogastric tubes are not used. Clear liquids, ice, and popsicles are allowed postoperatively, and the diet progresses as the patient requests. Laxatives or enemas are given if requested. Appendectomy is routine on the author's service, and does not influence management of the patient's gastrointestinal tract.

Prophylactic antibiotics are given as one dose preoperatively and one dose postoperatively. If a catheter is in place, oral antibiotics are given. Hormone replacement therapy, if indicated, is started at discharge or when the patient notes symptoms. Unopposed estrogen is given.

When the patient can ambulate with ease, tolerate a regular diet, and requires only oral analgesics, she is discharged. Pathology results are reviewed with the patient before discharge or at the first office visit. Home health nurses, clinic staff follow-up with the patient at home, and 24-hour phone access to her doctor, is available. Patients return to the office at 7 to 10 days for clip removal. Heavy lifting (takes two hands) is proscribed for 6 weeks. Walking and climbing stairs is encouraged, and the patient is told she may drive when she feels comfortable doing so, but is asked to have someone with her the first few times. Showers or tub baths are permissible. Douching

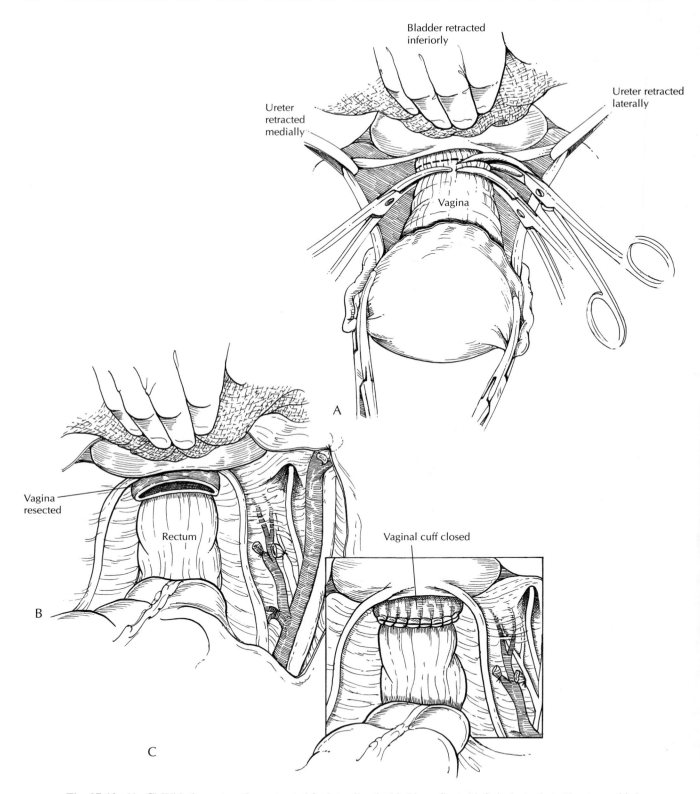

Fig. 27-10. (A–C) With the ureters then retracted far laterally, the bladder reflected inferiorly so that at least one-third to one-half of the vagina is visible anteriorly, and the posterior rectal space developed so that at least one-third to one-half of the vagina is visible posteriorly, the operative specimen is resected and the cuff either closed or dealt with by running the edge.

and intercourse are proscribed until the patient is seen and examined at the office.

There is no value to routinely ordering an intravenous pyelogram in the postoperative period in patients who are without complaints. If radiotherapy is planned, it is started approximately 4 weeks postoperatively. Should minor wound separation occur, this does not delay institution of radiation.

COMPLICATIONS

Radical hysterectomy with pelvic lymphadenectomy entails meticulous dissection near the bladder, rectum, ureters, and great vessels of the pelvis. Understandably, the more common complications relate to injuries to these viscera. Other complications, such as pulmonary embolus, myocardial infarction, bowel obstruction, pneumonia, or fluid or electrolyte imbalance are common to all gynecologic surgery. These latter topics are discussed elsewhere in the text; this section focuses on complications peculiar to, or at least often associated with, radical hysterectomy and pelvic lymphadenectomy. Although the range of complications associated with this operation are the same for all gynecologic oncologists, the incidence of various complications among different surgeons may be significantly different.[58] This physician factor will necessarily influence studies of patient outcome.

Hemorrhage

The average blood loss for this procedure is 900 to 1500 ml, with a range from as little as less than 100 ml to as much as several liters. Major vascular injuries can be encountered anywhere in the procedure. Usually, the bleeding vessel can be readily seen, grasped with pickups or a clamp, and controlled. However, bleeders, particularly venous ones, may be more difficult to identify. Here it usually helps to place direct pressure on the bleeding site with a finger, sponge stick, or laparotomy pad; to facilitate good exposure; to explain what is required of the assistants; to be sure clamps and suture materials are available; and to alert the anesthesiologist to the problem at hand. One wants to be sure there are adequate blood and blood products at hand to stabilize the patient. Frantic suturing or hemoclipping, or blindly clamping in a pool of blood will usually result in further blood loss, and may lead to ureteral or nerve injury.

Most injured pelvic vessels can simply be ligated, with the exception of the external and common iliac vessels, which are best repaired. This is accomplished by compressing the vessel above and below the injury, and closing the defect with a running small caliber permanent suture (i.e., 4–0 Prolene). Vascular clamps can also be used to temporarily occlude a vessel while the repair is done. After closure, patency should be confirmed by palpation of a pulse distal to the repair. The presence of a clot, absent pulse, or injury so severe as to be beyond one's scope, requires consultation with a vascular surgeon. Clips or cautery suffice for small vessels; however, cautery is inappropriate for the larger vessels and clips may either fall off or actually cut into larger vessels, particularly large veins. Placing multiple clips also makes it difficult to isolate and identify the bleeding site.

Occasionally, it will be necessary to firmly pack the bleeding site, usually on the pelvic side wall, while the remainder of the procedure is completed. At that time, when returning to the bleeding site, often the patient's clotting mechanism has resolved the problem. If not, with the additional room and exposure now available, repair can be undertaken. With venous injuries near the iliac bifurcation or behind the internal iliac artery, it may help to divide and remove the internal iliac artery to facilitate working on the vein. It also helps to resect the internal iliac artery when trying to control bleeders beneath the obturator nerve along the side wall.

With diffuse venous bleeding, bilateral hypogastric artery ligation may be useful. After ligating the vessels, which presumably lowers the pressure head of the pelvic vasculature, a firm pelvic pack is placed for at least 10 minutes, to allow the clotting mechanism to take effect. To reap the maximum benefit of hypogastric artery ligation, the uterus needs to be already removed, and both arteries need to be ligated. In these patients with massive blood loss, appropriate replacement fluids must include fresh frozen plasma in addition to packed red cells. There are synthetic materials available as powder and sheets that may serve as a nidus for clot formation. Their use in pelvic cancer surgery is of limited value.

Bleeders over the sacral area are particularly frustrating. After trying pressure, ligature, clips, bone wax, and cautery, this author has twice in over 15 years succeeded in controlling the bleeding by placing a sterile, steel thumbtack directly into the bleeding site. The thumbtack is placed with a curved Kelly clamp, and left in place.

Rarely—because the patient is unstable and the vascular injury not identified when the vessels retract into the side wall, or there is injury over the sacrum—it is necessary to place a firm pelvic pack, using whatever materials are at hand, and to close the patient. Laparotomy pads, towels, or packs of any sort may be used. This author favors a nylon pack filled with laparotomy pads and soaked in kanamycin solution; the nylon does not stick to soft tissue when it is removed. The plan is to stabilize the patient, correct any bleeding abnormalities, and then bring the patient back to the operating room in 24 to 48 hours. There may occasionally be a role for embolization by interventional radiologists. It is possible to bring the pack out through the incision and to remove it in a controlled setting, to eliminate the need for a second surgery. There is a selected role for embolization of bleeding sites by interventional radiology.

Being in the "Wrong Place"

When learning this procedure or operating on patients with endometriosis, chronic pelvic inflammatory disease, or prior surgery or radiation, identifiable anatomic landmarks become obliterated or compromised. As a rule, the retroperitoneal approach to the pelvis will minimize this event. However, endometriosis and cancer will invade through tissue planes, making even this approach uncertain. The more common errors appear to be failing to dissect out vessels for fear of injuring them, and consequently leaving significant soft tissue on the vessels. This leads to misidentification of planes, and vascular injury. Time spent cleaning a vessel is time saved.

When developing the perivesical and perirectal spaces, misidentification of the boundaries of these spaces can lead to bladder, rectal, or side wall vessel injury. Time, patience, and experience prevent this. Recognition of these spaces is essential to any pelvic surgeon.[59] The perivesical space is more easily dissected then the perirectal, as it is avascular and its margins (the bladder and superior vesical artery medially, and the pelvic side wall and external iliac vessels laterally) are easily identified. The perirectal space, by contrast, is best visualized by placing the uterus under anterior and medial traction and the infundibulopelvic ligament under traction, to allow the identification of the ureter on the medial leaf of the broad ligament, and to allow the plane to be dissected by beginning immediately lateral to the ureter, as opposed to over the iliac vessels.

Bladder Injuries

Injection of intravenous indigo carmine, instillation of methlene blue through the urethral catheter, or simply opening the dome of the bladder help localize bladder injuries. If located in the dome, one could simply use this as a suprapubic catheter site and place a Foley catheter, bringing it out through a stab wound in the lower abdomen. With cystotomies located lower in the bladder, it is necessary to ensure that the ureteral orifices are not compromised by the closure of the hole. If questions of the patency of the ureters exist, a stent may be passed retrograde from the bladder, or indigo carmine injected intravenously. A simple two-layered closure with absorbable suture should suffice to close the bladder. If the specimen has not been removed, the repair should, if possible, be delayed until the specimen is out, since other injuries may occur. Also, the bladder dissection can be done very speedily if the bladder is already open and able to be elevated during freeing of the vagina. If the patient has received prior radiation or the bladder injury is extreme, the author frees the omentum from the hepatic flexure over to the splenic flexure, leaving the most lateral left-sided attachments of the omentum in place, and then places the omentum over the bladder repair to provide neovascularity.

With bladder injuries, the catheter is left in for a prolonged time, usually over 2 weeks.

Ureteral Injuries

The ureteral dissection during a radical hysterectomy leads to significant damage to the ureters' blood supply. Although branches to the ureter arise from the aorta, common, ovarian, and internal iliac arteries, as well as from the hypogastric artery's terminal branches, the true blood supply runs in a web or sheath that runs along the outer ureteral surface. Therefore, nicks or holes in the body of the ureter are best treated as transections, by dividing the ureter on an angle, that is, spatulating it, and performing a ureteroneocystotostomy after completing the radical hysterectomy and pelvic lymphadenectomy. The bladder is freed by developing fully the prevesical space, and by dividing the avascular lateral peritoneal attachments of the bladder. This allows tremendous mobility for the bladder, and allows it to be placed at the bifurcation of the common iliac vessel. Thus, nearly any pelvic injury to the ureter can be managed by reimplantation. The ureter is mobilized high above the pelvic brim with blunt and sharp dissection. A stent is placed within the ureter, and gently passed several centimeters up the ureter, stopping when resistance is met. Then a fine single suture is placed several centimeters above the transected end of the ureter, passing through both ureter and the body of the stent, to prevent displacement of the stent by ureteral peristalsis. A tonsil clamp is placed inside the bladder and a site for reanastomosis selected, which minimizes tension on the anastomosis and is located in a spot convenient for sewing. The tonsil tents up the bladder, a small incision is made, and the stent and ureter brought into the bladder. Interrupted fine absorbable mucosa-to-mucosa sutures are then placed to anastomose the ureter to bladder. Usually four to six are required. Several interrupted sutures are then placed outside the bladder attaching ureteral serosa to bladder serosa. The bladder is then laid along the external iliac vessels, and an absorbable suture is used to secure the bladder to the tendon of the psoas muscle, the so-called psoas hitch to lessen tension on the anastomosis.

The stent may then be brought out through a stab wound in the lower abdominal wall, or is left curled in the bladder. Catheter drainage of the bladder is carried out as usual. If the stent is displaced or passed, or after 14 to 21 days, an IVP is done to confirm patency and absence of leak. The stent, if remaining, can then be removed. Occasionally the stent will be inadvertently removed earlier than planned. If an IVP then shows a ureteral leak, it will need to be drained and a new stent placed, either cystoscopically or in a retrograde fashion percutaneously. After a ureteral implantation, a closed-system pliable suction drain is placed, and removed when minimal drainage occurs.

Rarely, insufficient ureter is available to reach the bladder.

This seldom occurs with intraoperative ureteral injury or transection, but is found when reoperation is needed to repair late fistula or significant ureteral obstruction. In this circumstance, after freeing the bladder from its lateral attachments and developing the prevesical space, a flap, with its base aimed at the injured ureter, can be developed, the bladder closed, and the flap then closed as a tube to the end of which the ureter may be anastomosed, the so-called Boari flap. If the ureteral injury is out of the pelvis entirely, the end of the ureter can be burrowed retroperitoneally behind the bowel mesentery, and the injured ureter anastomosed to the side of the healthy ureter, a trans ureteroureterostomy. In this circumstance, both kidneys will share a common distal ureter that, if obstructed, will lead to bilateral renal failure.

Nephrectomy or ureterostomy is almost unheard of for management of ureteral injury, and should only be considered as a last resort after all other efforts have failed.

Ureteral Obstruction

Slight hydronephrosis is often present on IVPs done in the immediate postoperative period (the value of which is unclear), but by 3 months postoperatively, this has usually resolved. Hydronephrosis found after this is most often attributable to recurrent cancer.[60] However, hydronephrosis may very infrequently result from radiation therapy, and even more infrequently from radical hysterectomy alone. In these patients, after efforts are made to rule out recurrent malignancy, ureteral dilation at the site of obstruction may be attempted via cystoscope or percutaneously (Fig. 27-11). This author favors the latter approach. Should this fail, or ureteral obstruction recur, then laparotomy with reimplantation, as outlined above, is appropriate.

Neurogenic Bladder Dysfunction

With the interruption of the parasympathetic and sympathetic innervation of the bladder (which results from the resection of the uterosacral and cardinal ligaments) and the extensive dissection and mobilization of the bladder, it is actually amazing that women resume normal or nearly normal voiding patterns after radical hysterectomy. Urodynamic studies of women after radical hysterectomy present varied and inconsistent findings. There is usually a phase during which the bladder has increased resting tone and small vol-

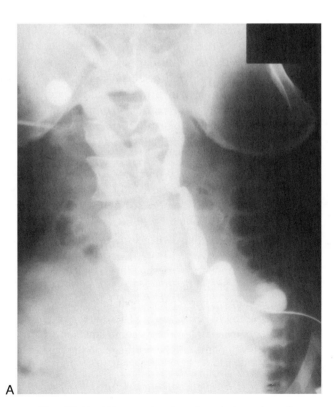

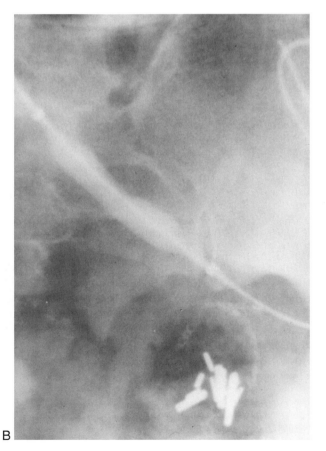

A B

Fig. 27-11. (A) Dye showing site of obturation of ureter; percutaneous catheter in place. **(B)** White ring indicating balloon that will dilate ureter (white clips in lower right).

ume, with intermittent uncontrolled contractions. This is usually followed by a period of decreased bladder tone, increased residual volume, and absence of bladder wall contractions. Fortunately, with constant drainage, the bladder usually resumes more normal function over several weeks or months, although some patients will always report decreased sensation and an inability to completely empty the bladder without increased abdominal pressure or suprapubic pressure. There have been suggestions that modifying the extent of parametrial excision would lessen urologic problems. This thinking would seem to risk compromising successful extirpation of the cancer.

If a suprapubic catheter is in place, the patient will usually report a few weeks after surgery that, when defecating, she is beginning to void small amounts of urine. Her bladder can be tested by instilling 200 to 250 ml of sterile saline through the suprapubic, clamping it and then allowing the woman to void. This may take up to an hour or longer. Residual urine can be measured after the patient voids, and if less than 75 ml, the catheter can be removed. If only small volumes of saline can be instilled (i.e., 100 to 125 ml or less), it is too early to consider removal. Testing at intervals of less than 1 to 2 weeks in not constructive.

If a transurethral catheter is used at an arbitrary time (i.e., 2 weeks postoperatively), sterile saline can be instilled into the bladder, the catheter removed, and the patient allowed to void and residual volume measured. If unable to void, depending on the patient, intermittent self-catheterization can be taught or another catheter placed. There are patients who can begin self-catheterization in the immediate postoperative period. Prevention of bladder distention and timed bladder emptying must be ensured.

With indwelling catheters, oral antibiotics are used, and the patient is encouraged to drink large amounts of fluids.

Rectal Injury

Small defects may be closed with a two-layered closure, such as a running absorbable layer for the mucosa, and interrupted silk for the serosa. One-layered closures and synthetic sutures with long tissue life suffice. For larger defects, a stapling device can be used. Colostomy is essentially never required. Copious irrigation is carried out after repairing the injury, and again prior to closing. Prophylactic antibiotics are used by this author for all radical hysterectomies, and no other antibiotics would be started because of a rectal injury. However, postoperatively, enemas and rectal probe temperatures would be proscribed.

Lymphedema/Lymphocyst

Unilateral or bilateral lymphedema of the lower extremities is rarely seen after radical hysterectomy, even if postoperative pelvic radiation is used. When encountered, it is a chronic problem for which there is little effective intervention. Support hose and leg wraps will minimize edema. Elevation of the extremities when sitting, and elevating the foot of the bed, help control the problem. When lymphedema is present, superficial infections such as insect bites or abrasions, can be troublesome. Patients should be warned to take care of their skin and pay special attention to the development of erythema or tenderness, which may suggest a need for systemic antibiotics.

Lymphocysts are also uncommon, probably occurring in 1 to 3 percent of patients, and they are seldom symptomatic. When symptoms do arise, patients usually complain of vague, colicy, lower abdominal pain. Most often, lymphocysts are detected when radiologic studies are done surveying the patient for recurrent disease. If found and symptomatic, or associated with hydronephrosis, they can be drained percutaneously.[61] Should they recur, they can be drained again and tetracycline instilled to sclerose the cavity. There is little, if any, role for laparotomy and drainage or marsupialization.

Neuropathies

Neuropathies in radical hysterectomy, although rare, are more commonly associated with patient positioning errors or malpositioned retractor blades than with operative injury.[62] When stirrups are used, pressure on the fibula head can lead to peroneal nerve palsy. Use of an improperly placed retractor can lead to the lateral blades placing excessive pressure on the femoral nerve with resultant injury. Both peroneal and femoral palsies lead to difficulty walking, and complete recovery is uncommon. Hyperflexion of the thigh could also theoretically lead to a femoral/sciatic nerve injury. All of these problems are preventable, by using care and gentleness in patient positioning.

During dissection of the obturator fossa, obturator nerve transection may occur. Occasionally, enlarged tumor-bearing nodes will encase the nerve. If unilateral injury occurs, minor ambulatory problems will be noted due to weakened adduction of the thigh. There will also be numbness of the inner thigh.

With dissection of the external iliac lymph nodes, the genitofemoral and lateral femoral cutaneous nerves may be cut, leading to numbness over the upper labia and groin, or the front of the thigh, respectively. These areas of paresthesia may, over considerable time, become smaller.

Attempts at controlling hemorrhage on the posterolateral pelvic side wall may lead to placement of clips or sutures into the nerve trunks of the femoral/sciatic nerve. Control of bleeding with pressure, followed by identification and, if necessary, dissection of the bleeding site, will minimize this source of nerve injury.

Infectious Morbidity

Febrile morbidity for radical hysterectomy ranges from 20 to 30 percent, with most of the infections attributable to the urinary tract, wound, or pelvic cellulitis.[42,58] Fever within the first 48 hours of surgery is almost always attributable to atelectasis, and is best treated with ambulation, incentive spirometry, and respiratory toilet. Blood and urine cultures are unnecessary. After 48 hours, a fever work up is reasonable, although usually, empiric antibiotics will be started. The most important part of the evaluation is a thorough inspection of the wound and good rectovaginal examination. Generic metronidazole and gentamycin will usually suffice as empiric therapy, although more cost-effective, single-agent regimens may be better. Blood cultures are seldom positive, and antibiotics have usually been started before results are available. When results of urine and blood cultures are positive, antibiotic management can be simplified based on bacterial sensitivities. Urinary tract infections occur approximately 20 percent of the time; ill-defined pelvic cellulitis (i.e., fever, negative cultures, leucocytosis) is equally common. Superficial wound infection/hematoma occurs in approximately 10 percent of patients.

If a patient remains febrile with no localizing signs of infection after 48 hours of broad-spectrum antibiotics, it has been our custom to diagnose septic pelvic thrombophlebitis and to begin heparin. We begin at 1,000 units per hour, without a bolus, and increase the rate based on partial thromboplastin time (PTT) levels. If the patient becomes afebrile, the heparin dose is held constant even if the PTT is not elevated. After the patient has been afebrile for 48 hours, heparin and antibiotics are discontinued. If the patient remains febrile with negative cultures and therapeutic PTT levels, then a CT scan of the pelvis with contrast is done, looking for occult fluid collections that can be percutaneously drained.

An IVP is appropriate in any patient febrile after 24 hours of antibiotics, to rule out occult ureteral obstruction. If present, percutaneous management with stent placement is performed.

Ileus/Bowel Obstruction

Ileus obstruction was seen in approximately 1 to 5 percent of patients in the past, but with early ambulation and feeding we seem to be seeing this less often. Patients usually present with nausea and vomiting, and examination reveals a nontender abdomen. When it occurs, the patient is placed NPO and kept well hydrated with attention to maintaining normal electrolytes. Bowel sounds may be normal, hyperactive, or decreased. Bowel movements may or may not be occurring. If vomiting is persistent, a nasogastric tube is placed, and left in place at least 24 hours. It is removed when drainage is consistently less than 500 ml in 8 hours. If the patient's symptoms are not improved after 48 hours of being NPO,

with or without nasogastric tube, then a chest x-ray and abdominal series are ordered. This is the baseline study for further comparison. We will usually allow 7 or more days of conservative management (i.e., NPO, nasogastric drainage, hydration, and electrolyte correction) before contemplating surgical intervention. However, should leucocytosis, fever, and peritoneal signs develop, surgery is indicated. Dye studies of the gastrointestinal tract have not been helpful. Parenteral nutrition is seldom needed, unless the patient was cachectic preoperatively and surgical intervention is considered likely.

Urinary Tract Fistula

Fistulas of the ureter, bladder, or both occur is less than 1 percent of patients. Localization of the fistula is accomplished by cystoscopy, IVP, and retrograde studies of the ureter. Simple vesicovaginal fistulae can be managed by prolonged drainage, to allow the opportunity for healing. If this fails, surgical correction by a Latzko procedure usually succeeds, with minimal morbidity. Repeated efforts may be appropriate. If ultimately unsuccessful, an abdominal approach is then indicated. This is discussed in Chapter 39.

A ureterovaginal fistula may be stented, preferably percutaneously. Healing usually occurs. If this fails, the patient can be explored and managed as discussed previously.

Complex ureterovesicovaginal fistulas require complex management by physicians experienced with the problem. Stenting and drainage until inflammation and infection have resolved will infrequently allow for healing, but more likely lead to optimization of the patient for a combined abdominopelvic repair.

There are surgeons who believe in immediate repair of urinary tract fistulas; this author does not find this unreasonable. However, stenting and drainage do allow a significant number of fistulas to heal, and are associated with minimal morbidity.

Gastrointestinal Fistula

Gastrointestinal fistulas are so rare as to be anecdotal. They tend to occur 10 to 14 days postoperatively, and may be heralded by spiking temperatures with no clear source and no response to antibiotics, and a tender, otherwise normal-appearing, incision. Management consists of resting the gastrointestinal tract by placing the patient NPO, and possibly by using inhibitors of pancreatic and gastric secretion. The site of the fistula is determined radiographically, usually by first injecting dye into the fistula (fistulogram) and then subsequently doing a small bowel and large bowel series. Healing occurs in weeks, not days. If there is an obstruction distal to the fistula, it will not heal. Parenteral nutrition may be of help, but that is not proved.[63] Because of the rarity of this complication, consultation with more experienced clinicians is reasonable.

Sexual Dysfunction

In theory, the vagina is a soft, pliable organ that should be able to stretch and accommodate during intercourse. However, the fibrosis that may result from radical hysterectomy, combined with the psychological adjustments the diagnosis of cancer of the cervix require, may lead to patients having problems with sexual intercourse and vaginal function. Thoughtful discussion of sexual function should precede and follow radical hysterectomy. If problems are identified with a patient's sex life, then appropriate counselling is warranted as soon as possible.

Management of the physical problems related to sexual dysfunction is multifaceted. Adequate endogenous hormones or exogenous therapy, is required. Vaginal lubrication can be augmented with commercial water-soluble lubricants. Sexual positons in which the female is on the bottom can be made more comfortable by having the woman keep her thighs slightly closer together to create a "longer" vagina. This will require her to guide the penis during entry. Female superior or side-by-side positions will allow the female more control over depth of penile penetration. Oral and anal sex may be reasonable considerations in women who find this acceptable. Masturbation by the patient or her sex partner may allow gradual adjustments to altered perceptions of sexual pleasure.

Failure of a physician to ask about the patient's sexual function does not prevent problems from arising; rather, it prevents the physician from identifying a problem that can usually be addressed. Speaking with the patient's sexual partner can be very informative and lead to identification of communication problems, which can be addressed by a thoughtful physician. If the physician is uncomfortable with this area, then those health care providers who are more adept at handling these problems should be allowed to work with the patient. Fulfilling sexual function is a major part of successful surgical rehabilitation.

Patients who are not sexually active may over many months or years suffer significant shortening of the vagina, which will later preclude establishing sexual relations. This perhaps can be prevented by using vaginal molds or dilators. If a patient is not sexually active, the physician should at least raise the question of potential future sexual relationships. Age is a factor in sexual activity only in the mind of the physician.

COMPLICATED RADICAL HYSTERECTOMIES

Pregnancy

When radical hysterectomy is proposed in a pregnant patient, involvement of colleagues in maternal fetal medicine and neonatology is vitally important. Most oncologists lack the sophistication to assess the optimal timing of pregnancy termination that would maximize the likelihood of a normal child. Clearly, pregnancies in the second and third trimesters should be allowed to proceed to a point where viability of an intact child is very likely. First trimester pregnancies should probably not be allowed to continue to viability; but, as our neonatal intensive care units progress, the likelihood of intact viability is seems to move to lower and lower gestational ages. However, there is an understandable paucity of data on allowing a pregnant woman to delay surgical treatment. Consultation with maternal fetal medicine colleagues also makes sense for medicolegal considerations.

Pregnant women have a higher pulse rate, lower mean blood pressure, and greater blood volume than nonpregnant women. These and other physiologic changes of pregnancy can confuse clinicians evaluating blood loss, fever, and other factors.

During the procedure, pregnancy does change some aspects of the surgical technique. The uterus becomes soft, "boggy," and hard to hold. After approximately 16-weeks size, the author finds the uterus more difficult to use to provide countertraction for pelvic side wall dissection. This, therefore, is one circumstance where performing the radical hysterectomy before the pelvic lymph node dissection may be advantageous. However, the perivesical and perirectal spaces should be well developed so that the hypertrophied blood supply to the pregnant uterus is well exposed. The ovaries will most likely be preserved in these patients, and individual vessels in the broad ligament may require individual ligation. The utero-ovarian ligament and mesosalpinx may require suture ligation, or double tying.

If cesarean section is performed, the incision (preferably low vertical) must be closed and hemostatic. If the fetus is being sacrificed, hysterotomy is not indicated, as it will increase blood loss and febrile morbidity.

Finally, when cutting across the vagina, the elasticity of the pregnant vagina must be taken into account to prevent removing excessive amounts of the vagina.

Prior Supracervical or Total Hysterectomy

Supracervical hysterectomy is now primarily of historical interest. However, a small number of women who have undergone this outdated procedure will present with cancer of the cervix.[64-67] In addition, despite efforts to properly evaluate women and provide routine cancer screening, a nonradical hysterectomy will be performed for benign indications, with the pathology specimen revealing invasive cancer of the cervix. Although many would prefer to manage these patients with radiotherapy, patients who would otherwise be good operative candidates can be offered radical hysterectomy in the absence of the uterus, or radical parametrectomy.

There are very few patients, fortunately, who fall into this group. Consequently, no controlled studies or large clinical series exist. However, certain guidelines seem appropriate. Radical parametrectomy and pelvic node dissection offer the advantage of possibly precluding the need for pelvic radiation, of preserving an ovary if indicated, and of providing information about the true extent of disease. The clinical studies cited above suggest no increase in operative morbidity with these procedures compared to radical hysterectomy, and survival rates seem equal to those of patients who are radiated.

However, in the absence of the uterine corpus, the radical procedure is made more difficult for several reasons. First, there is less tissue to use as a source of countertraction. Second, there is invariably more difficulty in establishing the anterior peritoneal plane between the bladder and "uterus," since there will have been some prior surgery in this area, often of uncertain extent. Third, if prior hysterectomy was recent, there will be some tissue reaction. Consequently, if approaching this operation, one should plan to address these problems.

When developing the perivesical and perirectal spaces, any connective tissue that can be swept towards the midline will provide more bulk for countertraction. After doing the node dissection, the bladder must be seperated from the stump of the cervix, or the cuff, to a sufficient extent that a good flap of viable vaginal tissue is freed. Right-angle clamps or large crushing clamps can then be placed on the cuff and then used for traction. The lateral pelvic dissection, in the absence of the uterine corpus, can be easily carried out. But, the anterior and posterior planes require that there be a means of applying vertical upward traction.

Tissue reaction or inflammation to prior hysterectomy is dealt with by ensuring that the lateral extent of the pelvic resection removes the involved tissue. Cutting through this tissue creates a potential problem; removing this tissue prevents the problem. This is the reason that prior conization does not affect morbidity for radical hysterectomy: the parametritis is removed, and cannot serve as a nidus for infection.[68]

Combining Pelvic Radiation and Radical Hysterectomy

Radiated tissue will undergo a progressive small vessel endarteritis, which compromises blood supply to the affected tissue. However, this is a slow and gradual process, not seen to be clinically significant for many months or years.

Yet, when approaching a patient with previous radiation, this fact is foremost in the surgeon's mind. In addition, the acute inflammatory or edematous effects of radiation are recognized to exist. Therefore, it is surprising to find little evidence to support the adverse effects of performing a radical hysterectomy on patients with prior radiation. If the radiation failed to control the tumor, and the radical hysterec-

tomy is performed to control persistent or progressing disease, prognosis is understandably bleak. Also, if pelvic nodes contain cancer after therapeutic doses of radiation, the advantage of resecting them is unclear.

Patients who undergo radical hysterectomy and pelvic lymphadenectomy for treatment of cervical cancer, and who then undergo pelvic radiation, represent a small, highly select group of women. In most patients, radical surgery is meant to be curative, total treatment. The need for postoperative radiation is based on a perception of operative or pathologic findings that dictate a need for something additional to surgical treatment alone.[69,70] Most often this reflects physician prejudice since this is such a small subset of cancer patients that double-blind, controlled studies are impractical. There are clearly patients with stage IB cervical cancer who appear to have tumors whose histologic criteria predict a high treatment failure rate. These poorly defined subsets of patients can then be radiated, with disagreement as to whether this is associated with significant complications or not.[71-73] Finally, it remains to show that radiating these controversial "high-risk" patients results in sufficiently improved survival to justify a potential increase in significant treatment-related morbidity. Undoubtedly, this problem is complicated by the lack of uniformity in patient selection, differences in the total dose of radiation delivered, time-dose interval of radiotherapy, and thoroughness and length of patient follow-up.

NEW TECHNIQUES AND INNOVATIONS

There has been a suggestion that stapling devices may be useful in shortening the length of radical surgery, and possibly lessening blood loss.[74] There remains the question as to whether these stapling devices allow as adequate a parametrial dissection as do scissors. There is also the larger question of whether this surgical approach can largely be supplanted by laparoscopic surgery or combined laparoscopic and open surgery. This is a provocative area, and much investigation is needed. Subsequent chapters deal with these topics, and also discuss the radical vaginal hysterectomy that might logically fit into the endoscopic surgeon's armamentarium.

Finally, there is the question of whether pelvic lymph node dissection might, in seleced circumstances, be a procedure that could stand on its own. In endometrial cancer, the currently adopted surgical staging relied heavily on findings of pelvic lymph node biopsy. One would expect a thorough dissection to provide more information than random, limited biopsies, although no data exist to support this. Nonetheless, one would certainly believe that if decisions to use or not to use postoperative radiation will be based largely on the presence or absence of metastases to the pelvic nodes, then there is a definite need to ensure an adequate sample. In this circumstance, the procedure would be identical to that already outlined.

Surgical staging of cervical cancer in advanced stages prior to instituting radiation is actually looking for extrapelvic disease. However, if for protocol or study purposes, lymph node dissection were required before radiation, one could approach this dissection retroperitoneally using a hockey stick incision that runs parallel to the inguinal ligament and then rises vertically into the abdomen. After dividing the muscles of the abdominal wall, the peritoneum is bluntly mobilized medially and the pelvic and midline abdominal vessels exposed. Lymph node dissection can then be done, although the bowel must be mobilized to beyond the midline to allow the contralateral nodes to be dissected. Alternately, a laparoscopic approach (see Ch. 29) might prove optimal.

SUMMARY

Radical hysterectomy with bilateral pelvic lymphadenectomy meets the broad definition of an adequate cancer operation: the cancer, the primary organ in which it arises, the first area of contiguous spread, and the regional lymphatics are resected. Good patient survival is achieved, although patients with a lesser likelihood of cure are identified. Unfortunately, the value to adjunctive treatment in these patients is unclear.

Intraoperative complications involve damage to pelvic vessels and viscera, and require the pelvic surgeon to be familiar with their management and repair. Postoperative complications are usually self-limited, if recognized and treated aggressively.

Radical hysterectomy and pelvic lymphadenectomy remains one of the more difficult and elegant procedures in the gynecologic oncologist's repertoire.

REFERENCES

1. Clark JG: Radical abdominal hysterectomy for cancer of the uterus. p. 718. In Kelly HA (ed): Gynecology and Abdominal Surgery. Vol. 1. WB Saunders, Philadelphia, 1907
2. Clark JG: A more radical method of performing hysterectomy for cancer of the uterus. Johns Hopkins Hospital Bulletin 52–53:120, 1895
3. Clark JG: Ten cases of cancer of the uterus operated upon by a more radical method of performing hysterectomy. Johns Hopkins Hospital Bulletin 59–60:37, 1896
4. Werder XO: Original communications. A new operation for the radical treatment of cancer of the cervix, consisting of the removal of the uterus and vagina en masse by the suprapubic method: with report of a case. Am J Obstet Dis Women Child 37:19, 1898
5. Wertheim E: A discussion on the diagnosis and treatment of cancer of the uterus. BMJ 2:689, 1905
6. Ries E: Recent developments in our knowledge of cancer of the uterus. Am J Obstet Dis Women Child 44:29, 1901
7. Wertheim E: The extended abdominal operation for carcinoma uteri (based on 500 operative cases). Am J Obstet Dis Women Child 66:169, 1912
8. Sampson JA: The importance of a more radical operation in carcinoma cervicis uteri as suggested by pathological findings in the parametrium. Johns Hopkins Hospital Bulletin 141:299, 1902
9. Sampson JA: The relation between carcinoma cervicis uteri and the ureters, and its significance in the more radical operations for that disease. Johns Hopkins Hospital Bulletin 156:72, 1904
10. Taussig FJ: Iliac lymphadenectomy with irradiation in the treatment of cancer of the cervix. Am J Obstet Gynecol 28:650, 1934
11. Taussig FJ: Original communications: iliac lymphadenectomy for group II cancer of the cervix. Am J Obstet Gynecol 45:733, 1943
12. Okabayaski H: Radical abdominal hysterectomy for cancer of the cervix uteri. Surg Gynecol Obstet 33:335, 1921
13. Yagi H: Treatment of carcinoma of the cervix uteri. Surg Gynecol Obstet 95:552, 1952
14. Bonney V: The treatment of carcinoma of the cervix by Wertheim's operation. Am J Obstet Gynecol 30:815, 1935
15. Bonney V: The results of 500 cases of Wertheim's operation for carcinoma of the cervix. Br J Obstet Gynaecol 48:421, 1941
16. Bonney V: Wertheim's operation in retrospect. Lancet 1:637, 1949
17. Meigs JV: Carcinoma of the cervix—the Wertheim operation. Surg Gynecol Obstet 78:195, 1944
18. Meigs JV: The Wertheim operation for carcinoma of the cervix. Am J Obstet Gynecol 49:542, 1945
19. Meigs JV: Radical hysterectomy with bilateral pelvic lymph node dissections. A report of 100 patients operated on five or more years ago. Am J Obstet Gynecol 62:854, 1951
20. Liu W, Meigs JV: Radical hysterectomy and pelvic lymphadenectomy: a review of 433 cases including 244 for primary cancer of the cervix. Am J Obstet Gynecol 69:1, 1955
21. Piver MS, Rutledge F, Smith JP: Five classes of extended hysterectomy for women with cervical cancer. Obstet Gynecol 44:265, 1974
22. Averette HE, Nguyen HN, Donato DM et al: Radical hysterectomy for invasive cervical cancer. Cancer 71:1422, 1993
23. Kelso JW, Funnell JW: Radical Wertheim hysterectomy. Am J Obstet Gynecol 99:106, 1967
24. Hoskins WJ, Ford JH, Lutz MH, Averette HE: Radical hysterectomy and pelvic lymphadenectomy for the management of early invasive cancer of the cervix. Gynecol Oncol 4:278, 1976
25. Langley II, Moore DW, Tarnasky JW, Roberts PHR: Radical hysterectomy and pelvic lymph node dissection. Gynecol Oncol 9:37, 1980

26. Lee YN, Wang KL, Lin MH et al: Radical hysterectomy with pelvic lymph node dissection for treatment of cervical cancer: a clinical review of 954 cases. Gynecol Oncol 32:135, 1989

27. Webb MJ, Symmonds RE: Wertheim hysterectomy: a reappraisal. Obstet Gynecol 54:140, 1979

28. Underwood PB, Wilson WC, Kreutner A et al: Radical hysterectomy: a critical review of twenty-two years' experience. Am J Obstet Gynecol 134:889, 1979

29. Morris M: Early cervical carcinoma: are two treatments better than one?, editorial. Gynecol Oncol 54:1, 1994

30. Baltzer J, Kopcke W, Lohe KJ et al: Die operative behandlung des zervixkarzinoms. Geburtsch u Frauenheilk 44:279, 1984

31. Rutlege S, Carey MS, Prichard H et al: Conservative surgery for recurrent or persistent carcinoma of the cervix following irradiation: is exenteration always necessary? Gynecol Oncol 52:353, 1994

32. Benedet JL, Turko M, Boyes DA: Radical hysterectomy in the treatment of cervical cancer. Am J Obstet Gynecol 137:254, 1980

33. Powell JL, Burrell MO, Franklin EW: Radical hysterectomy and pelvic lymphadenectomy. Gynecol Oncol 12:23, 1981

34. Shuster PA, Barter JF, Potkul RK et al: Radical hysterectomy morbidity in relation to age. Obstet Gynecol 78:77, 1991

35. O'Leary JA, Symmonds RE: Radical pelvic operations in the geriatric patient. Obstet Gynecol 28:745, 1966

36. Lawton FG, Hacker NF: Surgery for invasive gynecologic cancer in the elderly female population. Obstet Gynecol 76:287, 1990

37. Kinney WK, Egorshin EV, Potratz KC: Wertheim hysterectomy in the geriatric population. Gynecol Oncol 31:227, 1988

38. Fuchtner C, Manetta A, Walker JL et al: Radical hysterectomy in the elderly patient: analysis of morbidity. Am J Obstet Gynecol 166:593, 1992

39. Masterson JG: Radical surgery in early carcinoma of the cervix. Am J Obstet Gynecol 87:601, 1963

40. Geisler JP, Geisler HE: Radical hysterectomy in patients 65 years of age and older. Gynecol Oncol 53:208, 1994

41. Soisson AP, Soper JT, Berchuck A et al: Radical hysterectomy in obese women. Obstet Gynecol 80:940, 1992

42. Mann WJ, Orr JW, Shingleton HM et al: Perioperative influences on infectious morbidity in radical hysterectomy. Gynecol Oncol 11:207, 1981

43. Gauthier P, Gore I, Shingleton HM et al: Identification of histopathologic risk groups in stage IB squamous cell carcinoma of the cervix. Obstet Gynecol 66:569, 1985

44. Shingleton HM, Orr JW: Cancer of the Cervix. Churchill Livingstone, New York, 1987

45. Ferenczy A, Winkler B: Carcinoma and metastatic tumors of the cervix. p. 218. In Kurman RJ (ed): Blaustein's Pathology of the Female Genital Tract. 3rd Ed. Springer-Verlag, New York, 1987

46. Gallion HH, van Nagell JR, Donaldson ES et al: Combined radiation therapy and extrafascial hysterectomy in the treatment of stage IB barrel-shaped cervical cancer. Cancer 56:262, 1985

47. Alvarez RD, Gelder MS, Gore H et al: Radical hysterectomy in the treatment of patients with bulky early stage carcinoma of the cervix uteri. Surg Gynecol Obstet 176:539, 1993

48. Baltzer J, Koepcke: Tumor size and lymph node metastases in squamous cell carcinoma of the uterine cervix. Arch Gynecol 227:271, 1979

49. Clarke-Pearson DL, Synan IS, Hinshaw WM et al: Prevention of postoperative venous thromboembolism by external pneumatic calf compression in patients with gynecologic malignancy. Obstet Gynecol 63:92, 1984

50. Aster RH: Heparin-induced thrombocytopenia and thrombosis. N Engl J Med 332:1374, 1995

51. Kolbenstvedt A, Kolstad P: The difficulties of complete pelvic lymph node dissection in radical hysterectomy for carcinoma of the cervix. Gynecol Oncol 4:244, 1976

52. Roberts WS, Cavanagh D, Marsden DE, Roberts VC: Urinary tract fistulas following ligation of the internal iliac artery during radical hysterectomy. Gynecol Oncol 21:359, 1985

53. Jensen JK, Lucci JA, DiSaia PJ et al: To drain or not to drain: a retrospective study of closed-suction drainage following radical hysterectomy with pelvic lymphadenectomy. Gynecol Oncol 51:46, 1993

54. Patsner B: Closed-suction drainage versus no drainage following radical abdominal hysterectomy with pelvic lymphadenectomy for stage IB cervical cancer. Gynecol Oncol 57:232, 1995

55. Anderson B: Ovarian function after radical hysterectomy. Gynecol Oncol 56:1, 1995

56. Monk BJ, Tewari K, Gamboa-Vujicic G et al: Does perioperative blood transfusion affect survival in patients with cervical cancer treated with radical hysterectomy? Obstet Gynecol 85: 343, 1995

57. Benjamin I, Barakat RR, Curtin JP et al: Blood transfusion for radical hysterectomy before and after the discovery of transfusion-related human immunodeficiency virus infection. Obstet Gynecol 84:974, 1994

58. Covens A, Rosen B, Gibbons A et al: Differences in the morbidity of radical hysterectomy between gynecological oncologists. Gynecol Oncol 51:39, 1993

59. Knapp RC, Donahue VC, Friedman EA: Dissection of paravesical and pararectal spaces in pelvic operations. Surg Gynecol Obstet 137:758, 1973

60. Hatch KD, Parham G, Shingleton HM et al: Ureteral strictures and fistulae following radical hysterectomy. Gynecol Oncol 19:17, 1984

61. Mann WJ, Vogel F, Patsner B, Chalas E: Management of lymphocysts after radical gynecologic surgery. Gynecol Oncol 33:248, 1989

62. Hoffman MS, Roberts WS, Cavanagh D: Neuropathies associated with radical pelvic surgery for gynecologic cancer. Gynecol Oncol 31:462, 1988

63. Mann WJ: Nutritional complications in gynecologic surgery. p. 260. In Orr JW, Shingleton HM (eds): Complications in Gynecologic Surgery. JB Lippincott, Philadelphia, 1994

64. Mikuta JJ: Cervical stump cancer. Am J Obstet Gynecol 105: 490, 1965

65. Green TH, Morse WJ: Management of invasive cervical cancer following inadvertent simple hysterectomy. Obstet Gynecol 33:763, 1969

66. Orr JW, Ball CG, Soong SJ et al: Surgical treatment of women found to have invasive cervix cancer at the time of total hysterectomy. Obstet Gynecol 68:353, 1986

67. Chapman JA, Mannel RS, DiSaia PJ et al: Surgical treatment of unexpected invasive cervical cancer found at total hysterectomy. Obstet Gynecol 80:931, 1992

68. Orr JW, Shingleton HM, Hatch KD et al: Correlation of perioperative morbidity and conization to radical hysterectomy interval. Obstet Gynecol 59:726, 1982

69. Monk BJ, Cha D-S, Walker JL et al: Extent of disease as an indication for pelvic radiation following radical hysterectomy and bilateral pelvic lymph node dissection in the treatment of stage IB and IIA cervical carcinoma. Gynecol Oncol 54:4, 1994

70. Abdulhayoglu G, Rich WM, Reynolds J, DiSaia PJ: Selective radiation therapy in stage IB uterine cervical carcinoma following radical pelvic surgery. Gynecol Oncol 10:84, 1980

71. Remy JC, Fruchter RG, Choi K et al: Complications of combined radical hysterectomy and pelvic radiation. Gynecol Oncol 24:317, 1986

72. Jacobs AJ, Perez CA, Camel HM, Kao M-S: Complications in patients receiving both irradiation and radical hysterectomy for carcinoma of the uterine cervix. Gynecol Oncol 22:273, 1985

73. Barter JF, Soong SJ, Shingleton HM et al: Complications of combined radical hysterectomy-postoperative radiation therapy in women with early stage cervical cancer. Gynecol Oncol 32:292, 1989

74. Fanning J, Hilgers RD, Palabrica C: Surgical stapling technique for radical hysterectomy. Gynecol Oncol 55:179, 1994

INTERNATIONAL FEDERATION OF GYNECOLOGY AND OBSTETRICS (FIGO) STAGING OF CARCINOMA

CARCINOMA OF THE CERVIX UTERI

Stage 0	Carcinoma in situ, intraepithelial carcinoma
Stage I	Carcinoma is strictly confined to the cervix (extension to the corpus should be disregarded)
IA	Preclinical carcinomas of the cervix, that is, those diagnosed only by microscopy
IA1	Measured invasion of stroma no greater than 3.0 mm in depth and no wider than 7.0 mm
IA2	Measured invasion of stroma greater than 3 mm and no greater than 5 mm and no wider than 7 mm
IB	Clinical lesions confined to the cervix or preclinical lesions greater than stage IA
IB1	Clinical lesions no greater than 4.0 cm in size
IB2	Clinical lesions greater than 4 cm in size
Stage II	The carcinoma extends beyond the cervix but has not extended to the pelvic wall. The carcinoma involves vagina but not as far as the lower third
IIA	No obvious parametrial involvement
IIB	Obvious parametrial involvement
Stage III	The carcinoma has extended to the pelvic wall. On rectal examination, there is no cancer-free space between the tumor and the pelvic wall
The tumor invades the lower third of vagina
All cases with a hydronephrosis or non-functioning kidney are included unless they are known to be due to other causes
IIIA	No extension to the pelvic wall
IIIB	Extension to the pelvic wall and/or hydronephrosis or nonfunctioning kidney
Stage IV	The carcinoma has extended beyond the true pelvis or has clinically involved the mucosa of the bladder or rectum. A bullous edema as such does not permit a case to be alloted to stage IV
IVA	Spread of the growth to adjacent organs
IVB	Spread to distant organs

CARCINOMA OF THE CORPUS UTERI

Stage IA G123	Tumor limited to endometrium
IB G123	Invasion to less than one-half the myometrium
IC G123	Invasion to more than one-half the myometrium
Stage IIA G123	Endocervical glandular involvement only
IIB G123	Cervical stroma invasion
Stage IIIA G123	Tumor invades serosa and/or adnexa, and/or positive peritoneal cytology
IIIB G123	Metastases to pelvic and/or para-aortic lymph nodes
Stage IVA G123	Tumor invasion of bladder and/or bowel mucosa
IVB	Distant metastases including intra-abdominal and/or inguinal lymph nodes

CARCINOMA OF THE VAGINA

Stage 0	Carcinoma in situ, intraepithelial carcinoma
Stage I	Carcinoma is limited to the vaginal wall
Stage II	Carcinoma has involved the subvaginal tissue but has not extended to the pelvic wall
Stage III	The carcinoma has extended to the pelvic wall
Stage IV	Carcinoma has extended beyond the true pelvis or has clinically involved the mucosa of the bladder or rectum. Bullous edema as such does not permit a case to be allotted to stage IV
IVA	Spread of the growth to adjacent organs and/or direct extension beyond the true pelvis
IVB	Spread to distant organs

CARCINOMA OF THE OVARY

Stage I	Growth limited to ovaries
IA	Growth limited to one ovary; no ascites present containing malignant cells. No tumor on the external surface; capsule intact
IB	Growth limited to both ovaries; no ascites present containing malignant cells. No tumor on the external surfaces; capsules intact
IC*	Tumor classified as either stage IA or IB but with tumor in the surface of one or both ovaries, or with ascites containing malignant cells present, or with positive peritoneal washings
Stage II	Growth involving one or both ovaries, with pelvic extension
IIA	Extension and/or metastases to the uterus and/or tubes
IIB	Extension to other pelvic tissues
IIC*	Tumor either stage IIA or IIB but with tumor on the surface of one or both ovaries, or with capsule(s) ruptured, or with ascites containing malignant cells present, or with positive peritoneal washings
Stage III	Tumor invading one or both ovaries with peritoneal implants outside the pelvis and/or positive retroperitoneal or inguinal nodes. Superficial liver metastasis equals stage III. Tumor is limited to the true pelvis but with histologically proven malignant extension to small bowel or omentum
IIIA	Tumor grossly limited to the true pelvis with negative nodes but with histologically confirmed microscopic seeding of abdominal peritoneal surfaces
IIIB	Tumor of one or both ovaries with histologically confirmed implants of abdominal peritoneal surfaces, none exceeding 2 cm in diameter, nodes are negative
IIIC	Abdominal implants greater than 2 cm in diameter and/or positive retroperitoneal or inguinal nodes
Stage IV	Growth involving one or both ovaries, with distant metastases. If pleural effusion is present, there must be positive cytologic findings to allot a case to stage IV. Parenchymal liver metastasis equals stage IV

CARCINOMA OF THE VULVA

Stage 0	
Tis	Carcinoma in situ; intraepithelial carcinoma
Stage I	
T1N0M0	Tumor confined to the vulva and/or perineum; 2 cm or less in greatest dimension; nodes not palpable
Stage II	
T2N0M0	Tumor confined to the vulva and/or perineum; more than 2 cm in greatest dimension, nodes not palpable
Stage III	
T3N0M0	Tumor of any size with
T3N1M0	1) adjacent spread to the lower urethra and/or vagina, or the anus, and/or
T1N1M0	2) unilateral regional lymph node metastasis
T2N1M0	
Stage IVA	
T1N2M0	Tumor invades any of the following:
T2N2M0	Upper urethra, bladder mucosa, rectal mucosa, pelvic bone, and/or bilateral regional node metastasis
T3N2M0	
T4 any N M0	
Stage IVB	
Any T	Any distant metastasis including pelvic lymph nodes
Any N, M1	

TNM Classification of Carcinoma of the Vulva

T   **Primary tumor**

Tis   Preinvasive carcinoma (carcinoma in situ)

T1   Tumor confined to the vulva and/or perineum; more than 2 cm in greatest dimension

T2   Tumor confined to the vulva and/or perineum; more than 2 cm in greatest dimension

T3   Tumor of any size with adjacent spread to the urethra and/or vagina, and/or to the anus

T4   Tumor of any size infiltrating the bladder mucosa and/or the rectal mucosa, including the upper part of the urethral mucosa and/or fixed to the bone

N   **Regional lymph nodes**

N0   No lymph node metastasis

N1   Unilateral regional lymph node metastasis

N2   Bilateral regional lymph node metastasis

M   **Distant metastasis**

M0   No clinical metastasis

M1   Distant metastasis (including pelvic lymph node metastasis)

SCHAUTA PROCEDURE

ROBERT F. PORGES

The radical abdominal and radical vaginal hysterectomy for the treatment of invasive cancer of the cervix were described at the turn of the century.[1-3] At that time, the advantages of a lymph node dissection, in terms of survival, were balanced against the additional morbidity of any abdominal procedure. After 1940, when Meigs described his radical abdominal hysterectomy and lymph node dissection, the complications of the abdominal approach had been largely conquered by antibiotics, safer blood transfusions, and a better understanding of the physiology of fluid and electrolyte balance. During the 1930s and 1940s except for a few centers on the European continent, the Schauta procedure was in decline. Not until widespread cytologic screening allowed cervical cancer to be diagnosed more commonly in a microinvasive stage did an indication re-emerge for the performance of the radical vaginal operation. By that time, however, the number of radical operative procedures for invasive cancer had diminished to such an extent that even large cancer centers did fewer radical hysterectomies and could afford by then only to train gynecologic oncologists in one type of procedure. Given the choice, and the greater utility of the abdominal approach, teaching of the Schauta operation was sacrificed.

INDICATIONS

The ideal candidate for a Schauta operation is a young woman with an early stage I lesion of the cervix with a modest degree of vaginal relaxation in whom the abdominal approach may be compromised either by obesity, multiple previous laparotomies, or regional enteritis. The postoperative recovery of these patients is generally swift and usually uncomplicated. An additional benefit of performing this operation is the insight one receives into the relationship of the connective tissues of the pelvis to the uterus and levator muscles.

PARAVAGINAL SCHUCHARDT INCISION

Although a paravaginal Schuchardt incision is usually an accompaniment of the procedure, it is not a necessary step in the operation, as the levator muscle may be approached with a small bilateral vaginal helping incision. The disadvantage of the Schuchardt incision is that it exposes the fatty tissues of the ischiorectal fossa, provides a nidus for the implantation of tumor cells, and contributes significantly to postoperative pain. By contrast, the Schuchardt incision is an essential component of the gynecologic surgeon's armamentarim. There is no substitute for the exposure it provides to gain access to the upper vagina for the repair of fistulas, to do a dilation and curettage in a very elderly nulliparous woman suspected of having endometrial carcinoma, and occasionally for removal of an impacted pessary.

AIM

The aim of the Schauta operation is to excise a wide portion of the paravaginal and parametrial connective tissues lateral to the cervix, almost to the lateral pelvic sidewall. Consequently, the uterine artery must be ligated at least 2 to 4 cm proximal to its insertion in the uterus. To accomplish this step with safety, the ureter must be separately identified

and displaced laterally. The usual circular incision in a vaginal hysterectomy, at the junction of cervix and vagina, is made instead 2 to 4 cm lower in the vagina, toward the introitus. After a circular incision of the full thickness of vaginal wall, the upper vagina is formed into a sleeve that encloses the carcinomatous cervix.

INSTRUMENTATION

The instruments used are standard, with the possible exception of two lateral vaginal retractors whose blades are about 3 cm longer than the average spade retractor. One posterior weighted speculum with a blade about 3 in. in length also should be provided. For the initial incisions and for the help incision, the cautery knife is used. This device

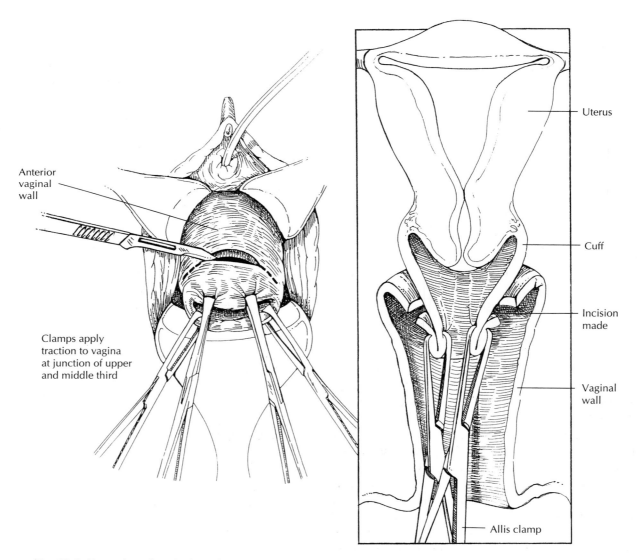

Anterior
vaginal
wall

Clamps apply
traction to vagina
at junction of upper
and middle third

Uterus

Cuff

Incision
made

Vaginal
wall

Allis clamp

Fig. 28-1. Formation of vaginal hood over the cervix. After initial incision, the Kocher clamps are reapplied to the upper cut edge of the vagina.

provides hemostasis and a clearer division of the different lines of cleavage.

OPERATIVE PROCEDURE

Formation of the Vaginal Cuff

At about the upper two-thirds of its length, the vaginal wall is grasped circumferentially with five or six Kocher clamps (Fig. 28-1). The cuff thus formed is then circularly incised with the cautery knife. The upper third of the vagina, which remains attached to the cervix, is freed by blunt dissection with a sponge stick in an upward direction and then closed with heavy silk sutures. The ends of these sutures are maintained long in order to enable the operator to exert a pull not only on the vaginal cuff, but also indirectly on cervix and uterus. At the same time, the suturing of the cuff conceals the malignancy and prevents spread.

The Help Incision

Using two Kocher clamps, the operator grasps the edge of the vaginal wall laterally, below the previously cut edge of the vagina. Using the cautery knife, an incision extending about 3 cm horizontally toward the pelvic wall is cut between the 2 forceps (Fig. 28-2). The surgeon then probes into the opening thus formed with the index finger. The finger is pushed laterally toward the pelvic wall, where it reaches the completely smooth surface of the levator muscle. At this level, a sweeping movement up and down mobilizes the paravaginal tissues completely (Fig. 28-3). This digital ex-

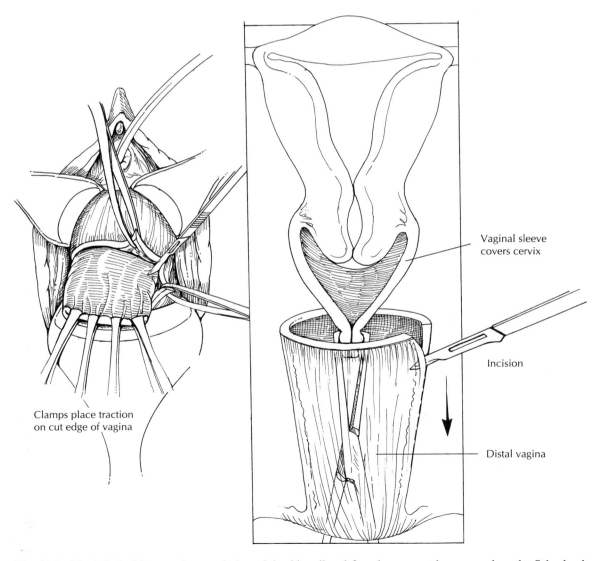

Clamps place traction on cut edge of vagina

Vaginal sleeve covers cervix

Incision

Distal vagina

Fig. 28-2. The help incision, used to reach the pelvic sidewall and free the parametria, may replace the Schuchardt incision.

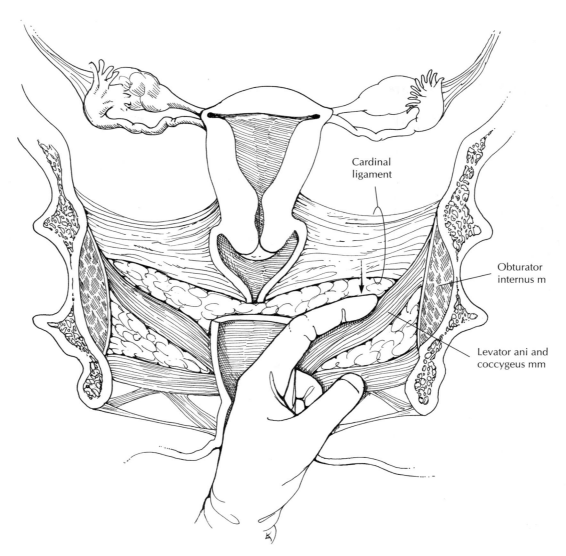

Cardinal ligament

Obturator internus m

Levator ani and coccygeus mm

Fig. 28-3. The index finger runs along the upper surface of the levator muscle, helping to mobilize the paravaginal tissue.

ploration extends posteriorly as far as the lateral rectal wall and anteriorly lateral to the bladder. Upward separation is limited by the dense parametrial tissue, which is found cephalad.

Separation of the Rectum and Opening of the Pouch of Douglas

With the silk traction sutures forcibly pulled upward, a long posterior retractor is used to retract and protect the rectum. The posterior peritoneum is opened and the uterosacral ligaments are identified. A lateral retractor is now inserted into the lateral space previously opened by finger exploration. This brings the connective tissues of the pararectal spaces into full view.

Dissection of Ligaments and Connective Tissue

Dissection of the uterosacral ligaments and pararectal connective tissue is now completed. Using large curved scissors, these structures are cut as close as possible to the levator ani fascia. No ligature need be placed before or after cutting, because the arterial blood supply for this part of the parametrial tissue will be controlled by lateral ligation of the uterine arteries.

Separation of Bladder and Ureter

The silk traction sutures are now drawn downward. The base of the bladder and its lateral attachments are separated, first from the vaginal tube and then higher up from the cer-

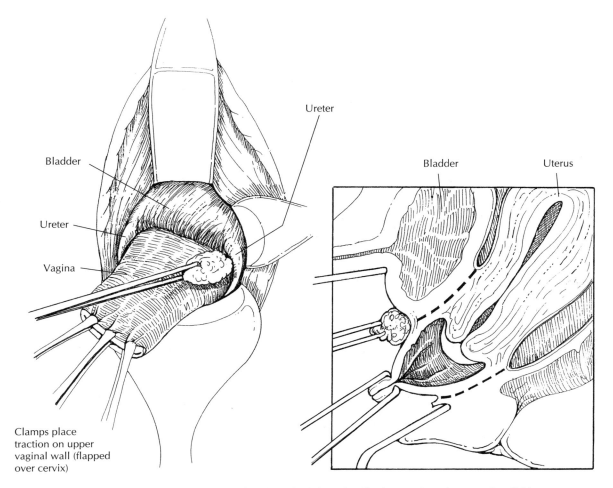

Fig. 28-4. Lateral advancement of the bladder brings the distal ureter into the operative field.

vix. The separation may be achieved for the most part by blunt dissection with a sponge stick. Only thicker strands, if encountered, require scissor dissection. An anterior retractor is inserted to lift the mobilized floor of the bladder, automatically bringing the ureteral aspect of the bladder into view (Fig. 28-4). With the ureters still attached to the parametrial tissue, the two pillars that contain the ureters become evident. With sponge stick dissection and occasional use of fine scissors, the ureters are pushed lateral and cephalad. At this time, the uterine artery comes into view. With continued dissection, the ureters are pushed upward and out of the operative field. The parametrial tissue can then be visualized in its entirety, and the full course of the uterine artery can be observed.

Ligation of Uterine Artery and Excision of Parametrium

With large curved scissors the parametrial tissue is divided as closely as possible to the pelvic wall without preliminary ligation. The uterine artery is then ligated as closely as possi-

ble to the lateral wall. Ligation close to the pelvic wall results in severance of the artery before arborization, and therefore, hemostasis is not a problem.

Opening of Vesicouterine Peritoneum and Removal of Specimen

These steps follow the usual sequence of an ordinary vaginal hysterectomy. The removal of the tubes and ovaries is optional, since cervical carcinoma spreads primarily by the lymphatics to the parametrial tissue and not to the adnexa.

Closure

The free vesical reflection of peritoneum anteriorly and the peritoneal fold over the rectum posteriorly are approximated in the midline with two sutures. The adnexal stumps on either side are religated with the ends of these sutures. This effects complete closure of the peritoneum, with all stumps remaining extraperitonealized. Lateral sutures into the vaginal wall, for hemostasis, are optional.

SUMMARY

The radical vaginal hysterectomy is well tolerated, even in patients with obesity and medical complications. It is an appropriate operation in a patient with an early stage invasive carcinoma of the cervix. As more patients are being diagnosed with microinvasive disease, it was anticipated that the number of Schauta operations would increase. This has not happened. Perhaps, if lymph node dissections are done more often laparoscopically, the popularity of the Schauta operation may return, as it meets many of the requirements of less invasive surgery.

REFERENCES

1. Porges JC: Radical vaginal hysterectomy. Clin Obstet Gynecol 4:217, 1961
2. Halban J: Gynaekologische Operationslehre. Urban & Schwartzenberg, Vienna, 1932
3. Schauta F: Die erweiterte vaginale Totalextirpation. Safar, Vienna 1908

CHAPTER TWENTY-NINE

PELVIC AND PARA-AORTIC LYMPHADENECTOMY

KEITH M. HARRIGILL

JOEL M. CHILDERS

In the United States last year, there were approximately 13,000 cases of invasive cervical carcinoma, 19,000 cases of ovarian carcinoma, and 33,000 cases of endometrial carcinoma.[1] Each of these diseases may spread from their respective sites of origin to the lymph nodes in the pelvic or para-aortic regions, and the presence of this metastatic disease carries implications for the prognosis and treatment of these cancers. For this reason, the International Federation of Gynecology and Obstetrics includes lymph node sampling in the surgical staging of ovarian and endometrial cancers. Although the staging of cervical carcinoma remains clinical, the surgical management of this disease also calls for removal of regional lymphatic tissue, and lymph node sampling/dissection may be used for treatment and planning.

The extent of the lymphadenectomy to be performed in each malignancy is a matter of philosophy, and is dependent on many factors. There is little worldwide consensus on this issue, unfortunately, and opinions differ on numerous issues, including

1. Whether para-aortic lymphadenectomy should be performed in patients with early cervical or endometrial cancer

2. Whether para-aortic lymphadenectomy should include the left side

3. Whether bilateral lymphadenectomy should be performed in unilateral adnexal malignancies

4. Whether para-aortic lymphadenectomy should include the lymph nodes between the inferior mesenteric and renal arteries for adnexal malignancies

5. Whether lymphadenectomies should be a sampling (selective) or be therapeutic (complete)

This debate is beyond the scope of this chapter; however, we believe these decisions should not be made based on the surgical technique employed.

Traditionally, lymphadenectomy has been carried out by laparotomy. However, recent improvements in laparoscopic techniques and equipment have led to increased interest in the performance of laparoscopic pelvic and para-aortic lymphadenectomy. It is now feasible and safe to perform these procedures laparoscopically with efficacy comparable to that of laparotomy, as well as the known benefits of diminished postoperative discomfort, shorter hospital stays, and reduced recuperative times. In this chapter, the authors present their current techniques for laparoscopic pelvic and para-aortic lymphadenectomy.

INDICATIONS

The indications for laparoscopic pelvic and para-aortic lymphadenectomy are listed in Table 29-1.

Cervical Cancer

Patients with stage IB or IIA cervical cancer may be candidates for radical hysterectomy, while patients with more advanced cancers are managed with radiotherapy. If lymph node sampling is carried out in a candidate for radical hysterectomy and metastatic disease is encountered on the frozen section, the surgeon has the option of selecting radiotherapy rather than continuing with the hysterectomy. Such an approach may save the patient unnecessary morbidity. If the lymph nodes are found to be free of disease, a hysterectomy may be performed laparoscopically or vaginally, thereby avoiding a laparotomy.

In patients with advanced cervical carcinoma for whom radiotherapy is planned, selective lymphadenectomy may be performed at the cephalad extent of the planned radiation field and just beyond. This sampling would include the proximal common and low para-aortic lymph nodes bilaterally. Traditionally, this procedure is performed using an extraperitoneal approach because of the known increase in radiation enteritis if both laparotomy and transperitoneal lymphadenectomy are performed.[2] Therefore, the use of laparoscopy in this setting remains controversial, because a transperitoneal technique is used for the para-aortic lymphadenectomy. There is animal evidence, however, that the laparotomy incision rather than the peritoneal incision is the culprit.[3]

Ovarian Carcinoma

Laparoscopic lymphadenectomy can be used in patients with ovarian carcinoma in two situations.[4] The first instance is the surgical staging of those patients with presumed early ovarian cancer (stage I or II). Unilateral or bilateral selective lymphadenectomy from the renal vessels to the pelvis is required and should include samples of the obturator, common iliac, external iliac, and internal iliac nodes as well as the para-aortic nodes both above and below the inferior mesenteric artery.

The second group of ovarian cancer patients eligible for laparoscopic lymphadenectomy include those with advanced disease who have undergone surgical debulking, platinum-based chemotherapy and have no evidence of disease following treatment. A thorough inspection should be carried out in this group, as lymphadenectomy is indicated only in the absence of any intraperitoneal disease.

Endometrial Carcinoma

A combined laparoscopic and vaginal approach may be used in patients with clinical stage I adenocarcinoma of the endometrium.[5,6] If a laparoscopic surgical staging procedure is to be carried out, a complete intraperitoneal inspection, pelvic washings, and lymphadenectomy should be performed in additon to the vaginal hysterectomy. Surgical staging may also be carried out in the patient who was not staged at the time of hysterectomy.[7] Adequate sampling of the obturator, external, internal, and common iliac nodes is particularly important in endometrial cancer. Para-aortic lymphadenectomy may be performed at the discretion of the surgeon but, when done, should involve only those nodes below the inferior mesenteric artery.

BACKGROUND

The use of operative laparoscopy in gynecologic oncology is a very recent development. Dargent and Salvat[8] introduced the concept of using laparoscopic lymphadenectomy in pelvic malignancies in 1989, when they reported a series of patients with early cervical carcinoma in whom they used an extraperitoneal approach to sample pelvic nodes prior to radical hysterectomy.

Querlou et al[9] further demonstrated the feasibility of a transperitoneal approach to the pelvic nodes in 1991 when they reported their technique of staging patients with early cervical carcinoma. The development of techniques for low para-aortic lymphadenectomy soon followed and patients

---

Table 29-1. Indications for Laparoscopic Lymphadenectomy in Gynecologic Oncology

Cervical cancer
   Radical hysterectomy candidate
      Prior to laparotomy to rule out positive nodes
      To convert abdominal procedure to
         Laparoscopic radical hysterectomy
         Laparoscopic-assisted radical hysterectomy
         Radical vaginal hysterectomy
   Radiotherapy candidate
      Before standard pelvic radiotherapy
      To assist transperitoneal interstitial needle placement
Ovarian cancer
   Staging early carcinoma
   Second-look laparoscopy
Endometrial cancer
   Staging in conjunction with laparoscopic-assisted vaginal hysterectomy for clinical stage I carcinoma
   Staging following hysterectomy in the patient who has not been surgically staged

with endometrial and ovarian carcinomas joined those with cervical carcinoma in published series.[5,10,11] Most recently, the performance of high para-aortic lymphadenectomy clearly showed that complete laparoscopic staging of pelvic malignancies is possible.[4,12–14] Given the shorter hospital stay, decreased postoperative discomfort, and shorter convalescent period associated with laparoscopy compared with laparotomy, one may assume that the use of laparoscopic lymphadenectomy will increase in the future.

This chapter outlines the transperitoneal technique of pelvic and para-aortic lymphadenectomy developed and used at the University of Arizona since 1990.

PREOPERATIVE CONSIDERATIONS

Laboratory Evaluation

The authors routinely obtain a complete blood count with differential, renal and liver panels, type and hold, and a urinalysis for our surgical patients. A chest radiograph is also obtained if the patient is over 50 years old and has had no prior radiographic pulmonary study in the preceding 6 months, has a significant pulmonary history, or is at risk of pulmonary metastasis. We also perform electrocardiograms in patients over 60 or patients with known cardiac disease. A baseline CA-125 is occasionally useful in patients with known or suspected ovarian or advanced endometrial carcinoma. A urine pregnancy test should be strongly considered in patients of reproductive age.

Bowel Preparation

The laparoscopic approach to pelvic and para-aortic lymphadenectomy is occasionally limited by inadequate exposure caused, in part, by poor bowel preparation. Therefore, all patients should receive an adequate preoperative bowel preparation. We currently favor placing the patient on a liquid diet during the 2 days before surgery and having the patient consume one 240-ml bottle of magnesium citrate on each of those days. Alternatively, a 1-day bowel preparation using Golytely provides acceptable results. We do not routinely use oral or intravenous antibiotics.

Anesthesia

After evaluation by an anesthesiologist, general anesthesia is implemented with subsequent placement of an endotracheal tube and an end-tidal carbon dioxide monitor. Pulse oximetry is indicated, and placement of a nasogastric or orogastric tube will minimize stomach distension. This decreases the likelihood of viscus perforation during insertion of the trocar or Veress needle and facilitates the placement of the omentum and small bowel into the upper abdomen.

A Foley catheter should be used to ensure continuous bladder drainage.

The supine position is used for all patients except those in whom vaginal surgery is anticipated; in those cases, the dorsal lithotomy position is more appropriate. If the dorsal lithotomy position is to be used, keeping the patient's knees at or below the plane of the body will maximize the available operative room for the surgeon, particularly if performing para-aortic lymphadenectomy. The authors also prefer to tuck both of the patient's arms to her sides, as this allows more mobility for the surgeons. The arms must be tucked with the hand in the neutral position, taking care to pad the ulnar nerve. Because of the inaccessability of peripheral intravenous sites with tucked arms, the anesthesiologist may prefer to place a central venous or arterial line. Temperature monitoring, heating blankets, and sequential compression devices are recommended. An electrocautery grounding pad should be placed.

Operating Room and Instrumentation

The patient is brought to the operating room, placed under general anesthesia, and positioned as mentioned above. If the dorsal lithotomy position is indicated, the authors favor the use of fiberglass bows or candy-cane stirrups, although Allen universal stirrups may also be used. Shaving is avoided except in the unusually hirsute patient, in which case it is performed immediately before the surgery. The abdomen is prepared using chlorhexadine gluconate or povidone-iodine, paying particular attention to the umbilicus. If vaginal surgery is anticipated, then vaginal preparation is performed as well. The patient is draped using a standard laparotomy drape, or a perineal/abdominal drape if a combined approach is planned.

Familiarity with instruments and troubleshooting equipment problems is as important as knowledge of the surgical techniques. The problems associated with a lack of familiarity with laparoscopic equipment are compounded if the surgeon works out of several hospitals, each with different equipment. Simple problems may result in long delays if troubleshooting skills are not acquired. We strongly recommend acquiring these skills as rapidly as possible, not relying on hospital personnel to solve video, insufflator, camera, and light source problems. Equipment, including video apparatus, should be checked prior to induction of anesthesia.

The instrument requirements for laparoscopic lymphadenectomy are relatively modest. Most of the instruments involved may be reusable; however, the authors use disposable scissors because they are invariably sharp. On occasion, a laparoscopic clip-applier may be needed. Specialized instruments such as laparoscopic needle-drivers, knot-pushers, pre-tied slipknots, staplers, and fascial closure devices are frequently useful and should be available.

Instruments Used in Laparoscopic Pelvic And Para-Aortic Lymphadenectomy

- One 12-mm, one 10-mm, and two five-mm disposable trocars and sleeves
- Four no. 0 silk sutures on cutting needles to sew the laparoscopic sleeves to the skin
- A 10-mm, zero-degree telescope
- A three-chip camera
- A Xenon light source
- An high-flow insufflator (at least 9 L/min)
- Two high-resolution video monitors on movable carts
- Electrocautery unit with monopolar and bipolar capabilities
- Videotape recording equipment
- An assortment of 5-mm laparoscopic graspers
- Large spoon or tripronged forceps to assist in the extirpation of nodal tissue
- Sharp blunt-tipped scissors with monopolar cautery capabilities
- An irrigation-suction apparatus
- Several minilaparotomy pads (4 × 16 cm)

OPERATIVE TECHNIQUE

Instrument Insertion

Most gynecologists are very comfortable obtaining access to the peritoneal cavity. Currently, the authors prefer the technique of direct trocar insertion through the umbilicus without the prior establishment of a pneumoperitoneum. This technique, when done properly, is safe and has the benefits of allowing faster access to the cavity as well as faster insufflation rates through the trocar sleeve compared to the Veress needle.

Perforating towel clips are used to grasp the skin on either side of the umbilicus and the anterior abdominal wall is elevated. A #11 blade is used to make a vertical incision through the base of the umbilicus, using a hemostat to provide visualization as needed. A 10-mm disposable trocar is then introduced through the skin incision directly downward. The authors believe that angling the trocar towards the pelvis, as is traditionally taught, is not necessary, increases the incidence of preperitoneal placement, and makes inspection of the upper abdomen more difficult. The use of marked upward traction on the anterior abdominal wall during insertion of the trocar is mandatory. Once the sleeve is in place, the 10-mm telescope is introduced

and intraperitoneal placement is confirmed before abdominal insufflation.

An alternative approach is preferred in those patients with umbilical hernias or previous abdominal surgeries in which the umbilicus was involved in the incision. The incidence of adhesions from the umbilicus to the underlying abdominal structure may be as high as 68 percent.[15] Therefore, the authors prefer a left upper quadrant approach in this type of patient.

The left upper quadrant approach involves placing a Veress needle in the 9th or 10th intercostal space between the left midclavicular and midaxillary lines. When inserted properly, two distinct pops will be felt; the first as the needle passes through the intercostal fascia and the second as the needle enters the peritoneal cavity. A pneumoperitoneum is established to an intraperitoneal pressure of 25 mmHg. A second incision is made in the left midclavicular line inferior to the costal margin; this incision should be larger than 5 mm to avoid skin resistance and unwanted downward displacement of the anterior abdominal wall during introduction of the primary trocar. A 5-mm trocar is introduced through this incision and a 5-mm laparoscope is then used to confirm intraperitoneal placement, as well as to assess the location of adhesions and plan the placement of ancillary ports. The intraperitoneal pressure may be reduced to 15 mmHg following successful introduction of the 5-mm trocar. If the surgeon is not comfortable with this approach, open laparoscopy is an acceptable alternative; however, a lateral insertion site affords better visualization if adhesiolysis is required.

The authors use three ancillary ports. Each of these ancillary ports is placed under direct laparoscopic visualization following establishment of an adequate pneumoperitoneum. Transillumination of the anterior abdominal wall to minimize the risk of laceration of superficial vessels should be carried out before port insertion. A 5-mm trocar is placed lateral to the rectus abdominis and inferior epigastric vessels bilaterally in the middle of the lower abdomen. The third ancillary port is placed two fingerbreadths above the symphysis in the midline and should be 10 to 12 mm in size.

Following satisfactory placement of these ports, the sleeves should be inserted to their desired depth in the abdominal cavity. Number 0 silk suture may then be used to fix the sleeves to the skin, thereby preventing inadvertent removal of the sleeves with concomitant loss of pneumoperitoneum during instrument changes (Fig. 29-1).

Inspection of the Peritoneal Cavity

Once the laparoscopic ports are in place, a systematic examination of the intraperitoneal cavity should be carried out. This examination must be thorough since any disease noted will be of prognostic importance. The authors examine the iliocecal region first and proceed in a clockwise fashion.

The patient should not be placed into the Trendelenburg

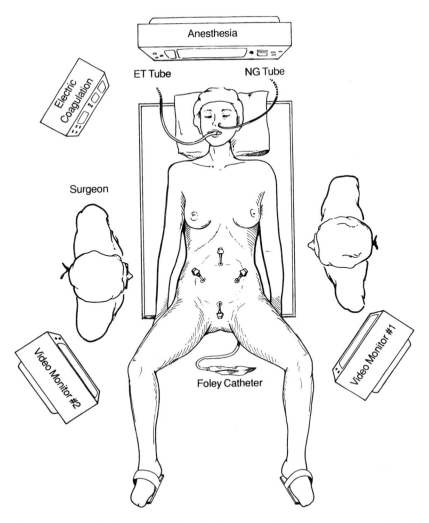

Fig. 29-1. Operating room set-up for laparoscopic lymphadenectomy. Note the arrangement of the lateral 5-mm ports and the midline 10- to 12-mm ports. All ports are affixed to the skin with silk suture. ET, endotracheal; NG, nasogastric. (From Childers,[19] with permission.)

position until the examination of the upper abdomen is completed. Following completion of the examination and before initiating the lymphadenectomy, intraperitoneal washings may be taken.

Before beginning the lymphadenectomy, identification of several landmarks should be carried out. The external and common iliac vessels are usually appreciable under the peritoneum at the pelvic sidewall. The bifurcation of the common iliac artery into the hypogastric and external iliac arteries may also be noted, and the right ureter can often be seen as it passes over this bifurcation. In the thin patient, the inferior mesenteric artery and left ureter may be seen adjacent to the aorta. The obliterated umbilical artery, which traverses the anterior abdominal wall from its origin from the distal hypogastric toward the umbilicus, is the most important structure in gaining access to the obturator lymph nodes.

Peritoneal Incision Considerations

The peritoneum may be incised in two locations to provide access to the pelvic and para-aortic lymph nodes. An incision over the external iliac vessels extending from the round ligament to the ovarian vessels will allow access to the external iliac, internal iliac, obturator, and low common iliac lymph nodes. Using this incision provides sufficient exposure to perform a pelvic lymphadenectomy. A separate incision is called for if para-aortic lymphadenectomy is indicated. This incision overlies the aorta and extends from the transverse duodenum or small bowel mesentery to the proximal common iliac artery; this incision provides access to the low para-aortic lymph nodes. To perform a complete bilateral pelvic and para-aortic lymphadenectomy, a total of three incisions is needed: one incision over the aorta and one incision over each of the external iliac arteries.

Intraperitoneal Structures Examined During the Abdominal Cavity Survey

- Iliocecal junction and appendix
- Right paracolic gutter
- Gallbladder
- Surface of the right lobe of the liver
- Right hemidiaphragm
- Falciform ligament
- Greater curvature of the stomach
- Anterior wall of the stomach
- Left hemidiaphragm
- Supracolic omentum
- Transverse colon
- Infracolic omentum
- Descending colon
- Left paracolic gutter
- Rectosigmoid and its mesentery

Laparoscopic Pelvic Lymphadenectomy

The laparoscopic pelvic lymphadenectomy involves sampling the obturator, external iliac, internal iliac, and common iliac lymph nodes. The surgeon stands on the side of the patient contralateral to the pelvic nodes to be dissected, placing graspers through the suprapubic port and the monopolar-capable scissors through the lateral port nearest to the surgeon. The assistant assumes control of the telescope in the umbilical port and places graspers through the remaining lateral port.

If a hysterectomy is to be performed, the round ligament is grasped and incised, with the incision extended superiorly and inferiorly. If the uterus is to be conserved, this peritoneal incision is made between the round ligament at its insertion into the inguinal canal and the infundibulopelvic ligament, overlying the external iliac artery and vein. Either of these incisions provides adequate access to the paravesical/obturator space, which is opened primarily with blunt dissection. This dissection is made considerably easier if the obliterated umbilical artery, lying near the external iliac vessels, is retracted medially; the paravesical space is located between the obliterated umbilical artery and the external iliac vein. This space is opened and the obturator nerve, artery, and vein are located; the obturator nodes lie between the obturator nerve and the external iliac vein.

The authors begin the pelvic lymphadenectomy with the obturator lymph nodes, since this area is the most dependent of the spaces to be dissected (Fig. 29-2). If this dissection is not done first, then blood, irrigant, and lymph fluid from less gravity-dependent areas may settle over the obturator space, obscuring the field. A minilaparotomy pad, initially placed through the 12-mm suprapubic port and left in the pelvis for most of the case, may be used to blot the operative field free of blood as needed.

Once the obturator nerve is identified, the obturator nodal bundle anterior and lateral to the nerve is gently grasped and freed from the obturator nerve using blunt and sharp

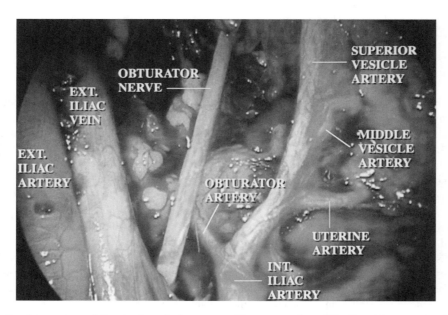

Fig. 29-2. Left pelvic anatomy following lymphadenectomy. Obturator nodes will be found between the obturator nerve and the external iliac vein. External, common, and internal iliac nodes lie ventral to those arteries. (From Hallum and Childers,[20] with permission.)

dissection. Next, the nodes are freed from the medial aspect of the external iliac vein along its length. Aberrant or accessory vessels emptying into the external iliac vein are frequently found in this area; caution must be exercised to avoid lacerations.

The nodal bundle is followed distally to the pelvic wall, where it is coagulated, then cut. Once this is done, the only remaining attachment of the obturator nodal bundle is at the junction of the internal and external iliac arteries; adequate visualization of this area is frequently limited as the nodal bundle begins to course laterally. These attachments are coagulated and cut as before, paying particular attention to the course of the ureter in this region. Once the nodes are free, they may be removed through the suprapubic midline port using spoon forceps.

External iliac lymph nodes are removed in a similar fashion through the same incision. This blunt and sharp dissection begins by finding the adventitial plane of the external iliac artery and following it to the circumflex iliac artery, using monopolar cautery as needed to maintain hemostasis. The genitofemoral nerve courses nearby and is susceptible to damage. This dissection is extended proximally to the point where the ovarian vessels or the ureter crosses the iliac vessels, and distally along the common iliac artery. In this way, the internal and common iliac nodes may be removed along with the external iliac nodes. The distal portion of this nodal dissection is greatly facilitated if the assistant retracts the ureter cephalad through the peritoneal incision.

When the pelvic lymphadenectomy is done on the left side, it may be necessary to take down the rectosigmoid from the left pelvic sidewall if the rectosigmoid is not sufficiently mobile. In this case, an incision along the white line of Toldt will provide access to the retroperitoneal space as well as mobilization of the rectosigmoid. If access to the retroperitoneal space is not limited by the rectosigmoid, then an incision between the ovarian vessels and the round ligament, as described above, may be made. The dissection proceeds as above, with the surgeon standing on the side contralateral to the nodes of interest.

At the end of the procedure, the operative site is irrigated and inspected for hemostasis. The peritoneum is left open, and no drains are used.

Laparoscopic Para-Aortic Lymphadenectomy

Proper placement of the small bowel into the upper abdomen will provide adequate visualization of the operative field and is the key to successful para-aortic lymphadenectomy. This packing of the bowel is accomplished by identifying the mesentery of the small bowel, flipping it cephalad, and carefully laying the small bowel into the upper abdomen. This process is greatly facilitated with a good bowel preparation, and the small bowel may be inspected for metastatic implants while it is positioned into the upper quadrants of the abdomen. Trendelenburg's—and, occasionally, left lateral tilt—positioning will assist in keeping the bowel out of the para-aortic area. In the grossly obese patient or in the patient with a poor bowel preparation, the addition of another port specifically to maintain the bowel's position in the upper abdomen may be necessary. The importance of properly packing the bowel is impossible to overstate, and any time lost during this portion of the surgery is more than made up later when the para-aortic field is visually unimpeded and the surgeon operates without constantly replacing recalcitrant bowel.

The transverse duodenum can often be seen as it crosses the aorta and vena cava. Elevating the small bowel mesentery at the aorta will aid the surgeon in visualizing the third portion of the duodenum; the aorta, right common iliac artery, and the ureter as it crosses the right iliac vessels should all be located before beginning the para-aortic lymphadenectomy.

Right-Side Para-Aortic Lymphadenectomy

The surgeon begins the procedure by standing on the left side of the patient, using a pair of graspers through the suprapubic port and scissors through the left lateral port. The assistant stands on the right side of the patient, using graspers in the right lateral port and assuming control of the camera and telescope that is placed through the umbilical port. The assistant's role is to provide exposure and visualization for the surgeon throughout the lymphadenectomy. The camera should be oriented so that the aorta and inferior vena cava are horizontal on the video screen, with the patient's head to the right of the screen. This allows the operating surgeon to be completely oriented.

The surgeon begins by incising the peritoneum over the aorta and right common iliac artery. This incision is extended inferiorly along the right common iliac to the right ureter, and superiorly along the aorta to the mesentery of the small bowel or transverse duodenum. The lateral peritoneal edges are then lifted, and blunt dissection is carried out laterally toward the psoas muscle. The right ureter must be identified. Lateral dissection is continued below the ureter and above the vena cava and psoas. The ureter is then elevated and moved out of the way by the assistant, who accomplishes this retraction using the grasper placed through the right lateral port. This improves exposure, prevents ureteral damage, and also creates a small tent, which helps prevent small bowel from slipping into the field.

The surgeon then sharply dissects the nodal bundle off the surface of the aorta by working in the adventitial plane of the aorta. This adventitial dissection is extended down the right common iliac artery and up the aorta as far as possible.

The process of unroofing the nodal bundle from the vena cava does not begin until the tissue has been freed from its vascular attachments. The separation of the nodal bundle from the vena cava can begin anywhere along the vena cava and is accomplished by grasping and elevating the nodal bundle. The cava will be tented upwards as well, so care must taken to stay in the proper plane. Small vessels should be cauterized with the tips of the scissors using monopolar electricity (coagulation current). Even a small amount of bleeding can stain the tissue, obscuring visualization. It is very uncommon to encounter a perforating vessel from the vena cava that cannot be controlled with monopolar electricity. Short bursts of current using a fulguration technique in which sparks are allowed to jump from the electrode to the tissue are completely safe, even using coagulation current.

The nodal bundle is easily separated from its lateral attachments to the cava and psoas using blunt dissection. The bundle is also easily transected at its cephalad and caudad extents with fulgurating monopolar electricity. Electrical effects are greatly enhanced if tension is kept on the tissue. Caution must be used during these transections, as the transverse duodenum and the right ureter could be easily damaged if they are not completely visualized. The bundle may then be extracted through the lower midline port using the spoon forceps. Hemostasis should be confirmed.

Right common iliac node sampling, if it is to be carried out, may be performed through the same peritoneal incision. The assistant retracts the ureter, atraumatically, toward the pelvis, exposing the nodal bundle over the right common iliac beyond its bifurcation. The dissection proceeds as before down the common iliac artery in the adventitial plane first (Fig. 29-3).

Left-Side Para-Aortic Lymphadenectomy

The surgeon, now standing on the right side of the patient, places graspers through the lower midline port and scissors through the left lateral port. The assistant holds the telescope and attached camera in the umbilical port, taking care to orient the camera properly with the major vessels horizontal on the monitor and the patient's head to the left of the screen. This positioning facilitates the actions of the surgeon, but the monitor image will be upside down for the assistant.

If the peritoneal incision has not already been made, incising the preaortic peritoneum is done in exactly the same manner as for the right-side para-aortic lymphadenectomy. This incision is carried as far cephalad as possible, and will eventually be limited by the small bowel mesentery or the transverse duodenum. The caudal terminus of the incision should be carried to the proximal left common iliac artery.

The surgeon then dissects in the adventitial plane along the aorta both cephalad and caudad. This dissection should be as extensive as possible to provide maximum room and visualization for the lymphadenectomy. On the left side, the cephalad extent of the nodal dissection will be limited by the origin of the inferior mesenteric artery. Since its origin from the aorta is frequently difficult to visualize, care should be taken to avoid injury to either the aorta or the inferior mesenteric artery. Again, the more extensive the dissection, the better the visibility will be during this portion of the procedure.

Only after the aortic adventitia has been adequately dissected free should lateral dissection along the psoas be car-

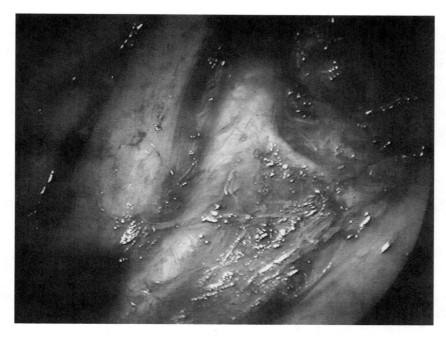

Fig. 29-3. Para-aortic anatomy following low right para-aortic lymphadenectomy. The vena cava lies to the left and the aorta to the right. The lymphatic tissue has been completely removed.

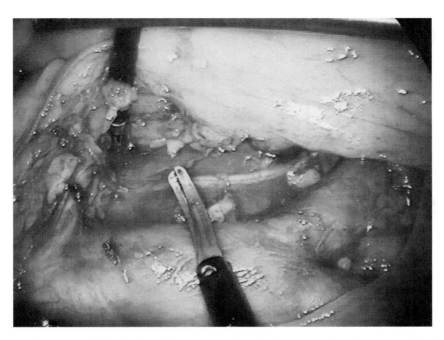

Fig. 29-4. Para-aortic anatomy following low left para-aortic lymphadenectomy. Note the aorta and its bifurcation. The inferior mesenteric artery is being retracted by the graspers.

ried out. By staying in the previously dissected adventitial plane, the surgeon will be able to safely dissect beneath the left ureter and rectosigmoid mesentery. Note that the sequence of the left-side dissection differs from that of the right, where the lateral dissection is done after the peritoneal incision is made but before the dissection of the aortic adventitia.

Lateral dissection is performed until the psoas muscle and its tendon are clearly identified. The assistant may then place either the irrigator or grasper into the dissected space beneath the rectosigmoid mesentery and left ureter, retracting to provide maximum exposure to the left-side para-aortic lymph nodes. This exposure is crucial because of the lateral position of the nodes with respect to the aorta.

Once adequate exposure is achieved, the nodal bundle is grasped near the aortic bifurcation and lifted anteriorly. A window should be created bluntly beneath the nodal chain at its caudal end; transection of the bundle may then be carried out using cautery and scissors. Dissection of the bundle then proceeds cephalad using sharp and blunt dissection, with cautery and clips used as needed for hemostasis. The cephalad end of the nodal chain is transected near the inferior mesenteric artery. The specimen is removed through the lower midline port, and hemostasis is again confirmed (Fig. 29-4).

Infrarenal Para-Aortic Lymphadenectomy

The vena cava and the aorta are separated from the transverse duodenum by blunt and sharp dissection. This dissection is carried cephalad, but lateral dissection is also carried out by sweeping the laparoscopic instruments bluntly toward the psoas muscles. The assistant maintains upward traction on the transverse duodenum. A fifth port may be needed to aid in the elevation of the duodenum. Anterior retraction is then accomplished through the right lower quadrant and left upper quadrant, with the surgeon facing cephalad. The monitors should be repositioned toward the patient's head. The authors find it much easier for the surgeon to remove the nodes contralateral to the side on which the surgeon is standing; however, this is not absolutely necessary.

After adequate cephalad exposure is obtained, the nodal dissection is continued. On the right side, one continues the previously performed lymphadenectomy to the origin of the ovarian vein, which typically enters the vena cava distal to or near the left renal vein (Figs. 29-5 and 29-6). On the left, the surgeon will be limited by the inferior mesenteric artery. By first extending the dissection caudad to the inferior mesenteric artery, enough of the nodal bundle may be freed to allow completion of the dissection of the chain by working cephalad to the artery.

On the left side, it is helpful to identify the left ovarian vein as it traverses toward the left renal vein. Blunt dissection between the nodal bundle and the left ovarian vein defines the lateral extent of the dissection. The left renal vein is usually found immediately after separating the transverse duodenum off the cava and aorta, but may not be found until dissecting the lymphatic tissue off the adventitia of the aorta. The renal vein defines the cephalad boundary. The medial boundary is the lymphatic attachments to the aortic adventitia. With the lymphatic bundle separated from the left ovarian vein and the left renal vein clearly visualized, the surgeon

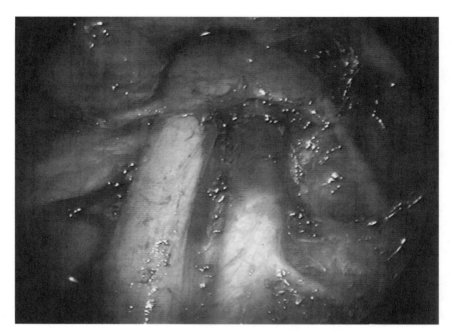

Fig. 29-5. The para-aortic area following high node dissection. Note the right ovarian vein entering the vena cava at the level of the left renal vein, which is seen crossing the aorta. The left ovarian vein enters the left renal vein directly.

separates the nodal bundle from the adventitia of the aorta up to the left renal vein. The bundle is bluntly separated from its inferior attachment, taking extreme care not to injure lumbar veins in the area. The authors usually pack the field with a minilaparotomy pad following this dissection.

The peritoneum is not closed, nor are retroperitoneal drains placed. The small bowel mesentery is repositioned over the para-aortic incision site at the end of the dissection and the fascia and skin are closed in the standard fashion.

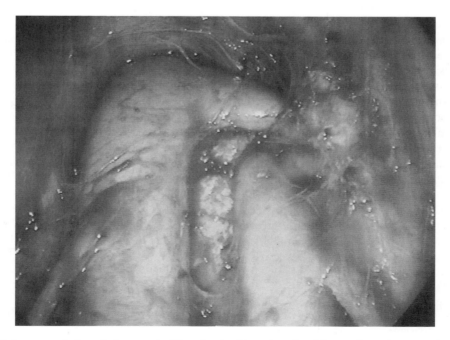

Fig. 29-6. High para-aortic lymphadenectomy. Note that in this patient the right ovarian vein enters the vena cava at a considerable distance below the insertion of the left renal vein.

COMPLICATIONS

Vascular Complications

The most commonly injured vein during a para-aortic lymphadenectomy is the vena cava. Vena cava injuries during the removal of nodal tissue can occur as a result of tearing perforating veins extending from the vena cava to the nodal bundle, or by direct trauma to the vena cava itself. The authors have had three such injuries in over 100 laparoscopic para-aortic lymphadenectomies. The first injury was managed with immediate laparotomy and repair. This patient recieved transfusions and developed a deep venous thrombosis postoperatively. The next two injuries were managed laparoscopically by placing clips over the caval injury; neither of these patients required transfusions or experienced postoperative deep venous thrombosis. The authors commonly place a minilaparotomy pad (4 × 16 cm) into the intraperitoneal cavity through a 10- or 12-mm sleeve. With this in place, pressure can be rapidly applied to the bleeding sites. Pressure alone stops many bleeding problems; however, clips may be required. Blood loss from venous injuries is probably less than with open procedures because of the increased intraperitoneal pressure of approximately 15 mmHg. Both the surgeon and the anesthesiologist should be aware that carbon dioxide embolism is possible during laparoscopy, particularly with large venous injuries. Should such an injury be encountered, blood pressure, heart rate, and carbon dioxide end-tidal values should be carefully followed. An esophageal stethoscope may be placed to listen for a mill wheel murmur.

The ovarian, renal, and lumbar veins are obviously at risk of injury during a para-aortic lymphadenectomy. The authors have yet to encounter this problem but are very concerned about the potential for injury to the left renal vein and to the lumbar veins emptying into the vena cava on the left side during this procedure. The morbidity of such an injury could be significant; furthermore, laparoscopic repair of these veins would be very difficult and perhaps impossible.

Vascular injuries during a pelvic lymphadenectomy are very uncommon. In well over 250 pelvic lymph node dissections, the authors encountered two potentially serious venous injuries. In one patient with a previous pelvic lymphadenectomy, the external iliac vein was cut when the retroperitoneal space was being opened. This was controlled laparoscopically with three clips. The second patient had a large vein below the obturator nerve torn while undergoing a pelvic lymphadenecetomy. This injury was also controlled laparoscopically with clips. Neither of these patients required transfusion or experienced postoperative cardiovascular complications.

In the authors' experience, the artery most likely to be damaged during the performance of para-aortic lymphadenectomy is the inferior mesenteric artery. The authors have partially transected this vessel on two occasions, managing both injuries with total occlusion using laparoscopic clips. Laparotomy and transfusions were not required and neither patient had postoperative bowel complications. Damage to the inferior mesenteric artery typically occurs when the surgeon performing the left-sided para-aortic lymphadenectomy has not dissected laterally toward the psoas muscle in the appropriate plane. The proper plane lies beneath the mesentery of the rectosigmoid, the ureter, and the inferior mesenteric artery; proper dissection will decrease the likelihood of damage to these structures.

The surgeon may encounter small arterial branches off of the aorta or common iliac arteries that are injured during lymphadenectomy. These bleeding vessels are usually controllable with monopolar fulgaration applied directly over the laceration site. Boitke et al[16] reported one such case during a para-aortic lymphadenectomy, which did not require transfusion, but did require conversion to laparotomy.

Genitourinary Complications

Ureteral injuries during laparoscopic pelvic lymphadenectomy have not occurred in the authors' practice; however, several have been reported in the urologic literature.[17,18] These injuries occurred where the ureter crosses the common iliac artery. Ureteral injuries during para-aortic lymphadenectomy appear to be uncommon as well. Boitke et al[16] reported one delayed left lumbar ureteral injury following a left para-aortic lymphadenectomy for endometrial cancer. They attributed this injury to thermal damage. The authors have partially transected one left lumbar ureter during the performance of a low para-aortic lymphadenectomy. This resulted from lateral dissection in the improper surgical plane. Recognition of this complication at the time of the injury allowed this patient to avoid laparotomy. After the injury was recognized, the authors placed a transurethral ureteral stent and repaired the injury laparoscopically with interrupted 4–0 sutures. This injury healed without complications despite postoperative para-aortic radiation to the field for microscopically positive lymph nodes. Her stent was not removed until her radiotherapy was completed. To avoid lumbar ureteral injury, the surgeon must visualize the ureter and retract it superiorly after dissecting laterally toward the psoas muscle.

Bladder lacerations most likely occur during insertion of the suprapubic port. Kavoussi et al[17] and Burney et al[18] both reported two lacerations in their group of men undergoing lymphadenectomy for prostate carcinoma. Bladder drainage before insertion of the suprapubic trocar should prevent this complication most of the time. Bladder lacerations may also occur during dissection of the paravesical space prior to obturator lymph node removal. Lacerations of the bladder may be repaired either laparoscopically or via laparotomy, depending on the skill level of the laparoscopist.

Gastrointestinal Complications

Gastrointestinal complications that may be encountered during the performance of lymphadenectomy generally occur as a result of trauma or postoperative herniation through a port site. Enterotomy is most likely to occur during trocar insertion or during adhesiolysis. With experience and caution, the vast majority of bowel injuries may be avoided. If a laceration occurs, repair may be accomplished laparoscopically or via a minilaparotomy incision. The most important issue related to laparoscopic enterotomy is intraoperative recognition.

The most common gastrointestinal complication that results from laparotomy is postoperative herniation. This virtually always occurs through a 10-mm or larger port site. This complication is essentially preventable if fascial closure is carried out at all 10-mm or larger port sites. Using a laparoscopic fascial closure device or a needle with a five-eights curvature will facilitate this closure.

SUMMARY

Proper surgical management of most gynecologic malignancies is dependent on adequate surgical staging, and sampling of pelvic and para-aortic lymph nodes remain integral components of surgical staging. Because laparotomy is the gold standard for gynecologic malignancy staging, laparoscopy must be comparable to laparotomy if it is to play a role in this surgical management. Initial reports indicate that laparoscopic lymphadenectomy is feasible, safe, and, in experienced hands, provides adequate results while offering several advantages to the patient. Because laparoscopy results in fewer hospital days, less postoperative discomfort, and shorter recovery time than does laparotomy, laparoscopic lymphadenectomy could revolutionize the staging of early gynecologic cancers. The role of pelvic and para-aortic lymphadenectomy via laparotomy varies from surgeon to surgeon, depending on philosophy of cancer management. This will certainly be true of laparoscopic lymphadenectomy as well. Nonetheless, with the emergence of para-aortic lymphadenectomy, adequate laparoscopic staging of gynecologic malignancies is finally within the reach of oncologists. The authors anticipate that the use of laparoscopic lymphadenectomy will increase into the 21st century as more gynecologic oncologists incorporate these techniques into their repertoires.

REFERENCES

1. Ca-A Cancer Journal for Clinicians: annual statistics issue. 42, 1994
2. Weiser ET, Bundy BN, Hoskins WJ et al: Extraperitoneal versus transperitoneal selective para-aortic lymphadenectomy in the pretreatment surgical staging of advanced cervical cancer (a G.O.G study). Gynecol Oncol 33:283, 1989
3. Fowler JM, Hartenbach H, Reynolds HT et al: Pelvic adhesion formation after pelvic lymphadenectomy: comparison between transperitoneal laparoscopy and extraperitoneal laparotomy in a porcine model. Gynecol Oncol 55:25, 1994
4. Childers JM, Surwit EA, Lang J et al: Laparoscopic staging of ovarian cancer. Gynecol Oncol 59:25, 1995
5. Childers JM, Surwit EA: A combined laparoscopic vaginal approach in the management of stage I endometrial cancer. Gynecol Oncol 45:46, 1991
6. Childers JM, Brzechffa PR, Hatch KD et al: Laparoscopic assisted surgical staging (LASS) of endometrial carcinoma. Gynecol Oncol 52:221, 1993
7. Childers JM, Spirtos NM, Brainard P et al: Laparoscopic staging of the patient with incompletely staged early adenocarcinoma of the endometrium. Obstet Gynecol 83:597, 1994
8. Dargent D, Salvat J: L'Envassement Ganglionnaire Pelvien. Medsci-McGraw-Hill, Paris, 1989
9. Querleu D, LeBlanc E, Castelain B: Laparoscopic pelvic lymphadenectomy in the staging of early carcinoma of the cervix. Am J Obstet Gynecol 164:579, 1991
10. Childers J, Hatch K, Surwit E: The role of laparoscopic lymphadenectomy in the management of cervical cancer. Gynecol Oncol 47:38, 1992
11. Nezhat C, Nezhat F, Burell M et al: Laparoscopic radical hysterectomy and laparoscopic-assisted vaginal radical hysterectomy with pelvic and para-aortic node dissection. J Gynecol Surg 9:105, 1993
12. Querleu D: Laparoscopic para-aortic node sampling in gynecologic oncology: a preliminary experience. Gynecol Oncol 49:24, 1993
13. Querleu D, LeBlanc E: Laparoscopic infrarenal para-aortic node dissection in the restaging of carcinomas of the ovary and fallopian tube. Cancer 73:1467, 1994
14. Childers J, Hatch K, Tran A et al: Laparoscopic para-aortic lymphadenectomy in gynecologic malignancies. Obstet Gynecol 82:741, 1993
15. Childers J, Brezchffa P, Surwit E: Laparoscopy using the left upper quadrant as the primary trocar site. Gynecol Oncol 50:221, 1993
16. Boitke G, Lurain J, Burke J: A comparison of laparoscopic management of endometrial cancer with traditional laparotomy, abstracted. Gynecol Oncol 52:105, 1994
17. Kavoussi L, Sosa E, Chandhoke P et al: Complications of laparoscopic pelvic node dissection. J Urol 149:322, 1993
18. Burney T, Campbell E, Naslund M et al: Complications of staging laparoscopic pelvic lymphadenectomy. Surg Laparosc Endosc 3:184, 1993
19. Childers JM: Laparoscopic approaches to uterine malignancy for endometrial cancer. p. 123. In Diamond M, Daniell J, Jones H III (eds): Hysterectomy. Blackwell Science, Cambridge, MA, 1995
20. Hallum AV, Childers JM: Laparoscopy in the treatment of early cervical carcinoma. Diagn Therap Endosc 1(1):19, 1994

CHAPTER THIRTY

EXENTERATIVE SURGERY OF THE FEMALE PELVIS

KEN HATCH

WILLIAM J. MANN, JR.

BACKGROUND

As surgical and radiation treatment for cancer of the cervix and other pelvic malignancies has evolved, there has also been a constant improvement in patient selection, individualization of patient management, and resulting long-term survival and patient cure. However, particularly with cancer of the cervix, patients are recognized who have extensive central pelvic disease that precludes initial radical hysterectomy, and that persists after therapeutic doses of pelvic radiation are given. Logically, if indeed the disease is confined to the pelvis, then an extended surgical resection might offer a chance of cure. Such a resection would require removal of the female reproductive organs, and an en bloc resection of the lower urinary tract and at least a portion of the rectosigmoid. This in fact was proposed and attempted in 1946 by Alexander Brunschwig.[1] He published the results following his first 22 patients in 1948. The text and figures that accompany the article are remarkable for their simplicity (Fig. 30-1). Brunschwig referred to this operation as ''a procedure of desperation,'' which he performed on unselected patients expecting little chance of success. He and his patients recognized the dire situation of these women, and he stated, de-

spite significant morbidity and mortality, ''of those surviving at this writing, not one has expressed the feeling that they would have preferred to have remained as they were and not to have had the operation.'' His goal in this paper was to show that immediate operative mortality (5 of 22) was acceptable, and that a wet colostomy, with both ureters anastomosed to the colon and brought out as a colostomy, would work.

As physician experience with exenterative surgery developed, more patients became long-term survivors. Clinicians soon realized that anastomosing the ureters to the colon led to recurrent pyelonephritis with subsequent loss of renal function, and also that constituents of the urine were absorbed through the colonic mucosa, leading to hyperchloremic acidosis.[2] Bricker[3] published the technique of isolating a loop of ileum, closing one end, and bringing the other out as a stoma, and then anastomosing the two ureters to this blind pouch. This was facilitated by the parallel development of external appliances that would provide water tight seals for stoma, a tremendously important aid to patients. Most patients undergoing exenteration for gynecologic cancer have received prior pelvic radiotherapy, with resulting damage, in varying amounts, to the distal ileum. This led to several surgeons advocating the use of segments of colon,

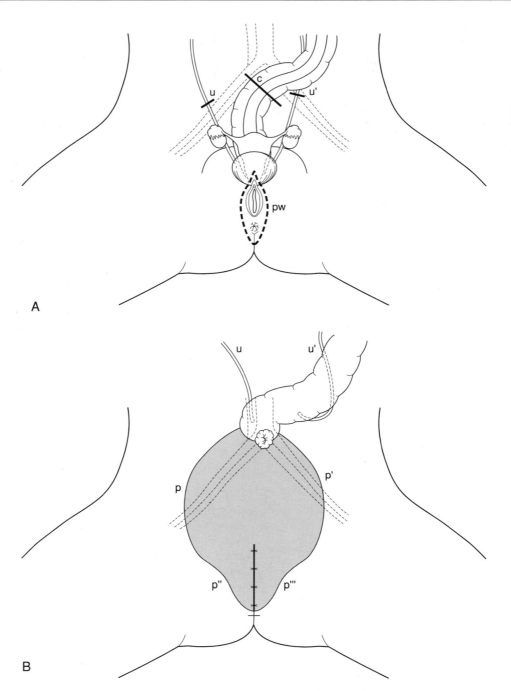

Fig. 30-1. Illustrations from Brunschwig's orginal paper describing the technique of pelvic exenteration. **(A)** Lines of resection are indicated. **(B)** Reconstruction with a wet colostomy is shown. (Adapted from Brunschwig,[1] with permission.)

usually the transverse colon, as their urinary conduit.[4] This lessens problems with healing attributable to prior radiation damage, and the colon stoma may also have fewer problems with stenosis.[5] When the sigmoid colon is used, an anastomosis in the colon is not needed, shortening operating time and saving a potential site of fistula formation. In addition, the introduction of surgical stapling devices significantly

shortens the operating time required for exenteration. The methods of urinary diversion described thus far all require that a patient continually wear an appliance. Efforts have been made to construct continent diversions, which could be intermittently catheterized by the patient. A continent ileal reservoir was developed, using a nipple valve mechanism.[6] However, stenosis often occurred and construction of the continent reservoir was difficult.[7] A continent, low pressure pouch that uses a narrowed segment of ileum as a valve has now been developed, with apparently good results in gynecologic oncology patients undergoing exenterative procedures.[8,9] This eliminates or minimizes a patient's need for an external drainage system.

When the cancer does not involve the lower vagina or vulva, the level of resection of the rectum may leave a sufficient length of distal bowel to allow a low rectal anastomosis.[10] A diverting colostomy does not improve results, while use of an omental wrap may lessen complications. When possible, the use of a low rectal anastomosis will save the patient from a colostomy.

Vulvar reconstruction and vaginal reconstruction are also now possible, using various flaps from the abdomen or leg, the omentum, and split-thickness skin grafts. These techniques are discussed in Chapter 31. These recent changes are aimed at improving the quality of life of patients who have undergone exenteration, essentially making the gynecologic oncologist a pelvic reconstructive surgeon.[11]

TERMINOLOGY

Pelvic exenteration has been also referred to as pelvic evisceration. A total exenteration refers to removal of the uterus, tubes, ovaries, parametrium, a portion of the levator muscles, the bladder, rectum or rectal segment, the vagina, and the urethra. In an anterior exenteration, the rectum is spared, while in a posterior exenteration, the bladder and urethra are preserved (Fig. 30-2).

A perineal phase may be required, in which the anus and portions of the vulva are also resected. The choice of which procedure to offer the patient is based on the location of the cancer, difficulties that may arise during the surgery, the type and location of previous radiotherapy, and the postoperative goals and expectations of the patient. Clearly, there is no such thing as a ''standard'' exenteration.

In the past, an anterior exenteration was termed a North American exenteration, a South American exenteration referred to a posterior exenteration, and a total exenteration was called an All American. These names have thankfully nearly been forgotten.

An extremely common error of young residents, students, and other health professionals is to refer to exenterative surgery as pelvic ''ex*on*eration.'' This is incorrect.

INDICATIONS

The extreme radical nature of exenterative surgery dictates that it be used only when all other treatment options have failed or cannot be used. Essentially all patients will have received prior pelvic radiation. Rarely, a woman will present with advanced vulvar or cervical cancer involving

---

Indications

- Cervical cancer
- Pelvic recurrence
- Severe radiation necrosis
- Vulvar cancer
- Endometrial or ovarian cancer
- Carcinomas, rhabdomyosarcomas, and other rare tumors
- Palliation

---

the bladder, urethra, anus, or rectum, which lends itself to primary exenterative surgery as definitive treatment. Before deciding, serious consideration must be given to brachytherapy (including interstitial placement of sources) and for combined chemotherapy and radiotherapy.

The curative potential of exenterative surgery is based entirely on the idea of resecting in entirety the patient's cancer. Hence, diseases that early in their course spread by lymphatic, blood, or peritoneal pathways will not lend themselves to ultraradical resection, such as exenteration. Cancer of the cervix, a disease that spreads by contiguous invasion of surrounding tissues is therefore the most common gynecologic cancer for which exenterative surgery is contemplated. Primary radiotherapy is used to treat nearly all patients with cervical cancer, except a few with early, localized disease who may undergo local resection or radical hysterectomy, as discussed in Chapter 27. The remainder of cervical cancer patients all receive primary radiotherapy, with curative intent.

Patients whose cancer recurs after radical surgery or radiation with metastasis outside of the pelvis, such as to the lung, liver, or para-aortic nodes, cannot be salvaged by exenterative surgery. Patients who have a pelvic recurrence after a radical hysterectomy usually then receive whole pelvic radiation. If disease persists, they rarely will then be candidates for exenteration. Unfortunately, most will by then evidence distant metastases, or have disease fixed to the pelvic sidewall. Patients who were initially treated with whole pelvic radiation, whose cancer persists or recurs, comprise the majority of patients considered for exenteration. Nearly one-half of these patients will be found to have distant metastasis, and therefore will be dropped from consideration. Of the remaining patients, at exploration, perhaps one-half will have unresectable or extrapelvic disease found, and the procedure will be aborted. The remaining patients will undergo exenteration, which will be curative for 30 to 50 percent, a few will die from complications of the surgery 3 to 5 percent, and the rest will die of recurrent cancer (Fig. 30-3). This is a small yield overall for patients failing primary therapy for

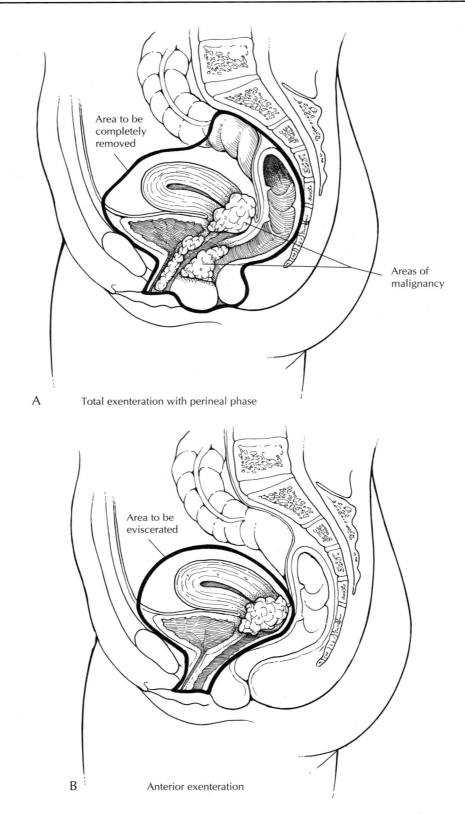

Area to be
completely
removed

Areas of
malignancy

A   Total exenteration with perineal phase

Area to be
eviscerated

B   Anterior exenteration

Fig. 30-2. Schematic representation of lines of resection for **(A)** total exenteration and **(B)** anterior exenteration.

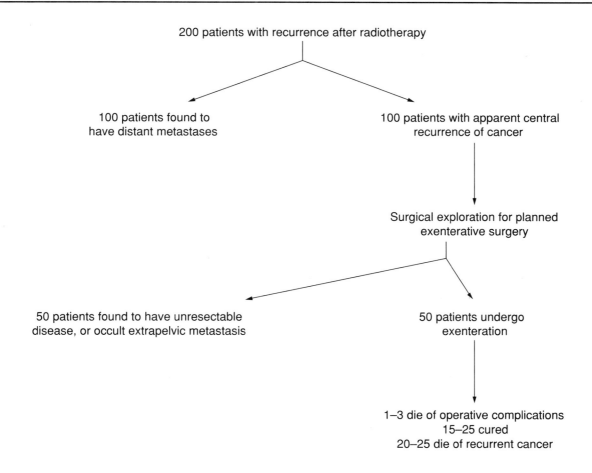

200 patients with recurrence after radiotherapy

100 patients found to
have distant metastases

100 patients with apparent central
recurrence of cancer

Surgical exploration for planned
exenterative surgery

50 patients found to have unresectable
disease, or occult extrapelvic metastasis

50 patients undergo
exenteration

1–3 die of operative complications
15–25 cured
20–25 die of recurrent cancer

Fig. 30-3. Algorithm showing theoretical outcome for patients diagnosed with recurrent cervical cancer.

cervical cancer, but for those fortunate few women it is an opportunity for cure when faced with certain death.

In the past, a few women would develop severe radiation necrosis of the pelvis after radiotherapy, with no proven persistence of their cancer. Total pelvic exenteration was used to relieve their severe pain and foul-smelling, necrotic perineal discharge.[11] Morbidity was high, and even when no cancer was found in the operative specimen, many patients later died of recurrence. Fortunately, with modern radiotherapy, this indication essentially no longer exists.

Vulvar cancer, like cervical cancer, often stays confined to the pelvis until late in its natural history. When patients present with large cancers involving the urethra or anus, or both, exenteration is often considered.[12] However, radiotherapy has been shown able to effectively eliminate or markedly shrink vulvar cancer, lessening the extent of surgery needed.[13] In addition, the combination of radiotherapy and chemotherapy has also been shown to markedly reduce the need for exenterative surgery.[14] Consequently, at this time, primary exenterative surgery would not seem appropriate for most patients presenting with advanced vulvar cancers. A limited role does exist for exenteration in patients whose cancer recurs.

Patients with either endometrial or ovarian cancer, both of which have a propensity to spread beyond the pelvis, seem poor candidates for exenterative surgery. Survival for patients with ovarian or endometrial cancer undergoing exenteration is less than 20 percent at 5 years.[15,16] There has been described in more recent times a "modified posterior exenteration," which is done for primary and secondary cytoreduction of ovarian cancer.[17] The operation described is an en bloc resection of the pelvic peritoneum, uterus, tubes, ovaries, and a segment of rectosigmoid. It is a supralevator ani resection, useful for dealing with a pelvis obliterated by ovarian cancer, in which attempting to develop planes between the pelvic organs is not feasible. It is done as part of a cytoreductive procedure that involves resecting cancer throughout the peritoneal cavity. Conceptually, it violates the principal that exenterative surgery is meant to be curative, by resecting cancer limited to the central pelvis. It is a nice addition to the surgical treatment of ovarian cancer, although probably more often referred to as resection of a frozen pelvis with segmental resection of the rectosigmoid.

Exenteration has also been used for vaginal carcinomas, rhabdomyosarcomas, and other miscellaneous rare tumors. Whenever ultraradical central resection of cancer is feasible, and lesser therapy not feasible, it is not unreasonable to consider exenteration.

More controversial is the use of exenterative surgery for palliation. Traditionally, the associated morbidity, complications, risk of death, and long hospitalization were considered too great a price to pay for a palliative procedure. When first described, the extended dissections done to determine operability often led to significant morbidity, even if the procedure was subsequently aborted and the integrity of the gastrointestinal tract and urinary tract maintained. Our increasing sophistication with postoperative care may lead a few to reconsider this option. However, for the present, significant palliation can be obtained for terminal cancer patients using diverting procedures when needed, which are often feasible percutaneously. There is also a much more successful and broad range of approaches to chronic cancer pain. Hence, intentional palliative exenteration is probably not indicated. However, in a retrospective review of patients who underwent exenteration for the intention of cure, patients identified to have operative findings that in retrospect made the procedure futile, nontheless had a median survival of 19 months, and a mean hospital stay of only 22 days. There was acceptable morbidity. Use of exenterative surgery for palliation remains controversial, and "considered surgical judgment and discretion must be exercised in the selection of those patients who can tolerate the palliative operative procedures without excessive morbidity . . . and who can enjoy in comfort the additional survival potentially provided by operation."[18]

PATIENT SELECTION

A woman is not a candidate for pelvic exenteration if she cannot accept the major changes in body image that will occur despite best efforts at reconstruction. She needs a caring family support system, intact mental faculties, and access to continued medical care. Extended conversations with other women who have undergone this surgery, in the absence of medical staff, are invaluable. Nurses who deal with this woman need a positive, frank, and understanding manner.

Clearly, no other potentially fatal disease should coexist, and the patient's general medical condition must be adequate for a prolonged operative procedure (i.e., 4 to 8 hours) with probable extensive fluid shifts, transfusion, and nutritional support. She must understand there is a 3 to 5 percent operative mortality, that she will spend several days in the intensive care unit, and likely have a prolonged hospitalization measured in weeks. Sexual function will be altered, and she may need to become adept at caring for one or two stoma. In addition, she must accept that even after all this, there is no guarantee of cure. It is also necessary to discuss the possibility of an aborted procedure, if unresectable disease is found. The range of complications must be explained. Often, a patient will cry and verbalize considerable anguish

---

Contraindications to Exenterative Surgery

- Absolute
  - Patient unable to accept change in body image
  - Mental disease preventing adequate consent, and/or sufficient independence to care for herself postoperatively
  - Lack of continued access to knowledgeable medical care
  - Concurrent fatal medical diseases
  - Inadequate medical condition to withstand exenterative procedure
  - Evidence of distant metastasis
  - The presence of unilateral leg edema, ipsilateral hydronephrosis, and ipsilateral sciatic pain
  - Inability to obtain a surgical margin intraoperatively (resectability cannot be reliably determined by physical examination or radiologic imaging)
- Relative
  - Age over 65
  - Refusal to accept blood or blood products

---

when these discussions occur. This, however, is preferable to the patient who cheerfully demands that one proceed immediately, and only begins to deal with her emotions postoperatively. The woman in tears truly is beginning to understand what is proposed. In one sense, this is a terrible operation to offer someone; it is justified by desperation and a chance for cure, but must be approached thoughtfully and carefully. The surgeon discussing the procedure with the patient needs to have considerable maturity and experience, and must be able to honestly answer the questions that are asked and relay the uncertainty of the operative result.

Age over 65 may increase the operative mortality of exenteration, although this probably reflects concurrent medical problems. Biologic age is clearly more important than simple chronological age.

The medical evaluation begins by first confirming histologically that the cancer is present. The authors rarely, if ever, accept slides from another institution, and never accept only a pathology report. Next, the workup proceeds by trying to show that the patient is *not* a suitable candidate for exenteration because of unresectable or metastatic disease.

If, in taking a review of systems and history, the patient indicates any signs or symptoms suggestive of metastatic disease (i.e., dry hacking cough), this may help to focus the radiologic workup. Also, a history of significant weight loss, particularly if verified by family or by comparison with prior photographs of the patient, can suggest cachexia secondary to metastatic cancer. Unilateral leg swelling and unilateral or bilateral sciatic pain are worrisome, as they suggest metastatic disease to the posterolateral pelvis. The triad of unilateral leg swelling, ipsilateral sciatic pain, and unilateral hydronephrosis on intravenous pyelogram (IVP) contraindicates exenteration, and indicates unresectable cancer metastatic to the posterolateral side wall. Patients with one or two of the triad have a high likelihood of metastatic disease, but should not be precluded from exploration unless metastasis can be documented.

As in any surgical patient, a careful examination also looks for concurrent medical problems that would impact on the proposed procedure. Before planning exenteration, new murmurs must be explained, lungs should be clear, and the breasts should be without masses. The general principles outlined in Chapter 1 must be closely followed. Physical examination focuses on looking for evidence of cachexia, palpable supraclavicular or inguinal adenopathy, hepatomegaly, or intra-abdominal masses. Rarely, skin metastasis is found.

Routine biopsy of nonpalpable supraclavicular lymph nodes is not recommended, as the yield is vanishingly low. Palpable supraclavicular nodes, by contrast, almost always represent metastatic disease and preclude exenteration. Aspiration is usually adequate to confirm cancer.

Laboratory studies screen for chronic active hepatitis or human immunodeficiency virus positivity, which probably contraindicate exenteration. Elevated liver enzymes obviously direct one to rule out liver metastasis, anemia must be corrected preoperatively, and one expects normal clotting parameters. Severe bleeding disorders that cannot be readily corrected are a relative contraindication to exenteration.

A normal chest radiograph is sufficient to rule out metastatic disease, but a computed tomography (CT) scan is favored by many. Should any lesions be found, needle aspiration of biopsy by thoracoscopy should document cancer and conclude the evaluation. If the evaluation of the chest is negative, then a CT scan with contrast is done of both the abdomen and pelvis. If liver lesions or retroperitoneal adenopathy are seen, needle aspiration should be done to confirm cancer spread. Patients who have undergone exenteration, with pathology subsequently revealing metastasis to pelvic or para-aortic nodes, have a small chance of cure (i.e., approximately 5 to 10 percent), so documentation of enlarged nodes containing cancer suggests an even worse prognosis. Any intraperitoneal fluid should be aspirated for cytology. The role of diagnostic laparoscopy with node sampling, peritoneal cytologies, and biopsy as indicated remains undefined. However, this is certainly a promising option for evaluating a patient for exenteration, *in the hands of a skilled laparoscopist.*

One should not rely on CT scanning for determining re-

sectability, on the basis of apparent absence of fatty planes lateral to tumor. But neither CT nor magnetic resonance imaging (MRI) are able to assess parametrial or levator extension accurately. Radiation fibrosis, with or without superimposed endometriosis, chronic inflammation, or foreign body reaction, cannot be differentiated from cancer with current imaging techniques. Ureteral obstruction on IVP or CT is not a contraindication to exenteration. Obstruction at the ureteral vesical junction is resectable; however, obstruction by enlarged pelvic or para-aortic nodes is unresectable. Similarly, ureteral obstruction by extrinsic masses does not influence resectability; only the nature of the mass is important. Bone scans are usually not done unless the patient gives a history of recent onset of pain in a given area.

Pelvic examination is extremely inaccurate in assessing resectability. It is just not possible to differentiate radiation fibrosis, endometriosis, or igneous cellulitis from cancer. Fixation to the side wall on examination is not a contraindication to exploration. If a total exenteration is planned, cystoscopy and sigmoidoscopy are not necessary. However, if either the bladder or rectum are to be preserved, then they must be carefully examined to ensure the absence of occult metastasis. In patients undergoing exenteration following radiotherapy for cervical cancer, the bladder is usually removed, as its preservation leads to increased risk of recurrence and urinary tract fistula or stricture in most patients.

PREOPERATIVE PATIENT PREPARATION

Concurrent medical problems are dealt with as described in Chapter 1. A mechanical bowel preparation is given, consisting of a clear liquid diet and oral hyperosmotic solutions to induce diarrhea. Intravenous fluids are started at the time of the bowel preparation to avoid dehydration. The patient is taught incentive spirometry preoperatively, and given prophylactic antibiotics. The sites of stoma are marked by the ostomy team the morning of surgery, and checked when the patient sits, stands, and lies down. Care is taken to avoid skin creases, scars, and the site where the patient normally wears her belt and elastic waistlines. If the patient is severely malnourished, total parenteral nutrition (TPN) may be started in advance of surgery. Usually these patients will remain NPO (nothing by mouth) for a week or longer. A central line can be placed in the operating room during the procedure, and TPN started postoperatively. Central lines with multiple ports facilitate postoperative fluid management. Line placement and principles of nutritional support are discussed in Chapters 1 and 2. Usually, 6 U of packed red blood cells are ordered, and electrolytes checked early in the morning before surgery.

Consent for surgery is obtained before admission, after all of the extensive discussions concerning the nature of the surgery, risks, complications, and possible outcomes are reviewed in detail.

OPERATIVE TECHNIQUE

The patient is placed in a low dorsal lithotomy position, using stirrups that support the hips, knees, and things (Fig. 30-4). This allows assistants on each side of the table, as well as between the legs. The instrument stand is placed over the leg opposite the primary surgeon. The lithotomy position also aids in allowing simultaneous abdominal-pelvic examination when the abdomen is open and resectability being assessed. Finally, the lithotomy position is helpful with the perineal phase of the procedure, or if myocutaneous grafts are planned for reconstruction. It also allows for double team approach to the procedure. The patient is prepared and draped from nipples to knees, and a catheter is placed after the draping is completed.

Intermittent pneumatic compression devices are applied as prophylaxis for deep vein thrombosis (Fig. 30-5). Although general anesthesia is adequate, combined epidural and general anesthesia allows the epidural to be maintained in the immediate 72 hours after surgery, giving good pain control while keeping the patient alert and able to comply with respiratory toilet.

A midline incision adequate for exploring upper and lower abdomen is made, and later extended upward as needed. In a systematic manner, the diaphragm, liver, gallbladder, stomach, spleen, omentum, large and small bowel, and abdominal and pelvic peritoneum are examined for metastatic disease, secondary primary lesions, or unexpected or known incidental pathology (i.e., gallstones, hepatic cysts). The pelvis is inspected, looking for evidence of tumor breakthrough into the peritoneal cavity, or metastasis to pelvic peritoneum or adnexae. The retroperitoneum and para-aortic areas are carefully palpated, looking for masses. Any suspicious findings are biopsied and sent for frozen section to confirm unre-

sectability. If no evidence of metastasis outside of the pelvis is found, the peritoneum over the para-aortic area is incised and a para-aortic biopsy obtained and sent for frozen section. If negative, the pelvic exploration begins.

It is not uncommon to encounter small bowel adhesions, and these must be lysed to allow adequate exploration of the abdomen. However, on occasion, a loop of small bowel will be found densely adherent to the uterus. Rarely, there will be actual invasion directly into the loop of small bowel. Although most would resect or bypass the involved loop, reanastomose the bowel, and abort the procedure, there have been reported a few patients who underwent exenteration with resection of the small bowel and survived more than 5 years (6 of 49 patients).[19]

The round ligaments can be divided at the side wall and the prevesical and pararectal spaces developed. Alternately, the prevesical space can be opened, dissected to the urethra, then extended laterally to both side walls, where the round ligaments can then be divided retroperitoneally, the lateral pelvic peritoneum reflected medially, and the spaces then developed. Biopsy of the pelvic nodes is done if suspicious areas are seen. Routine lymphadenectomy is not done, as it would, at best, be of prognostic value in the postoperative period, and of no therapeutic value. However, in the infrequent event of exenteration being done as primary therapy without prior radiation, lymphadenectomy may be believed to be appropriate by some surgeons. The infundibulopelvic ligaments are divided well above the common iliac vessels. The ureters are dissected free for several centimeters past their point of crossing the common iliac vessels. If preoperative studies showed hydronephrosis, the point of obstruction is identified, and biopsies taken to determine if unresectable cancer is causing the blockage. If the ureter is obstructed below the bifurcation of the iliac vessels, but medially, this

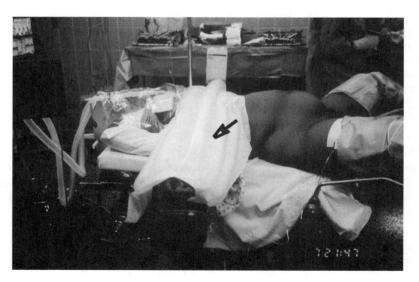

Fig. 30-4. Patient in modified dorsal lithotomy position. Arrow indicates thermal drape used to prevent excessive heat loss during procedure.

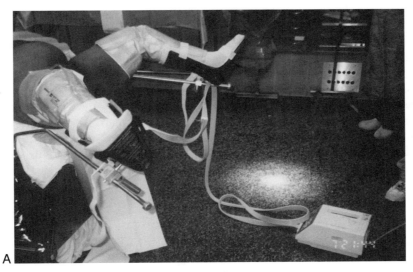

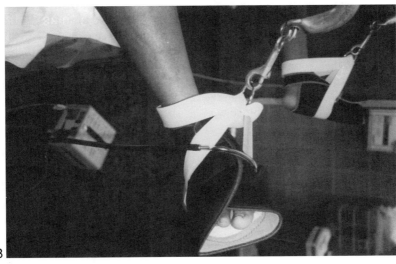

Fig. 30-5. Intermittent pneumatic compression devices are applied before draping, and the power units placed well out of the way of the surgeons and assistants. Devices may wrap around (**A**) the entire leg or alternately (**B**) just the feet.

is not a contraindication to resection and does not need to be dissected out, as this area will be included in the major specimen. The ureters are not divided until resectability is determined, and then, on an angle to facilitate anastomosis to bowel. There is no point in trying to gain an extra centimeter or two in dividing the ureter; rather, it is important to ensure an adequate margin from cancer. The spaces lateral to the rectum are sharply developed and carried across the midline, where blunt dissection can be used to develop the potential space posterior to the rectum. At this point, the anterior tissue planes will have been developed down to the levator ani muscles, as will the bilateral perivesical and perirectal spaces, and the rectum will be freed posteriorly down to the sacral curve. This is usually a relatively bloodless dissection.

Beginning on the side most likely to contain cancer, the parametrium is sharply divided at the side wall, taking the internal iliac artery just after it crosses the internal iliac vein. This sacrifices the uterine artery, vesicle arteries, and the obliterated umbilical artery. The remainder of the hypogastric artery is left intact. It carries the internal pudendal and inferior hemorrhoidal arteries, which are important to maintain vascularity to the anal canal and lower rectum, a potential site of anastomosis. It also carries the obturator artery, which provides significant blood supply to the gracilis muscle, and is necessarily preserved if planning a gracilis muscle neovagina. The cardinal ligament is divided and ligated at the side wall, and the broad attachments of the rectum to the sacrum are also divided. The vaginal attachments to the tendonus arch are divided and the vaginal arteries and vein are located on the lateral margin of this pedicle. The specimen is now completely mobilized, and the penetration of the rectum and vagina through the pubococcygeus muscle can be identified. A combined abdominal-pelvic examination can be carried out at any point, to identify areas suspicious for cancer, which can then be biopsied.

When performing a biopsy to establish resectability, the specimen should be reflected medially, and the biopsy taken from tissue that will be left behind if the exenteration proceeds. The biopsy is meant to tell one what cannot be removed, so it is necessary to have one's planes of dissection well formed before performing a biopsy. Particularly difficult to biopsy are anterolateral and posterolateral areas where tumor may extend to the side wall along the fascia or muscle fibers of the levator muscles. Kevorkian biopsy forceps, which are excellent for colposcopy, are also superb for biopsy of hard-to-reach areas (and for the diaphragm and liver). The operative specimen makes visualizing this area difficult. Occasionally, troublesome bleeding will be encountered and is best handled with pressure or by placing figure-of-eight sutures.

If a biopsy comes back positive for metastatic cancer, the procedure is terminated. The planes developed are copiously irrigated, and hemostasis confirmed. No attempt is made to close these planes or to approximate peritoneal edges. Drains are not placed. A bulk closure of the abdomen is used, and the central line left in for fluid replacement. If stable in the recovery area, the patient can usually be returned to the gynecology floor. The surgeon needs to be available to deal with the obviously difficult questions that the patient will ask when she awakens.

If all biopsies return negative, then the exenterative specimen can begin to be removed. The ureters are now divided and placed into the upper abdomen, and anesthesia is notified that there will no longer be any measurable urine output, and that urine will be mixed with blood loss.

Anterior Exenteration

Anterior exenteration is suitable for lesions confined to the cervix and the anterior upper vagina. The plan is to removed the bladder, urethra, and anterior vagina, and to save the posterior vagina and rectum. Bimanual palpation, with the pelvic hand inserting one finger into the vagina and another into the rectum, while the abdominal hand palpates the cul-de-sac and retracts the rectum posteriorly, will confirm the initial impression that an anterior resection is advisable. If the space posterior to the cervix feels free, than an incision can be made in the cul-de-sac to allow the rectum to drop away with sharp dissection from the upper vagina, giving at least a 4 cm margin on the vagina. The potential space between the rectum and posterior vagina is developed abdominally, and adequacy of margin confirmed by direct vision vaginally. The posterior vaginal incision is made from below, with the cancer in view, to ensure adequate margin. Biopsies of the vagina, which will be left intact over the rectum, are sent for frozen section if any question remains about cancer involvement. The perineal incision is made,

removing the urethra and surrounding soft tissue, but preserving the clitoris and labia. Cautery reduces blood loss while doing this.

A pointed clamp such as a long tonsil is passed from the abdomen beneath the pubis and directed out superior to the urethra. The clamp is spread to open the space, and then widened from below with the two index fingers. Clamps are then passed under the pubic arch to allow the pubococcygeal muscles attached to the vagina at the 3 and 9 o'clock positions to be divided. Clamps may also need to be passed from below upward to be sure the whole pedicle is taken. Large suture ligatures are used for hemostasis. The posterior vaginal wall is then separated from the rectum, and this posterior space (which communicates with the cul-de-sac) is joined with the anterior space, thus totally mobilizing the specimen, which can be delivered through the perineal opening. Warm laparotomy pads are then placed abdominally into the defect, and pressure applied from above and below. Cautery and ligature are used to obtain hemostasis. The specimen is then carefully inspected to be sure all margins are acceptable. It is often useful to place long sutures into the specimen to aid in orienting the pathologist, who must fix and section this specimen (Fig. 30-6). Many surgeons prefer to be present when the pathologist begins the gross examination of the specimen, to be sure it is done appropriately.

If at any time during the exenterative procedure there is difficulty separating the rectum and posterior vagina from the cancer, it is prudent to resect the piece of rectum to ensure an adequate margin.

Reconstruction of the vagina is done, as described in Chapter 31. If no vaginal reconstruction is planned, the omentum can be mobilized from the hepatic flexure to the splenic flexure, leaving 3 to 4 cm intact, and then loosely sewn over the pelvic defect. The perineal opening will close rapidly by granulation. Irrigations are usually started after 72 hours to keep the perineum clean, if no reconstruction is done.

Urinary diversion is then accomplished.

Total Exenteration With Perineal Phase

If a total exenteration is planned and resectability determined, the sigmoid and descending colon are mobilized, and the sigmoid transected at the pelvic brim after dividing the ureters. The proximal end of the bowel, which will become the stoma, is packed into the upper abdomen. The rectosigmoid is elevated by an assistant and the posterior attachments of the colon freed down to the levator muscles. The sigmoid mesenteric arteries and the superior rectal artery are divided.

The perineal phase begins by making an incision sufficient to remove the urethra and entire vagina, and to include the anus. Cautery is used. The subcutaneous tissues are divided around the rectum, and then the urethra and anterior vagina freed as in an anterior exenteration. In addition, the pubococ-

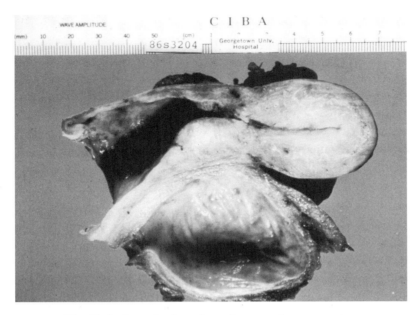

Fig. 30-6. Gross fixed specimen from anterior exenteration.

cygeal attachments to the perineal body are identified, as is the anococcygeal ligament, and they are clamped, divided, and suture ligated. The specimen is removed through the perineal defect and hemostasis attained with ligature and cautery (Fig. 30-7).

This leaves a huge pelvic defect, best filled with myocutaneous flaps of either gracilis or rectus abdominis muscles. These are discussed in Chapter 31.

Alternately, after hemostasis has been attained, a large pelvic pack may be placed. A nylon or similar fabric pouch is filled with laparotomy pads and placed with the opening coming out through the perineum, and the pouch is closed with a pursestring suture. The omentum can be mobilized and used to cover the pelvis. It can then be loosely sewn over the pelvic pack, as a floor. The colostomy and urinary diversion can then be constructed. If a pack is placed, the pursestring suture is cut after 48 to 72 hours, and one-half of the laparotomy pads removed. The remainder of the pack is removed 24 hours later, and twice daily irrigations begun of the pelvic defect. Warmed saline and peroxide, lactated Ringer's, or similar solutions may be used. Care is taken to ensure that fluid does not collect in the curve of the sacrum.

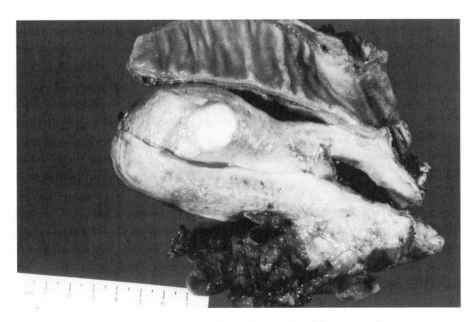

Fig. 30-7. Gross fixed specimen from total pelvic exenteration.

It is usually sufficient to have the patient stand after each irrigation. With considerable time, the entire pelvic defect will granulate in and close.

Supralevator Total Exenteration With Low Rectal Anastomosis

Women with disease extending posteriorly from the cervix onto the vaginal mucosa or into the rectal wall are candidates for this procedure, provided that the cancer does not extend to the lower third of the vagina posteriorly. After the bladder, urethra, and anterior vagina are mobilized, as previously described, the posterior vaginal wall incision is made 4 cm below the tumor. The vaginal epithelium is mobilized for 1 to 2 cm away from the rectal muscularis. The hand then encircles the mobilized rectum and pulls it cephalad. The specimen side is clamped to reduce spillage of feces and divided, leaving an anal and rectal stump. The length of the anal rectal stump from the anal sphincter is ideally 6 cm or greater. If less than 6 cm in length, the risk of fistula and incontinence are greater.

After mobilization of this lower specimen, the sigmoid colon is divided along with the sigmoidal arteries and the superior rectal artery. Ample mobilization for reanastomosis is accomplished by incising the lateral attachments of the sigmoid and descending colon, mobilizing it, and if necessary, sacrificing some of the sigmoidal vessels. The major blood supply is from the inferior mesenteric artery, which has significant anastomoses between it and the middle colic artery. After the sigmoid and left colon are mobilized, it will be observed for adequacy of blood supply and viability while the urinary diversion is done and the flaps for neovaginal construction are harvested. If the appearance of both cut edges is satisfactory, then the anastomosis can be carried out. If there is lack of vascularity to either stump, they should be trimmed back until bleeding is encountered. The anastomosis is accomplished by using 28- or 31-mm diameter circular staplers. Following anastomosis, the omentum is mobilized and brought into the pelvis as an omental graft. It is used to wrap the low rectal anastomosis and to fill the presacral space (Fig. 30-8).

A neovagina can then be made. The type of neovagina selected depends on the amount of space to be filled and the patient's anatomy. The easiest flap is a bulbocavernosus neovagina. It is limited in the amount of skin and muscle that can be harvested. It is most successful when a significant portion of posterior vaginal mucosa can also be preserved. The gracilis and rectus abdominis grafts are the most successful when a large skin area is needed. The gracilis muscles are most successful for total exenteration with a large perineal phase, but they can be used with other types of exenterative procedures, if there is sufficient room in the anterior pelvis.

Posterior Exenteration

Posterior exenterations are rarely performed, except for primary stage IVA cancers of the cervix invading the rectum. When a cervical cancer recurs after radiotherapy, even if it is confined to the posterior vagina and rectum, one should remove the distal ureters, bladder, and urethra in order to avoid the very significant morbidity and mortality of a urinary tract fistula. The technique of posterior exenteration differs from those described so far in that the bladder and ureters are preserved. This of course means that the anterior vagina will be preserved as well. After posterior exenteration, these women will have significant bladder dysfunction resulting from the extensive removal of the hypogastric plexus that enervates the bladder. Patients have a high likelihood of requiring long-term catheter drainage or self-catheterization.

The posterior exenteration differs from the low anterior resection of the rectosigmoid that general surgeons perform, in that they do not remove the uterus or cardinal ligaments, and thus the ureters and bladder are not disturbed. It is the radical en bloc excision of the uterus, cardinal ligaments, rectum, and rectal pillars that removes the hypogastric plexus and severely injures bladder function. Before planning a posterior exenteration, radiotherapy must be seriously considered. For patients who have had recurrence following radiotherapy, a total exenteration with low rectal anastomosis should be the first option.

After dividing the round ligaments and developing the perivesical and perirectal spaces, the peritoneum between bladder and uterus is incised and the bladder reflected as inferiorly as possible with sharp dissection. The ureters are then mobilized and dissected free of their soft tissue attachments, similar to the technique for radical hysterectomy. The uterine arteries are divided at their origin and reflected medially, trying to preserve the other branches of the internal iliac arteries. The cardinal ligaments are then divided laterally, the ureteral dissection completed to the bladder, and the anterior vagina entered. The rectosigmoid is freed posteriorly, the parametrium mobilized medially, and the dissection carried down to the levator muscles, identical to the posterior dissection in a total exenteration. The perineal incision will involve only the posterior aspect of the vulva and anus. An omental flap and small pack can be used to complete management of the defect, and colostomy performed (Fig. 30-9).

Urinary Diversion

The standard urinary diversion for several decades was the urinary conduit. A segment of ileum 12 to 15 cm in length was isolated using staplers, and the distal end brought out as a stoma. Bowel continuity was usually re-established by performing an ileoascending colon enteroenterostomy. Both ureters were transected, spatulated, and stented. A tonsil was then placed down the stoma of the isolated loop of

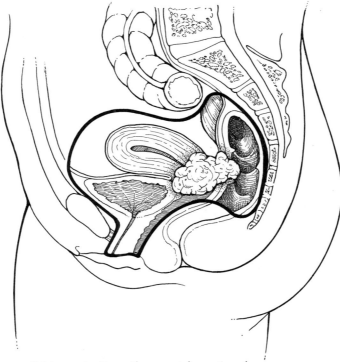

A   Pelvic exenteration with segmental resection of
rectosigmoid and low rectal anastomosis

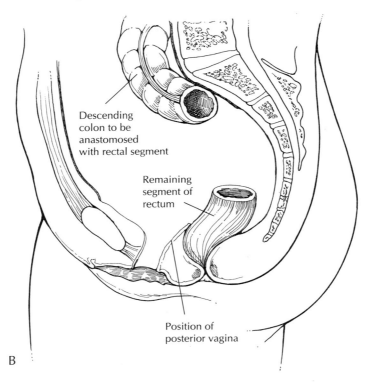

Descending
colon to be
anastomosed
with rectal segment

Remaining
segment of
rectum

Position of
posterior vagina

B

Fig. 30-8. (A–E) Schematic representation of low rectal anastomosis as part of exenterative procedure. *(Figure continues.)*

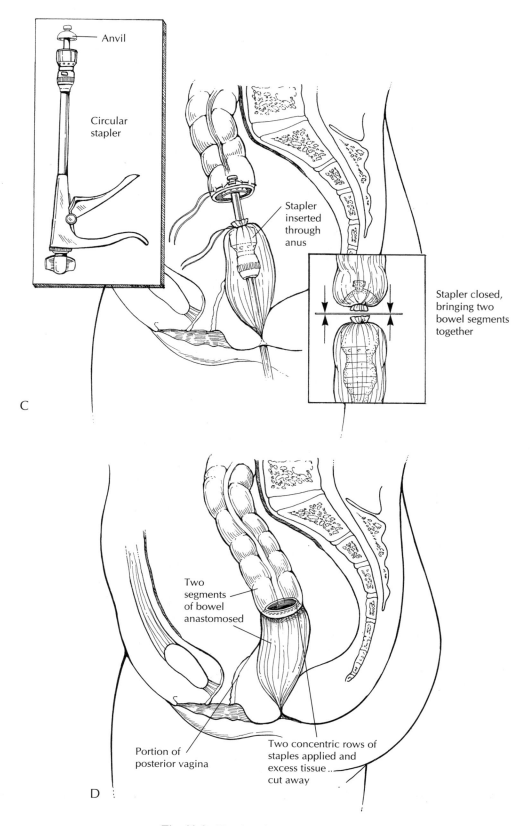

Anvil

Circular
stapler

Stapler
inserted
through
anus

Stapler closed,
bringing two
bowel segments
together

C

Two
segments
of bowel
anastomosed

Portion of
posterior vagina

Two concentric rows of
staples applied and
excess tissue
cut away

D

Fig. 30-8 *(Continued). (Figure continues.)*

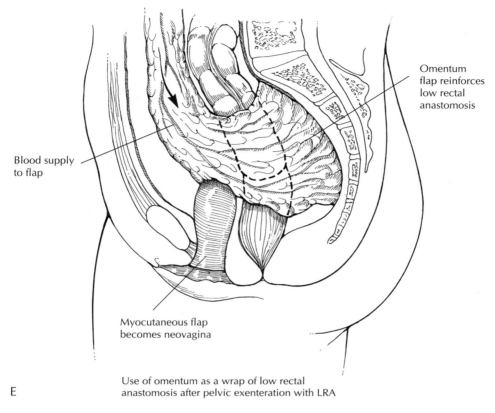

Omentum
flap reinforces
low rectal
anastomosis

Blood supply
to flap

Myocutaneous flap
becomes neovagina

E

Use of omentum as a wrap of low rectal
anastomosis after pelvic exenteration with LRA

Fig. 30-8 *(Continued).*

ileum, a small incision made in the wall of the loop, and the ureteral stent delivered into the loop and out the stoma. The edges of the ureter were then sewn, mucosa to mucosa full thickness, to the loop of ileum. Interrupted sutures were used, and knots placed exterior to the mucosa. A similar procedure would then be carried out with the second ureter. The stoma was located in the right lower abdomen, and the left ureter tunneled beneath the bowel mesentery to reach the loop. The ileum had usually received part or all of the pelvic radiation given to the patient; consequently healing was impaired, and fistulas and anastomotic leaks were a major problem (Fig. 30-10).

As previously mentioned, use of the transverse colon avoids offering an acceptable conduit using bowel that had not been radiated. In addition, the stoma seemed to stenose less with colon than ileum. The surgical technique involves freeing the omentum from the transverse colon, selecting a 12- to 15-cm segment of transverse colon fed by the middle colic artery, and isolating it from the gastrointestinal tract. The colon was reanastomosed to restore bowel patency, and the conduit carried out essentially the same as for the ileal procedure.

Currently, when feasible, the preferred method of urinary diversion is a continent pouch, created from the distal ileum, ascending colon, and a portion of the transverse colon[8] (Fig. 30-11). The ileum is divided 10 to 12 cm proximal to the

ileocecal valve, and the transverse colon just distal to the middle colic artery. An ileotransverse colon enteroenterostomy is performed to restore continuity to the gastrointestinal tract. The isolated segment of bowel is opened with cautery along the tenia. The bowel is then folded on itself in a U shape and the edges closed with staples. This division and closure of the bowel is believed to prevent subsequent peristalsis and generation of intermittent high pressures, which would overcome the continence mechanism.

The ureters are brought through stab wounds into the bowel reservoir, and the spatulated ends anastomosed mucosa to mucosa. The left ureter is brought through the sigmoid mesentery to reach the reservoir. A 14 French catheter is placed into the ileum, and passed through into the reservoir. Excess ileum is excised from the antimesenteric edge with a stapling device, and three pursestring sutures placed at the ileocecal valve to tighten the ileum. The tapered end of the ileum is brought out as a stoma. The ureters are stented and, with a Malecot catheter, are brought out through the anterior wall of the reservoir and through a separate opening in the abdominal wall. Stents and catheter are removed at 2 weeks. This operation provides a low pressure reservoir, which the patients can catheterize as needed. Results have been very encouraging, with most patients maintaining continence, and catheterizing their stoma every several hours.

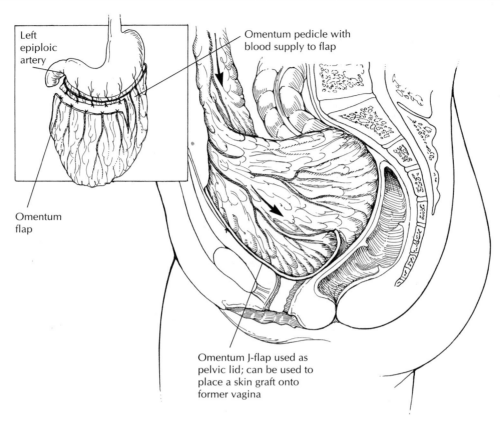

Left epiploic artery

Omentum pedicle with blood supply to flap

Omentum flap

Omentum J-flap used as pelvic lid; can be used to place a skin graft onto former vagina

Use of omentum as carpet to cover pelvic defect after anterior exenteration

Fig. 30-9. Omentum is freed starting at the hepatic flexure, with a 4- to 6-cm band left attached at the splenic flexure, and the freed omentum is then placed along the left paracolic gutter into the pelvis, where it is stitched into place as a ''lid'' to keep small bowel out of the pelvic defect.

POSTOPERATIVE CARE

Patients are best managed in a surgical intensive care unit, with Swan-Ganz catheter monitoring. For younger patients with no concurrent medical diseases, this may not be necessary. However, Swan-Ganz monitoring facilitates administration of blood products, colloid, and crystalloid, particularly in those patients whose urine output is not a reliable predictor of fluid status, and who have a pelvic defect, a huge area devoid of peritoneum that will weep serum in large amounts comparable to a burn patient. Concealed hemorrhage and inadequate fluid replacement are constant considerations. It is advisable to keep the hematocrit stable (a level of 30 percent allows a reserve should bleeding occur) and, to keep the prothrombin and partial thromboblastin time values normal with fresh frozen plasma and vitamin K as needed. Most inexperienced surgeons underestimate the amount of colloid needed in these patients, and measurement of serum protein levels may help appreciate the magnitude of loss. Frequent blood counts and electrolyte measurements are needed, until the patient is believed to be stable, euvolimic, and has normal clotting parameters.

Prompt extubation is preferred, with serial measurements of oxygen saturation used to ensure adequate pulmonary function. A postoperative chest film is needed to ensure that both lungs are expanded, and to rule out pneumothorax from central line insertion. Since delayed pneumothorax can occur, a repeat film at 24 hours is useful. Vigorous respiratory toilet, including use of incentive spirometry and patient positioning, is an integral part of postoperative care. Acute respiratory distress must always be addressed as potential pulmonary embolus, myocardial infarction, or congestive heart failure. Appropriate evaluation is discussed in Chapter 1. The intermittent pneumatic compression devices, begun in the operating suite, are continued until discharge, and are removed only when the patient is ambulating.

A first-generation cephalosporin is given immediately preoperatively for prophylaxis. If febrile episodes occur postoperatively, and no cause is easily identified, antibiotics are empirically started. Blood and urine culture results are used to select antibiotics as they become available. Most postoperative febrile episodes remain unexplained and respond to antibiotic therapy. Fecal spill during surgery is frequently treated by beginning antibiotics that cover anaerobic and gram-negative organisms. There are little hard data, if any, on which to base intelligent decisions concerning antibiotic usage after

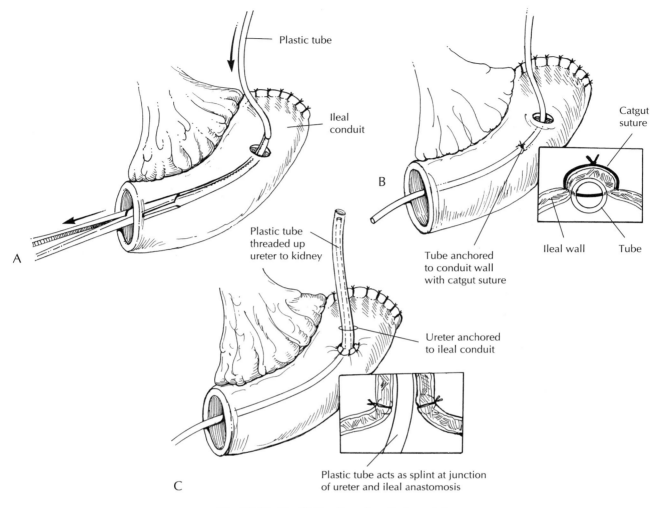

Fig. 30-10. (A–C) Creation of an ileal conduit.

exenterative surgery. These patients have undergone complicated, extended surgery, and personal bias and past experience influence choice of agents. The presence of central lines and the use of TPN complicate the situation even further.

With the gastrointestinal surgery that is so integral a part of exenterative surgery, it is not unusual for patients to go 14 days or longer without adequate oral intake. Therefore, TPN is started immediately after surgery and continued until the clinician feels the integrity of the bowel is confirmed, and oral intake is adequate to support the patient. Chronically malnourished patients may actually be started on nutritional support well in advance of their exenterative surgery. The implementation and monitoring of TPN is discussed in Chapter 2.

The role of drains, and what to drain, is unclear. There seems to be a gradual but definite move away from the use of drains in gynecologic surgery. Again, personal bias and past experience will determine whether drains are placed and when they should be removed. Rarely does a surgeon regret having a drain in place, provided it is not in contact with an anastomosis. With extensive urinary diversion procedures, occasionally questions will arise as to whether drainage is serum or urine. Measuring the blood urea nitrogen creatinine level of the fluid will often answer this question.

Patients who have a pelvic pack are usually kept at bedrest until it is removed, but the upper body can be elevated to improve respiratory toilet. With reconstructive surgery, patients can be ambulated or at least out of bed within 48 hours. Adequate pain control must be maintained. Physical therapists are most useful in ensuring good range of motion and gradual increases in physical activity levels.

The continent reservoir is irrigated several times a day to remove mucus and clots. The mucus gradually disappears, but irrigations are necessary for up to 6 weeks. Self-catheterization is ideally taught before discharge, and further schooling is provided by home health care nurses.

For patients with a low rectal anastomosis, oral feedings are started at 14 to 21 days. Initial stooling will be frequent, since rectal storage capacity is limited. Lomotil and Immodium can be used to decrease peristalsis. The goal is to have

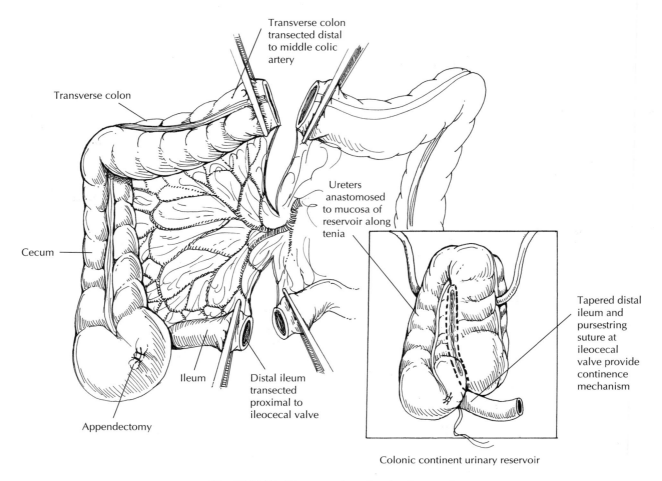

Transverse colon transected distal to middle colic artery

Transverse colon

Cecum

Appendectomy

Ileum

Distal ileum transected proximal to ileocecal valve

Ureters anastomosed to mucosa of reservoir along tenia

Tapered distal ileum and pursestring suture at ileocecal valve provide continence mechanism

Colonic continent urinary reservoir

Fig. 30-11. Performance of continent colon pouch.

the patient pass stools three to six times a day. Gradually, the patient's lower rectum accommodates, and after 4 to 6 months, a more normal stooling pattern is usually achieved and antiperistaltics may be discontinued. When anastomoses are less than 6 cm accommodation is more difficult and incontinence and frequent stooling are more of a problem.

Frequent opportunities to speak with other patients who have successfully undergone exenteration help keep the patient's spirits high and attitude positive. Stomal therapists and home health care nurses are also important in aiding the patient in the immediate postoperative period and after discharge.

COMPLICATIONS

With such extensive surgery, the range of potential complications is legion. As many as 50 percent of patients may suffer a major complication.[20–22] Those relating to prior medical problems and those seen with more commonly performed gynecologic procedures are discussed elsewhere in the text. The need for strict fluid management, and hence the need for a central line, cannot be overemphasized. Pro-

phylactic antibiotics and intermittent pneumatic compression stockings for prevention of pulmonary embolus are always used. Death in the perioperative period now occurs in fewer than 5 percent of patients, with patients over the age of 65 perhaps at increased risk. Sepsis, adult respiratory distress syndrome, heart failure, pulmonary embolus, and multiorgan system failure are usual terminal events.

Intraoperative complications are predominantly related to hemorrhage and problems related to the mechanics of the reconstructive phase of the procedure. Blood loss of 6 U or more is not unusual.[21–23] Management of intraoperative hemorrhage is discussed in Chapter 27. Rarely, in patients with an infected pelvic defect, delayed hemorrhage may be encountered. This is best handled with percutaneous embolization by interventional radiology, as re-exploration is extremely morbid. During bowel anastomoses, segments of bowel may infarct, turn out to be too short, or ureteral anastomoses may tear. Patience and diligent attention to technique will minimize these occurrences.

Gastrointestinal complications requiring surgical re-exploration, are usually attributable to problems with healing of the anastomosis in previously irradiated bowel. Bowel obstruction is managed conservatively, with decompression and fluid replacement. Similarly, fistulas that may be entero-cutaneous or through the perineal defect are given a chance to heal, maintaining the patient NPO and continuing TPN. Low output fistulas, in the absence of distal obstruction, occasionally heal. Usually, re-exploration and surgical correction, with high patient morbidity and mortality, is required. Surprisingly, significant concurrent medical dis-

eases, prior laparotomies, and severe malnutrition do not seem to be associated with major complications of exenteration that require surgical correction.[23] In anterior exenterations, difficult extended dissections to preserve the rectum frequently lead to fistula. In these situations, a total exenteration or low rectal anastomosis may be preferable.

Use of colon conduits or reservoirs, thereby avoiding

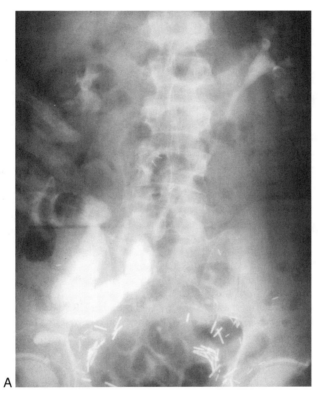

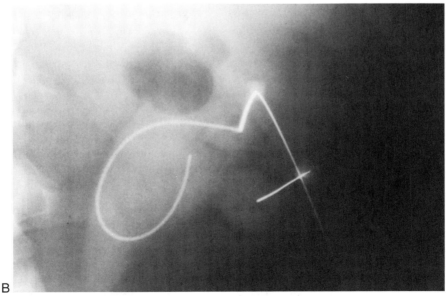

Fig. 30-12. (A) Conduit leak at urethral anastomosis. (B) Percutaneous stent into conduit, which allowed drainage and subsequent healing.

anastomosis in radiated bowel, lessens problems with anastomotic leaks. When leaks are encountered, management with percutaneous stenting and drainage is preferable to reoperation with attempts at reconstruction[24] (Fig. 30-12). Percutaneous catheters can also be used to dilate areas of ureteral stenosis.

Unexplained fevers are frequently encountered and treated empirically with broad-spectrum antibiotics. Before assuming that there is no identifiable source, the presence of ureteral obstruction, leaking anastomosis, or pelvic defect abscess must be ruled out.

Delayed complications consist of bowel obstruction, bowel or urinary fistula, ureteral obstruction with renal compromise, and stomal stenosis. Recurrent cancer must always be considered. Attempts at conservative management, to avoid laparotomy, are always wise.

Having run the gauntlet of all of these complications and risks, survival and presumptive cure is possible in approximately one-half of patients undergoing exenteration as salvage therapy for pelvic cancers.

SUMMARY

Pelvic exenteration is an operation of last resort, performed to hopefully save women otherwise doomed to die of their cancer. Most procedures are done for recurrent cancer of the cervix, although in certain patients with other cancers or cancer-related problems, exenteration has a limited role. A successful outcome requires careful pre operative optimization of the patient, meticulous intraoperative attention to surgical technique, and diligent postoperative surveillance. Despite this, many patients will experience major surgical complications that are best managed by avoiding re-exploration. Fortunately, the improved sophistication of our colleagues in radiation is making this operation less and less necessary, although it remains a part of every gynecologic oncologist's armamentarium.

REFERENCES

1. Brunschwig A: Complete excision of pelvic viscera for advanced carcinoma. Cancer 1:177, 1948
2. Bricker EM: The evolution of the ileal segment bladder substitution operation. Am J Surg 135:834, 1978
3. Bricker EM: Bladder substitution after pelvic evisceration. Surg Clin North Am 30:1511, 1950
4. Orr JW, Shingleton HM, Hatch KD et al: Urinary diversion in patients undergoing pelvic exenteration. Am J Obstet Gynecol 142:883, 1982
5. Hancock KC, Copeland LJ, Gershenson DM et al: Urinary conduits in gynecologic oncology. Obstet Gynecol 67:680, 1986
6. Kock ND, Nilson AE, Nilson LO et al: Urinary diversion via a continent ileal reservoir: clinical results in 12 patients. J Urol 128:469, 1982
7. Montie JE, Mac Gregor PS Fazio VW, Lavery L: Continent ileal urinary reservoir (Kock Pouch). Urol Clin North Am 13: 251, 1986
8. Penalver MA, Bejany DE, Averette HE et al: Continent urinary diversion in gynecologic oncology. Gynecol Oncol 34:274, 1989
9. Mannel RS, Braly PS, Buller RE: Indiana pouch continent urinary reservoir in patients with previous pelvic irradiation. Obstet Gynecol 75:891, 1990
10. Hatch KD, Gelder MS, Soong S-J et al: Pelvic exenteration with low rectal anastomosis: survival, complications, and prognostic factors. Gynecol Oncol 38:462, 1990
11. Barber HRK, Brunschwig A: Pelvic exenteration for extensive necrosis following radiation therapy for gynecologic cancer. Obstet Gynecol 25:575, 1965
12. Phillips B, Buschbaum HJ, Lifshitz S: Pelvic exenteration for vulvo vaginal carcinoma. Am J Obstet Gynecol 15:141, 1981
13. Boronow RC, Hickman BT, Reagam MT et al: Combined therapy as an alternative to exenteration for locally advanced vulvo vaginal cancer. II. Results, complications and dosimetric and surgical considerations. Am J Clin Oncol 10:171, 1990
14. Thomas G, Dembo A, Depetrillo A et al: Concurrent radiation and chemotherapy in vulvar carcinoma. Gynecol Oncol 36: 181, 1990
15. Barber HRK, Brunschwig A: Pelvic exenteration for advanced and recurrent ovarian cancer. Surgery 58:935, 1965
16. Barber HRK, Brunschwig A: Treatment and results of recurrent cancer of the corpus uteri in patients receiving anterior and total pelvic exenteration 1947–1963. Cancer 22:949, 1968
17. Eisenkop SM, Nalick RH, Teng NN: Modified posterior exenteration for ovarian cancer. Obstet Gynecol 78:879, 1991
18. Stanhope CR, Symmonds RE: Palliative exenteration—what, when, and why? Am J Obstet Gynecol 152:12, 1985
19. Brunschwig A, Barber HRK: Extended pelvic exenteration for advanced cancer of the cervix. Cancer 17:1267, 1964
20. Rutledge FN, Smith JP, Wharton JT, O'Quinn AG: Pelvic exenteration: analysis of 296 patients. Am J Obstet Gynecol 129: 881, 1977
21. Soper JT, Berchuck A, Creasman WT, Clarke-Pearson DL: Pelvic exenteration: factors associated with major surgical morbidity. Gynecol Oncol 35:93, 1989
22. Morley GW, Hopkins MP, Lindenauer SM, Roberts JA: Pelvic exenteration, University of Michigan: 100 patients at 5 years. Obstet Gynecol 74:934, 1989
23. Orr JW, Shingleton HM, Hatch KD et al: Gastrointestinal complications associated with pelvic exenteration. Am J Obstet Gynecol 145:325, 1983
24. Bladou F, Houvenaeghel G, Delpero J-R, Guerinel G: Incidence and management of major urinary complications after pelvic exenteration for gynecological malignancies. J Surg Oncol 58:91, 1995

CHAPTER THIRTY-ONE

GRAFTS AND FLAPS IN GYNECOLOGIC SURGERY

JOHN T. SOPER

Gynecologic surgery, especially gynecologic oncology and vulvar procedures, often produces loss of tissue, scarring, and distortion of normal pelvic, vaginal, or vulvar anatomy. This is especially true when these procedures are performed on women who have received prior pelvic radiotherapy, which produces loss of tissue vascularity. Radical pelvic surgery often results in loss of significant tissue and alterations in both functional pelvic anatomy and sexual response. Recent studies have focussed on the effects of radical pelvic procedures upon the patient's body self-image and psychosocial interactions.[1-3] Recognition of these issues has led to the recommendation for appropriate individualization of the radicalness of major resections for some diseases[4] and an increasing recognition of the need to pay attention to principles of reconstructive surgery at the time of the primary radical pelvic procedure.

This chapter reviews common principles of reconstructive surgery, with special emphasis on the features unique to their application in pelvic reconstructive procedures. Several of these principles can be applied to less radical pelvic procedures and are often used in reconstructions after complications of benign gynecologic procedures, necrotizing fasciitis, pelvic trauma, and in conjunction with general surgical or urologic procedures. Because many texts devoted to reconstructive and gynecologic surgery illustrate a wide variety of pelvic reconstructive techniques,[5-10] this chapter does not present an encyclopedic review of techniques. Rather, the procedures most frequently used by the gynecologic oncology service at Duke University Medical Center are discussed in detail.

In general, the most simple repair of a surgical defect that accomplishes the goals of reconstruction will usually be the most effective and least likely to incur major morbidity (Table 31-1). Direct closure of a surgical defect is to be preferred if there is minimal tissue loss, mobility and laxity of the surrounding tissues, and if local factors favor primary wound healing. Factors adversely affecting wound healing include infection, malnutrition, cardiovascular disease, smoking, diabetes, and prior radiotherapy. Fortunately, the pelvis is well vascularized and adjacent tissues can often be mobilized to cover a surgical defect.

Simple vulvar incisions should be planned to take advantage of the native lines of tissue stress (Fig. 31-1), and closed parallel to these lines to avoid contractures. It should be remembered that circular incisions tend to produce progressive contracture with healing, a factor that might produce stenosis at the introitus or in the vagina. Finally, important surgical principles of hemostasis, debridement of poorly vascularized adipose tissue, irrigation of surgical defects before closure, and obliteration of dead space will improve the chances of healing for any wound.[11] Specific reconstructive techniques are discussed below.

SKIN GRAFTS

Skin grafts are frequently used as adjuncts to reconstructive procedures of the vulva and vagina. Split-thickness skin grafts, consisting of the thin layer of epidermis and

Table 31-1. Relative Complexity of Reconstructive Surgical Techniques

Complexity	Example	Technique
Simple	Vulvar incision	Direct closure
	Skinning vulvectomy	Split-thickness skin graft
Intermediate	Radical vulvectomy	Local ''random'' rotational flap
	Vulvovaginal defect at exenteration	Myocutaneous flap
Complex	Massive tissue loss from necrotizing fasciitis	Free flap with microvascular reanastomosis

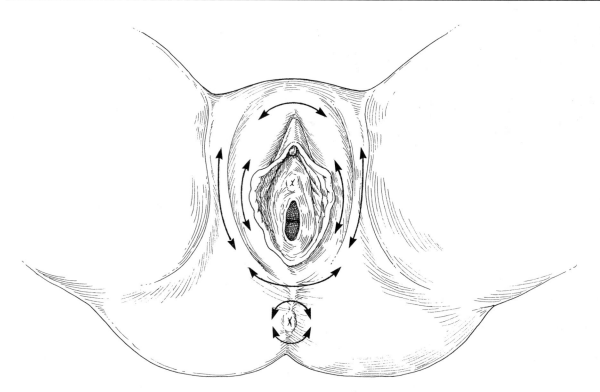

Fig. 31-1. Tissue "wrinkle lines" of the vulva. Closure of defects parallel to these lines will reduce scarring and contracture.

reticular dermis, are used most frequently because of the thin vulvar skin and vaginal mucous membrane that they replace.

The donor site is usually selected from the thigh, buttocks, lower abdomen, or mons. The donor sites noted above have skin of a similar consistency to the vulva. If cosmesis is desired, buttock or mons is selected as the donor site. A Brown dermatome is used to harvest a 0.16- to 0.20-mm thickness of skin, approximately 4 to 5 cm in width. More than one strip of skin can be harvested for grafting, or the skin graft can be expanded with a skin mesher to fit virtually any size defect. The skin donor site is a raw surface consisting of reticular dermis, epidermal rete pegs, and skin adnexal structures. It is dressed with any of a variety of dressings, such as scarlet red gauze or dermoplast, to allow healing and re-epithelialization from the rete pegs and skin adnexa, a process that usually takes several weeks to complete. Often, the patient's major pain is derived from the donor site; therefore, the lower abdomen or thigh is used as the donor site unless cosmesis is of major concern to the patient.

The split-thickness skin graft heals to its bed in stages over the first 4 to 7 days after grafting.[11] Over the first 24 to 48 hours, the graft is oxygenated and nourished by plasmatic imbibition from the underlying raw surface, similar to growth of cells in cell culture. Immobility of the graft on the bed is critical for graft survival, as the graft adheres to the bed by fibrin bonding. Over the next several days the graft is revascularized by connecting existing small vessels in the graft to vessels in the bed (inosculation), or by ingrowth of vessels from the underlying bed (neovascularization).[11] During revascularization, it is important that the graft be immobilized on its bed to prevent shearing of the immature vascular bed.

Several local factors are required for successful skin graft take. The recipient bed must have sufficient vascularity to support the graft. Fascia, muscle, vascularized adipose tissue, perineurium, peritoneum, pericardium, and intact periosteum are tissues that can support a skin graft.[11] Because the periosteum is usually partially stripped away from the symphysis during radical surgery, and because a split-thickness skin graft provides no cushion of underlying fat, these grafts are usually not applied directly onto the exposed pubic bone. Denuded tendon, nerve, cartilage, and bone will not directly support a skin graft.[11] Radiated tissues also may be poor tissues to serve as the recipient bed for a skin graft because of late obliterative endarteritis produced by radiation. The recipient bed must not be heavily contaminated with bacteria, because infection can interfere with the early stages of graft revascularization. Finally, it is of critical importance that the graft remain in contact during the early phases of healing. Hemostasis must be excellent before the graft is placed on the recipient bed. Making "pie crust" incisions or meshing the graft will allow blood and serum to escape from beneath the graft during the critical first few days after grafting, so that the graft will not ''float'' and can be nourished from the recipient bed. Immobilization should continue for several days thereafter to allow establishment of the immature vascular bed of the graft. Because the vagina and vulva have irregular contours, flexible pressure dressings are used to immobilize the graft.

After the split-thickness skin graft has become established, some contracture of the underlying recipient bed will occur. This is usually not a problem when it is used for vulvar reconstruction, but should be kept in mind when the split-thickness skin graft is used for vaginal reconstruction.

Split-Thickness Skin Graft for Vulvar Reconstruction

Split-thickness skin grafts are often used for repair of large vulvar and perianal defects produced by surgical resection of multifocal preinvasive intraepithelial neoplasia, or in conjunction with radical resections for invasive vulvar carcinoma. The procedure was first described for this indication by Rutledge and Sinclair[12] in 1968 and remains a valuable option for the management of vulvar intraepithelial neoplasia despite the introduction of laser vaporization and other techniques. Skinning vulvectomy with split-thickness skin grafting results in more normal postoperative functional and cosmetic results than simple vulvectomy.[12-14] A single surgical procedure may be preferable to multiple laser vaporizations for the treatment of extensive multifocal vulvar intraepithelial neoplasia.

In contrast to laser vaporization, a tissue specimen will be available for histology after skinning vulvectomy. Approximately 5 to 10 percent of women with extensive multifocal disease will have occult invasive carcinoma.[14] Fortunately, the majority will have minimally invasive (less than 1 mm stromal invasion) lesions. However, all patients should undergo a careful evaluation with acetic acid and hand lens, or low-power colposcopy combined with liberal biopsies to exclude invasive disease before the procedure. Patients should be evaluated for vaginal and cervical involvement. The perianal region must also be carefully examined to exclude involvement by intraepithelial neoplasia extending into the anal canal. Disease in the vagina, perianal region, and anal canal can be resected and grafted along with the vulvar disease,[14-16] or can be treated concurrently with laser vaporization.

All patients are treated with a mechanical bowel preparation before surgery. Perioperative first-generation cephalosporins are used for antibiotic prophylaxis. Low-dose heparin or intermittent calf compression are used throughout hospitalization, because patients will be at bed rest for at least 5 to 7 days postoperatively and are at an increased risk of thromboembolism. If skin is to be harvested from the mons or buttocks, patients are instructed to develop a ''tan line'' using their customary swimming suit, so that a hidden donor site can be selected.

The patient is positioned in the lithotomy position. The perineum and donor site are prepared for surgery and draped. The split-thickness skin graft is harvested after the extent of the operative defect has been mapped out to determine the amount of skin needed. If the graft is harvested before performing the skinning vulvectomy, it is kept moist in gauze saturated in physiologic saline until it is used.

The skinning vulvectomy is initiated by incising the lateral margins of the dissection at right angles to the skin. This prevents burying of partially transected hair follicles at the margin of the graft. If frozen section margins are critical, these are usually obtained *before* resecting the specimen, so that results will be available before the graft is deployed.

Dissection proceeds from lateral to medial and anterior to posterior when developing the vulvar specimen. The deep plane of resection is Buck's fascia, a continuation of Camper's superficial fascia over the vulva, just below the dermis. This is a relatively avascular plane perforated by small vessels that are easily controlled with electrocautery. The fascia will have a glistening white sheen and the vulvar skin will usually be easily dissected away from this in the anterior and lateral vulva using blunt dissection with the handle of the scalpel. Traction/countertraction will aid in dissection along this plane. Preservation of the subcutaneous tissues for the bed of the graft results in a relatively normal postoperative contour and texture of the vulva.[13,14]

The clitoris is preserved if no invasive disease is involved. If the skin of the clitoris is involved with intraepithelial neoplasia (Fig. 31-2A), de-epithelialization can be performed with the scalpel or laser. The clitoris can either be covered with the split-thickness graft or left uncovered and allowed to re-epithelialize. By leaving the shaft and glans of the clitoris intact, most patients will have no alteration in clitoral sensation.[13,14]

The medial and perianal margins are developed last. Most often the medial margin is at the hymeneal ring. Hemostasis is ensured and the resection bed irrigated. If necessary, windows are made in the central graft for the introitus and/or anus. The graft is trimmed to fit the defect and anchored to the margins with peripheral fine absorbable sutures (Fig. 31-2B). Excess skin is trimmed so that the graft fits the defect without wrinkles or undue tension. Small, 5-mm ''pie crust'' incisions are made into the graft at approximately 2 to 3-cm intervals to allow escape of serum during the first few days of healing. A bolus dressing is tied down over the graft with medial and lateral stay sutures to provide constant and even pressure to immobilize the operative site (Fig. 31-2C). A Foley catheter is placed in the bladder, and a large Foley catheter is placed in the anus if the anal canal has been grafted.

The introital and anal openings in the skin graft must be large enough to prevent stenosis. Occasionally, two or more grafts are required to cover a large defect, but expansion of the graft with a mesher is usually not needed.

The patient is kept at bed rest for 5 to 7 days to prevent

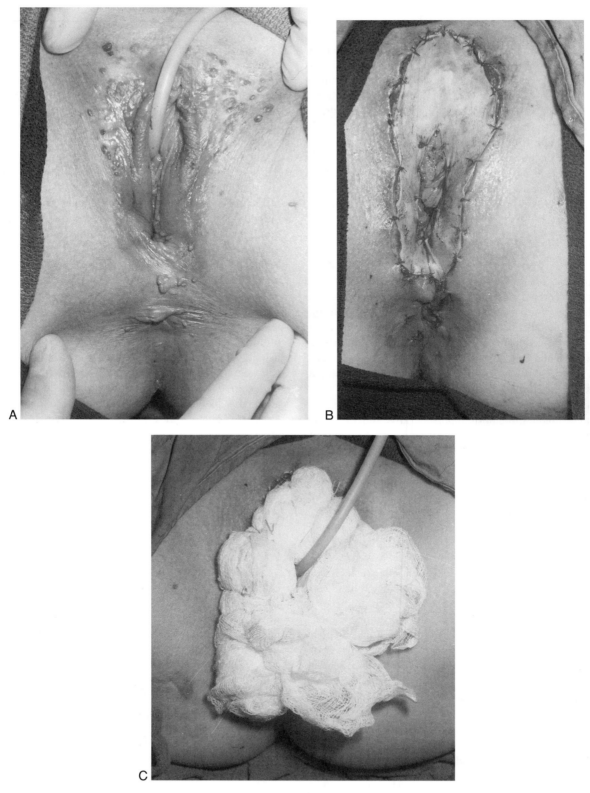

Fig. 31-2. **(A)** Extent of multifocal vulvar intraepithelial neoplasia to be treated with skinning vulvectomy. **(B)** The vulvar defect has been covered with split-thickness skin graft. Several ''pie crust'' incisions will be made into the graft to allow escape of serum. Additional sutures will be placed at the lateral and medial margins of the graft to secure the bolus dressing. **(C)** Bolus dressing is secured to the operative site by tying down the long lateral and medial sutures. The dressing is removed on the sixth postoperative day.

the graft from being sheared off of the immature vascular bed. The patient is kept constipated until the dressing is removed. The dressing can be irrigated with clindamycin if odor from the packing becomes offensive. On the sixth or seventh postoperative day, the bolus dressing is removed. In the absence of infection, more than 95 percent of the graft will take. Patients are instructed in frequent sitz baths or irrigation of the operative site, followed by gentle drying with a hair dryer on a low heat setting.

Intercourse is permissible after 4 to 6 weeks. The skin graft will develop slight concentric shrinkage as it matures but will retain a relatively normal texture. No hair growth occurs within the graft, because hair follicles are not transferred with the split-thickness skin graft.

Vulvar intraepithelial neoplasia often recurs. Almost one-third of patients with involved margins will develop a recurrence during short-term follow-up.[14] However, free margins are associated with almost a 25 percent incidence of recurrence.[14] Although rare recurrence has been reported within the skin graft, most occur at the margins of the graft and can be managed with simple excision or laser vaporization.

The major disadvantages of the skinning vulvectomy with split-thickness skin graft include possible morbidity due to the prolonged bed rest. Thromboembolic prophylaxis and aggressive pulmonary toilet should be employed until the patient is fully ambulatory. Patients also have prolonged discomfort during healing of the donor site.

Split-Thickness Skin Graft for Neovaginal Construction

Split-thickness skin grafting can be used for vaginal construction in surgical correction of congenital vaginal agenesis (McIndoe procedure)[17,18] (Fig. 31-3), repair of vaginal stenosis after surgery or radiotherapy,[18,19] and for neovaginal reconstruction after radical vulvovaginal procedures.[18,20–22] The split-thickness graft serves as a vaginal mucosa, lining the vaginal tube that has been created surgically. Because the skin graft does not provide vascularized tissue bulk, it must be combined with other procedures to construct a recipient bed when it is used for neovaginal reconstruction after exenteration.

The principles of split-thickness skin graft formation of a vagina are similar to other skin grafting procedures. After forming the vascularized recipient bed, the neovaginal skin graft must be immobilized with vaginal packing or a vaginal stent for 5 to 7 days to allow establishment of microcirculation. Because the split-thickness neovagina will stricture during late healing, mechanical dilatation or sexual activity is required to retain vaginal patency.

In all split-thickness vaginal procedures, the skin grafts are harvested as 4- to 5-cm wide by 8- to 10-cm long strips with a thickness of 0.3 to 0.5 mm. Two or three strips expanded with a skin mesher are sutured together with fine absorbable sutures. The skin graft is sutured over a vaginal mold with the epidermal surface toward the mold to create the vaginal tube (Fig. 31-3B). The neovaginal tube can be created by one member of the team while others are preparing the recipient bed. The skin graft should be kept moist with physiologic saline until use.

In the McIndoe procedure, a semicircular or H-shaped incision is made in the posterior vaginal dimple, sufficient to create a 3- to 4-cm wide introitus.[17,18] The potential space between the rectum and bladder is carefully developed with sharp and blunt dissection (Fig. 31-3A). Near the perineum, the loose areolar tissues lateral to the midline raphe can be easily opened, but the midline septum must be divided with sharp dissection until the looser tissues of the upper rectovaginal space are encountered. Palpation of the urethral catheter and frequent rectal examinations are used to monitor the progress of the dissection. The vaginal space should extend at least 12 cm in depth and 4 cm in diameter. After ensuring hemostasis, the vaginal stent covered with the graft is placed in the vaginal cavity and sutured to the labia majora (Fig. 31-3C). The patient is kept at bed rest with continuous bladder drainage for 5 to 7 days before removing the vaginal stent.

In patients with vaginal stenosis resulting from radiotherapy, it is usually preferable to dilate the vagina using serial dilators and estrogen cream. Patients who have received pelvic radiotherapy are routinely instructed in vaginal dilation to prevent total vaginal coaptation. Occasionally, however, total obliteration of the vagina will result from combined radical external beam radiation/brachytherapy techniques, and a patient will desire vaginal reconstruction. In these cases, the scarred vagina must be carefully dissected from the bladder and rectum using sharp dissection.[18] Care must be taken to avoid entry into these structures, as these patients are at high risk of fistula formation. After development of the recipient bed, the graft and stent are placed as in the McIndoe technique.

When split-thickness skin grafting is used for primary neovagina formation at exenteration the author usually performs this concurrently to avoid a second procedure; however, others have utilized delayed grafting after a bed of granulation tissue has developed in the pelvis.[20,21] Vascularized tissue such as omentum, peritoneum, muscular flap, or bowel serosa should be used as recipient bed and to create the walls of the neovaginal space.[22] If a rectosigmoid anastomosis is performed, an interposed vascularized pedicle of omentum or muscular flap is used to protect the anastomosis. The vaginal tube can be formed over a sigmoidoscope[22] and packed into the pelvic bed with clindamycin-saturated gauze, rather than using a rigid vaginal mold.

In all situations, the vaginal stent or packing is removed 5 to 7 days after surgery and inspected for take. A vaginal dilator is used daily for at least 6 weeks to prevent the development of stenosis, which is the biggest disadvantage to using this technique for vaginal reconstruction. Estrogen

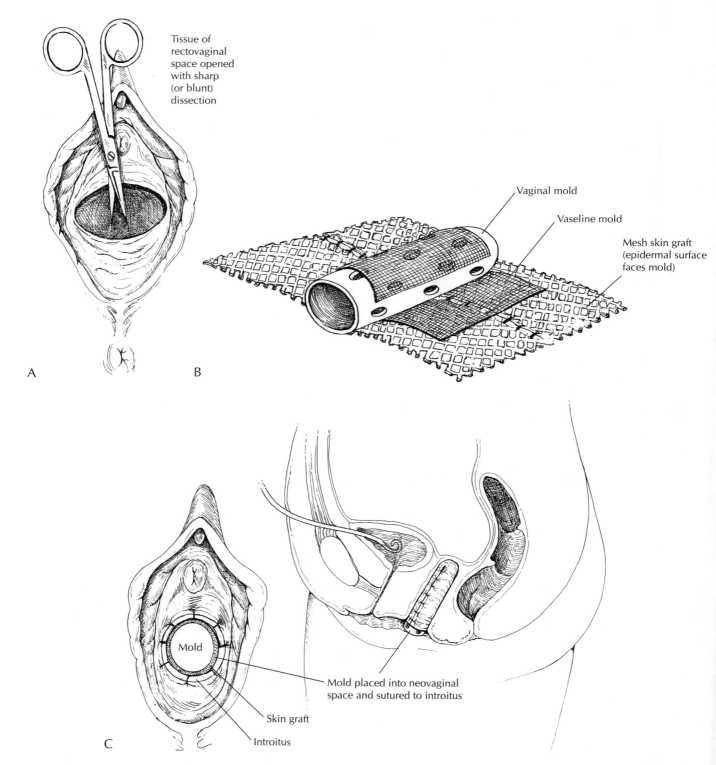

Tissue of rectovaginal space opened with sharp (or blunt) dissection

Vaginal mold

Vaseline mold

Mesh skin graft (epidermal surface faces mold)

A

B

Mold

Mold placed into neovaginal space and sutured to introitus

Skin graft

Introitus

C

Fig. 31-3. **(A)** In the McIndoe procedure for vaginal agenesis, the loose tissues of the rectovaginal space are dissected using sharp and blunt dissection to form the vaginal space. This should measure at least 12 cm in depth and more than 4 cm in width. **(B)** The skin graft is sutured over a vaginal mold with the epidermal surface oriented towards the mold. **(C)** The mold is placed into the neovaginal space and sutured into place at the introitus. A suprapubic catheter is often used to drain the bladder until the mold is removed on the sixth or seventh postoperative day.

vaginal cream should be used for lubrication. If the patient is not sexually active, a stent should be used at night to maintain vaginal patency. If vaginal mucosa is retained at the introitus the split-thickness skin graft will eventually assume the characteristics of vaginal epithelium, including response to estrogen and production of glycogen.[18]

FLAPS

Many different types of tissue flaps are available for pelvic reconstructive surgery (Fig. 31-4). The majority of flaps are designed to bring vascularized subcutaneous adipose tissue and skin with or without underlying muscle into the operative defect, although some of the myosubcutaneous and muscular flaps can be used to provide only vascularized soft tissue to fill a large defect. To be clinically useful, flaps must have an arc of rotation that will allow the flap to be mobilized to fill the tissue defect without jeopardizing the blood supply to the flap. Unlike skin grafts, tissue flaps do not develop contracture during the course of healing if they are properly vascularized.

A basic knowledge of the vascular tree leading to the microcirculation of the skin is needed to understand the principles of flap construction. The major arterial branches off of the aorta form segmental or axial arterial systems (e.g., femoral-posterior tibial/anterior tibial/peroneal system). These arteries branch off further to form named and unnamed perforator arteries that can course in the deep subcutaneous tissues (direct cutaneous), along the fascial septa between muscle bellies (fasciocutaneous), and along or through the muscle bellies myocutaneous or musculocutaneous) before terminating in the dermal and subdermal anastomotic plexus.[11]

Random skin flaps are vascularized through the dermal-subdermal plexus and are composed of skin with a margin of underlying fat (Fig. 31-4A). These are formed without intentional inclusion of major vessels, and must be kept relatively short, with the length usually restricted to less than twice the width.[11] Because of compromised microvascularization of the skin after radiotherapy, random skin flaps should be used with caution in previously radiated tissues. In their simplest form, random flaps are used when adjacent skin and fat are mobilized to fill a tissue defect without tension. Advancement flaps, lateral transposition or rhomboid flaps, rotational flaps, and Z-plasty procedures are other frequently performed examples of random flaps. Limberg has extensively described the mathematics behind the geometry of random flaps.[23]

Axial or arterial flaps (Fig. 31-4B) are widely used for head and neck reconstructions, but have limited applications in the pelvis. These include a direct cutaneous artery in the deep subcutaneous fat that supplies a reliable territory of overlying skin.[11]

In fasciocutaneous flaps (Fig. 31-4C), the vessels course along the septa between muscle bellies and supply a predictable territory of overlying skin.[11] Fasciocutaneous flaps from the labia[24] and inner thigh[25] can be used for vulvovaginal reconstruction.

Myocutaneous or musculocutaneous flaps (Fig. 31-4D) consist of a unit comprised of muscle and fascia with an overlying island of subcutaneous fat and skin supplied by a musculocutaneous perforator that runs through the belly of the muscle.[11] Occasionally, flaps consisting of muscle alone (muscular) or of muscle and overlying subcutaneous fat (myosubcutaneous) are used to provide vascularized tissue to obturate dead space. Individual variations in the vascular supply and skin territory supported by the myocutaneous perforator are usually minimal. The most versatile flaps have an arc of rotation that allows the flap to be employed for a variety of reconstructive procedures. A major advantage of myocutaneous flaps lies in their mobilization of a large bulk of vascularized tissue to provide obliteration of dead space after radical pelvic procedures. Gracilis, rectus abdominis, bulbocavernosus, tensor fascia lata, and gluteus maximus flaps are examples of myocutaneous flaps that are often used for pelvic reconstructions.

Free tissue flaps with microvascular anastomosis can be used to transplant a myocutaneous unit from virtually any body site.[11] Serial tissue expansion using an inflatable implant can also be used to increase the amount of skin and underlying fat available for tissue transfer. Specific flap techniques frequently used for pelvic reconstructions are discussed below.

Random Skin Flaps

Axial Translocation Flaps

Axial translocation or advancement flaps can be used to fill rectangular defects occurring on a relatively flat surface (Figs. 31-5 and 31-6). The entire flap and tissues adjacent to the base of the flap must be mobilized adequately to allow the flap to fill the defect.[11] The flap should not exceed twice the width of the base. Excision of paired equilateral triangles of skin adjacent to the base, measuring approximately one-quarter the length of the flap, will allow forward mobility. Alternatively, the flap can be mobilized and the redundant dog-ear cone of skin lateral to the mobilized flap can be excised.

Lateral Transposition Flaps

Lateral transposition flaps are versatile for filling defects of virtually any configuration (Fig. 31-7). They are especially useful for vulvar (Fig. 31-8) and vaginal reconstruction procedures.[26] The flap and surrounding tissues must be mobilized adequately, and the flap width should not be more than twice the length.[11] Lateral transposition flaps should

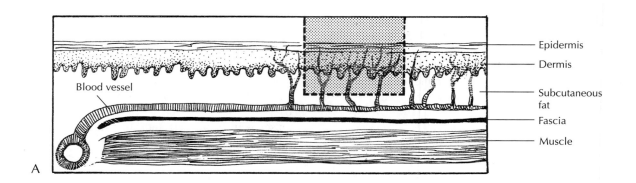

Epidermis

Dermis

Subcutaneous fat

Fascia

Muscle

Blood vessel

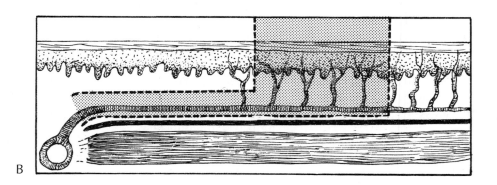

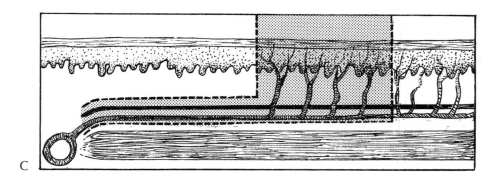

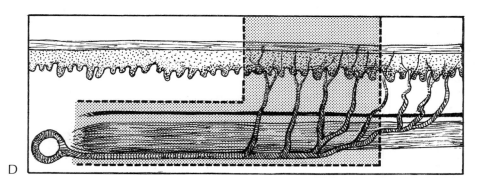

Fig. 31-4. Representation of the vascular supply of various tissue flaps used in reconstructive tissue. **(A)** Random flap, **(B)**) axial or arterial flap, **(C)** fasciocutaneous flap, and **(D)** myocutaneous flap.

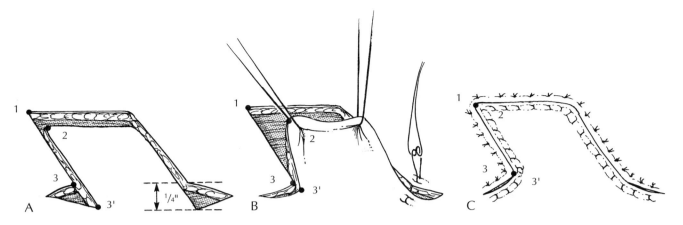

Fig. 31-5. Axial translocation (advancement) flap to fill rectangular skin defects on a relatively flat surface. **(A)** A random skin flap below the broad side of the defect is mobilized. The length should be twice the width and the flap length (3:2) should be two to three times as long as the defect (1:2). Equilateral triangles are excised lateral to the base of the flap, with each side (3–3) approximately one-quarter the length of the flap. **(B)** Skin and subcutaneous fat are mobilized widely to allow advancement of the flap into the defect. **(C)** The flap is sutured into place.

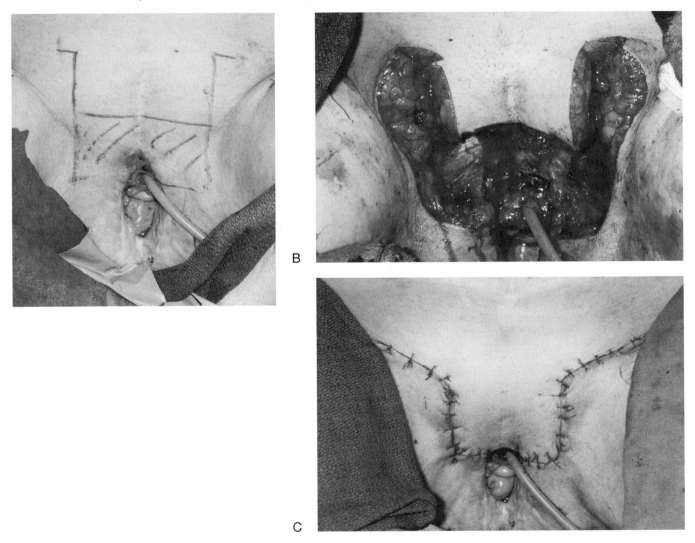

Fig. 31-6. Axial translocation flap to repair anterior vulvar defect. **(A)** Flap and defect are planned before resection. **(B)** Flap raised and widely mobilized. **(C)** Flap advanced to fill defect.

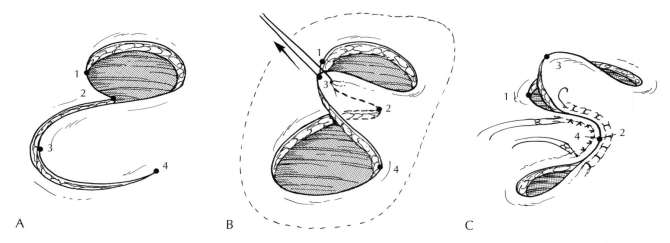

A   B   C

Fig. 31-7. Lateral transposition flap development. **(A)** Flap (2–3–4) is designed so that is will be rotated 45 to 90 degrees into the defect and is slightly larger than the defect. The flap length with ratio should be less than 2:1. **(B)** The flap and adjacent tissues are mobilized widely, allowing rotation of the apex of the flap (3) to the apex of the defect (1). **(C)** The small wedge at point 2 is brought to the base of the flap (4) and the flap is sutured into position.

be rotated in a direction approximately perpendicular to the skin tension lines (wrinkles).[27,28]

Limberg described rhomboid lateral transposition flaps to close rhomboidal defects having a narrow angle of less than 60 degrees[23,26–28] (Fig. 31-9A). Four potential mirror-image Limberg flaps exist around any rhomboidal defect of this

configuration. Paired flaps close parallelogram defects and 3 to 4 symmetrical flaps can close circular defects.[23,27]

The Dufourmental flap was designed to close rhomboidal defects having a narrow angle of 60 to 90 degrees[28] (Fig. 31-9B). These have a larger base and better blood supply than Limberg flaps. Four potential mirror-image Dufour-

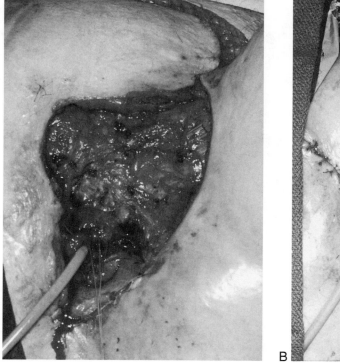

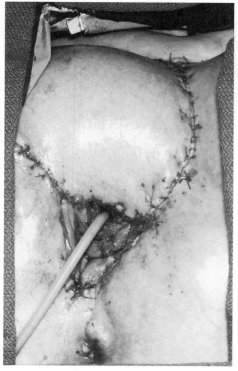

A   B

Fig. 31-8. Use of mons lateral transposition flap to close larger anterior vulvar defect. **(A)** A flap is developed from the mons that will be rotated 80 to 90 degrees into the vulvar defect. **(B)** Flap rotated and sutured into position.

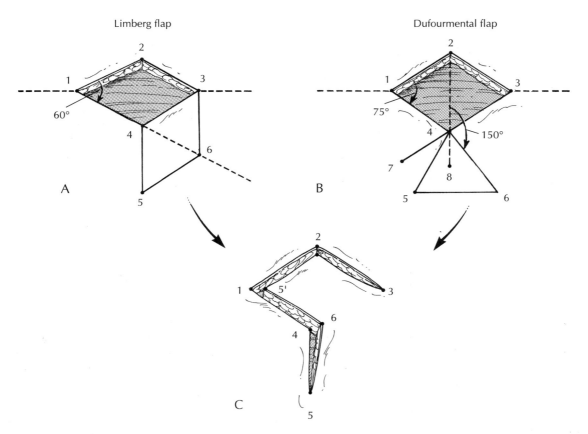

Limberg flap

Dufourmental flap

60°

75°

150°

A

B

C

Fig. 31-9. Design of the (**A**) Limberg and (**B**) Dufourmental flaps to (**C**) close a rhomboidal defect.

mental flaps can close a rhomboid, while 8 can be constructed around a square defect.[28] Rectangular or parallelogram defects can be closed with paired flaps.[28]

Rotational Skin Flaps

Rotational skin flaps can be used to fill large round or triangular defects (Fig. 31-10). The skin of the anterior and lateral abdominal wall, with its richly anastomotic blood supply, is able to support large flaps of this type, and of filling abdominal wall or groin defects of up to 10 to 15 cm in diameter.[29]

Z-Plasty Flaps

Z-plasty flap techniques allow substitution of vertical and horizontal dimensions (Fig. 31-11). These flaps are particularly useful in relieving contractures at the vaginal introitus or in the vagina. Limberg illustrates multiple examples of simple and combined Z-plasty procedures.[23] Small Z-plasties can be used at the introitus of a myocutaneous flap neovagina at primary surgery to prevent a stenosis from developing during healing.

Myocutaneous Flaps

Gracilis Myocutaneous Flap

In 1976, McGraw et al[30] first described the application of the gracilis myocutaneous flap technique for neovaginal reconstruction after pelvic exenteration (Fig. 31-12). This versatile flap has become widely used for both vulvar and vaginal reconstructions after radical pelvic surgery.[31-38]

The thin strap-like gracilis muscle is the most medial adductor of the thigh. It normally functions to stabilize the knee but can be sacrificed without loss of function. It originates from the pubic tubercle and runs posterior to the adductor longus to insert into the medial tibial plateau (Fig. 31-12A). The classic gracilis flap derives its major blood supply from a vascular pedicle that is derived from branches of the medial femoral circumflex artery and supports a large territory of skin extending along the medial thigh extending to the distal one-third of the thigh posterior to the adductor longus[30] (Fig. 31-12B). The dominant vascular pedicle is constant in location, entering the deep gracilis with paired venae comitantes and nerve approximately 6 to 8 cm distal to the pubic tubercle after passing between the adductor longus and brevis muscles. An accessory blood supply, derived from anastomotic terminal branches of the obturator and pu-

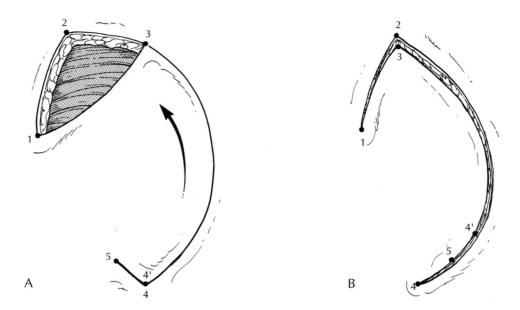

Fig. 31-10. Design of rotational flap to close triangular defect on a flat surface. **(A)** Mobility of flap (5–4–3) is obtained by back-cutting the base of the flap (5–4). The flap should be 2.5 to 3 times the size of the defect. The flap length should be 1.5 times the width (3–2/1–5). **(B)** After mobilization and rotation, point 3 is moved to point 2, forming the apex of the suture line. Points 5 and 4 are advanced along the convexity of the closure, increasing the circumference of the flap by the distance 4–5.

dendal arteries, enters within the proximal 1 to 3 cm of the gracilis.[35,36,38] Although these accessory vessels are not as well defined as the dominant vascular pedicle, they have been used by Copeland et al[35] and Soper et al[36,38] to support a short gracilis flap that can be successfully used for vulvovaginal reconstructions (Fig. 31-12C).

The gracilis flap can be rotated either anterior or posterior within a wide arc of rotation, allowing it to be deployed for anterior vulvar or groin reconstructions, neovaginal formation, or repair of posterior vulvar and perianal defects. The arc of rotation of the classic flap is around the mobilized dominant vascular pedicle, while the short flap is rotated around the origin of the muscle from the pubic tubercle (Fig. 31-12D). If a classic long gracilis flap is developed, the proximal muscle can be divided to facilitate rotation,[33] but usually there is sufficient mobility to preclude division of the

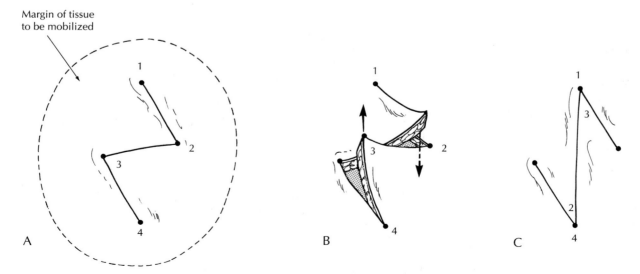

Fig. 31-11. **(A–C)** Design of the Z-plasty flap. Z-plasty allows the exchange of the length of the line 2–3 for the length of line 1–4.

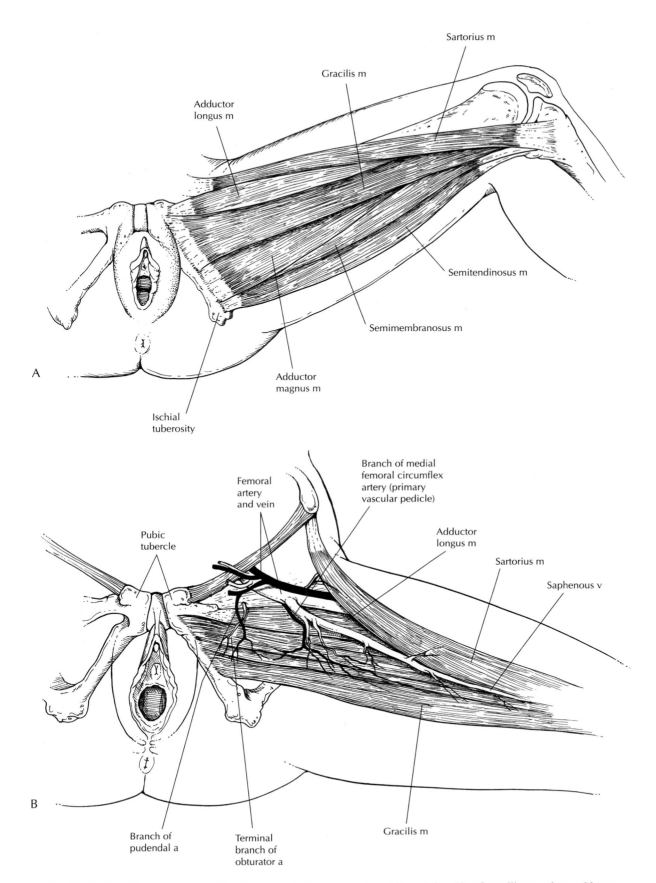

Fig. 31-12. Gracilis myocutaneous flap for neovaginal reconstruction. **(A)** Relationship of gracilis muscle to adductor muscles of the inner thigh. **(B)** Vascular supply of the gracilis muscle. *(Figure continues.)*

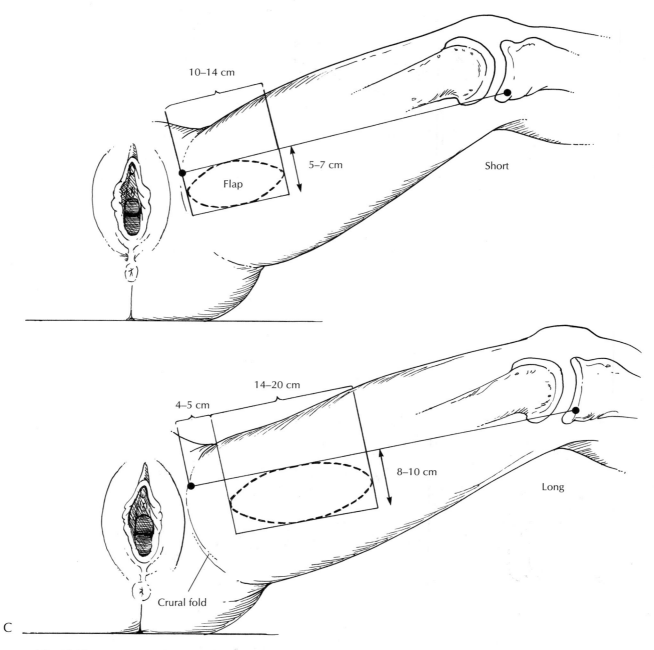

Fig. 31-12 *(Continued).* **(C)** Relative size and location of short and long gracilis myocutaneous flaps. *(Figure continues.)*

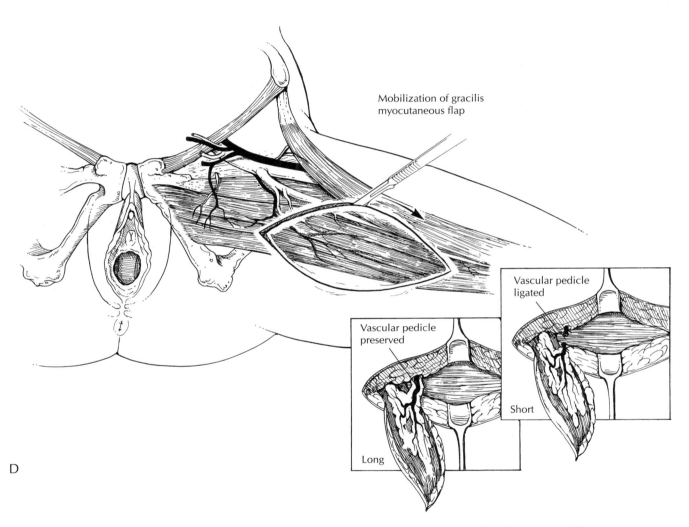

Mobilization of gracilis myocutaneous flap

Vascular pedicle preserved

Vascular pedicle ligated

Long

Short

D

31-12 *(Continued).* **(D)** Mobilization of gracilis myocutaneous flaps and rotation through perineal tunnel. When short gracilis flaps are employed, the dominant vascular pedicle is deliberately sacrificed (inset). **(E & F)** Formation of neovaginal tube and closure of thigh donor sites. The gracilis neovagina will be rotated posteriorly into the pelvis and anchored to the levator plate, symphysis and/or sacral hollow to prevent prolapse of the flap. *(Figure continues.)*

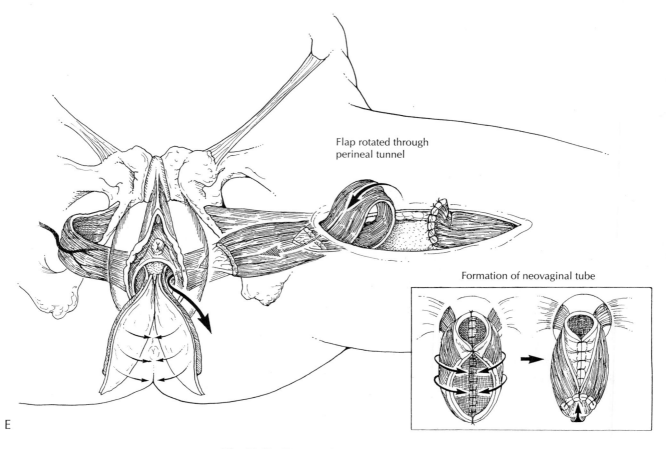

Flap rotated through perineal tunnel

Formation of neovaginal tube

E

Fig. 31-12 *(Continued). (Figure continues.)*

muscle. Furthermore, division of the proximal muscle deprives the flap of its secondary blood supply.

Figure 31-12 illustrates the use of a gracilis flap for neovaginal formation during pelvic exenteration. The patient is positioned in the modified Whitmore position using Allen stirrups (Edgewater Medical Systems, Inc., Mayfield Heights, OH), with the hips adducted approximately 45 degrees and flexed sightly. The medial thighs are prepared to the knees to allow access to the full skin island if needed. A guideline is drawn on the medial thigh from the pubic tubercle to the medial tibial plateau along the margin of the adductor longus. The skin island supplied by the gracilis will be located posterior to this line. If a long flap is to be employed, a 14- to 20- cm long and 6- to 10- cm wide ellipsoid skin island will be developed with the proximal margin 4 to 6 cm distal to the crural fold. Skin islands up to 25 cm in length can be developed, but the distal third of the skin in the medial thigh is supplied via the sartorius perforators, with a variable watershed of blood supply beyond the midthigh. A 10- to 14- cm long and 5- to 8- cm wide ellipsoid with the proximal margin at the crural fold will be used for a short flap (Fig. 31-12C).

A full-thickness incision is made along the anterior and distal margin of the skin island through the fascia lata. It is

important that the incision be either straight to the fascia or slightly flared at its base so that the skin will not be undermined and lose vascularity. The skin is loosely anchored to the fascia with temporary interrupted sutures to prevent shearing of the fat way from the underlying fascia during manipulation of the flap. The belly of the gracilis muscle is identified at the distal margin of the flap posterior to the adductor longus, isolated, and divided. The remainder of the full-thickness incision to the fascia is completed around the margin of the skin island.

The gracilis is mobilized from its bed with sharp and blunt dissection. It is important to work from the distal tip of the flap toward the origin so that the dominant vascular pedicle can be identified. The dominant vascular pedicle enters the deep anterior belly of the gracilis muscle approximately 6 to 8 cm from the pubic tubercle, emerging from underneath the belly of the adductor longus (Fig. 31-12D). With its paired venae comitantes, it is easily distinguished from the loose areolar tissue between the muscles. The nerve usually enters with, or just proximal to, the dominant vascular pedicle. If a classic long flap is to be employed, the pedicle is mobilized. If a short flap is to be used, the pedicle is cross-clamped, divided, and ligated (Fig. 31-12D). The nerve can usually be spared to provide muscular innervation and sensa-

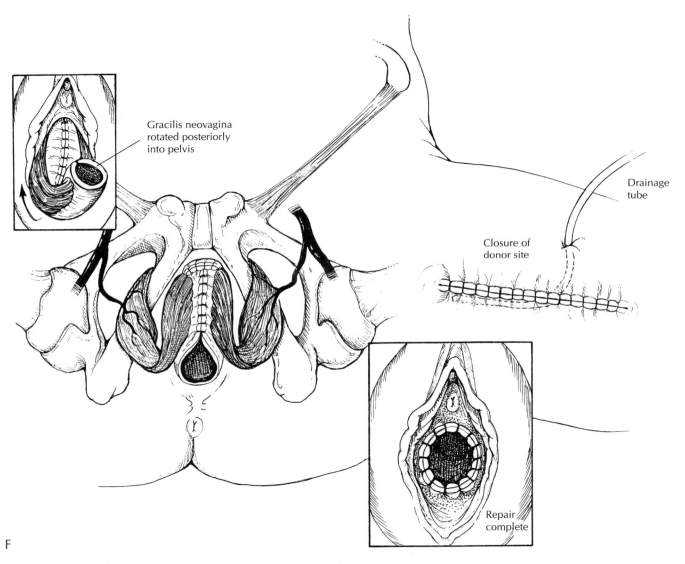

Gracilis neovagina rotated posteriorly into pelvis

Drainage tube

Closure of donor site

Repair complete

F

Fig. 31-12 *(Continued).*

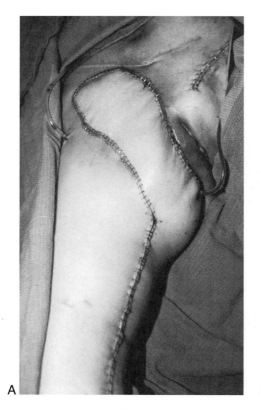
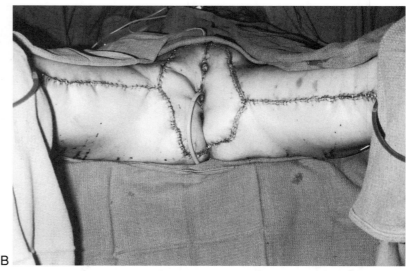

A   B

Fig. 31-13. Use of gracilis myocutaneous flaps to close (**A**) groin and (**B**) vulvar defects.

tion to the skin island in the short flap, but may be sacrificed. The remainder of the gracilis flap is mobilized to its origin. If a short flap is used, the 2 to 3 cm of the proximal gracilis muscle should not be aggressively skeletonized so that the small accessory vessels are not stripped away.

For neovaginal construction, a subfascial tunnel is constructed to the vaginal introitus with sharp and blunt dissection. The tunnel should allow passage of the gracilis flap freely without pressure. Bilateral flaps are rotated posteriorly through the tunnels and allowed to hang freely between the patient's legs (Fig. 31-12E). The neovaginal tube is constructed by approximating the skin edges with interrupted absorbable suture, beginning at the distal tips of the flaps (Fig. 31-12E). The temporary sutures anchoring the skin to the fascia are cut. The proximal skin margins are left open to form the introitus, an opening sufficient to allow passage of two to three fingers (Fig. 31-12F). The neovaginal tube is then rotated posteriorly into the pelvis and anchored to the levator plate and symphysis or sacral hollow with interrupted sutures. Redundant skin is trimmed and the proximal skin of the flap is sutured to the introitus with absorbable sutures.

When unilateral or bilateral flaps are employed for vulvar reconstructions, the flaps are rotated either anteriorly or posteriorly, depending on the defect, without use of the subfascial tunnels (Fig. 31-13). The muscle is achored to the deep tissues of the defect with loose interrupted sutures, and the skin approximated with interrupted absorbable sutures.

The thigh incisions are irrigated and closed in layers over closed suction drains. Each patient is allowed to ambulate within 24 to 48 hours of surgery.

If gracilis flaps are used to create a neovagina during an exenteration, the neovagina can be constructed by a second team without interrupting the abdominal procedure. This results in minimal prolongation of the operative time and no added blood loss.[34,35,37] Several investigators have reported a decrease in gastrointestinal or urologic complications among patients receiving the gracilis flap neovagina at exenteration, compared to historical or contemporary controls.[34,35,37,39]

Complications

Complications specific to the gracilis flap are frequently encountered,[31–38] but the majority can be prevented using careful planning of the reconstruction and flap design. Fortunately, most flap-specific complications are relatively minor. Most series report survival rates of more than 80 percent for gracilis flaps, with major flap loss encountered in 10 to 15 percent of patients.[30–38] Minor loss of skin from the margins of the flap is encountered more frequently. The author has not found that flourescein improves prediction of flap survival, but frequently observes the cut skin margin for red bleeding during development and manipulation of the flap. Other complications include donor site hematoma or abscess, introital stenosis, and vault prolapse.

Copeland et al[35] and Soper et al[38] reported no difference in the incidence of major flap loss, among patients receiving long versus short gracilis flaps. However, short flaps should not be employed when the hypogastric artery has been ligated because this will result in loss of the secondary proximal perforators that vascularize the short flap. Because major flap loss results in prolonged healing and frequently results in secondary morbidity, potential causes of this complication should be considered before performing a gracilis myocutaneous flap reconstruction.

In obese patients, sagging of the medial thigh fat may make identification of the skin territory supplied by the gracilis difficult, resulting in inclusion of skin anterior to the adductor longus and outside of the territory supplied by the gracilis perforators. In these patients, it is best to make the distal incision first, identify and isolate the distal gracilis, and place it on traction. The skin folds of the medial thigh are then elevated, and identification of the correct skin island is facilitated. It is also important to anchor the skin to the fascia to prevent shearing of the fat from the fascia and producing devascularization of the skin island.[36,40] The anchoring sutures should be released only after the flap has been rotated into position.

During rotation of the flap, the vascular pedicle or proximal muscle should not be traumatized or stretched to the point of developing vascular spasm.[40] Furthermore, the vulvar tunnels should be capacious enough to allow for the development of postoperative edema without producing obstruction of venous return and congestion of the flap, which can result in loss of a flap that has an adequate arterial supply.[40]

In an analysis of a series of patients receiving gracilis flap reconstructions, the author and colleagues reported that the only clinical factor significantly associated with major flap loss was performance of a gracilis neovaginal reconstruction in association with rectosigmoid anastomosis during exenteration.[38] Four of eight patients (50 percent) developed major loss of one or both flaps in this situation compared to only 3 of 38 patients (8 percent) who received gracilis flap reconstructions without concurrent rectosigmoid anastomosis ($P < 0.05$).[38] It is likely that this combination produces venous congestion of the gracilis flaps by crowding tissues into the pelvis. Alternative methods of neovaginal reconstruction should be considered in these patients. Other factors, such as obesity, prior chemoirradiation, or pelvic abscess or fistula after exenteration were not associated with statistically significant increases in the risk of major flap loss, although the power of the study was limited for measuring the relative effects of other clinical factors because of the relatively low incidence (15 percent) of major flap loss.[38]

Prolapse of a gracilis neovagina is a rare occurrence in the author's experience.[38] Copeland et al[35] reported that 12 percent of 103 patients experienced severe vault prolapse of gracilis neovaginas. The incidence decreased in patients with short flaps and those with reconstructions performed during the later years of the study.[35] The gracilis neovagina should be anchored to the levator plate and either the sacral hollow or symphysis with several interrupted sutures to prevent this complication.

Introital stenosis of a gracilis neovagina is rare in the absence of major flap loss.[38] This can be prevented by performing small Z-plasties at the introitus and partially removing the perineal body if the rectum is preserved. The Z-plasties break up the circular introital scar, which has a tendency to shrink as the scar tissue matures.

In general, myocutaneous flaps, unlike skin grafts, do not require mechanical dilation to prevent stenosis of the upper vagina. Patients report that neovaginas created from the short gracilis flaps are mechanically satisfactory for coitus, although many women are not sexually active after radical pelvic procedures. Because the keratinized skin of a myocutaneous flap does not convert to nonkeratinized vaginal mucous membrane, vaginal lubrication is poor. The author usually uses vaginal estrogen cream to promote vaginal lubrication. Most patients will report a scant malodorous watery discharge. Dilute vinegar douches can be used to decrease the amount of vaginal discharge and odor.

Inferior Rectus Abdominis Flap

A variety of vertical or transverse inferior rectus abdominis flaps can be constructed to provide myocutaneous flaps for vaginal, vulvar, and groin or abdominal wall reconstructions.[41] The inferior rectus abdominis flap can provide a large skin island, or can be used as either a muscular or myosubcutaneous flap without skin if only tissue bulk is needed for reconstruction. It is supplied by a very reliable vascular pedicle that can be mobilized with an extremely wide arc of rotation, making this one of the most versatile flaps for pelvic reconstruction procedures.

The vascular supply of the inferior rectus abdominis flap is from the deep inferior epigastric artery[41] (Fig. 31-14A). The deep inferior epigastric artery originates from the distal external iliac artery, coursing upwards and medially to the lateral border of the rectus abdomini. The artery travels with paired venae comitantes to enter the rectus sheath at approximately the level of the arcuate line, and ascends along the deep belly of the muscle. It divides into two or three branches below the level of the umbilicus and travels within the belly of the muscle to anastomose with branches of the superior epigastric system above the level of the umbilicus. Peritoneal, muscular, and cutaneous branches extend off of all portions of the deep inferior epigastric system, usually radiating away from the umbilical region.[41] These anastomose cranially with branches of the superior epigastric, laterally with intercostal and lumbar vessels, caudally with superficial and deep vessels from the groin, and across the midline with branches of the contralateral deep inferior epigastric system.[41] The largest cutaneous perforators are located in the periumbilical region. The entire rectus muscle and overlying abdominal skin can be supported by the deep inferior epigastric system, even if the superior epigastric artery and secondary vessels are divided. The richly anastomotic blood supply of the anterior abdominal wall will allow the inferior rectus abdominis flap to support both vertical and transverse skin islands that extend far beyond the level of the underlying strip of anterior rectus fascia[41] (Fig. 31-14A).

The inferior rectus abdominis myocutaneous flap consists of mobilized rectus muscle, a strip of anterior rectus sheath, and a skin island. The inferior rectus abdominis flap can be developed either above or below the level of the arcuate line. Because of the lack of posterior sheath in the inferior abdomen, transverse skin islands should be used below the arcuate line in order to limit the defect in the anterior rectus

fascia to 3 to 4 cm in length so that the anterior fascia can be closed transversely.[42,43] Above the arcuate line, either vertical or transverse islands can be developed.[41,44,45] The posterior sheath should be left intact, and an attempt should be made to close the anterior fascial defect in order to prevent herniation.

The principles of inferior rectus abdominis flaps are similar for vertical or transverse flaps. The skin island is defined and incised along the superior border through the anterior rectus sheath. The belly of the rectus muscle is mobilized with blunt dissection proceeding from the rectus diastasis off of the posterior sheath to define the lateral margin of the muscle, and the anterior fascial incision is extended to this point. The muscle is divided and anastomotic vessels con-

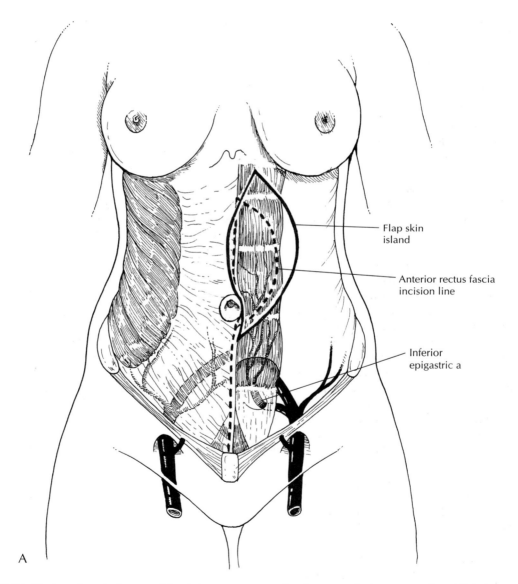

Flap skin island

Anterior rectus fascia incision line

Inferior epigastric a

A

Fig. 31-14. Design of vertical rectus abdominis myocutaneous flap for neovaginal reconstruction. **(A)** Relationship of muscle, vascular pedicle, and flap. Dotted line indicates approximate extent of resection of anterior rectus sheath. *(Figure continues.)*

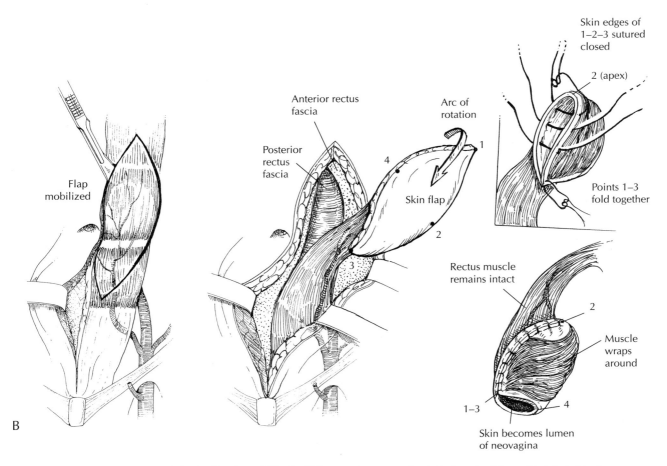

Fig. 31-14 *(Continued).* **(B)** The flap is mobilized off the anterior rectus fascia below the falp and intubated to form the neovaginal tube. The muscle is not divided. *(Figure continues.)*

necting to the superior epigastric system are ligated. The remaining borders of the skin island are incised to the level of the anterior fascia and the subcutaneous fat is mobilized back to the lateral and medial margins of the rectus muscle. After the anterior rectus fascia is incised along the medial border, the muscle and fascia are elevated. The inferior margin of the fascial strip is incised. It is important to retain the fascia over at least 1 to 2 segments of the rectus, so that several perforating vessels will supply the skin island.[42]

The rectus muscle inferior to the skin island is mobilized from both the posterior and anterior sheaths using sharp and blunt dissection (Fig. 31-14B). If the flap is being raised in conjunction with a midline incision, this can be performed very rapidly, working from the medial to lateral aspect of the muscle. If an isolated skin island is being raised for repair of a superficial defect, a small transverse incision can be made at the base of the muscle to facilitate identification of the vascular pedicle and mobilization of the inferior half of the muscle. In the inferior portion of the rectus, peritoneal branches from the deep inferior epigastric system should be isolated and individually controlled. The lateral tendinous insertions and segmental neurovascular bundles of the mus-

cle are also isolated and divided. The deep inferior epigastric pedicle is dissected free, if necessary, and can be isolated to the external iliac vessels to facilitate mobilization of the rectus muscle. In lower transverse flaps, the inferior base of the rectus is usually separated from the pubis and can be used to re-enforce the neovaginal skin tube.[42,43]

The inferior rectus flap can be rotated posteriorly into the pelvis either through the midline peritoneal defect below the arcuate line or through a separate lateral peritoneal defect (Fig. 31-14C). If it is to be transferred to the groin or vulva, it can be passed through a subcutaneous tunnel (Fig. 31-15). During rotation of the flap, the vascular pedicle should be observed to determine that there is no twisting or tension on the vessels.

If a rectus flap is used for neovaginal creation, a 12- to 14-cm wide skin island will provide an introitus approximately 4 cm in diameter. The neovaginal tube is formed by approximating skin edges with absorbable sutures, rotating the tube into the pelvis (Fig. 31-14C), and suturing the open end of the neovagina to the introitus.[42–45] In morbidly obese patients with bulky subcutaneous tissues, a bulky rectus myocutaneous flap might place enough pressure to produce ve-

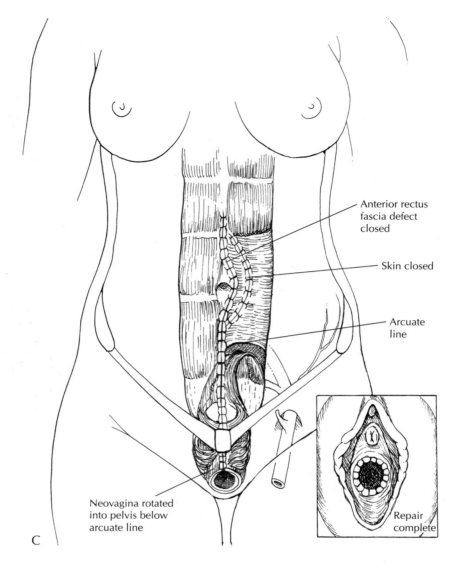

Anterior rectus
fascia defect
closed

Skin closed

Arcuate
line

Neovagina rotated
into pelvis below
arcuate line

Repair
complete

C

Fig. 31-14 *(Continued)*. **(C)** The neovagina is rotated into the pelvis through the peritoneal incision below the arcuate line. The anterior rectus fascia defect is closed to prevent hernia formation.

nous congestion and skin slough. In these patients, use of a muscular flap or myosubcutaneous flap with split-thickness skin graft may be preferable.

Because of the extremely predictable vascular pedicle and richly anastomotic blood supply of the anterior abdominal wall skin, most series of patients with inferior rectus abdominis flap pelvic and groin reconstructions have reported very satisfactory results, with close to 100 percent flap viability.[42–45] In patients with severe atherosclerosis of the lower extremities, preoperative angiography should be used to ensure patency of the inferior epigastric arteries before developing the flap.[41]

Making no effort to close upper abdominal anterior rectus sheath defects might predispose to herniation, even though the posterior rectus sheath is intact. However, no hernias occurred during short follow-up in several series when the

anterior fascia was not closed.[44,45] The author attempts to repair the anterior fascial defect using either a primary closure or synthetic mesh, but is reluctant to use synthetic materials in the abdominal wall during exenteration because of the potential for infectious morbidity. Use of a 4- to 5-cm strip of anterior fascia results in a defect that can usually be closed transversely.

A minor disadvantage of the inferior rectus flap for neovaginal reconstruction during exenteration is interruption of the operative "flow" of the exenteration while the flap is being raised. Unlike the gracilis flap, construction of the rectus flap adds extra operative time because the flap construction takes place within the abdominal operative field.

Similar to the gracilis flap, the rectus abdominis flap provides adequate tissue bulk to obturate the denuded pelvis after exenteration or provide soft tissue contour after radical

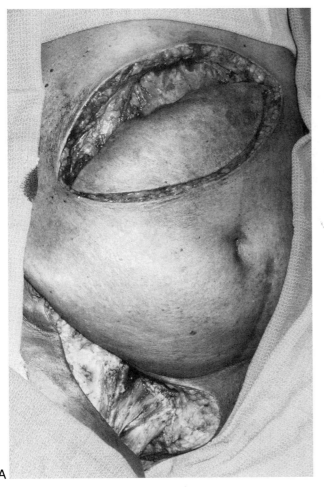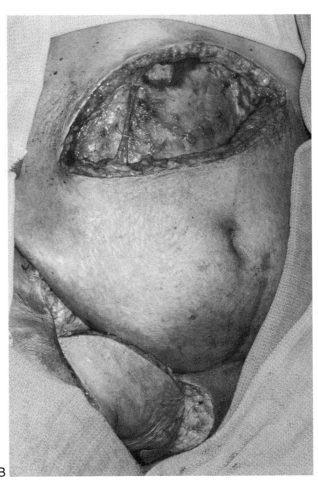

A   B

Fig. 31-15. (A) Development of a transverse rectus abdominis flap to fill a large ipsilateral groin defect. (B) The flap is rotated through a subfascial tunnel into the groin. All skin and fascial defects were closed primarily.

vulvar surgery. The neovagina is satisfactory for coitus and is not prone to develop stenosis. Because the abdominal skin will not convert into nonkeratinized vaginal mucosa, lubrication is poor and a chronic watery discharge is frequently observed.

Bulbocavernosus Flap

The bulbocavernosus or Martius flap was originally described as a myosubcutaneous flap to repair large urinary tract fistulas[46] and was subsequently used to repair rectovaginal fistulas resulting from radiotherapy.[47] The bulbocavernosus muscle supports a stable skin island supplied from the perineal branch of the pudendal artery, which enters at the posterior aspect of the muscle. Hatch[48] has described use of the bulbocavernosus myocutaneous flap for neovaginal construction after exenteration. The author also has used unilateral bulbocavernosus myocutaneous flaps to repair defects in the inferior vagina.

The skin island is 4 to 7 cm wide, extending from the interlabial fold medially to the lateral labia majora laterally, and 8 to 10 cm in length, extending approximately from the level of the clitoris posteriorly to approximately the level of the posterior fourchette (Fig. 31-16). Pinching and elevating the labia majora essentially identifies the muscle and fat pad. After incising the skin island, the dissection is carried through the subcutaneous tissues between the muscle and the introitus to the level of the pubic arch. The muscle is elevated off of the deep tissues with sharp and blunt dissection proceeding from the medial and superior aspect of the muscle in a lateral and inferior direction (Fig. 31-16B). The introital skin is dissected off of the pubic arch to create a short tunnel. The flap is rotated medially into the vagina to fill the tissue defect (Fig. 31-16C).

A partial neovaginal tube can be formed by suturing paired bulbocavernosus flaps together in the posterior midline and using omentum to form the anterior wall of the vagina[48] (Fig. 31-16D). The omentum can either undergo split-thickness skin grafting or be allowed to epithelialize from the introitus and flaps.

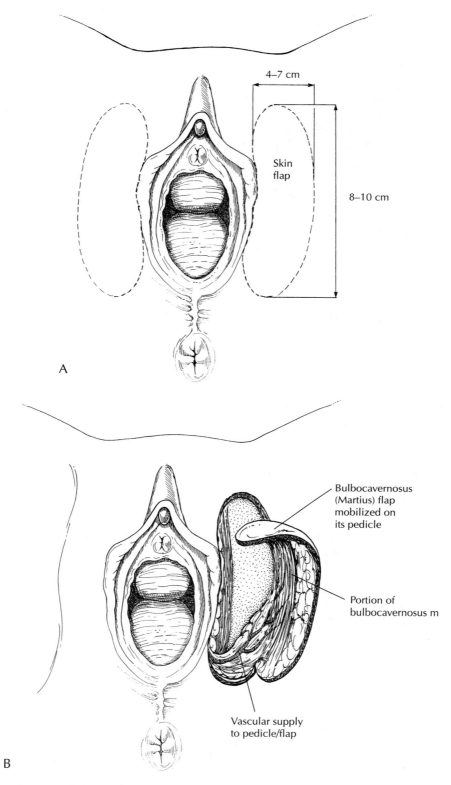

A

B

Fig. 31-16. Development of bulbocavernosus flap for vaginal reconstruction. **(A)** Location and approximate dimensions of bulbocavernosus flap. Dual blood supply to the bulbocavernosus muscle arises from the deep pudendalartery (posterior) and superficial pudendal artery (anterior). **(B)** The flap is elevated off of the deep tissues by outlining the skin island and pinching the muscle and subcutaneous tissues. The muscle is divided anteriorly and dissected off of the deep tissues towards the posterior portion of the muscle. *(Figure continues.)*

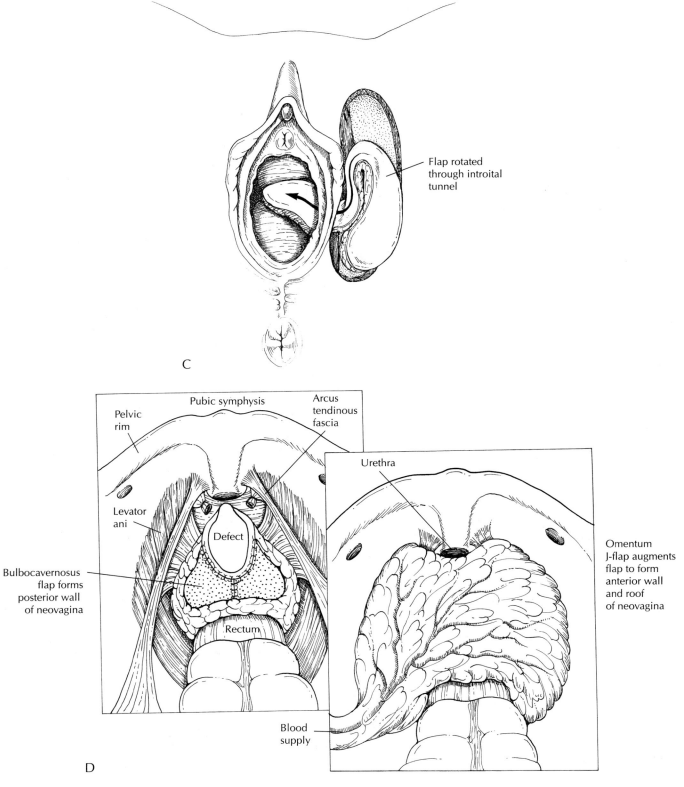

C

Fig. 31-16 *(Continued)*. **(C)** The flap is rotated into the vagina under a subcutaneous tunnel. **(D)** The bulbocavernosus flaps form the posterior wall of the neovagina, which can be augmented with an omental J-flap to form the anterior wall of the vagina.

The bulbocavernosus flap is best suited for vaginal reconstruction after partial exenteration or exenteration with rectosigmoid anastomosis. It does not provide much tissue to obliterate the denuded pelvis, but does allow transfer of vascularized tissue to protect irradiated rectosigmoid colon.[48] Unlike skin transferred from the inner thigh and abdomen with the gracilis and rectus flaps, vulvar skin transferred with the bulbocavernosus flaps will have a significant amount of persistent hair growth during short-term follow-up. Despite these limitations, it is a useful flap for vaginal reconstruction.

Tensor Fascia Lata Flap

The tensor fascia lata muscle originates laterally to the sartorius muscle on the iliac crest and the anterior superior iliac spine (Fig. 31-17A). It is a thin, broad muscle that inserts distally into the fascia lata along the lateral thigh. Its dominant vascular pedicle, derived from the lateral femoral circumflex artery, enters the muscle approximately 6 to 8 cm below the iliac spine after coursing between the rectus femoris and vastus lateralis muscles. The cutaneous branches from this muscular perforator support a lateral skin island approximately 25 to 30 cm in length and 5 to 6 cm in width.[49–51] The arc of rotation of the flap allows it to be used for groin and anterior vulvar reconstructions (Fig. 31-17B).

The patient's lateral thigh is prepared to the knee. The extent of the defect is measured. The tensor fascia lata flap is usually not tunnelled, and will rotate about the point of entry of its vascular supply, so the length of the flap is judged from this point. The anterior margin of the flap is a line running from the anterior superior iliac crest to the lateral condyle of the tibia. The posterior margin of the muscle and potential posterior border of the skin island run from the greater trochanter to the knee, but most tensor fascia lata flaps are 6 to 8 cm in width. The skin territory extends to within approximately 5 cm of the knee, resulting in a potential flap length of approximately 40 cm.

The anterior and distal margins of the flap are dissected first to below the tensor fascia lata. The skin is anchored to the fascia with temporary stay sutures. Elevation of the flap proceeds from distal to proximal, lifting the muscle off of the vastus lateralis. After identifying the vascular pedicle, the flap is rotated to close the defect and skin closed similar to a lateral transposition flap (Fig. 31-17C & D). Drains under the flap should run parallel to the length of the flap to avoid kinking the vessels, which run in the direction of the muscle fibers. The flaps can be long enough to cover both groin and vulvar defects after radical vulvectomy.[51] Because of changes in philosophy toward the management of primary vulvar carcinoma, the author rarely employs this flap during primary resections for vulvar malignancy, but recently has used rectus or gracilis flaps for repairs of groin defects because of increasing familiarity with these flaps.

Gluteus Maximus Flap

The gluteus maximus originates from the dorsal pubic ramus, the posterior sacrum, and the sacrotuberous ligament, inserting into the posterior upper femur (Fig. 31-18A). The muscle is easily identified overlying the medial aspect of the ischial tuberosity when the patient is in lithotomy position.[52,53] The inferior gluteal branch of the hypogastric artery supplies the muscle and skin of the posterior thigh, extending to approximately 8 cm above the popliteal fossa. This flap can be used to cover large defects of the posterior vulva, perineum, and sacral hollow but cannot be used when the hypogastric artery has been ligated near its origin.[52,53]

With the patient in lithotomy position, a line extending from the ischial tuberosity to the midpopliteal fossa is used to center the skin island, which can extend up to 8 cm wide and more than 20 cm long (Fig. 31-18B). The margins of the skin island are circumscribed, and deep subcutaneous tissues are mobilized working distal to proximal. The muscle fibers of the gluteus maximus are carefully divided longitudinally at the lateral margin of the skin flap, after identifying the medial branches of the inferior gluteal artery. The resulting flap uses only the proximal and medial portion of the gluteus maximus to support the skin island (Fig. 31-18C). After good mobilization, the pelvic defect is filled by rotating in the flap medially (Fig. 31-18D). Although this flap can reach portions of the anterior vulva, its main utility is for reconstruction of posterior pelvic defects.[52,53] The author does not often use this flap because of the need to position the patient in lithotomy or prone jack knife position to harvest the flap and frequent sacrifice of the hypogastric artery during exenteration.

Omental J-Flap

The omentum can be utilized as a vascularized pedicle that functions essentially as a nonepithelialized subcutaneous flap for abdominal wall reconstructions,[49] to provide neovascularization and tissue bulk to the pelvis after pelvic exenteration,[22,39] and to interpose as a layer of vascularized tissue during repair of complicated intestinal or urinary fistulas.[54] It can also be used as a partial or complete tube for split-thickness skin graft neovaginal construction.[22,49]

The omentum has a richly anastomotic blood supply with dual dominant vascular pedicles. The right gastroepiploic artery branches from the gastric artery, while the left gastroepiploic is a branch of the splenic artery. Accessory blood supply is derived from the greater curvature of the stomach, but the entire omentum can be supported by a single gastroepiploic artery pedicle.

In creating an omental J-flap, either the complete omen-

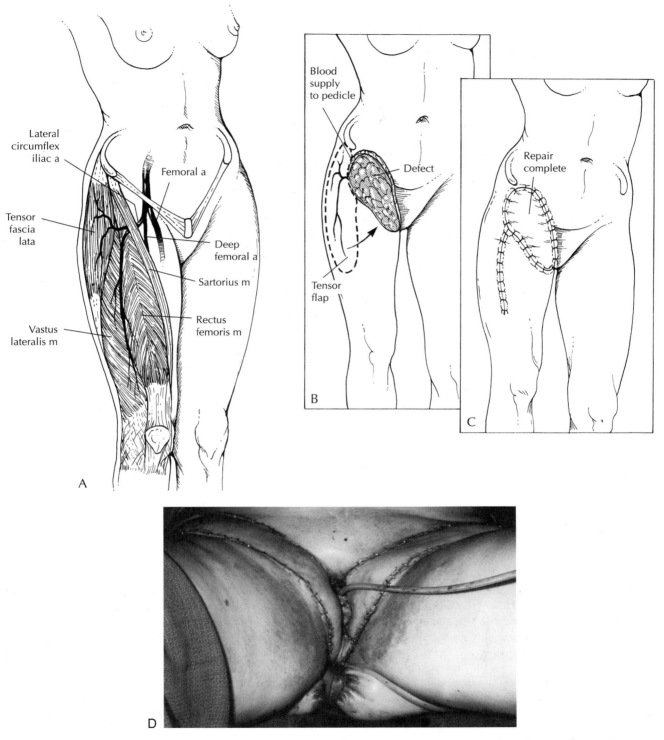

Fig. 31-17. Development of the tensor fascia lata flap. **(A)** Anatomy of the anterior/lateral thigh. The vascular supply of the tensor fascia lata flap is deveined from branches of the lateral circumflex femoral artery. **(B)** Tensor fascia lata flap (dashed line) developed to fill ipsilateral groin/vulvar defect. **(C)** Rotation of tensor fascia lata flap into groin/vulvar defect. **(D)** Reconstruction of bilateral groin/vulvar defect with bilateral tensor fascia lata myocutaneous flaps.

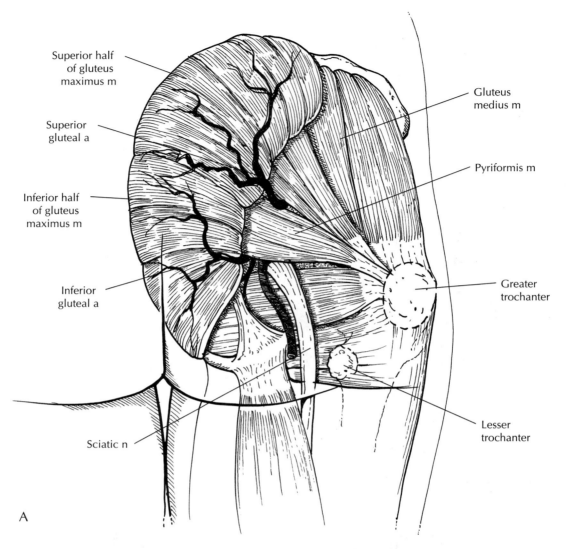

Superior half of gluteus maximus m

Superior gluteal a

Inferior half of gluteus maximus m

Inferior gluteal a

Sciatic n

Gluteus medius m

Pyriformis m

Greater trochanter

Lesser trochanter

A

Fig. 31-18. Development of gluteus maximus myocutaneous flap. **(A)** Anatomy of gluteal region—posterior view. *(Figure continues.)*

tum or the omentocolic omentum alone can be used, depending on the size and location of the tissue defect and the size and mobility of the omentum. Most frequently, the omentocolic ligament is divided, mobilizing the omentum completely, and a left-sided pedicle is developed. The right gastroepiploic artery is divided and the omentum mobilized off of the greater curvature of the stomach. Care must be taken to not traumatize the gastric serosa and muscularis during ligation of the perforators. The mobilized omentum is inspected for hemostasis and viability.

Although Valle[55] first proposed that the omentum be used as a sling to elevate the bowel out of the pelvis after exenteration, the author prefers to use the omentum as a carpet over the denuded pelvis. This avoids the potential complication of internal herniation and obliterates dead space with vascularized tissue.

The omentum is passed laterally down the pericolic gutter into the pelvis and gently draped into the pelvis or sutured into a neovaginal tube. The omental carpet is loosely sutured into place with interrupted sutures. Closed suction drains are usually placed under the omental carpet to drain the operative defect.

The most serious potential complication of the omental flap is failure to ensure hemostasis. The omental flap is often performed at the end of an exenteration, when the patient is frequently hypothermic and vasoconstricted. Release of vasoconstriction postoperatively is a potential cause of intra-abdominal hemorrhage. Internal herniation has not been a significant problem when the omentum is passed lateral to the colon and the free edges sutured into the pelvis after it emerges from the pericolic gutter.

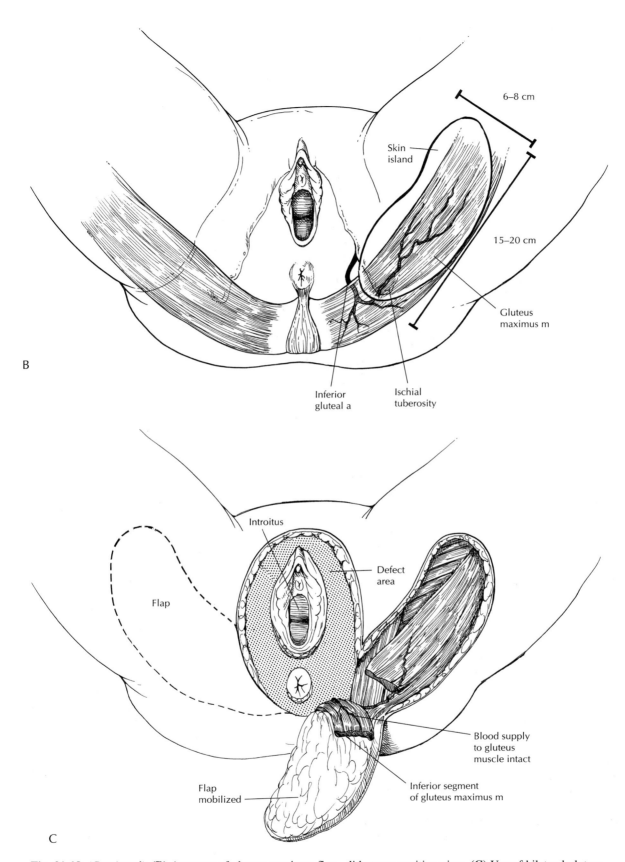

Fig. 31-18 *(Continued).* **(B)** Anatomy of gluteus maximus flap—lithotomy position view. **(C)** Use of bilateral gluteus maximus flaps to close vulvo perineal defect. The inferior half of the gluteus maximus muscle is divided to allow medial rotation of the myocutaneous unit. *(Figure continues.)*

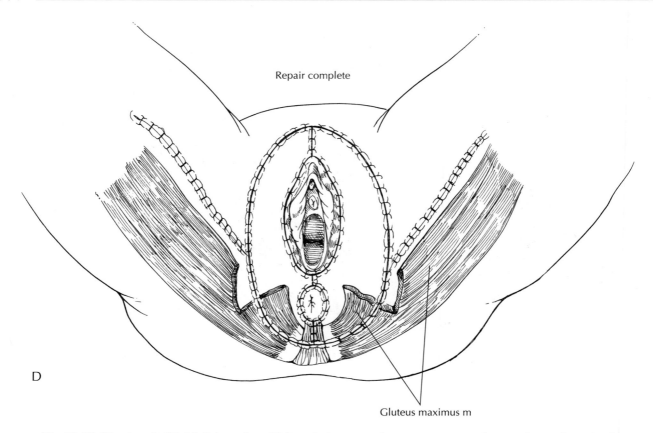

Repair complete

Gluteus maximus m

Fig. 31-18 *(Continued).* **(D)** Medial rotation of bilateral gluteus maximus myocutaneous flaps to close vulvoperineal defect. The partially divided inferior portion of the gluteus maximus muscle is rotated medially to provide adequate blood supply to the myocutaneous unit.

SUMMARY

The gynecologist who performs pelvic reconstructive procedures has a large armamentarium of techniques that are useful adjuncts to routine wound closure for the treatment of large pelvic defects. It is essential to have an adequate knowledge of several options for reconstruction of any single type of defect, so that the most appropriate procedure can be selected for individual patients.

REFERENCES

1. Anderson BL, Hacker NF: Psychosexual adjustment following pelvic exenteration. Obstet Gynecol 61:331, 1983

2. Anderson BL, Hacker NF: Psychosexual adjustment after vulvar surgery. Obstet Gynecol 62:457, 1983

3. Anderson BL: Sexual functioning complications in women with gynecologic cancer. Outcomes and directions for prevention. Cancer 60:2123, 1987

4. DiSaia PJ, Creasman WT, Rich WM: An alternate approach to early cancer of the vulva. Am J Obstet Gynecol 133:825, 1979

5. McCraw JB, Arnold PJ (eds): McCraw and Arnold's atlas of Muscle and Musculocutaneous Flaps. Hampton Press, Norfolk, VA, 1986

6. Strauch B, Vasconez LO, Hall-Findlay EJ: Grabb's Encyclopedia of Flaps. Little, Brown, Boston, 1990

7. Knapstein PG, Frieberg V, Sevin BU (eds): Reconstructive Surgery in Gynecology. Thieme Medical Publishers, New York, 1990

8. Kaser O, Ikle FA, Hirsch HA, Friedman EA (eds): Atlas of Gynecological Surgery. Thieme-Stratton, New York, 1985

9. Wheeless CR Jr: Atlas of Pelvic Surgery, 2nd Ed. Lea & Febiger, Philadelphia, 1988

10. Lee RA: Atlas of Gynecologic Surgery. WB Saunders, Philadelphia, 1992

11. Rens WF, Matches SJ: Wound closure. p. 7. In Jurkewicz MJ, Krizek TJ, Mathes SJ, Ariyan SJ (eds): Plastic Surgery Principles and Practice. CV Mosby, St Louis, 1990

12. Rutledge F, Sinclair M: Treatment of intraepithelial carcinoma of the vulva by skin excision and graft. Am J Obstet Gynecol 135:185, 1979

13. DiSaia PJ, Rich WM: Surgical approach to multifocal carcinoma in situ of the vulva. Am J Obstet Gynecol 140:136, 1981

14. Rettenmaier MA, Berman ML, DiSaia PJ: Skinning vulvec-

tomy for the treatment of multifocal vulvar intraepithelial neoplasia. Obstet Gynecol 69:247, 1987

15. Strauss RJ, Fazio VW: Bowen's disease of the anal and perianal area. A report and analysis of twelve cases. Am J Surg 137:231, 1979

16. Schlaerth JB, Morrow CP, Nalick RH, Gaddis O: Anal involvement with carcinoma in situ of the perineum in women. Obstet Gynecol 64:406, 1984

17. McIndoe AH, Bannister JB: An operation for the cure of congenital absence of the vagina. Br J Obstet Gynecol 45:490, 1938

18. Magrina JF, Masterson BJ: Vaginal reconstruction in gynecologic oncology: a review of techniques. Obstet Gynecol Surv 36:1, 1981

19. Berek JS, Hacker NF, Lagasse LD, Smith ML: Delayed vaginal reconstruction in the fibrotic pelvis following radiation or previous reconstruction. Obstet Gynecol 61:743, 1983

20. Morley GW, Lindenauer SM, Young SD: Vaginal reconstruction following pelvic exenteration: surgical and psychological considerations. Am J Obstet Gynecol 116:996, 1973

21. Watring WG, Lagasse LD, Smith ML et al: Vaginal reconstruction following extensive treatment for pelvic cancer. Am J Obstet Gynecol 125:809, 1976

22. Berek JS, Hack NF, Lagasse LD: Vaginal reconstruction performed simultaneously with pelvic exenteration. Obstet Gynecol 63:318, 1984

23. Limberg AA (Wolfe SA, translator): The Planning of Local Plastic Operations on the Body Surface: Theory and Practice. Collamore Press, Lexington, MA, 1984

24. Morton KE, Davies D, Dewhurst J: The use of the fasciocutaneous flap in vaginal reconstruction. Br J Obstet Gynaecol 93:970, 1986

25. Wang T, Whetzel T, Mathes SJ, Vasconez LO: A fasciocutaneous flap for vaginal and perineal reconstruction. Plast Reconstr Surg 80:95, 1987

26. Julian CG, Callison J, Woodruff JD: Plastic management of extensive vulvar defects. Obstet Gynecol 38:193, 1971

27. Borges AF: Choosing the correct Limberg flap. Plast Reconstr Surg 62:542, 1978

28. Jervis W, Salyer KE, Busquets MAV, Atkins RW: Further applications of the Limberg and Dufourmental flaps. Plast Reconstr Surg 54:335, 1974

29. Rayment R, Evans DM: Use of an abdominal rotation flap for inguinal lymph node dissection. Br J Plast Surg 40:485, 1987

30. McCraw JB, Massey FM, Shanklin D, Horton CE: Vaginal reconstruction with gracilis myocutaneous flaps. Plast Reconstr Surg 58:176, 1976

31. Becker DW Jr, Massey FM, McCraw JB: Musculocutaneous flaps in reconstructive pelvic surgery. Obstet Gynecol 54:178, 1979

32. Ballon SC, Donaldson RC, Roberts JA, Lagasse LD: Reconstruction of the vulva using a myocutaneous graft. Gynecol Oncol 7:123, 1979

33. Morrow CP, Lacey CG, Lucas WE: Reconstructive surgery in gynecologic cancer employing the gracilis myocutaneous pedicle graft. Gynecol Oncol 7:176, 1979

34. Lacey CG, Stern JL, Feigenbaum S et al: Vaginal reconstruction with use of gracilis myocutaneous flaps: the University of California, San Francisco experience. Am J Obstet Gynecol 158:1278, 1988

35. Copeland LJ, Hancock KC, Gershenson DM et al: Gracilis myocutaneous vaginal reconstruction concurrent with total pelvic exenteration. Am J Obstet Gynecol 160:1095, 1989

36. Soper JT, Larson D, Hunter VJ et al: Short gracilis myocutaneous flaps for vulvovaginal reconstruction after radical pelvic surgery. Obstet Gynecol 74:823, 1989

37. Cain JM, Diamond A, Tamimi HK et al: The morbidity and benefits of concurrent gracilis myocutaneous graft with pelvic exenteration. Obstet Gynecol 74:185, 1989

38. Soper JT, Rodriguez G, Berchuck A, Clarke-Pearson DL: Gracilis myocutaneous flaps for vulvovaginal reconstruction after radical pelvic surgery. Presented at Poster Session, 25th Annual Meeting of Society of Gynecologic Oncology, Orlando, Florida, 1994

39. Soper JT, Berchuck A, Creasman WT, Clarke-Pearson DL: Pelvic exenteration: factors associated with major surgical morbidity. Gynecol Oncol 35:93, 1989

40. Vasconez LO, McCraw JB, Hall EJ: Complications of musculocutaneous flaps. Clin Plast Surg 7:123, 1980

41. Taylor GI, Corlett RJ, Boyd JB: The versatile deep inferior epigastric (inferior rectus abdominis) flap. Br J Plast Surg 37:330, 1984

42. McCraw J, Kemp G, Given F, Horton CE: Correction of high pelvic defects with the inferiorly based rectus abdominis myocutaneous flap. Clin Plast Surg 15:449, 1988

43. Benson C, Soisson AP, Carlson J et al: Neovaginal reconstruction with a rectus abdominis myocutaneous flap. Obstet Gynecol 81:62, 1988

44. Tobin GR, Day TG: Vaginal and pelvic reconstruction with distally based rectus abdominis myocutaneous flaps. Plast Reconstr Surg 81:62, 1988

45. Pursell SH, Day TG, Tobin GR: Distally-based rectus abdominis flap for reconstruction in radical gynecologic procedures. Gynecol Oncol 37:234, 1990

46. Martius J: Operations for urinary incontinence. In McCall M, Bolton KA (eds): Operative Gynecology. Little, Brown, Boston, 1956

47. White AJ, Buchsbaum HJ, Blythe JG, Lifshitz S: Use of the bulbocavernosus muscle (Martius procedure) for repair of radiation-induced rectovaginal fistulas. Obstet Gynecol 60:114, 1982

48. Hatch KD: Construction of a neovagina after exenteration using the vulvobulbocavernosus myocutaneous graft. Obstet Gynecol 63:110, 1984

49. Bostwick J, Hill HL, Nahai F: Repairs in the lower abdomen, groin, or perineum with myocutaneous or omental flaps. Plast Reconstr Surg 63:186, 1979

50. Nahai F, Hill HL, Hester TR: Experiences with the tensor fascia lata flap. Plast Reconstr Surg 63:788, 1979

51. Chafe W, Fowler WC Jr, Walton LA, Currie JL: Radical vulvectomy with use of tensor fascia lata myocutaneous flap. Am J Obstet Gynecol 145:207, 1983

52. Hurwitz DI, Swartz WM, Mathes SJ: The gluteal thigh flap: a reliable, sensate flap for the closure of buttock and perineal wounds. Plast Reconstr Surg 68:521, 1980

53. Achauer BM, Turpin IM, Furnas DW: Gluteal thigh flap in reconstruction of complex pelvic wounds. Arch Surg 118:18, 1983

54. Kiricuta J, Goldstein AMB: The repair of extensive vesicovaginal fistulas with pedicled omentum: a review of 27 cases. J Urol 180:724, 1972

55. Valle G, Ferraris G: Use of the omentum to contain the intestines in pelvic exenteration. Obstet Gynecol 33:772, 1969

CHAPTER THIRTY-TWO

TUBAL AND OVARIAN ANATOMY

THOMAS G. STOVALL
FIDEL A. VALEA

SURGICAL ANATOMY OF THE FALLOPIAN TUBE

The fallopian tube extends from the urine fundus to an area that approximates the ovary on the corresponding side. The tube lies within a peritoneal fold (mesosalpinx), which is the superiormost aspect of the broad ligament. The arterial blood supply of the fallopian tube is supplied by tubal branches of the uterine artery, along with tubal branches of the ovarian artery. The venous blood supply and the lymphatic drainage is similar to and accompanies the ovarian vessels. The vascular supply enters the tube laterally, with all of the vasculature lying within the mesosalpinx (Fig. 32-1).

The fallopian tube is approximately 9 to 12 cm in length, and is divided into five segments histologically: the fimbria or fimbriated end, which overlies the ovary; the infundibulum, which is approximately 1 cm in length (Fig. 32-2); the ampullary portion, which extends about 6 cm (Fig. 32-3); the isthmic portion, which is approximately 2 to 3 cm in length (Fig. 32-4); and the intramural segment, which extends about 1 cm and transverses the myometrium to approximate the endometrial cavity. The histologic segments of the fallopian tube are important from a surgical standpoint, especially when one considers the various methods of sterilization. As one quickly notices, the diameter of the tubal lumen narrows progressively as one moves from the distal to proximal tubal segments.

SURGICAL ANATOMY OF THE OVARY

The normal adult ovary is one-half of a paired organ that is usually the size and shape of a large almond. Its surface is grayish white and quite irregular. The various pits and indentations seen on its surface are from numerous ovulations and the subsequent scarification that results. Although there is a great deal of individual variation, the dimensions of a normal premenopausal ovary are approximately 4 cm long, 2.5 cm wide, 1.5 cm thick, and weighing 3 to 8 g. As the woman ages, the ovaries tend to become smaller and firmer in consistency. In a menopausal woman, they may even look like streaks.

The position of the ovary in the pelvis is also variable. It can change with parity or with the enlargement of any pelvic organ. In a patient with an enlarged uterus, the ovaries may actually be found outside of the pelvis and in the upper abdomen. Classically, it rests in a depression of the peritoneum named the ovarian fossa. This depression can be found on either pelvic sidewall medial to the vessels and inbetween the ureter and the external iliac vein (Fig. 32-5). It is this close relationship between the ovary and the ureter that make it easy to injure the ureter when dissecting the ovary from the ovarian fossa.

The ovary is suspended in the pelvis by three conspicuous ligaments that determine its mobility and its position in the pelvis. The first is the utero-ovarian ligament, which is a short fibrous cord that extends from the lateral aspect of the uterus to the medial or lower pole of the ovary. In order to preserve the ovary when performing a hysterectomy, this ligament must be divided. Next is the suspensory ligament of the ovary, or infundibulopelvic ligament. This structure originates from the pelvic sidewall at the level of the pelvic brim and contains the ovarian artery, vein, lymphatics, and accompanying nerves. It represents the most superior aspect of the broad ligament, and is divided when performing an oophorectomy. It is in dividing this ligament at hysterectomy that the ureter is most commonly injured, due to its close proximity to the ovarian vessels at the level of the pelvic brim. There is only a potential space, which can be devel-

587

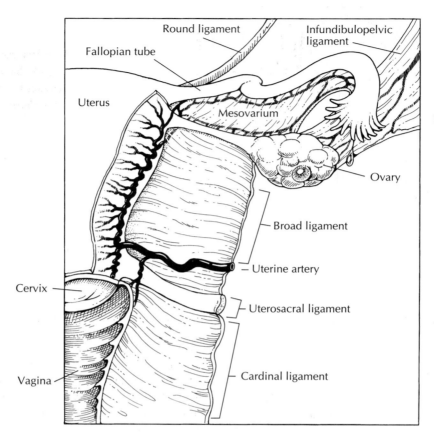

Fig. 32-1. Anatomic relationship of the uterus, ovary, and fallopian tube.

oped by elevating this pedicle, and separating the ureter from the ovarian vessels. The last support structure is the mesovarium, an extension of the posterior aspect of the broad ligament that attaches to the anterior border of the ovary. It contains the anastamotic branches of the ovarian and uterine arteries, as well as a plexus of veins and crossing vessels that either supply or originate from the ovary.

The arterial blood supply to the ovaries originates from the abdominal aorta, just below branching off to the renal vessels. The ovarian artery descends in the retroperitoneum and crosses the ureter obliquely in its midportion, and parallels its course before crossing anterior to the psoas muscle. It enters the infundibulopelvic ligament at the pelvic brim, crosses over the iliac bifurcation, and enters the mesovarium, where it branches off to the fallopian tube and the ovary before anastamosing with the uterine artery in the broad liga-

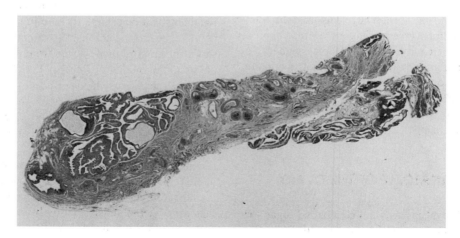

Fig. 32-2. Histology of the infundibular portion of the fallopian tube.

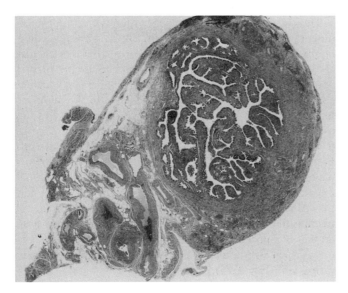

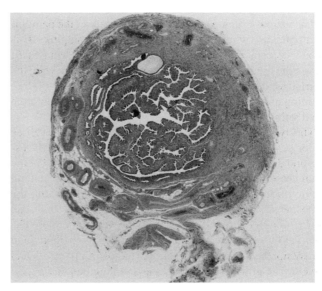

Fig. 32-3. Histology of the ampullary portion of the fallopian tube.

Fig. 32-4. Histology of the isthmic portion of the fallopian tube.

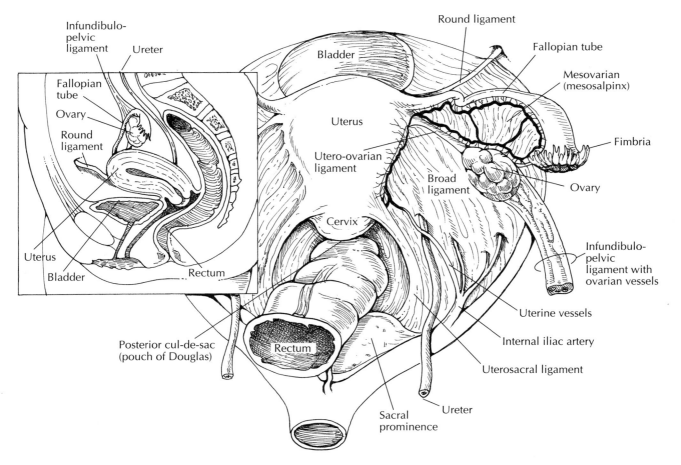

Fig. 32-5. Normal pelvic anatomy.

ment. The ovarian blood supply enters through the hilum of the ovary.

The venous drainage of the ovary is by way of the pampiniform plexus, which is situated in the mesosalpinx. This plexus of veins combines to form several large veins as it leaves the hilum and ultimately forms a single large vein, the ovarian vein, which accompanies the ovarian artery before draining directly into the vena cava on the right and into the renal vein on the left.

The lymphatic drainage of the ovaries occurs via three major pathways. The first is via the infundibulopelvic vessels and drains primarily to the aortic nodes at the level of the renal vessels. Second, the ovaries can drain to the ipsilateral pelvic nodes or cross the uterine fundus and drain into the opposite side via the ovarian ligament. Finally, they can drain through the round ligament to the inguinal nodes. The innervation of the ovary comes from both sympathetic and parasympathetic fibers that parallel the ovarian vessels and travel in the infundibulopelvic ligament. Segmental innerva-

tion from the T10 and T11 nerve roots supply motor and sensory fibers to the ovaries as well.

The close anatomic relationship to the ureter is of paramount importance when considering any surgical procedure on the ovary. The ureter crosses over the pelvic vessels just above the bifurcation of the common iliac artery. At this point it is just below the infundibulopelvic ligament and then courses deep into the pelvis. It is attached to the posterior leaf of the broad ligament and is in close proximity to the ovarian fossa. This relationship is important when trying to remove an ovary that is adherent to the pelvic sidewall. Frequently, the ureter must be dissected free in order to completely remove all the ovarian capsule and avoid injury to the ureter. This can easily be accomplished with blunt dissection between the ureter and the posterior leaf attachments, retracting the ureter laterally with an atraumatic vessel loop around it. Special care must be taken so that the ureter is not grasped with forceps or any other potentially traumatic instrument (Fig. 32-5).

CHAPTER THIRTY-THREE

DIAGNOSIS AND SURGERY FOR ECTOPIC PREGNANCY

THOMAS G. STOVALL

BACKGROUND

The first reported surgical intervention for ectopic pregnancy was by Bard in 1759.[1] In 1884, Lawson Tait[2] described the first salpingectomy done for a ruptured ectopic pregnancy, and this report began the modern era of surgical management of this condition. During the past 30 years, the development of radioimmunoassay for human chorionic gonadotropin (hCG), combined with the development and refinement of abdominal and endovaginal ultrasound have changed our approach to ectopic pregnancy diagnosis. These advances have allowed us the opportunity to make the diagnosis before rupture in most cases. Our ability to make the diagnosis at an earlier gestational age, the development and expanded use of diagnostic and operative laparoscopy, and the introduction of nonsurgical therapy have combined to change our approach to ectopic pregnancy management. In the past, our goal was to prevent the patient's death, which could result from diagnosis late in the clinical course; now our goal is more frequently to develop a minimally morbid management plan, often attempting to preserve the involved tube. This chapter covers the diagnosis and medical treatment of ectopic pregnancy, but concentrates on the surgical management of this condition.

EPIDEMIOLOGY AND RISK FACTORS

Data collected since 1970 by the Centers for the Disease Control demonstrates a rate of 19.7 ectopic pregnancies per 1,000 reported pregnancies, with ectopic pregnancy accounting for approximately 15 percent of all maternal deaths, with the rates for blacks being significantly higher than for whites.[3–5]

Several risk factors have been shown to independently increase one's risk of ectopic pregnancy. These risk factors include (1) previous laparoscopically proven pelvic inflammatory disease, (2) previous tubal pregnancy, (3) current intrauterine device use, and (4) previous tubal surgery, including tubal sterilization. Other risk factors that are commonly associated include progestin-only contraception, prior surgery, a history of infertility, and smoking.[6–8]

DIAGNOSIS

A patient presenting for care with an ectopic pregnancy may be completely asymptomatic or may have an acute abdomen with associated hemodynamic shock. The ultimate goal is for the patient to present and the diagnosis be confirmed before rupture of the tube. However, this is not always practical, since at times the patient may not even know that she is pregnant. Most commonly, the patient presents with the complaint of abnormal vaginal bleeding or lower abdominal cramping or pain. The nature and severity of the pain varies greatly, and may be unilateral or bilateral. The physical examination is of little help, except to make certain that the patient is hemodynamically stable, and that an acute abdomen is not present.[9,10] Therefore, one or more diagnostic modalities must be used to make the diagnosis. A variety of diagnostic tests have been studied, and a number of diagnostic algorithms have been published. Virtually all of these algorithms use a combination of quantitative hCG β-subunit assays (Fig. 33-1).

hCG Titers

Serum and urine hCG assays are virtually always positive in the patient with an ectopic pregnancy, although it is possible to have an ectopic pregnancy in the face of a negative hCG titer.[11-13] There are three reference standards for hCG measurement. The First International Standard was introduced in the 1930s by the World Health Organization. The assays were modified and the Second International Standard was introduced in 1964. The assays most commonly used today are the Third International Standard. Although it has its own scale, as a general rule, the Second International Standard is approximately one-half of the Third International Standard.[14]

A single hCG titer has limited usefulness, and therefore, serial titers are necessary. A 66-percent rise in the hCG titer over 48 hours (85 percent confidence interval) represented the lower limit of normal for viable intrauterine pregnancies in one study. However, at this level, approximately 15 percent of patients with a viable intrauterine pregnancy will have less than a 66-percent rise over 48 hours, and a similar percentage of ectopic pregnancies will be associated with a greater than 66 percent rise over 48 hours.[15] In our series of patients, there have been no patients with a normal intrauterine pregnancy who had a less than 50 percent rise in their hCG titer over 48 hours associated with a level of less than 2,000 mIU/ml. Above this level, the rate of rise is not important, because an intrauterine pregnancy can be excluded by endovaginal ultrasound. It is necessary to use serial levels above this level to make certain that the hCG is rising.

Serum Progesterone Titers

Serum progesterone titers are generally lower in patients with an ectopic pregnancy when compared to patients with a viable intrauterine pregnancy. Statistically, the best progesterone cutoff for distinguishing ectopic pregnancy from an intrauterine pregnancy is 10 ng/ml. Clinically, this level is not helpful, since there is considerable overlap between abnormal and normal pregnancies.[16] In other studies, a serum progesterone of less than 5.0 ng/ml was never associated with a viable pregnancy.[17,18] At least two patients with a serum progesterone of less than 5.0 ng/ml have been identified in association with a viable intrauterine pregnancy. When calculated, the risk of a normal pregnancy with a serum progesterone of less than 5.0 ng/ml is approximately 1 in 1,500. Thus, as a screening test for normal and abnormal pregnancy, serum progesterone is an excellent test. The clinician must remember, however, that a serum progesterone level of less than 5.0 ng/ml is highly suggestive, but is not 100 percent predictive of an abnormal pregnancy. Because of this, a single serum progesterone titer is not recommended as a method to determine pregnancy nonviability (McCord ML, unpublished data, 1993).

Transvaginal Ultrasound

Endovaginal scanning has replaced transabdominal scanning for ectopic pregnancy diagnosis and early screening of an intrauterine pregnancy, because it can visualize an intrauterine sac at an earlier gestational age. A gestational sac should always be seen in the patient with a viable intrauterine pregnancy when the hCG titer reaches a level of 2,000 mIU/ml. In many cases, the gestational sac can be seen at a level of about 1,000 mIU/ml.[19-21] Although not mandatory, the addition of Doppler evaluation increases the sensitivity of ectopic pregnancy diagnosis.[22]

Culdocentesis

The presence of nonclotting blood within the peritoneal cavity (positive culdocentesis) in association with a positive pregnancy test is highly suggestive of an ectopic pregnancy. However, only about 50 percent of patients with a positive culdocentesis have a ruptured tube.[23] Because of this, culdocentesis is of no benefit if one is going to rely on nonsurgical diagnosis and medical treatment. By contrast, if one is going to use laparoscopic diagnosis and operative treatment, culdocentesis combined with hCG testing may be beneficial.

Suction Curettage

When the pregnancy has been confirmed to be nonviable using hCG testing, suction curettage is useful in determining whether the pregnancy is intrauterine or extrauterine. This is most useful when the hCG titer is rising, is less than 2,000 mIU/ml, and endovaginal scanning demonstrates no evidence of an intrauterine gestational sac. If the endovaginal scan does not show a gestational sac when the hCG titer is rising and is greater than 2,000 mIU/ml, suction curettage is not necessary before proceeding with surgical or nonsurgical management, because ultrasound can eliminate the possibility of an intrauterine pregnancy. The use of endometrial sampling to diagnose ectopic pregnancy has not been shown to be equivalent to suction curettage for recovery of intrauterine chorionic villi and is not recommended.

Laparoscopy

Laparoscopy is a relatively safe tool and is widely used to visualize the pelvis and make the diagnosis of ectopic pregnancy. However, it should not be forgotten that in 3

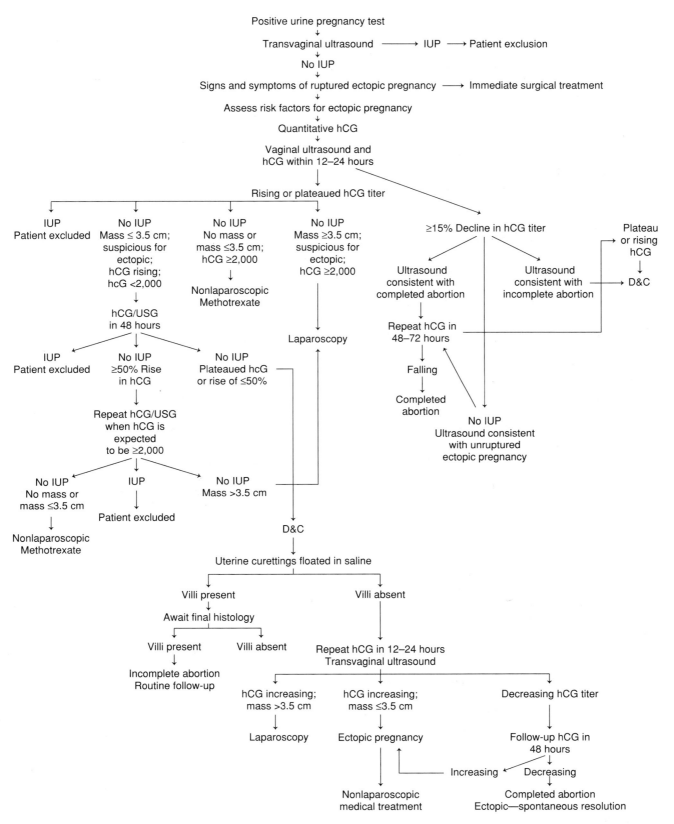

Fig. 33-1. Diagnostic algorithms showing modalities and end result. IUP, intrauterine pregnancy; hCG, human chorionic gonadotropin; USG, ultrasonography; D&C, dilation and curettage.

to 4 percent of patients, the ectopic pregnancy cannot be visualized by laparoscopy. Tubal dilation or discoloration may be misinterpreted as being an ectopic pregnancy. If surgical treatment is selected, laparoscopy is an expedient and accurate means of diagnosis. If nonsurgical therapy is appropriate, laparoscopy, with its associated risk, should be avoided so that the patient is not exposed to the risks of both surgical and medical therapy. In either situation, a nonsurgical diagnostic algorithm can be used to confirm the diagnosis in the patient who is hemodynamically stable (Fig. 33-1). When this methodology is combined with medical therapy, surgery can be avoided in many patients.

TREATMENT

There are three approaches to the management of a patient in whom an ectopic pregnancy has been diagnosed. Allowing for spontaneous resolution, initiation of medical management, or surgical intervention are all possible treatment alternatives. Certainly if spontaneous resolution could be guaranteed, it would be the treatment of choice. Although the best predictor of spontaneous resolution is a declining hCG titer, this does not always guarantee success. Since this is not possible, surgical or medical treatment is used in most patients. Medical treatment has proven successful in many patients with a small unruptured ectopic pregnancy, but whether this treatment is better than surgical treatment has not been shown in a randomized clinical trial. Thus, at present, it seems appropriate for the physician to discuss all treatment options with the patient and select the treatment that is most appropriate in any given situation.

Nonsurgical Treatment

Various pharmacologic agents have been studied in search of the perfect drug for ectopic pregnancy treatment. Most of the work centers around the use of methotrexate, a folic acid analogue that inhibits dehydrofolate reductase and thereby blocks DNA synthesis. Although potential side effects of methotrexate include leukopenia, thrombocytopenia, bone marrow suppression, stomatitis, and gastrointestinal upset, few such effects have been reported with the doses necessary for ectopic pregnancy treatment.

Initially, methotrexate was reported for treatment of trophoblastic tissue left in situ after surgical management of abdominal pregnancy.[24,25] Tanaka and colleagues[26] were the first to report intramuscular methotrexate for the treatment of an unruptured tubal pregnancy. These reports were followed by other case reports and then larger case series, so that now, over 400 cases have been reported using various treatment regimens.

Two treatment schedules are currently used by most gynecologists. The multidose regimen requires that patients re-

Table 33-1. Multidose Methotrexate/Citrovorum Factor Treatment Schedule for Unruptured Ectopic Pregnancy

Day	Time	Therapy
1	Variable	CBC, SGOT, MTX, hCG, blood type + Rh, BUN, creatinine
2	8:00 AM	CF, hCG
3	8:00 AM	MTX, hCG
4	8:00 AM	CF, hCG
5	8:00 AM	MTX, hCG
6	8:00 AM	CF, hCG
7	8:00 AM	MTX, hCG
8	8:00 AM	CF, hCG

Abbreviations: CBC, complete blood count with differential and platelet count; SCOT, serum glutamic oxalacetic transaminase (U/L); MTX, intramuscular methotrexate (1.0 mg/kg); hCG, quantitative β-human chorionic gonadotropin (mIU/ml); CF, intramuscular citrovorum (0.1 mg/kg); BUN, blood urea nitrogen.

ceive methotrexate alternated with citrovorum factor on a daily basis until the hCG titer begins to drop[27,28] (Table 33-1). Using this protocol, approximately 18 percent of patients required only one methotrexate/citrovorum dose. As a result, a treatment strategy was defined in which patients receive only a single intramuscular injection of methotrexate without citrovorum rescue (Table 33-2). Although no randomized trial has been done that directly compares the two treatment schedules, the results using the same treatment criteria in the same population indicate that single-dose treatment is equivalent to multidose treatment.[29,30] Single-dose methotrexate offers several advantages compared with multidose treatment: less total methotrexate is required, less patient follow-up is necessary, fewer methotrexate side effects are encountered, and the cost of treatment is decreased.

Table 33-2. Single-Dose Intramuscular Methotrexate Treatment for Unruptured Ectopic Pregnancy Treatment

Day	Therapy
0	hCG, D&C, CBC, SGOT, BUN, creatinine, blood type + Rh[a]
1	MTX, hCG[b]
4	hCG
7	hCG

Abbreviations: hCG, quantitative β-human chorionic gonadotropin (mIU/mL); D&C, dilation and curettage; CBC, complete blood count; SGOT, serum glutamic oxalacetic transaminase (U/L); BUN, blood urea nitrogen; MTX, intramuscular methotrexate (50 mg/m²).

[a] In those patients not requiring D&C prior to MTX initiation (hCG ≥2,000 mIU/ml and no gestational sac on transvaginal ultrasound), day 0 and day 1 are combined.

[b] If <15% decline in hCG titer between day 4 and 7, give second dose of methotrexate 50 mg/m² on day 7. If ≥15% decline in hCG titer between day 4 and 7, follow weekly until hCG <10 mIU/mL.

Ultrasound and laparoscopy have been used to aid with injection of various agents, including methotrexate, into the ectopic pregnancy. The success of this treatment approach has not been as favorable as that of intramuscular methotrexate.[31–36] In addition, patients require injection through the cul-de-sac with laparoscopy. These are significant drawbacks when compared to intramuscular injection.

Surgical Treatment

Because medical management of ectopic pregnancy is relatively new, surgical management is the mainstay of ectopic pregnancy treatment. The optimum surgical approach has changed over the years, from one in which the tube and ovary were removed, to the present day, in which tubal-sparing surgery is generally recommended.[37,38] Stromme,[39] in 1953, was the first to report the use of salpingotomy in the English literature.

Laparotomy Versus Laparoscopy

The operative approach for ectopic pregnancy treatment can be either laparotomy or laparoscopy. Because salpingotomy and salpingectomy or segmental resection can be done using either approach, the procedure chosen should not dictate the operative approach. Likewise, whether the tube is intact or ruptured does not determine in and of itself whether laparoscopy or laparotomy is needed. Rather, this decision depends on the hemodynamic stability of the patient, the size and location of the ectopic mass, and the surgeon's expertise.

When laparoscopy was first used for operative treatment of ectopic pregnancy, a number of authors published results of retrospective and prospective studies in which a series of patients were treated using the laparoscopic technique. These reports established the safety and efficacy of using operative laparoscopy for ectopic pregnancy treatment.[40–45] Once the safety and efficacy of the approach was established, the next step was to compare laparoscopic management to laparotomy.

All other factors being equivalent, several studies support the use of laparoscopy over laparotomy in any particular clinical situation. In a case-controlled study, Brumsted et al[46] compared 25 patients undergoing laparoscopy to 25 patients undergoing laparotomy. In this study, hospital stay was significantly shorter in the laparoscopy group (1.34 ± 0.8 versus 3.02 ± 1.1 days). Operative time was shorter (77.5 ± 26.1 versus 103.6 ± 26.7 minutes) as were convalescence days (8.7 ± 7.9 versus 25.7 ± 16.2). Patients undergoing laparoscopy also required less postoperative analgesia (0.84 + 2.3 versus 4.6 + 2.9 doses; $P < .01$). Using a randomized format, 60 patients undergoing salpingostomy were reported by Vermesh and colleagues.[47] Laparoscopic salpingostomy was associated with less estimated blood loss and a shorter hospital stay. Two patients in the laparoscopy group required laparotomy for hemostasis, and two patients had a wound infection following laparotomy. Postoperatively, tubal patency rates were equivalent as were intrauterine pregnancy rates. Only one patient in each group developed a persistent ectopic pregnancy. In another study, patients undergoing laparoscopy (n = 26) were compared with patients undergoing laparotomy (n = 37) using a prospective format in which patients were assigned to a treatment method on alternating months. Patients undergoing laparoscopy had similar operative times compared with laparotomy, along with a significant decrease in estimated blood loss, postoperative hospital stay, narcotic requirement, and time to return to normal activity. These advantages were produced with less cost when compared to laparotomy ($5,528 ± 1,586 versus $6,793 ± 155).[48] In the largest study reported, Lundorff et al[49] studied the surgical outcome of 105 patients randomized to laparoscopy or laparotomy after being stratified for age and other risk factors. Of 73 patients who underwent a second-look laparoscopy, significantly more patients who had previously undergone laparotomy had adhesions at the surgical site than patients treated by laparoscopy. Bauman et al[50] compared laparoscopy (n = 65) to laparotomy (n = 27) in a prospective manner in which the treatment was chosen by the surgical preference and experience of the operating surgeon. This study also showed that laparoscopy was associated with a shorter postoperative hospital stay and a faster return to work. These advantages were associated with an overall decrease in cost. In the laparoscopy group, two patients required laparotomy and two patients required reoperation for persistent trophoblastic growth. If taken together, it appears that laparoscopy has the advantage when compared with laparotomy for ectopic pregnancy management. A word of caution must be emphasized here, in that much of the advantage of laparoscopic management is the reduced postoperative stay and shorter convalescence period. Now that similar postoperative stays for laparoscopy and laparotomy have been reported in patients undergoing various types of gynecologic surgery, the advantages of laparoscopy over laparotomy become less obvious.[51]

Following salpingotomy, trophoblastic tissue may continue to proliferate, giving rise to persistent growth of trophoblastic tissue. When this occurs, the patient must have additional surgery (usually salpingectomy) or be treated with methotrexate. Obviously, this increases the potential for morbidity and adds to the cost of treatment. The incidence of persistent trophoblastic growth is generally thought not to be related to surgical approach. However, Seifer et al[52] reviewed medical records of 157 patients following salpingostomy for unruptured ampullary ectopic pregnancies. The incidence of persistent trophoblastic growth in patients undergoing laparoscopic salpingostomy was 15.5 percent compared with only 1.8 percent in patients treated by laparotomy. These authors found that risk factors for development of this condition include surgical approach, initial hCG titer duration of amenorrhea, and ectopic size. In addition, few studies report the number of failed laparoscopic salpingostomies, that is, the number of procedures in which salpingostomy is thought to be the procedure of choice, but because of technical difficulty, adhesive disease, or bleeding, the procedure is converted to salpingectomy. Each of the studies comparing laparoscopy with laparotomy report a shorter hospital stay with laparoscopic surgery. However, the postoperative care was not standardized in any of these studies. Thus, it is possible that a study bias exists in which patients undergoing laparotomy are not allowed to be discharged as early as those undergoing laparoscopy. Outpatient and 1-day hospitalization following laparotomy for a variety of reproductive procedures has been reported.[53,54] Thus, it appears from these studies that it is possible to perform laparotomy for gynecologic surgery on an outpatient basis. These issues call into question the advantages of the laparoscopic approach.

Washington and Katz[55,56] have shown that there has been and will continue to be an increasing burden of the expense for ectopic pregnancy treatment falling on public payers. This fact, along with the overall increasing cost of health care, has forced the discussion of cost-containment and cost-effectiveness and is an ever-increasing factor in the practice of obstetrics and gynecology.

Maruri and Azziz[57] performed a technology assessment and reviewed the cost-effectiveness and cost-benefit of laparoscopic surgery as compared with laparotomy for the surgical treatment of ectopic pregnancy. Their findings suggest that at least 80 percent of patients could have their ectopic pregnancy treated by laparoscopy. They estimated that if this were done nationally, there would be a savings of $105.6 million in direct medical costs along with a $65 million dollar savings by employers' or patients' income because of a more rapid return to work. However, the use of laparoscopic surgery would result in increased expenditure for equipment and for treatment of patients with persistent ectopic pregnancy following laparoscopy. Given these findings, there would be a $1.4 million dollar annual savings for ectopic pregnancy treatment.

Creinin and Washington[58] studied the cost of methotrexate treatment in a retrospective fashion. In their study, it was estimated that 30 percent of patients would have been eligible for methotrexate treatment with an annual national cost savings in excess of $280 million. Stovall et al[59] compared the immediate direct medical expenses for medical and surgical approaches to ectopic pregnancy treatment using a retrospective review of 60 consecutive patients. The mean direct cost of methotrexate treatment ($1,563; range, $1,169 to $2,300) was significantly lower than either laparoscopic treatment ($6,626; range, $5,683 to $10,429; $P < .00001$) or laparotomy ($8,001; range, $6,834 to $22,082; $P < .00001$). In this study it was found that approximately 45 percent of patients were eligible for methotrexate treatment.

Taken together, these data support the cost-benefits of laparoscopic surgery in candidates for surgical management, and supports the use of methotrexate for patients who are eligible for medical treatment. A word of caution must be added, since to date, there are no prospective randomized trials comparing methotrexate management to that of laparoscopic surgery.

Salpingectomy Versus Salpingotomy

Tubal-sparing surgery (salpingotomy) is advocated by most surgeons when an ectopic pregnancy is encountered. DeCherney and Kase[60] compared tubal-sparing surgery with salpingectomy and found no difference in the subsequent intrauterine pregnancy rate (40 percent), and no increase in the rate of repeat ectopic pregnancies (8 percent). Although there was no difference in pregnancy rates, the authors believe that conservative surgery should be used whenever possible. This approach has also be championed by other investigators.[61–63] Tuomivaara and Kauppila[64] studied a group of 323 patients who desired fertility after surgical treatment of ectopic pregnancy. These authors performed a salpingectomy if the tube was ruptured or the contralateral tube appeared grossly normal. If the patient had a history of infertility or the tube was not ruptured, salpingotomy was considered the procedure of choice. Patients were followed for 1 to 11 years (mean 5.1 years). The conception rate was 82 percent, with 79 percent delivering a full-term infant and 13 percent having a recurrent ectopic gestation. Whether the ectopic pregnancy was treated with salpingotomy or salpingectomy had no effect on the subsequent fertility if the patient had an intact contralateral tube. Nulliparous women had a significantly lower conception rate than parous women (74 percent versus 83 percent), and a higher risk of repeat ectopic pregnancy (9 percent versus 22 percent). This suggests that a history of infertility or difficulty in achieving pregnancy is a predictor of subsequent fertility following surgical treatment of ectopic pregnancy. These findings were confirmed by Ory et al.[65] This group reported a series of patients who had previously undergone surgery for an ectopic pregnancy. Patients were followed for a period of 3 to 12.5 years. In these patients, no difference in the rate of future intrauterine pregnancies was found whether the patient underwent salpingectomy or salpingostomy. The most important determinant of future fertility was a history of infertility before the ectopic pregnancy. In patients who had a history of infertility, those who had a salpingectomy had equivalent rates of intrauterine pregnancies and a decreased incidence of recurrent ectopic pregnancies. Thus, patients who have an ectopic pregnancy and have a history of infertility are probably better served by having a salpingectomy rather than undergoing salpingostomy if surgery is chosen as the treatment method.

Salpingectomy

Salpingectomy is the procedure of choice for the patient who has rupture of the tube, especially if the patient is hemodynamically unstable, or the tube has been damaged beyond the point of repair or ability to function. The ovary should not be removed unless it is involved in a tubo-ovarian complex, in which dense adhesions surround the tube and make it impractical to separate it from the adjacent fallopian tube.

If performed by laparotomy, salpingectomy is accomplished by placing a clamp across the mesosalpinx, followed by placement of a second clamp across the proximal portion of the fallopian tube (Fig. 33-2A). The tip of the first clamp is approximated to the tip of the second clamp so that the mesosalpingeal vessels are completely occluded. More than two clamps can be used if necessary, but this is generally not needed. The tube is then excised, and the pedicles are ligated using a 2–0 or 3–0 synthetic absorbable suture material (Fig. 33-2B). The clamp should be placed as close as possible to the uterine cornu, so that as much as possible of the fallopian tube can be removed. Cornual resection is not necessary as it does not eliminate the possibility of a future interstitial pregnancy.[66] It is also probable that resection of the cornual portion of the uterus would weaken the uterine wall and predispose the patient to uterine rupture in the event of a future pregnancy.

Salpingectomy can also be performed using operative laparoscopic techniques. Generally, two or three laparoscopic ports are established, with a periumbilical and one or two lower quadrant ports. Before beginning the actual procedure, the pelvis is visualized and accessed for the presence or absence of hemoperitoneum or adhesive disease. As necessary, suction/irrigation is used to remove excess blood so that the affected fallopian tube can be visualized. The anatomy of the fallopian tube is then normalized by lysing any adhesions so that the fallopian tube is mobile. Several methods have been described for removing the tube. One method is to use a pre-tied surgical loop. The cornual portion of the fallopian tube is cauterized as close as possible to the uterus (Fig. 33-3). A pre-tied loop is inserted through a lower laparoscopic port of the affected side. The fallopian tube is then brought through the loop using grasping forceps. The knot is tightened and the suture cut. A second loop is placed in a similar fashion. The fallopian tube is then resected and removed. Once hemostasis has been ensured, the remaining suture loop is cut and removed. An alternate and equally effective method is to use bipolar electrosurgical forceps and scissors (Fig. 33-4). Graspers are used to grasp and stabilize the fimbriated end of the tube. The bipolar forceps are then used to coagulate the distal portion of the mesosalpinx. Once fulgurated, scissors are used to divide the coagulated portion. These steps are repeated in successive fashion until the entire mesosalpinx has been coagulated. The cornual portion of

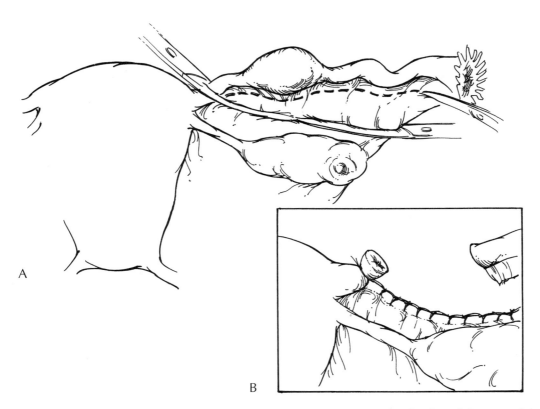

A

B

Fig. 33-2. (A) Technique of salpingectomy at laparotomy. **(B)** Excision and suture ligation of the mesosalpinx at laparotomy.

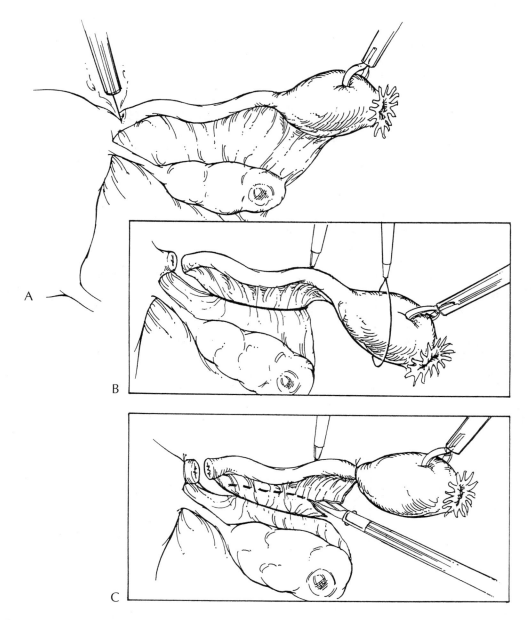

Fig. 33-3. Technique of laparoscopic salpingectomy. **(A)** Bipolar cautery is used to fulgurate the tube at its insertion into the uterus. **(B)** Pre-tied surgical loops are placed over the fallopian tube. **(C)** Fallopian tube is excised.

the tube is then desiccated as close to the uterus as possible and the tube cut and removed. One must be certain that the tube is adequately elevated before it is desiccated, in order not to inadvertently coagulate the ovarian vasculature. Yet another method that has been described uses the laparoscopic linear staplers to ligate and divide the mesosalpinx. However, the cost of these instruments makes this a less attractive option than using the suture or electrosurgical methods.

Additional suction/irrigation is used to remove as much intra-abdominal blood as possible. Sometimes, not all blood can be removed. If this is the case, it can be left in situ and it will reabsorb over time.

Salpingotomy

The goal of salpingotomy is to remove the products of conception while causing as little damage as possible to the affected tube. The surgical technique for salpingotomy (Fig. 33-5) is the same whether performed by laparotomy or laparoscopy. If present, any adhesions are lysed and the tubal anatomy restored as nearly to normal as possible. It is often difficult to obtain hemostasis at the tubal incision site and in the placental attachment site. Therefore, many surgeons infiltrate the incision site with a dilute solution of vasopressin in saline in an effort to decrease bleeding from the serosal

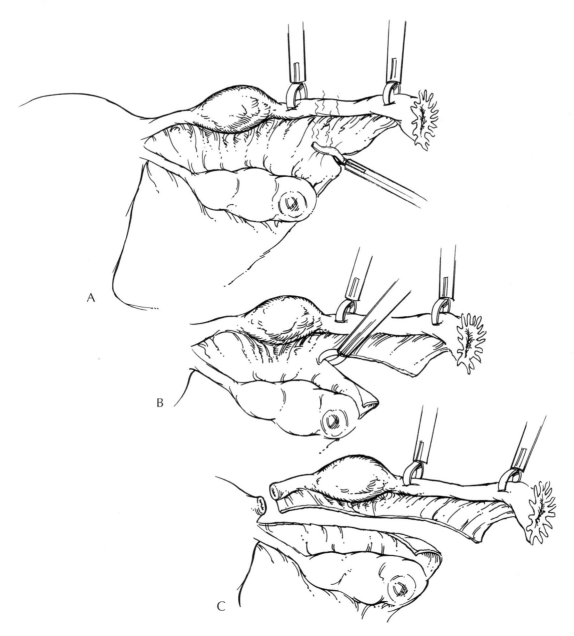

Fig. 33-4. **(A–C)** Laparoscopic salpingectomy using electrosurgery. Bipolar forceps are used to fulgurate the mesosalpinx, which is followed by using scissors to cut the mesosalpinx.

surface. This solution is made by mixing 10 U of vasopressin in 50 to 100 ml of saline. This can be done using a laparoscopic needle placed through the laparoscope or using a 20-gauge spinal needle placed directly through the abdominal wall and injected into the tube where the incision is to be made. An incision is made on the antimesenteric border of the tube over the point of maximal distension. An electrosurgical needle electrode, laser, or scissors can be used to make this incision. The products of conception are removed using smooth forceps. Once removed, the placental bed should be copiously irrigated, and hemostasis is obtained using electro-

surgery. Every effort should be made to avoid damage to the tube. The tubal incision site does not require closure and can be left to heal by secondary intention. Nelson et al[67] compared primary closure of the incision with closure by secondary intention using a rabbit model. No difference was observed in adhesion formation, subsequent pregnancy rate, or the rate of fistula formation. Suture reapproximation may be helpful for obtaining hemostasis and can be used for this purpose.

Another method to assist with obtaining hemostasis is that of mesosalpingeal vessel ligation. This can be done by plac-

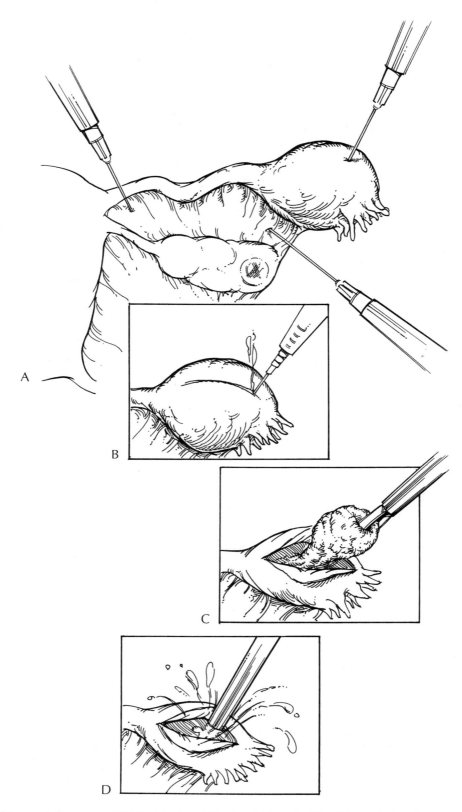

Fig. 33-5. Linear salpingostomy. **(A)** The tube is stabilized and injected with a dilute solution of vasopressin. **(B)** An incision is made on the antimesenteric border overlying the ectopic. **(C)** The products of conception are removed using atraumatic forceps. **(D)** The implantation site is irrigated and hemostasis obtained.

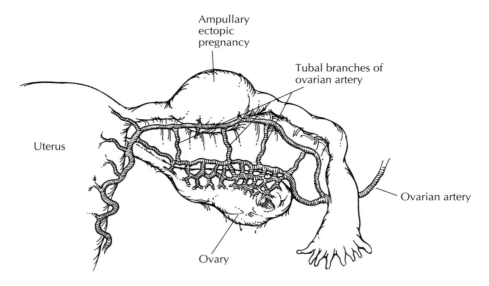

Fig. 33-6. Mesosalpingeal vessel ligation.

ing the tube on tension so that the mesosalpingeal vessels can be visualized. The mesosalpingeal vessels at the ectopic site as well as those proximal and distal to the ectopic are ligated (Fig. 33-6). If individual vessels can not be identified, a running-locked suture can be placed in the mesosalpinx, or the vessels fulgurated.

Segmental Resection

Another type of conservative surgical management is segmental resection, in which only the affected portion of the fallopian tube is removed. Once removed, the patient must undergo immediate or future anastomosis. As with salpingotomy, the technique for segmental resection is similar whether performed by laparoscopy or laparotomy. The bipolar electrocautery forceps are used to fulgurate the tube distal and proximal to the affected site. The tube is incised and the attached mesosalpinx is desiccated and cut. The ectopic pregnancy and its surrounding tubal segment is removed (Fig. 33-7). Electrosurgery should be used sparingly so that as little damage as possible is done to the tube. In an effort to conserve as much tube as possible for later anastomosis, a pre-tied surgical loop can be used (Fig. 33-8). The ectopic pregnancy is stabilized with graspers and a pre-tied loop is passed over it and tightened. A second loop is placed just beneath the first. The ectopic pregnancy is excised and removed.

Treatment of Interstitial Pregnancy

The presence of a cornual or interstitial pregnancy represents a challenging surgical procedure. Traditional treatment consist of cornual resection or hysterectomy. More recently,

laparoscopic management and medical management have been described.[26,28,30,68–72]

If laparoscopic surgery is used, the mesosalpinx is first coagulated and incised. A dilute vasopressin solution is injected into the wall of the ectopic gestation and into the surrounding myometrium. The myometrium proximal to the gestation is coagulated and cut circumferentially in a repeated and deliberate fashion. Once completely resected, the specimen is then removed. The uterine incision is repaired with interrupted sutures (Fig. 33-9). The potential problem with this technique is that hemorrhage may be encountered and difficult to control at laparoscopy. Also, it is often very difficult to obtain complete closure of the myometrium, and the potential for subsequent uterine rupture exists. Thus, it may be more appropriate to manage these patients via laparotomy if surgical treatment is chosen. Yet another school of thought would suggest that medical therapy should be used for the interstitial or cornual pregnancy that is less than 3.5 cm in greatest dimension, with surgery reserved for the larger cornual or interstitial pregnancy.

Potential Surgical Complications

Patients undergoing surgical treatment of ectopic pregnancy can suffer any of the complications that are known to occur with either laparotomy or laparoscopy. The only postsurgical complication that is specific to ectopic pregnancy management is the potential for the development of persistent trophoblastic growth following salpingotomy.

Persistent ectopic pregnancy is defined as the continued growth of trophoblastic tissue after incomplete removal of the ectopic pregnancy during conservative surgical treatment. The occurrence of persistent ectopic pregnancy was first described in 1979.[73] Following salpingotomy, the hCG

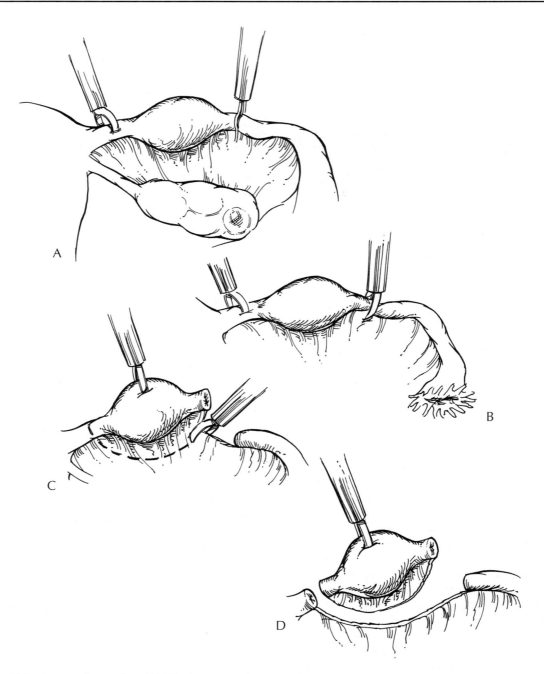

Fig. 33-7. Segmental resection. **(A)** Bipolar cautery is used to fulgurate the tube distal and proximal to the ectopic pregnancy. **(B)** The tube is then cut, and **(C)** the mesosalpinx coagulated and cut. **(D)** The ectopic pregnancy and affected tubal segment is then removed.

titer must be followed until it is negative to ensure that there is no residual trophoblastic tissue remaining in situ. Risk factors for persistent ectopic pregnancy include less than 42 days of amenorrhea, ectopic size less than 2.0 cm, and an hCG titer of less than 3,000 mIU/ml.[52,74,75] Trophoblastic implants in the pelvis have also been reported following salpingostomy.[75] The preoperative hCG titer has also been associated with persistence of trophoblastic growth. A retro-spective study of 98 patients found a 22 percent persistence rate when the hCG titer was greater than 3,000 mIU/ml, compared with only 1.4 percent when the hCG titer was less than 3,000 mIU/ml.[74] The etiology of this condition is probably multifactorial, and may result from dissection of trophoblastic tissue through the endosalpinx and into the tubal muscularis, or following incomplete removal during surgery.[76,77] Because of the possible development of this

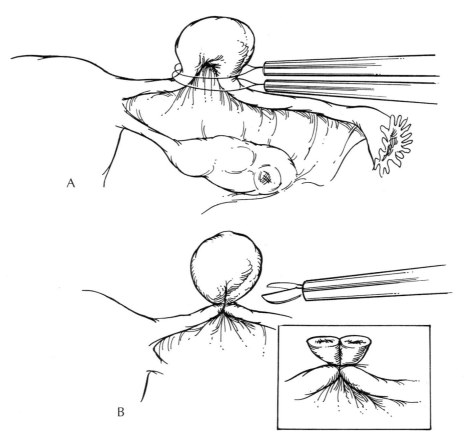

Fig. 33-8. (A & B) Laparoscopic partial salpingectomy using a pre-tied surgical loop.

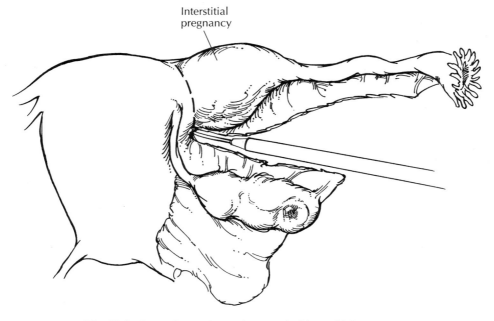

Fig. 33-9. Cornual resection and removal of interstitial pregnancy.

condition, patients who have undergone salpingotomy should have their hCG level monitored until negative. This can generally be done on a weekly basis. If the hCG level begins to plateau or rise, treatment must be undertaken. The optimum treatment for this condition is not known. Like treatment of primary ectopic pregnancy, expectant management has been described for the asymptomatic patient. However, the mainstay of treatment is either medical or surgical treatment. Surgical treatment consists of repeat salpingotomy or, more commonly, salpingectomy. The medical treatment that is most commonly used is methotrexate.[28–30,78–80] Because this condition is specific to salpingotomy, patients should be counseled preoperatively regarding this possibility. By doing so, they will better understand the need for hCG follow-up after surgery.

MANAGEMENT OF RECURRENT ECTOPIC PREGNANCY

For the patient who has previously been treated for an ectopic pregnancy, nothing is more distressing than being told that she has another tubal pregnancy. This occurs in 6 to 27 percent of patients who have previously been treated for an ectopic pregnancy. Little scientific data are available to guide the clinician's decision-making process when faced with this situation. DeCherney et al[81] reviewed 32 patients who had two ectopic pregnancies. Of 13 patients trying to conceive, 4 (30.8 percent) had a term intrauterine gestation. These authors suggested that the subsequent intrauterine pregnancy rate was not sufficiently high to consider tubal-sparing surgery if the second ectopic pregnancy occurred in the same tube. For the patient who has previously undergone salpingectomy, it seems prudent to make every effort to save the remaining tube, especially if the patient will not be able to undergo in vitro fertilization. Otherwise, the patient has no chance of conceiving. If both tubes are present, and the ectopic pregnancy occurs in the ipsilateral tube, it is probably best to remove the tube. If the recurrent ectopic occurs in the contralateral tube, the tube should probably be conserved if possible, although this is controversial.

SURGICAL MANAGEMENT OF OVARIAN PREGNANCY

Implantation of a pregnancy into the ovary accounts for only about 1 percent of all ectopic gestations. The criteria for diagnosis of an ovarian pregnancy were established by Spiegelberg[82] in 1878 and include

1. The fallopian tubes must be intact and separate from the ovary
2. The pregnancy must occupy the normal position of the ovary

3. The pregnancy must be connected to the uterus by the utero-ovarian ligament
4. There must be ovarian tissue present with the gestational sac

In the past, laparotomy with oophorectomy was the procedure of choice for ovarian pregnancy treatment. Now, however, laparoscopic treatment or medical therapy using methotrexate can be used. Several surgical techniques may be used including oophorectomy, cystectomy, or wedge resection of the ovary. If wedge resection or cystectomy are used, the hCG titer should be monitored until negative to make certain that there is no residual trophoblastic tissue remaining.

CERVICAL PREGNANCY

Implantation of the pregnancy within the cervix ranges from 1 in 2,400 to 1 in 50,000 pregnancies.[83] Until recently, the diagnosis was generally not made until the patient underwent hysterectomy because of profuse vaginal bleeding. In many instances, cervical pregnancy is suspected when the patient presents early in pregnancy with vaginal bleeding. In such cases, cervical pregnancy can be diagnosed using ultrasound and conservative surgical therapy can be used. In others, cervical pregnancy is not suspected until the patient develops profuse bleeding while undergoing a suction curettage for a presumed incomplete abortion.

If diagnosed before surgery, conservative surgical options may be used for the patient who desires future fertility. If the patient does not desire future fertility, consideration should be given to hysterectomy, as this is definitive treatment and conservative treatment options carry the potential for significant morbidity. Consideration should also be given to treatment with methotrexate.[84–86]

Various techniques have been described to control the bleeding that may be associated with cervical pregnancy, including uterine packing, lateral cervical suture placement, placement of a cervical cerclage, or insertion of a 30-ml Foley catheter in an attempt to tamponade the bleeding. Angiographic arterial embolization has also been successful in some patients.[87–92]

ABDOMINAL PREGNANCY

Abdominal pregnancy is defined as an intraperitoneal implantation excluding tubal, ovarian, or intraligamentous implantation. The incidence of abdominal pregnancy varies from 1 in 372 to 1 in 9,714 live births.[93,94] The patient with an abdominal pregnancy is at risk of marked morbidity and possible mortality, with the risk of death being 7 to 8 times greater than that of tubal ectopic pregnancy. The infant is also at risk of marked morbidity if it survives, with the risk of congenital anomalies ranging from 20 to 40 percent.[95–97]

The clinical presentation of patients with an abdominal pregnancy varies depending on the gestational age at the time the patient becomes symptomatic. In the first trimester, symptoms are similar to those of tubal ectopic pregnancy, while in the second and third trimesters, the diagnosis may be suspected because of abnormal fetal presentation, displaced uterine cervix, or easily palpable fetal parts. Diagnostic aids include abdominal radiographs or ultrasound, computed tomography scanning, and magnetic resonance imaging.[98,99] A markedly elevated α-fetoprotein level (four to five times the mucoid otitis media) may also be a sign of abdominal pregnancy.[100,101]

For several reasons, most gynecologists recommend surgical intervention when an abdominal pregnancy is diagnosed. First, it is unlikely that an abdominal pregnancy will continue to term. Second, if it does and the infant survives, there will almost certainly be significant deformity and morbidity, if not mortality. At surgery, the umbilical cord is clamped and the fetus or infant removed. If reasonably possible, the placenta should be removed if its vascular supply can be identified and ligated, and its other attachments can be isolated and removed. The most significant event that can occur with placental removal is massive hemorrhage. When this occurs, the abdomen can be packed and the packs left in place and removed in 24 to 48 hours. During this time the patient can be stabilized, and angiographic arterial embolization can be considered.[102,103] If placental removal cannot be safely accomplished, it can be left it situ and allowed to absorb. Its involution can be followed using serial ultrasounds, hCG titers, or gallium scans. The major risks of leaving the placenta in place include bowel obstruction or fistula formation, and sepsis as the tissue begins to degenerate. Methotrexate treatment is not helpful.

REFERENCES

1. Longo LD: Classic pages in obstetrics and gynecology. A case of an extra-uterine foetus by John Bard from medical observation and inquiries (London), Vol. 2, p. 367–372, 1764. Am J Obstet Gynecol 123:305, 1975

2. Tait RL: Five cases of extrauterine pregnancy operated upon at the time of rupture. BMJ 1:1250, 1884

3. Goldner TE, Lawson HW, Xia Z, Atrash HK: Surveillance for ectopic pregnancy—United States, 1970–1989. MMWR CDC Surveillance Summary 42:(SS-6)73, 1993

4. National Center for Health Statistics: Annual summary of births, marriages, divorces and deaths: United States, 1989, Hyattsville, MD. U.S. Department of Health and Human Services, Public Health Service. CDC 38:23, 1990

5. Coste J, Job-Spira N, Fernandez H et al: Risk factors for ectopic pregnancy: a case-control study in France, with spe-cial focus on infectious factors. Am J Epidemiol 133:839, 1991

6. Ectopic Pregnancy—United States, 1990–1992. MMWR CDC, Current Trends 44:46, 1995

7. Westrom L, Bengtsson LPH, Mardh PA: Incidence, trends, and risks of ectopic pregnancy in a population of women. BMJ 282:15, 1981

8. DeStefano F, Peterson HB, Layde PM, Rubin GL: Risk of ectopic pregnancy following tubal sterilization. Obstet Gynecol 60:326, 1982

9. Stabile I, Grudzinskas JG: Ectopic pregnancy: a review of incidence, etiology, and diagnostic aspects. Obstet Gynecol Surv 45:335, 1990

10. Stovall TG, Kellerman AL, Ling FW, Buster JE: Emergency department diagnosis of ectopic pregnancy. Ann Emerg Med 19:1098, 1990

11. Maccato ML, Estrada R, Faro S: Ectopic pregnancy with undetectable serum and urine beta hCG levels and detection of beta HCG in the ectopic trophoblast by immunocytochemical evaluation. Obstet Gynecol 81:878, 1993

12. Lonky NM, Sauer MV: Ectopic pregnancy with shock and undetectable beta human chorionic gonadotropin: a case report. J Reprod Med 32:559, 1987

13. Uribe MA, Dunn RC, Buttram VC: Tubal pregnancy with normal hysterosalpingogram and negative serum pregnancy test. Obstet Gynecol 75:483, 1990

14. Storring PL, Gaines-Das RE, Bangham DR: International reference preparation of human chorionic gonadotropin for immunoassay: potency estimates in various bioassays and protein binding assay systems; and international reference preparations of the alpha and beta subunits of human chorionic gonadotropin for immunoassay. J Endocrinol 84:295, 1980

15. Kadar N, Caldwell BV, Romero R: A method of screening for ectopic pregnancy and its indications. Obstet Gynecol 58:162, 1981

16. Stovall TG, Ling FW, Andersen RN, Buster JE: Improved sensitivity and specificity of a single measurement of serum progesterone over serial quantitative beta-human chorionic gonadotropin in screening for ectopic pregnancy. Hum Reprod 7:723, 1992

17. Stovall TG, Ling FW, Carson SA, Buster JE: Serum progesterone and uterine curettage in the differential diagnosis of ectopic pregnancy. Fertil Steril 57:456, 1992

18. Stovall TG, Ling FW: Ectopic pregnancy: diagnostic and therapeutic algorithms minimizing surgical intervention. J Reprod Med 38:807, 1993

19. Emerson DS, Cartier MS, Altieri LA et al: Diagnostic efficacy of endovaginal color Doppler flow imaging in an ectopic pregnancy screening program. Radiology 183:413, 1992

20. Nyberg DA, Mack LA, Laing FC, Jeffery RB: Early pregnancy complications: endovaginal sonographic findings correlated with human chorionic gonadotropin levels. Radiology 167:610, 1988

21. Bree RL, Edwards M, Bohm VM et al: Transvaginal sonogra-

phy in the evaluation of normal early pregnancy: correlation with hCG level. Am J Roentgenol 53:75, 1989

22. Bernaschek G, Rudelstorfer R, Csaicsich P: Vaginal sonography versus serum human chorionic gonadotropin in early detection of pregnancy. Am J Obstet Gynecol 158:608, 1988

23. Vermesh M, Graczykowski JW, Sauer MV: Reevaluation of the role of culdocentesis in the management of ectopic pregnancy. Am J Obstet Gynecol 162:411, 1990

24. Hreshchyshyn MM, Naples JD Jr, Randall CL: Amethopterin in abdominal pregnancy. Am J Obstet Gynecol 93:286, 1965

25. St. Clair JT, Whealer DA, Fish SA: Methotrexate in abdominal pregnancy. JAMA 208:529, 1969

26. Tanaka T, Hayashi H, Kutsuzawa T et al: Treatment of interstitial ectopic pregnancy with methotrexate: report of a successful case. Fertil Steril 37:851, 1982

27. Stovall TG, Ling FW, Buster JE: Outpatient chemotherapy of unruptured ectopic pregnancy. Fertil Steril 51:435, 1989

28. Stovall TG, Ling FW, Gray LA et al: Methotrexate treatment of unruptured ectopic pregnancy: a report of 100 cases. Obstet Gynecol 77:749, 1991

29. Stovall TG, Ling FW, Gray LA: Single-dose methotrexate for treatment of ectopic pregnancy. Obstet Gynecol 77:754, 1991

30. Stovall TG, Ling FW: Single-dose methotrexate: an expanded clinical trial. Am J Obstet Gynecol 170:1840, 1993

31. Fernandez H, Pauthier S, Saimerc S et al: Ultrasound-guided injection of methotrexate versus laparoscopic salpingotomy in ectopic pregnancy. Fertil Steril 63:25, 1995

32. Fernandez H, Benifla JL, Lelaidier C et al: Methotrexate treatment of ectopic pregnancy: 100 cases treated by primary transvaginal injection under sonographic control. Fertil Steril 59:773, 1993

33. Lang PF, Tamussino K, Honigel W, Ralph G: Treatment of unruptured tubal pregnancy by laparoscopic instillation of hyperosmolar glucose solution. Am J Obstet Gynecol 166:1378, 1992

34. Kooi S, Kick HCLV: Treatment of tubal pregnancy by local injection of methotrexate after adrenaline injection into the mesosalpinx: a report of 25 patients. Fertil Steril 54:580, 1990

35. Mnottla GL, Rulin MC, Guzick DS: Lack of resolution of ectopic pregnancy by intratubal injection of methotrexate. Fertil Steril 57:685, 1992

36. O'Shea RT, Thompson GR, Harding A: Intra-amniotic methotrexate versus CO_2 laser laparoscopic salpingotomy in the management of tubal ectopic pregnancy—a prospective randomized trial. Fertil Steril 62:876, 1994

37. Schenker JG, Eyal F, Polishuk WZ: Fertility after tubal surgery. Surg Gynecol Obstet 135:74, 1972

38. Jeffcoate TN: Salpingectomy or salpingo-oophorectomy. J Obstet Gynaecol Br Emp 62:214, 1955

39. Stromme WB: Salpingostomy for tubal pregnancy: report of a successful case. Obstet Gynecol 1:472, 1953

40. Silva PD, Schaper AM, Rooney B: Reproductive outcome after 143 laparoscopic procedures for ectopic pregnancy. Obstet Gynecol 81:710, 1993

41. Wagner J, Droesch J, Mann WJ: Laparoscopic management of ectopic pregnancy in a resident training program. South Med J 86:619, 1993

42. Bruhat MA, Manhes H, Mage G, Pouly JL: Treatment of ectopic pregnancy by means of laparoscopy. Fertil Steril 33:411, 1980

43. DeCherney AH, Robero R, Naftolin F: Surgical management of unruptured ectopic pregnancy. Fertil Steril 35:21, 1981

44. Zouves C, Urman B, Gomel V: Laparoscopic surgical treatment of tubal pregnancy: a safe, effective alternative to laparotomy. J Reprod Med 37:205, 1992

45. Reich H, Johns DA, DeCaprio J et al: Laparoscopic treatment of 109 consecutive ectopic pregnancies. J Reprod Med 33:885, 1988

46. Brumsted J, Kessler C, Gibson C et al: A comparison of laparoscopy and laparotomy for the treatment of ectopic pregnancy. Obstet Gynecol 71:889, 1988

47. Vermesh M, Silva PD, Rosen GF et al: Management of unruptured ectopic gestation by linear salpingostomy: a prospective, randomized clinical trial of laparoscopy versus laparotomy. Obstet Gynecol 73:400, 1989

48. Murphy AA, Nager CW, Wujek JJ et al: Operative laparoscopy versus laparotomy for the management of ectopic pregnancy: a prospective trial. Fertil Steril 57:1180, 1992

49. Lundorff P, Hahlin M, Kallfelt B et al: Second-look laparoscopy after ectopic pregnancy. Fertil Steril 55:911, 1991

50. Baumann R, Magos AL, Turnbull SA: Prospective comparison of videopelviscopy with laparotomy for ectopic pregnancy. Br J Obstet Gynaecol 98:765, 1991

51. Seifer DB, Gutmann JN, Grant WD et al: Comparison of persistent ectopic pregnancy after laparoscopic salpingostomy versus salpingostomy at laparotomy for ectopic pregnancy. Obstet Gynecol 81:378, 1993

52. Seifer DB, Gutmann JN, Doyle MB et al: Comparison of persistent ectopic pregnancy after laparoscopic salpingostomy versus salpingostomy at laparotomy for ectopic pregnancy. Obstet Gynecol 81:378, 1993

53. Fayez JA, Dempsey RA: Short hospital stay for gynecologic reconstructive surgery via laparotomy. Obstet Gynecol 81:598, 1993

54. Berger GS: Outpatient pelvic laparotomy. J Reprod Med 39:569, 1994

55. Washington AE, Katz P: Ectopic pregnancy in the United States: economic consequences and payment source trends. Obstet Gynecol 81:2565, 1991

56. Washington AE, Katz P: Costs of payment and source for pelvic inflammatory disease. Trends and projections 1983–2000. JAMA 266:287, 1993

57. Maruri F, Azziz R: Laparoscopic surgery for ectopic pregnancies: technology assessment and public health implications. Fertil Steril 59:487, 1993

58. Creinin MD, Washington AE: Cost of ectopic pregnancy management: surgery versus methotrexate. Fertil Steril 60:963, 1993

59. Stovall TG, Bradham DD, Ling FW, Naughton M: Cost of

treatment of ectopic pregnancy: single-dose methotrexate versus surgical treatment. J Women Health 3:1, 1996

60. DeCherney A, Kase N: The conservative surgical management of unruptured ectopic pregnancy. Obstet Gynecol 54:451, 1979

61. Stromme WB: Conservative surgery for ectopic pregnancy. Obstet Gynecol 41:251, 1973

62. Langer R, Bukovsky I, Herman A et al: Conservative surgery for tubal pregnancy. Fertil Steril 38:427, 1982

63. Thorburn J, Philipson M, Lindblom B: Fertility after ectopic pregnancy in relation to background factors and surgical treatment. Fertil Steril 49:595, 1988

64. Tuomivaara L, Kauppila A: Radical or conservative surgery for ectopic pregnancy? A follow-up study of fertility of 323 patients. Fertil Steril 50:5803, 1988

65. Ory SJ, Nnadi E, Herrmann R et al: Fertility after ectopic pregnancy. Fertil Steril 60:231, 1993

66. Kalchman GG, Meltzer RM: Interstitial pregnancy following homolateral salpingectomy. Am J Obstet Gynecol 96:1139, 1966

67. Nelson LM, Margara RA, Winston RML: Primary and secondary closure of ampullary salpingostomy compared in the rabbit. Fertil Steril 45:292, 1986

68. Tulandi T, Vilos G, Gomel V: Laparoscopic treatment of interstitial pregnancy. Obstet Gynecol 85:465–467, 1995

69. Gleicher N, Karanda V, Rabin D, Pratt D: Laparoscopic removal of twin cornual pregnancies after in vitro fertilization. Fertil Steril 61:1161, 1994

70. Pasic R, Wolfe WM: Laparoscopic diagnosis and treatment of interstitial ectopic pregnancy: a case report. Am J Obstet Gynecol 163:587, 1990

71. Karsdorp Vh, Van der Venn F, Schats R et al: Successful treatment with methotrexate of five vital interstitial pregnancies. Hum Reprod 7:1164, 1992

72. Goldenberg M, Bider D, Oelsner G et al: Treatment of interstitial pregnancy with methotrexate via hysteroscopy. Fertil Steril 58:1234, 1992

73. Kelly RW, Martin SA, Strickler RC: Delayed hemorrhage in conservative surgery for ectopic pregnancy. Am J Obstet Gynecol 133:225, 1979

74. Lundorff P, Hahlin M, Sjoblom P, Linblom B: Persistent trophoblast after conservative treatment of tubal pregnancy: prediction and detection. Obstet Gynecol 77:129, 1991

75. Thatcher SS, Grainger DA, True LD, DeCherney AH: Pelvic trophoblastic implants after laparoscopic removal of a tubal pregnancy. Obstet Gynecol 74:514, 1989

76. Senterman M, Jibodh R, Tulandi T: Histopathologic study of ampullary and isthmic tubal ectopic pregnancy: prediction and detection. Obstet Gynecol 77:129, 1991

77. Stock RJ. Persistent tubal pregnancy. Obstet Gynecol 77:267, 1991

78. Pastner B, Kenigsberg D: Successful treatment of persistent ectopic pregnancy with oral methotrexate therapy. Fertil Steril 50:982, 1988

79. Higgins KA, Schwartz MB: Treatment of persistent trophoblastic tissue after salpingostomy with methotrexate. Fertil Steril 45:427, 1986

80. Hoppe DE, Bekkar Be, Nager CW: Single dose systemic methotrexate for the treatment of persistent ectopic pregnancy after conservative surgery. Obstet Gynecol 83:51, 1994

81. DeCherney AH, Silidker JS, Mezer HC, Tarlatzis BC: Reproductive outcome following two ectopic pregnancies. Fertil Steril 43:82, 1985

82. Spiegelberg O: Sur Cosuistik der Ovarialschwager schalt. Arch Gynaekol 13:73, 1878

83. Parente JT, Ou CS, Levy J, Legatt E: Cervical pregnancy analysis: a review and report of five cases. Obstet Gynecol 62:79, 1983

84. Farabow WS, Fulton JW, Fletcher V Jr et al: Cervical pregnancy treated with methotrexate. NC Med J 44:91, 1983

85. Stovall TG, Ling FW, Smith WC et al: Successful nonsurgical treatment of cervical pregnancy with methotrexate. Fertil Steril 50:672, 1988

86. Oyer R, Rarakjian D, Lev-Toaff A et al: Treatment of cervical pregnancy with methotrexate. Obstet Gynecol 71:469, 1988

87. Sheldon RS, Aaro LA, Welch JS: Conservative management of cervical pregnancy. Am J Obstet Gynecol 87:504, 1963

88. Ratten GJ: Cervical pregnancy treated by ligation of the descending branch of the uterine arteries: case report. Br J Obstet Gynaecol 90:367, 1983

89. Wharton KR, Gore B: Cervical pregnancy managed by placement of a shirodkar cerclage before evacuation: a case report. J Reprod Med 33:227, 1988

90. Nolan TE, Chandler PE, Hess LW, Morrison JC: Cervical pregnancy managed without hysterectomy: a case report. J Reprod Med 34:241, 1989

91. Patchell RD: Cervical pregnancy managed by balloon tamponade, letter. Am J Obstet Gynecol 149:107, 1984

92. Nelson RM: Bilateral internal iliac artery ligation in cervical pregnancy: conservation of reproductive function. Am J Obstet Gynecol 134:145, 1979

93. Beacham WD, Hernquist WC, Becham DW, Webster HD: Abdominal pregnancy at Charity Hospital in New Orleans. Am J Obstet Gynecol 84:1257, 1962

94. Atrash HK, Friede A, Hogue CJR: Abdominal pregnancy in the United States: frequency and maternal mortality. Obstet Gynecol 69:333, 1987

95. Rahman MS, Al-Suleiman SA, Rahman J, Al-Sibai MH: Advanced abdominal pregnancy observations in 10 cases. Obstet Gynecol 59:366, 1982

96. Cartwright PS, Brown JE, Davis RJ et al: Advanced abdominal pregnancy associated with fetal pulmonary hypoplasia: report of a case. Am J Obstet Gynecol 155:396, 1986

97. Tan KL, Goon SM, Wee JH: The paediatric aspects of advanced abdominal pregnancy. J Obstet Gynaecol Br Commonw 76:1021, 1969

98. Stanley JH, Horger EO III, Fagan CJ et al: Sonographic findings in abdominal pregnancy. AJR 147:1043, 1986

99. Harris MB, Angtuaco T, Franzer CN, Mattison DR: Diagnosis

of a viable abdominal pregnancy by magnetic resonance imaging. Am J Obstet Gynecol 159:150, 1988

100. Tromans PM, Coulson R, Lobb MO, Abdulla U: Abdominal pregnancy associated with extremely elevated alpha-fetoprotein: case report. Br J Obstet Gynaecol 91:296, 1984

101. Nelson LH, Benson J, Burton BK: Outcomes in patients with unusually high maternal serum alpha-fetoprotein levels. Am J Obstet Gynecol 157:575, 1987

102. Martin JN Jr, Ridgway LE III, Connors JJ et al: Angiographic arterial embolization and computed tomography-directed drainage for the management of hemorrhage and infection with abdominal pregnancy. Obstet Gynecol 76:941, 1990

103. Kivikoski AI, Martin C, Weyman P et al: Angiographic arterial embolization to control hemorrhage in abdominal pregnancy: a case report. Obstet Gynecol 71:456, 1988

CHAPTER THIRTY-FOUR

TUBAL RECONSTRUCTIVE SURGERY

Zev Rosenwaks

Isaac Kligman

Claudio A. Benadiva

Owen K. Davis

Reconstructive surgery of the fallopian tubes has evolved considerably since the first report of a unilateral ampullary cuff salpingostomy by Schroeder[1] in 1884. The emergence of microsurgical techniques for tubal reconstruction—state-of-the-art in the 1970s—was soon eclipsed by technological advances such as operative laparoscopy and laser surgery. These advances were in short order complemented by the advent of in vitro fertilization (IVF). This revolutionary method brought therapeutic options to patients previously deemed sterile because of severe tubal disease, and has rendered many tubal surgery procedures virtually obsolete. However, despite major refinement and advances in IVF, many of the original surgical procedures can still be applied when appropriate selection criteria are met. The gynecologic surgeon is, therefore, obligated to carefully screen and counsel patients with tubal factor infertility about all available treatment options.

ETIOLOGIC ASPECTS OF TUBAL FACTOR INFERTILITY

Fallopian tube physiology plays a critical role in the reproduction process. Conception requires tubal orchestration of oocyte pickup, egg and sperm transport, fertilization, and finally, transport of the early embryo to the endometrial cavity. These steps must be temporarily synchronized so that the early embryo arrives when the endometrium is most receptive. The concert of these functions requires normal tubal and ovarian anatomy. The goal of reconstructive surgery is to restore the anatomic architecture of the pelvis in the hope of re-establishing normal physiologic function.

Infections

Tubal abnormalities account for 40 percent of all female infertility. Although multiple etiologies have been implicated in tubal disease, most are a consequence of infection.

Neisseria gonorrhea has long been recognized as a causative agent of pelvic inflammatory disease (PID).[2] Salpingitis may result in tubal occlusion at various sites (cornua to fimbria), tuboinflammatory masses, or hydrosalpinx. Although infection with *N. gonorrhea* remains a major causative factor, infection with *Chlamydia trachomatis* is also important. Mardh et al,[3] in studies using laparoscopic-directed cultures and tubal biopsies, were the first to suggest that infections with *C. trachomatis* were responsible for one-third of PID cases. Westrom[4,5] was the first to demonstrate a relationship between PID and obstructive infertility. He reported a 13 percent incidence of tubal obstruction after an initial episode of acute salpingitis, a 39 percent incidence after two episodes, and a 75 percent incidence after three episodes.

Salpingitis Isthmica Nodosa

Salpingitis isthmica nodosa (SIN) is a well-described pathologic entity of unknown etiology that appears to be associated with tubal obstruction and ectopic pregnancy. It is a lesion of the proximal fallopian tube characterized by the presence of isthmic diverticula, outpouchings of tubal epithelium with secondary hypertrophy of the surrounding muscularis. It is diagnosed by the typical appearance on hysterosalpingogram (HSG) of 2-mm contrast medium accumulations in close approximation to the isthmic portions of the oviducts bilaterally.[6] The cause of SIN has been debated; some believe it to be a neoplastic phenomenon,[7] while others suggest it is infectious.[8] Its association with tubal factor infertility and ectopic pregnancy has been substantiated by several studies. Fortier[9] found a 24 percent incidence of microscopic evidence of SIN in 42 patients undergoing tubal surgery to correct proximal tubal obstruction and Honor[10] found the disease in three of six tubal specimens obtained from patients undergoing tubal surgery for infertility.

Previous Abdominal Surgery

Peritoneal surface exposure and injury during laparotomy and manipulation of the tubes and adjacent structures are known factors in the genesis of adhesions. Ovarian cystectomy or ovarian wedge resection are examples of surgical interventions that might cause adhesions and consequently alter the anatomic relationship between the tubes and the ovaries. Similarly, appendicitis associated with perforation or abscess formation (or both) can involve the reproductive organs. Similarly, inflammatory bowel disease or bowel surgery may produce periadnexal adhesions.

Endometriosis

Endometriosis is a major cause of tuboperitoneal disease. The severity of the disease can range from pinpoint powder burn lesions to extensive adhesions that completely distort the pelvic anatomy. Although not included in the conventional classifications, endometriosis should be considered as a cause of tubal obstruction and infertility. Peritubal adhesions with impaired tubal motility can be present in as many as 30 percent of patients with endometriosis and infertility, even in the presence of demonstrable tubal patency.[11]

Ectopic Pregnancy

Tubal surgery for ectopic pregnancy, either partial salpingectomy or salpingostomy, can distort pelvic anatomic integrity or result in pelvic adhesion formation. Indeed, ectopic pregnancies can result from previous tubal surgery. Women with a history of previous ectopic pregnancy resulting in the removal of a portion of the fallopian tube, or with adhesions as a consequence of the disease, are candidates for surgical repair. Ectopic pregnancy as a consequence of prior tubal surgery is a well-recognized entity. The risk of ectopic pregnancy after reconstructive surgery varies greatly and depends on the previous condition of the tube, the nature of the surgical procedure performed, and the specific techniques employed.[12] By contrast, an ectopic pregnancy may signal the presence of a damaged tube. Here, reconstructive surgery should be entertained only after careful analysis of the likelihood for recurrence. Oelsner[13] reported a recurrent ectopic pregnancy rate of 15.4 percent in 1,087 patients who underwent previous salpingectomies and DeCherney et al[14] reported a 20 percent ectopic pregnancy rate in 15 such patients with one remaining patent tube.

Previous Tubal Ligation

Reanastomosis of previously ligated tubes remains an important indication for reconstructive surgery; indeed, approximately 1 percent of all patients who undergo sterilization by tubal ligation undergo tubal reanastomosis.[15] Success of tubal reanastomosis depends on the original method of sterilization as well as the degree of tubal destruction. Methods employing monopolar or bipolar tubal coagulation yield the greatest anatomic destruction and distortion, while clips, silastic rings, or the Pomeroy procedure produce only local obstruction with little distortion.

Treatment Options According to Etiology

Many surgical procedures have been described for the treatment of tubal pathology; the specific surgical technique is determined by the anatomic location of the damage. Thus, salpingolysis refers to the lysis of peritubal adhesions. Correction of proximal tubal obstruction can be accomplished by hysteroscopic cannulation, uterotubal implantation (mentioned for historic reasons), and cornual-tubal anastomosis. Midsegment obstruction requires end-to-end anastomosis, while distal obstruction mandates salpingostomy or fimbrioplasty. In general, the term *salpingoplasty* describes any surgical procedure involving the distal portion of the oviduct.

Outcome Reporting

A major pitfall in reporting tubal reconstructive surgery results has been the lack of a uniform classification of pelvic pathology and of the surgical procedures involved. In an effort to achieve consistent reporting, a number of classification systems have been devised. Similarly, classification systems for adnexal adhesions and tubal occlusive diseases have been proposed.[16] As no studies to date have used these classification systems, their usefulness remains to be established.

PREOPERATIVE EVALUATION

Three methods are currently available for studying the anatomy and function of the fallopian tubes,[17] these include HSG, laparoscopy, and salpingoscopy (falloposcopy). The most complete evaluation includes laparoscopy with either HSG or salpingoscopy.

Hysterosalpingography

The first step in evaluating the structure and function of the fallopian tube is the HSG (Fig. 34-1); it is performed as an outpatient procedure and has very low associated morbidity. In fact, Acton[18] reported only 5 cases of pelvic inflammatory disease requiring hospitalization in 3,631 patients undergoing HSG. The HSG should be scheduled in the follicular phase of the cycle, after the menstrual flow has ceased but before ovulation. Patients with known risk factors for PID should receive antibiotic prophylaxis with doxycycline (100 mg twice daily beginning 12 hours before the procedure) for 3 days. Antibiotic coverage for anaerobic bacteria is indicated for patients with suspected or diagnosed distal tubal obstruction. Some clinicians administer antibiotic prophylaxis for all HSGs.

In order to obtain maximal visualization, cervical reflux of contrast media must be avoided. An adequate cervical seal can be accomplished by using a Jarco cannula with a disposable acorn tip (Fig. 34-2). In the presence of cervical stenosis Rosenwaks et al[19] have devised a method utilizing a Tomcat catheter pulled through the acorn to facilitate insertion through the stenotic cervical canal (Fig. 34-3). The HSG is then performed under fluoroscopic visualization. The total volume of contrast medium should not generally exceed 10 ml; small volumes injected slowly under image intensification will provide the most information while causing the least discomfort. Discomfort is the most common problem associated with HSG.[20] The use of a nonsteroidal anti-inflammatory agent administered to the patient 1 hour before the procedure can minimize discomfort. Two basic types of contrast media are currently available: oil based and water soluble. The authors prefer the latter, as it provides greater detail of tubal mucosal anatomy and visualization of the fimbrial spill. The authors consider two to four films necessary for a complete assessment. An early film visualizes the uterine cavity, followed by a tubal film that observes tubal fill. In this film, it is very important to evaluate the distal rugal folds and the diameter of the distal portion of the tube. A third film is obtained to ascertain tubal patency under fluoroscopic guidance. The last film can document free dispersion of media through the pelvis, as evidenced by outlining of the pelvic viscera; occasionally loculations and adhesions surrounding the fallopian tubes can be visualized. Although the dynamics of tubal filling, spill, and mobility are best seen during the fluoroscopic examination, the details of uterine and tubal anatomy are best seen in the spot films.

Radionuclide Scintigraphy

Another less frequently employed procedure to test uterine normality and tubal patency is radionuclide HSG (RN-HSG). The procedure is performed by depositing human albumin microspheres labeled with technetium-99m over the exocervix and external cervical os and evaluating subsequent transport to the peritoneal cavity via the uterus and oviducts by gamma ray imaging. The transport of microspheres depends not only on the anatomic integrity of the uterus and oviducts but also on their function. The dose of radioactivity delivered to the ovaries with this method may be comparable to or higher than traditional HSG.[21] The major disadvantage of RN-HSG is its inability to provide anatomic information on the uterus and tubes.

Laparoscopy

Laparoscopy plays a critical role in assessing the degree of tubal disease and providing accurate prognosis for future fertility. It is particularly useful when an abnormal hysterogram or a history of PID is present. Moreover, tubal reconstructive procedures can be performed via the laparoscopic approach.

Salpingoscopy

Salpingoscopy (falloposcopy) has been recently introduced as a method for evaluating the tubal mucosa. Venezia et al[22] studied 18 patients using a linear everting falloposcope introduced through the cervix under direct vision, and found a 40 percent difference when comparing this method with HSG. They propose that salpingoscopy provides more complete information about tubal status than an HSG. De-Bruyne et al[23] suggest that endosalpingeal adhesions, agglu-

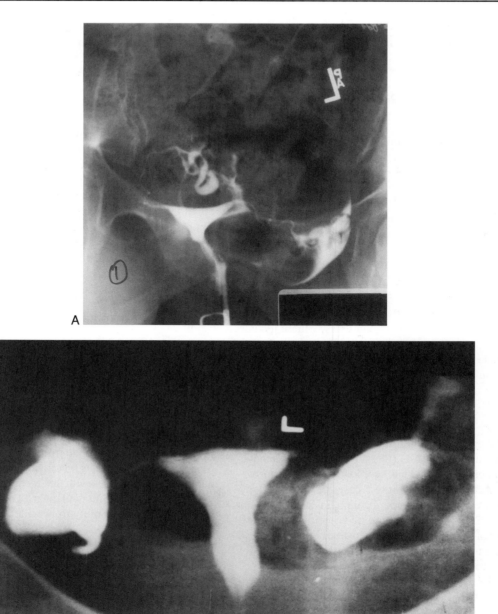

Fig. 34-1. (A) Normal hysterosalpingogram. The uterine cavity is well visualized. There is a complete tubal fill, the rugal folds are clearly seen, and both tubes are patent, as demonstrated by the spill of the contrast media into the peritoneal cavity. **(B)** Abnormal hysterosalpingogram. Bilateral hydrosalpinges are noted.

tination, and flattened mucosa correlate with poor pregnancy outcome. In spite of these preliminary studies, this method is not widely used in the preoperative evaluation.

The ultimate proof of success of tubal reconstructive surgery is an intrauterine pregnancy; however, postoperative HSG and laparoscopy (termed *second-look laparoscopy*) have been used to evaluate the success of surgery or to explain the absence of conception after the procedure. HSG has traditionally been performed 2 to 4 months after the operative procedure to assess tubal patency and, in the absence of pregnancy, a second-look laparoscopy can be per-

formed 12 to 18 months after surgery to evaluate the results of the original surgical procedure.[24] With the advent of assisted reproductive technologies and because of the relatively poor outcome in repeat tubal reconstructive procedures, second-look laparoscopy has been largely abandoned and these patients are now referred for IVF. Young et al[25] followed 23 women within 2 to 28 months after tubal surgery with postoperative HSGs and found that, although tubal patency could indeed be demonstrated in 32 of the 39 tubes analyzed (82 percent), the pregnancy rate was eventually 35 percent (8 of 23 patients), confirming that even in the pres-

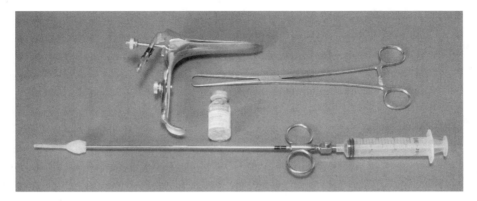

Fig. 34-2. Instruments used to perform a hysterosalpingogram.

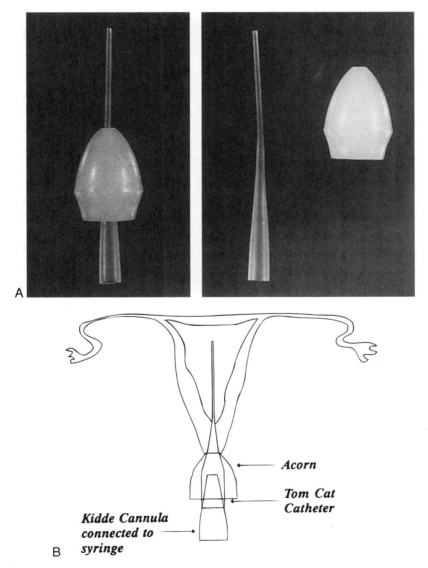

Fig. 34-3. **(A)** Tomcat catheter and acorn cannula. **(B)** Demonstration of the method of insertion of the assembled unit. (From Rosenwaks et al,[19] with permission.)

ence of a high patency rate there are other factors such as intrinsic tubal function or previous damage to the mucosa that can alter the outcome. Letterie[26] followed 25 patients who underwent microsurgical tubal reanastomosis and distal fimbrioplasties with postoperative HSGs and laparoscopies 12 months after the surgical procedure and found that HSG was more reliable in detecting tubal patency than pelvic adhesions (sensitivity of 96 percent and 12 percent, respectively) when confirmed by laparoscopy. Schnack Peen et al[27] found preoperative laparoscopy more valuable than HSG when comparing both methods, claiming that in 115 patients studied, only 5 percent had findings on HSG not detected by laparoscopy and neither of those needed surgical correction. In his study, 70 patients underwent second-look laparoscopy resulting in minor lysis of adhesions. Second-look laparoscopy did not affect the pregnancy rates when comparing these patients with the 45 that did not have the procedure.

Evaluation of Candidates for Tubal Reanastomosis

The preoperative evaluation of patients desiring tubal reanastomosis should include both physical and psychosocial considerations. A careful medical and social history should be taken from both partners, with special attention to prior reproductive history. Meticulous preoperative screening will lead to improved pregnancy rates by discouraging couples with little chance of success and leading them toward other alternatives such as assisted reproduction. It has been shown that after the initial interview, up to 25 percent of the couples elected not to continue with the evaluation for several reasons, including a more realistic understanding of what was actually involved in the preoperative evaluation and surgical procedure itself, as well as a realization of lower chances of success in cases of advanced reproductive age, where the type of sterilization procedure precludes reversal or the chances of success fall short of the couple's expectations.[28] Gomel[29] analyzed the factors that led to request of reversal of tubal sterilization in 100 consecutive patients and found that 63 percent of the patients claimed change in marital status; 17 percent had a child who died of crib death; 10 percent desired more children even without change in their marital status; 4 percent had one or more children; and 6 percent alleged psychological reasons.

The most important factor in determining the success of tubal reanastomosis is the length and quality of the remaining fallopian tube or tubes;[11,30–32] therefore, it is crucial to review the operative record of the initial sterilization procedure and the pathology report on resected segments of fallopian tubes when available. In general, sterilization procedures performed without coagulation, such as the rings or bands or the Pomeroy technique, have a greater chance of success. A Pomeroy ligation destroys 3 to 4 cm of fallopian

tube, in contrast to electrocoagulation, which destroys significantly more tube, especially if the multiple burn technique is used.[28] Seiler[33] laparoscopically evaluated 94 patients desiring tubal reanastomosis and found that 91 percent of the patients who had undergone tubal ligation with noncoagulation techniques had at least 4 cm or more of residual fallopian tube, whereas only 58 percent of patients who had the procedure performed with electrocoagulation had similar residual tubal length. Other aspects of the preoperative assessment should include a semen analysis and, depending on the specific cases, a postcoital test, charting of basal body temperature, endometrial biopsy, serum progesterone evaluation, and an HSG or laparoscopy (or both). The HSG provides information about the condition of the uterine cavity, the length and internal patency of the proximal tubal segments, and the internal architecture of these segments. Karasick[34] evaluated 127 HSGs retrospectively and found that in all cases the proximal tubal segment could be evaluated. Tuboperitoneal fistulas were found in five patients and, in 16 patients, a small area of extravasation of the contrast medium next to the site of ligation was found. Laparoscopy provides a thorough evaluation of the pelvis and the distal tubal segments. The findings at laparoscopy are not infrequently at odds with those described in the original sterilization procedure and pathology report. However, extensive pelvic adhesions and fimbrial occlusion may be associated with any type of sterilization procedure. The length of the proximal and distal tubal segments should also be evaluated in the procedure using a graduated blunt probe inserted through the suprapubic puncture site. Some authors question the use of laparoscopy in the preoperative evaluation of the patient undergoing tubal reanastomosis. DeCherney and Mezer[35] limit preoperative diagnostic laparoscopy to cases in which the patient has a history of pelvic pathology (such as endometriosis or pelvic inflammatory disease), when there is suspicion of inadequate residual tubal length after sterilization with a multiple burn technique, or when the operative note of the previous procedure and the pathology report provide conflicting information. DeCherney et al[36] reported a series of 131 patients undergoing tubal reanastomosis, two of whom would have benefited from preoperative laparoscopy. Opsahl and Klein[37] followed an algorithm by which laparoscopy would be bypassed if the patient had a sterilization procedure with clips, bands, Pomeroy, or single burn technique. If the patient had an unknown procedure, or one in which multiple burn technique was used, then preoperative laparoscopy was performed. Using this approach, they studied 259 patients undergoing sterilization reversals and found that in the group without preoperative laparoscopy (n = 185), Seven (3.8 percent) had inoperable tubes at laparotomy. Opsahl and Klein[37] concluded that given their criteria for proceeding with tubal reanastomosis, laparoscopy may be unnecessary in properly selected candidates. The authors, even after carefully reviewing the previous operative records, routinely perform laparoscopy before the reanastomosis procedure, and not infrequently have found that the degree of tubal damage is greater than that described in the original operative report. The patient is counseled extensively about the possibility of an aborted procedure if the tubes are found to be inoperable at the time of laparoscopy.

ASSESSMENT OF OPERATIVE FEASIBILITY

Assessing operative feasibility is the ultimate step in the evaluation of the patient with tubal factor infertility. A delicate balance exists in deciding whether to proceed with surgery or with IVF. After performing a complete evaluation of a particular patient, the gynecologic surgeon must decide on the most expeditious approach for the patient and whether or not surgery is indicated. To make that decision, the surgeon must be familiar with the success rates obtained through IVF and other assisted reproduction procedures. The most recent survey of the Society for Assisted Reproductive Technology (SART) IVF-ET (embryo transfer) registry describes a delivery rate (per retrieval) in 33,001 stimulation cycles for IVF, gamete intrafallopian (tube) transfer (GIFT), and zygote intrafallopian (tube) transfer (ZIFT) of 15.2 percent, 26.6 percent, and 19.7 percent respectively, for the year 1991.[38] Benadiva et al[39] analyzed the cumulative pregnancy rates for couples with tubal factor infertility undergoing IVF, in relation to factors such as age and other pathology associated with tubal disease. The overall delivery rate per ET in 771 patients with a primary diagnosis of tubal factor infertility who underwent 1,068 oocyte retrievals was 28.9 percent (303 deliveries in 1,048 ETS). Cumulative pregnancy rates for four cycles studied with sole tubal factor were 32 percent, 59 percent, 70 percent, and 77 percent, respectively. Delivery rates of 28 percent, 55 percent, 62 percent and 75 percent, which did not significantly differ, were found in couples who had additional associated infertility factors such as endometriosis, diethylstibestrol (DES) exposure, immunologic or male factors, as well as tubal disease. It is interesting to note, as pointed out by Oehringer et al,[40] that neither the severity of the tubo-ovarian disease nor the extent of pelvic adhesions have an impact on the success of IVF. However, there was a significant decline in success rates per ET with advancing age in this group of patients (less than 30 years of age, 48.4 percent; 30 to 34, 44 percent; 35 to 38, 28 percent; 39 to 40, 20 percent; 41 to 42, percent; and older than 42, 4.3 percent). These findings suggest that a young patient with mild tubal disease may benefit initially from reconstructive surgery, whereas an older patient should proceed directly to IVF. In the presence of severe tuboperitoneal disease—at any age—IVF should be considered as the first line of treatment.

TECHNICAL ASPECTS OF MICROSURGERY

The advent of microsurgery of the fallopian tube was marked by the introduction of magnification techniques by Swolin[45] in 1967, who used either loupes or the operating

---

Contraindications to Attempted Tubal Repair

1. Evidence of genital tuberculosis (in this case a tubal biopsy is of great value in confirming the diagnosis[41,42])
2. The tubes are sclerotic or there are dense adhesions not amenable to surgical repair[41]
3. There is a great danger of bowel injury
4. The total length of the repaired tube is 4 cm or less[11,31]
5. There is a large discrepancy in the diameters of the segments to be anastomosed[43]
6. Bilateral fimbriectomy has been performed, leaving as the only option ampullary or isthmic neosalpingostomy[11,44]
7. There is bipolar occlusion of the tube[11,30,31]
8. Less than optimal circumstances such as the emergency removal of an ovarian cyst[41] or end-to-end anastomosis during the surgical management of ectopic pregnancy[31]
9. Age older than 38 years[41]
10. Absolute azoospermia, if the couple does not wish to undergo insemination by donor
11. Where there are medical contraindications for surgery or pregnancy (or both)

---

microscope for salpingolysis and salpingostomy. As it stands, microsurgery is a principle of tissue handling and operative technique that uses delicate instruments, fine needles, and sutures; continuously irrigates the operative field with an emphasis on providing meticulous hemostasis; and avoids electrodesiccation of tissue. It is generally defined as surgery requiring the use of an operating microscope. Gomel[46] expanded the concept to include surgery performed under any magnification with loupes, hoods, or operating microscopes.

Magnification

Magnification of the operative field ranging from $\times$ 1 to $\times$ 20 may be provided with a microscope, operating hood, or binocular lenses, depending on the optical system.[47] Binocular lenses yield magnifications between $\times$ 2 and $\times$ 6. Proper lighting can be delivered by a fiberoptic cable covered with a sterile plastic sheath. The operating microscope offers the advantage of a wider range of magnification along with a coaxial light system, as well as a manual zoom system for the control of magnification and focusing. Photographic

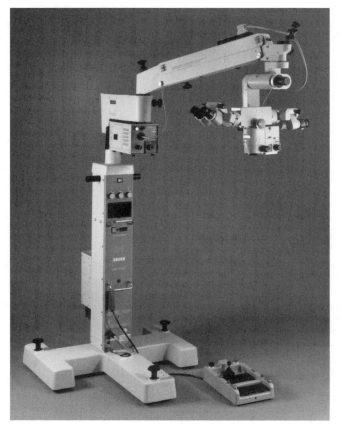

Fig. 34-4. Zeiss operating microscope ZMS-414 System (OPMI CS-I on S4 Stand). (Courtesy of Carl Zeiss, Inc., Thornwood, NY.)

attachments and an assistant binocular observation system are also available. In general, microsurgical procedures are performed under magnifications of × 6; however, greater magnifications may be needed for procedures such as cornual-isthmic anastomosis. The authors prefer the Zeiss OpMI-7 with a magnification of × 6 for tubal reanastomosis procedures (Fig. 34-4). Special sterile plastic sheaths are available for wrapping the microscope when using it in the sterile operating field.

Instrumentation

Several specialized instruments are available for microsurgery. However, the standard set includes jeweler's forceps, spring-handled scissors, and a needle holder (Fig. 34-5). In principle, microsurgical instrumentation facilitates the procedure while minimizing hand movement. Rounded handles in the needleholders aid in the placement of fine needles through the tissue with minimal rotational finger movements. Locks are usually cumbersome and may impede smooth motion when tying knots. Microelectrode monopolar or bipolar cautery is useful for obtaining hemostasis with minimal tissue trauma.

Heparinized saline solution irrigation may be provided with a bulb-tipped syringe or with a 16- to 18-gauge Teflon tip attached to a regular syringe. Glass or Teflon rods are useful for gentle tissue manipulation and to elevate adhesions before excision.

Straight iris scissors and lacrimal duct probes may be helpful when performing tubal reanastomosis procedures.

Suture Material

When choosing the appropriate suture material for tubal reconstructive surgery the main concern is tissue reactivity. There are many nonreactive sutures available today. Stangel et al[48] demonstrated that 9–0 Polyglycolic acid suture resulted in minimal reactivity for anastomosis when used for reanastomosis procedures in the muscular layers or endosalpingeal folds. Delbeke et al[49] assessed the histologic reaction to nylon, polypropylene, polyglactin-910, and polydioxanone in the uterine horn of the rabbit. Eighty days after the insertion of the suture, the polydioxanone was almost entirely absorbed and the reaction to polyglactin-910 was minimal, whereas moderate histiocytic infiltration and fibrosis persisted around nylon and polypropylene sutures. Winston[50] showed the superiority of 10–0 nylon suture as compared with 8–0 catgut in the rabbit oviduct. To date, however, there have been no studies demonstrating a correlation between suture type and pregnancy outcome.

The optimal surgical technique requires the use of a fine

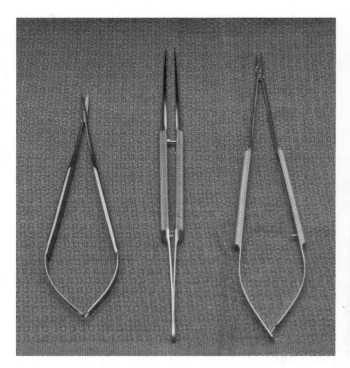

Fig. 34-5. Microsurgical instruments. Note the rounded handles, which help to reduce hand movements when placing the sutures.

suture with minimal reactivity, keeping in mind that the fewer sutures used the less foreign body reaction. When performing tubal reanastomosis, a 7–0 or 8–0 absorbable nonreactive suture such as polyglactin (Vicryl, Ethicon, Inc., Somerville, NJ), with a 4- to 6-mm reverse cutting needle should be used. This type of needle can be passed through the tissue with minimal trauma or suture drag. Care should be taken in manipulating the suture under the microscope, since the small needle can be easily lost in the peritoneal cavity and cause damage and foreign body reaction.

OPERATIVE PROCEDURES

Salpingolysis

Mechanical peritoneal injury or infection triggers the outpouring of polymorphonuclear leukocytes, platelets, and fibrinogen, forming a fibrin clot that eventually becomes organized by fibroblast proliferation, and finally results in collagenous adhesions. Peritubal adhesions are usually a consequence of postabortal or puerperal infection, PID, previous appendicitis (especially with perforation), endometriosis, or previous gynecologic or bowel surgery. The infundibulum is by definition uninvolved, but careful inspection of the fimbria under magnification must be performed to look for fimbrial adhesions; if present, lysis can be accomplished with a lacrimal duct probe.

With the advent of laparoscopy, salpingolysis by laparotomy is not commonly performed, especially since isolated peritubal adhesions are very uncommon. However, when these are found during concurrent procedures (e.g., myomectomy), employing microsurgical principles of careful tissue handling, hemostasis, and irrigation will minimize further adhesion formation.

When opting for the abdominal approach, a Pfannenstiel incision can achieve maximum exposure of the pelvic area. Careful rinsing of gloves will avoid powder (talc)-induced peritoneal reactions. A universal retractor is used for the incision. The patient is placed in the Trendelenburg position and the bowel is retracted using either lint-free laparotomy pads or regular pads contained in small plastic bags. To facilitate access to the adnexa for proper hand support, Gomel[41] recommends packing the vagina in order to elevate the uterus; however, these authors have obtained good exposure of the operative field and elevation of the uterus by packing the cul-de-sac. Tubal patency before and after the procedure can be demonstrated by chromoinsufflation through a previously placed Humi catheter or via a Teflon cannula placed in the fundus through a #16 Jelco needle after clamping the cervix with a cervical clamp (Fig. 34-6).

Careful inspection of the landmarks for tubo-ovarian relationship are necessary before starting adhesiolysis, in order to avoid inadvertent incision of the fimbria or a portion of the tube or vasculature; delicate digital blunt dissection may

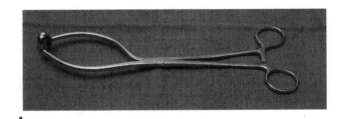

A

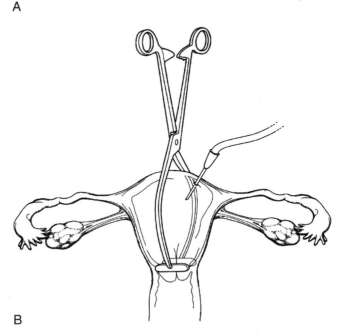

B

Fig. 34-6. (A) Cervical clamp. **(B)** Application of the clamp to the cervix allows infusion of Methilene blue through the uterine fundus, facilitating the demonstration of tubal patency before and after the reconstructive procedure.

detach an adnexa adhered to the pelvic sidewall. Once mobilized, all the adhesions should be carefully excised using scissors or a fine needle insulated microelectrode with cutting or blend current. Care should be taken to excise all adhesions at their origin and insertion. Plastic or insulated metal rods can be used for gentle traction, but the authors prefer using smooth pickups for tissue manipulation and traction (Fig. 34-7). When using scissors for dissection, care should be taken to transilluminate the tissue before cutting in order to avoid large vessels, and to cut one layer at a time, especially when dealing with thick adhesions. Small bleeders should be individually coagulated. When using monopolar or bipolar current for cutting, care should be taken to avoid thermal injury to adjacent structures, particularly when dealing with adnexae that are adherent to the pelvic side wall or bowel.

Even when using careful operative technique, inadvertent peritoneal denudation may result. Small serosal defects should be reperitonealized by approximation with 5–0 or 6–0 polyglactin sutures for larger defects, or size 7–0 or 8–0 for smaller ones.[51] When appropriate, the denuded areas

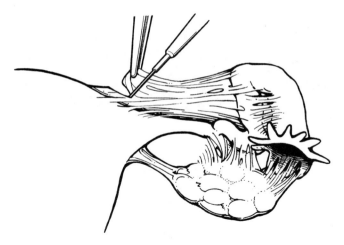

Fig. 34-7. Salpingolysis, open technique. Adhesions are excised by exerting gentle traction with smooth pickups and dissecting with scissor or a fine needle insulated microelectrode with cutting or blend current.

can be covered with oxidized methylcellulose (Interceed, Johnson & Johnson, Raritan, NJ). Best results are obtained when the Interceed is applied over a dry surface and moistened with irrigating solution. Needless to say, meticulous hemostasis is the hallmark of microsurgery.

Laparoscopy

The use of laparoscopy in fertility surgery was first introduced by Gomel[52] in 1975. Based on the procedures performed with the open microsurgical technique, this operation is carried out through the laparoscopic ports. The three-puncture technique is used with an umbilical puncture for the laparoscope and two smaller puncture sites in the lower quadrants. A Humi catheter is placed transcervically before surgery to facilitate mobilization of the uterus and can serve as a test for and assessment of tubal patency.

The key to safe dissection of adhesions is to correctly identify and avoid the ureters, urinary bladder, and intestines, thus ensuring that vital structures are not encroached.[53] Dissection should begin in the posterior cul-de-sac. It is best accomplished by placing the adhesions under traction either by manipulating the uterus with the Humi cannula or by countertraction with a probe or forceps inserted through one of the secondary puncture sites. After cutting the end of an adhesion, it can be rolled on a grasper for better access to the other end. Adhesions are usually multilayered and should be divided one layer at a time to prevent trauma to the organs or peritoneal surfaces to which they are attached. Vascular adhesions are coagulated next to the uterus and sharply divided. Broad adhesions should be totally excised by dividing and removing them[54] (Fig. 34-8). Systematic dissection of the pelvic floor is followed by adhesiolysis of the lateral pelvic sidewall. The ovary and the fallopian tubes are freed

from the sidewall and bowel. When using the carbon dioxide laser, the beam is adjusted to the smallest spot size possible and applied in superpulse mode to vaporize the edge of the adhesion using a sweeping motion. Care should be taken to apply gentle traction on the tissue to avoid tearing. A blunt probe or a pool of fluid in the pelvis should be used as a backstop to avoid burning adjacent structures. Once the procedure is complete, the pelvis is thoroughly lavaged with warm heparinized lactated Ringer's solution; this helps to identify any persisting bleeding points that may need to be cauterized.

On occasion, thick, vascular adhesions involving omentum, apendicae epiploica, or bowel serosa are so extensive that they may not be amenable to laparoscopic correction. In such cases, laparotomy is indicated. When the preliminary laparoscopic evaluation reveals such severe adhesions, the patient should be counseled and advised to consider an alternative method such as IVF.

Results

Success of adhesiolysis is directly related to the severity of the adhesions.[41,55] Irrespective of adjunctive procedures, pregnancy rates are quite satisfactory following salpingolysis either by laparotomy or laparoscopy. Wallach and coworkers[56] reported a pregnancy rate of 45.7 percent following macroscopic adhesiolysis, with an ectopic pregnancy rate of 7 percent. The time interval from surgery to conception ranged from 1 to 46 months postoperatively. Rock[11] reported on 72 patients following salpingolysis, of which 58 (80 percent) became pregnant. There was a total of 72 pregnancies, which resulted in 49 term infants, 11 spontaneous abortions, and 12 ectopic pregnancies (16 percent). Others report success rates ranging from 39 to 69 percent using a macroscopic approach by laparotomy.[57,58] By contrast, studies by Caspi,[59] Donnez and Cassanas-Roux,[60] and Tulandi,[61] using mi-

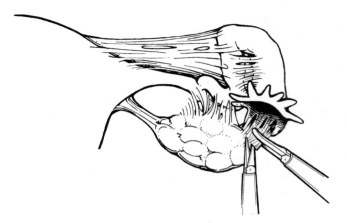

Fig. 34-8. Adhesiolysis by laparoscopy. The procedure follows the same surgical principles as the open technique; adhesions should be excised one layer at a time to prevent bleeding or trauma.

crosurgical techniques report success rates between 38 and 64 percent. Reported rates of ectopic pregnancies between micro- and macrosurgical techniques reveal no major differences; these rates range from to 2 to 6 percent.[41] Gomel[62] reported on a series of 92 women who underwent salpingoovariolysis for moderate to severe adnexal adhesions; 57 (62 percent) achieved a term pregnancy with a 5 percent ectopic pregnancy rate. Fayez[63] reported a 67 percent pregnancy rate with laparoscopic tubolysis, 72 percent with ovariolysis, and 50 percent with salpingoovariolysis. Other reports by Bruhat et al[64] and by Donnez[66] employing laparoscopic technique showed pregnancy rates ranging between 30 and 60 percent.

Salpingoplasty

In general, the term *salpingoplasty* implies a surgical procedure that involves the tubal infundibulum. It includes procedures such as fimbrioplasty, which consists of disagglutination or dilation of the tubal ostium and salpingoneostomy, entailing the creation of a new ostium.

Fimbrioplasty

Fimbrioplasty covers a spectrum of operative procedures that includes disagglutination of the fimbria and incision of any adhesive peritoneal ring that can partially obstruct the distal portion of the fallopian tube. Before establishing patency, the tubo-ovarian anatomic relationship must be restored. Occasionally, a peritoneal adhesive ring can cause relative obstruction of the distal fallopian tube. Lysis of these strands can uncover healthy fimbrial tissue and relieve the obstruction. Fimbrial agglutination can be corrected by introducing a fine closed mosquito forceps through the ostium after distending the tube by chromotubation. The forceps is repeatedly opened and closed until the fimbria has been disagglutinated (Fig. 34-9A). Extensive bleeding, although rare, can be stopped with a microelectrode tip. Occasionally, incising scar tissue may be necessary. To maintain the fimbrial eversion, a few sutures of 8–0 polyglactic acid suture (Vicryl) can be placed to secure the fimbrial edges. Magnification is rarely required for this procedure.[41]

Laparoscopy

Fimbrioplasty may be performed through the laparoscope when the distal portion of the tube is free of adhesions. The tube is distended to identify the lumen and is then stabilized with atraumatic forceps. Occasionally the anterior cul-de-sac may be used to create a platform for dissection. As in laparotomy, the principle of restoring the anatomy and relationships before establishing patency also applies to this procedure. The peritoneal adhesive bands that surround the terminal end of the fallopian tube are divided with laparoscopic

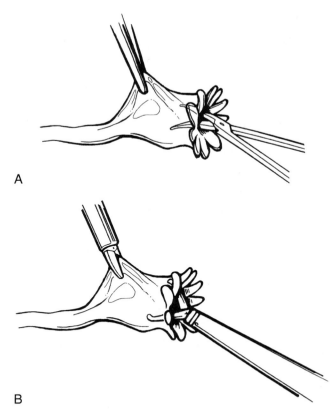

Fig. 34-9. (A) Fimbrioplasty open technique. A fine mosquito forceps is introduced through the ostium and repeatedly opened and closed until the fimbria has been deagglutinated. **(B)** Fimbrioplasty laparoscopic technique. Following the same principle, a 3-mm alligator forceps is gently introduced into the tube. The jaws of the forceps are then opened within the oviduct and the forceps is withdrawn in the opened position.

scissors, fine point unipolar cautery, or laser. To release the agglutinated fimbria, the tube is aligned with the long axis of a 3-mm alligator forceps. The forceps in closed position is gently introduced into the tube. The jaws of the forceps are then opened within the oviduct and the forceps gently withdrawn in the opened position. The procedure is repeated several times, changing the direction of the jaws of the forceps until the partially agglutinated fimbria is opened and tubal patency is demonstrated[52] (Fig. 34-9B). At times, the tube may be obstructed at the apex of the infundibulum, a condition also known as prefimbrial phimosis.[53] It is best corrected by placing an incision over the antimesosalpingeal aspect of the tube, starting at the fimbriated end and extending beyond the constriction site into the distal ampulla; a pointed electrode scissors or laser can be used for this purpose. Eversion of the flaps, if needed, can be accomplished by light electrocoagulation of the serosal aspect of the tube or by gentle application of a defocused carbon dioxide laser beam.

Results

Fimbrioplasty results are difficult to compare because of the diverse pathology and grades of tubal obstruction associated; findings may range from discrete bands to severe pelvic adhesions. Pregnancy rates following these procedures are reported in the range of 30 to 70 percent.[66] Intrauterine pregnancy rates between 20 and 50 percent have been reported for laparoscopic fimbrioplasty, with an ectopic pregnancy rate of 5 percent after both laparotomy and laparoscopy series.[62,63]

Neosalpingostomy (Salpingoneostomy)

By definition, neosalpingostomy denotes the creation of a new tubal ostium, a procedure required when total occlusion of the fimbria is present. Because of poor clinical results, ampullary and isthmic neosalpingostomy are no longer used and are noted only for historical interest. The aim of neosalpingostomy is to re-establish tubal patency at the level of the fimbria while maintaining a normal anatomic condition. For this purpose, it is very important to identify the fimbria ovarica and the relationship of the tube with the ovary. The normal tubo-ovarian relationship must be restored as much as possible and the fimbria ovarica—always present—is a helpful landmark in establishing the normal axis of the oviduct. On entering the abdomen, adhesions are lysed as previously described and the ovaries are mobilized. The cul-de-sac is packed to elevate the uterus and the adnexae are placed on an appropriate platform before the tubo-ovarian relationships are established.

Terminal neosalpingostomy may be performed with or without magnification. In most cases, preliminary salpingolysis is required as described above. The conventional technique was originally described by Kistner and Pattone.[67] The tube is distended by chromotubation and the "dimple" at the distal end is identified. Two incisions are made at a 90-degree angle with the intersection at the dimple. Redundant portions of the distal sac are trimmed. Hemostasis is secured and the flaps thus formed are sutured to the serosa with fine interrupted sutures.

Several alternative microsurgical approaches have been described by Swolin,[68] Gomel[41] and Winston.[69] The tube is distended in the same fashion, noting the finer detail of the central dimple. From the dimple, white avascular lines can be seen, radiating like spokes from the hub of a wheel. Using the monopolar electrode, the hub is punctured, allowing fluid to escape. A glass rod or fine forceps can be introduced into the tube to explore the ampullary portion. Occasionally, normal-appearing fimbriae may protrude through the opening. More often, the fimbriae are severely damaged and confined to the tubal lumen. Using forceps or a glass rod as a backstop, radial incisions are made along the avascular areas. The epithelium is gently everted and, where it remains tethered, additional small incisions are made. Another approach

is to perform an initial incision at the 6-o'clock position in the direction of the fimbria ovarica, everting the edges with 7–0 or 8–0 Vicryl sutures. The mucosa is then everted using a minimal number of sutures. The microscope assists in avoiding damaging blood vessels that may result in profuse bleeding. If bleeding occurs, the capillaries may be identified under continuous irrigation and coagulated using a microtip bipolar coagulator at a low setting.

Laparoscopy

The principles of laparoscopic tubal surgery are similar to those observed at laparotomy.[51,70] Magnification during laparoscopic procedures is provided by the video monitor. Two to three secondary suprapubic puncture sites might be necessary to properly manipulate the tubes. The tube is initially distended with dye via a Humi catheter inserted through the cervix; this procedure helps in the identification of the tubo-ovarian relationships and the scarred ostium. After any necessary salpingolysis, the tube is stabilized. The dimple at the end of the hydrosalpinx is identified and is entered either electrosurgically with needle point cautery with laser, or with laparoscopic scissors. The edge of this initial incision is held with 3-mm grasping forceps and the incision is extended toward the ovary using the same instruments in order to form a new fimbria ovarica. The incision is now large enough to permit working from within the tube. To complete the neostomy, further incisions are made along the circumference of the tube along the avascular lines located between the folds. Eversion of the edges can be achieved by light electrocoagulation of the serosa of the flaps using an electrode with a ball-shaped tip.[54] Alternatively, the edges can be everted by application of a defocused carbon dioxide laser beam of low power density to the serosa proximal to the fimbria. Clips or endoscopic polydioxanone sutures of 4–0 may also be used to keep the flaps in place[71] (Fig. 34-10).

Results

It is difficult to compare and contrast the results of neosalpingostomy procedures mainly due to inadequate detailing of the surgical techniques employed as well as the lack of consistent documentation of the degree and nature of tubal disease and pelvic adhesions encountered at the time of surgery. The different classification systems further confuse the issue. A clear example is the classification of procedures proposed by the 10th World Congress of Fertility and Sterility[45]; it was suggested that the term *salpingoneostomy* be used only for those operations performed on the distal portion of the fallopian tubes when no fimbria could be identified. However, the condition of the fimbria may be seen to vary once patency is established and hence should be taken into consideration in patients requiring creation of a new tubal ostium.

Beside the condition of the fimbria, many other prognosti-

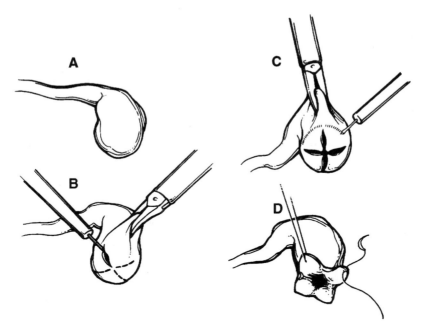

Fig. 34-10. (A) Neosalpingostomy. The tube is distended with dye via a Humi catheter inserted through the cervix. **(B)** After identifying the dimple at the end of the hydrosalpinx, incisions are made along avascular lines. **(C)** Eversion of the edges can be achieved by electrocoagulation with electrode or application of defocused carbon dioxide laser beam. **(D)** Alternatively, the flaps are kept in place by using endoscopic polydioxanone sutures of 4–0.

cators of the success of neosalpingostomy have been studied. Shirodkar[72] found that the presence of a hydrosalpinx greater than 2.5 cm in diameter decreased the postoperative success rate from 50 to 10 percent. Other pertinent factors were the condition of the tubal wall, ciliary epithelium (established by biopsy), and fimbria. The presence of rugae in the preoperative hysterogram was found by Young and co-authors[73] to be of positive prognostic value. A pregnancy rate of 61 percent was observed when rugae were present, and decreased to 7 percent where rugae were not demonstrated. A practical classification system for tubal disease was proposed by Rock et al,[74] using parameters known to influence the pregnancy rate, such as the size of the hydrosalpinx, the condition of the fimbria, the presence or absence of rugae documented by HSG, and the extent of pelvic adhesions. This system classifies tubal disease with distal fimbrial occlusion as mild, moderate, or severe (Table 34-1). Schlaff et al[75] confirmed the usefulness of this classification in a study that included 95 patients who underwent microsurgical neosalpingostomy. They found an overall pregnancy rate of 80 percent for those patients with mild disease, 31 percent for patients with moderate disease, and 16 percent for those with severe disease. Furthermore, they did not find any statistical significance when comparing this to a previously studied group in which no microsurgical techniques were used. In the same study, 75 percent of the patients who conceived did so in the first year after the procedure and 25 percent in the second year. Boer-Meisel et al[76] analyzed the

Table 34-1. Classification of Tubal Disease With Distal Fimbrial Obstruction

Extent of Disease	Observations
Mild	Absent or small hydrosalpinx ≤15 mm diameter
	Inverted fimbriae easily recognized when patency is achieved
	No significant peritubal or periovarian adhesions
	Rugal pattern on preoperative hysterogram
Moderate	Hydrosalpinx 15–30 mm diameter
	Fragments of fimbriae not readily identified
	Periovarian or peritubular adhesions without fixation, few cul-de-sac adhesions
	Absence of a rugal pattern on preoperative hysterogram
Severe	Large hydrosalpinx ≥30 mm diameter
	No fimbriae
	Dense pelvic or adnexal adhesions with fixation of the ovary and tube to broad ligament, pelvic sidewall, omentum, or bowel
	Obliteration of the cul-de-sac
	Frozen pelvis (adhesion formation so dense that limits of organs are difficult to define)

(Modified from Rock et al,[74] with permission.)

importance of additional factors for the prediction of success of the technique. In addition to the diameter of the hydrosalpinx, the extent of the adhesions, and macroscopic aspect of the fimbria, they incorporated the thickness of the tubal wall into the classification. The combination of these factors resulted in the creation of three prognostic groups in terms of pregnancy outcome: good (77 percent intrauterine pregnancy rate and 4 percent ectopic), intermediate (21 percent pregnancy rate), and poor (3 percent intrauterine pregnancy rate and 16 percent ectopic). The condition of the cilia on microscopic examination has not been correlated with pregnancy rates. However, Vasquez et al,[77] using scanning electron microscopy, demonstrated a significant reduction of ciliated cells from hydrosalpinges. There are few reports comparing the laparoscopy versus laparotomy approach. Nevertheless, it appears that both approaches offer similar results. Laparoscopic series have described pregnancy rates between 0 and 44 percent,[78,79] and laparotomy-based series (either microsurgical or conventional) indicated pregnancy rates ranging between 5 and 41.6 percent.[80,81] A study by Russell et al[81] (utilizing microsurgical approach) described a 41.6 percent pregnancy rate with an ectopic pregnancy rate of 17 percent. This was the highest pregnancy rate reported with this technique when compared with other series cited in their study. Bruhat and Mage[64] compared the outcome of neosalpingostomy by laser to a group of historical controls treated with microcautery and found no significant difference in pregnancy rates. Tulandi et al[82] also compared different approaches in the treatment of 91 patients with distal tubal occlusion. Salpingostomy with the carbon dioxide laser was compared with that employing a microneedle electrode. They found no significant difference in the pregnancy rates (21.7 percent versus 22.7 percent) at 1-year follow-up. The surgery-to-conception interval was shorter in the group treated with the carbon dioxide laser, suggesting that the healing interval might be reduced with this technique.

CONGENITAL TUBAL ANOMALIES

On occasion, infertile patients may be found to have congenital anomalies of otherwise normal-appearing oviducts. Some authors have studied the alteration of the tubo-ovarian relationships related to the presence of congenital accessory ostia, elongated fimbria ovarica, and distal distortion caused by paratubal cysts.[83] Defects in the canalization of the mullerian system can cause duplication of the ostia in the oviducts. Elongation of the fimbria ovarica has been attributed to polycystic ovaries (possibly due to stretching).

To repair accessory tubal ostia, sutures of 8–0 nylon are placed in the proximal and distal edges and held with forceps. Elevation of the angle sutures permits the invagination of the accessory endosalpingeal tissue into the lumen of the ampulla and the borders are then brought together with 8–0 interrupted nylon or Vicryl sutures to close the gap. Serosal sutures may then be placed if desired. To repair an elongated fimbria ovarica, care should be taken in examining the fimbria to ensure that there are no interfimbrial bridges or adhesions. The fimbria ovarica is then attached to a chosen point on the outer surface of the ovary. Using a 7–0 Vicryl suture, the fimbria ovarica is plicated and anchored to the ovary; this results in its relocation closer to the ovarian surface. Cysts resulting in tethering of the tube may be excised. Bipolar cautery is used to coagulate any vessels transversing the mesosalpinx over the intended lines of incision. An incision is then made over the anterior portion of the mesosalpinx and once the correct plane is identified, the cyst is dissected out either bluntly or with the assistance of scissors. Vascular pedicles are then clamped and tied or coagulated. The mesosalpinx may be left open or sutured with a fine absorbable suture.

TUBAL ANASTOMOSIS

When an isolated segment of the tube is occluded, it is possible to excise the occluded portion and anastomose the patent proximal and distal segments. The classification of these procedures is based on the location of the proximal and distal segments; an intramural-isthmic anastomosis describes the joining of the proximal intramural with the isthmic distal portion of the tube.

The most common cause of midtubal occlusion is surgical sterilization. Conservative surgery for ectopic pregnancy (in which a small segment of the tube that has been destroyed by the invading trophoblast is resected followed by end-to-end anastomosis) is seldom performed and has been largely replaced by linear salpingostomy. Endometriosis and tuberculosis can also result in midtubal occlusion.[55,84] In a study by Madelenat et al,[85] the causes of proximal obstruction in 131 patients were salpingitis isthmica nodosa (34 percent), a sclerosing process (32 percent), endometriosis (19 percent), unruptured ectopic pregnancy (4.5 percent), latent tuberculosis (3.5 percent) and idiopathic factors (6 percent).

Surgical Technique

Tubal reanastomosis should preferably be performed in the follicular phase of the cycle to take advantage of the proliferation that occurs in the tubal mucosa.[66] Magnification of the operative field is obtained by means of a loupe or a microscope. Some surgeons prefer using magnifying loupes during the process of undermining the mesosalpinx, lysing adhesions, dissecting the proximal and distal segments of the tube, and then switching to the operating microscope at the time of the actual reanastomosis procedure. The authors perform this surgery using the operating microscope under a magnification of ×3 throughout the procedure.

Isthmic-Isthmic Anastomosis

The tube is isolated; any periadnexal adhesions should be lysed. A small incision is performed in the underlying mesosalpinx to allow mobilization of the proximal and distal ends. The proximal end of the fallopian tube is identified, and the tip is resected with iris scissors cutting perpendicularly to the tube. Patency is confirmed by observing the spillage of indigo carmine through the proximal end. If the tip is still occluded, successive proximal cuts can be made until patency is observed. With the help of a lacrimal duct probe, the distal end is catheterized until its occluded tip is identified. Using the same technique the tip is resected. At this point, both resected ends are of similar diameter. A 2–0 nylon suture stent is passed through the proximal segment into the uterine cavity and the other end through the distal segment toward the fimbria. The mesosalpinx is carefully approximated to avoid tension of the anastomotic site. The lumina of the anastomotic ends are approximated with a 7–0 or 8–0 Polygalactin (Vicryl) suture on a three-eighths in circle taper needle in four quadrants, taking care to place the first suture at the 6-o'clock position followed by 3 o'clock, 9 o'clock and leaving the 12-o'clock position for last. The needle is only passed through the muscularis of the proximal segment and then through the muscularis of the distal segment. After these sutures are securely tied, the serosa is sutured using three sutures of 6–0 Vicryl. The nylon stent is then removed from the fimbriated end (Fig. 34-11A).

Isthmic Ampullary Anastomosis

This type of anastomosis is encountered when the original sterilization procedure involves the distal tube. The proximal segment is approached as described earlier. To overcome the discrepancy in the diameters of the two segments the following technique is employed: a no. 16 Teflon obturator from an intravenous catheter is inserted through the fimbriated end to the occluded site of the oviduct. The needle is inserted into the obturator and the occluded end is perforated by the needle and the Teflon sheath and once through, the needle is removed. A 2–0 nylon suture is introduced through the Teflon obturator and the obturator is removed. The mesosalpinx is then approximated to reduce tension at the anastomotic site. In order to place the tip of the needle into the ampullary lumen, it is placed on the tip of the lumen of the Teflon obturator. The tip of the obturator is then withdrawn

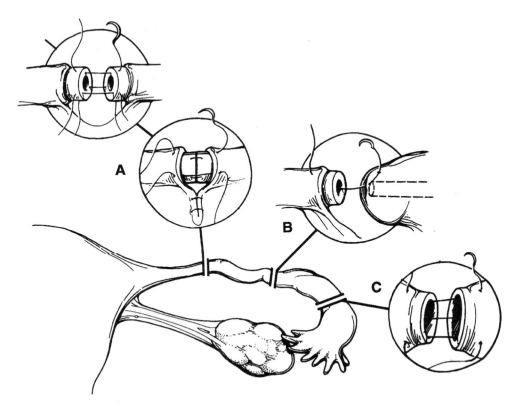

Fig. 34-11. (**A**) Isthmic isthmic anastomosis–anastomotic ends are sutured with four sutures of 7–0 or 8–0 Vicryl placed through the muscularis of both segments. Serosa is then sutured using three sutures of 6–0 Vicryl. (**B**) Isthmic ampullary anastomosis. A teflon obturator with a needle is employed to overcome the discrepancy in diameters of the two segments. (**C**) Ampullary ampullary anastomosis. Six to eight sutures of 7–0 or 8–0 Vicryl are placed involving the three layers of the segments to be anastomosed.

into the ampullary portion of the tube. Four sutures of 7–0 or 8–0 polyglactic acid (Vicryl) are placed between the serosa, muscularis, and endosalpinx of the proximal isthmic end to the endosalpinx, muscularis, and serosa of the distal (ampullary) portion of the tube in four quadrants, placing the 6-o'clock suture first and the 12-o'clock suture last (Fig. 34-11B). The sutures are then securely fastened. Occasionally, a two-layer closure is possible, in which case three or four 6–0 interrupted polyglactic acid sutures can be placed in the serosa.

Other methods of overcoming the diameter discrepancy between the two ends have been suggested. Winston[87] proposed circumcising the tip of the ampulla over a bulbous end of a probe inserted through the fimbria in a similar way as the Teflon obturator, stripping back the serosa and then incising the mucosa in order to facilitate a two-layer closure. Using this technique, the two-layer closure is possible. However, care should be taken, as the wall of the oviduct at this site is thin and extensive bleeding can occur, as well as inadvertent widening of this end of the oviduct. A single-layer closure is necessary in this area due to the width of the lumen.

Ampullary-Ampullary Anastomosis

Since the muscularis in this area is delicate and the lumina are quite large, a suture through all layers easily approximates the tubal lumina. Six to eight 7–0 or 8–0 polyglactic acid sutures are placed around the circumference of the ampulla—from serosa, muscularis, and endosalpinx of the proximal segment to endosalpinx, muscularis, and serosa of the distal portion of the tube (Fig. 34-11C).

Cornual-Isthmic Anastomosis

If a small proximal portion of the oviduct is occluded, cornual isthmic anastomosis can be undertaken. A serosal flap is developed over the proximal segment; a small knife is used to core out the obstructed segment as disks. Patency is confirmed by the spillage of dye through the proximal segment. The isthmic portion is then approximated to the intramural portion of the fallopian tube. This is the only procedure that requires high magnification and in which the microscope is most useful. Magnifications of $\times 10$ to $\times 20$ are recommended. Hemostasis is achieved by using high-frequency fine needle cautery. A two-layer closure, as described above, with 7–0 or 8–0 polyglactic suture is used (Fig. 34-12). This procedure has replaced uterotubal reimplantation, which has become obsolete.

Cornual-Ampullary Anastomosis

The cornual-ampullary anastomosis procedure is infrequently performed. Special attention has to be paid to the large disparity in the lumen diameter. The proximal segment is cored out as described earlier and the ampullary region is

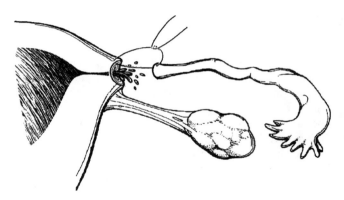

Fig. 34-12. Cornual isthmic anastomosis. After patency is confirmed by spillage of the dye through the segment, a two-layer closure with 7–0 or 8–0 Vicryl suture is employed.

prepared using either the Teflon catheter or circumcision technique described earlier for isthmic ampullary anastomosis. A two-layer closure may not be possible and each case must be approached individually, based on the ampullary or cornual segment of the oviduct. A 2–0 nylon splint is placed through the proximal segment as described above in order to facilitate suture placement in the oviduct.

Laparoscopic Tubal Anastomosis

This procedure is performed through an intraumbilical incision for a 10-mm laparoscope and right and left suprapubic secondary incisions for 5-mm trocar ports. A Humi catheter is inserted through the cervix to mobilize the uterus and instill dye. The pelvis and tubal segments are evaluated and periadnexal adhesions are lysed. The proximal end of the tube is mobilized and the occluded end placed under tension with a biopsy forceps. This end is opened using scissors that cut at right angles with the longitudinal axis of the tube until free flow of dye is obtained. Hemostasis is obtained with careful cauterization of the bleeding vessels. A stent is made using a 6-cm segment of a 12 French urethral dilator divided from its tapered tip and passed through the fimbria to the occluded end of the distal segment. This end is then opened using laparoscopic scissors. A 4–0 polydioxanone suture or a 4–0 polypropylene suture is placed at the 6 o'clock position of the tubal muscularis and endosalpinx; a second suture is placed at the 12-o'clock position. The knots are tied using the extracorporeal technique.

Using this approach in 22 patients, Reich[88] obtained a pregnancy rate of 35 percent, with an ectopic pregnancy rate of 18 percent. Laparotomy reversals yield a birth rate of between 48 and 78 percent and a tubal pregnancy rate of 1.7 to 6.5 percent.[16] With current technology and experience, the results of laparoscopic tubal anastomosis fall short of those achieved via laparotomy. In an attempt to decrease hospital stay, Silva et al[89] studied prospectively 17 patients treated with a combined approach of laparoscopy (to assess feasibility of the anastomosis and to lyse adhesions) and minilaparotomy. A 6-cm transverse suprapubic incision was made and the uterus and adnexa were exteriorized assisted with a Somers clamp; the procedure was performed using the described microsurgical technique. Patients were discharged 6 hours after the procedure and followed up in the office 3 days later. With this approach, 12 of the 17 patients (71 percent) conceived and one ectopic pregnancy occurred.

Results

The overall success rate following tubal reanastomosis is in the range of 60 to 80 percent live births (with a 3 to 4 percent ectopic pregnancy rate) (Table 34-2). Prognosis can be predicted by parameters indicating the tubal length after reanastomosis, site of reanastomosis, type of sterilization procedure performed, and interval since the sterilization procedure. Fallopian tube length has been found to be the most important factor in predicting the outcome. Gomel[28] noted that fallopian tubes of less than 3 cm in total length were associated with a long interval between reconstructive surgery and pregnancy; with oviducts over 6 cm in length, pregnancy often occurred within three to four cycles. Rock[11] determined a significant decrease in pregnancy rates following the procedure if the final fallopian tube length was less than 4 cm. Paterson[90] found a significant difference both in pregnancy rates and in the interval between surgery and conception (by life table analysis), when comparing tubal lengths of less than 4 cm (37.5 percent) to those 4 cm or longer (63 percent). In this same study, the site of anastomosis was also of importance in assessing chances for success. Isthmic-isthmic anastomosis was associated with the highest pregnancy rate, whereas intramural-ampullary anastomosis yielded reduced pregnancy success rates. According to Rock[11] the site of anastomosis was not a factor in subsequent

pregnancy success when studying reanastomosis after Falope ring sterilization. In the group sterilized with cautery, tubal length and site of anastomosis influenced the pregnancy rate. All women with 4 cm or less of oviductal length in this group required an ampullary-isthmic anastomosis, which might in part explain the reduced rate observed.

The specific sterilization procedure has a direct influence on the success rate after reversal. When the sterilization procedure is performed with electrocautery, a relatively large segment of tube is destroyed (more so if the triple burn technique is employed). Reanastomosis after this type of procedure carries the lowest pregnancy rate and the highest rate of ectopic pregnancy when compared to Falope ring and clip procedures. Furthermore, tubal reanastomosis following partial salpingectomy has a higher pregnancy rate than that following monopolar cautery. In a series reported by Rock et al[91] reflecting pregnancy success in 246 patients after reanastomosis following different sterilization procedures, 86 percent of the patients with previous Falope ring sterilization became pregnant, whereas only 54 percent of the patients previously sterilized with monopolar cautery achieved pregnancy. The ectopic pregnancy rate was also the highest in the later group (8.3 percent versus 2.2 percent). The extent to which normal physiologic function returns to the fallopian tubes after cauterization is unknown; the increased incidence of ectopic pregnancy in this group suggests some degree of irreversible damage to the transport mechanism of the tube. Donnez[92] showed that the deciliation of the oviduct extends 2 cm from the site of cautery. For this reason, one has to ensure at the time of anastomosis that a sufficient margin of the obliterated tube is excised so that once patency is established, healthy, well-vascularized tissue is present at the site of anastomosis.

The time interval between sterilization and reversal appears to play a role in the success rates achieved with the procedure. Associated tubal pathology increases with an increased interval from previous sterilization. Loss of cilia becomes significant and the presence of tubal polyps increases 4 years after sterilization. The pathogenesis of these tubal polyps is not clear but chronic inflammation has been implicated. The pregnancy rate is lower in patients who have been sterilized for 4 years or more. Vasquez et al[93] confirmed that the interval from sterilization to reversal has a significant impact on results—the longer the interval the lower the pregnancy rate. Putman,[94] however, found no association of sterilization interval and pregnancy rates. Seiler[95] studied 73 patients undergoing sterilization reversal. He obtained a 64 percent overall pregnancy rate with an ectopic rate of 4.4 percent. In his study, the final tubal length, the time interval between sterilization and reversal, and the site of anastomosis did not play a significant role in the outcome. Sterilization procedures performed with electrocoagulation, however, were only reversible 58 percent of the time due to the extent of tubal damage compared with 91 percent of the non coagulation procedures. It also took longer for the patients with

Table 34-2. Success Rates Following Tubal Reanastomosis

Author	Cases	Live Births (%)	Ectopic Pregnancies (%)
Chang, Kim (1986)	250	44	5
Rock et al (1987)	246	53	4
Paterson (1985)	147	59	5
Seiler (1983)	73	64	2
Grunert et al (1981)	40	57	3
Gomel (1980)	118	64	1
Winston (1980)	126	58	2
Patterson (1980)	50	40	4
Silber, Cohen (1980)	25	56	4
Total	1,075	55	3

(From Rock,[11] with permission.)

electrocoagulation to conceive, an average of 13 months versus 6.7 months for the noncoagulation group.

TRANSCERVICAL FALLOPIAN TUBE CATHETERIZATION

The transcervical approach may be attempted in the presence of proximal obstruction not due to tubal ligation, as an alternative to tubointerstitial anastomosis. The procedure may be performed under fluoroscopic guidance or with the hysteroscope and simultaneous laparoscopy.[96,97] The catheter set is comprised of coaxial catheters 9, 5.5, and 3 French in diameter, which are introduced into the cervix either with a vacuum adapter or with hysteroscopic guidance. The 5.5-French catheter is wedged into the cornua, the 3-French catheter with wire guide is introduced, and the wire guide is advanced through the obstruction. The 3-French soft tube is then advanced over the wire. Simultaneously, the laparoscopic operator assists in maintaining the tube in a straight line while it is being cannulated and can identify any tubal perforation that might occur. Balloon-tip catheters have also been developed and are used to dilate the proximal segment of the tube once cannulation is achieved.

PREVENTION OF POST OPERATIVE ADHESIONS

Mechanical injury or infection of the peritoneum results in an outpouring of polymorphonuclear leukocytes, platelets, and fibrinogen, which form a fibrin clot that eventually becomes organized by fibroblast proliferation, resulting in collagenous adhesions.[98] Clotted blood is thought to constitute a fibrinous network on which fibroblasts may proliferate, resulting in adhesion. Therefore, it is of the utmost importance to remove as much blood as possible from the operative field, especially clotted blood, when performing pelvic reconstructive surgery.[99] The most effective way to minimize the formation of postoperative adhesions is through the use of meticulous microsurgical technique, minimizing operative trauma.

Many adjuvants have been proposed to help prevent postoperative adhesions, as shown in Table 34-3. The use of lasers, particularly the carbon dioxide laser, was initially suggested to reduce the incidence of adhesion formation. In theory, its use in reparative surgery posed several advantages over traditional methods, including the precision achieved with the laser beam, which enables the experienced operator to vaporize adhesions close to the ureter or the bowel with the additional benefit of the magnification obtained via laparoscope. Tulandi[100] also failed to document a difference in the degree of adhesion reformation when following 19 women who underwent tubal surgery with carbon dioxide lasers and 20 who underwent similar procedures using the

Table 34-3. Surgical Adjuvants to Minimize Postoperative Adhesions

Fibrinolytic agents
    Fibrinolysin
    Papain
    Streptokinase
    Urokinase
    Hyaluronidase
    Chymotrypsin
    Trypsin
    Pepsin
Anticoaglants
    Heparin
    Citrates
    Oxalates
Anti-inflammatory agents
    Corticosteroids
    Ibuprofen
    Antihistamines
Antibiotics
    Tetracyclines
    Cephalosporins
Mechanical separation
    Intra-abdominal instillates
        Dextran
        Silicone
        Povidone
        Crystalloid solutions
        Carboxymethylcellulose
    Barriers
        Endogenous tissue
            Omental grafts
            Peritoneal grafts
            Bladder strips
            Fetal membranes
        Exogenous material
            Polytetrafluoroethylene
            Goretex surgical membrane
            Oxidized regenerated cellulose (Interceed TC7)
            Fibrin gel glue
            Rubber sheets
            Metal foils
            Plastic hoods

microdiathermy needle with second-look laparoscopy. In experiments conducted in rabbits, Pittaway et al[101] and Filmore et al[102] did not find a reduction in the incidence of postoperative adhesion formation when comparing the carbon dioxide laser with electrocautery.

Irrigation of the operative field is used as an adjuvant measure in tubal surgery. Saline solutions are commonly employed to wash irritants such as blood and tissue fragments from the pelvis. However, the lavage solution itself may be damaging to the serosal surface of the peritoneum by causing chemical irritation. Blandau[103] observed edema and formation of a plasma membrane over fallopian tubes bathed with saline. Because of these findings, authors such as Wallach and others introduced the use of lactated Ringer's instead of saline so that the mesothelium is exposed to physiologic concentrations of potassium, calcium, and lactate.[101] In addition to washing away blood, crystalloid solutions have other actions that reduce the incidence of posttraumatic serosal adhesions.[104,105] When left in the abdominal cavity, they aid in separating raw surfaces and dilute clotting factors contained in exudates from injured tissue. The rationale behind the use of anticoagulation as an adjuvant in the prevention of postoperative adhesions is the preclusion of the formation of a fibrin matrix for the proliferation of fibroblasts. Based on these principles, anticoagulants also have been evaluated in adhesion prevention. Anticoagulation with heparin, citrates, and dicumarol in animal studies have been shown to effectively reduce the incidence of adhesions following intestinal manipulation.[105] However, full systemic anticoagulation is necessary in order for the adhesion-reducing properties of anticoagulation to be expressed; this carries an unacceptable risk. Currently, heparinized solutions are used locally for continuous irrigation during the open procedures, avoiding the possible complications of the systemic use of these agents.

Oxidized regenerated cellulose (Interceed TC7, Johnson & Johnson, New Brunswick, NJ) is currently being employed as an adjuvant for the prevention of adhesion formation, based on the results of prior animal[106] and clinical studies.[107] Pagidas and Tulandi[108] compared the effects of Interceed, Gore-Tex surgical membrane (W. L. Gore and Assoc., Flagstaff, AZ), and lactated Ringer's on postoperative adhesion formation in a rat uterine horn model. Following a standardized injury, the animals were assigned to control and the above mentioned adjuvant groups. The extent of adhesion formation was evaluated 2 weeks later; the lactated Ringer's group had significantly fewer adhesions when compared to the Interceed and control groups. Although the Gore-Tex surgical membrane group also had a reduction in adhesions when compared to the other two groups, the lactated Ringer's group fared the best. There was no significant difference in the adhesion scores between the control and Interceed groups. Other studies failed to support the advantage of using Interceed as an adhesion prevention adjuvant over other agents.[109–111]

Tulandi[112] evaluated the impact of fibrin glue (Tiseel, Immuno Canada Ltd., Toronto, Canada) on subsequent adhesion formation in 12 women undergoing bilateral isthmic-isthmic anastomosis for reversal of sterilization. One side was approximated using the conventional suturing technique and the other using the fibrin glue. He did not find a significant difference in adhesion formation between the two sides.

The use of 32 percent dextran 70 has also been advocated by some authors for the prevention of adhesions.[113,114] Administered intraperitoneally, dextran induces an osmotically mediated transudation of serum into the peritoneal cavity; it is then slowly eliminated from the peritoneal space in approximately 10 days. Evidently, dextran separates raw surfaces and inhibits coagulation of fibrin over an exceptionally long period following instillation. The potential risks associated with use of this preparation include anaphylaxis and, theoretically, infection, as dextran might act as a culture medium within the peritoneal cavity.

The use of adjuvants for adhesion prevention is widespread. The literature is replete with conflicting results for most adjuvants and efficacy is not well established. The difficulty in determining their efficiency might be due to differences in the pathology being treated, the various classification systems for extent of the disease, and the follow-up methods employed for these patients.

REFERENCES

1. Schroeder C: Die excision von ovarientumoren mit erhaltung des ovarium. Zentralbl Gynak 8:716, 1884
2. Peterson H, Galaid EI, Cates W: Pelvic inflammatory disease. Med Clin North Am 74:1603, 1990
3. Mardh P-A, Ripa T, Svensson L et al: Chlamydia trachomatis infections in patients with acute salpingitis. N Engl J Med 296:1377, 1977
4. Westrom L: Pelvic inflammatory disease; bacteriology and sequelae. Contraception 36:111, 1987
5. Westrom L: Effect of acute pelvic inflammatory disease on infertility. Am J Obstet Gynecol 121:707, 1975
6. Jenkins CS, Williams SR, Schmidt GE: Salpingitis isthmica nodosa: a review of the literature, discussion of clinical significance, and consideration of patient management. Fertil Steril 60:599, 1993
7. Bundey JG, Williams JD: Salpingitis isthmica nodosa with tumor formation resembling torsion of an ovarian cyst. J Obstet Gynecol Br Commonw 70:519, 1963
8. Punnonen R, Sodestrom KO: Inflammatory theory of salpingitis isthmica nodosa: a clinical, histological and ultrastructural study. Acta Eur Fertil 17:199, 1986
9. Fortier KJ, Haney AF: The pathologic spectrum of uterotubal junction obstruction. Obstet Gynecol 65:93, 1985
10. Honore LH: Salpingitis isthmica nodosa in female infertility and ectopic tubal pregnancy. Fertil Steril 29:164, 1978
11. Rock JA: Reconstruction of the fallopian tube. p. 437. In Thompson JD, Rock JA (eds): Te Linde's Operative Gynecology. JB Lippincott, Philadelphia, 1992
12. Lavy G, Diamond MP, DeCherney AH: Ectopic pregnancy: its relationship to tubal reconstructive surgery. Fertil Steril 47:543, 1987
13. Oelsner G, Tarlatzis BC: Radical surgery for extrauterine pregnancy. p. 127. In DeCherney AH (ed): Ectopic Pregnancy. Aspen Publishers, Rockville, MD, 1986
14. DeCherney AH, Maheaux R, Naftolin F: Salpingostomy for ectopic pregnancy in the sole patent oviduct: reproductive outcome. Fertil Steril 37:619, 1982

15. Weisberg E, Fraser IS: Fertility following reversal of male and female sterilization. Contraception 26:361, 1982

16. The American Fertility Society: The American Fertility Society classifications of adnexal adhesions, distal tubal occlusion, tubal occlusion secondary to tubal ligation, tubal pregnancies, mullerian anomalies and intrauterine adhesions. Fertil Steril 49:944, 1992

17. Johnston I, Speirs I, Hoult J, Lopata A: Preoperative assessment for tubal surgery and in vitro fertilization. Aust NZ J Obstet Gynaecol 21:153, 1981

18. Acton CM, Devitt JM: Hysterosalpingography in infertility—an experience of 3631 examinations. Aust NZ J Obstet Gynaecol 28:127, 1988

19. Rosenwaks Z, Sultan KM, Davis OK: A novel technique for cervical cannulation during hysterosalpingography. Fertil Steril 59:1329, 1993

20. James C, Gomel V: Surgical management of tubal factor infertility. Curr Opin Obstet Gynecol 2:200, 1990

21. Gurgan T, Kisnisci HA, Yarali H et al: Radionuclide hysterosalpingography: a simple and potentially useful method of evaluating tubal patency. J Reprod Med 36:789, 1991

22. Venezia R, Zangara C, Knight C, Cittadini E: Initial experience of a new linear everting falloppscopy system in comparison with hysterosalpingography. Fertil Steril 60:771, 1993

23. DeBruyne F, Puttemans P, Boeckx W et al: The clinical value of salpingoscopy in tubal infertility. Fertil Steril 51:339, 1989

24. Polan ML: Endoscopy in infertility. p. 1. In Sciarra JJ (ed): Obstetrics and Gynecology. JB Lippincott Philadelphia, 1990

25. Young GP, Ott DJ, Chen MY et al: Postoperative hysterosalpingography: radiographic appearances and clinical results following tubal surgery. J Reprod Med 38:924, 1993

26. Letterie GS, Haggerty MF, Fellows DW: Sensitivity of hysterosalpingography after tubal surgery. Arch Gynecol Obstet 251:175, 1992

27. Schnack Peen UB, Pelle J, Bostofte E, Felding IC: Hysterosalpingography, pre- and postoperative laparoscopy in operative treatment of infertility. Acta Eur Fertil 20:355, 1989

28. Gomel V: Microsurgical reversal of female sterilization: a reappraisal. Fertil Steril 33:587, 1980

29. Gomel V: Profile of women requesting reversal of sterilization. Fertil Steril 30:39, 1978

30. Alvarez A: Reconstructive surgery of the oviduct. p. 146. In Rock JA, Alvarez A, Murphy M, Jones HW (eds): Female Reproductive Surgery. Williams & Wilkins, Baltimore, 1992

31. Taylor PJ: Tubal surgery. Obstet Gynecol Annu 11:253, 1982

32. Silber SJ, Cohen R: Microsurgical reversal of female sterilization: the role of tubal length. Fertil Steril 6:598, 1980

33. Seiler JC: Factors influencing the outcome of microsurgical tubal ligation sterilization reversals. Am J Obstet Gynecol 146:292, 1983

34. Karasick S, Ehrlich S: The value of hysterosalpingography before reversal of sterilization procedures involving the fallopian tubes. AJR 153:1247, 1989

35. DeCherney A, Mezer H: Current approach to tubal anastomosis. Obstet Gynecol Annu 11:277, 1982

36. DeCherney AH, Mezer HC, Naftolin F: Analysis of failure of microsurgical anastomosis after midsegment, non coagulation tubal ligation. Fertil Steril 39:618, 1983

37. Opsahl MS, Klein TA: The role of laparoscopy in the evaluation of candidates for sterilization reversal. Fertil Steril 48:546, 1980

38. Society for Assisted Reproductive Technology, The American fertility Society: Assisted Reproductive Technologies in the United States and Canada: 1991 Results from the Society for Assisted Reproductive Technology generated from the American Fertility Society registry. Fertil 59:956, 1993

39. Benadiva CA, Kligman I, Rosenwaks Z: Assisted reproductive technologies versus tubal surgery. (in press)

40. Oehringer S, Scott R, Muasher SJ et al: Effects of the severity of tubo-ovarian disease and previous tubal surgery on the results of in vitro fertilization and embryo transfer. Fertil Steril 51:126, 1989

41. Gomel V: Recent advances in surgical correction of tubal disease producing infertility. p. 100. In Kistner RW (ed): Current Problems in Obstetrics and Gynecology. Vol. 1. Year Book Medical Publishers, Chicago, 1978

42. Mottashaw ND, Alookar S, Ambani L et el: Laparoscopy and laparoscopic gonadal biopsy in the management of primary amenorrhea. In Phillips JM Endoscopy in Gynecology. American Association of Gynecologic Laparoscopists, Downey, CA 1978

43. Hoffman JJ: A practical classification of the risk factor in restorative surgery of the fallopian tube. Fertil Steril 28:1006, 1977

44. Pauerstein CJ: From fallopius to fantasy. Fertil Steril 30:133, 1978

45. Swolin K: Fertilitratsoperatronen, Teil I and II. Acta Obstet Gynecol Scand 46:204, 1967

46. Gomel V: Classification of operations for tubal and peritoneal factors causing infertility. Clin Obstet Gynecol 23:1259, 1980

47. Jones H, Rock J: Surgery of the oviduct. In Jones HW, Rock JA (eds): Reproductive and Constructive Surgery of the Female Generative Tract. Williams & Wilkins, Baltimore, 1980

48. Stangel J, Settles H, Reyniak J et al: Microsurgical anastomosis of the rabbit oviduct using 9−0 monofilament polyglycolic acid suture. Fertil Steril 30:210, 1978

49. Delbeke LO, Gomel V, McComb PF, Jetha N: Histologic reaction to four synthetic microsutures in the rabbit. Fertil Steril 40:248, 1983

50. Winston RML: Microsurgical reanastomosis of the rabbit oviduct and its functional and pathological sequelae. Br J Obstet Gynaecol 2:513, 1975

51. Gomel V: Salpingostomy by microsurgery. Fertil Steril 29:380, 1978

52. Gomel V: Laparoscopic tubal surgery in infertility. Obstet Gynecol 46:47, 1975

53. Hunt RB: Therapeutic laparoscopy. p. 89. In Martin DC (ed): Manual of Endoscopy. The American Association of Gynecologic Laparoscopists, Downey, CA, 1992

54. Gomel V: Operative laparoscopy: time for acceptance. Fertil Steril 52:1, 1989
55. Hulka JF, Omram R, Berger GS: Classification of adnexal adhesions: a proposal and evaluation of its diagnostic value. Fertil Steril 30:661, 1978
56. Wallach E, Manara L, Eisenberg E: Experience with 143 cases of tubal surgery. Fertil Steril 39(5):609, 1983
57. O'Brien JR, Arronet GH, Edulijee SY: Operative treatment of the fallopian tube pathology in human fertility. Am J Obstet Gynecol 103:520, 1969
58. Betz G, Engel T, Penney LL: Tuboplasty: comparison of the methodology. Fertil Steril 534:34, 1980
59. Caspi E, Halperin Y, Bukovsky I: The importance of periadnexal adhesions in tubal reconstructive surgery for infertility. Fertil Steril 31:296, 1979
60. Donnez J, Casanas-Roux F: Prognostic factors of fimbrial microsurgery. Fertil Steril 46:200, 1986
61. Tulandi T: Salpingo-ovariolysis: a comparison between laser surgery and electrosurgery. Fertil Steril 45:489, 1986
62. Gomel V: Salpingo-ovariolysis by laparoscopy in infertility. Fertil Steril 40:607, 1983
63. Fayez JA: An assessment of the role of operative laparoscopy in tuboplasty. Fertil Steril 39:476, 1983
64. Bruhat MA, Mage G, Manhes H et al: Laparoscopic procedures to promote fertility. Ovariolysis and salpingolysis. Results of 93 selected cases. Acta Eur Fertil 14:113, 1983
65. Donnez J: CO_2 laser laparoscopy in infertile women with endometriosis and women with adnexal adhesions. Fertil Steril 48:390, 1987
66. Patton GW: Pregnancy outcome following microsurgical fimbrioplasty. Fertil Steril 37:150, 1982
67. Kistner RW, Patton GW Jr: Atlas of infertility surgery. Little, Brown, Boston, 1975
68. Swolin K: Fifty fertility operations. I. Literature and methods. Acta Obstet Gynecol Scand 46:234, 1967
69. Winston RML: Microsurgery of the fallopian tube: from fantasy to reality. Fertil Steril 34:521, 1980
70. Gomel V: Microsurgery in Female Infertility. Little, Brown, Boston 1983
71. Nezhat C, Winer WK, Cooper JD et al: Endoscopic infertility surgery. J Reprod Med 34:127, 1989
72. Shirodkar VN: Factors influencing the results of salpingostomy. Int J fertil 2:361, 1966
73. Young PE, Egan JE, Barlow JA et al: Reconstructive surgery for infertility at the Boston Hospital for women. Am J Obstet Gynecol 108:1092, 1970
74. Rock JA, Katayama KP, Martin EJ et al: Factors influencing the success of salpingostomy techniques for distal fimbrial obstruction. Obstet Gynecol 52:591, 1978
75. Schlaff W, Hassiakos DK, Damewood MD, Rock JA: Neosalpingostomy for distal tubal obstruction: prognostic factors and impact of surgical technique. Fertil Steril 54:984, 1990
76. Boer-Meisel ME, TeVelde ER, Habbena JDF et al: Predicting the pregnancy outcome in patients treated for hydrosalpinx: a prospective study. Fertil Steril 45:23, 1986
77. Vasquez G, Winston RML, Boeckx W et al: Tubal lesion subsequent to sterilization and their relation to fertility after attempts at reversal. Am J Obstet Gynecol 138:86, 1980
78. Daniell JF, Herbert CM: Laparoscopic salpingostomy utilizing the CO_2 laser. Fertil Steril 41:558, 1984
79. Fayez JA: An assessment of the role of operative laparoscopy in tuboplasty. Fertil Steril 39:476, 1983
80. Betz G, Engel T, Penney LL: Tuboplasty: comparison of the methodology. Fertil Steril 34:534, 1980
81. Russell JB, DeCherney AH, Laufer N et al: Neosalpingostomy: comparison of 24 and 72 month follow up time shows increased pregnancy rate. Fertil Steril 45:296, 1986
82. Tulandi T, Farag R, McInnes RA et al: Reconstructive surgery of hydrosalpinx with and without the carbon dioxide laser. Fertil Steril 42:839, 1984
83. Cohen BM: Microsurgical reconstruction of congenital tubal anomalies. Microsurgery 8:68, 1987
84. Urman B, Gomel V, Mc Comb, Lee N: Midtubal occlusion: etiology, management and outcome. Fertil Steril 57:747, 1992
85. Madelenat P, De Brux J, Palmer R: L'etiologie des obstructions tubaires proximales et son role dans le pronostic des implantations. Gynecologie 28:47, 1977
86. Jones HW, Rock JA: On the reanastomosis of fallopian tubes after surgical sterilization. Fertil Steril 29:702, 1978
87. Winston RML: Reversal of sterilization. Clin Obstet Gynecol 23:1261, 1980
88. Reich H, Mc Glynn F, Parente C et al: Laparoscopic tubal reanastomosis. J AAGL 1:16, 1993
89. Silva PD, Schaper AM, Meisch JK, Schauberger CW: Outpatient microsurgical reversal of tubal sterilization by a combined approach of laparoscopy and minilaparotomy. Fertil Steril 55:696, 1991
90. Paterson PJ: Factors influencing the success of microsurgical tuboplasty for sterilization reversal. Clin Reprod Fertil 3:57, 1985
91. Rock JA, Guzick DS, Katz et al: Tubal anastomosis: pregnancy success following reversal of Falope ring or monopolar cautery sterilization. Fertil Steril 48:13, 1987
92. Donnez J, Casanas-Roux F, Ferin J: Macroscopic and microscopic studies of fallopian tubes after laparoscopic sterilization. Contraception 20:498, 1979
93. Vasquez G, Winston RML, Boeckx W et al: Tubal lesions subsequent to sterilization and their relation to fertility after attempts of reversal. Am J Obstet Gynecol 138:86, 1980
94. Putman JM, Holden AEC, Olive DL: Pregnancy rates following tubal anastomosis: Pomeroy partial salpingectomy vs. electrocautery. J Gynecol Surg 6:173, 1990
95. Seiler JC: Factors influencing the outcome of microsurgical tubal ligation reversals. Am J Obstet Gynecol 146:292, 1983
96. Confino E, Friberg J, Gleicher W: Preliminary experience with transcervical balloon tuboplasty. Am J Obstet Gynecol 159:370, 1988
97. Novy MJ, Thurmond AS, Patton P et al: Diagnosis of cornual obstruction by transcervical fallopian tube cannulation. Fertil Steril 50:434, 1988

98. DiZerega GS: The peritoneum and its response to surgical injury. p. 1. In DiZerega GS, Malinak LR, Diamond MP, Linsky CB (eds): Treatment of Post Surgical Adhesions. Proceedings of the First International Symposium for the Treatment of Post Surgical Adhesions. Phoenix, Arizona, September 15–17, 1989. Wiley-Liss, New York, 1989

99. Pfeffer W: Adjuvants in tubal surgery. Fertl Steril 33:245, 1980

100. Tulandi T: Adhesion reformation after reproductive surgery with and without the carbon dioxide laser. Fertil Steril 47:704, 1987

101. Pittaway DE, Maxson WS, Daniell JF: A comparison of the CO_2 laser and electrocautery on postoperative intraperitoneal adhesion formation in rabbits. Fertil Steril 40:366, 1983

102. Filmore S, Gomel V, McComb P: The effectiveness of CO_2 laser and electrocautery adhesiolysis: a comparative study? Fertil Steril 45:407, 1986

103. Blandau RJ: Comparative aspects of tubal anatomy and physiology as they relate to reconstructive procedures. J Reprod Med 21:7, 1978

104. Boys F: The prophylaxis of peritoneal adhesions. Surgery 11:118, 1942

105. Ellis H: The cause and prevention of postoperative intraperitoneal adhesions. Surg Gynecol Obstet 133:497, 1971

106. Linski CB, Diamond MP, Cunningham T et al: Adhesion reduction in a rabbit uterine horn model using TC-7. J Reprod Med 32:17, 1987

107. Interceed (TC-7) Adhesion Barrier Study Group: Prevention of post surgical adhesion by Interceed (TC-7), an absorbable adhesion barrier: a prospective, randomized, multicenter clinical study. Fertil Steril 51:933, 1989

108. Pagidas K, Tulandi T: Effects of Ringer's Lactate, Interceed (TC-7) and goretex surgical membrane on post surgical adhesion formation. Fertil Steril 57:199, 1992

109. Best CL, Rittenhause D, Vasquez C et al: Evaluation of Interceed (TC-7) for reduction of postoperative adhesions in rabbits. Fertil Steril 58:817, 1992

110. Haney AF, Doty E: Expanded-polytetrafluorethylene but not oxidized regenerated cellulose prevents adhesion formation and reformation in a mouse uterine horn model for surgical injury. Fertil Steril 60:550, 1993

111. Rice VM, Shanti A, Moghissi K, Leach RE: A comparative evaluation of Poloxamer 407 and oxidized regenerated cellulose (Interceed, TC-7) to reduce post operative adhesion formation in the rat uterine horn model. Fertil Steril 59:901, 1993

112. Tulandi T: Effects of a fibrin sealant on tubal anastomosis and adhesion formation. Fertil Steril 56:136, 1991

113. Holtz G, Baker E, Tsai C: Effect of thirty two percent dextran 70 on peritoneal adhesion formation-reformation after lysis. Fertil Steril 33:660, 1980

114. Holtz G, Baker ER: Inhibition of peritoneal adhesion reformation after lysis with thirty two percent dextran 70. Fertil Steril 34:394, 1980

CHAPTER THIRTY-FIVE

STERILIZATION

THOMAS G. STOVALL

Background
Preoperative
Evaluation
Informed Consent • Timing
of Sterilization • Regret
After Sterilization
Sterilization Methods
Laparotomy • Laparoscopic
Sterilization • Vaginal
Sterilization
Teaching/Learning
 Laparoscopic
 Sterilization
Sterilization Failure
Sterilization Safety
Complications

I t would be ideal if a nonsurgical method of sterilization were available that would bypass the potential problems encountered with surgical sterilization. A host of nonsurgical methods have been tried, including chemical agents that induce sclerosis and occlusive methods such as tubal plugs. Unfortunately, the chemical methods studied to date have been toxic or ineffective, or both. As these methods are not widely available, this chapter deals only with surgical methods to accomplish sterilization.

BACKGROUND

The first tubal sterilization was performed at the time of cesarean section by Lungren in 1880.[1] Anderson[2] is credited with performing the first laparoscopic electrocoagulation procedure in the United States in 1937. Steptoe[3] in 1967 reported the first large series of laparoscopic sterilizations and Wheeless[4] in 1972 reported the first single-puncture laparoscopic technique. Numerous methods for achieving permanent sterilization have been described. The various procedures were introduced for a variety of reasons. Irving[5] in 1924 described a technique in which the proximal end of the fallopian tube was buried in the myometrium. This technique was introduced as a way to decrease the reported 20 percent failure rate of the Pomeroy procedure. This failure rate was later revised to 3 in 1,000 after Husbands et al[6] reviewed the previously published data. In 1948, Boyson and McRae recommended that the vaginal approach was the procedure of choice, although they had a reported failure rate of 0.6

percent. During the 1960s, vaginal colpotomy was widely used as a method to reduce hospital stay, and the need for laparotomy.

The refinement of laparoscopy and the widespread availability of laparoscopic equipment forever changed gynecology and the approach to sterilization. The use of laparoscopy allowed the procedure to be done on an outpatient basis and even allowed for easy completion with local anesthesia. Thus, the procedure became commonplace even in underdeveloped countries. Because many of the techniques that were used at laparotomy were not suitable for use at laparoscopy, new occluding methods had to be developed. The initial technique involved unipolar electrocoagulation. Because of accidents that occurred with this technique, physicians Rioux[7] and Corson designed bipolar forceps. It is no surprise that several manufacturers designed their own systems as the popularity of this technique grew. Richard Kleppinger designed a complete electrical system, which is currently the system used by most gynecologists. This system uses specifically designed forceps combined with a generator designed only for bipolar surgery.

The Hulka clip is another popular method for laparoscopic sterilization, initially publicized in 1972.[8] The tubal ring was designed and published some 3 years later by Yoon and colleagues.[9] Both methods are still widely used.

PREOPERATIVE EVALUATION

Tubal sterilization should be available to any woman who desires permanent sterilization, assuming that she has proper informed consent and knowledge regarding the procedure.

631

The procedure should be considered purely elective. There are virtually no absolute contraindications to tubal sterilization except for gynecologic malignancy or gynecologic disease that requires hysterectomy or bilateral oophorectomy. There are circumstances that require specific mention. For example, if the patient has known extensive intra-abdominal adhesions, the potential for intraoperative morbidity may be so great as to consider another form of contraception. For the patient with a severe medical problem, it is probably advisable to consult with a specialist in the particular disease-related area or a maternal medicine specialist to determine exactly how pregnancy would affect the condition in question. Often, patients have been told by a well-meaning health care provider that pregnancy is contraindicated when in fact it is not. The family of a severely mentally retarded patient may request sterilization, but these are special circumstances that require discussion with the family and most often require a second opinion, an ethics committee recommendation, or at times, a court order.

Informed Consent

Proper informed consent is the cornerstone to preoperative counseling and aids in the reduction of poststerilization regret. In order to fully inform the patient, her decision to undergo sterilization must first be voluntary and noncoerced. A discussion of informed consent includes a review of alternative methods of contraception as well as male sterilization. The permanence of the procedure should be emphasized, although not guaranteed, since the procedure, if done correctly, has a known failure rate. The patient should also be given a description of the planned operative technique along with a discussion of specific risk of laparotomy or laparoscopy. Since many patients have concerns about side effects, the patient should be reassured that there is no evidence that abnormal bleeding or uterine cramping is increased after sterilization. Following this discussion, the patient should have an opportunity to ask questions and express any concerns that might exist. Finally, the use of continued contraception before sterilization should be emphasized. This will help to decrease the occurrence of luteal phase pregnancies. Although not mandatory, some surgeons provide the information to the patient in booklet form, which may aid with patient understanding. It should also be remembered that patients whose sterilization will be federally funded must sign a special consent document, and must be at least 21 years of age.

The patient's husband is not required to give consent before performing the procedure. Obviously, it is best if both partners have an understanding of the procedure as well as the benefits and potential risks of it. Thus, if a problem is encountered, the patient's family is in a better position to deal with the problem.

Timing of Sterilization

There are four times when the performance of a sterilization procedure seems appropriate. First, for the patient who decides during her pregnancy that she desires permanent sterilization, the procedure can be done within a short time following delivery. For the patient who has had conduction anesthesia for labor, the immediate postpartum period is an excellent time for sterilization, as the method for anesthetic administration has already been performed. A number of investigators have shown that patients can undergo sterilization immediately following delivery without any increased risk of complications.[10–12] The longest period that the patient may wait before undergoing sterilization is controversial. In some circumstances, a delay of 12 to 24 hours may be needed to assess the infant's condition, or delays secondary to staffing patterns or availability of anesthesia may be encountered. Studies done show no increased risk of morbidity if the sterilization was delayed for the first postpartum day.[13–14] If it is not feasible during this time period to perform the sterilization, the patient should probably wait at least 6 weeks so that the uterine architecture will be back to normal. Before this time, the uterus may be enlarged, making laparoscopy more difficult, and there may be an increased risk of infection during the postpartum period. The patient who has a postpartum endometritis, or has had premature rupture of the membranes, intrapartum fever, or manual placental removal is probably at increased risk of a postsurgical infection. Therefore, it may be prudent for this patient to wait and undergo interval sterilization. If cesarean section is required, and the patient desires sterilization, the two procedures should be performed concurrently. The addition of sterilization to cesarean section adds little to the operative risk of the procedure or to the postoperative morbidity. Also, performance of the sterilization procedure at the time of cesarean section or shortly following vaginal delivery also allows the patient to recover from the two procedures simultaneously, and therefore does not add to the patient's hospitalization or convalescence period.

Elements of Informed Consent for Sterilization

- Review of alternative methods of permanent sterilization (e.g., vasectomy)
- Indicate that the procedure is considered permanent
- Review failure rate of procedure
- Description of the planned operative technique
- Discuss potential surgical risk

Interval sterilization, or sterilization after the immediate postpartum period should be delayed for 6 or 8 weeks. Most of these procedures are performed by laparoscopy and can be done using local, conduction, or general anesthesia. Performance of the procedure during the menstrual or proliferative phase of the cycle reduces the chance of pregnancy at the time of the procedure. However, if this is not practical, a sensitive urine or serum pregnancy test can be done on the day the procedure is performed. This too has been shown to decrease the risk of luteal phase pregnancy.[15] Finally, sterilization can be performed in conjunction with other surgical procedures such as cholecystectomy or plastic surgical procedures.

Regret After Sterilization

Sterilization is the most prevalent method of contraception among married women in the United States, and as a result, if only a few of these women experience regret following sterilization, it becomes an important problem. It is estimated that regret after tubal sterilization occurs in approximately 3 to 25 percent of women. However, only about 1 to 2 percent of all women who have undergone sterilization seek tubal ligation reversal.[16-19] Numerous studies have been conducted and a variety of populations have been studied. The data are somewhat confused, but is summarized in Table 35-1. Wilcox and associates[20] reported data from the Collaborative Review of Sterilization, a prospective, multicenter study enrolling 7,590 women. In this report, women were followed for up to 5 years. Young age at the time of sterilization was the strongest predictor of regret, regardless of parity or marital status. For women 20 to 24 years of age at sterilization, 4.3 percent reported regret compared with 2.4 percent for women 30 to 34 years of age. Other researchers have not found such an association.[21]

The most common factor associated with regret is a change in marital status.[22,23] Some studies also report an association between regret and marital discord at the time

of sterilization, although other studies do not report this association. Factors not generally associated with regret include religious, socioeconomic, and educational background, and low parity at the time of sterilization.

STERILIZATION METHODS

In excess of 100 sterilization procedures have been described in the gynecologic literature. A discussion of the risks, benefits, technical aspects, and failure rates of each of these procedures is beyond the scope of this chapter. Therefore, only those techniques that are currently popular or are widely used are discussed. For the most part, interval sterilizations are performed by laparoscopy and postpartum sterilizations are done by minilaparotomy. The advantages of interval sterilizations being done by laparoscopy are widely accepted and include decreased operative time and postoperative pain, along with shorter hospital stays and more rapid return to normal functional activities.[24]

Laparotomy

A minilaparotomy can be used for interval sterilization, but is most commonly used for postpartum sterilization. Minilaparotomy for sterilization can be performed under general, regional, or local anesthesia.[25,26] A potential advantage of laparotomy is that a tissue specimen is commonly removed and can provide histologic documentation. However, if this is important, this can also be accomplished at laparoscopy. Potential disadvantages include a higher complication rate, greater need for postoperative analgesia, longer recovery time, and a larger surgical incision. Although most commonly used postpartum, laparotomy may also be used by the surgeon not trained in laparoscopy, when the patient is morbidly obese, or when severe tubal adhesive disease is present. It may also be used in remote areas where laparoscopic equipment is not available.

Pomeroy Method

In 1930, Bishop and Nelms[27] first reported the sterilization procedure that was developed by their late associate Pomeroy. The Pomeroy method can be completed through a suprapubic incision if performed as an interval procedure, through a colpotomy incision, or with a subumbilical incision in the immediate postpartum visit. Regardless of the type of incision that is performed, the fallopian tube is identified and grasped with a Babcock clamp in the midportion (Fig. 35-1A). The "knuckle" of tube is then double ligated with 0 or 2–0 plain catgut suture (Fig. 35-1B). The open blade of Metzenbaum scissors is used to puncture the mesosalpinx within the knuckle. The ligated segment of the fallopian tube is excised (Fig. 35-1C). Once cut, the ligated ends

Table 35-1. Factors That Have and Have Not Been Associated With Regret Following Sterilization

Factors Associated With Regret	Factors Not Associated With Regret
Marital status change	Religion
Family stress (e.g., death of a child)	Socioeconomic level
Desire for additional children as the "baby" grows up	Education level
	Low parity
Post-tubal ligation syndrome symptoms	Decision made with husband's
Post-partum timing	approval
Sterilization before age 30	Interval procedure

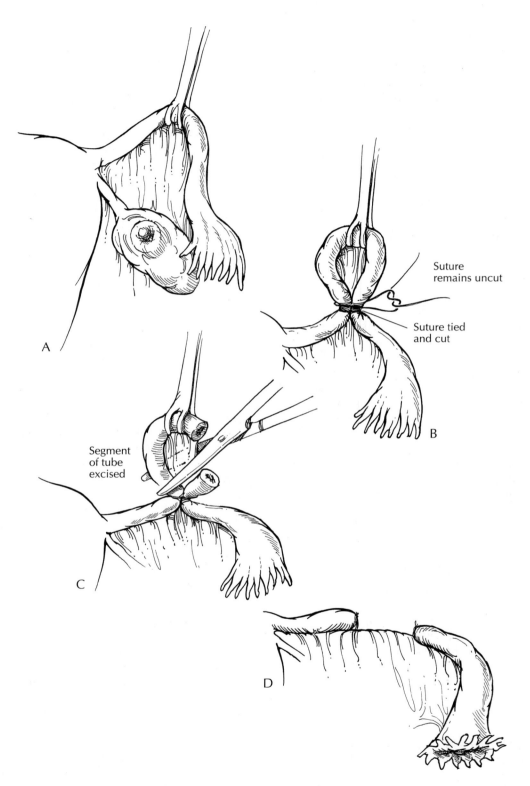

Suture
remains uncut

Suture tied
and cut

Segment
of tube
excised

A

B

C

D

Fig. 35-1. (A–D) Pomeroy technique of sterilization.

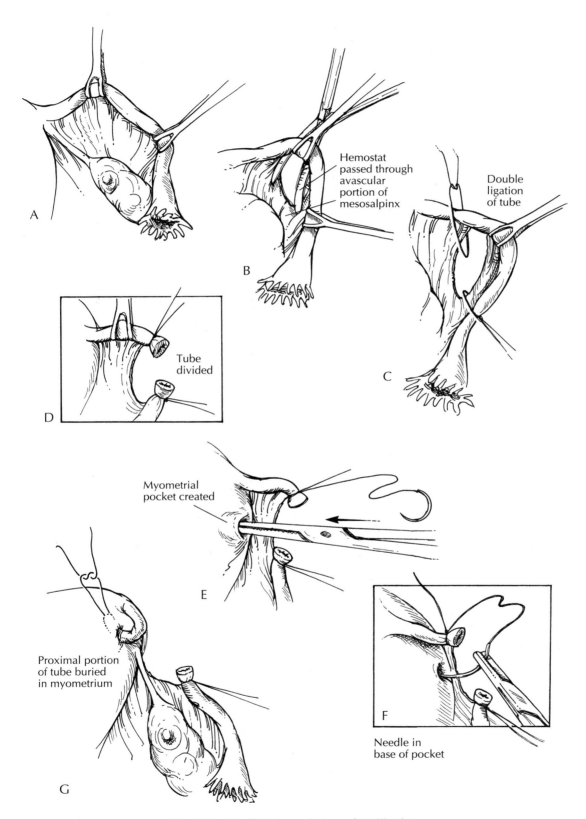

Fig. 35-2. (A–G) Irving technique of sterilization.

should be inspected for hemostasis and the presence of the tubal lumen visualized. Once the tube has been cut, the muscularis retracts, causing protrusion of the tubal lumen. The same procedure is completed on the contralateral side. The plain catgut suture resorbs in 3 to 4 days, and the tubal lumina separate (Fig. 35-1D). Use of a suture material that takes longer to resorb or one that is permanent increases the chance of fistula formation and sterilization failure. The tubal segments from the right and left tubes are labeled and sent in separate containers for histologic analysis. The pathologist should be able to document complete resection of a tubal segment. It is the surgeon's responsibility to review the pathologist's report to make certain that both tubal lumina were transected.

The most common complication with this method of sterilization is slippage of the suture ligatures with retraction of the tube. The fallopian tube must be grasped and ligated to ensure proper hemostasis. The potential for this can be minimized by placement of two sutures and placing traction only on the distal suture. Proper identification of the fallopian tube will prevent inadvertent ligation of the round ligament or mesosalpingeal veins.

Irving Method

The Irving technique was developed as a method of sterilization at the time of cesarean section.[5] Because it requires an incision that is large enough to expose the uterus and broad ligament, it is not generally used as a method for interval sterilization. It has an extremely low failure rate of less than 1 per 1,000 cases, but is generally associated with greater intraoperative blood loss. The original description buried the proximal tubal stump within the myometrium and buried the ligated distal tubal segment in the broad ligament. Burying the distal tubal end does not appear to increase the effectiveness of the procedure and is generally omitted. Following completion of the cesarean section, the fallopian tube is grasped with a Babcock clamp (Fig. 35-2A). A hemostat is passed through an avascular portion of the mesosalpinx near the ampullary-isthmic junction (Fig. 35-2B). Two 0 synthetic absorbable sutures are passed through this opening in the mesosalpinx and the tube is doubly ligated (Fig. 35-2C). If one desires, a portion of the tube can be removed and sent for histologic confirmation (Fig. 35-2D). A hemostat is used to pierce a hole approximately 1 cm deep into the posterior

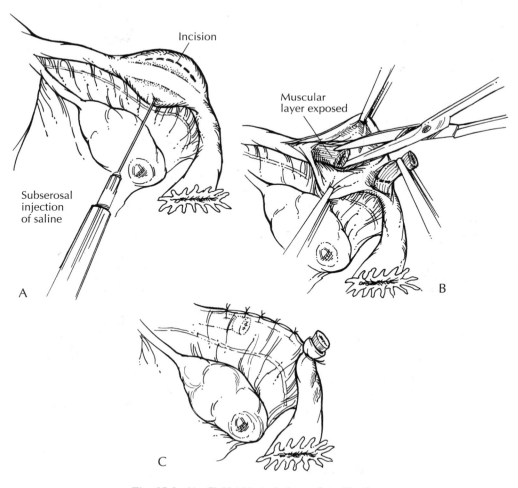

Fig. 35-3. (A–C) Uchida technique of sterilization.

aspect of the myometrium (Fig. 35-2E). The sutures attached to the proximal tubal segment are threaded into a curved needle and passed through the base of the myometrial hole to exit the uterine surface 1 to 2 cm apart (Fig. 35-2F). These two sutures are then tied together and the tubal stump is buried in the uterine muscularis. An absorbable suture is then used to reapproximate the uterine serosa (Fig. 35-2G). A similar procedure can be accomplished at laparoscopy. The advantage of this technique is that it provides a surgical specimen that can be confirmed histologically. A plain catgut suture should be used, so that resorption of the suture material is rapid.[28,29]

The most common complication of this method of sterilization is bleeding from the myometrium. Bleeding, if encountered, can usually be controlled with a figure-of-eight suture.

Uchida Method

The Uchida method is probably the most complex method of tubal sterilization. It was described as a method of interval sterilization and performed through a suprapubic minilaparotomy incision.[30] Its advantage is that it has an extremely low failure rate, with Uchida reporting no failures after completing more than 20,000 procedures.

A uterine manipulator is used to maneuver the uterus toward the suprapubic incision. The fallopian tube is identified and grasped with a Babcock clamp and elevated through the incision. A 25-gauge needle is used to inject saline into the subserosal layer in an area approximately 2 cm distal to the uterine cornu. The saline functions to balloon the serosa away from the muscularis (Fig. 35-3A). A scalpel is used to incise the tubal serosa longitudinally to free a 2- to 3-cm segment of serosa. Two pieces of plain 0 or 2-0 absorbable suture are passed under the freed segment of tube and tied at both ends of the isolated tubal segment. Both sutures are held with hemostats and the isolated tubal segment is excised and inspected to make certain that the tubal lumen has been interrupted (Fig. 35-3B). The excised tubal segment is sent for histologic confirmation. The proximal suture is cut and the tube retracts into the mesosalpinx. Tension is placed on the distal segment to elevate it above the mesosalpinx. A 3-0 synthetic absorbable suture is used to reapproximate

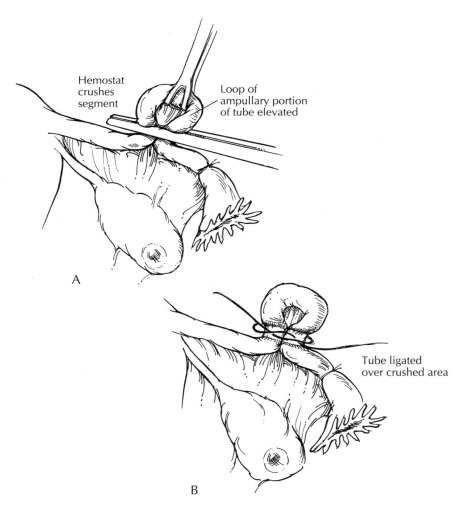

Fig. 35-4. (A & B) Madlender technique of sterilization.

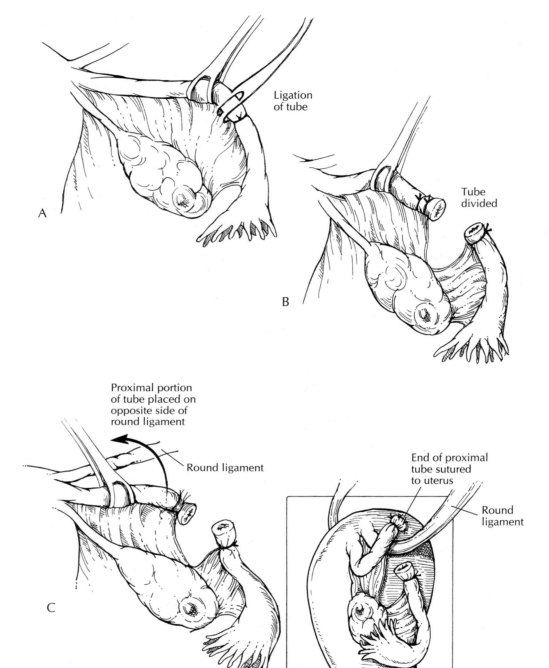

Ligation
of tube

A

Tube
divided

B

Proximal portion
of tube placed on
opposite side of
round ligament

Round ligament

C

End of proximal
tube sutured
to uterus

Round
ligament

D

Fig. 35-5. (A–D) Oxford technique of sterilization.

the serosa so that the proximal stump is buried within the mesosalpinx and the distal stump is exteriorized. The distal tube and fimbria can also be excised (Fig. 35-3C).

Like the Irving method, the most common complication of this method of sterilization is bleeding. Retraction of the distal segment can occur and can be prevented by placing traction on the distal segment, or by placing a suture around the distal tubal stump and attaching it to the serosa before closure of the serosa is completed.

Other Tubal Sterilization Techniques

A variety of other techniques have been described for tubal sterilization, although they are less frequently used. These methods include the Madlinger technique, Oxford technique, Kroener procedure, and Aldridge procedure.

The Madlener technique is similar in concept to laparoscopic tubal occlusion using a banding technique. However, it is employed using a laparotomy incision. In this technique, a loop of the ampullary portion of the tube is elevated and crushed with a hemostat. The tube is then ligated with a nonabsorbable suture material, and the tubal segment is not excised (Fig. 35-4). The failure rate of this technique is higher as a result of fistula formation beneath the permanent suture material. Therefore, it should not be used.

The Oxford technique is similar in concept to the Irving procedure in that the fallopian tube is divided at the ampullary-isthmic junction. Instead of burying the proximal tubal segment in the myometrium, it is carried under the round ligament and secured in place. The distal tube is then tied on the opposite side of the round ligament (Fig. 35-5).

Kroener described the use of fimbriectomy by sterilization in 1969.[31] This is one of the easiest methods to perform. The fimbriated end of the fallopian tube is grasped with a Babcock clamp. The mesosalpinx and outer third of the tube are clamped, and doubly ligated with synthetic absorbable suture. The tube is then excised to make certain that the entire fimbriated end of the tube is removed. This method removes the fimbriated end as well as a portion of the ampulla (Fig. 35-6). The most common complication associated with this method of sterilization is incomplete excision of the fimbriae. If done correctly, the failure rate is reported to be low, although most investigators believe that this form of sterilization should not be used, as more effective alternatives are available. Kroener reported a series of 200 fimbriectomies with no failures.

The Aldridge procedure involves burying the fimbriated end in the broad ligament with a series of nonabsorbable sutures. The series of sutures incorporates the serosal and

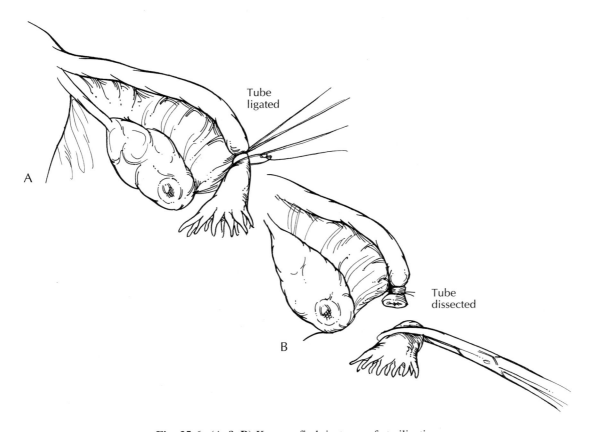

Fig. 35-6. (A & B) Kroener fimbriectomy of sterilization.

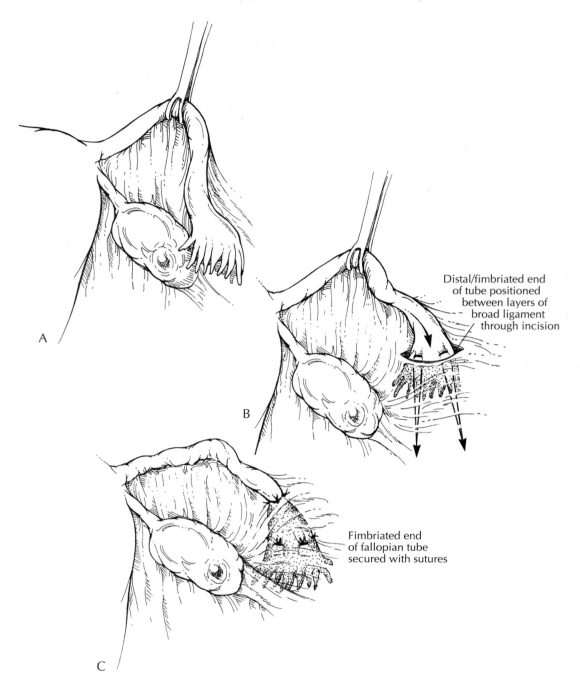

Distal/fimbriated end
of tube positioned
between layers of
broad ligament
through incision

Fimbriated end
of fallopian tube
secured with sutures

Fig. 35-7. (A–C) Aldridge technique of sterilization.

muscular layers of the tube in the broad ligament. The tube remains uninterrupted[32] (Fig. 35-7).

Laparoscopic Sterilization

Laparoscopic sterilization is the most widely used surgical approach for accomplishing interval sterilization. The most commonly used methods of laparoscopic tubal occlusion in-clude Falope ring application, electrocoagulation, and Hulka clip application. When correctly performed, these three tech-niques have essentially identical failure rates. It is generally accepted that there are no absolute contraindications to lapar-oscopic sterilization other than the desire for future fertility. Authors debate the relative contraindications but generally include severe cardiac or pulmonary disease, severe bleeding diathesis, severe adhesive disease, and massive obesity that would preclude obtaining laparoscopic access.

Bipolar Electrocoagulation

Unipolar electrocoagulation is the oldest technique and was originally described by Palmer in 1947.[33] This method of sterilization was widely used until reports of bowel burns begin to surface.[34,35] When these cases were reviewed, the injuries were the result of faulty technique or the use of high-voltage grounded generators delivering thousands of volts of current. To reduce this risk, only low-voltage generators with a maximum peak of 600 volts and a maximum power of 100 watts should be used. An isolated output system should be used rather than the grounded system.[36]

For bipolar electrodesiccation, it is important to remember that the forceps used must be compatible with the generator and that the current settings are appropriate for the procedure. The operating forceps of the bipolar system carries both the active and return electrode. The jaws are completely isolated from one another, so that high-frequency current passes through one jaw and is retrieved and returned to the generator through the other jaw. Thus, the current selectively passes through the grasped tissue and has to travel only the short distance between the jaws and the forceps. The danger of sparking is consequently eliminated. A cutting current with a power setting of 25 to 35 W should be used. An ammeter, optical meter, or sound meter should be used to make certain that the tissue grasped has been completely desiccated to the point that the tissue can no longer transmit an electrical current (Fig. 35-8). Most commonly, when failures occur, it is as a result of incomplete destruction of the endosalpinx (Fig. 35-9). This problem can be avoided with the use of these devices.

After the laparoscope is inserted, the pelvis is examined and any pelvic pathology noted. At times it will be necessary to cut and remove adhesions from around the tube so that the fallopian tube can be fully visualized. The fallopian tube is grasped and maneuvered until the fimbriated end can be identified. This step will ensure that the tube is the structure to be desiccated, as opposed to round ligament or utero-ovarian ligament. The tube is then grasped with the bipolar forceps approximately 2 to 3 cm from the uterine cornu. The tube is placed on tension to ensure that the forceps are not in contact with any other structures, and the current is then applied until the ohmmeter demonstrates complete tubal desiccation (Fig. 35-10A). The tube is then regrasped and desiccated at immediately adjacent sites (Fig. 35-10B) to coagulate 3 cm of contiguous tube (Fig. 35-10C). It is suggested that the desiccation begin distal and move proximal so that the uterus can function as a heat "sink." If this is done, no current flow can pass through the previously destroyed tubal segment, so that all electrical flow would have to go toward the uterus. The same procedure is repeated on the opposite side. It is not necessary to transect the tube following desiccation. In fact, it is thought that this might increase the risk of fistula formation.[37]

The most common serious complication specific to electrodesiccation is inadvertent electrical injury to adjacent organs or structures. This risk can be essentially eliminated by making certain that the tube has been mobilized and then placed on tension away from adjacent organs before the gen-

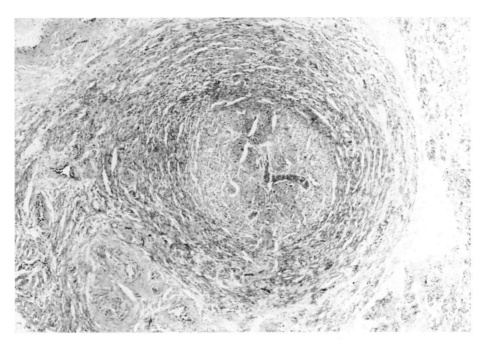

Fig. 35-8. Histologic cross-section of a fallopian tube demonstrating complete destruction of the endosalpinx. (Courtesy of Richard Soderstrom, M.D., Seattle, WA.)

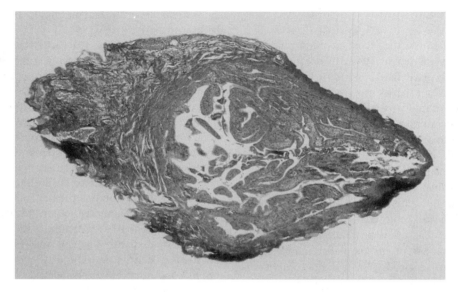

Fig. 35-9. Histologic cross-section of fallopian tube demonstrating an intact serosa with a coagulated muscularis layer. The endosalpinx remains viable. (Courtesy of Richard Soderstrom, M.D., Seattle, WA.)

erator is activated. Another risk inherent in this technique is incomplete destruction of the tubal mucosa. This problem can also be essentially eliminated by use of an ohmmeter. The electrical injury is applied until no flow of current is recorded. A timed coagulation of at least 10 seconds for each tubal segment has been used in the past. However, this method is less precise than using the ohmmeter.

Banding

Yoon et al[9,38] were the first to publish the use of a silicone rubber banding technique for tubal occlusion through the laparoscope. The technique was modified slightly in a subsequent report and emphasis was placed on the fact that the ring should be applied in the proximal tubal segment as described below.[39]

The tubal band applicator has two concentric cylinders, the inner of which contains grasping prongs that grasp and elevate the fallopian tube (Fig. 35-11). The movement of these cylinders is controlled by a single ring grip (Fig. 35-12). The handle of the applicator allows the surgeon to extend the grasping prongs beyond the inner cylinder, grasp the tube, and bring it inside the inner cylinder. One or two

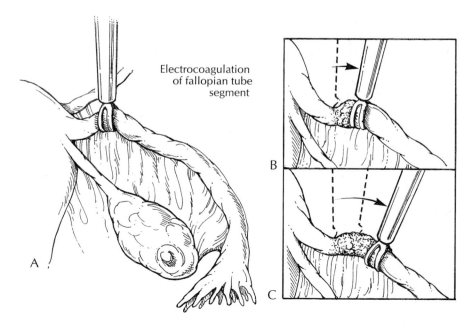

Electrocoagulation
of fallopian tube
segment

Fig. 35-10. (A–C) Bipolar Electrodesiccation of laparoscopic sterilization.

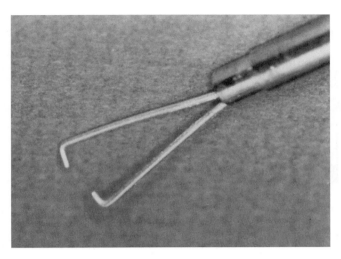

Fig. 35-11. Distal end of tubal ring applicator showing grasping prongs.

Falope rings can be placed on a conical device that stretches them sufficiently to permit transfer to the applicator. The handle is then squeezed slowly, which causes the outer cylinder to push the ring over the tubal segment that has been drawn within the inner cylinder. The applicator is designed to draw a 2.5-cm tubal segment into the inner cylinder.

The Falope ring (Falope Ring Band, Cabot Medical, Langhorne, PA) is made of a nonreactive silicone rubber that incorporates a solution of 5 percent barium sulfate to permit radiologic identification. The ring is 2.2 mm thick with an outer diameter of 3.6 mm and an inner diameter of 1 mm (Fig. 35-13). If not stretched to more than 6 mm, it possesses a specific elastic power with a recovery of 90 to 100 percent.

After the laparoscope has been inserted, the pelvis visualized, and the tubes identified, the preloaded ring applicator is placed through the operating channel of an operating laparoscopic or through a suprapubic puncture. The grasping forceps is extended, and the fallopian tube is grasped approximately 2 to 3 cm distal to the uterotubal junction (Fig. 35-14A). The tube should not be grasped next to the uterus because the lack of tubal mobility may cause a laceration of the tube or formation of an inappropriate knuckle of tube. If the distal third of the tube is grasped, incomplete tubal occlusion may occur, as the tubal diameter in this area is larger. Because of the larger diameter it is also more difficult to obtain a complete knuckle of tube above the ring. Once the tube is drawn into the inner sleeve the handle is squeezed slowly and the ring is pushed off the applicator and onto the tube (Fig. 35-14B). If the tubal ring has been applied correctly, a 1.0-cm high knuckle of tube will be seen above the ring, and both the distal and proximal tubal segments can be seen entering the tubal ring (Fig. 35-14C). The ring functions to occlude the blood supply to the tubal knuckle and, over a period of several days, necrosis takes place and the tubal segments separate.

If the tube is drawn into the inner cylinder too quickly, tubal transection can occur. This is usually signaled by a clicking sound. If this occurs, a tubal band can be placed on

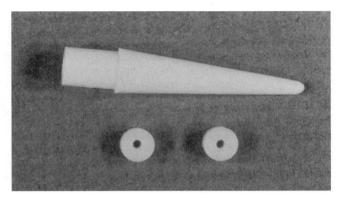

Fig. 35-13. Tubal band.

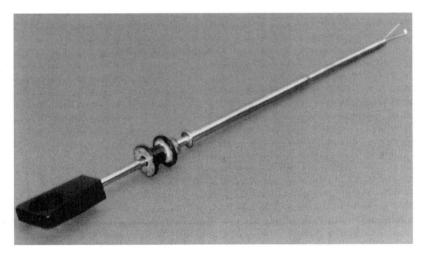

Fig. 35-12. Tubal ring applicator showing piston grip.

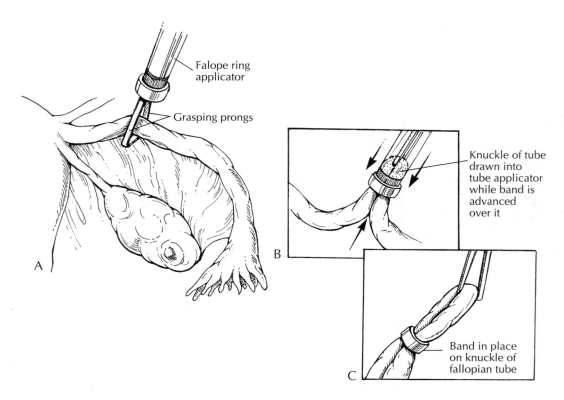

Falope ring applicator

Grasping prongs

Knuckle of tube drawn into tube applicator while band is advanced over it

Band in place on knuckle of fallopian tube

Fig. 35-14. (A–C) Tubal ring sterilization by laparoscopy.

the proximal and distal tubal segments or electrocoagulation can be used to destroy both the proximal and distal tubal segments. On occasion, a tubal band may fall off the applicator before it has been applied to the tube. If this occurs, the band can be retrieved. However, if the band cannot be visualized, it can be left in the abdominal cavity and will cause not problems. Yoon[40] has described a three-grasp technique, which was designed to compensate for the thickened fallopian tube. The tube is grasped as it normally is and retracted toward the applicator. It is then released and regrasped 1 cm proximal and distal to the original area and retracted partially into the applicator. This will bend the edematous tube so it can be grasped in its normal position and retracted fully into the applicator.

Clip

Several types of clips have been used for tubal occlusion. Currently, the only clip that is approved by the Food and Drug Administration for use in the United States is the Hulka-Clemens clip (Hulka-Clemens, Richard Wolf, Rosemont, IL). The spring-loaded clip was devised in an effort to have a simpler and more reversible method of sterilization.[38] After completion of the initial studies, the clips were distributed to several clinics throughout the world. One thousand patients underwent this form of sterilization and were followed for 6 months. Of 24 pregnancies reported, 11 were

due to clip misapplication and 3 were due to a defect in clip manufacturing.[41] This series was later updated to include a 1-year follow-up, and the report emphasized the importance of clip placement.[42] In another study, women were followed for up to 3.5 years. The failure rate in this study was 3.7 percent, with three of the failures occurring after 1 year.[43]

Two methods for clip application are available. An operating laparoscope is available that has been designed espe-

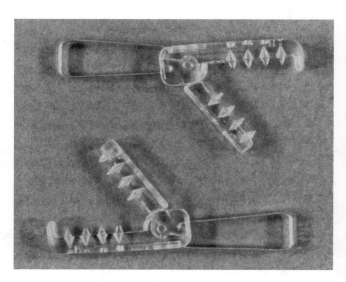

Fig. 35-15. Hulka-Clemens clip.

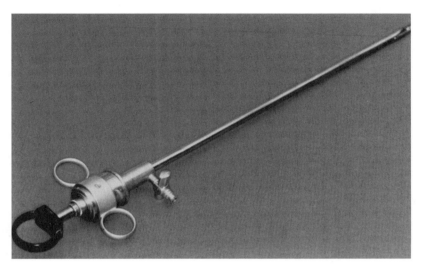

Fig. 35-16. Spring-loaded clip applicator.

cially for clip application. Alternatively, and just as effectively, the clip applier can be placed through a secondary trocar site. The Hulka clip consists of two toothed jaws made of lexan plastic, joined by a metal hinge pin. The lower jaw possesses a distal hook. A gold-plated spring maintains the clip in an open position. When completely advanced, the spring closes and locks the jaws (Fig. 35-15). The applicator is 7 mm in diameter with a three-ring configuration at the handle. At the end of the applicator, there is a fixed lower jaw to accommodate the clip. When the handle is retracted, a mobile upper jaw permits placement of the open clip, and when advanced, closes the clip. A center piston, when totally advanced, locks the spring. Until that point, the jaws may be opened and closed as many times as needed (Fig. 35-16).

The Hulka clip was designed to be applied at a right angle to the isthmic portion of the tube, or about 2 to 3 cm from the cornu. If the clip is placed in a more distal tubal segment, there is a higher chance that the clip will not be effective, due to the increased volume of tissue and the larger tubal lumen that must be occluded. The clip should be placed at a right angle to the tube, and across the complete diameter of the tube (Fig. 35-17A). Once secured in place and released from the applicator, its position should again be verified (Fig. 35-17B). If the clip is not properly placed, a second clip can be applied adjacent to the first (Fig. 35-17C).

Chromopertubation After Laparoscopic Tubal Occlusion

Chromopertubation is a method of transcervcial injection of dye to assess tubal patency, and is advocated by some authors after laparoscopic sterilization.[44] In addition, some surgeons have performed hysterosalpingograms in an effort to document tubal occlusion.[45,46] Hysterosalpingography, although generally well tolerated, is expensive and has been implicated in the development of fistulas, sterilization failure, and the development of pelvic inflammatory disease. Paper[47] documented recovery of bacteria from the peritoneal cavity in 90 percent of women undergoing chromopertubation during laparoscopy. However, none of the patients developed a postoperative infection. It is thought by some that chromopertubation might lead to an increase in the development of endometriosis, as endometrial cells can be recovered from the peritoneal cavity following chromopertubation.[48–50] Jordan et al[46] reported 22 patients who had chromopertubation at sterilization, 6 of whom had intraoperative dye spill and additional electrocoagulation. Five patients still had patent tubes at follow-up hysterosalpingography. These authors were the first to state that chromopertubation was contraindicated following electrocoagulation and that any test of tubal patency should be delayed for a minimum of 12 weeks. A real problem with hysterosalpingogram is that the tubes may indeed be patent, yet the hysterosalpingogram demonstrates occlusion because of tubal spasm or lack of tubal filing. Even if the follow-up hysterosalpingogram demonstrates tubal patency, some authors haven shown the risk of subsequent pregnancy to be very low, suggesting that anatomic distortion and tubal dysfunction, or delayed tubal fibrosis may be partially responsible for the action of the tubal sterilization.[51–53] In fact, the tube may be patent following ring application once the tube necrosis and the segments separate. A potential advantage of chromopertubation at the time of sterilization is that if there is dye spill, corrective action can be taken to ensure tubal occlusion. At the time of chromopertubation, there does not appear to be an associated dislodgement of the occluding devices, or a change in position of these devices, or dye spillage from the occlusion sites. However, in a study of 500 consecutive patients, there was no difference in the overall failure rate whether the patient did or did not undergo chromopertubation.[54]

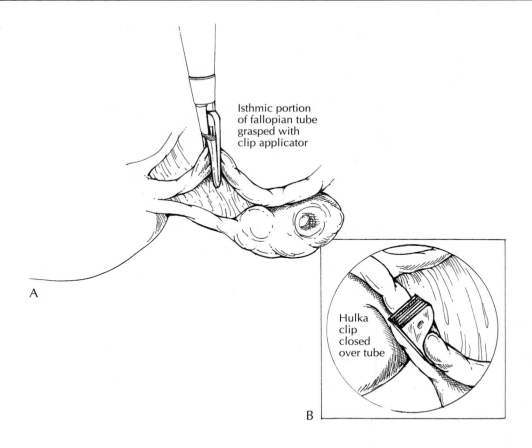

Isthmic portion
of fallopian tube
grasped with
clip applicator

A

Hulka
clip
closed
over tube

B

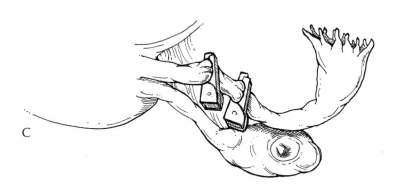

C

Fig. 35-17. (A) Clip method of laparoscopic sterilization. (B) Correct placement of spring-loaded clip. (C) Placement of a second clip if first clip does not completely occlude the tube.

Laparoscopic Sterilization Under Local Anesthesia

The largest series of sterilization procedures was reported by Mehta[55] in which 250,136 procedures were performed by a single operator using Fallope rings applied by laparoscopy under local anesthesia. The procedures were performed in India in sterilization camps and represent an incredible report. The author says that with good teamwork, the number of women sterilized was generally 40 to 50/hr. There were 12 deaths, not all attributable to the procedure, for a mortality rate of 4.8 per 100,000; eight major complications required laparotomy for a major complication rate of 3.2 per 100,000.

The use of local anesthesia has also been described by numerous other investigators.[56–58] Local anesthesia offers important advantages over general anesthesia, such as avoidance of risks associated with general anesthesia, decreased anesthesia time, lower cost, rapid recovery, earlier awareness

Table 35-2. Drugs Used During Laparoscopic
Sterilization Under Local Anesthesia

Drug	Dose	Time of Administration
Ibuprofen	800 mg	Oral 30 min before procedure
Atropine	0.4–0.6 mg	Intravenous on arrival in operating room
Midazolam HCl	2.5 mg	Intravenous in divided doses during preparation
Fentanyl	0.05–0.1 mg	Intravenous during preparation
Fentanyl or alfentanil	0.5–1.0 mg	Intravenous as needed for pain during procedure

of complications, and less nausea and vomiting. Patients who desire to can actually observe her procedure and therefore will have a better understanding of what is being done. Although most patients undergoing laparoscopy can have the procedure done under local anesthesia, it can also be used for patients in whom general anesthesia is a relative contraindication. Certain patients may be less suitable candidates for sterilization under local anesthesia, including those with known adhesive disease or massive obesity, since these patients may require longer operative time, more tissue dissection, or the surgeon may encounter difficulty placing the laparoscopic trocar. Local anesthesia may also not be ideal for the patient who is excessively anxious or nervous for obvious reasons.

The key to a successful procedure is the use of proper preoperative and intraoperative medication so that the procedure remains relatively painless. Table 35-2 outlines the dose and time of administration of the various medications used. The procedure is similar to the procedure performed when using general anesthesia. The patient is placed in the lithotomy position, and a warmed single-hinged speculum is placed in the vagina and the cervix is cleaned with a prewarmed povidone-iodine solution. A Hulka uterine manipulator is inserted into the uterine cavity and attached to the anterior cervical lip. If the uterus is retroverted, the manipulator is placed along the uterine axis and then rotated 180 degrees (Fig. 35-18). A 25-gauge, 1-in. needle is used to injected 5 ml of 0.5 percent bupivacaine hydrochloride (HCl) into the infraumbilical skin (Fig. 35-19A). Once the skin has been anesthetized, a 22-gauge, 3.5-in. spinal needle is used to create a diamond-shaped fascial block. One milliliter of 0.5 percent bupivacaine HCl is injected at each corner and in the center of the diamond, which will be the point of fascial entry (Fig. 35-19B). The skin incision is made using a #11 scalpel, and a hemostat is used to enlarge the incision slightly. The periumbilical trocar is inserted using either an indirect or direct technique. The abdomen is insufflated using a rate of 1 L/min, and the uterus is slowly manipulated to expose the right fallopian tube. Although some investigators are of the opinion that nitrous oxide is associated with less intraoperative and postoperative pain, a randomized comparison of nitrous oxide and carbon dioxide pneumoperitoneum showed no difference.[59] Once visualized, 5 ml of 0.5 percent bupivacaine HCl is sprayed over and under the tube and round ligament. Using this amount of bupivacaine is not associated with toxic or near toxic serum levels.[60] The use of intraperitoneal lidocaine has been shown to reduce postoperative pain and provides long-lasting analgesia.[61] This procedure is repeated on the opposite side. The sterilization procedure is then completed using either electrocoagulation, a Falope ring, or a Hulka clip. If electrocoagulation is used, the current is applied in an intermittent fashion to prevent heat buildup and pain. Electrocoagulation has been thought to be associated with less pain.[62,63] Again, using a randomized trial format, the pain associated with the use of electrocoagulation and silastic rings was compared when both procedures were performed under local anesthesia. Silastic rings were preferable. This group had a shorter operating time and required less intraoperative anesthesia. There was no difference in the report of pain following sterilization.[64] Following the procedure, the patient is asked to cough or bear down (the Valsalva Maneuver) to remove as much

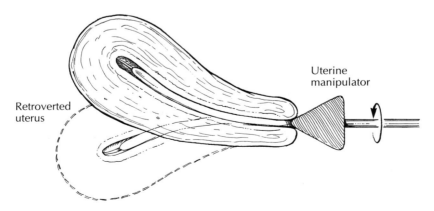

Fig. 35-18. Placement of uterine manipulator.

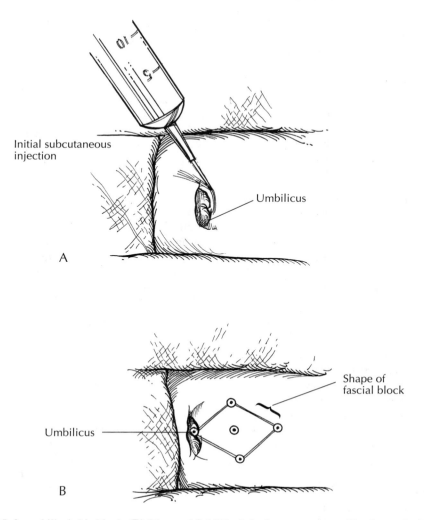

Initial subcutaneous injection

Umbilicus

A

Shape of fascial block

Umbilicus

B

Fig. 35-19. (**A**) Infraumbilical skin block. (**B**) Diamond field block for laparoscopic sterilization under local anesthesia.

gas as possible. The trocar valve should only be opened when the patient is increasing her intra-abdominal pressure so that atmospheric air does not enter the abdomen and cause peritoneal irritation.

Care should be taken not to oversedate the patient, as it may lead to loss of the gag reflex and airway control, as well as increase the potential for aspiration. Pain can be diminished by using adequate preoperative medication and sedation, a good fascial and field block, and gentle uterine and pelvic organ manipulation. During the procedure it is helpful to talk the patient and provide reassurance, and to tell the patient when she might feel uterine movement or experience discomfort.[64–66]

The cost of the procedure has also been analyzed and compared with the cost of the procedure using general anesthesia. The average cost of the procedure performed under general anesthesia was nearly twice the cost of the procedure performed using local anesthesia. The procedure is even less expensive if performed in an office setting, which has been advocated by some investigators.[67]

Vaginal Sterilization

The development of laparoscopy led to a virtual disappearance of the vaginal route for tubal sterilization. The reported increase of postoperative pelvic infections following vaginal sterilization when compared with laparoscopic methods also contributed to the decreased use of this technique.[68,69] This study was done before the time when prophylactic antibiotics were recommended. Smith et al[70] found comparable rates of morbidity with laparoscopic and vaginal sterilization when prophylactic antibiotics were used routinely. The vaginal approach is particularly helpful in very obese patients or patients who have an umbilical hernia or previous umbilical hernia repair. Relative contraindications include multiple pelvic surgical procedures, endometriosis, known pelvic adhesive disease, or uterine immobility on examination.

The patient is placed in the dorsal lithotomy or knee-chest position. A right-angle or Dever retractor is used to expose the cervix, which is grasped on its posterior lip with a single-

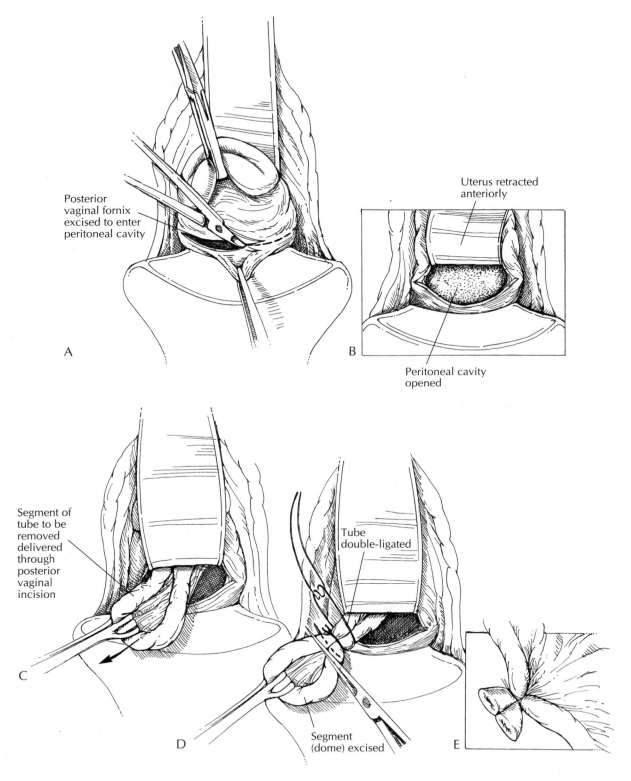

Posterior vaginal fornix excised to enter peritoneal cavity

A

Uterus retracted anteriorly

B

Peritoneal cavity opened

Segment of tube to be removed delivered through posterior vaginal incision

C

D

Tube double-ligated

Segment (dome) excised

E

Fig. 35-20. (A–E) Vaginal tubal sterilization.

tooth tenaculum (Fig. 35-20A). The posterior cul-de-sac is exposed, and a colpotomy incision is performed using Mayo scissors (Fig. 35-20B). The tips of the scissors are placed in the peritoneal opening and spread to enlarge the incision. The anterior retractor is placed posterior to the cervix just inside the incision and is elevated (Fig. 35-20C). This maneuver results in retroflexion of the uterus. The fallopian tube is grasped with a Babcock clamp and brought into the operative field (Fig. 35-20D). The sterilization can be accomplished using tubal bands, electrocautery, or clips.[71] However, the most common method described is the use of the Pomeroy technique[72] (Fig. 35-20E). Once completed, the colpotomy incision is closed using interrupted figure-of-eight sutures or a single running suture of an absorbable suture material.

Intraoperatively, the most common problem encountered is difficulty in exposing the fallopian tube. Placing the anterior retractor too deeply into the incision will antevert the uterus rather than cause uterine retroflexion. Suprapubic pressure can be used to facilitate uterine retroversion. Postoperatively, pelvic infection is the most serious potential complication following vaginal sterilization. Therefore, a single dose of a prophylactic antibiotic should be administered approximately 30 minutes before the procedure.

TEACHING/LEARNING LAPAROSCOPIC STERILIZATION

There is no question that if the methods of sterilization are applied incorrectly, the subsequent failure rate will be increased. There is then a certain knowledge base that is necessary to ensure that the operator is familiar with the prescribed methods of sterilization. If the surgeon does not know these facts, it has been shown to be correlated to the overall sterilization failure rate.[73,74] A training model was developed, which included an instructional videotape with an accompanying monograph that detailed basic laparoscopic techniques and sterilization techniques. When residents were required to complete this training module and demonstrate their knowledge by completing a written test, the sterilization failure rate decreased.[75] When this same multiple choice test was administered to a group of practicing obstetrician/gynecologists who routinely perform the procedure, none of the practitioners performed at the level required by the residents before performing the procedure.[76] Although this information does not mean that practicing gynecologists should not be performing laparoscopic tubal sterilization, it does suggest that a formalized teaching module is helpful.

STERILIZATION FAILURE

Few other events are more distressing for the surgeon and the patient than a surgical procedure that does not result in its anticipated outcome. Although all of the methods of sterilization have an inherent risk of failure, it is important to understand why such failures might occur. If this is known, then the failures themselves might be preventable. Soderstrom[77] performed 47 laparoscopic sterilization procedures on patients who had previously been sterilized. At laparoscopy, chromopertubation was used to document tubal patency. The resection methods failed most frequently because of spontaneous reanastomosis or fistula formation. All nine failures following fimbriectomy failed because a remnant of fimbriaovarica was left and spontaneous reanastomosis occurred. All bipolar failures demonstrated intact serosa, coagulated muscularis, and a viable endosalpinx. All the unipolar sterilization failures were found to have fistulas. The tubal ring failures showed lack of separation of the tubal segments with fistula formation. There were also two cases of operator failure in which the occluding device was placed on the round ligament. There were six Weck clip sterilization failures. These clips were not designed for sterilization and should not be used for this purpose. In an analysis of 32 failures, Thompson and Wheeless[78] reported similar findings.

Technical failures or failures associated with the equipment or the inability to complete the procedure by laparoscopy can occur. Risk factors associated with technical failure include obesity, prior use of an intrauterine device, and previous pelvic surgery.[79]

An ectopic pregnancy can occur following tubal sterilization. Kjer and Knudsen[80] reviewed a group of 10,104 sterilization procedures. A total of 54 pregnancies occurred during the 5-year follow-up period, 41 (76 percent) of which were ectopic pregnancies. Thus, when a pregnancy occurs following sterilization it is important to determine the location of the pregnancy as soon as practical. This is also an important aspect of patient education. All patients undergoing a sterilization procedure should be warned about the possibility of ectopic pregnancy and should be told that they should seek medical care as soon as they realize that they are pregnant.

Luteal phase pregnancy, or a pregnancy that is diagnosed after a tubal sterilization is performed in the luteal phase but in which conception occurred before the sterilization, is another form of sterilization "failure." Actually, this is not a sterilization failure. To reduce the number of such occurrences, the procedure can be performed in the follicular or menstrual phase of the cycle. Since this is not always possible, the use of a sensitive pregnancy test on the day of the procedure has also been shown to decrease the number of luteal phase pregnancies.[81] The use of concurrent dilation and curettage at the time of sterilization does not lower the risk of luteal phase pregnancy.[82] If called on to perform a repeat sterilization after a previous sterilization has failed, it is helpful to document the findings carefully. If photographs can be taken, these can be very helpful. It is most helpful to resect the tube and subject it to careful histologic analysis to determine whether a fistula has formed. If an occluding method was used, it is helpful to measure the tubal length and determine which portion of the tube was destroyed. If electrocoagulation was used as the primary sterilization method, a Mallory trichrome stain should be performed to document the extent of previous coagulation. If the Hulka clip was used, its correct placement (2 to 3 cm from the cornu and at a 90-degree angle to the tubal axis) should be documented.

SAFETY OF TUBAL STERILIZATION

Large reviews of sterilization procedures have documented the safety of the procedure.[83,84] Deaths secondary to tubal sterilization were reviewed by Peterson et al[85] between 1977 and 1981. During this time 29 deaths occurred; 11 followed complications of general anesthesia, 7 were due to sepsis, 4 were due to hemorrhage, 3 were due to myocardial infarction, and 4 deaths were related to other causes.

COMPLICATIONS

Cohen[86] followed all women undergoing tubal ligation in 1974 in one Canadian province to determine the rates of subsequent hysterectomy. At 2 years, there was no increase in adverse gynecologic outcomes. After 2 years, there was a 1.6 percent rise in the hysterectomy rate for women aged 25 to 29. For women age 30 and over at the time of sterilization, tubal ligation was not a risk factor for subsequent hysterectomy.[87] This was confirmed by Rulin[88] who noted a higher hysterectomy rate among previously sterilized women. The reason for this association is unclear. There were no long-term effects on menses or pelvic pain. In general, there appears to be no change in duration of menstrual bleeding, menstrual cycle length, cycle regularity, amount of menstrual bleeding, menstrual pain, or intermenstrual bleeding.[88–90]

REFERENCES

1. Lungre SS: A case of cesarean section twice successfully performed on the same patient with remarks on the time, indications, and details of the operation. Am J Obstet Gynecol 14: 76, 1881
2. Anderson ET: Peritoneoscopy. Am J Surg 35:136, 1937
3. Steptoe PC: Laparoscopy in Gynaecology. E. and S. Livingston Ltd., Edinburgh, 1967
4. Wheeless CR Jr: Elimination of second incision in laparoscopic sterilization. Obstet Gynecol 39:134, 1972
5. Irving FC: A new method of insuring sterility following cesarean section. Am J Obstet Gynecol 8:335, 1924
6. Husbands ME, Pritchard JA, Pritchard SA: Failure of tubal sterilization accompanying cesarean section. Am J Obstet Gynecol 107:966, 1970
7. Rioux JE, Cloutier D: A new bipolar instrument for laparoscopic tubal sterilization. Am J Obstet Gynecol 119:737, 1974
8. Hulka JF, Omran KF: Comparative tubal occlusion: rigid and spring loaded clips. Fertil Steril 23:633, 1972
9. Yoon IB, Wheeless CR, King T: A preliminary report of a new laparoscopic sterilization approach: the silicone rubber band technique. Am J Obstet Gynecol 120:132, 1975
10. Whitcare FE, Loeb WM, Loeb L: The timing for postpartum sterilization. Am J Obstet Gynecol 52:1041, 1946
11. Rozier JR: Immediate postpartum tubal ligation. Am J Obstet Gynecol 117:226, 1973
12. Lu T, Chun D: A long-term follow-up study of 1055 cases of postpartum tubal ligation. J Obstet Gynaecol Br Emp 74:875, 1967
13. Black WP, Sclare EBB: Sterilization by tubal ligation—a follow-up study. J Obstet Gynaecol Br Commonw 75:219, 1968
14. Green LR, Laros RK: Postpartum sterilization. Clin Obstet Gynecol 23:647, 1980
15. Lipscomb GH, Spellman JR, Ling FW: The effect of same-day pregnancy testing on the incidence of luteal phase pregnancy. Obstet Gynecol 82:411, 1993
16. Grubb GS, Peterson HB, Layde PM, Rubin GL: Regret after decision to have a tubal sterilization. Fertil Steril 44:248, 1985
17. Henshaw SK, Singh S: Sterilization regret among U.S. couples. Fam Plann Perspect 18:238, 1986
18. Phillips JM, Hulka JF, Hulka B et al: 1979 American Association of Gynecologic Laparoscopists membership survey. J Reprod Med 26:529, 1981
19. Allyn DP, Leton DA, Westcott NA et al: Presterilization counseling and women's regret about having been sterilized. J Reprod Med 31:1027, 1986
20. Wilcox LS, Chu SY, Eaker ED et al: Risk factors for regret after tubal sterilization: 5 years of follow-up in a prospective study. Fertil Steril 55:927, 1991
21. Vessey M, Huggins G, Lawless M et al: Tubal sterilization: findings in a large prospective study. Br J Obstet Gynaecol 90:203, 1983
22. Divers WA: Characteristics of women requesting reversal of sterilization. Fertil Steril 41:233, 1984
23. Wiston RML: Why 103 women asked for reversal of sterilisation. BMJ 2:305, 1977
24. Sherman PA, Burigo JA: Comparison of laparoscopic falope-ring and minilaparotomy sterilization. Obstet Gynecol 63:71, 1984
25. Penfield AJ: Minilaparotomy for female sterilization. Obstet Gynecol 54:184, 1979
26. Lee RB, Boyd JAK: Minilaparotomy under local anesthesia for outpatient sterilization: a preliminary report. Fertil Steril 33:129, 1980
27. Bishop E, Nelms WF: A simple method of tubal sterilization. NY State J Med 30:214, 1930
28. Fox MD, Long CA, Meeks GR et al: Laparoscopic pomeroy tubal ligation as a teaching model for residents. J Reprod Med 39:862, 1994
29. Murray JE, Hibbert ML, Heth SR, Letterie GS: A technique

for laparoscopic pomeroy tubal ligation with endoloop sutures. Obstet Gynecol 80:1053, 1992

30. Uchida H: Uchida tubal sterilization. Am J Obstet Gynecol 121:153, 1975

31. Kroener WF: Surgical sterilization by fimbriectomy. Am J Obstet Gynecol 104:247, 1969

32. Aldridge AH: Temporary surgical sterilization with subsequent pregnancy. Am J Obstet Gynecol 27:741, 1934

33. Palmer R: Instrumentation et technique de la coelioscopie gynecologique. Gynecol Obstet (Paris) 46:420, 1947

34. Rioux JE, Quesnel G, Blanchet J et al: Laparoscopie: sterilisation tubaire: etude de 1,000 cas et evaluation globale de la methode. Union Med Can 102:1865, 1973

35. Yuzpe AA, Rioux JE, Lofer FD, Pent D: Laparoscopic tubal sterilization by the 'burn only' technique. Obstet Gynecol 49:106, 1977

36. Soderstrom RM: Electrical safety in laparoscopy. p. 306. In Philips JM (ed): Endoscopy in Gynecology. American Association of Gynecologic Laparoscopists Downey, CA, 1967

37. Black WP: Sterilization by laparoscopic tubal electrocoagulation: an assessment. Am J Obstet Gynecol 111:979, 1971

38. Yoon IB, King TM, Parmley TH: A two-year experience with the Falope ring sterilization procedure. Am J Obstet Gynecol 127:109, 1977

39. Yoon I, Poliakoff SR: Laparoscopic tubal ligation: a follow-up report on the Yoon falope ring methodology. J Reprod Med 23:76, 1979

40. Poliakoff SR, Yoon IB, King TM: A four year experience with the Yoon Ring. In Phillips JM (ed): Endoscopy in Gynecology. American Association of Gynecologic Laparoscopists, Downey, CA, 1978

41. Hulka JF, Omran KF, Phillips JM et al: Sterilization by spring clip: a report of 1000 cases with a 6-month follow-up. Fertil Steril 26:1122, 1975

42. Hulka JF, Mercer JP, Fishburne JI et al: Spring clip sterilization: one-year follow-up of 1,079 cases. Am J Obstet Gynecol 125:1039, 1976

43. Griffin WT, Mandsager NT: Spring clip sterilization: long-term follow-up. South Med J 80:301, 1987

44. Aubert JM, Garcia A: Improving Falope-ring application in laparoscopic training. J Reprod Med 32:340, 1987

45. Steptoe PC: Recent advances in surgical methods of control of fertility and infertility. Br Med Bull 26:60, 1970

46. Jordan JA, Edwards RL, Person J, Maskery PJK: Laparoscopic sterilization and follow-up hysterosalpingogram. J Obstet Gynaecol Br Commonw 78:460, 1971

47. Paper RJD, Ahmet Z, Houang ET: Bacteriological contamination during laparoscopy with dye injection. Br J Obstet Gynaecol 95:367, 1988

48. Kulenthran A, Jeyalakshmi N, Path M: Dissemination of endometrial cells at laparoscopy and chromopertubation—a preliminary report. Int J Fertil 34:256, 1989

49. Peterson EP, Behgrman SL: Laparoscopic tubal sterilization. Am J Obstet Gynecol 110:24, 1972

50. Sheikh HH: Hysterosalpingographic follow-up of laparoscopic sterilization. Am J Obstet Gynecol 126:181, 1976

51. Ayers JW, Johnson RS, Ansbacher R et al: Sterilization failures with bipolar cautery. Fertil Steril 42:526, 1984

52. Cook CL: Evaluation of ring sterilization by hysterosalpingogram. J Reprod Med 27:243, 1982

53. Grunert GM: Late tubal patency following tubal ligation. Fertil Steril 35:406, 1981

54. Lipscomb GH, Stovall TG, Summitt RL Jr, Ling FW: Chromopertubation at laparoscopic tubal occlusion. Obstet Gynecol 83:725, 1994

55. Mehta PV: A total of 250,136 laparoscopic sterilizations by a single operator. Br J Obstet Gynaecol 96:1024, 1989

56. Poindexter AN, Abdul-Malak M, Fast JE: Laparoscopic tubal sterilization under local anesthesia. Obstet Gynecol 75:5, 1990

57. Bordahl PE, Raeder JC, Nordentoft J et al: Laparoscopic sterilization under local or general anesthesia? A randomized study. Obstet Gynecol 81:137, 1993

58. Peterson HB, Hulka JF, Spielman FJ et al: Local versus general anesthesia for laparoscopic sterilization: a randomized study. Obstet Gynecol 70:903, 1987

59. Lipscomb GH, Summitt RL Jr, McCord ML, Ling FW: The effect of nitrous oxide and carbon dioxide pneumoperitoneum on operative and postoperative pain during laparoscopic sterilization under local anesthesia. J Am Assoc Gynecol Laparosc 2:57, 1994

60. Lipscomb GH, Summitt RL Jr, McCord ML, Ling FW: Serum bupivacaine levels during laparoscopic sterilization using local anesthesia. J Am Assoc Gynecol Laparosc 2:27, 1994

61. Benhamou D, Narchi P, Mazoit JX, Fernanadez H: Postoperative pain after local anesthetics for laparoscopic sterilization. Obstet Gynecol 84:877, 1994

62. Pelland PC: The application of lidocaine to the fallopian tubes during tubal fulguration by laparoscopy. Obstet Gynecol 47:501, 1976

63. Gordon AC: Laparoscopy under local anesthesia. J R Soc Med 77:540, 1984

64. Lipscomb GH, Stovall TG, Ramanatha JA, Ling FW: Comparison of silastic rings and electrocoagulation for laparoscopic tubal ligation under local anesthesia. Obstet Gynecol 80:645, 1992

65. Fishburne JI: Office laparoscopic sterilization with local anesthesia. J Reprod Med 18:233, 1977

66. Penfield AJ: Laparoscopic sterilization under local anesthesia. Obstet Gynecol 49:735, 1977

67. Handa VL, Berlin M, Washington AE: A comparison of local and general anesthesia for laparoscopic tubal sterilization. J Women Health 3:135, 1994

68. Lee JG, Randal JH, Keettel WC: Tubal sterilization: a review of 1,169 cases. Am J Obstet Gynecol 62:568, 1951

69. Miesfield RR, Giarratano RC, Moyers TG: Vaginal tubal ligation: is infection a significant risk? Am J Obstet Gynecol 137:183, 1980

70. Smith RP, Maggi CS, Nolan TE: Morbidity and vaginal tubal cautery: a report and review. Obstet Gynecol 78:209, 1991

71. Hartfield VJ: Female sterilization by the vaginal route: a positive reassessment and comparison of four tubal occlusion methods. Aust NZ J Obstet Gynaecol 33:408, 1993

72. Hartfield VJ: Day care Pomeroy sterilization by the vaginal route. NZ Med J 85:223, 1977

73. Stovall TG, Ling FW, Henry GM, Ryan GM Jr: Method failures of laparoscopic tubal sterilization in a residency training program: a comparison of the tubal ring and spring-loaded clip. J Reprod Med 36:283, 1991

74. Stovall TG, Ling FW, O'Kelley KR, Coleman SA: Gross and histologic examination of tubal ligation failures in a residency training program. Obstet Gynecol 76:46, 1990

75. Stovall TG, Ling FW, Lipscomb GH et al: A model for resident surgical training in laparoscopic sterilization. Obstet Gynecol 83:470, 1994

76. Lipscomb GH, Stovall TG, Ling FW: Basic laparoscopic knowledge among gynecologic laparoscopists. Am J Obstet Gynecol 171:1455, 1994

77. Soderstrom RM: Sterilization failures and their causes. Am J Obstet Gynecol 152:395, 1985

78. Thompson BH, Wheeless CR: Failures of laparoscopy sterilization. Obstet Gynecol 45:659, 1975

79. Chi I, Mumford SD, Laufe LE: Technical failures in tubal ring sterilization: incidence, perceived reasons, outcome and risk factors. Am J Obstet Gynecol 138:307, 1980

80. Kjer JJ, Knudsen LB: Ectopic pregnancy subsequent to laparoscopic sterilization. Am J Obstet Gynecol 160:1202, 1989

81. Lipscomb GH, Spellman JR, Ling FW: The effect of same-day pregnancy testing on the incidence of luteal phase pregnancy. Obstet Gynecol 82:411, 1993

82. Grubb GS, Peterson HB: Luteal phase pregnancy and tubal sterilization. Obstet Gynecol 66:784, 1985

83. Peterson HB, Lubell I, DeStefano F, Ory HW: The safety and efficacy of tubal sterilization: an international overview. Int J Gynaecol Obstet 21:139, 1983

84. Peterson HB, DeStefano F, Greenspan JR, Ory HW: Mortality risk associated with tubal sterilization in United States hospitals. Am J Obstet Gynecol 143:125, 1982

85. Peterson HB, DeStefano F, Rubin GL et al: Deaths attributable to tubal sterilization in the United States, 1977 to 1981. Am J Obstet Gynecol 146:131, 1983

86. Cohen MM: Long-term risk of hysterectomy after tubal sterilization. Am J Epidemiol 125:410, 1987

87. Rulin MC, Davidson AR, Philliber SG et al: Long-term effect of tubal sterilization on menstrual indices and pelvic pain. Obstet Gynecol 82:118, 1993

88. DeStefano F, Huezo CM, Peterson HB et al: Menstrual changes after tubal sterilization. Obstet Gynecol 62:673, 1983

89. Bhiwandiwala PP, Mumford SD, Feldblum PJ: Menstrual pattern changes following laparoscopic sterilization with different occlusion techniques: a review of 10,004 cases. Am J Obstet Gynecol 145:684, 1983

90. Bhiwandiwala PP, Mumford SD, Feldblum PJ: Menstrual pattern changes following laparoscopic sterilization: a comparative study of electrocoagulation and the tubal ring in 1,025 cases. J Reprod Med 27:249, 1982

CHAPTER THIRTY-SIX

DIAGNOSIS AND SURGERY FOR BENIGN OVARIAN DISEASE

FIDEL A. VALEA

OOPHORECTOMY

Oophorectomy may be indicated for a wide variety of pathologic conditions, depending on the patient's age and the specific concerns. The role of prophylactic oophorectomy at the time of hysterectomy continues to be a controversial issue. The most recent statement by the American College of Obstetricians and Gynecologists on this topic is that it should be individualized and that dogmatic recommendations should be avoided.[1] The mean age of menopause in the United States is about 51 years of age, with 95 percent confidence intervals between ages 45 and 55 years.[2] Coulam et al[3] report that only 3.8 percent of patients that were still premenopausal by age 40 became menopausal by age 45. Despite this, there are still gynecologists that offer prophylactic oophorectomy at the time of a hysterectomy after the age of 40. Advantages to the prophylactic removal of the ovaries include the potential reduction in the number of deaths due to ovarian cancer and the number of reoperations for ovarian pathology, as well as a decrease in the potential symptomatology of continued ovarian function. The disadvantages of routine removal include the need for hormone replacement to relieve the associated symptoms of surgical castration such as vasomotor symptoms, a potential decrease in self image, osteoporosis, increased cardiovascular risk, and possibly a decrease in libido attributed to a decrease in testosterone normally produced by the ovary. If one considers the complexity of postmenopausal hormone replacement and problems with patient compliance, it is clear that the prophylactic removal of the ovaries should be individualized.

Advantages of Prophylactic Oophorectomy

The major argument in favor of prophylactic oophorectomy is decreasing the risk of ovarian cancer. The American Cancer Society estimates that in 1996 there will be 26,700 new cases of ovarian cancer, and 14,800 deaths attributable to this disease.[4] It is still estimated that the lifetime risk of developing ovarian cancer is 1 in 70, and most of these

Possible Indications for Oophorectomy

- Ovarian malignancies
- Adnexal torsion with necrosis
- Tubo-ovarian abscess unresponsive to antibiotics
- Postmenopausal solid or complex mass
- Definitive surgery for endometriosis
- Prophylactic removal
- Male pseudohermaphrodites (gonadectomy)

Table 36-1. Reoperation on Residual Ovaries

Study (Year)	No. of Hysterectomies With Retained Ovaries	No. Reoperated	Percentage Reoperated
Ranney (1977)	1,557	14	0.9
Grogan (1955)	391	19	5.1
Funt (1977)	922	13	1.4
Bukovsky (1988)	329	6	1.8
Christ (1975)	6,188	202	3.3
Total	9,387	254	2.7

women present with advanced disease.[5] However, outside of age, there may be other risk factors that can influence the decision to prophylactically remove the ovaries.

It has been proposed that either a high fat diet or exposure to talc may increase the relative risk of developing ovarian cancer.[6-9] In addition, hereditary conditions such as site-specific ovarian cancer syndrome, Lynch II cancer family syndrome, and breast-ovarian cancer syndrome can be associated with risks as high as 50 percent.[10,11] If a woman has two first-degree relatives that developed early onset ovarian cancer, she should be considered at high risk and have her ovaries removed prophylactically after childbearing is complete. It is more common for a patient to have only one first-degree relative, or several other relatives with ovarian cancer, and her risk is probably elevated, although how much is not known. Of interest is that true hereditary ovarian cancer probably represents less than 4 percent of all ovarian cancers. In addition, a history of breast, colon, or endometrial cancer also increases the risk of developing ovarian cancer.[5]

Another situation in which prophylactic oophorectomy should be considered is when dealing with colonic cancer. Barber[5] states that ovarian metastases were encountered in 25 percent of patients with an adenocarcinoma of the gastrointestinal tract when they were carefully examined, and in about 50 percent of these, the metastases were occult. Given these figures, it seems that oophorectomy should be considered in these patients, especially as they approach the perimenopausal years.

Although it seems logical that oophorectomy would decrease the possibility of developing ovarian cancer, it does not offer full protection from this type of malignancy. Tobacman et al[12] followed 28 high-risk women after prophylactic oophorectomies and noted the occurrence of intraperitoneal carcinomatosis that was indistinguishable from ovarian cancer in 3 of them. In these patients, it is believed that the entire coelomic cavity is at risk and they may represent cases of primary peritoneal carcinoma. These cancers are histologically very similar to ovarian cancers, but appear to arise in an extraovarian site.[13-15] Hence, oophorectomy alone may

not completely eliminate the risk. In the 5 years between 1988 and 1993, 19 such cancers were treated at this author's hospital (University Medical Center at Stony Brook).

The final advantage of prophylactic oophorectomy is to decrease the risk of future surgery or treatment of symptomatology related to the retained ovary. The incidence of reoperation on a residual ovary varies from 0.9 to 5.1 percent.[16-20] These data suggest that approximately 2.7 percent of patients who have one or both ovaries preserved at the time of a hysterectomy will require reoperation for symptoms related to the ovary (Table 36-1). Most of patients who require surgery do so because of pain, a pelvic mass, or dyspareunia. Over one-half of these patients will require the second operation within 5 years of the hysterectomy.[20] Although prophylactic removal of the ovaries at the time of a hysterectomy may have its advantages, patients must participate in the decision to remove apparently normal ovaries.

Disadvantages of Prophylactic Oophorectomy At Hysterectomy

Clearly, in a postmenopausal woman undergoing a hysterectomy, prophylactic removal of both ovaries has many of the advantages listed above. However, prophylactic removal in a premenopausal woman may have shortcomings. Once a premenopausal woman has undergone oophorectomy, she will require the initiation of hormonal therapy earlier than usually expected in order to treat the symptoms of menopause. Although these symptoms can be disabling at times, it is the long-term risks such as coronary artery disease, osteoporosis, and its associated fractures that require long-term therapy. However, which estrogen and in what dosage it should be given is far from uniform. In fact, there is evidence that the addition of a progestin and sometimes even an androgen may be beneficial. There is no clear benefit to adding a progestin in a woman who has had a hysterectomy, but there are physicians who still do so because of the theoretical risk of breast cancer. Estrogen replacement therapy does not increase the risk of breast cancer.[21]

Other potential problems with the use of postmenopausal

hormonal therapy include the various contraindications to their use. Patients with acute and chronic liver disease and acute vascular thrombosis are not the best candidates for hormonal therapy. Despite prior fears, most patients with endometrial and many patients with breast cancer can safely receive estrogen replacement therapy. One must weigh the advantages of preventing osteoporosis and coronary artery disease against the theoretical risk of estrogens increasing the risk of recurrent disease. However, patients who will not comply with the potential therapy may best be served by preservation of ovarian function to provide as much protection from osteoporosis and coronary artery disease as possible.

The decision to perform elective oophorectomy is a complex one. Many factors should be evaluated, including the patient's age, parity, associated medical problems, various risk factors, family history, and most importantly, her desires. Usually it is the patient's age and proximity to natural menopause that dictate this practice. Although the decision ultimately rests with the patient, it is important that the physician adequately educate the patient and prepare her for the sequelae of her decision.

Surgical Technique

Oophorectomy, either unilateral or bilateral, is a fairly straightforward procedure as long as the pelvic anatomy is well known. The classical oophorectomy is performed through an abdominal incision, although more recently, the laparoscopic approach has gained wide acceptance.

Open Technique

After entering the abdominal cavity with either a transverse or midline incision, the infundibulopelvic ligament and the ureter are identified. The peritoneum is incised parallel to the ovarian vessels and the retroperitoneal space is entered. Alternatively, the round ligament can be divided to enter the retroperitoneal space. Using blunt dissection with a finger or preferably, meticulous sharp dissection with Metzenbaum scissors, the broad ligament is opened and the ureter identified on its medial, or posterior, leaf. Once its relationship to the ovarian vessels is confirmed, the ovarian vessels are elevated, doubly clamped, and divided, and the pedicles are doubly ligated to ensure hemostasis (Fig. 36-1). Elevating the ovarian vessels, which lie in close proximity to the ureter at the level of the pelvic brim, allows for good visualization of the ureter before dividing the vessels.

If the ovary is to be removed alone and the fallopian tube is to be preserved, the multiple tubal branches of the ovarian artery should be clamped and ligated inferior and parallel to the fallopian tube in a systematic fashion. This separates the ovary from the fallopian tube and allows clear visualization of the ovarian branch of the uterine artery. Finally, this too

should be clamped, divided, and ligated. If the tube is to be preserved, special care must be taken to avoid postsurgical tubal adhesions by using microsurgical techniques and fine absorbable suture material.

More commonly, the fallopian tube is removed with the ovary, and in this case, both the ovarian and fallopian tube branches of the uterine artery are clamped parallel and just lateral to the uterus. Once the ovary and tube has been excised, the pedicle is ligated. Some surgeons advocate performing a wedge resection of the fallopian tube stump and approximating the surrounding cornual edge of myometrium over the stump with a mattress stitch. This latter procedure is performed to decrease the chances of a uteroperitoneal fistula, to ensure hemostasis, and to prevent the theoretical risk of a cornual ectopic pregnancy if the patient is in her reproductive years.

Laparoscopic Technique

The recent advancements in laparoscopic surgery have uncovered a new frontier for abdominal surgery. The appropriately skilled surgeon is now able to perform procedures that, in the past, could only be performed via laparotomy. Oophorectomy is one of these procedures. There are several ways to perform an oophorectomy via the laparoscope. The most common of these is to use a pre-tied loop that can be introduced through a separate puncture site. The ovary is "slipped" through the loop, which is then cinched down around its vascular pedicles (Fig. 36-2). Usually, one uses 2 to 3 pre-tied loops around the pedicles and the adnexae is then excised distal to the cinched down loops. Before the placement of the loop, the adnexae must be free of adhesions and mobile. Occasionally, one must free the adnexae of adhesions and actually incise the mesosalpinx to allow for easy placement of the loop.

Another common method uses bipolar electrocautery. With this method the ovarian vessels are identified in the infundibulopelvic ligament, and with the ureter identified and clear of the ovarian vessels, the infundibulopelvic ligament is grasped with bipolar forceps and desiccated. The ligament is then transected with endoscopic scissors and the broad ligament incised up to the utero-ovarian ligament, or alternatively, the broad ligament can be electrocoagulated as well and then incised. The medial attachments of the adnexae to the uterus, including the blood supply, can also be dessicated with the bipolar forceps or tied off using endoscopic loop ties. The adnexae can now be safely excised. It is possible to preserve the fallopian tube with this method if one is careful not to injure it, and the mesosalpinx is divided, thus freeing up the ovary from the attachments to the fallopian tube. Another less popular method to perform laparoscopic oophorectomy is the use of endoscopic stapling devices to control the various attachments. Unfortunately, these are usually more difficult to manage and tend to be more expensive due to the cost of the stapling devices.

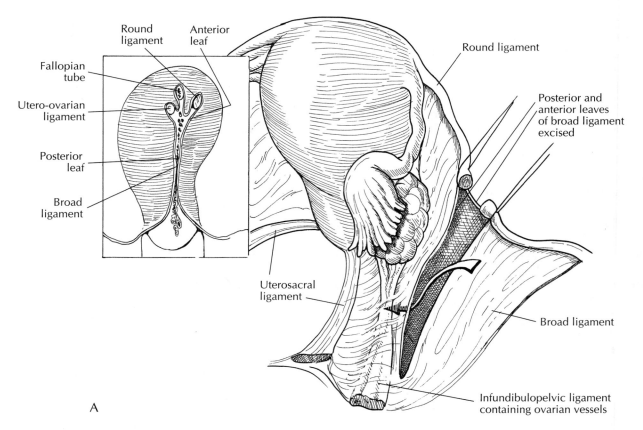

Fig. 36-1. Open oophorectomy. **(A)** The round ligament is divided and the retroperitoneal space entered. *(Figure continues).*

Laparoscopic oophorectomy is safe and offers the patient a quicker recovery time. However, one must not lose sight of the indications for oophorectomy when choosing the surgical approach. There are times when the more traditional open method is safer and more appropriate. In addition, operative laparoscopy can be technically more difficult than the open procedure and should only be attempted by those individuals with the appropriate training in operative laparoscopy. Ureteral injuries have been reported with laparoscopic oophorectomy when ureteral identification was either not performed, or performed incorrectly. Although the ureter can be seen through the peritoneum in many patients, in others, the peritoneum must be opened and varying degrees of dissection carried out to expose the ureter.

Open Versus Laparoscopic Management

One of the most debated issues in operative gynecology is the surgical management of the adnexal mass. Traditionally, these cases were managed with a laparotomy or at times a minilaparotomy. However, with the advances in laparoscopic surgery, more and more patients are being evaluated laparoscopically despite the lack of randomized clinical trials comparing the two procedures. The advantages of the laparoscopic technique are decreased recovery time and a theoretical decrease in the incidence of postoperative pelvic adhesive disease, especially if the oxidized regenerated cellulose membrane is used.[22] The disadvantages are potential spill if the mass is malignant and the inability to predict which masses are malignant on the basis of laparoscopic appearance.

The laparoscopic removal of a benign mass is as appropriate as the use of laparotomy to remove a malignant mass. How does one decide which approach should be used for a particular patient? At the current time there is no unequivocal way to determine the exact nature of an adnexal mass. Ultrasonography, and more specifically, vaginal probe ultrasonography has been used to determine the malignant potential of adnexal masses with mixed results. In their series, Herrmann et al[23] had a positive predictive value of 73 percent, but also had a 4.4 percent false-negative rate. However, of the 48 patients with a simple cystic mass that was less than 10 cm, none of these were malignant. This supports the beliefs of Rulin and Preston[24] who, after a retrospective evaluation of patients undergoing surgery for an adnexal mass, reported that not all postmenopausal women with simple cystic adnexal masses required surgery. In fact, in this select group of patients, the risk of malignancy was low. Parker

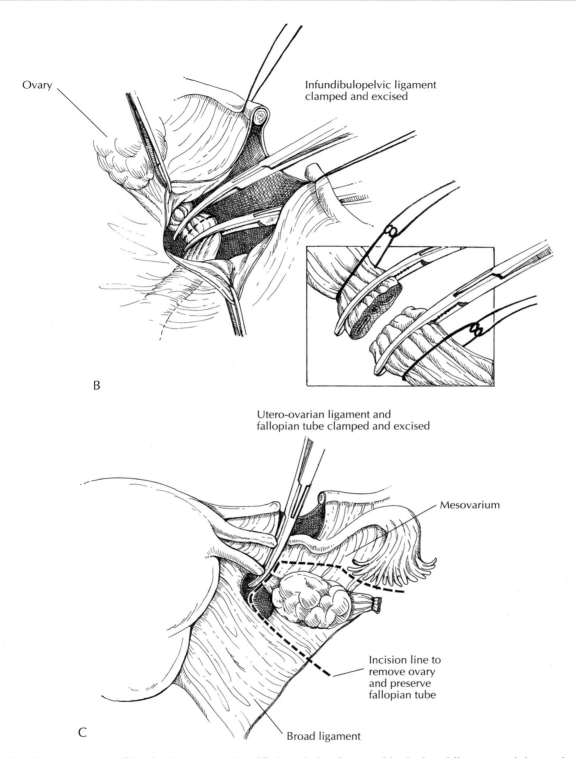

Ovary

Infundibulopelvic ligament
clamped and excised

B

Utero-ovarian ligament and
fallopian tube clamped and excised

Mesovarium

Incision line to
remove ovary
and preserve
fallopian tube

C

Broad ligament

Fig. 36-1 *(Continued).* **(B)** After the ureter is identified, a window is created in the broad ligament and the ovarian vessels are doubly clamped and divided. **(C)** The infundibulopelvic ligament (ovarian vessels) is then doubly ligated. **(D)** The medial attachments of the ovary are clamped and the adnexa is removed.

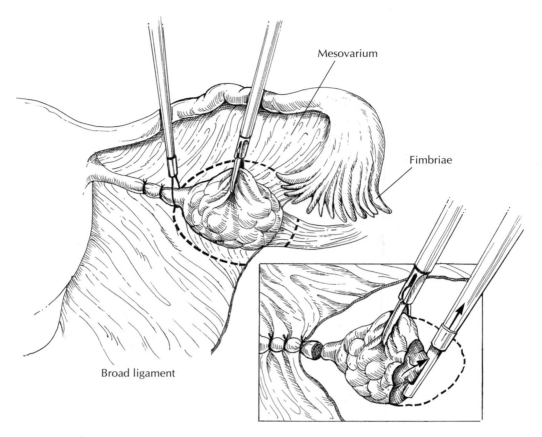

Mesovarium

Fimbriae

Broad ligament

Fig. 36-2. Laparoscopic oophorectomy. Two to three loops are placed around the ovary and cinched down across the ovarian vessels and the utero-ovarian ligament. The ovary is then excised distal to the last loop.

and Berek[25] took this one step further and performed laparoscopy on postmenopausal patients with simple cystic masses less than 10 cm with no other features suggestive of malignancy and CA-125 values of less than 35. In this series, all 25 patients were accurately predicted to have benign pathology and 22 were safely managed laparoscopically. This certainly supports the notion that some select patients can be managed laparoscopically.

What about the patients with noncystic masses or cysts that are not simple; how should these patients be approached? In the past, these patients underwent laparotomy. However, there is increasing sentiment to evaluate some of these with the laparoscope, with the assumption that most of them are benign. There should be no dogmatic recommendations for this group of patients and clinicians must individualize treatment according to their index of suspicion. The concerns associated with the use of laparoscopy in this setting are that, if a malignancy is encountered, the prognosis may be worsened by cyst rupture. This stems from the report of Webb et al[26] that cited cyst rupture as one of the factors that worsened the prognosis in early stage ovarian cancer. More recently, this has been questioned by Dembo et al.[27] They did not find that cyst rupture increased the risk of relapse in the early stage patient. In their series, tumor grade,

large volume ascites, and dense adhesions were the only predictive factors of relapse. However, a series of 79 stage I ovarian cancers was evaluated; 20 of these patients were stage Ic on the basis of tumor rupture at the time of surgery.[28] There were 36 patients with stage Ia tumors and 17 stage Ic patients on the basis of capsular invasion-serosal disease or positive ascites or washings. The overall recurrence rates were 20, 3, and 18 percent, respectively, for patients with stage Ic-ruptured, Ia, and Ic-capsular invasion-serosal disease. The authors concluded that intraoperative rupture of malignant epithelial neoplasms may worsen the prognosis in these patients. Hence, the theoretical risk of tumor spread by rupture of a malignant cyst appears to have some validity.

One must take into account the patient's age, medical condition, appearance of the mass, tumor markers, and the likelihood of malignancy when deciding on the proper operative management. Until laparoscopy has undergone the appropriate scientific evaluation, it should be reserved for those cases where the risk of malignancy is very low. Unfortunately, because of its popularity, this has not been the case. In addition, surgeons must know their limitations and should be well trained in operative laparoscopy before resorting to this treatment option. Finally, if a malignancy is encountered, the patient should either have the appropriate open surgical procedure or prompt access to a gynecologic oncologist for definitive care.

OVARIAN CYSTECTOMY

Ovarian cystectomy is the treatment of choice for a variety of pathologic and even some physiologic conditions that affect the ovary. It offers an advantage over oophorectomy in that it allows for preservation of ovarian function. However, cystectomy, either laparoscopic or as an open procedure, should be reserved for those cases that are clearly not malignant.

Indications

Follicular cysts represent one of the most common functional cysts of the ovary. In the rare situation that they do not resolve spontaneously, cystectomy (not oophorectomy) is the treatment of choice. Surgical intervention is usually reserved for those cysts that are 8 cm or greater or a cystic mass from 5 to 8 cm that persists for more than 8 weeks. In the properly chosen situation, laparoscopic cystectomy may be used. In a series of simple follicular cysts averaging 6 cm in diameter, DeWilde et al[29] found a 2 percent recurrence rate after laparoscopic fenestration as opposed to cystectomy.

Although less common than follicular cysts, corpus luteum cysts can be a critical reason for ovarian cystectomy because of their propensity to cause serious intra-abdominal hemorrhage.[30] Of concern is that 14 percent of persistent corpus luteum cysts treated with fenestration alone recurred.[29] Hence, fenestration of all physiologic cysts is discouraged.

Cystic teratomas represent the most common benign ovarian neoplasm in young women and are another common indication for ovarian cystectomy. These neoplasms may present as a solid or cystic mass, or as a combination. Although they can be fairly large at times, cystectomy is still the procedure of choice with preservation of as much ovarian cortex as possible. If the diagnosis of a dermoid is certain, laparoscopic cystectomy has been evaluated and is believed to be a safe alternative to an open cystectomy.[31] It is inappropriate to perform oophorectomy in a young woman with a cystic teratoma, as ovarian cortex can always be saved.

Lastly, ovarian endometriomas represent another condition that is best treated by cystectomy rather than oophorectomy. Except for the very small endometriomas, medical therapy is of little value in their management. They can frequently become rather large and bilateral; however, they remain amenable to ovarian cystectomy.

Surgical Technique

Open Cystectomy

Before actually performing the cystectomy, the normal relationship between the ovary and the other pelvic structures should be restored. All adhesions should be carefully divided to allow proper mobilization of the ovary. An elliptical incision is made over the thin ovarian cortex in the axis of the ovary and over its most dependent area (Fig. 36-3). The area adjacent to the fallopian tube and the fimbria ovarica should be avoided to limit potential injury to the fallopian tube. In addition, excessive handling of the ovary should be avoided, and the operative field should be kept moist to minimize the risk of adhesion formation.

After the initial incision, the back of the knife handle or dissection with Metzenbaum scissors can be used to develop the plane between the cyst wall and the ovarian cortex to shell out the cyst. Countertraction can be applied by placing an Allis clamp on the cortex. Every attempt should be made to remove the cyst intact, but if the cyst is ruptured, care should be taken to control the spill and avoid gross contamination of the abdominal cavity. This can usually be achieved by packing the surrounding areas with surgical packs and the defect in the cyst can be controlled with a carefully placed Kelly clamp. In the event of a cyst rupture, copious irrigation of the abdominal cavity is performed to decrease the risk of both pseudomyxoma peritonei and chemical peritonitis.

Occasionally the base of the cyst is very adherent to the ovarian stroma and requires sharp excision with Metzenbaum scissors or alternatively with electrocautery. After removal of the cyst, the deep tissues of the ovary can be reapproximated with interrupted fine absorbable mattress sutures (4–0 or 5–0) to obliterate the dead space, or left open if hemostasis is adequate. Special care should be taken to avoid sutures on the ovarian surface to decrease the risk of postoperative adhesion formation.

The ovarian cortex may appear thin and the natural tendency is to trim the cortex. This may remove viable ovarian tissue and should be avoided if at all possible. Alternatively, if the defect is hemostatic, it can be left to heal by secondary intention. Reoperation of these cases has revealed ovaries that have resumed normal shape and anatomic relationships despite their appearance at the initial surgery.

Recently, modified oxidized regenerated cellulose membranes (Interceed, TC7) applied over the ovarian defects have shown significant reductions in the incidence and severity of postoperative adhesion formation.[22]

Occasionally, large or multiple cysts may need to be resected and represent an interesting challenge to the surgeon. The same good surgical principles apply. The ovarian incision should be placed in the axis of the ovary preserving the anatomic relationships and avoiding proximity to structures such as the fimbria ovarica and the utero-ovarian ligament. The least number of incisions possible should be made and if sutures are placed they should not be exposed on the ovarian

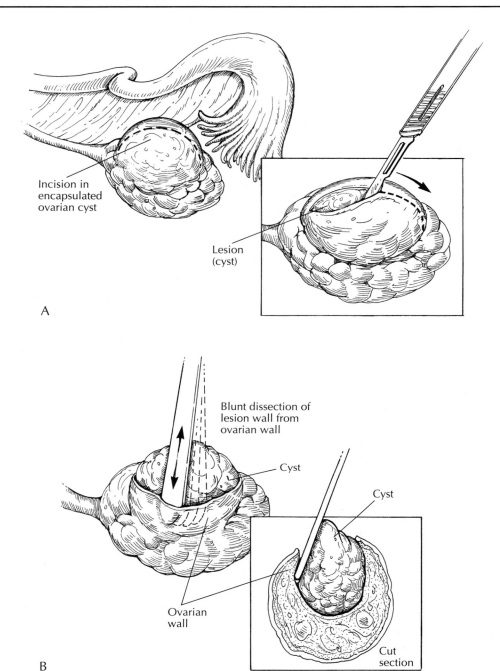

Incision in
encapsulated
ovarian cyst

Lesion
(cyst)

A

Blunt dissection of
lesion wall from
ovarian wall

Cyst

Cyst

Ovarian
wall

Cut
section

B

Fig. 36-3. Open cystectomy. **(A)** A thin incision is made in the axis of the ovary over its most dependent area. **(B)** The back of the knife handle is used to separate the cyst wall from the ovarian cortex. *(Figure continues.)*

surface. Even if the major portion of an ovary is removed, an oophorectomy should not be performed. Pregnancies have been reported in women with less than 25 percent of one ovary remaining.

Laparoscopic Cystectomy

Laparoscopic cystectomy can be performed in the appropriately selected patient. After induction of pneumoperitoneum, the laparoscope is inserted infraumbilically and other punc-

ture sites are placed in the midline suprapubically and 5 to 6 cm laterally on either side. The infraumbilical site is reserved for the camera, the midline suprapubic puncture site is generally used for suction/irrigation, and the lateral sites are used for stabilization of the ovary.

After a thorough inspection of the abdominal cavity and the ovarian cyst itself to confirm no suspicions of malignancy on gross visualization, the utero-ovarian ligament is grasped and the ovary stabilized. The cyst is then punctured

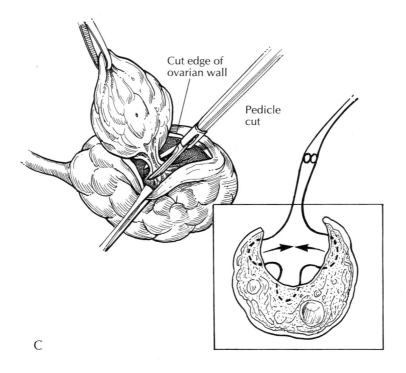

C

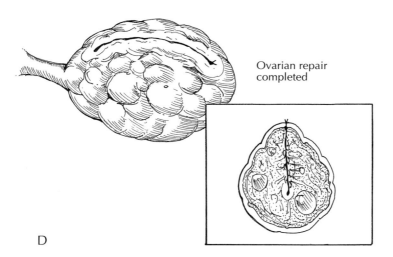

D

Fig. 36-3 *(Continued).* **(C)** Sharp excision to separate the base of the cyst from the ovary. **(D)** The deep tissues of the ovary are reapproximated using fine absorbable sutures avoiding the surface of the ovary. **(E)** The ovarian cortex is approximated with no visible sutures.

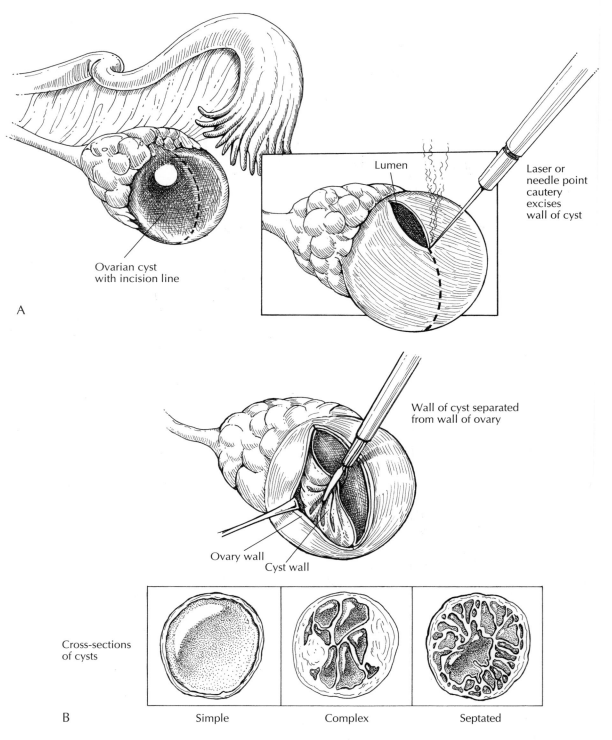

Ovarian cyst
with incision line

Lumen

Laser or
needle point
cautery
excises
wall of cyst

A

Wall of cyst separated
from wall of ovary

Ovary wall

Cyst wall

Cross-sections
of cysts

Simple

Complex

Septated

B

Fig. 36-4. Laparoscopic cystectomy. The cyst is punctured with a 16- to 18-gauge needle and the contents are aspirated (not shown). **(A)** The ovarian cortex is incised in the direction of the ovarian axis. **(B)** The cyst wall is grasped and blunt dissection used to separate the cyst wall from the ovarian cortex. *(Figure continues.)*

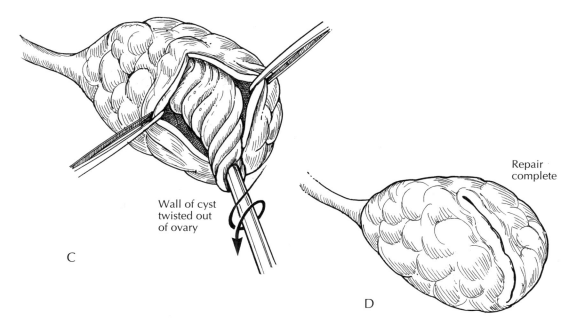

Wall of cyst
twisted out
of ovary

C

Repair
complete

D

Fig. 36-4 *(Continued).* **(C)** Alternatively, the cyst wall can be grasped and rotated to separate it from the ovarian cortex. **(D)** The cyst is removed and the ovary is left to heal by secondary intention.

with a 16- to 18-gauge needle and the cyst contents are aspirated, not only to control the contents of the cyst, but to facilitate its removal. The cystotomy is extended to allow introduction of a suction/irrigator and the cyst cavity is irrigated thoroughly. The cystotomy is then extended once again in the direction of the ovarian axis and the internal walls of the cyst are inspected. If no suspicious areas are encountered, the cyst wall is grasped and it is dissected off the ovarian stroma with blunt or sharp dissection using endoscopic scissors, a blunt probe, or even a laser. The forceps grasping the cyst wall can be rotated to assist in the dissection and actually peel away the cyst wall from the surrounding ovary (Fig. 36-4). Incomplete areas of excision can either be sharply excised or simply fulgurated to destroy the lining cells.

If the cyst bed is hemostatic it can be left to heal by secondary intention. As is the case with the open cystectomy, any suturing that is done should avoid the surface of the ovary. Oxidized regenerated cellulose (Interceed, TC7) can also be applied through the laparoscope in an attempt to deter adhesion formation.[32]

Open Versus Laparoscopic Cystectomy

With the advent of multiple puncture surgical laparoscopy, many patients previously requiring an open cystectomy can now be managed laparoscopically. The major advantages to laparoscopy are the decrease in recovery time, hospital stay, and possibly, adhesion formation, although these entities are poorly studied and little solid data confirm these statements. Certainly the removal of most benign

masses laparoscopically may be appropriate; however, it is difficult to predict which masses are benign before pathologic evaluation.[33] Clearly, the simple persistent cyst is likely to be benign and as such can be managed safely through the laparoscope. However, there is much debate as to what lesions can be safely managed through the laparoscope. Although Nezhat[31] reported on nine patients with dermoid cysts who were safely treated with laparoscopy, this does not justify this procedure as safe or as a standard of care. This presumes that the preoperative diagnosis of a dermoid cyst is accurate. The classical ultrasound findings of dermoids were found to occur in only one of three dermoids in the series of Laing et al.[34] Additionally, the percentage of patients undergoing a laparoscopic cystecomy that end up with oophorectomy because of the difficulty of this procedure is not known at this time. Calcified areas are particularly hard to remove laparoscopically.

Clearly, the laparoscopic approach to the adnexal mass should be investigated in prospective controlled trials to determine its safety and efficacy compared with the standard open procedures. Until the appropriate studies have been performed, surgeons must continue to use good judgment and be selective in the cases chosen for laparoscopic treatment. In the meantime, the criteria listed in the box are a reasonable guideline.

SURGERY FOR TUBO-OVARIAN/OVARIAN ABSCESS

The surgical treatment of acute pelvic inflammatory disease, including tubo-ovarian abscesses, although the mainstay of therapy for many years, has decreased immensely in

Criteria Used for the Operative Management of Ovarian Cystectomy

1. Simple physiologic cysts should be observed for 8 weeks before operative intervention, and laparoscopy is a reasonable treatment choice
2. Cysts that are complex should be removed and not fenestrated, given the possibility of malignancy and high recurrence rates
3. Cysts should not be drained into the peritoneal cavity
4. Findings suspicious for malignant warrant an open and not a laparoscopic evaluation
5. A solid adnexal mass that is small enough to be removed intact via colpotomy or via a laparoscopic bag can be evaluated by laparoscopy
6. A smooth appearance on the surface of the cyst does not exclude the possibility of a malignancy

recent years. With the various improvements in antibiotics and the enhanced concern about infertility, conservative management of the unruptured tubo-ovarian abscess has gained popularity.[35] Surgical treatment is reserved for ruptured tubo-ovarian abscesses, medical failures, and life-threatening infections when the diagnosis is unclear. Because of the various advancements of in vitro fertilization and other assisted reproductive technologies, conservative surgery with preservation of ovarian and uterine function has gained wide acceptance in women who have not completed childbearing. As such, unilateral removal of a tubo-ovarian abscess, colpotomy drainage of a cul-de-sac abscess, percutaneous drainage, and open drainage are all fairly common conservative therapies that preserve the reproductive organs.

Conservative Versus Extirpative Surgery

Approximately 50 percent of all patients admitted with a tubo-ovarian abscess will eventually require surgical treatment for the disease.[35,36] Despite this high rate of surgical intervention, no consensus exists as to the appropriate type of surgical intervention. In addition to the conservative surgical therapies listed above, total abdominal hysterectomy with bilateral salpingo-oophorectomy and even laparoscopic drainage have been used for the surgical treatment of this disease.

The drainage of a tubo-ovarian abscess through a posterior colpotomy is considered an effective method of treating patients presenting with a midline fluctuant collection that is dissecting the rectovaginal septum, when combined with appropriate antimicrobial therapy.[37–39] However, in Rivlin's series[39] of 59 patients, there were 2 (3 percent) deaths, both related to septic abortions, and 13 (22 percent) patients required further surgery during that same admission. This procedure is performed less frequently now because of the many treatment-related complications, and because most tubo-ovarian abscesses do not meet the criteria for vaginal drainage (i.e., midline fluctuant mass dissecting the rectovaginal septum). In addition, the high incidence of unilateral tubo-ovarian abscesses that are amenable to conservative surgery with preservation of fertility preclude its frequent use.

The colpotomy procedure itself requires general anesthesia with the patient in the dorsal lithotomy position. Generous exposure is also necessary to be able to adequately explore the abscess cavity. After the bladder is emptied and an examination confirms a fluctuant midline mass dissecting the rectovaginal septum, the posterior lip of the cervix is grasped with a tenaculum for adequate traction, and the vaginal mucosa is incised transversely. The cul-de-sac is entered and a Kelly clamp is used to bluntly enter the abscess and extend the vaginal incision. Appropriate cultures are obtained, the abscess cavity is explored (usually with the surgeon's finger), and all adhesions are broken down. A closed suction catheter or a mushroom catheter is left indwelling in the cavity and brought out through the vagina. For the more difficult cases, real-time ultrasonography may offer additional guidance. In Rivlin's series,[39] 12.5 percent of the potentially fertile patients were able to have successful pregnancies after colpotomy drainage of tubo-ovarian abscess.

Pedowitz and Bloomfield[40–42] reported that one-third of the patients thought to have unilateral disease had microscopic abscesses on the contralateral ovary, leading many authors to advocate the use of extirpative surgery with removal of both ovaries, tubes, and uterus. Although the complete extirpation of the reproductive organs is frequently curative, the more conservative unilateral salpingo-oophorectomy has gained acceptance because it offers the potential for future fertility. Recently, the reported incidence of unilateral disease has approached 70 percent in some cases—much higher than previously believed.[35,36] As such, more consideration has been given to conservative surgery with preservation of reproductive function. The big issue is whether these benefits outweigh the potential risks of reoperation and other complications.

Conservative surgery for unilateral tubo-ovarian abscesses has been evaluated by several authors.[35,36,43,44] Approximately 21 percent of patients with clinical evidence of tubo-ovarian abscess initially treated with antibiotics will require surgical intervention in the acute phase. In addition, 19 percent of the patients initially treated with conservative surgery will require a second procedure at a later date (Table 36-2). For comparison, none of the patients that had definitive surgery with hysterectomy and salpingo-oophorectomy in the series of Ginsberg et al[35] required subsequent surgery. However, 8.4 percent had bowel injuries. Clearly there is

Table 36-2. Summary of Conservative Surgery for
Tubo-ovarian Abscess

Study (No. of Patients)	No. With Conservative Surgery	No. Requiring Subsequent Surgery (%)
Landers (35)	19	1 (10.5)
Ginsberg (34)	5	1 (20)
Mickal (42)	8	1 (12.5)
Rivlin (43)	27	7 (26)
Total	59	11 (19)

morbidity from extirpative treatment as well as risk of subsequent surgery in the group treated conservatively. However, the conservative approach does offer potential for future fertility and preservation of hormonal function. In the series of Lander and Sweet,[36] approximately 14 percent of the patients with long-term follow-up achieved intrauterine pregnancies after conservative surgery. Unfortunately, the data on conservative surgical therapy for tubo-ovarian abscess are retrospective and have poor long-term follow-up. However, conservative surgery appears acceptable in the selected cases with unilateral involvement and when the patient desires future fertility.

Surgical Technique

Surgery for a tubo-ovarian abscess is frequently complicated by numerous inflammatory adhesions involving loops of bowel, bladder, and other pelvic structures. Often the normal tissue planes are distorted and the dissection can be both bloody and difficult. However, adhering to certain principles can minimize the difficulty of this operation.

First and foremost is the incision. A Pfannensteil incision, although aesthetically pleasing, is probably one of the more difficult incisions to use for this type of surgery. Exposure is paramount to dissect free the pelvic structures adequately and safely and to evaluate the abscess cavity properly. This incision has the disadvantage of limiting exposure both to the pelvis and the abdominal organs. A Maylard incision can still offer aesthetics, and allow for adequate exposure in the pelvis as well as the lower portion of the upper abdomen. More importantly, it allows for excellent pelvic sidewall exposure. A possible concern associated with this incision is the potential for subfascial fluid collections in an already infected scenario; however, this has not been a major problem. A vertical incision offers excellent exposure and the ability to easily extend the incision if necessary. The final decision as to which incision to chose should be individualized, taking into account the patient's body habitus, previous incisions, and the proposed operation.

Given the high likelihood of pelvic, as well as abdominal, adhesions in this type of surgery, careful restoration of normal anatomy should be undertaken before removal of any of the pelvic organs. At times, it is often useful to enter the retroperitoneal space and trace out the path of the ureter to prevent it from being injured. Before closing the abdomen, and preferably at the beginning of the case (to minimize potential contamination of the upper abdomen), the entire abdominal cavity should be explored to look for concealed collections of purulent fluid. Just before closing, copious amounts of irrigation with a warm saline solution should be used to dilute any possible contaminants. If a hysterectomy is performed, some believe it should be standard practice to suture the vaginal cuff open to allow adequate drainage of this area. Others advocate the use of a closed suction drain brought out through the vagina to improve the drainage of this area. The usefulness of these procedures has never been proved, and in the era of modern antibiotics, may be limited. Clearly, if an abscess cavity is just unroofed, it is not unreasonable to leave a closed suction drain in the cavity and bring it out through a separate stab incision. However, the routine use of a single closed suction device to drain the entire peritoneal cavity in the absence of an obvious pocket is suspect at best.

Many of these patients have gross contamination at the time of surgery, with subsequent poor or delayed healing of the skin and underlying fascia. As such, the fascia should be closed with a permanent monofilament suture such as nylon, Prolene, or even surgical wire to minimize the tissue reactivity in this area and offer long-lasting strength while the incision heals. More recently, the author and colleagues have used a long-lasting absorbable monofilament suture, Maxon, with excellent results. A delayed primary closure of the skin and underlying subcutaneous tissues is the best way to handle the grossly contaminated cases. Simple 3–0 nylon or Prolene sutures are placed in the skin edges approximately 1 cm back from the edge and 2 cm apart. These sutures are not tied, but are merely left long, and fine-mesh gauze is used to cover the subcutaneous tissues and the skin edges. This is then covered with a sterile dressing and left intact for 3 to 4 days, at which time the wound is uncovered and inspected. If the incision is clean, the loose sutures are tied and the edges reapproximated. In one series of 146 patients who had delayed primary closure, there were only 3 (2 percent) wound infections compared with a matched group of 146 patients who had immediate closure and subsequently 34 (23 percent) patients developed a wound infection.[45]

Percutaneous Drainage

Recently, there have been several reports of ultrasound-guided percutaneous drainage or aspiration of tubo-ovarian abscesses with excellent results.[46–48] In a series by Worthen and Gunning,[46] 35 patients underwent ultrasound-guided aspiration drainage or catheter drainage with a percutaneous technique. The success rate of aspiration alone was 94 percent and that of catheter drainage was 77 percent, although the catheter-drained patients tended to have larger and more complex abscesses. This is in agreement with the results of Tyrrel et al.[47] who had nine patients with tubo-ovarian abscesses who underwent computed tomography-guided percutaneous catheter drainage with an 88 percent success rate. In Teisala et al's series[48] of 10 patients, the ultrasound was used to guide the vaginal aspiration of the abscess cavities with complete resolution in all of the patients. Unfortunately, long-term sequelae, fertility rates, and ectopic pregnancy rates have not been adequately evaluated. However, this technique has shown promising results and, with further evaluation, may have a major role in the future.

Laparoscopic Approach

The laparoscopic treatment of tubo-ovarian abscesses has been used infrequently at this time. In Adducci's series[49] of nine patients, all were successfully managed with colpotomy drainage during laparoscopy. In another series 45 of 50 patients (40 percent) were adequately treated laparoscopically with drainage and irrigation of the abscess cavity.[50] In a recent series, Reich and McGlynn[51] used laparoscopy to lyse adhesions, excise necrotic tissue, and drain purulent fluid laparoscopically in 21 patients with tubo-ovarian abscess. One patient subsequently required an abdominal hysterectomy and bilateral salpingo-oophorectomy, for a success rate of 95 percent. In the few reported series, laparoscopic management of the tubo-ovarian abscess has shown good results. Laparoscopy requires copious irrigation (2 to 3 L) of the peritoneal cavity after draining the abscess. No drains are placed, but antibiotics are given for a prolonged period. This may become the standard of care. Subsequent laparoscopic "second looks" to lyse adhesions and ensure tubal patency may be indicated if fertility is desired.

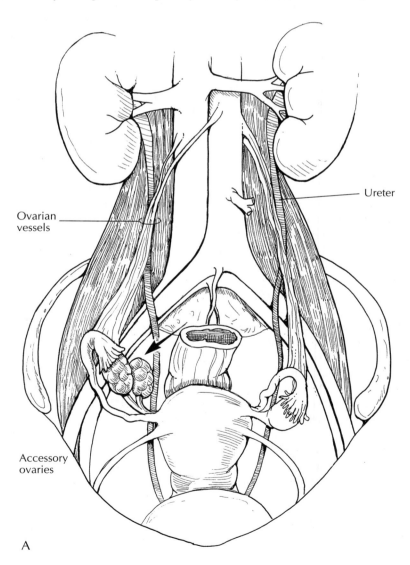

Ovarian vessels

Ureter

Accessory ovaries

A

Fig. 36-5. Disorders of normal ovarian development. **(A)** Accessory ovary with its medial attachments to the uterus. *(Figure continues.)*

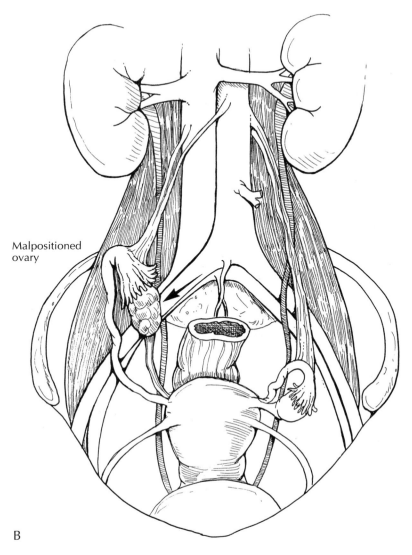

Fig. 36-5 *(Continued).* **(B)** Malpositioned ovary situated above the pelvic brim with an associated elongation of the fallopian tube and the utero-ovarian ligament. *(Figure continues.)*

OVARIAN REMNANT SYNDROME

The ovarian remnant syndrome should be considered a complication of oophorectomy. It occurs in patients who have undergone bilateral oophorectomy and subsequently present with a constellation of symptoms related to the ovulatory function of ovarian tissue inadvertently left behind. It should be distinguished from the residual ovary syndrome, which can present with similar symptoms, but here, the ovary was intentionally preserved and subsequently developed pathology. The typical patient presents with pelvic pain and a mass. The pain at times is cyclic, although many times it is persistent with acute flare-ups. Occasionally, a patient may present with an asymptomatic mass either on pelvic examination or on ultrasound examination of the pelvis. The most commonly associated conditions are endometriosis followed by pelvic inflammatory disease.

In one series, the authors suggest that there are three conditions that complicate the initial surgery and predispose to incomplete removal of all the adnexal tissue.[52] First is the existence of adhesive disease, which distorts the normal anatomy and makes the surgery tedious and difficult. The second condition is a neoplasm, and the third condition is increased pelvic vascularity at the time of initial surgery, which can predispose to hemorrhage, difficulty obtaining hemostasis, and timid attempts at resection.

The most ideal way to make the diagnosis is to check an follicle stimulating hormone (FSH) level. If it is in the premenopausal range and combined with a mass, an ovarian remnant probably exists. The surgical treatment of this dis-

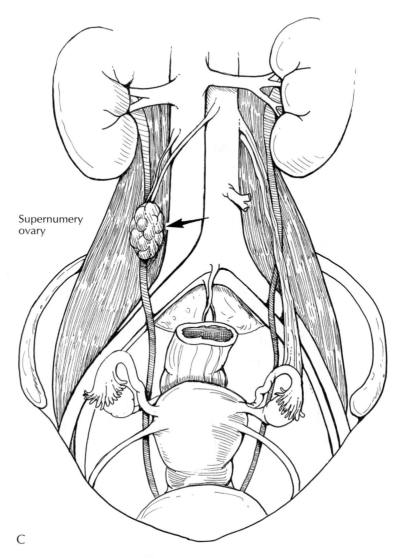

Supernumery ovary

Fig. 36-5 *(Continued).* **(C)** A supernumerary ovary situated near the midline with no attachments to the uterus.

ease is to excise the remaining ovarian tissue and its surrounding attachments. However, this procedure is usually difficult and requires meticulous dissection to delineate the normal anatomy in an otherwise abnormal pelvis. Perhaps the best approach is through the retroperitoneum. The ureter must be identified and dissected out depending on where the remnant is located. In addition, one may have to mobilize the bowel adequately to allow safe and easy access to the pelvic side wall. The remnant is usually encased in adhesions and frequently is retroperitoneal. Unless there is a definite mass or cyst present, the remnant may be difficult to delineate from the surrounding tissues. After several attempts, one such case was referred to the author and the remnant was superovulated before the operation, facilitating identification and successful excision. Laparoscopy should be considered by only the very skilled laparoscopists.

SURGICAL APPROACH TO THE MALDEVELOPED GONAD

Disorders of normal ovarian development can lead to a variety of conditions that include accessory, malpositioned, and supernumerary ovaries (Fig. 36-5), as well as complete failure of gonadal development (Fig. 36-6). An accessory ovary is usually found close to the normally positioned ovary, and it is attached to either the utero-ovarian ligament or the suspensory ligament of the ovary. By contrast, a malpositioned ovary is usually attached to the uterus by the utero-ovarian ligament and to the fallopian tube by the fimbria ovarica. Because this is usually a problem of ovarian descent, the ovary can be found anywhere along its usual path of anatomic descent. As such, the attachments to the ovary can be quite long at times. Fallopian tubes have been

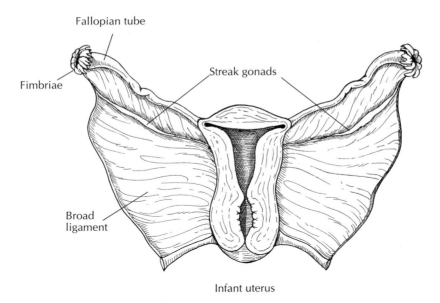

Fig. 36-6. Pelvic organs in a patient with complete failure of gonadal development. The bilateral streak ovaries can be found attached to the posterior broad ligament.

reported in excess of 20 cm in length.[53] A supernumerary ovary can be found anywhere but is usually found near the midline or lateral inbetween the normal position of the ovary and the kidney. The implications of the abovementioned conditions on reproductive life are not known at this time and routine removal is not recommended.

Failure of gonadal development is the most common cause of primary amenorrhea. It is most frequently due to a chromosomal disorder or deletion of parts of an X chromosome, in which case it is usually not inherited, but it can also be attributed to a genetic defect. For many years, it was believed that individuals with gonadal dysgenesis were at high risk of the development of ovarian tumors. After several reports, it is now known that the increased risk of malignancy is confined to individual with a Y chromosome in their karyotype.[54–57] Clearly, any phenotypic female with gonadal tissue that contains any component from the Y chromosome should have the gonads removed to avoid the risk of malignant tumors arising in this tissue (which has been reported to occur in 20 to 30 percent of patients).[57–60] The only exception to this rule is the patient with complete androgen insensitivity in which it is rare to develop a malignancy before 20 years of age. In one series, the risk of developing a malignancy before age 10 was estimated at no more than 3 percent.[61] It is usually recommended that the gonads in these patients be left in place until after puberty to allow for normal sexual development. After puberty, they should be removed.

The patient with gonadal dysgenesis associated with a Y chromosome should undergo bilateral gonadectomy or bilateral removal of the gonadal streaks. Occasionally, the gonadal streaks can be difficult to see (Fig. 36-6), making laparotomy the standard approach because of ease and

safety. Recently, there have been reports of laparoscopic management of the gonadal streaks, as well as the testes, in androgen insensitivity.[62–64] This clearly requires laparoscopic expertise and should not be attempted by those less experienced. As is the case with androgen insensitivity, the gonads can be very close to the external iliac artery, and can even be herniated into the inguinal canal. Special care must be taken to remove the gonad completely from the inguinal canal to ensure its complete excision. Occasionally, a small abdominal incision or a culdotomy is necessary to remove the gonad intact. There is no need to remove the uterus or the fallopian tubes. These organs can be preserved for the possibility of future fertility using donor-directed oocytes.

OOPHOROPEXY

Oophoropexy is a procedure that surgically secures the ovary in a fixed anatomic location so that it cannot freely return to its normal position. It is used in very few specific situations.

Oophoropexy is performed in an attempt to shield the normal premenopausal ovary from the damaging effects of radiation. The normal ovary does not tolerate a great deal of radiation, and the closer a woman is to menopause, the less radiation the ovary can tolerate before becoming permanently sterilized.[65–67] Thus, minimizing the dose of radiation received by the ovaries without altering the efficacy of tumor control is the primary goal of this procedure. In patients undergoing the standard inverted Y irradiation for Hodgkin's disease, reports of oophoropexy either lateral or medial to the treatment field have had reasonable success.[68,69] In one

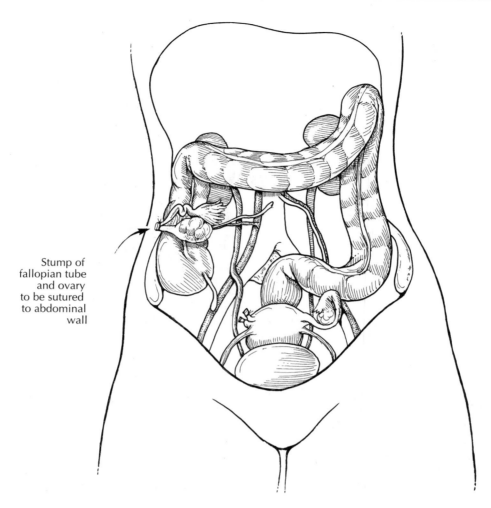

Stump of
fallopian tube
and ovary
to be sutured
to abdominal
wall

Fig. 36-7. Ovarian transposition (lateral oophoropexy). Final location of the transposed ovary brought out of the pelvis above and lateral to the psoas muscle.

series, 87 percent of the females undergoing treatment for Hodgkin's disease retained ovarian function.[70] In the series by Stillman et al,[71] of 182 survivors of childhood cancers, the only risk factor identified for subsequent ovarian failure was the location of the ovaries relative to the radiation treatment field.

Oophoropexy is used frequently in the surgical management of cervical cancer, either at the time of radical hysterectomy or at the time of lymph node dissection. In a recent series of 82 patients who received oophoropexy at the time of surgical management for cancer of the uterine cervix, only 33 percent of the patients who received postoperative radiation had continued ovarian function despite oophoropexy.[72] This is in contrast to the 84 percent who had continued ovarian function in the nonirradiated group. However, 17 percent of the patients who had oophoropexy and no radiation required removal of the ovary for persistent, severe pain, leaving only 65 percent with ovarian function. In another series of patients undergoing radical hysterectomy and

oophoropexy, 88 percent retained ovarian function but an additional 16 percent required surgery to remove the ovary.[67] When radiation is used after oophoropexy, persistence of ovarian function appears to be related to the final position of the ovary and the amount of radiation received. Clearly, the ovary separated from its attachments and blood supply from the uterus can survive, with perhaps a shorter life span than the ovary that is not transposed.

Another situation in which oophoropexy is used to preserve ovarian function is in the setting of torsion. If the ovary is salvageable, it should be oophoropexed to try and prevent recurrence of the torsion. Some believe that the contralateral ovary should have oophoropexy to prevent it from torsion as well.[73]

Recently, the use of oophoropexy to maintain access to the ovaries in the pelvis has been considered, especially for the patient considering oocyte retrieval. By fixing ovaries to the posterior aspect of the uterus, they can be easily accessed using endovaginal sonography and percutaneous aspiration.

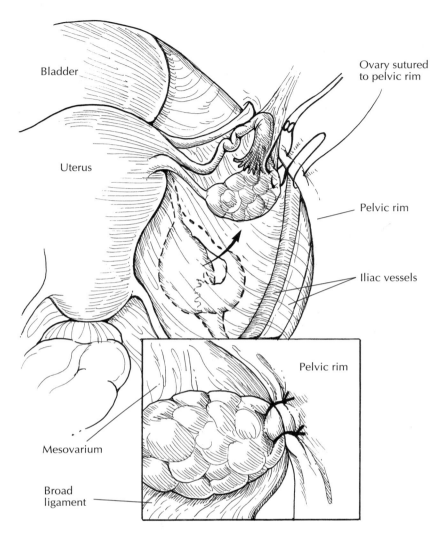

Fig. 36-8. Lateral oophoropexy for ovarian torsion. The ovary is sutured to the peritoneum of the pelvic sidewall with permanent sutures to prevent torsion.

However, the utility of this procedure and the long-term effects on the ovary are still not known.

There are numerous ways to perform oophoropexy, depending on the indication for the procedure. Oophoropexy is usually performed to move the ovaries either laterally or medially away from the radiation field.[68] The technique of medial oophoropexy involves placement of one or both ovaries and their vascular supply in the pelvic midline. This is accomplished by suturing the ovaries to the serosal surface of the posterior uterus as low as possible, after the medial attachments to the uterus have been divided.[68,69] Use of a stainless steel wire as the suture material allows good visualization of the ovaries and their relationship to the radiation field. Alternatively, the ovary can be marked with metalic surgical clips to allow for its easy identification on routine abdominal films. In the lateral oophoropexy, the ovaries and their attached vascular supply from the ovarian vessels are brought out of the pelvis and sutured lateral and perhaps

above the psoas muscle to get them out of the field of radiation (Fig. 36-7). Some would recommend using permanent suture for this procedure and not dividing any of the attachments.[74] This latter technique is best saved for the ovary at risk of torsion where the issue of pelvic irradiation is not present (Fig. 36-8).

An alternative approach for the ovary at risk of torsion is to shorten the supportive ligaments, thus creating a shorter limb for the ovary to "dangle" from and minimizing the risk of torsion in the process (Fig. 36-9). This latter approach avoids suturing the ovary directly, and, it is hoped, would minimize adhesion formation.

The procedures described above are usually performed using an open procedure, necessitating laparotomy. Although laparoscopy is not contraindicated, its role in this capacity has not been well studied. Clearly, in the hands of an experienced laparoscopist, many of these procedures can be done safely and probably with less recuperation time for

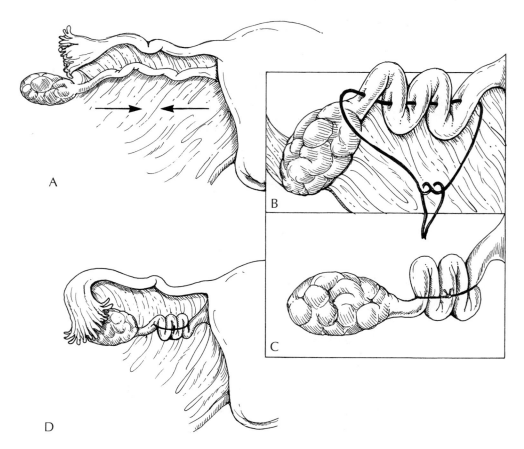

Fig. 36-9. Shortening of the utero-ovarian ligament. **(A–D)** The utero-ovarian ligament is sutured in a fashion that gathers it and effectively shortens its length in an attempt to prevent torsion.

the patient. The role of laparoscopic oophoropexy continues to evolve.

REFERENCES

1. American College of Obstetricians and Gynecologists: Technical Bulletin, No. 11, December 1987

2. Stanford JL, Hartage P, Brinton LA et al: Factors influencing the age at natural menopause. J Chron Dis 40:996, 1987

3. Coulam CB, Adamson SC, Annegers JF: Incidence of premature ovarian failure. Obstet Gynecol 67:604, 1986

4. Packer SL, Tong T, Bolden S, Wingo PA: Cancer statistics 1996. CA Cancer 46:8, 1996

5. Barber HRK: Ovarian cancer. Cancer 36:149, 1986

6. Cramer DW, Welch WR, Hutchinson GB et al: Dietary animal fat in relation to ovarian cancer risk. Obstet Gynecol 63:833, 1984

7. Byers T, Marshall J, Graham S et al: A case-control study of dietary and nondietary factors in ovarian cancer. J Natl Cancer Inst 71:681, 1983

8. Cramer DW, Welch WR, Scully RE et al: Ovarian cancer and talc: a case-control study. Cancer 50:372, 1982

9. Hartge P, Hoover R, Lesher LP et al: Talc and ovarian cancer, letter. JAMA 250:1844, 1983

10. Piver MS, Mettlin CJ, Tsukada Y et al: Familial ovarian cancer registry. Obstet Gynecol 64:195, 1984

11. Lynch HT, Guirgis HA, Albert S et al: Familial association of carcinoma of the breast and ovary. Surg Gynecol Obstet 138:717, 1974

12. Tobacman JK, Greene MH, Tucker MA et al: Intraabdominal carcinomatosis after prophylactic oophorectomy in ovarian-cancer-prone families. Lancet 2:795, 1982

13. Hertig AT: Case 14;49. Proceedings of the Eighteenth Seminar of the American Society of Clinical Pathology, Chicago, 1952

14. Swerdlow M: Mesothelioma of the pelvic peritoneum resembling papillary cystadenocarcinoma of the ovary. Am J Obstet Gynecol 77:197, 1959

15. Kannerstein M, Churg J, McCaughey WTE et al: Papillary tumors of the peritoneum in women: mesothelioma or papillary carcinoma. Am J Obstet Gynecol 127:306, 1977

16. Ranney B, Abu-Ghazaleh S: The future function and fortune of ovarian tissue which is retained in vivo during hysterectomy. Am J Obstet Gynecol 128:626, 1977

17. Grogan RH, Duncan CJ: Ovarian salvage in routine abdominal hysterectomy. Am J Obstet Gynecol 70:1277, 1955

18. Funt MI, Benigno BB, Thompson JD: The residual adnexa—asset or liability? Am J Obstet Gynecol 129:251, 1977

19. Bukovsky I, Liftshitz Y, Langer R et al: Ovarian residual syndrome. Surg Gynecol Obstet 167:132, 1988

20. Christ JE, Lotze EC: The residual ovary syndrome. Obstet Gynecol 46:551, 1975

21. Kaufman DW, Miller MS, Rosenberg L et al: Noncontraceptive estrogen use and the risk of breast cancer. JAMA 252:63, 1984

22. Interceed (TC7) Barrier Adhesion Study Group: Prevention of postsurgical adhesions by Interceed (TC7), an absorbable adhesion barrier: a prospective randomized multicenter clinical study. Fertil Steril 51:933, 1989

23. Herrmann UJ, Locher GW, Goldhirsch A: Sonographic patterns of ovarian tumors: prediction of malignancy. Obstet Gynecol 69:777, 1987

24. Rulin MC, Preston AL: Adnexal masses in postmenopausal women. Obstet Gynecol 70:578, 1987

25. Parker WH, Berek JS: Management of selected cystic adnexal masses in postmenopausal women by operative laparoscopy: a pilot study. Am J Obstet Gynecol 163:1574, 1990

26. Webb MJ, Decker DG, Mussey E et al: Factors influencing survival in stage I ovarian cancer. Am J Obstet Gynecol 116:222, 1973

27. Dembo AJ, Davy M, Stenwig AE et al: Prognostic factors in patients with stage I epithelial ovarian cancer. Obstet Gynecol 75:263, 1990

28. Sainz de la Cuesta R, Goff BA, Fuller AF et al: Prognostic importance of intraoperative rupture of malignant ovarian epithelial neoplasms. Obstet Gynecol 84:1, 1994

29. DeWilde R, Bordt J, Hesseling M et al: Ovarian cystostomy. Acta Obstet Gynecol Scand 68:363, 1989

30. Hallatt JG, Steele CH, Snyder M: Ruptured corpus luteum with hemoperitoneum: a study of 173 surgical cases. Am J Obstet Gynecol 149:5, 1984

31. Nezhat C, Winer WK, Nezhat F: Laparoscopic removal of dermoid cysts. Obstet Gynecol 73:279, 1989

32. Diamond MP, Cunningham T, Linsky CB et al: Laparoscopic application of Interceed (TC7) in the pig. J Gynecol Surg 5:145, 1989

33. Schwartz LB, Seifer DB: Diagnostic imaging of adnexal masses: a review. J Reprod Med 37:63, 1992

34. Laing FC, Van Dalsem VF, Marks WM et al: Dermoid cysts of the ovary: their ultrasonographic appearances. Obstet Gynecol 57:99, 1981

35. Ginsberg DS, Stern JL, Hamod KA et al: Tubo-ovarian abscess: a retrospective review. Am J Obstet Gynecol 138:1055, 1980

36. Landers DV, Sweet RL: Tubo-ovarian abscess: contemporary approach to management. Rev Infect Dis 5:876, 1983

37. Rubenstein PR, Mishell DR, Ledger WJ: Colpotomy drainage of pelvic abscess. Obstet Gynecol 48:142, 1976

38. Rivlin ME, Golan A, Darling MR: Diffuse peritoneal sepsis associated with colpotomy drainage of pelvic abscess. J Reprod Med 27:406, 1982

39. Rivlin ME: Clinical outcome following vaginal drainage of pelvic abscess. Obstet Gynecol 61:169, 1983

40. Pedowitz P, Bloomfield RD: Ruptured adnexal abscess (tuboovarian) with generalized peritonitis. Am J Obstet Gynecol 88:721, 1964

41. Nebel WA, Lucas WE: Management of tuboovarian abscess. Obstet Gynecol 32:381, 1968

42. Kaplan AL, Jacobs WM, Ehresman JB: Aggressive management of pelvic abscess. Am J Obstet Gynecol 98:482, 1967

43. Mickal A, Sellmann AH: Management of tubo-ovarian abscess. Clin Obstet Gynecol 12:252, 1969

44. Rivlin ME, Hunt JA: Ruptured tuboovarian abscess: is hysterectomy necessary? Obstet Gynecol 50:518, 1977

45. Brown SE, Allen HH, Robins RN: The use of delayed primary wound closure in preventing wound infections. Am J Obstet Gynecol 127:713, 1977

46. Worthen NJ, Gunning JE: Percutaneous drainage of pelvic abscesses: management of the tubo-ovarian abscess. J Ultrasound Med 5:551, 1986

47. Tyrrel RT, Murphy FB, Bernardino ME: Tubo-ovarian abscesses: CT-guided percutaneous drainage. Radiology 175:87, 1990

48. Teisala K, Heinonen PK, Punnonen R: Transvaginal ultrasound in the diagnosis and treatment of tubo-ovarian abscess. Br J Obstet Gynaecol 97:178, 1990

49. Adducci JE: Laparoscopy in the diagnosis and treatment of pelvic inflammatory disease with abscess formation. Int Surg 66:359, 1981

50. Henry-Souchet J, Soler A, Laffredo V: Laparoscopic treatment of tuboovarian abscesses. J Reprod Med 29:579, 1984

51. Reich H, McGlynn F: Laparoscopic treatment of tuboovarian and pelvic abscess. J Reprod Med 32:747, 1987

52. Symmonds RE, Petit P: Ovarian remnant syndrome. Obstet Gynecol 54:175, 1979

53. Rock JA, Parmley TP, Murphy AA et al: Malposition of the ovary associated with uterine anomalies. Fertil Steril 45:561, 1986

54. Scully R: Gonadoblastoma. Cancer 6:455, 1953

55. Teter J, Boczkowski K: Occurrence of tumors in dysgenetic gonads. Cancer 20:1301, 1967

56. Andrews J: Streak gonads and the Y chromosome. J Obstet Gynaecol Br Commonw 78:448, 1971

57. Dewhurst C, et al: Gonadal malignancy in XY females. J Obstet Gynaecol Br Commonw 78:1077, 1971

58. Simpson JL, Christakos AC, Horwith M et al: Gonadal dysgenesis in individuals with apparently normal chromosomal complements: tabulation of cases and compilation of genetic data. Birth Defects 7:215, 1971

59. Barr M, et al: Male pseudohermaphroditism and pure gonadal dysgenesis in sisters. Am J Obstet Gynecol 99:1047, 1967

60. Simpson JL, Photopulos G: The relationship of neoplasia to disorders of abnormal sexual differentiation. Birth Defects 12:15, 1976

61. Manuel M, Katayama KP, Jones HW Jr: The age of occurrence

of gonadal tumors in intersex with a Y chromosome. Am J Obstet Gynecol 124:293, 1976

62. Droesch K, Droesch J, Chumas J et al: Laparoscopic gonadectomy for gonadal dysgenesis. Fertil Steril 53:360, 1990

63. Shalev E, Zabari A, Romano S et al: Laparoscopic gonadectomy in 46XY female patient. Fertil Steril 57:459, 1992

64. Gililland J, Cummings D, Hibbert ML et al: Laparoscopic orchiectomy in a patient with complete androgen insensitivity. J Laparoendosc Surg 3:51, 1993

65. Ash P: The influence of radiation on fertility in man. Br J Radiol 53:271, 1980

66. Peck WS, McGreer JT, Kretzschmar NR et al: Castration of the female by irradiation: the results in 334 patients. Radiology 34:176, 1940

67. Chambers SK, Chambers JT, Kier R et al: Sequelae of lateral ovarian transposition in irradiated cervical cancer patients. Int J Radiat Oncol Biol Phys 20:1305, 1991

68. Ray GR, Trueblood HW, Enright LP et al: Oophoropexy: a means of preserving ovarian function following pelvic mega-voltage radiotherapy for Hodgkin's disease. Radiology 96:175, 1970

69. Thomas PRM, Winstanly D, Peckham MJ et al: Reproductive and endocrine function in patients with Hodgkin's disease: effects of oophoropexy and irradiation. Br J Cancer 33:226, 1976

70. Ortin TTS, Shostak CA, Donaldson SS: Gonadal status and reproductive function following treatment for Hodgkin's disease in childhood: the Stanford experience. Int J Radiat Oncol Biol Phys 19:873, 1990

71. Stillman R, Schinfield J, Schiff I et al: Ovarian failure in long term survivors of childhood malignancy. Am J Obstet Gynecol 139:62, 1981

72. Anderson B, LaPolla J, Turner D et al: Ovarian transposition in cervical cancer. Gynecol Oncol 49:206, 1993

73. Davis AJ, Feins NM: Subsequent asynchronous torsion of normal adnexa in children. J Pediatr Surg 25:687, 1990

74. Elkins T, Stock R: Recurrent massive edema of the ovary. South Med J 75:478, 1982

CHAPTER THIRTY-SEVEN

DIAGNOSIS AND SURGERY FOR MALIGNANT OVARIAN DISEASE

EVA CHALAS
FIDEL A. VALEA

Therapeutic Goals
Staging Procedure •
Cytoreductive Surgery
Operative Technique
Laparoscopic Approach •
Laparotomy
Secondary Surgery
Second-Look Laparotomy/
Secondary Cytoreduction •
Exploration for Recurrence
Postoperative
 Management
Ovarian Cancer
 Screening
Surgery for Germ Cell
 Tumors of the Ovary
Primary Surgery • Second-
Look Surgery

The American Cancer Society estimates that 26,600 women will develop ovarian cancer and 14,500 women will die of the disease in 1995.[1] Because most are epithelial malignancies, the ensuing discussion focuses on these tumors, which classically present as advanced (stage III or IV) disease. Symptoms can be quite nonspecific, such as gastrointestinal disturbances that are not alarming in nature. Medical attention is usually not sought, and when it is, comprehensive workup is often not performed. Weight loss is not appreciated because, although the woman's appetite and oral intake diminish, the accumulation of ascites may actually cause a net weight gain. Signs such as fluid wave and decreased breath sounds on auscultation of right lung base imply that metastatic lesions are present in the abdomen and pleural space. Thus, at evaluation, these women are suffering with respiratory complaints and symptoms of partial or complete bowel obstruction, and are malnourished.

Occasionally, ovarian masses can cause pain, and early stage malignancy will be diagnosed. Women undergoing pelvic evaluation for other disease processes, or those having regular ultrasound screening will also be diagnosed earlier in the course of the disease.[2]

THERAPEUTIC GOALS

To offer a woman with epithelial ovarian cancer the best possible chance at long-term survival and limited morbidity, the extent of her disease must be accurately assessed. Addi-

tionally, the disease-free interval is inversely related to the size of the largest residual tumor nodule before the start of induction chemotherapy. Therefore, staging procedure and cytoreductive surgery (also known as debulking) represent crucial factors in determining the success of management of this malignancy.

Staging Procedure

Adequate assessment of potential tumor spread requires an appreciation of routes of metastasis. Exfoliation of malignant cells could result in implants representing clockwise peritoneal circulation of fluid: right paracolic gutter, right diaphragm, omentum, left diaphragm, left paracolic gutter, and the cul-de-sacs. Although any peritoneal surface is at risk, the most common sites are the right diaphragm and omentum, due to absorption of fluid through the diaphragm and by the omentum. Direct extension can cause involvement of uterus, tubes, bladder, bowel and its mesentery, or appendix. Hematogenous spread can result in parenchymal liver metastases, and rarely in lung, brain, and bone lesions. Lymphatic metastases affect primarily pelvic and para-aortic nodes, and represent advanced disease, occasionally causing marked inguinal and supraclavicular adenopathy. The final theoretical cause of advanced disease is an unrest in multipotential peritoneal cells that results in synchronous develop-

Table 37-1. Ovarian Carcinoma Staging

Stage	Extent of Disease
Stage IA	Growth limited to one ovary; no tumor on the external surface; capsule intact; no ascites present containing malignant cells
Stage IB	Growth limited to both ovaries; no tumor on the external surface; capsule intact; no ascites present containing malignant cells
Stage IC	Stage IA or IB disease with tumor on the external surface; ruptured capsule; ascites or washings containing malignant cells
Stage IIA	Extension and/or metastases to uterus and/or tubes
Stage IIB	Extension to other pelvic tissue
Stage IIC	Stage IIA or IIB disease with tumor on the external surface; ruptured capsule; ascites or washings containing malignant cells
Stage IIIA	Tumor grossly limited to the true pelvis with negative nodes but with histologically confirmed microscopic seeding of abdominoperitoneal surfaces
Stage IIIB	Histologically confirmed tumor implants of abdominal peritoneal surfaces not exceeding 2 cm each; negative nodes
Stage IIIC	Abdominal implants >2 cm in diameter and/or positive retroperitoneal or inguinal nodes
Stage IV	Parenchymal liver disease; malignant cells in pleural effusion, or other cytologic or histologic confirmation of extra-abdominal disease

ment of ovarian and peritoneal malignancy, with multiple lesions arising throughout the peritoneal mesothelium.

The staging procedure includes a thorough exploration of the pelvis and the abdomen (Table 37-1). If gross metastatic disease is present, the focus of the surgery shifts toward cytoreduction, which is addressed later in this chapter. In the absence of evidence of carcinomatosis, the affected ovary must be removed and evaluated by frozen section. A full staging procedure should be performed if the diagnosis of malignancy is confirmed or equivocal. If the frozen section yields a benign diagnosis, limited surgery, as appropriate for that patient, may be performed. The clinician should be aware that a 5- to 10-percent false-negative rate exists for frozen sections, particularly in mucinous tumors, which are notoriously difficult to assess.

The staging operation, as previously indicated, can be individualized. In postmenopausal patients, pelvic and abdominal washings, total hysterectomy, bilateral salpingo-oophorectomy, appendectomy, omental biopsy, pelvic and para-aortic node sampling, multiple peritoneal biopsies (including both diaphragms) and biopsies of all adhesions are performed. The rationale is to remove disease, the tissue at risk of developing malignancy (the other ovary), and to randomly sample all possible sites for micrometastases. In premenopausal women who have not completed childbearing, a more limited operation is performed. The unaffected ovary is biopsied, and uterus is allowed to remain in situ. Individuals wishing to preserve childbearing when both ovaries are involved may retain their uterus for future donor egg in vitro fertilization.

The prognosis and recommendation on whether chemotherapy is indicated depends greatly on accurate staging. Women with stage IA, grade I and II ovarian cancer can expect 5-year survival rates in excess of 90 percent and do not benefit from additional treatment. Women with stage IC, grade III and all stage II disease are be advised to receive limited local (intraperitoneal P32) or systemic therapy, possibly short in duration. Women with microscopic metastases outside of the pelvis will have a 5-year survival rate of 40 percent, with a recommended duration of adjuvant chemotherapy exceeding four courses, or alternatively, may receive whole abdominal and pelvic radiation.[4,5]

Cytoreductive Surgery

In 1975, Griffiths[6] published a landmark paper describing the impact of residual disease on survival. He demonstrated that the duration of median survival was inversely related to the size of the largest residual nodule at the completion of initial debulking. The acceptance of this clinical evidence coincided with the widespread use of cisplatinum-based chemotherapy, which yielded response rates ranging from 60 to 80 percent. The combination of optimal cytoreductive surgery and the highly effective cisplatinum-based chemotherapy resulted in median survivals exceeding 2 years.[7]

Optimal cytoreductive efforts have become accepted by gynecologic oncologists as an integral part of first-line treatment of ovarian carcinoma. The definition of *optimal resection* in publications varies, but generally now reflects residual disease of less than 1.0 cm, although resection of all macroscopic disease is desirable. The initial surgery is followed by aggressive multiagent chemotherapy; recently, Taxol and cisplatinum were chosen as first-line chemotherapy.[8]

Critics of aggressive surgical debulking have observed a number of findings that should be incorporated into clinical decision-making. Technically, it is usually more feasible to perform resections of well-differentiated tumors and their metastases as compared with the less differentiated lesions. Thus, one could argue that the patients whose lesions could be optimally resected represent a selected population with more differentiated tumor and better prognosis. Less differentiated tumors tend to present as advanced lesions and be aggressive in their behavior; when completely resected, the 5-year survival rate is not comparable to well-differentiated lesions; and finally, even if no disease is found at laparotomy at the completion of chemotherapy (second look), a recurrence rate of up to 50 percent is seen.[9] Given this information, what is the justification for aggressive surgical management? First, removal of the bulk of tumor quickly results in a significantly improved quality of life. Symptoms of advanced disease, such as difficulty breathing and eating, are related to tumor burden. Second, with advances in chemotherapy, a prolonged survival exceeding 2 years can be offered to women who would likely die of their disease within months. Currently available techniques of drug resistance testing of the malignant tissue allow for a more individualized selection of chemotherapeutic agents.[10] Introduction of maintenance therapy, such as oral alkylating agents following initial chemotherapy, or the use of prophylactic treatment, such as intraperitoneal P32 following a negative second-look laparotomy, represents attempts to decrease the risk of recurrence and increase the disease-free interval.[11,12] Most gynecologic oncologists believe that the success of these attempts is tumor burden dependent. That is, the larger the amount of residual disease to be treated, the greater the chance of sublethal cellular damage and risk of emergence of multidrug resistant clones. Clearly, optimal cytoreduction represents an all-out effort at a possible cure or prolonged disease-free interval and increased quality of life.[13]

Ovarian cancer patients, particularly those presenting with advanced disease, are often depleted of resources. They exist in a highly catabolic state due to metabolic demands of the tumor and decreased oral intake. Metabolic demands related to aggressive surgical efforts further shift the balance away from favorable outcome for the patient. Thus, the gynecologic oncologist must consider all of these factors when planning debulking surgery, and must be familiar with the techniques and interventions, such as minimizing blood loss and providing nutritional support, to improve the benefit/risk ratio of the procedure.

The goal of optimal cytoreduction is achieved in up to 60 to 75 percent of patients explored by gynecologic oncologists.[14,15] Factors limiting the extent of surgery include parenchymal liver disease and mesenteric or extra-abdominal metastases. Under these conditions, the ability to resect disease while preserving function is compromised. Resection of mesenteric involvement requires resection of a large segment of intestine, and the risk/benefit ratio is unfavorable when liver parenchyma metastases are present.

Other principles of cytoreductive surgery address metastatic lesions involving the intestine. Bowel surgery is usually not performed unless it significantly adds to cytoreductive efforts and optimal resection is then possible, or if obstruction is present. In the presence of other unresectable disease, bowel surgery is of little value, except in patients with a gastrointestinal obstruction. Ultraradical surgery, including complex or multiple bowel resection, is associated with high morbidity and potential perioperative mortality, particularly in nutritionally depleted patients. Thus, at exploration, a thorough assessment of intra-abdominal findings will aid in determining the extent of cytoreductive efforts (Table 37-2).

OPERATIVE TECHNIQUE

Laparoscopic Approach

A laparoscopic approach to surgical management of ovarian cancer is technically possible, but is not considered prudent by many authorities and clinicians. Most often, it is selected in patients with adnexal disease believed to be be-

Table 37-2. Surgical Procedures For Treatment of Ovarian Carcinoma

Staging Procedure for Minimal Disease	Intra-abdominal Metastases <2 cm, No Lymphadenopathy	Cytoreductive Surgery for Metastases >2 cm

Postmenopausal patient
  Washings, TAH, BSO, appendectomy, omental biopsy, bilateral pelvic and para-aortic node biopsies, multiple peritoneal biopsies, including both diaphgrams, biopsies of any adhesions
Preservation of fertility
  Unilateral salpingo-oophorectomy with preservation of the uterus and biopsy of unaffected ovary
Full staging procedure as above
Planned adnexectomy of unaffected ovary on completion of childbearing
	For all patients (optimal cytoreduction feasible in majority)
	  TAH, BSO, appendectomy, omentectomy with aggressive effort to resect all visible disease
	Node sampling must be performed to rule out miscroscopic disease
	Bowel resection should be performed if optimal cytoreduction can be achieved, or if bowel obstruction is present
		Patients without liver parenchymal, extra-abdominal, bulky mesenteric or retroperitoneal disease
		  TAH, BSO, appendectomy, omentectomy, resection of all visible disease, bowel resection, splenectomy or other ultraradical procedures to achieve optimal cytoreduction as the medical status of the patient allows
		Nodal sampling not necessary unless it significantly contributes to cytoreduction
		Patients with unresectable disease
		  Limited surgery for palliation or chemotherapy preceding debulking surgery

Abbreviations: TAH, total abdominal hysterectomy; BSO, bilateral salpingo-oophorectomy.

nign, only to discover an unsuspected ovarian cancer. Intact removal of an ovarian mass is often not possible; spillage of malignant cells is associated with a possibility of rapid intra-abdominal dissemination via the peritoneal circulation. The controversy regarding the effect of a spill on the patient's prognosis remains unresolved. However, a recent publication supports a negative outcome.[16] Additionally, tumor seeding of access sites, particularly the umbilicus, have been documented by clinicians. Because young patients are more likely to have benign disease, a laparoscopic approach to management of adnexal mass is often used in this population. If malignancy is diagnosed, borderline lesions or early stage invasive disease is often present. To prevent a tragic mistake and potentially compromise the outcome for these patients, who would otherwise enjoy an excellent prognosis, some useful sonographic criteria have been developed.[17] The use of these criteria, incorporated into the clinical picture and combined, as indicated, with serum CA-125 marker, can minimize the chance of choosing laparoscopic approach in patients at high risk of having a malignant lesion. A minority of clinicians argue that these criteria are imprecise, and favor aggressive laparoscopy combined with access to a gynecologic oncologist who can rapidly intervene if malignancy is found.[18]

Laparotomy

Debulking is best accomplished by laparotomy, utilizing a vertical midline incision. This approach provides potentially unlimited exposure to pelvis and abdomen, with placement of incision in a relatively avascular plane. Access to the peritoneal cavity is gained rapidly and with ease. Alternatively, a pre-existing paramedian incision can be chosen to avoid the presence of parallel vertical abdominal incisions and devascularization of tissue between these incisions. However, access is more difficult. The rectus muscle on the side of the incision may be split or reflected to reach the midline. Closure of this paramedian incision is more complex, the appearance is less cosmetic, and patients generally experience more postoperative incisional discomfort.

If a Pfannenstiel incision was chosen because of erroneous expectations of benign findings, several options exist. In a slim patient, particularly with a mobile abdominal wall, the Pfannenstiel incision can be converted to a Maylard or Cherney incision, providing that the resulting exposure does not compromise the extent of surgery performed. In all other patients, a midline vertical incision should be performed (''anchor''). The foremost concerns are minimizing technical limitations and maximizing the possibility of optimal cytoreductive effort.

Once the peritoneal cavity is entered, any ascites should be collected and a representative sample sent for cytologic evaluation. Washings of the pelvis, paracolic gutters, and both diaphragms are obtained for staging purposes, if ascites

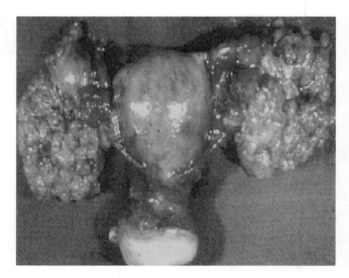

Fig. 37-1. Uterus with bilateral ovarian malignancies.

or extrapelvic tumor nodules are not identified. The umbilicus should be carefully palpated, as metastasis to the peritoneal side can occur, and excision simple. Exploratory laparotomy is then carried out in a systematic manner, assessing the status of the pelvic organs, small and large intestine, stomach, liver, gallbladder, pancreas, spleen, kidneys, omentum, and both diaphragms. The purpose of a thorough evaluation is to determine the site of origin of the cancer, extent of disease spread, presence or absence of organs (i.e., appendix or gallbladder), presence of other coexisting conditions, and feasibility of cytoreductive surgery. Visual assessment combined with palpation is useful; however, malignant lesions are often friable and care must be taken not to place traction on the tissue.

If a thorough exploration reveals only gross involvement of one or both ovaries (Fig. 37-1), a staging procedure is carried out to determine by histologic assessment the possibility of microscopic metastases. Multiple biopsies of peritoneal surfaces, including the anterior and posterior cul-de-sacs, the paracolic gutters, and both diaphragms, are obtained by elevating the peritoneum with the help of the Allis clamp or a pickup, and sharply resecting a subcentimeter section. Any adhesions are also sampled, as tumor may be associated with an inflamatory or desmoplastic reaction and may result in adhesion formation. Omental sampling is usually accomplished by removing a segment of the infracolic omentum, isolating the vascular pedicles with Kelly (or equivalent) clamps, or by using an automatic stapler, such as the LDS (ligate-staple-divide). Pelvic and para-aortic node sampling must be performed to rule out the possibility of microscopic stage III disease, which can occur in up to one-third of apparent stage I disease cases.[13] The retroperitoneum may be accessed by dividing the round ligament if a hysterectomy is planned, and then developing the pararectal and paravesical spaces. The pararectal space is developed by blunt dissection between the medial leaflet of the broad ligament and the external and internal iliac vessel, taking care to protect the ureter on the medial leaflet and avoiding dissection lateral to the internal iliac artery, which lies inferior and medial to the external iliac vessel. The paravesical space is created by blunt dissection toward the pelvic floor between the superior vesical artery and the external iliac vessels. Using clips, clamps, or cautery, selective sampling of the pelvic nodes can be performed. The para-aortic nodes can be sampled through an incision in the peritoneum overlying the right common iliac artery and blunt dissection to develop the retroperitoneal space with biopsies of right (paracaval) and left para-aortic nodes. Hysterectomy and bilateral adnexectomy is performed in all postmenopausal patients and premenopausal women no longer interested in childbearing, because the risk of developing malignancy in the remaining ovary in patients with stage IA disease is thought to be approximately 15 percent. Thus, even young women with well-differentiated lesion of one ovary, who have had a full staging operation but do not have the normal ovary or their uterus removed to preserve childbearing, are advised to have the ovary removed on completion of their families or by the age of 35.

Routine appendectomy is performed as part of the staging procedure, because the appendix is a pelvic organ and frequently is involved with disease. The mesentery is clamped, cut, and ligated, and the appendix is clamped closed to the cecum. After it is removed, the stump is ligated. The use of absorbable sutures is acceptable if the selected material has delayed absorption to prevent leakage from the stump. Complex procedures involving manipulation of the stump are unnecessary. At the completion of the staging operation, the involved organs, as well as the regions most at risk of metastatic disease have been removed or sampled.

Bulky disease detected at laparotomy usually presents with the majority of cancer distributed in the pelvis, the omentum, and the right diaphragm. Resection of disease in these locations results in prolonged palliation. Thus, even when unresectable disease, as previously described, is detected, extirpation of omentum and pelvic disease can be attempted for palliation, histologic confirmation of diagnosis, and identification of primary tumor site. If resection of the bulk of disease appears technically feasible, an aggressive surgical approach aimed at resection of all or most visible disease is warranted.

Resection of the omentum, even when replaced by densely packed metastases (so-called omental cake), is not particularly challenging (Fig. 37-2A). Performance of omentectomy early in the operation results in significant debulking, thus serving several functions: it facilitates packing of the bowel to improve pelvic exposure, provides an adequate sample for frozen section, and assures the surgical team of visible success. After the peritoneal reflection is separated off the transverse colon, the mesentery of the colon is identified and preserved. An infracolic or a complete omentectomy is then performed by dividing the gastroepiploic vessels. If necessary, hepatic and splenic flexures can be mobilized to allow for removal of all of the omentum. If tumor nodules extend into the splenic hilum, a splenectomy can be contemplated if optimal cytoreduction is then possible (Fig. 37-2B). The spleen is mobilized and the splenic vessels are ligated, taking care to avoid injury to the tail end of the pancreas. Rarely, it may be necessary to resect the tail if involved by contiguous cancer spread. Similarly, if hepatic disease is present and affects only a segment of a lobe, a partial hepatectomy can be performed if optimal cytoreduction results. Generally, this can be performed with the help of intense cautery heat, which dissects the liver parenchyma. The parenchyma can be finger fractured along cautery dissection, and intact blood vessels ligated as they become accessible during this process. The use of argon beam coagulator in obtaining hemostasis after a partial hepatectomy is highly effective. Diaphragmatic disease can be approached with stripping or scraping of the peritoneal surface. Alternatively, the liver can be partially retracted, the hepatic ligament divided, and an ultrasonic dissection system can be carried out.

Pelvic anatomy is frequently bizarre in patients with ovarian carcinoma (Fig. 37-3). A very useful approach to resection of disease, which minimizes the risk of injury to bladder or ureters and results in excellent access to blood supply, is by a retroperitoneal technique (previously described for pelvic node sampling). The round ligaments are identified, suture ligated, and divided. The peritoneum overlying the psoas muscle is incised and the pararectal spaces are bluntly developed. The ureters are thus exposed and can be mobilized. Infundibulopelvic ligaments are identified, clamped, cut, and ligated. Should it be necessary, access to the uterine artery at its origin is also possible. The anterior cul-de-sac peritoneum is incised at the reflection and the bladder is mobilized off the lower uterine segment. If there are implants on the anterior cul-de-sac peritoneum, the peritoneum can be stripped off. The space of Retzius can be developed, the bladder elevated, and dissected off. The remainder of the hysterectomy can then be carried out in a routine fashion. If the posterior cul-de-sac is obliterated by cancer, disease-free bowel can be identified below the peritoneal reflection, since ovarian cancer implants are generally on the peritoneal surface or bowel serosa, leaving retroperitoneal structures intact. In extreme cases, the peritoneum overlying the paracolic gutters may be incised, the retroperitoneum entered, the ureters and vessels identified, and the pelvis entered from above.

Bowel resections are performed on 10 percent of women having surgery for gynecologic malignancies.[19] Most of these procedures are for patients with ovarian carcinoma. Most commonly, the rectosigmoid implants constitute the bulk of intestinal involvement. Small-volume disease can be

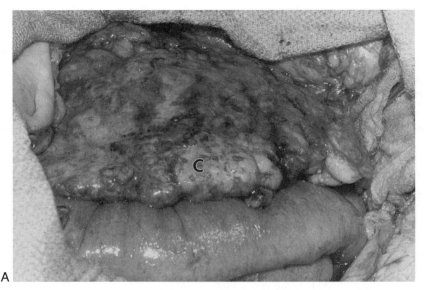

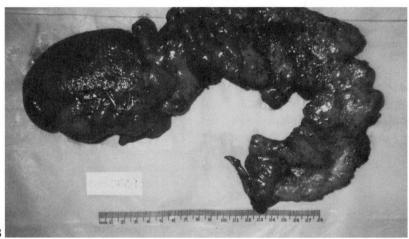

Fig. 37-2. (A) Large omental cake (C) overlying small bowel. (B) Gross specimen.

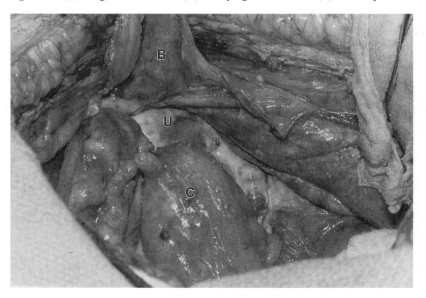

Fig. 37-3. Example of frozen pelvis demonstrating the urinary bladder (B) and the uterine fundus (U) surrounded by tumor plaque. Redundant rectosigmoid colon (C) is seen on the left.

simply shaved off, taking advantage of the fact that these implants are often only superficially invasive. Bulkier implants may require that resection and reanastamosis be performed; the surgery should be carried out only if optimal cytoreduction is possible or if obstruction is present. In circumstances in which the patient is not stable, or a bowel resection is contraindicated, an intestinal bypass procedure can be performed instead. Proximal and distal bowel is simply approximated without resection of the involved segment, thus bypassing the area of resistance to permit flow of gastrointestinal contents. The procedure is well tolerated and results in palliation, but may be associated with blind loop syndrome with bacterial overgrowth or potential perforation.

Intestinal resections can be performed most rapidly with the aid of stapling devices such as the gastrointestinal anastomosis and transverse anastomosis stapling devices. The continuity of the bowel can be re-established by aligning the proximal and distal ends of the bowel and stapling the antimesenteric sides to each other in a so-called side-to-side,

functional end-to-end anastomosis, using the gastrointestinal anastomosis stapler. The enterotomies necessary for placement of gastrointestinal anastomosis are then closed using the transverse anastomosis gun (Fig. 37-4). The advantage of stapled anastomoses over the traditional hand-sewn include speed, improved blood supply at the site, and ease of technique. The procedure can be applied to any segment of the bowel, except when low rectal anastomosis is performed. The end-to-end anastomosis stapler avoids the need for a colostomy in this situation (Fig. 37-5).

An alternative technique employs biofragmentable rings (Valtrac), which allows direct end-to-end anastomosis by simply snapping the rings together (Fig. 37-6). This procedure can also be performed more rapidly and with ease as compared to hand-sewn anastomoses, which are usually performed as a double-layer closure (Fig. 37-7). The issue of speed arises in patients having cytoreductive surgery, because multiple procedures are often required to achieve optimal cytoreduction, and the entire operation can be quite

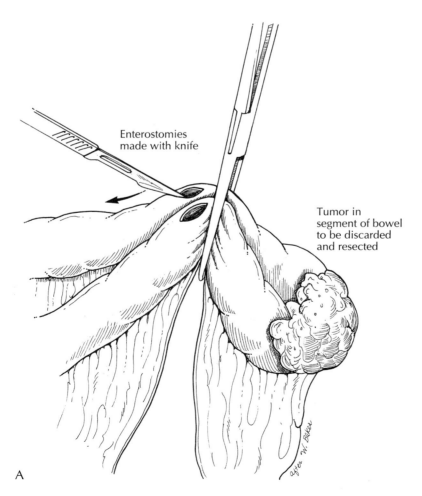

Enterostomies
made with knife

Tumor in
segment of bowel
to be discarded
and resected

A

Fig. 37-4. (A) Enterotomies. *(Figure continues).*

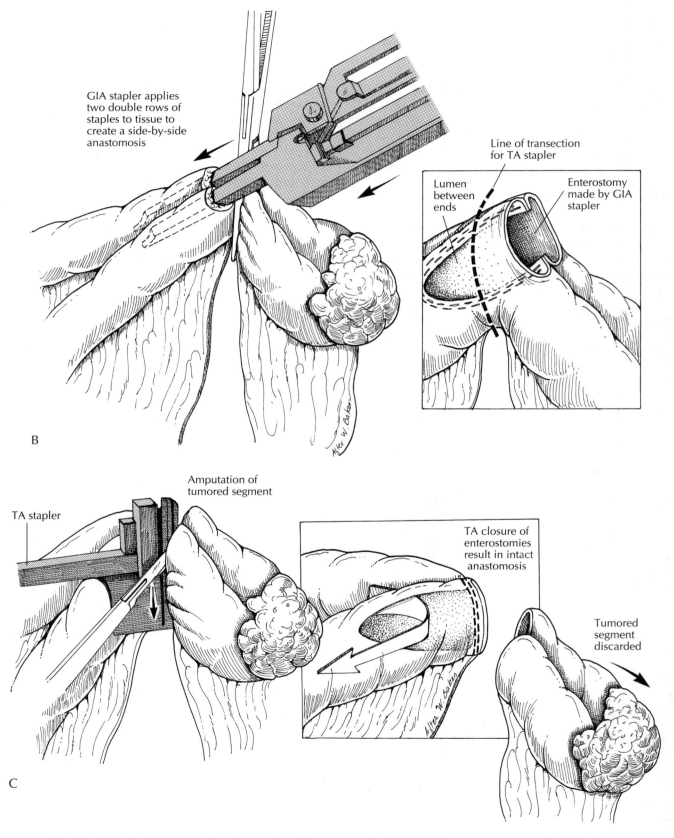

GIA stapler applies
two double rows of
staples to tissue to
create a side-by-side
anastomosis

Line of transection
for TA stapler

Lumen
between
ends

Enterostomy
made by GIA
stapler

B

Amputation of
tumored segment

TA stapler

TA closure of
enterostomies
result in intact
anastomosis

Tumored
segment
discarded

C

Fig. 37-4 *(Continued).* **(B)** Side-by-side gastrointestinal anastamosis (GIA). **(C)** Transverse anastomosis (TA) closure of enterotomies, amputation of resected segment, and intact anastamosis.

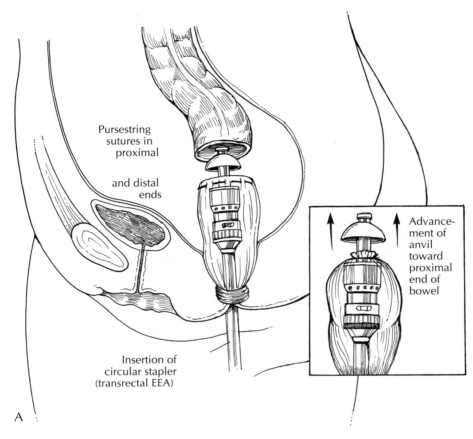

Pursestring
sutures in
proximal

and distal
ends

Insertion of
circular stapler
(transrectal EEA)

A

Advance-
ment of
anvil
toward
proximal
end of
bowel

Fig. 37-5. (A) Transrectal end-to-end anastomosis (EEA) insertion and ligature of distal pursestring around stapler and advancement of anvil toward the proximal end of the bowel (inset). *(Figure continues).*

lengthy. Regardless of the choice of technique, the surgeon must check for patency, hemostasis, and intactness of the anastomotic site. To prevent the risk of internal hernia or entrapment of the bowel, the mesentery must be approximated after the completion of the anastomosis. It is desirable to close only one side, as through-and-through mesenteric sutures can interfere with the blood supply to the respective segments of the anastomosis.

Stapling devices can also be used to remove a Meckel's diverticulum and the appendix. However, if only the appendectomy is planned, the use of automatic stapler will not be cost-effective. A traditional ligation or suture ligation of the appendix is then appropriate.

The need for stomas is quite limited in ovarian cancer surgery. Adequate amount of uninvolved intestine, which can be reapproximated, is usually available at the time of primary cytoreduction. However, if a stoma is required, an effort should be made to place it in the lower abdominal quadrants. Upper abdominal sites limit the type of clothing that can be worn. The best location is in the left lower abdomen, approximately in the middle of a triangle drawn between the pubic symphysis umbilicus, and the anterior supe-

rior iliac spine. Care should be taken to avoid placing the stoma near incisions or skin creases. If possible, the site should be selected before surgery with the patient placed in different positions to minimize the chance of poor adherence of the stoma bag. Many surgeons believe the bowel should be secured to the fascia and the peritoneum to minimize the risk of hernia or prolapse. Liquid output, such as would be expected from transverse colon or proximally, would require a creation of a spout-like stoma (Fig. 37-8). Stomas with solid output can be flush with the skin.

Resection of bladder or ureters is rarely necessary to achieve optimal debulking initially, unless the tumor has invaded the bladder or has obstructed the ureter. Resection of these structures may require complete mobilization of the bladder to accommodate the decreased length of the remaining ureter. Reapproximation with delayed absorbable suture results in good healing if there is no tension on the anastomosis site and the blood supply is adequate. Initially, these anastomoses are not watertight, and drainage of the pelvis by closed suction is prudent. Placement of ureteral stents is based on the surgeon's preference, since there is no scientific support for either method of management.

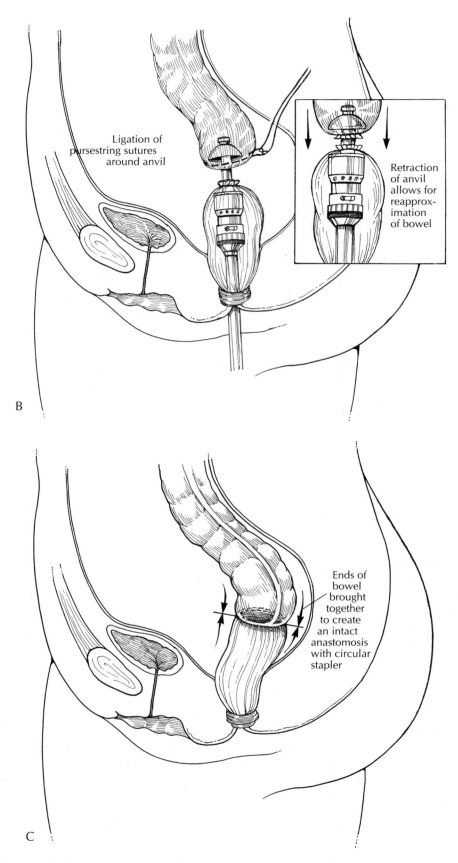

B

Ligation of
pursestring sutures
around anvil

Retraction
of anvil
allows for
reapprox-
imation
of bowel

C

Ends of
bowel
brought
together
to create
an intact
anastomosis
with circular
stapler

Fig. 37-5 *(Continued).* **(B)** Ligature of proximal pursestring around the anvil and retraction of anvil to allow for reapproximation of bowel and stapling (inset). **(C)** Intact anastomosis.

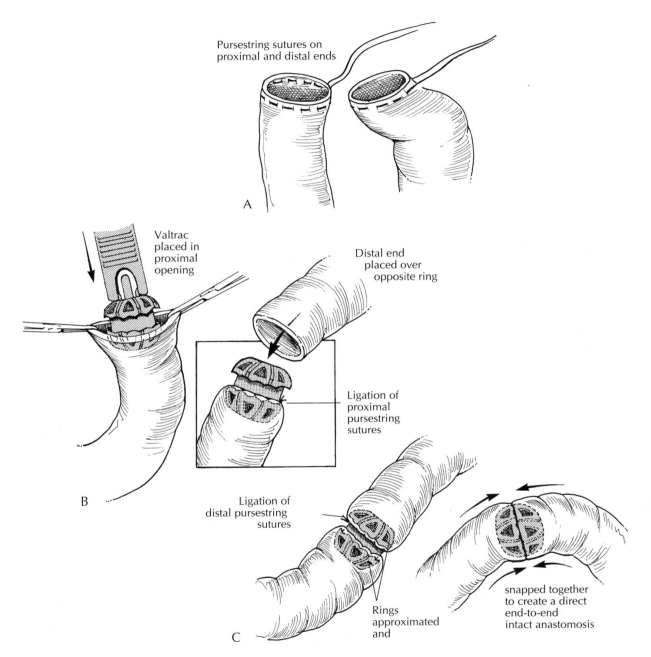

Fig. 37-6. **(A)** Pursestring suture on proximal and distal ends. **(B)** Placement of Valtrac and ligation of proximal pursestring sutures. **(C)** Ligation of pursestring distally and approximated rings and intact anastomosis.

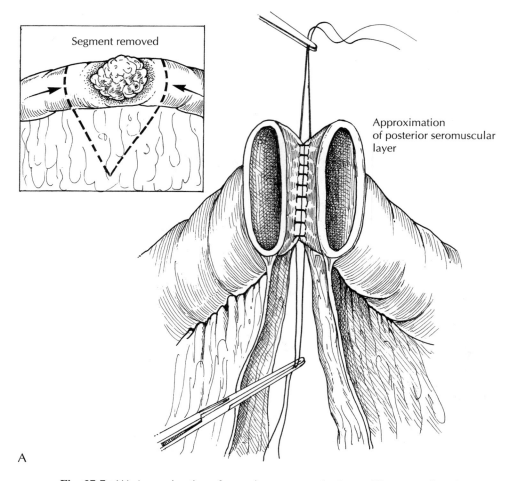

Fig. 37-7. (A) Approximation of posterior seromuscular layer. *(Figure continues).*

SECONDARY SURGERY

The issue of surgical management after primary cytoreductive surgery is extremely controversial, and continues to evolve. Several opportunities for surgery exist, and are discussed separately. They are second-look laparotomy, or secondary cytoreduction, and exploration for recurrence.

Second-Look Laparotomy/Secondary Cytoreduction

The purpose of this procedure is to assess response after completion of first-line chemotherapy. With the widespread application of serum CA-125 testing, detection of subclinical disease has become possible, allowing for better counseling of patients offered a second-look laparotomy, but not eliminating the need for the procedure.[20] At exploration, up to 60 percent of patients who were clinically disease-free had histologic or gross evidence of disease. Secondary cytoreduction has been shown to be associated with prolonged survival.[21–23] Further, patients found to have no histologic

evidence of disease experienced 30- to 50-percent recurrence rates with continued follow-up.[9] Studies have shown that if these patients receive prophylactic therapy, lower recurrence rates are noted.[11] Thus, up to 80 percent of candidates for second-look laparotomy could benefit from additional chemotherapy.

The role of second-look laparotomy is slowly being redefined by the data accumulated in the literature. The high rate of positive findings and the significant risk of recurrence decrease the benefit of the procedure. One recommendation would be to use maintenance chemotherapy in patients who are clinically without disease at completion of primary, or induction, chemotherapy. Women who could benefit from second-look procedure would include those who had significant residual disease but enjoyed at least a partial response to first-line chemotherapy, or in whom the planned treatment would be altered by the laparotomy findings. Laparoscopy might also be a helpful tool to triage patients immediately before second-look laparotomy.

At second-look operations, any gynecologic organs not previously removed are resected. Secondary cytoreduction is attempted or, in the abscence of gross evidence of disease,

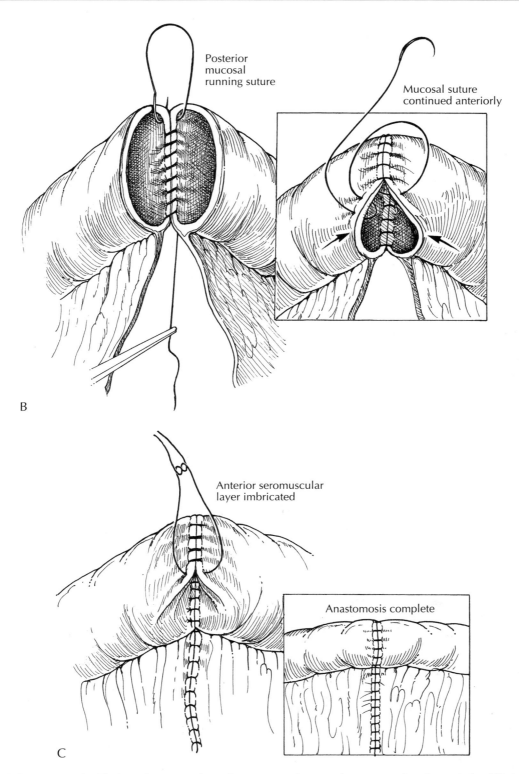

Posterior
mucosal
running suture

Mucosal suture
continued anteriorly

B

Anterior seromuscular
layer imbricated

Anastomosis complete

C

Fig. 37-7 *(Continued).* **(B)** Posterior mucosal running suture and mucosal suture continued anteriorly. **(C)** Anterior seromuscular imbricating layer.

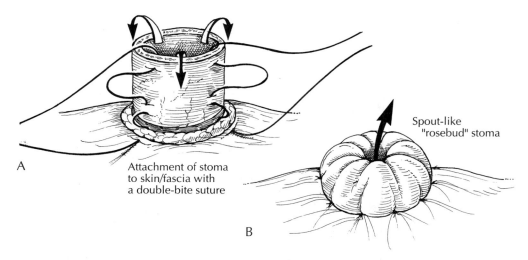

Fig. 37-8. (A) Attachment of stoma at skin and fascia (B) Spout-like stoma.

multiple biopsies are taken. Although the pelvic peritoneum and surface of the diaphragm are the most likely sites of persistent disease, one must also sample the abdominal peritoneum, mesentery of the small and large bowel, and remove all apparently benign adhesions. Pelvic and para-aortic nodes should also be sampled, if not previously done.

Exploration for Recurrence

Recurrences are unfortunately common in women with ovarian cancer. With recurrent or persistent disease, cancer implants are no longer superficial, but rather grow into tissue and cannot be easily scraped off (Fig. 37-9). If the patient has been clinically free of disease for more than 12 months, redebulking may be of value.[24] Earlier recurrences are often

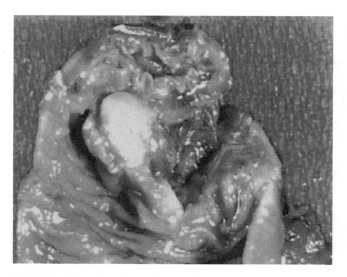

Fig. 37-9. Example of rectosigmoid with nodule of cancer growing into the lumen of the colon.

associated with a lack of adequate response to second-line agents, thus limiting the benefit of redebulking. The overall response rates to chemotherapy are 20 to 30 percent, with issues of quality of life gaining emphasis. Surgical procedures for patients presenting with obstruction are associated with a very high morbidity and mortality as well as a short median survival.[19] Bowel obstruction in ovarian cancer may result from a combination of factors. It may be purely mechanical, with kinking or external compression of the bowel, or it may occur due to massive mesenteric involvement by cancer. At exploration it is not always possible to resect the site of obstruction and there may be no loops free of disease to allow bypassing of the obstruction. Placing a gastrotomy tube for decompression may be all that can be accomplished. Even if the obstruction is relieved, it may recur as disease progresses. The risk of the procedure occasionally outweighs any potential benefit. Palliation by percutaneous route, intravenous hydration, and hospice care are generally of greatest benefit to the patient and her family.

POSTOPERATIVE MANAGEMENT

Patients with advanced ovarian carcinoma undergoing primary or extensive secondary cytoreduction experience significant fluid shifts. Blood loss during the procedure and the extent of the operation further tax the individual patient's resources. The use of volume expanders, including blood products or colloids, may be necessary, with fluid resuscitation being an integral part of the management in the first 24 to 48 hours postoperatively. Invasive monitoring may be necessary to administer fluid safely. Thus, some of these patients will clearly benefit from being transferred to the intensive care unit, where staff is knowledgeable in the management of surgical patients. Fluid shifts, including reaccumulation of ascites, will continue to occur for some time.

Close monitoring of intake and output is important until the patient has established competent gastrointestinal function. Danger of fluid overload is greatest 48 to 72 hours postoperatively, when mobilization of third-spaced fluid results in increased intravascular volume. The physician in charge must understand the natural physiologic postoperative progress to avoid iatrogenic complications.

OVARIAN CANCER SCREENING

The concern of the public and of clinicians with the number of patients presenting with advanced stage disease has resulted in intense research efforts in screening techniques for detection of ovarian carcinoma. The development of a cost-effective screening test has been limited by the relatively low incidence of ovarian cancer and the lack of a premalignant phase in the development of this malignancy. Transvaginal sonogram, alone or combined with CA-125 or color doppler flow, is highly sensitive and has acceptable specificity. The utilization of these tests, in view of the low incidence of malignancy and a relatively high incidence of benign ovarian neoplasms and functional lesions, has resulted in numerous operations to detect one malignancy.[25] Preventive measures, such the use of oral contraceptives, and further testing of screening techniques are currently recommended. Application of screening techniques to individuals with strong family histories improves yield.

SURGERY FOR GERM CELL TUMORS OF THE OVARY

Most germ cell tumors of the ovary are stage I at initial presentation. They are rarely bilateral, except for dysgerminomas, which can be bilateral in 10 to 15 percent of cases.[26–28] Although there are several types of germ cell neoplasms, surgical management is similar for all types. The same basic surgical principles used for the management of epithelial cancers of the ovary apply, namely, thorough exploration of the abdomen, surgical staging, and cytoreductive surgery when safe and feasible. However, most patients can be safely treated with conservative surgery and preservation of fertility.

Malignant germ cell tumors of the ovary spread either by lymphatic drainage or by peritoneal surface dissemination. In fact, nodal involvement is more common in these tumors than the epithelial cancers of the ovary. In addition, it has a slightly greater predilection to metastasize hematogenously to the parenchyma of the liver and lung. Fortunately, many germ cell tumors have the ability to produce biologic markers (in addition to CA-125) that can be detected in the

Table 37-3. Ovarian Germ Cell Tumors and Their Respective Serum Makers

Tumor	HCG	AFP	LDH
Dysgerminoma	+	−	+ +
Immature Teratoma	−	+	+
Embryonal Carcinoma	+ +	+ +	+
Endodermal Sinus Tumor	+	+ +	+

Abbreviations: HCG, human chorionic gonadotropin; AFP, α-fetoprotein; LDH, lactate dehydrogenase. Key: −, not usually elevated; +, occasionally elevated; + +, frequently elevated.

serum, such as human chorionic gonadotropin, lactate dehydrogenase, and even α-fetoprotein (Table 37-3).

Primary Surgery

The surgical treatment for germ cell neoplasms of the ovary is not only therapeutic; it is also diagnostic. A generous midline vertical incision is usually recommended to allow for adequate exposure and a thorough evaluation of the upper abdomen, which is crucial to the staging of these neoplasms. Because these tumors tend to occur in a younger age group than the epithelial cancers, preservation of fertility is usually important and can safely be accomplished in properly selected patients. For women beyond reproductive age, removal of the uterus, both ovaries, and tubes is warranted. In the younger patient, unilateral oophorectomy with preservation of fertility is appropriate. Wedge biopsy of the normal-appearing contralateral ovary should only be routinely performed if the tumor is a dysgerminoma or immature teratoma; it is less useful with other cell types.

Ascites, if present, should be collected and sent for cytologic evaluation. If none is noted, cytologic washings of the pelvis, both gutters, and the diaphragm should be performed using a cool saline solution. If the disease appears to be limited to the pelvis, random peritoneal biopsies of the areas at risk of spread should be performed. These include the omentum (where one should take a generous sample), both paracolic gutters, pelvic cul-de-sac and sidewalls, vesicouterine fold, and the diaphragm. In addition, if adhesions are present, these should also be sent for histologic review.

Given the propensity for nodal metastasis, it is important to adequately sample pelvic and para-aortic nodes. If no suspicious nodes are encountered, a representative sample of the nodes in these areas should be obtained. A complete lymphadenectomy is not necessary and may only add to the potential for complications.

In the event that advanced disease is encountered, it should be debulked according to the principles of cytoreductive surgery mentioned in the discussion of epithelial cancer. Because of their rarity, the data surrounding the issue of cytoreductive surgery are not clear, especially when one considers that these neoplasms, in general, are much more chemosensitive than other neoplasms of the ovary. In one Gynecologic Oncology Group series, patients with complete resection of the tumor had fewer chemotherapy failures than did those with incomplete resection (28 versus 68 percent).[28] Similarly, patients who had been optimally debulked did better than those who were not optimally debulked, but not as well as those who did not require debulking to have minimal residual disease.[30] The surgeon must keep in mind the biologic behavior of these tumors and that, even in advanced disease, a cure is possible and occasionally even a contralateral ovary can be preserved. The overall prognosis of patients with germ cell neoplasms has dramatically improved with the advent of modern multiagent chemotherapy. All cases of nondysgerminomatous germ cell malignancies, except unruptured stage 1A, grade 1 immature teratomas, require postoperative chemotherapy. The two most widely accepted regimens include VAC (vincristine, actinomycin-D, and cytoxan) and BEP (bleomycin, etoposide, and cisplatin). In the Gynecologic Oncology Group trials, both of these regimens had good activity against the various germ cell malignancies.[31] After completion of therapy most patients will resume normal ovarian function, and childbearing can even be preserved. In a series of 40 patients treated with combination chemotherapy for germ cell malignancies, 27 (68 percent) resumed normal menstrual function, and 12 of the 16 patients that attempted to conceive did so, resulting in 11 women giving birth to 22 healthy infants.[32]

Second-Look Surgery

The issue of second look or even secondary cytoreduction is even less clear. As a routine, second-look laparotomy is usually not done for this disease. However, there are exceptions. For example, a patient with an isolated focus of disease after completion of first-line chemotherapy may benefit from resection of this focus before altering the chemotherapy. Similarly, patients with early-stage disease and positive serum markers at the completion of therapy may benefit from surgical exploration. Fortunately, these situations are fairly rare.

REFERENCES

1. Wingo PA, Tong T, Bolden S: Cancer Statistics 1995. CA Cancer J Clin 45:71, 1995
2. Campbell S, Bhan V, Royston P et al: Transabdominal ultrasound screening for early ovarian cancer. BMJ 299:1363, 1989
3. Young RC, Walton LA, Ellenberg SS et al: Adjuvant therapy in stage I and stage II epithelial ovarian cancer: results of two prospective randomized trials. N Engl J Med 322:1021, 1990
4. Nguyen HN, Averette HE, Hoskins W et al: National Survey of Ovarian Carcinoma IV. Critical assessment of current International Federation of Gynecology and Obstetrics staging system. Cancer 72:3007, 1993
5. Thomas GM, Dembo AJ: Integrating radiation therapy into the management of ovarian cancer. Cancer 71:1710, 1993
6. Griffiths CT: Surgical resection of tumor bulk in primary treatment of ovarian carcinoma. Natl Cancer Inst Monogr 42:101, 1975
7. Hoskins WJ: The role of cytoreductive surgery in ovarian cancer. Cancer Principles and Practice of Oncology, 1987
8. Thigpen T, Vance R, Puneky L, Khansur T: Chemotherapy in advanced ovarian carcinoma: current standards of care based on randomized trials. Gynecol Oncol 55:S97, 1994
9. Rubin SC, Hoskins WJ, Saigo PE et al: Prognostic factors for recurrence following negative second-look laparotomy in ovarian cancer patients treated with platinum-based chemotherapy. Gynecol Oncol 42:137, 1991
10. Kern DH, Weisenthal LM: Highly specific prediction of antineoplastic drug resistance with an in vitro assay using suprapharmacologic drug exposures. J Natl Cancer Inst 82:582, 1990
11. Spencer RT, Marks RD, Fenn JO et al: Intraperitoneal P32 after a negative second-look laparotomy in ovarian carcinoma. Cancer 63:2434, 1989
12. Manetta A, MacNeill C, Lyter JA et al: Hexamethylmelamine as single second-line agent in ovarian cancer. Gynecol Oncol 36:93, 1990
13. Hoskins WJ: Epithelial ovarian carcinoma: principles of primary surgery. Gynecol Oncol 55:S91, 1994
14. Hacker NF, Berek JS, Lagasse LD et al: Primary cytoreductive surgery for epithelial ovarian cancer. Obstet Gynecol 61:413, 1983
15. Piver MS, Baker T: The potential of optimal (less than 2 cm) cytoreductive surgery in advanced ovarian carcinoma at a tertiary medical center. A prospective study. Gynecol Oncol 28:1, 1986
16. Sainz de la Cuesta R, Goff BA, Fuller AF et al: Prognostic importance of intraoperative rupture of malignant ovarian epithelial neoplasms. Obstet Gynecol 84:1, 1994
17. Sassone AM, Tomor-Tritsch IE, Artner A et al: Transvaginal sonographic characterization of ovarian disease: evaluation of a new scoring system to predict ovarian malignancy. Obstet Gynecol 78:70, 1991
18. Mann WJ, Reich H: Laparoscopic adnexectomy in postmenopausal women. J Reprod Med 37:254, 1992
19. Chalas E, Mann WJ, Westermann CP et al: Morbidity and mortality of stapled anastomoses on a gynecologic oncology service: a retrospective review. Gynecol Oncol 37:82, 1990
20. Potter ME, Moradi M, To ACW et al: Value of serum CA 125 levels: does the result preclude second look? Gynecol Oncol 33:201, 1989
21. Hoskins WJ, Rubin SC, Dulaney E et al: Influence of secondary cytoreduction at the time of second-look laparotomy on survival of patients with epithelial ovarian carcinoma. Gynecol Oncol 34:365, 1989
22. Creasman, WT: Second-look laparotomy in ovarian cancer. Gynecol Oncol 55:S122, 1994
23. Podratz KC, Cliby WA: Second-look surgery in the management of epithelial ovarian carcinoma. Gynecol Oncol 55:S128, 1994

24. Janicke F, Holscher M, Kuhn W et al: Radical surgical procedure improves survival time in patients with recurrent ovarian cancer. Cancer 70:2129, 1992

25. Karlan BY, Platt LD: The current status of ultrasound and color doppler imaging in screening for ovarian cancer. Gynecol Oncol 55:S28, 1994

26. Mueller CW, Topkins P, Lapp WA: Dysgerminoma of the ovary: an analysis of 427 cases. Am J Obstet Gynecol 60:153, 1950

27. Asadourian LA, Taylor HB: Dysgerminoma: an analysis of 105 cases. Obstet Gynecol 33:370, 1969

28. De Palo G, Pilotti S, Kenda R et al: Natural history of dysgerminoma. Am J Obstet Gynecol 143:799, 1982

29. Slayton RE, Park RC, Silverberg SG et al: Vincristine, dactinomycin, and cyclophosphamide in the treatment of malignant germ cell tumors of the ovary: a Gynecologic Oncology Group study. Cancer 56:243, 1985

30. Williams SD, Blessing JA, Moore DH et al: Cisplatin, vinblastine, and bleomycin in advanced and recurrent ovarian germ-cell tumors. Ann Intern Med 111:22, 1989

31. Williams SD, Blessing J, Slayton R et al: Ovarian germ cell tumors: adjuvant trials of the Gynecologic Oncology Group (GOG), abstracted. J Clin Oncol 8:150, 1989

32. Gershenson DM: Menstrual and reproductive function after treatment with combination chemotherapy for malignant ovarian germ cell tumors. J Clin Oncol 6:270, 1988

CHAPTER THIRTY-EIGHT

DIAGNOSIS AND MANAGEMENT OF URINARY INCONTINENCE

DEIRDRE ROBINSON
PEGGY A. NORTON

There has been a tremendous surge of interest in the evaluation and treatment of women with urinary incontinence in both lay and academic circles. The current phenomenon of the aging American population, combined with the commercial advertising of anti-incontinence products, has aided in the gradual destigmatization of female incontinence. Unfortunately, patient embarrassment continues to deter women from seeking care. The burden of identifying women with incontinence remains on the care providers.

A systemic approach to the management of urinary incontinence has become a necessity as the array of surgical and nonsurgical interventions continues to expand. Each patient must be carefully negotiated through the appropriate testing modalities and treatment options to optimize outcome. This chapter provides an overview of the etiology and evaluation of female incontinence, with emphasis on conservative and surgical management.

PATHOPHYSIOLOGY

The ability to maintain normal bladder function throughout the entire life span is a surprisingly complex achievement. The possibilities for failure are great and it is not surprising that one in four women will develop incontinence at some time in their lives. The continence mechanism relies on coordination between neurologic, smooth, and striated muscle, and depends on the continued integrity of connective, vascular, and mucosal components.[1] Overriding all these must be an intact sensorium. Alterations in one or more of these factors can lead to lower urinary tract dysfunction or incontinence, or both. Attention must be paid to each of these components and their interactions while evaluating the patient and planning incontinence therapy.

Incontinence Types

Urinary incontinence can derive from one or more of several etiologies. The most common of these are genuine stress incontinence (GSI), detrusor instability (DI), mixed incontinence, and urinary retention with overflow incontinence. GSI occurs when the intravesical pressure exceeds the urethral resistance in the absence of a detrusor contraction. This can be caused by increased mobility of the bladder or by loss of urethral sphincteric function. DI is identified when uncontrolled detrusor contractions are present during the filling phase while the patient is trying to avoid urination. The presence of both GSI and DI is termed mixed incontinence. A less common type of incontinence is overflow incontinence, which results from incomplete bladder emptying and the persistence of an abnormally large amount of residual urine. The leakage from the overdistended bladder may present as a symptom of stress incontinence due to the persistence of high bladder pressure, or as urge incontinence due to unstable detrusor contractions from the weakened detrusor muscle.

Although it is tempting to forge ahead with surgical therapy for incontinence based on a complete history and physical examination, the physician must use caution. Prospective comparison of urinary symptoms and multichannel urodynamic testing has clearly shown that the patient's history does not always correlate well with cystometric diagnosis.[2] Although inappropriate conservative management of incontinence may only lead to failure or delayed improvement, the incorrect choice of surgical management can lead to disastrous results and a "cure" much worse that the original disease. A directed history and physical examination with identification of the patient's primary symptoms, combined with thoughtful selection of appropriate urodynamic testing is required to understand the etiology and management of incontinence.

BASIC INCONTINENCE EVALUATION

History

Utmost in the historical evaluation of urinary incontinence is an understanding of the patient's perspective of the severity of incontinence. The International Continence Society has defined urinary incontinence as "urinary leakage which is a social or hygienic *problem.*"[3] Urinary leakage that is of little or no concern to a sedentary older woman may be devastating to the young, active, professional. Identification of the patient with truly problematic incontinence remains a challenge. Societal taboos and lack of public education have perpetuated incontinence as a relatively hidden disease. The lack of awareness of treatment options, embarrassment, and a sense of futility toward incontinence therapy dissuade women from seeking help.[4] It remains the obligation of the physician to probe for the presence of incontinence symptoms and their impact on the patient.

Elicitation of incontinence symptoms is best obtained by asking general questions such as "Do you have trouble with your bladder?" or "Do you have trouble holding your urine (water)?" Positive responses can then prompt more specific questions such as "Do you ever lose urine when you don't want to?" and "Do you ever wear a pad or other protective device to collect your urine?"[5]

Once the presence of incontinence has been elicited, the patient can be probed for symptoms associated with her urinary leakage. The classical symptoms of stress incontinence include leakage associated with activities that increase intra-abdominal pressure, such as coughing, sneezing, lifting, or walking. Urge incontinence is loss of urine associated with a sudden, urgent need to urinate, often with frequency and nocturia. Overflow incontinence may present with a variety of symptoms, including hesitancy or incomplete emptying. Although helpful, symptoms associated with incontinence can be misleading, particularly when urgency or frequency is reported. These symptoms are as likely to be reported by women with stress incontinence as those with DI.[6] In addition, incontinence due to detrusor contractions can be provoked by sudden movements or coughing, and may be falsely assumed to be due to GSI. No matter what the etiology, the importance of determining the impact of each symptom on the patient's lifestyle cannot be overemphasized. It is of no use to cure mild leakage with coughing only to find that the patient's primary concern centers on urgency and frequency symptoms.

The assessment of the severity of incontinence begins with a determination of the usual pattern of voluntary and involuntary micturitions and fluid consumption. Although the simplest means of obtaining these data is by direct patient recall, self-reporting of health status has been shown to be unreliable due to inaccurate recall and abnormal perception of disease severity.[7] The most effective means of symptom reporting is to ask the patient to keep a diary in which events are recorded as they occur. This can provide reproducible data that are helpful in both baseline assessment and evaluation of treatment outcomes.[6] Several different types of urinary diaries have been developed, all of which require the subject to record episodes of voluntary and involuntary voids. Some diaries are also designed to record an estimation of the volume of urine voided or lost with incontinent episodes and space may be present to record comments about aggravating factors (Fig. 38-1). In addition to determining voiding and leakage patterns, a urinary diary can identify abnormal timing or volume of fluid intake. A surprising number of women consume ab-

NAME _____ PHONE(H) _____ (W) _____

| | DAY ONE | | | | DAY TWO | | |
TIME	INTAKE	OUTPUT	SYMPTOMS	TIME	INTAKE	OUTPUT	SYMPTOMS
TOTAL							

Fig. 38-1. Frequency/volume bladder chart.

normally large quantities of fluids under the assumption that water will aid dieting or that good health is maintained by ''flushing the kidneys.'' Simple re-education as to normal urinary tract function and fluid consumption can dramatically reduce or eliminate symptoms.

The remainder of the directed history should focus on the identification of transient causes of urinary incontinence. Acute changes in health that should be specifically addressed include urinary tract infections, constipation, or alteration in mental acuity. In particular, elderly patients may develop limitations of cognition, mobility, or physical strength that will exacerbate or precipitate incontinence. Simple alterations in the living environment, such as a commode or modifications of a bathroom, can be helpful. Most importantly, a wide variety of pharmaceuticals, including antihypertensives, diuretics, antipsychotics, and antidepressants, can induce retention or incontinence[5] (Table 38-1).

Directed Physical Examination

The directed physical examination of the woman with urinary incontinence should focus on the causes of incontinence, conditions that may exacerbate incontinence (e.g., diabetes or edema), and sequelae of persistent urinary leakage. Confounding factors such as limited cognition, poor manual dexterity or poor mobility should be noted. In addition to the general physical examination, a neurologic examination, should be performed with emphasis on the sacral nerve roots. Motor function can be assessed by strength testing of the lower extremities, and sensory function of S2–S4 is determined by evaluating light and sharp sensation over the perianal and genital dermatomes (Fig. 38-2). The presence of intact sacral reflex arcs can be verified by identifying an ''anal wink'' or bulbocavernosus reflex (Fig. 38-3). Asymmetry of pelvic or perineal muscles may suggest neuromuscular damage.

Table 38-1. Pharmaceutical Causes of Transient Urinary Incontinence

Potential Causes	Comments
Sedative hypnotics	Benzodiazepines, especially long-acting agents such as flurazepam and diazepam, may accumulate in elderly patients and cause confusion and secondary incontinence Alcohol, frequently used as a sedative, can cloud the sensorium, impair mobility, and induce a diuresis, resulting in incontinence
Diuretics	A brisk diuresis induced by loop diuretics can overwhelm bladder capacity and lead to polyuria, frequency, and urgency, thereby precipitating incontinence in a frail older person The loop diuretics include furosemide, ethacrynic acid, and bumetanide

Anticholinergic agents
    Antihistamines
    Antidepressants
    Antipsychotics
    Disopnamide
    Opiates
    Antispasmodics (dicyclomine and donnatal)
    Antiparkinsonian agents (trihexyphenidyl and benztropine mesylate)
	Nonprescription (over-the-counter) agents with anticholinergic properties are taken commonly by older patients for insomnia, coryza, pruritus, and vertigo, and many prescription medications also have anticholinergic properties
	Anticholinergic side effects include urinary retention with associated urinary frequency and overflow incontinence
	Besides anticholinergic actions, antipsychotics such as thioridazine and haloperidol may cause sedation, rigidity, and immobility

α-Adrenergic agents
    Sympathomimetics (decongestants)
    Sympatholytics (e.g., prazosin, terazosin, and doxzaosin)
	Sphincter tone in the proximal urethra can be decreased by α-antagonists and increased by α-antagonists.
	An older woman whose urethra is shortened and weakened with age may develop stress incontinence when taking an α-antagonist for hypertension
	An older man prostate enlargement may develop acute urinary retention and overflow incontinence when taking multicomponent cold capsules that contain α-agonists and anticholinergic agents, especially if a nasal decongestant and a nonprescription hypnotic antihistamine are added

Calcium channel blockers	Calcium channel blockers can reduce smooth muscle contractility in the bladder and occasionally can cause urinary retention and overflow incontinence

(Modified from Agency for Health Care Policy and Research,[5] with permission.)

Particular attention is given to a detailed genital and pelvic examination. The initial external inspection may reveal severe vulvar excoriation from continual dampness, and a gaping introital hiatus may signify previous pelvic floor trauma or neurologic deficit. The vaginal tissue should be inspected for signs of atrophy, stenosis, and bladder neck mobility (see below). Attention to the anterior vaginal wall can reveal urethral diverticula. Assessment of pelvic muscle strength can be easily performed during the bimanual examination by asking the patient to contract her pelvic muscles. This presents an excellent opportunity for patient education on the correct technique of pelvic muscle exercises. An abnormally large postvoid residual may be evidenced during the pelvic examination by palpation of a distended bladder. Finally, a rectal examination should be included to evaluate rectal sphincter tone or the presence of fecal impaction.

Basic Urodynamic Evaluation

After characterization of incontinence and identification of abnormal physical findings, all women should undergo a basic evaluation consisting of urinalysis (with culture if indicated), determination of postvoid residual and a cough stress test. Routine urinalysis can identify asymptomatic bacteriuria, infection, glycosuria, or hematuria as causative or exacerbating factors for incontinence. The presence of a large residual after voiding is a significant indicator of abnormal detrusor function or, less commonly, urinary outflow obstruction. Although the definition of an abnormal postvoid residual remains controversial, a residual of over 200 ml is generally considered abnormal, 50 to 199 ml is possibly abnormal, and less than 50 ml is normal. As the stress of the laboratory situation may not be conducive to optimal detrusor function, an abnormal postvoid residual should always be re-evaluated. Persistence of a high residual should prompt the investigator to proceed to more complex urodynamic testing.

Documentation of urinary incontinence is most simply accomplished by a cough stress test. This is optimally performed with a comfortably full bladder by asking the patient to cough forcefully while the urethra is visualized, in order to observe urinary leakage. The cough stress test can be performed in either the lithotomy or sitting positions but is most likely to be positive with the patient standing. Although leakage with coughing is suggestive of stress incontinence,

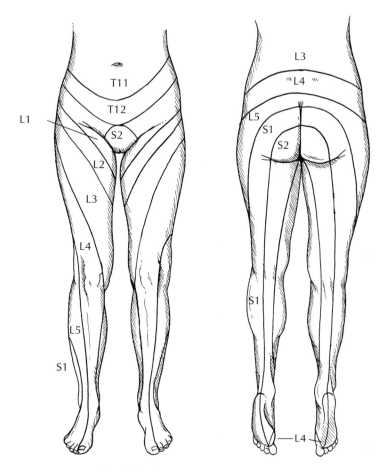

Fig. 38-2. Sacral sensory dermatomes.

urinary loss several moments after coughing may indicate cough-induced unstable detrusor contractions.[8]

Urethral Mobility

Evaluation of urethral mobility aids in the assessment of genital prolapse and the differentiation between GSI due to intrinsic sphincter deficiency (ISD) and stress incontinence due to urethral hypermobility. The cotton swab or "Q-tip" test was designed as a simple means to measure urethral mobility. The rotational descent of the urethra is measured by placing the cotton-tipped swab into the urethra up to the level of the bladder neck with the patient in the supine position. Using a protractor or goniometer, the angle of the swab, in degrees from the horizontal axis, is measured at rest and at maximal Valsalva effort. Although measuring urethral rotation can assist in describing the presence of bladder neck hypermobility, the cotton swab test is not diagnostic for the presence of GSI or DI.[9] Alternatives to using a cotton swab include the use of a semirigid catheter such as those used for intermittent catheterization. After the patient is catheterized for a post-

void residual, it is convenient to reposition the catheter into the urethra and ask her to strain in order to test urethral mobility. Simple direct visualization or manual reduction during the pelvic examination may also provide significant information about urethral mobility. Although there is no absolute definition of hypermobility, a urethral axis rotation of over 30 degrees is commonly accepted as abnormal. The presence of hypermobility does not exclude the possibility of concurrent intrinsic sphincter deficiency.

Simple Urodynamics

Urodynamics are a group of tests designed to aid in determining the etiology of lower urinary tract dysfunction. Each test should only be employed to add additional information to the diagnostic evaluation. The "shotgun" approach of ordering a large battery of tests is not cost-effective nor encouraged. The most widely used urodynamic tests include cystometry and uroflowmetry. Both of these tests can be performed with a wide range of equipment varying greatly in the amount of data and cost generated. Fortunately, most patients can be evaluated using simple techniques.

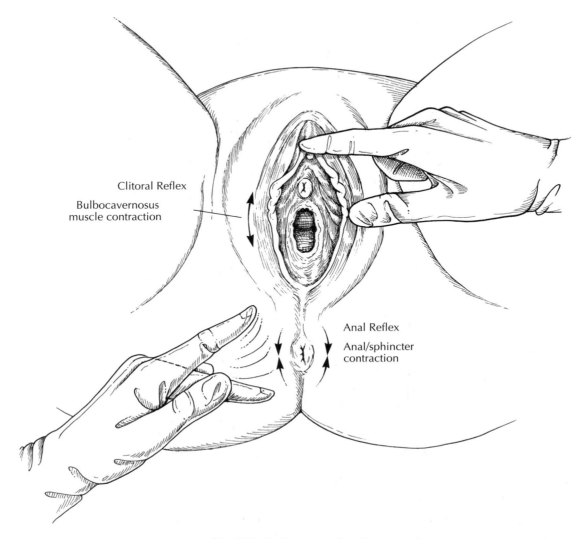

Clitoral Reflex

Bulbocavernosus
muscle contraction

Anal Reflex

Anal/sphincter
contraction

Fig. 38-3. Bulbocavernosis reflex.

Simple Cystometry

Simple cystometry involves gradual bladder filling with sterile water or normal saline while observing for evidence of detrusor contractions. The simplest form, "eyeball cystometrics," requires only a red rubber catheter and an attached graduated funnel, or the barrel of a 60-ml syringe, and involves the slow instillation of fluid into the bladder (Fig. 38-4). Detrusor contractions are evidenced by a rise in water level during filling due to back pressure from the detrusor contraction associated with urge symptoms. A slightly more complex version involves the attachment of a manometer, such as those used for central venous pressure measurements, to the filling catheter to allow a numeric measurement of the rise in bladder pressure[10] (Fig. 38-5). Normal values for cystometry include a first sensation to void of at least 150 ml and a bladder capacity of 400 to 600 ml. Simple cystometry is best suited to the uncomplicated patient be-

cause of a limited ability to detect small detrusor contractions and the inability to account for the contributions of abdominal pressures.[11]

Simple Uroflowmetry

Simple uroflowmetry is used to determine the urinary flow rate and flow time in order to screen for the presence of outflow obstruction and abnormal detrusor contractility. Available equipment ranges from a stopwatch and graduated collecting container to electronic collecting devices that rely on a weight displacement transducer. Normal uroflowmetry is generally accepted as a peak flow rate of at least 15 to 20 ml/sec with a voided volume of 150 to 200 ml. Nomograms are available for maximum and mean flow rates based on voided volumes.[12] An abnormal flow rate should always be repeated, as voiding in the laboratory situation may be difficult for many women. Persistently abnormal uroflowmetry

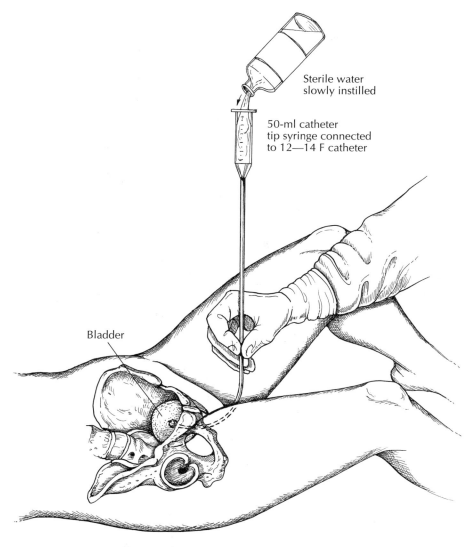

Sterile water
slowly instilled

50-ml catheter
tip syringe connected
to 12—14 F catheter

Bladder

Fig. 38-4. Simple cystometry.

requires further investigation with complex uroflowmetry.[13] Possible etiologies include outflow obstruction or poor detrusor contraction. These can only be differentiated by simultaneous measurement of voiding pressures and flow rates.

DETAILED EVALUATIONS

Complex Urodynamics

Complex urodynamic testing encompasses a wide range of testing modalities, including complex cystometry, complex uroflowmetry, urethral pressure profilometry, leak point pressures, cystourethrography, videocystourethrography, voiding cystourethrography, and electromyography. Such tests allow for the in-depth evaluation of lower urinary

tract dysfunction and are indicated for a variety of reasons, including the following[5]:

- Inability to determine diagnosis by simple urodynamics
- Urgency and frequency with negative simple cystometry
- Mixed incontinence symptoms with anticipated surgical intervention
- Previously failed incontinence surgery
- Failure of conservative therapy
- Previous pelvic irradiation
- Lower urinary tract obstruction
- Urinary retention
- Voiding dysfunction
- Neurologic abnormalities

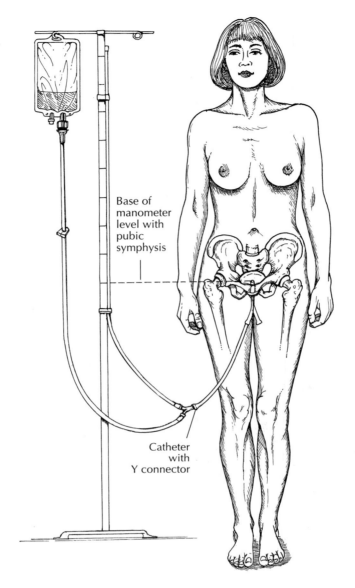

Base of
manometer
level with
pubic
symphysis

Catheter
with
Y connector

Fig. 38-5. Simple cystometry with manometry.

Complex Cystometry

Complex cystometry requires the placement of an intravesical catheter to measure detrusor pressures and a vaginal or rectal catheter to indirectly measure intra-abdominal pressures throughout the filling phase. It is particularly designed to detect the presence of DI, abnormal bladder capacity, and abnormal changes in detrusor pressure during the filling phase. The addition of a rectal or vaginal transducer permits subtraction of the intra-abdominal pressure from the vesical pressure to reduce artifact and, produce a measure of the true detrusor pressure.

Complex Uroflowmetry

Complex uroflowmetry is essential to evaluate outflow obstruction and urinary retention, and requires simultaneous measurements of intravesical and intra-abdominal pressures while studying spontaneous voiding. The differentiation of these two causes of abnormal flow patterns is particularly important when contemplating a potentially obstructive surgical treatment for stress incontinence. Outflow obstruction usually entails a low flow rate associated with a high detrusor pressure while urinary retention is often associated with poor detrusor contractility.

Intrinsic Sphincter Deficiency Indentification

Stress incontinence can be categorized into two subsets, urethral hypermobility and ISD. The urethra is surrounded by longitudinal and circular muscles that maintain urethral tone (Fig. 38-6). Damage to the periurethral tissue can result from trauma or denervation from surgery, childbirth, or neu-

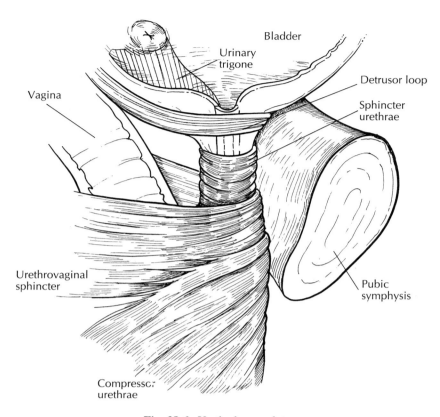

Fig. 38-6. Urethral musculature.

rologic disease, resulting in poor urethral function previously referred to as a ''lead pipe urethra'' or type III incontinence, now better described as ISD. Simple retropubic suspension is less likely to improve incontinence due to urethral dysfunction; more complex procedures such as slings, collagen injections, or artificial sphincters are needed. The presence of a positive cough stress test combined with reduced urethral mobility, or a history of previous incontinence surgery warrants further investigation for the possibility of ISD. The optimal means of diagnosing ISD is controversial and involves the documentation of sphincteric dysfunction by urethral pressure profilometry (UPP) or by leak point pressure (LPP) tests, or both.

Urethral Pressure Profilometry

UPP is performed by slowly withdrawing the intravesical catheter through the length of the urethra while measuring the amount of force exerted against the catheter transducer. This maneuver produces a measurement of the maximum urethral closure pressure, a reflection of the urethral resting tone, and a determination of the functional length of the urethra (Fig. 38-7). When performed during repetitive coughing, the ratio of pressure transmission to the urethra and bladder can be determined. Maximum urethral closure pressures of less than 20 cmH$_2$O have been associated with

poor success of standard retropubic urethropexy surgery and are suggestive of ISD.[14]

Leak Point Pressure

The LPP test is a more recently described evaluation of the urethra, and is a means of determining the amount of pressure required to overcome the resistance of the urethra.[15] LPP are presumed to reflect urethral tone and have been described in a variety of manners that have not yet been standardized. The bladder is generally filled with a specified amount of fluid (250 to 300 ml) and the patient is placed in the sitting or standing position. The woman is asked to cough using increasing amounts of force until stress incontinence is demonstrated. The intra-abdominal or intravesical pressure required to induce stress incontinence is designated as the LPP. Most studies identify an LPP of less than 60 cmH$_2$O as being associated with ISD, and values of 60 to 90 cmH$_2$O may indicate hypermobility or ISD. Further testing is needed to determine whether the LPP or UPP is the more specific indicator of sphincteric dysfunction.[16]

Additional Specialized Tests

Specialized tests may be helpful in selected situations to identify the etiology of incontinence. Videocystourethrography combines the use of fluoroscopy with filling cystometry

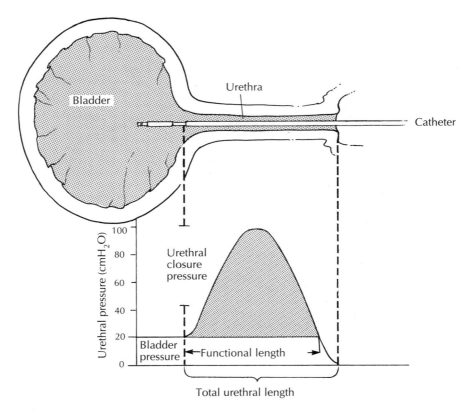

Fig. 38-7. Urethral pressure profile.

and is particularly useful to identify stress incontinence in women who have failed multiple surgical procedures or to detect anatomic defects or ureteral reflux. Voiding cystourethrography combines fluoroscopy with complex uroflowmetry to identify voiding dysfunction or structural abnormalities of the urethra, including fistulas or diverticula. Cystourethroscopy is used to identify structural abnormalities of the bladder or urethra, interstitial cystitis, urethritis, stones, polyps, and tumors. Its use in the evaluation of stress incontinence or DI is limited.

NONSURGICAL MANAGEMENT

Pelvic Muscle Exercises

Pelvic muscle exercise regimens were initially described by Dr. Arnold Kegel.[17] He hypothesized that the pelvic floor could be rehabilitated after childbirth in a way similar to other muscles that are rehabilitated after acute injury. Since Kegel's original article, a wide variety of exercise programs have been developed, with authors advocating 25 to 100 exercises per day. The foremost problems in attaining success with exercise remain the correct education of the patient in the identification and contraction of the pelvic floor, and motivation for long-term commitment. Devices such as vagi-

nal cones are commercially available to aid in the correct technique for pelvic muscle exercises[18,19] (Fig. 38-8).

Women with extremely weak muscles may benefit from biofeedback, a method of utilizing a pressure measurement device that notifies the patient when correct muscle contraction is performed and reinforces correct technique. Another alternative to strengthen pelvic muscles is electrical stimulation, which applies an electrical current to the muscle and induces a contraction. The repetitive use of electrical stimulation can increase muscle mass and strength. This technique may be particularly helpful in the patient with severe muscle weakness and denervation[20] (Fig. 38-9).

Mechanical Devices

Several attempts have been made to develop occlusive devices to reduce leakage due to stress incontinence. Intravaginal pessary-type devices have been developed that compress the urethra against the symphysis to increase resistance against urine loss[21] (Fig. 38-10). Similar results can be achieved with the use of a tampon in the vagina. Devices in the development stages include a small catheter-type device with an inflatable balloon, which is placed at the bladder neck, and a small occlusive device that adheres to the urethral opening with a hydrophilic gel. Most mechanical devices are best suited for women with smaller amounts of leakage.

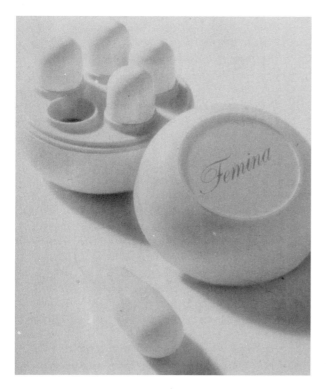

Fig. 38-8. Femina vaginal cones (Dacomed Corporation).

α-Agonist Therapy

Pharmaceutical therapy options for stress incontinence primarily consist of α-agonists and estrogen. The rational for α-agonist therapy is based on the high concentration of α-adrenergic receptors in the bladder neck and proximal ure-

thra. Stimulation of urethral musculature may decrease severity of incontinence in 30 to 60 percent of patients, but cures only 1 to 14 percent. The most commonly used medication is phenylpropanolamine in doses of 50 mg twice daily, which can induce a variety of side effects, including anxiety, respiratory difficulty, headache, hypertension, or cardiac arrhythmias. Caution should be used when treating women with hypertension or cardiovascular disease.

Estrogen therapy may provide some help for women with stress incontinence but is more likely to aid in treatment of urge incontinence. The variable response to estrogen therapy suggests that treatment should be considered on an individual basis.

SURGICAL MANAGEMENT

Preoperative Considerations

The inherent failure rate of incontinence surgery suggests that caution should be used when planning surgical interventions. All management options, including their likelihood of success, should be discussed preoperatively. In theory, nonsurgical management should be used initially, reserving surgery for women with more severe incontinence and those who fail conservative trials. Women with mild to moderate GSI due to urethral hypermobility should be considered for a trial of pelvic muscle exercises. Education and positive feedback during the initial pelvic examination will help the patient understand when she is correctly contracting her pelvic floor. Suitable candidates include those subjects who are motivated to avoid surgery and who are able to identify and

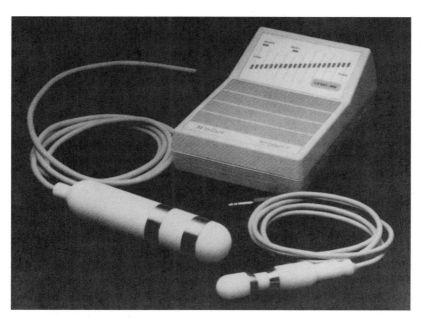

Fig. 38-9. Electrical stimulators (Hollister Corporation, Empi Corporation).

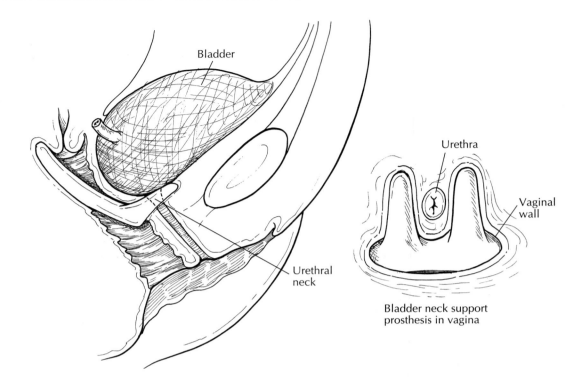

Fig. 38-10. Introl bladder neck support prosthesis in place (Johnson and Johnson Medical).

contract their pelvic muscles. In daily practice, surgery is often used as a first-line intervention in those women who are unlikely to comply with conservative therapies.

Coexisting DI should be preoperatively addressed. Despite complex urodynamics, it is often difficult to determine if most incontinent episodes are due to unstable contraction or stress incontinent events. Correction of DI through bladder training and pharmaceuticals before GSI surgery will clarify the impact of the component on the patient's symptoms and the amount of improvement that can be expected from corrective surgery.

Selection of Appropriate Operative Procedure

Surgical procedures are available to correct stress incontinence due to hypermobility, ISD, and DI. Unlike stress incontinence for which surgery is used as a primary treatment modality, surgery for DI is considered a last resort.

The choice of surgical procedure is made based on the degree of severity of incontinence, the risks and complications associated with surgery, long-term success rates, and expectations of the patient. A more aggressive approach is indicated in the younger, healthier, active woman who will demand the best long-term success rates. The older, frail, or sedentary woman may be better served by a less aggressive operation with a faster and easier recovery. Inherent in the choice of surgery is the anticipated long-term and short-term

success rates (Table 38-2). Despite decades of refinement in diagnosis and surgical technique, the inherent failure rate of incontinence surgery persists, and will vary from surgeon to surgeon depending on individual modification of techniques, experience level, and patient selection. Differences in tissue quality, individual anatomy, and associated prolapse requires that each operation be individualized to each

Table 38-2. Success Rates for Anti-incontinence Procedures

Procedure	Cure or Improvement (%)	Complications (%)
Burch colposuspension/ MMK	84 (27–100)	18 (6–57)
Needle urethropexy	85 (50–100)	21 (20–60)
Pubovaginal sling		
Fascia	89 (64–100)	31
Synthetic	83 (60–85)	17[a]
Periurethral bulking agents	61 (18–100)	6 (0–12)

Abbreviation: MMK, Marshall-Marchetti-Krantz.

[a] Although the overall complication rate for fascial slings was high, synthetic slings were associated with more severe complications.

(Modified from the AHCPR Clinical Practice Guidelines,[5] with permission.)

patient's particular needs. These variations are particularly important in incontinence surgery, as over- or undercorrection of anatomic defects can lead to surgical failure or increased postoperative complications, including voiding dysfunction.

Tailoring the choice of surgery to the patient's needs also includes a definition of surgical success. The absence of incontinence under usual daily activities, but the persistence of a positive stress test in the urodynamic lab, may be considered a "success" by the patient but a "failure" by laboratory definitions. Likewise, complete resolution of incontinence with postoperative urinary retention may constitute a "failure" to the patient, who is burdened with long-term intermittent catheterization. Preoperative discussions of expectations will help both the physician and patient achieve a "successful" outcome.

Anterior Colporrhaphy

The oldest described method of surgical therapy for incontinence is the anterior repair as described by Howard Kelly. The original intent of the anterior colporrhaphy was to narrow the bladder neck, as incontinence was thought to originate from funneling of the vesical neck. Subsequent modifications have placed further emphasis on the identification of endopelvic fascia and utilization of paraurethral fascia in re-establishing urethral support. Despite decades of experience with this operation, the long-term success rates of the anterior colporrhaphy for urinary incontinence are poor and range from 36 to 65 percent.[22–24] The anterior repair has now been replaced by needle and retropubic suspension procedures, which have significantly higher success rates.

Needle Suspension Procedures

Needle suspension procedures were developed by the gynecologist Armand Pereyra as an alternative to the Marshall-Marchetti-Krantz (MMK) operation, to decrease morbidity by minimizing the size of the abdominal wall incision. The key to this new type of procedure was the development of a suture carrier that allowed the passage of a ligature through the vaginal wall to the space of Retzius and finally, through the abdominal wall. Since Dr. Pereyra's original work, many attempts have been made to modify the needle suspension procedure, including changes in the techniques of vaginal dissection, method of suture placement through the vagina and endopelvic fascia, method of suture passage through the space of Retzius, and the use of intraoperative cystoscopy.[25]

Pereyra Procedure

The original Pereyra procedure was designed without vaginal dissection and used #30 silver wire for suture and a small transverse abdominal skin incision. The double-pronged ligature carrier was passed blindly through the space of Retzius and into the vagina. The suture was then threaded through each arm of the carrier, withdrawn through the rectus muscle, and tied against the abdominal wall. Concern for the possibility of bladder injury with a blind procedure led to the development of the modified Pereyra procedure. Unlike the original method, this technique involves a midline incision in the anterior vaginal wall, with dissection and identification of the endopelvic fascia. Sharp dissection is then used to remove the endopelvic fascia from its attachment to the pubic ramus to allow the placement of a helical suture into the fascia just lateral to the urethra (Fig. 38-11). The ends of the polypropylene sutures are then passed through the rectus fascia using the ligature carrier, and secured to the contralateral sutures[26] (Fig. 38-12).

Stamey Procedure

Stamey was the first to report the use of the endoscope in conjunction with a needle suspension procedure. Using a technique similar to the original Pereyra procedure, the endoscope was placed at the bladder neck while the ligature carrier was blindly passed. Lateral motion of the ligature carrier against the urethra could be seen through the cystoscope, and the correct placement of the carrier at the level of the bladder neck could be confirmed. The suture was then loaded on the carrier and withdrawn through the abdominal wall. The process was then repeated by passing the carrier through the abdominal wall to the vagina again, this time 1 to 2 cm lateral to the original punctures. The remaining end of the suture was passed through the abdominal wall and tied to the free end of the same suture. In order to decrease the likelihood that the sutures would pull through the fascial wall, Stamey described the inclusion of 1-cm Dacron buttresses, which were threaded on the suture and positioned against the endopelvic fascia[27] (Figs. 38-13 and 38-14).

Raz Procedure

The Raz modification of the needle suspension procedure is very similar to the modified Pereyra. Instead of a midline incision, Raz recommended an inverted U-shaped incision to maximize the exposure of the lateral vaginal wall (Fig. 38-15). Following the passage of one end of the ligature through the space of Retzius, the free end is used to place the helical suture into the detached endopelvic fascia. The most notable modification is that the lateral turns of the suture also incorporate the lateral aspect of the vaginal mucosa. The suture is then passed through the abdominal wall and secured to the contralateral sutures. The addition of the incorporation of the vaginal mucosa into the helical suture was designed to limit the amount of bladder elevation that could be achieved when the sutures were secured, and thus decrease the likelihood of postoperative urinary retention.[28]

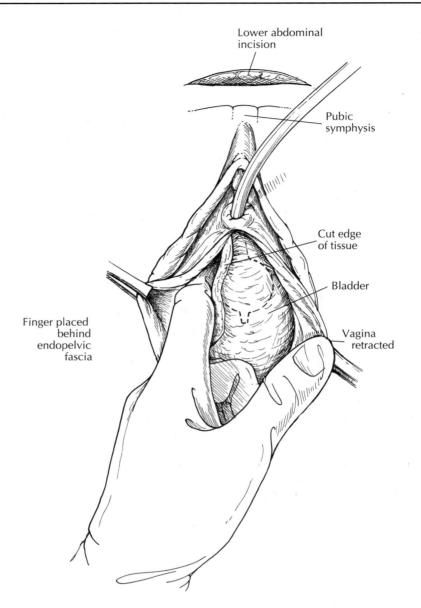

Fig. 38-11. Detachment of endopelvic fascia for helical suture placement.

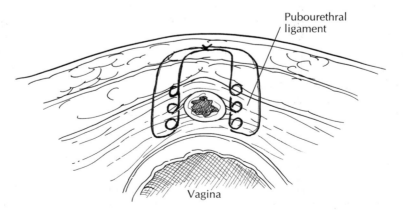

Fig. 38-12. Modified Pereyra procedure.

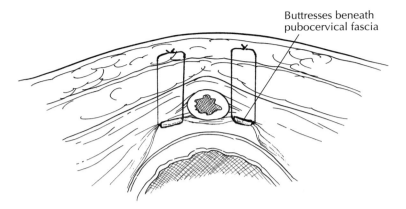

Fig. 38-13. Stamey procedure.

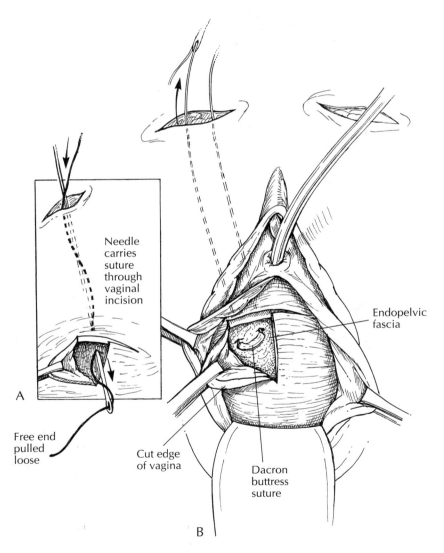

Fig. 38-14. (A & B) Stamey procedure with Dacron buttress.

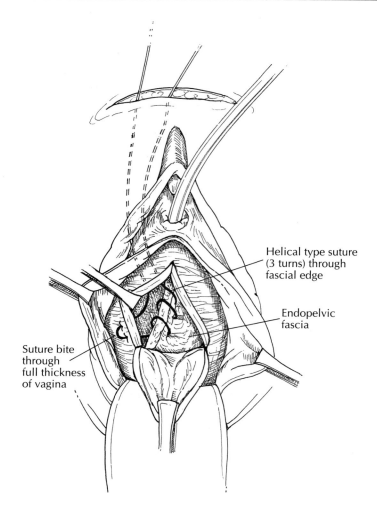

Fig. 38-15. Raz procedure.

Other Procedures

There have been several other reported modifications of the needle suspension procedure, including two "no-incision" techniques by Gittes and Benderev, which are very similar to Pereyra's original procedure. The Gittes technique begins with two small abdominal incisions through which the ligature carrier is passed. A 2 nylon suture is then withdrawn from the vagina to the abdominal wall. A free needle is used to make helical suture in the anterior vaginal wall and the suture is withdrawn through a second vaginal puncture site. The suture is tied to the free end across a small bridge of rectus fascia. The procedure is repeated on the remaining side and cystoscopy is used to confirm the absence of bladder injury (Fig. 38-16).

Another no-incision technique has been described by Benderev, using specially designed commercial products.[29] Unlike other described needle procedures, this method uses an orthopaedic anchor to fix the suture to the pubic symphysis. A small incision is made over the superior aspect of the pubic tubercle to allow placement of the anchor, with at-

tached suture, into the symphysis (Fig. 38-17). The free end of the suture is passed through the abdominal wall to the vagina using a specially designed suture carrier that can grasp and release the suture to allow placement into the intact vaginal wall in a similar fashion to the original Pereyra procedure.

Success Rates

Reported success rates for needle suspension procedures have varied widely. Success rates in the initial year postsurgery have been reported as low as 40 percent and as high as 90 percent.[30,31] As with every type of surgical procedure, it is difficult to achieve the ideal of the randomized controlled trial with pre- and postoperative urodynamics. Bergman et al[23] have provided the most longitudinal data available thus far. A randomized trial of a Burch retropubic urethropexy, needle suspension, and an anterior colporrhaphy revealed a 1-year success rate of 98 percent with the Burch method, as compared with an 85-percent success rate

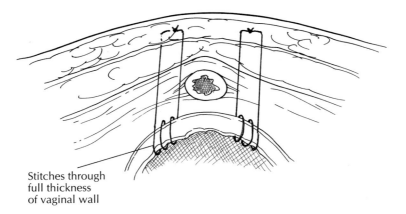

Stitches through
full thickness
of vaginal wall

Fig. 38-16. Gittes procedure.

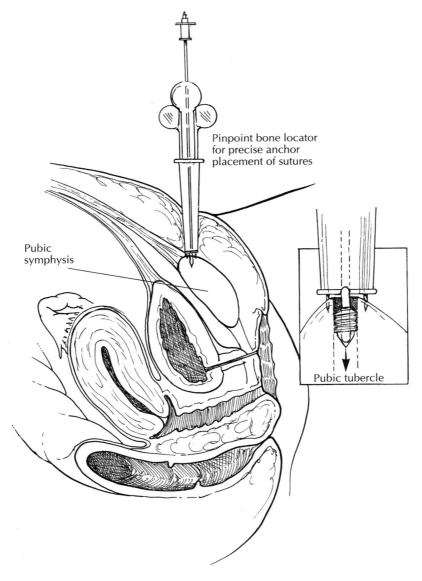

Pinpoint bone locator
for precise anchor
placement of sutures

Pubic
symphysis

Pubic tubercle

Fig. 38-17. Vesica bladder neck suspension with anchor fixation.

with the modified Pereyra method. A 5-year follow-up of this patient group has since shown a significant decline in success rates, to 82-percent for the Burch and 43 percent for the modified Pereyra procedure.[24] The significant advantage of reduced operative morbidity with a minimal incision technique should be carefully weighed against the possibility of reduced long-term success.[32] The choice of surgical technique must incorporate an understanding of the patient's outcome goals and the surgeon's expertise and individual success rates.

Urethropexy Procedures

Several types of retropubic urethropexy procedures have been described, all of which begin with dissection of the space of Retzius. Marshall et al[33] initially described a retropubic procedure for stress incontinence in 1949. They sutured the periurethral tissue to the periosteum of the pubic symphysis in a man who developed severe incontinence after radical pelvic surgery, and subsequently applied the technique to women with stress urinary incontinence. Since that time, retropubic procedures have been widely used in the treatment of hypermobile-type stress incontinence in women with a proven record of success.

The retropubic approach allows direct visualization of the bladder neck and periurethral fascia, allows precise suture placement, and reduces injury to the bladder and surrounding structures. The strength of the anchoring tissue, whether endopelvic fascia, iliopectineal ligament, periosteum, or arcus tendineus, can be assessed and used at its optimal point. The bladder is easily accessible for intentional cystotomy to assess bladder injury or ureteric patency. The major disadvantage of all types of retropubic urethropexies is the required abdominal incision, which increases postoperative pain and the duration of hospitalization. In cases in which an abdominal incision is part of the planned procedure, a retropubic approach to the surgical correction of stress incontinence is favored. In cases in which most of the planned procedure involves vaginal surgery without an abdominal incision, the surgeon must carefully weigh the advantages and disadvantages of needle procedures compared to retropubic procedures. The reduced long-term success rates reported with needle procedures may be significantly outweighed by the advantages of reduced operative morbidity for individual patients.

Retropubic Techniques

Access to the vagina is facilitated by placing the patient in low universal adjustable stirrups. The practice of "froglegging" the patient should be avoided, as this maneuver promotes stretch nerve injury due to the extreme external rotation at the hip and torque on the knee and ankle. The use of a perineal "condom drape" (3M TUR 1071 Steri-Drape)

with the condom inserted into the vagina allows the operator's vaginal hand to also be used abdominally and avoids repetitive glove changes. The adhesive portion of the drape is placed against the mons pubis before the sterile overdrapes are hung, with the hole above the condom used for insertion of the Foley catheter. Lubrication, such as KY Jelly or Betadine, facilitates insertion and removal of one or two fingers into the condom. As the diameter of this drape is only approximately 2.5 cm, surgeons with larger hands may find it awkward. Another alternative to regloving is the use of a stent or large Pratt dilator to elevate the vagina. However, the use of a stent makes it more difficult to assess tissue and quality.

A Pfannenstiel incision generally provides excellent exposure. Once the rectus abdominis has been opened in the midline, attention should be directed toward any intra-abdominal surgery that is to be accomplished in conjunction with the incontinence surgery. Elevation of the anterior compartment, which results from a retropubic urethropexy, is known to increase the occurrence of postoperative enterocele, with up to 20 percent of women developing an enterocele after retropubic urethropexy. Although the prophylactic plication of the cul-de-sac takes but a few minutes, a Moschcowitz or Halban procedure does require packing of the bowel; the patient may need more anesthetic, and may have more of an ileus than is usually seen with retropubic dissection alone. A prophylactic closure of the cul-de-sac should be considered in the following patients: women with coexisting genital prolapse in whom recurrent prolapse is more likely to occur; women with risk factors for genital prolapse, including a strong family history of prolapse or hernia; women with a history of heavy lifting or constipation; or women already undergoing an intraperitoneal procedure at the time of the retropubic procedure. The addition of hysterectomy to incontinence surgery does not improve cure rates and should be performed only when there is an indication for hysterectomy.

Following intraperitoneal procedures, the peritoneum is usually closed to keep bowel out of the surgical field. The placement of a self-retaining retractor beneath the rectus muscles will aid in exposure. The space of Retzius is a potential space, which lies just under the distal rectus abdominis and above the peritoneum. Blunt dissection beginning at the pubic symphysis and proceeding toward the pelvic sidewalls will expose the bladder, urethra, vagina, obturator vessels, and the arcus tendineum fascia pelvis.

Entry into the space of Retzius can be more difficult if there has been previous surgery or dissection. If the bladder wall was sutured instead of the periurethral fascia, sharp dissection may free this tissue and reveal previously untouched periurethral fascia. Scarring of the periurethral tissues to the symphysis and sidewalls should be carefully taken down to allow elevation of the endopelvic fascia into a more favorable position. In many cases of previous anti-incontinence surgery, the bladder may be so adherent to the symphysis and sidewalls as to prevent safe dissection without thinning or tearing of the anterior bladder wall and urethra. The surgeon may choose to perform an intentional cystotomy in the dome of the bladder. A small midline vertical bladder incision allows extension of the incision if necessary, and is simple to close. The surgeon then places the index finger of the nondominant hand into the bladder to differentiate bladder wall from its attachment to the symphysis and pelvic side wall. Dissection should always begin at the bladder neck and carry laterally. Extensive lateral dissection is unnecessary if the fascia can be identified and used more medially. The intentional cystotomy should be closed in two layers with absorbable suture and a suprapubic catheter placed if desired. Because of its nondependent position, continuous bladder drainage for 2 to 5 days after cystotomy should be sufficient to allow healing before voiding trials.

Once the bladder and adjacent tissues have been mobilized, the endopelvic fascia is identified by using the surgeon's finger to elevate the vagina on either side of the bladder neck. Several techniques have been described for mobilization of the bladder. Most commonly, the bladder and surrounding tissues are gently pulled medially and cephalad using sponge forceps for traction. Alternatively, the areolar and adipose tissue can be sharply removed, but this is more commonly associated with increased bleeding. Occasionally, large vessels running through the adventitia will require ligation. The dissection is sufficient when a space of 1 to 2 cm of shiny white fascia is visible on either side of the bladder neck. A transurethral Foley catheter with a

5- to 10-ml balloon is sufficient to identify the position of the bladder neck, while larger balloons of up to 30 ml may hinder dissection and mobilization of the bladder neck.

Once elevating sutures have been placed satisfactorily, the surgeon must ensure that bladder wall has not been breached. If any question remains, cystoscopy with a 30- or 70-degree scope through the urethra, or a stab wound into the bladder dome is helpful.

Burch Colposuspension

In 1961, Dr. John Burch of Nashville, Tennessee described a technique of suturing the periurethral fascia to Cooper's ligament for the correction of stress incontinence and cystocele. Burch sought an alternative anchoring site to the periosteum used with the MMK procedure. He first attempted to use the fascia covering the obturator internus, but abandoned this as it lacked sufficient strength. In 1968 he reported a long-term success rate of 90 percent using the iliopectineal ligament (Cooper's ligament), with the major postoperative complications being enterocele and DI. Since his first paper, there have been over 70 reports of surgical experience with the Burch retropubic urethropexy.[34]

Operative Procedure

The Burch colposuspension creates a shelf of endopelvic fascia to support the bladder neck and attaches this tissue to the iliopectineal ligament, or Cooper's ligament. The ap-

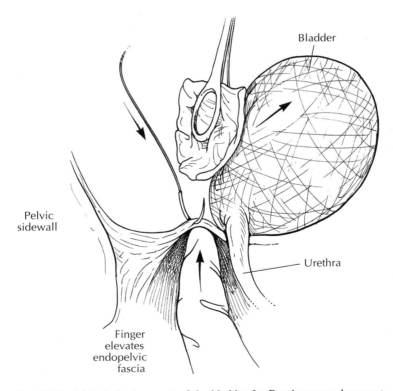

Fig. 38-18. Medial displacement of the bladder for Burch suture placement.

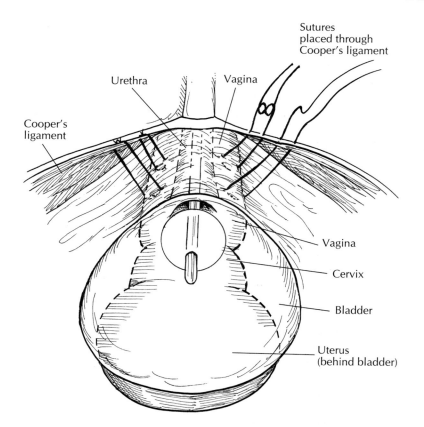

Fig. 38-19. Suture placement through Cooper's ligament.

proach to the space of Retzius is as described above. The endopelvic fascia is identified by placing the surgeon's nondominant hand into the vagina, and the vagina is stabilized by elevating a finger in one of the lateral fornices. A spongestick is used to gently pull the bladder edge medially while continuing to elevate the anterior vaginal wall (Fig. 38-18). Caution is used to avoid damaging the perivesical vessels. If bleeding does occur, upward pressure with the vaginal finger will control the hemorrhage until the vessel can be cauterized or sutured from above. Care should be taken to visualize the shiny white endopelvic fascia through which the sutures are to be placed, as opposed to the muscular bladder edge. Medial displacement of the bladder and surrounding tissues is maintained by an assistant while the operator places the sutures.

The placement of sutures in relation to the bladder neck varies; the authors prefer placement at the bladder neck by using the Foley balloon as the upper and lower limits of the sutures. Others prefer to place all of the sutures just below the bladder neck, alongside the urethra, thus producing a relative kinking effect (Fig. 38-19). This type of suture placement is more likely to produce postoperative voiding difficulties. A semicircle (MO-4, Ethicon) or five-eighths needle (UR-5, Ethicon) with 0 nonabsorbable braided suture facilitates placement. Sutures are placed through the vaginal fascia just lateral to the urethra. However, placement too lat-

erally results in inadequate support of the urethra and elevation of the posterior vaginal wall, causing dyspareunia (Fig. 38-20). The needle is first introduced into the fascia at the level of the bladder neck, encompassing a good piece of the endopelvic fascia but excluding the bladder edge. Entry into the vaginal skin should be avoided, but if it occurs, the tissue usually reepithelializes and is not a problem. The vaginal finger should briefly be moved to ensure that the needle has not perforated the surgeon's glove or condom drape (if used). A figure-of-eight suture or one or two knots (or both) can be thrown to reduce bleeding from the perivesical vessels and stabilize the suture to the vaginal tissue. The suture may be passed through Cooper's ligament at this time, or tagged until all of the periurethral sutures have been placed. The second suture is placed approximately 1.5 to 2 cm caudad to the first suture just below the bladder neck. The Foley balloon is then palpated to confirm the placement of the first two sutures at the bladder neck and, if necessary, a third suture can be placed to assure adequate bladder neck support. Caution should be used not to place undue traction on the Foley catheter; it can be pulled into the proximal urethra and distort the anatomy. Suture placement is then repeated on the contralateral side.

Cooper's ligament is approximately 5 cm below the pelvic brim and begins 4 to 5 cm lateral to the midline fusion of the pubic symphysis. The ligament is an inverted pyramid

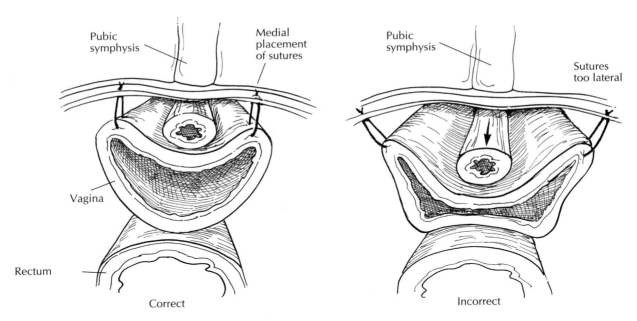

Fig. 38-20. Burch suture placement in endopelvic fascia.

in shape; therefore, the suture should be passed into the base of the ligament and brought out through its broad ventral surface. The sutures should be passed through the ligament above and slightly lateral to their placement in the endopelvic fascia. If the periosteum is encountered when inserting the needle, the surgeon should replace the suture slightly more ventrally. Some surgeons pass both ends of the suture behind or through Cooper's ligament and tie them on the ventral base of the ligament. This offers little additional security and may fray the ligament unnecessarily. The surgeon may find access to Cooper's ligament awkward, as there is often little space for the operator's hand and the needle-driver. This can be overcome by placing the suture through Cooper's ligament using the needle loaded left-handed, or tilting the operating table to improve visualization of the tissues. Retraction of the skin and subcutaneous tissues by the operator or an assistant can also be helpful. Occasionally a vessel runs the course of the ligament and should either be ligated or encompassed in the suture.

The degree of elevation and tightness of the sutures is only determined by experience. The operator may use a vaginal finger to support the bladder neck while the assistant ties the suture to help achieve the desired elevation. Support may be sufficient, even with a suture bridge or "bowstring" between the perivesical fascia and Cooper's ligament. The periurethral fascia should be elevated on either side to support the bladder neck without compressing or obstructing the urethra, and there should be room to insert a finger between the back of the symphysis and the bladder neck. Some surgeons have suggested the use of a cotton swab or cystoscopy to document bladder neck elevation and closure. No evidence is available to indicate that these methods improve

success rates. When using nonabsorbable suture, there is no reason to overcorrect by attempting to place the endopelvic fascia in direct approximation with Cooper's ligament. Overcorrection only induces postoperative voiding dysfunction and DI. The use of absorbable suture for the Burch colposuspension is strongly discouraged.

Any bleeding in the space of Retzius after tying the suspending sutures is controlled with cautery or absorbable sutures. If bleeding is excessive, the surgeon may wish to drain the space of Retzius through a separate stab wound with a #10 Jackson-Pratt or a similarly closed suction drain for 24 to 48 hours. If sutures are placed deeply and laterally, there is a possibility of ureteral obstruction. If the dissection was difficult or more extensive laterally, cystoscopy and intravenous indigo carmine can assess ureteral patency.

Advantages and Disadvantages

The success of the Burch procedure in the hands of many surgeons has been well documented, and has been subjected to the strictest surgical review of all anti-incontinence procedures. However, the procedure is poorly suited to women with small vaginal size and poor vaginal mobility. There is up to a 20-percent predilection to enterocele due to the alteration in the vaginal axis anteriorly, and consideration should be given to a prophylactic enterocele procedure in women at risk of developing genital prolapse. Overcorrection can lead to obstructive voiding dysfunction retention or DI. The Burch colposuspension has the advantage of being able to correct a coexisting cystocele, unlike the MMK or needle urethropexy. The complication of osteitis pubis is avoided, as is bowel perforation and rectus abdominis pain due to sutures, as seen with needle procedures.

Marshall-Marchetti-Krantz Procedure

In 1949 Marshall et al[33] described the MMK, a simple retropubic procedure for stress incontinence. Since that time, the MMK has been a popular retropubic procedure with a proven record of success. Its major drawback is a low (5 to 10 percent) incidence of osteitis pubis because of suture placement into the periosteum of the pubic symphysis. The MMK elevates and stabilizes the bladder neck by suturing the periurethral fascia to the periosteum of the pubic symphysis, but does not attempt to correct any cystocele. Therefore the dissection is aimed at the periurethral tissue, with less dissection along the bladder edge.

Operative Procedure

Access to the space of Retzius is described above in the general approach to retropubic procedures. With a vaginal finger, the surgeon identifies the periurethral tissue by elevating from the vagina and palpating the Foley catheter balloon at the bladder neck. A sponge stick may be used to help retract the bladder medially, or the surgeon may use manual retraction of the bladder. Because the dissection in the space of Retzius is carried underneath the symphysis,

gentle cephalad retraction of the bladder may bring the bladder neck more into the field of vision. Sharp or blunt dissection is used to identify the white periurethral fascia 1 to 2 cm laterally on either side of the urethra.

The original description of the MMK called for the placement of several elevating sutures through the periurethral fascia and the lateral aspect of the urethra as well as in the anterior surface of the bladder. This technique has been modified for fear of significant urethral injury, and subsequent descriptions recommend placement of one or more sutures just at the bladder neck and proximal urethra, taking care to exclude the urethra from the suture (Fig. 38-21). As in the Burch colposuspension, sutures are placed through the full thickness of the periurethral fascia. The MMK differs from the Burch, as often only one nonabsorbable suture is placed on either side of the bladder neck; for this reason, a figure-of-eight suture through the fascia may offer more security. The strength of this anchoring tissue should be tested before attaching the suture to the periosteum. The sutures are then passed through the periosteum of the pubic symphysis above and slightly medial to their placement in the endopelvic fascia and secured. As with the Burch, the surgeon should be certain that no suture material is inside the bladder cavity.

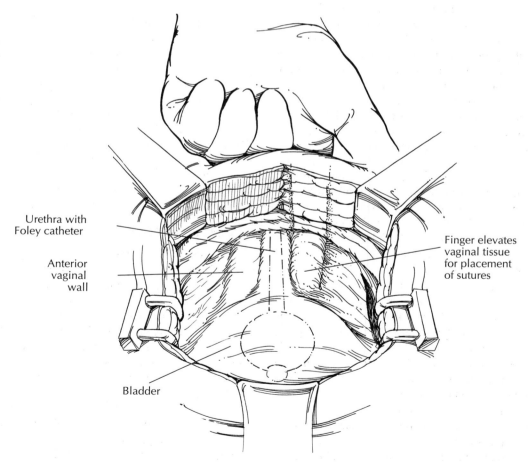

Urethra with
Foley catheter

Anterior
vaginal
wall

Bladder

Finger elevates
vaginal tissue
for placement
of sutures

Fig. 38-21. Marshall-Marchetti-Krantz procedure.

Advantages and Disadvantages

Compared with a Burch retropubic urethropexy, the MMK has the advantage of an easier dissection, which may be particularly important in the face of extensive scarring. The disadvantages of the MMK are that a cystocele is not corrected; the emphasis on urethral elevation may produce more of a bladder neck kinking effect than with the Burch colposuspension; and the possibility exists of osteitis pubis.[35] This is an inflammatory reaction set up by a foreign body in the periosteum, which is characterized by pain in the pubic symphysis 2 weeks to 6 months following an MMK and seems to be unrelated to the type of suture used. The diagnosis is one of exclusion—one must evaluate the patient for other causes of pain in this area, including abdominal trigger points, musculoskeletal pain, suture material in the bladder, or urgency reported as pain. Osteitis pubis is partially relieved by the administration of nonsteroidal anti-inflammatory agents, and occasionally by an injection of cortisone into the periosteum. Experienced surgeons have shown similar success and complication rates with both the MMK and Burch procedures. The difficulty and frustration seen with osteitis pubis, although uncommon, may ultimately make the MMK a less popular procedure.

Laparoscopic Approach to Retropubic Urethropexy

The laparoscope has become a widely used tool in the field of gynecology. The advantages of smaller abdominal incisions and the possibility of rapid hospital discharge has prompted the development of a myriad of new techniques, including the laparoscopic approach to retropubic urethropexy.

The laparoscopic bladder neck suspension was originally reported in 1991 by Vancaillie and Schuessler[35] using a conventional intraperitoneal approach to initiate dissection into the space of Retzius. Suture placement into the paravaginal fascia and Cooper's ligament was then performed laparoscopically to complete the Burch procedure. Subsequent modifications of this technique have included using an extraperitoneal approach to the dissection of the space of Retzius. In contrast to the intraperitoneal procedure, this method deliberately inserts a trocar into the preperitoneal space, into which a small balloon is placed. Distension of the balloon bluntly opens the space of Retzius before suture placement.

The use of polygalactin mesh and endostaples have also been advocated as time-saving techniques for the laparoscopist. The appropriate length of mesh is stapled or sutured to the paravaginal fascia and then secured to Cooper's ligament with staples, using enough tension to appropriately elevate the vagina. The long-term complication rate of the placement of mesh in the space of Retzius is unknown.[37]

All of the methods of laparoscopic retropubic urethropexy provide a means of utilizing the vaginal fascia and Cooper's ligament to resuspend the bladder. As these techniques continue to be developed, critical appraisal of both long- and short-term success rates will be needed before this method can be embraced as an improvement of standard operations. Preliminary data from the only reported randomized trial have suggested that subjective and objective outcomes are significantly lower with an intraperitoneal laparoscopic urethropexy than a standard Burch procedure.[38] The laparoscopic approach to retropubic urethropexy remains to be defined and should neither be abandoned nor promoted based on limited preliminary data. Ongoing randomized trials should provide a comparison between the advantages of a minimal incision procedure versus any alteration in long-term continence success.

Retropubic and Vaginal Paravaginal Repair

The paravaginal repair is indicated for the surgical correlation of a cystocele due to lateral detachment of the pubocervical fascia from the arcus tendineus fascia pelvis[39] (Fig. 38-22). As detachment of the endopelvic fascia from the "white line" has been implicated in the etiology of hypermobile type stress incontinence, the paravaginal repair has also been advocated by some authors as a primary treatment of stress incontinence (Fig. 38-23). The success of using a classical paravaginal repair for treatment of stress incontinence has varied widely among surgeons. When utilized in women with cystocele and stress urinary incontinence, the paravaginal repair is said to avoid postoperative voiding dysfunction, although there are no randomized comparison trials available to study the advantages of this procedure against other anti-incontinence procedures. A possible alternative for women with both a lateral defect and GSI may be the combination of Burch-type sutures at the level of the bladder neck and lateral sutures to repair the paravaginal defect.

The vaginal approach to the paravaginal repair was designed to reduce operative morbidity by avoiding the abdominal incision. Vaginal dissection is begun by making a midline or lateral mucosal incision and reflecting the vaginal mucosa off the underlying fascia, as is done with an anterior repair. The endopelvic fascia is broken through to give exposure to the space of Retzius. The arcus tendineous fascial pelvis is identified from its origin at the inferior aspect of the pubic ramus through its course along the pelvic sidewall. As with the abdominal approach, defects in the paravaginal tissue are sequentially identified and repaired by the placement of permanent suture. Judicious suture placement is required to avoid entrapment of the nearby ureter, obturator vessels, and nerves. The procedure may be performed on one or both sides of the vagina, as indicated by the presence of fascial defects. The inherent limitations on exposure, the possibility for significant injury to nearby structures and limited data on outcome makes it difficult to define the role of the vaginal paravaginal repair in the correction of genital prolapse.

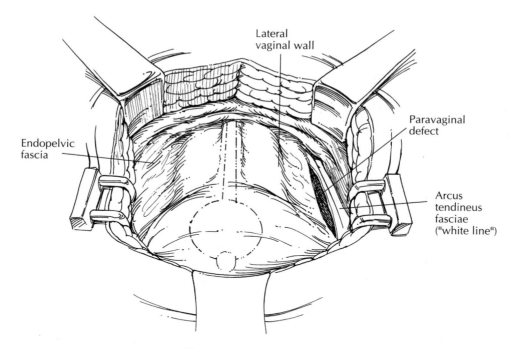

Fig. 38-22. Paravaginal defect.

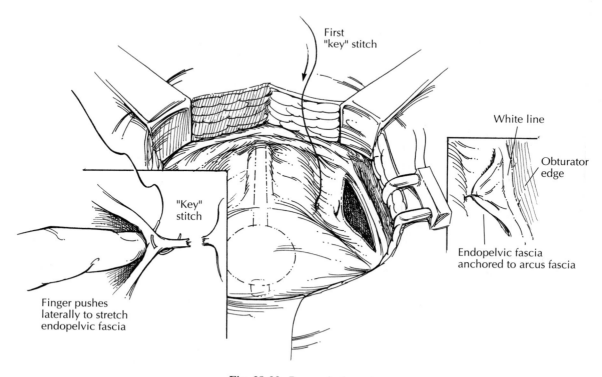

Fig. 38-23. Paravaginal repair.

Pubovaginal Slings

Sling procedures have two mechanisms of action—bladder neck support and, depending on how tightly the sling is attached, urethral obstruction. Suburethral slings are primarily used for the treatment of ISD.[40] As they both elevate and compress the urethra, slings are the procedure of choice for patients with bladder neck hypermobility and ISD as the etiologies of their stress incontinence. A sling may also be considered in women who have failed several previous urethropexies, or in whom the perivaginal fascia is deemed inadequate (such as after a vaginectomy and neovagina). Because a sling is considered for more complex patients, complex urodynamic testing is mandatory to (1) understand the etiology of the incontinence and therefore confirm the appropriate treatment, and (2) to identify women who are at risk of complications such as voiding dysfunction and DI. Suburethral slings are technically more difficult procedures than retropubic procedures and are best managed by the experienced surgeon.

Previously, slings were performed entirely in the retropubic space. This was to avoid the possibility of vaginal contamination and a presumed elevated risk of infection. Dissection through the space of Retzius under a previously operated bladder neck and scarred urethra was often difficult, and trauma to the bladder and urethra was common. More recently, a combined vaginal/abdominal approach has been favored. The vaginal approach facilitates the dissection between the bladder neck and the vaginal skin, while the abdominal dissection secures the sling to the rectus fascia.

Sling Material

A variety of sling material is available, including autologous fascia (fascia lata or rectus fascia) and artificial materials (Marlex, silastic, Gore-Tex). Autologous fascia requires harvesting and relies on the intrinsic strength of the patient's own fascia, but has the advantage of avoiding graft infection. Artificial materials have proven strength and are easily formed to the correct shape and size, but increase the risk of infection, with a removal rate as high as 23 percent in one series using polytetrafluoroethelene.[41] One compromise that allows the ease of artificial material and that shows some promise for limited tissue reaction is donor fascia, which has been rendered nonimmunogenic and is available from several central tissue banks.

Autologous Fascia

Autologous fascia is most easily obtained from rectus fascia during the approach to the retropubic space. The presence of previous incisions in this fascia does not seem to compromise the integrity of the graft. The fascia is obtained during a Pfannenstiel incision by making two parallel incisions 1 to 2 cm apart (1 cm laterally, 2 cm centrally where the sling would sit at the bladder neck) (Fig. 38-24). Normally, a sling 15 to 20 cm in length is sufficient, but less may be taken. Because any deficiency in length may be overcome by using a permanent monofilament suture to bridge the gap to the anchoring fascia, some surgeons take only 5 to 7 cm length of fascia when creating a sling. The graft should be cleaned of any fat or areolar tissue, and placed into sterile saline until used. Fascia lata is also a good source of autologous material. The authors prefer fascia lata in women with previous abdominoplasty or abdominal incisional hernia, where removal of additional fascia may make closure difficult. A small incision is made transversely at the lateral condyle down to fascia. A fascial stripper is then inserted and advanced cephalad in order to obtain a piece of fascia of similar proportions to those described above. An upper incision may be made if necessary to facilitate removal of the graft. A closed drain may be placed, and the incisions closed. Younger women may complain of discomfort in the leg for several weeks after this procedure.

Synthetic Slings

Many different synthetic materials have been used for suburethral slings. Their advantages are that the materials are readily available and have a known tensile strength. The success rates of operations performed with artificial materials have been reported to range from 60 to 92 percent. There are several significant disadvantages with all materials used. Because the material is heterologous, there is an increased chance of graft infection, sling erosion into the urethra, development of a fistula (as high as 20 percent), or sinus formation. With this in mind, autologous fascia or donor cadaveric fascia is considered to be the material of choice for use with a suburethral sling.

Operative Procedure

The vaginal approach allows for an easier, safer dissection of the bladder neck. In the dorsal lithotomy position, the bladder neck is identified by palpation of the Foley catheter balloon. An inverted U-shaped or midline incision is made through the anterior vaginal mucosa. Using sharp scissors, the dissection is carried laterally toward the pubic rami. Care should be taken to ensure that the scissors are directed laterally with tips away from the bladder, staying superficial to endopelvic fascia as much as possible. Once the underside of the pubic ramus is reached, blunt and sharp dissection is used to enter the retropubic space. The surgeon's index finger gently retracts the bladder medially, while advancing under the ramus. Although finger dissection may be adequate, perforation of the endopelvic fascia to enter the space of Retzius is best accomplished using Metzenbaum scissors (Fig. 38-25). Sharp entry is particularly helpful in women who have had previous anti-incontinence procedures and scarring in this area. The scissors should be placed flat

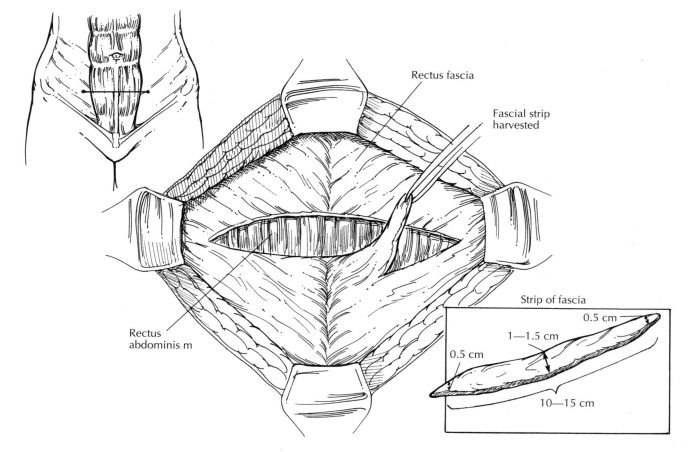

Fig. 38-24. Harvesting of rectus fascia for pubovaginal sling.

against the lateral pubic ramus, while retracting the bladder and overlying fascia medially with the index finger. If the plane of dissection is still difficult to achieve, little is lost by entering the retropubic space and assisting the dissection from above.

Once the space of Retzius has been entered, the surgeon's index finger sweeps the bladder medially while advancing toward the abdominal wall. An assistant must now choose a site on the rectus fascia for graft attachment. Ideally, this site should be 2 to 3 cm lateral from the midline and between the fascial incision (if rectus fascia was used) and its insertion into the symphysis. A 1-cm incision is made with scalpel into this site, and a long curved clamp is guided by the vaginal finger from the upper incision through the space of Retzius into the vaginal incision. The ends of the graft or the attached sutures are then grasped and pulled back up into the abdominal incision, and held while a similar procedure is performed on the contralateral side (Fig. 38-26). It is ideal to have fascial graft meet the perforated rectus fascia, but the suture bridge is adequate and acts in a manner similar to a needle urethropexy.

The sling is settled into place at the vesical neck, taking care to keep the graft flat and untwisted. Some surgeons

prefer to use absorbable or nonabsorbable sutures to fix the sling in place at the vesical neck before it is tied. Cystoscopy is performed to ensure bladder and urethral integrity. The graft or suture ends are then secured to the rectus fascia (Fig. 38-27).

When securing the sling, attention is directed to the graft tightness and degree of elevation. Recall that with hypermobility of the bladder neck, the surgical goal is to stabilize the bladder neck without obstruction. A sling that is secured without tension is optimal for most patients. In patients with ISD, adequate urethral compression will be achieved during times of increased intra-abdominal pressure. Sudden tension on the rectus fascia anteriorly, due to coughing or movement, will tighten the sling against the bladder neck at the moment when tension is most needed. Occasionally the goal of surgery is to totally obstruct the urethra and rely on intermittent catheterization. In these unusual cases, the sling may be tied under some degree of tension. Elevation of the ends of the sling and palpation of the vaginal side of the sling as it passes under the bladder neck will reveal the amount of tension that is present on the bladder neck. There should be only slight elevation of the bladder neck when no tension is present by the supporting sling. Sling tension should be con-

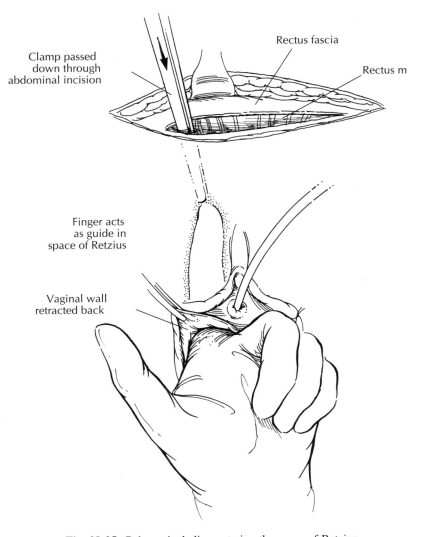

Clamp passed down through abdominal incision

Rectus fascia

Rectus m

Finger acts as guide in space of Retzius

Vaginal wall retracted back

Fig. 38-25. Pubovaginal sling entering the space of Retzius.

stantly checked as all the sutures are tied. The vaginal incision and the abdominal incision are then closed.

Collagen Injections

Periurethral injection of collagen are designed as a treatment for stress urinary incontinence resulting from ISD. The concept of an injectable cure for incontinence began with the use of a sclerosing agent to permanently scar and narrow the bladder neck.[42] Until recently, the most widely used compound was a polytetrafluoroethylene paste (Polytef). Although successful, reports of compound fragmentation and distant particle migration with granuloma formation eventually lead to withdrawal of the product. The compound currently in use is a glutaraldehyde cross-linked collagen (Contigen, Bard). Unlike collagen designed for plastic surgery augmentation procedures, the collagen used for incontinence has been modified into a cross-linked matrix to retard breakdown and improve stability.

The decision to use periurethral injections of collagen rather than a sling or artificial sphincter as treatment for ISD is based on the extent of surgery, complications, and success rates that the patient and physician are willing to assume. Collagen injections have the distinct advantage of being performed as an outpatient procedure with few complications and low risk of urinary retention. There appears to be no evidence of urethral erosion or delayed infection. Initial success rates have been reported as high as 60 to 80 percent, although objective cure rates may decline to as low as 48 percent after 2 years.[43]

Collagen has an allergic response rate of approximately 3 percent and thus preoperative screening by placement of 0.1 ml on the volar surface of the forearm is required 30 days before the procedure. Injection can be performed as an outpatient by using either a local or general anesthetic. Be-

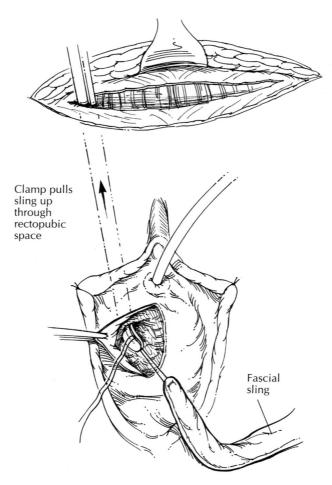

Clamp pulls
sling up
through
rectopubic
space

Fascial
sling

Fig. 38-26. Pubovaginal sling placement.

fore injection, routine cystoscopy is performed to confirm normal anatomy. The cystoscope is then used to identify the bladder neck during the procedure to aid in correct placement of the collagen. The most popular technique for injection in women is the periurethral approach. Local anesthetic, if desired, is placed around the urethral meatus and a fine gauge needle is then passed beneath the urethral mucosa to the level of the bladder neck (Fig. 38-28). Correct needle placement is essential to avoid rupture of the urethra or bladder mucosa with spillage of collagen or insufficient narrowing of the lumen. Collagen is gradually injected under direct visualization at both the 3-o'clock and 9-o'clock positions. The needle can be repositioned during injection as needed to ensure correct collagen placement. Enough material is injected to cause sufficient bulging of the submucosa to occlude the urethral lumen without causing rupture. If needed, reinjection can be carried out at a later date.

Alternatives to the injection of collagen have included the use of autologous fat. Liposuction of the lower abdomen can provide quantities of fat for processing and injection into the periurethral tissue, using similar techniques as for collagen injection. The possible advantages include a reduction in

cost and allergic response. Because of the likelihood of fat reabsorption, long-term success rates may be reduced.

Other Surgical Procedures

Urethral Diverticula

Up to 2 percent of all women have a clinically detectable urethral diverticulum. The etiology of these masses is unknown, but probably arise from occlusion of the periurethral glands through infection or inflammation. Urethral diverticula usually present as a painful mass protruding into the vagina. Occasionally, a diverticulum may be painless but symptomatic because urine may fill the sac during voiding, only to dribble out once the patient stands and ambulates. They also can be uncommon but significant causes of recurrent urinary tract infection or dyspareunia (or both).

Identification

Diverticula can be detected in some cases on simple inspection of the anterior vaginal wall. The mass underlies the vaginal skin and endopelvic fascia, and occasionally may be

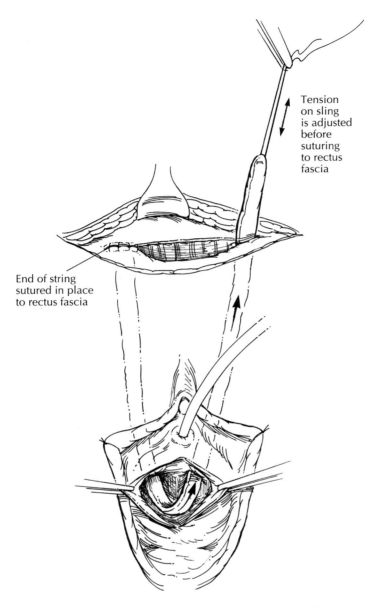

Tension on sling is adjusted before suturing to rectus fascia

End of string sutured in place to rectus fascia

Fig. 38-27. Adjusting the tension for a pubovaginal sling.

mistaken for an enlarged Skene's gland. Urethral diverticula are usually located in the posterior wall of the urethra, but may have complex, even "corkscrewing," connections to other diverticula. Palpation and "milking" of the anterior vaginal wall will sometimes produce purulence from the urethra as sac contents are expressed. Previously it was thought that all urethral diverticula were infectious and that the patient should be treated for sexually transmitted diseases; this has not been proven to be the case. Cystoscopy is occasionally helpful in visualizing the neck of the diverticulum as it opens into the urethral lumen, but there is usually insufficient pressure with this technique to forcefully open the neck of the diverticulum and allow for its identification. Adequate pressure may be produced using a double balloon-triple

lumen catheter (Trattnor or TeLinde catheter). One balloon of a catheter is placed in the bladder and pulled snugly down to the bladder neck. A second balloon is inflated at the external urethral orifice. The urethral portion of the catheter has a separate port to allow instillation of radiopaque dye under positive pressure, forcing dye into the diverticula and allowing visualization under fluoroscopy.

Indications

Urethral diverticula should not be operated on unless (1) the mass is painful or causing dyspareunia, (2) the diverticulum is suspected to be the etiology of recurrent cystitis that has not responded to usual therapy such as prophylactic antibiot-

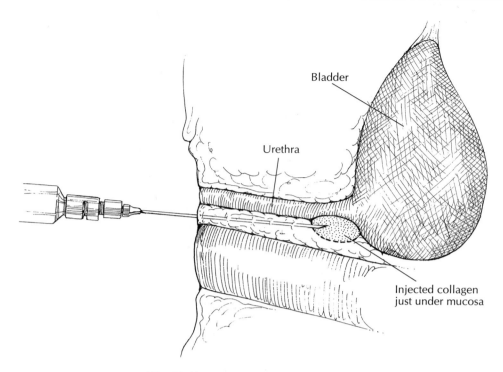

Fig. 38-28. Periurethral collagen injection.

ics, or (3) the diverticulum is producing postvoid dribbling that is reproducible, bothersome to the patient, and is not due to other causes of urinary incontinence. Urethral diverticula presenting during pregnancy usually do not cause problems at delivery and may spontaneously resolve or decrease within months of parturition. They should not be repaired until it is clear that resolution is not occurring, and then only if the mass is causing symptoms.

Extensive dissection and repair of symptomatic urethral diverticula may cause ISD-type stress incontinence or urinary fistula. Therefore, knowledge of the exact position of the diverticula and the periurethral structures is critical. Two main types of repair should be considered: (1) marsupialization of the sac into the vagina (the Spence procedure), or (2) complete excision of the sac. The Spence procedure is suitable only for single distal diverticula; otherwise excision is preferable.

Spence Procedure

Spence described a simple procedure for the permanent marsupialization and drainage of distal urethral diverticula.[44] A Foley catheter is placed in the bladder and a midline incision is made in the vaginal skin and underlying fascia over the diverticulum. The sac is then carefully inspected and confirmed to be a single diverticulum. The diverticulum is then entered sharply, and the walls of the sac sutured with 00 chromic catgut to the vaginal skin in a fashion similar to that when marsupialization is performed for a Bartholin's gland cyst. The total aperture of the opened sac should be

approximately 1 cm. Because the continence mechanism is above the distal fourth of the urethra, these patients usually do not experience stress incontinence related to the procedure. The sac cannot reaccumulate fluid, drains only during voiding, and remains otherwise asymptomatic. Bladder drainage is not needed after a Spence procedure, and the patient may be discharged the same day (Fig. 38-29).

Excision

For any other urethral diverticula—whether multiple, complex, or above the lowest quarter of the urethra—the procedure of choice is excision. A U-shaped or midline incision is made in the anterior wall of the vagina over the mass and the vagina mucosa reflected away. The periurethral fascia is gently incised over the diverticulum. Blunt and sharp dissection are used to isolate the diverticular sac, taking care to stay just outside its epithelial lining to minimize damage to the urethra. Dissection is facilitated by leaving the diverticulum intact. If rupture occurs, a pediatric Foley may be placed into the defect and inflated to further assist the dissection. In the authors' experience, the neck and lumen of the sac is rarely apparent until the dissection is almost complete. Once the entire sac is isolated, the neck of the diverticulum is divided and the sac inspected for any epithelial abnormalities. Any excess epithelium has the potential to re-form a sac and should be excised. Likewise, extensive dissection may devascularize the area and lead to fistula formation. In the case of a corkscrewing diverticula, the epithelium must be removed in its entirety while keeping the integrity of the urethral wall. Once

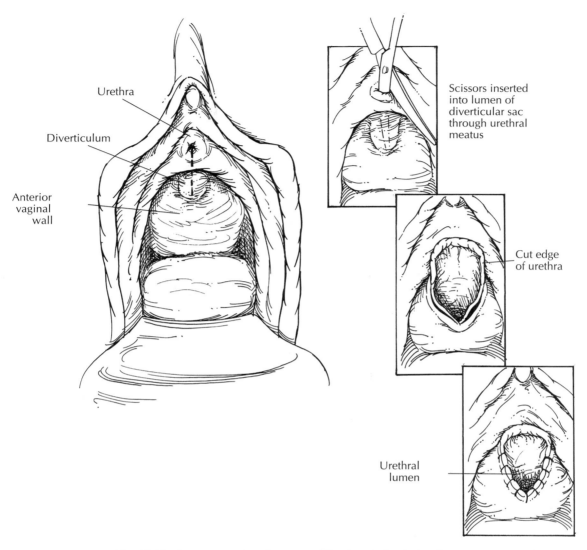

Urethra

Diverticulum

Anterior
vaginal
wall

Scissors inserted
into lumen of
diverticular sac
through urethral
meatus

Cut edge
of urethra

Urethral
lumen

Fig. 38-29. Spence procedure for marsupialization of distal diverticulum.

the diverticular epithelium is removed, the defects in the urethral wall are repaired using a double-closure of 000 delayed absorbable suture. Urethroscopy is used to ensure a watertight closure. The periurethra fascia is brought over the epithelial closure site and closed with delayed absorbable suture. If a large diverticulum has been excised, a vest-over-pants closure may be possible (Fig. 28-30). The U-shaped vaginal skin incision is finally closed, taking care to avoid crossing suture lines. If there is concern about the extent of the dissection and integrity of underlying tissues, a Martius graft can be used. A suprapubic catheter can be placed for 4 to 7 days to allow healing before voiding. The patient usually can be discharged the same day of surgery.

Bladder Augmentation

Augmentation of the urinary bladder with cecum or other isolated bowel is another alternative for intractable bladder storage dysfunction. The procedure is indicated in patients with small capacity bladders (200 ml or less) and urge incontinence that has failed all other therapies. Bladder augmentation has been described for use in patients with interstitial cystitis, although the bowel augmentation may develop the same condition as the bladder wall. Urodynamic testing is a prerequisite to bladder augmentation, to confirm the abnormal sensation and bladder function. Cystoscopy under general anesthetic will further distinguish patients with sensory abnormalities (whose bladder is structurally capable of holding normal volumes, and who would not benefit from bladder augmentation) from patients with true small capacity, noncompliant bladders.

Similar to a diversion, a segment of bowel is isolated and mobilized with its mesentery. The dome of the bladder is opened transversely, and the bowel used as a new roof to augment the bladder, similar to two bowls placed face to face. The augmented bladder is capable of holding larger volumes, and the new bladder wall is less prone to contrac-

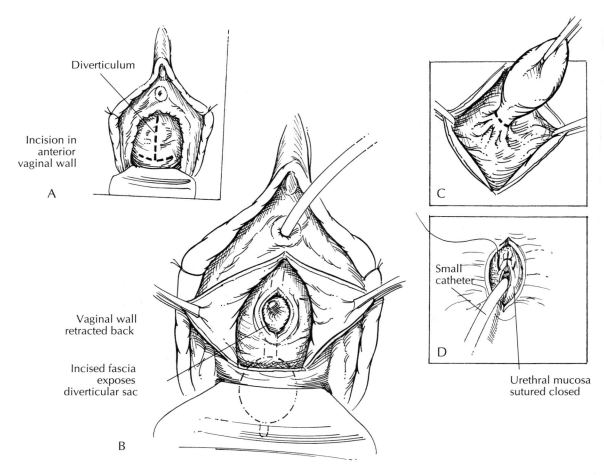

Diverticulum

Incision in
anterior
vaginal wall

A

Vaginal wall
retracted back

Incised fascia
exposes
diverticular sac

B

C

D

Small
catheter

Urethral mucosa
sutured closed

Fig. 38-30. (A–H) Diverticulectomy. *(Figure continues.)*

tion than its detrusor neighbor. Many patients will have postoperative retention and require intermittent self-catheterization. The procedure should not be expected to treat stress incontinence, and is a procedure of last resort after all medical and surgical therapy has failed for the treatment of severe DI.

POSTOPERATIVE INCONTINENCE

Surgical correction of urinary incontinence fails for a number of reasons that fall into two major groups: persistence or exacerbation of incontinent conditions that coexist with stress incontinence, and true surgical failures.

Many patients do not understand that there may be several causes of urinary incontinence. The patient may have had other urinary complaints preoperatively that were not intended to be treated by the stress incontinence surgery. For example, the patient who gets up every hour at night with urge incontinence may also leak from stress incontinence when she has a bad cold. Surgical correction of the stress incontinence will not significantly improve her quality of

life because it only addresses one minor component of her condition. Patients should clearly understand what the surgical procedure is expected to correct and what it will not correct. Women may also develop new lower urinary tract problems after surgical correction of the stress incontinence. For example, a severe voiding dysfunction or DI may develop as a result of excessive elevation of the bladder neck.

Patients who have failed prior procedures should have complex urodynamic testing performed by a specialist. Such testing is aimed at identification of the cause of incontinence, including new DI, voiding dysfunction, and ISD or hypermobile stress incontinence. Often several or all of these entities coexist in one patient. Examination of prior operative reports may reveal the use of absorbable suture or conditions in which an adequate dissection or evaluation of the bladder after suture placement was not accomplished.

If DI is identified as the cause of postoperative urinary incontinence, it should be determined whether the condition was present preoperatively. Such persistent DI may be transiently exacerbated in the postoperative period and only require brief intervention. Correct diagnosis of this coexistent incontinence condition preoperatively and awareness that DI

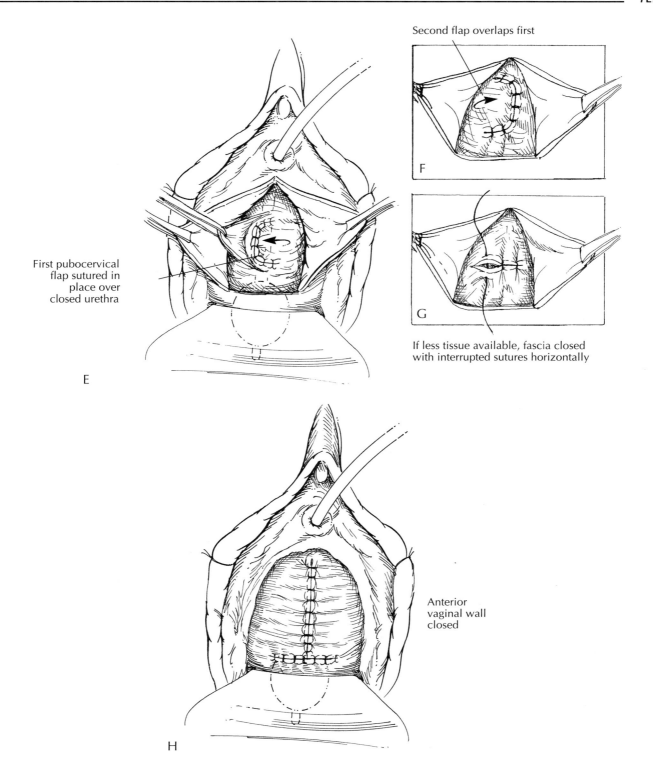

Second flap overlaps first

First pubocervical flap sutured in place over closed urethra

If less tissue available, fascia closed with interrupted sutures horizontally

Anterior vaginal wall closed

Fig. 38-30 *(Continued).*

may be exacerbated postoperatively will reassure the patient that her procedure for stress incontinence has not failed. De novo DI is sometimes associated with irritation from a suture in the bladder, from perioperative swelling, or with prolonged voiding dysfunction. The presence of pain or recurrent urinary tract infection together with urge incontinence is more suspicious for the presence of a suture in the bladder and cystoscopy should be performed. Most often, de novo urge incontinence is idiopathic and should be treated as such.

If voiding dysfunction persists after anti-incontinence surgery, the patient may develop urge incontinence as part of overflow incontinence. Evaluation of voiding may reveal high-pressure detrusor voiding pressures as the bladder generates these pressures in an effort to overcome the relative obstruction of the surgical procedure. If pressures remain high with each void, upper tract dilation and damage may occur over time. A takedown procedure to relieve the relative obstruction should be considered in very symptomatic patients.

Finally, recurrent hypermobile-type stress incontinence may be corrected with a repeat procedure if the patient chooses a surgical option. The surgeon should never assume that the problem will be corrected if only the second procedure is done ''correctly.'' Although technical errors do occur—such as the use of absorbable suture, suturing bladder wall instead of fascia, or overcinching sutures—the source of failure is not always easy to identify. Patients with postoperative ISD can benefit from either a sling or periurethral collagen injections, while those with both hypermobility and intrinsic defects should be considered for a sling procedure.

POSTOPERATIVE MANAGEMENT AND SURGICAL COMPLICATIONS

If the procedure was limited to the space of Retzius, most patients can take fluid orally the night of surgery, with advancement of the diet the next day. Procedure-specific complications are outlined in their specific sections (see above); only general complications are outlined here.

Bleeding in the space of Retzius is almost always self-limited and can generally be controlled with pressure, absorbable sutures, or cautery. Brisk bleeding from perivesical veins is best initially controlled by elevation of the vagina with the internal hand. The pressure will generally compress the vessel sufficiently to allow placement of hemostatic sutures. Caution must be used near the obturator complex, as injury to the obturator artery or vein can result in massive, difficult-to-control hemorrhage. Injury is usually the result of overzealous dissection or inappropriate retractor placement. The proximity of the obturator nerve makes hemostasis difficult to achieve without injury. After hemostasis is achieved, a #10 Jackson Pratt drain-to-bulb suction may be placed to take care of any residual bleeding in the space of Retzius, and may be removed 24 to 48 hours later.

A single dose of prophylactic antibiotics should be used for anti-incontinence procedures. Infection in the space of Retzius is relatively uncommon, but usually responds to intravenous antibiotics. Likewise, suture or bolster abscess are unusual but may require surgical excision and debridement. Cystitis is a common complication of bladder neck surgery, but is readily treatable.

Postoperative bladder drainage is a matter of surgeon preference. Depending on the preoperative risk factors for voiding dysfunction and patient ability, the decision is between suprapubic drainage and intermittent self-catheterization. For women in whom voiding dysfunction is expected to be limited, or who are unable to learn clean intermittent self-catheterization preoperatively, the suprapubic catheter is a good choice. If there is no bleeding from the bladder, a narrow catheter (Bonanno) is more comfortable and is easy to remove. Care must be taken to tape the catheter securely to ensure good drainage, as narrow catheters are prone to kink with patient movement. Wider suprapubic catheters should be placed if there is bleeding from the bladder, which may block a narrow catheter. A Foley or Malecot catheter placed suprapubically is commonly used in this situation.

The alternative to suprapubic placement is a transurethral Foley catheter. The catheter can be removed after 1 to 2 days and then clean intermittent self-catheterization is used. When the Foley catheter is ready to be removed, the bladder can be filled with approximately 250 ml of warm saline or water. The catheter is then removed and the patient asked to void. Because the bladder volume is known, the nursing staff can immediately assess adequacy of voiding and determine whether there is a need for self-catheterization. Clean intermittent self-catheterization is best performed with 14 French ''in and out'' type catheters. These catheters are stiffer and may be held at the far end, avoiding the need to touch the ''business end'' of the catheter.

Suprapubic clamping and voiding trials are usually initiated on the second postoperative day. Voiding trials or intermittent catheterizations are continued until voids are significantly greater than residuals and postvoid residuals are under 100 to 150 ml. Prophylactic antibiotics are not routinely needed and urinary tract infections are treated as indicated. Preoperative education about catheters, voiding trials, and expectations greatly reduce postoperative anxiety.

A few patients may encounter postoperative urgency and frequency. This is generally a self-limited problem related to bladder irritation. Other etiologies, including infection or intravesical suture placement, should be considered if the problem persists. Although anticholinergics may compromise bladder emptying, these indications can be prescribed with good symptomatic relief.

REFERENCES

1. DeLancey JO: The anatomy of the pelvic floor. Curr Opinion Obstet Gynecol 6:313, 1994
2. Summitt RL Jr, Stovall TG, Bent AE, Ostergard DR: Urinary

incontinence: correlation of history and brief office evaluation with multichannel urodynamic testing. Am J Obstet Gynecol 166:1835, 1992

3. Abrams P, Blavias JG, Stanton SL, Andersen JT: Standardization of terminology of lower urinary tract function. Neurourol Urodyn 7:403, 1988

4. Norton PA, MacDonald LD, Sedgwick PM, Stanton SL: Distress and delay associated with urinary incontinence, frequency, and urgency in women. BMJ 297:1187, 1988

5. Agency for Health Care Policy and Research: Urinary incontinence in adults clinical practice guideline. Bethesda, MD, 1996

6. Wyman JF, Elswick RK Jr, Ory MG et al: Influence of function, urological, and environmental characteristics on urinary incontinence in community-dwelling older women. Nursing Res 42:270, 1993

7. Verbrugge LM: Health diaries. Med Care 18:73, 1980

8. Kadar N: The value of bladder filling in the clinical detection of urine loss and selection of patients for urodynamic testing. Br J Obstet Gynaecol 95:698, 1988

9. Walters MD, Shields LE: The diagnostic value of history, physical examination, and the Q-tip cotton swab test in women with urinary incontinence. Am J Obstet Gynecol 159:145, 1988

10. Sand PK, Brubaker LT, Novak T: Simple standing incremental cystometry as a screening method for detrusor instability. Obstet Gynecol 77:453, 1991

11. Ouslander JG, Leach GE, Staskin DR: Simplified tests of lower urinary tract function in the evaluation of geriatric urinary incontinence. J Am Geriatr Soc 37:706, 1989

12. Haylen BT, Ashby D, Sutherst JR et al: Maximum and average urine flow rates in normal male and female populations—the Liverpool nomograms. Br J Urol 64:30, 1989

13. Fantl JA, Smith PJ, Schneider V et al: Fluid weight uroflowmetry in women. Am J Obstet Gynecol 145:1017, 1983

14. Sand PK, Bowen LW, Ostergard DR: The prognostic significance of augmentation of urethral closure and functional length. Int J Gynaecol Obstet 33:135, 1990

15. McGuire EJ, Fitzpatrick CC, Wan J et al: Clinical assessment of urethral sphincter function. J Urol 150:1452, 1993

16. Wan J, McGuire EJ, Bloom DA, Ritchey ML: Stress leak point pressure: a diagnostic tool for incontinent children. J Urol 150: 700, 1993

17. Kegel A: Progressive resistance exercise in the functional restoration of the perineal muscles. Am J Obstet Gynecol 56:238, 1948

18. Rose M, Baigis-Smith J, Smith D, Newman D: Behavioral management of urinary incontinence in homebound older adults. Home Health Nurse 8:10, 1990

19. Ferguson K, McKey PL, Bishop KR et al: Stress urinary incontinence: effect of pelvic muscle exercise. Obstet Gynecol 73: 671, 1990

20. Laycock J, Oreen RJ: Interferential therapy in the treatment of incontinence. Physiotherapy 74:161, 1988

21. Davila GW, Ostermann KV: The bladder neck support prosthesis: a nonsurgical approach to stress incontinence in adult women. Am J Obstet Gynecol 171:206, 1994

22. Stanton SL, Hilton P, Norton C, Cardozo L: Clinical and urodynamic effects of anterior colporrhaphy and vaginal hysterectomy for prolapse with and without incontinence. Br J Obstet Gynaecol 89:459, 1982

23. Bergman A, Ballard CA, Koonings PP: Comparison of three different surgical procedures for genuine stress incontinence: prospective randomized study. Am J Obstet Gynecol 160:1102, 1989

24. Elia G, Bergman A: Prospective randomized comparison of three surgical procedures for stress urinary incontinence: five year follow-up. Neurourol Urodyn 13:498, 1994

25. Karram MM, Bhatia NN: Transvaginal needle bladder neck suspension procedures for stress urinary incontinence: a comprehensive review. Obstet Gynecol 73:906, 1989

26. Pereyra AJ, Lebherz TB: The revised Pereyra procedure. p. 208. In Buchsbaum H, Schmidt JD (eds): Gynecologic and Obstetric Urology. WB Saunders, Philadelphia, 1978

27. Stamey TA: Endoscopic suspension of the vesical neck for urinary incontinence in females. Report on 203 consecutive patients. Ann Surg 192:465, 1980

28. Raz S: Modified bladder neck suspension for female stress incontinence. Urology 17:82, 1981

29. Benderev TV: A modified percutaneous outpatient bladder neck suspension system. J Urol 152:2316, 1994

30. Peattie AB, Stanton SL: The Stamey operation for correction of genuine stress incontinence in the elderly woman. Br J Obstet Gynaecol 96:983, 1989

31. Leach GE, Yip CM, Donovan BJ: Mechanism of continence after modified Pereyra bladder neck suspension. Urology 29: 328, 1987

32. Mundy A: A trial comparing the Stamey bladder neck suspension procedure with colposuspension for the treatment of stress incontinence. Br J Urol 55:687, 1983

33. Marshall V, Marchetti A, Krantz K: The correction of stress incontinence by simple vesicourethral suspension. Surg Gynecol Obstet 88:509, 1949

34. Burch JC: Cooper's ligament urethrovesical suspension for stress incontinence. Nine years' experience—results, complication, technique. Am J Obstet Gynecol 100:764, 1968

35. Lee R, Symmonds R, Goldstein R: Surgical complications and results of modified Marshall-Marchetti-Krantz procedure for urinary incontinence. Obstet Gynecol 53:447, 1979

36. Vancaillie TG, Schuessler W: Laparoscopic bladder neck suspension. J Laparoendosc Surg 1:169, 1991

37. Ou CS, Presthus J, Beadle E: Laparoscopic bladder neck suspension using hernia mesh and surgical staples. J Laparoendosc Surg 3:563, 1993

38. Burton G: A randomized comparison of laparoscopic and open colposuspension. Neurourol Urodyn 13:497, 1994

39. Richardson AC, Edmonds PB, Williams NL: Treatment of stress urinary incontinence due to paravaginal fascial defect. Obstet Gynecol 57:357, 1981

40. Summitt RL Jr, Bent AE, Ostergard DR, Harris TA: Stress incontinence and low urethral closure pressure. Correlation of preoperative urethral hypermobility with successful suburethral sling procedures. J Reprod Med 35:877, 1990

41. Bent A, Ostergard D, Zwick-Zaffuto M: Tissue reaction to expanded polytetrafluoroethylene suburethral sling for urinary incontinence: clinical and histologic study. Am J Obstet Gynecol 169:1198, 1993

42. Politano VA, Small MP, Harper JM, Lynne CM: Periurethral teflon injection for urinary incontinence. J Urol 111:180, 1974

43. Monga AK, Robinson D, Stanton SL: Periurethral collagen injections for genuine stress incontinence: 2 year followup. Br J Urol (in press)

44. Spence HM, Duckett JW Jr: Diverticulum of the female urethra: clinical aspects and presentation of a simple operative technique for cure. J Urol 104:432, 1970

CHAPTER THIRTY-NINE

MANAGEMENT OF VESICOVAGINAL, URETHROVAGINAL, AND URETEROVAGINAL FISTULAS

THOMAS E. ELKINS
ALAN GARELY

ETIOLOGY

Developed Versus Underdeveloped Countries

The etiology of urogenital tract fistulas today varies sharply between those fistulas seen in developed countries and those seen in underdeveloped countries. The urogenital fistula in the United States and other developed countries may correctly be termed the *gynecologic fistula*. By contrast, urogenital fistulas in developing countries are almost always secondary to "obstetric" problems.

In the recently published large series of fistula repairs from the United States, both Lee et al[1] and Tancer[2] underscore the above comments. In Lee's study, it is notable that obstructed labor was not an etiologic factor in the 300-plus cases reported.[1] Obstetric trauma was related to fistula formation in 8 percent of the cases, but these were all secondary to the use of forceps, or cesarean hysterectomy. By contrast, a Mayo Clinic review done 60 years earlier by Judd,[3] found obstructed labor to be a causative factor in 39 percent of patients. This change is due to the steady improvement in obstetric care seen in the United States over the past 50 to 75 years. In countries where obstetric care is scarce or nonexistent, obstructed labor is the most common cause of urogenital fistulas. In a recent study of 775 consecutive fistulas in Northern Nigeria (where 1 doctor is present for every 200,000 persons), Waaldijk[4] noted that 98 percent were secondary to obstructed labor. In the study by Elkins[5] of urogenital fistulas in West Africa, obstructed labor was the only cause of injury in 100 consecutive fistula operations. In contrast to cases followed in least developed nations, 20 patients were referred in the United States with urogenital fistulas, all of which followed gynecologic surgery or radiotherapy. Two cases occurred in patients who had refused obstetric care despite the presence of obstructed labor.

In reality, the etiology of the obstetric fistula in developing countries goes beyond the heading of "obstructed labor." The obstruction of labor is only the first hurdle that must be overcome for a successful delivery. It is a reflection of a social system that demands early childbearing of young adolescents. Additionally, the problem is partly hereditary. The presence of an anthropoid or android pelvis contributes directly to outlet obstruction. The local health care system often provides few doctors with surgical skills adequate to compliment the efforts of the village-level traditional birth attendants. At the village level, lack of knowledge and skill may become barriers to highly technical care. Poor roads and the lack of transport vehicles are the next obstacle. Tradi-

Table 39-1. Tissue Injury Levels from Radiation

Tissue	Approximate Tolerance Dose
Bladder	6,000–7,000 rads
Rectum	6,000–7,000 rads
Vaginal mucosa	7,000 rads
Bowel	6,000 rads
Cervix	>12,000 rads
Kidney	2,000–3,000 rads
Liver	2,500–3,500 rads

tional customs such as the necessity of a home birth often make it difficult for a woman to seek even emergency health care. Finally, illiteracy and dire poverty become the ultimate barriers to health care in developing countries. This broad definition of obstructed labor implies a neglected woman with cephalopelvic disproportion who has active contractions for over 48 hours.[6] In West African teaching hospitals, this leads to a maternal mortality rate of 7 to 10 per 1,000 deliveries, with even higher rates in rural areas, and 1 to 3 urogenital fistulas per 1,000 deliveries.[7]

In developed countries, urogenital fistulas are often unavoidable as a consequence of pelvic radiation. At one time, radiation fistulas were frequently found after cobalt therapy for carcinoma of the cervix or carcinoma of the endometrium. With refined radiotherapy techniques, urogenital fistulas have decreased significantly.[8] The tissue injury levels from radiation are shown in Table 39-1.[9] The remainder of the gynecologic urogenital fistulas seen in the United States are secondary to severe pelvic pathology, surgical misadventure, or injuries incurred in the healing process.

Ureteral Injuries

In many studies looking at ureteral injuries,[10–12] the surgical treatment of multiple leiomyomata, broad ligament myomas, and cervical myomas are common etiologic factors. The preoperative intravenous pyelogram has fallen out of favor as a diagnostic tool for chronic pelvic pain, and has almost been forgotten. However, it may be a very helpful test in identifying preoperative ureteral compression or deviation of ureteral placement due to pelvic masses, or rarely, invasion of the ureter by endometriosis. Some surgeons advocate the use of intraluminal ureteral catheters to assist with identification and dissection of the ureter.[13] This may be helpful in finding the ureter in instances when retroperitoneal fibrosis is a factor, as in cases of ovarian remnant syndrome, severe pelvic inflammatory disease, severe endometriosis, or pelvic carcinoma. However, stents may injure the ureter by direct physical trauma or infection, or make the ureter stiff and easily injured during dissection.[13,14] It is important to note that most instances of ureteral or vesical injury follow routine abdominal hysterectomies, when no risk factors are present.

Bladder Injuries

Bladder injuries associated with gynecologic surgery are most commonly seen after routine, benign surgery complicated by pelvic hemorrhage. Unfortunately, bladder injuries also occur in straightforward cases due to the lack of ''first'' and ''final'' sharp dissection in creating the bladder flap at abdominal hysterectomy. The first sharp dissection occurs at the level of the internal cervical os. The final sharp dissection should be done routinely at the level of the vaginal cuff, just before placement of angle clamps and sutures. This final dissection ensures that the bladder is safely away from the vaginal cuff before clamping and suturing of that tissue begins.

New Injuries With Improved Technology

The advent of pelviscopic/endoscopic pelvic surgery (i.e., laparascopically assisted vaginal hysterectomy and removal of ovaries, etc.) appears to have increased the incidence of bladder and ureteral injuries, at least initially. Laser procedures have also added to the incidence of injuries—especially to the ureter. Grainger et al[15] noted eight previous cases and added five others in a report in 1990. The operations were done for sterilization (4), endometriosis (5), adhesions (2), pelvic pain (1), and uterosacral ligament transection (1). The sterilization injuries occurred even with bipolar instruments—simply by touching the ureter with hot equipment. Presenting symptoms are abdominal pain, leukocytosis, and early postoperative fever.

A method of dissecting the cervix during an abdominal hysterectomy designed to protect the ureters and bladder is termed the *intrafascial* hysterectomy technique. It involves an incision into the pubocervicovesico fascia with lateral displacement of the fascial layer off of the anterior cervical tissue. All clamps from the level of the internal cervical os to the vaginal cuff are placed inside the endopelvic fascia.

Despite the best efforts of the surgeon, injuries to the urinary tract may still occur as part of the healing process in pelvic surgery. The mechanism of injury is always the same: tissue necrosis follows tissue ischemia, which can be secondary to external pressure (crush or clamp injury), kinking of urinary tract tissue (proximity to a ligated pedicle), or marked inflammation with tissue fibrosis.[11] Direct injury to the urinary tract by laceration or puncture usually results in immediate urine leakage. Delayed injury from retroperitoneal fibrosis, tissue pressure, or partial obstruction may not result in fistula formation and urine leakage for days or weeks.[16] Endarteritis obliterans, the ongoing process associated with radiotherapy, has been reported in fistula formation even years after initial radiation therapy.[17]

Urethrovaginal fistulas may follow urethral diverticulum repair attempts, obstetric forceps deliveries, or anterior repairs for cystocele reduction. The diverticulum repairs have an 18 percent fistula development rate, thought to result from attempting the repair in the presence of inflamed, chronically infected tissue.

DIAGNOSIS

Intraoperative Diagnosis

The diagnosis of a urogenital fistula is relatively straightforward. At surgery, there can be no substitute for direct visualization of the ureters to check for peristalsis, gross dilation (obstruction), or urine leakage. Intraoperative intravenous pyelograms (IVPs) may be helpful. Because of the high volume of body fluid seen in general anesthesia, most recommend using IVP dye at twice the strength in order for it to be seen clearly. Intravenous indigo carmen will identify intraperitoneal leakage from the urinary tract. Given with 20 to 40 mg of lasix, leakage of blue urine can rapidly lead to diagnosis of injury, or reassurance of its absence for an anxious surgeon. The use of methylene blue intravenously must be avoided because of the risk of methemoglobinemia. If ureteral obstruction is suspected, and retroperitoneal dissection is difficult, ureteral stents may be placed cystoscopically, or by direct insertion after opening the dome of the bladder to visualize the trigone. Filling the bladder with sterile milk through a Foley catheter will identify small bladder wall defects at surgery.

Thompson and others have encouraged the cystoscopic evaluation of the bladder, with special attention being paid to the spurting of urine from the ureters bilaterally. The authors routinely use this at Louisiana State University to check urogenital integrity after difficult vaginal surgery or urogynecologic procedures. Finally, there is nothing wrong with opening the bladder during abdominal surgery to check for bladder integrity. Small pediatric feeding tubes or ureteral stents may be passed under direct visualization to check ureteral integrity and patency.

Under the best circumstances, when an injury or defect is identified and repaired during the initial surgery, fistula formation may still occur. In a recent paper by Tancer,[2] 10 of 24 patients who had bladder repair at surgery went on to develop vesicovaginal fistulas.

Postoperative Diagnosis

Postoperatively, urogenital fistulas may be more difficult to identify. One office diagnostic procedure that has been reliable over the years is the Moir test.[18] In this test, three cotton swabs are placed into the vagina, and methylene blue is instilled into the bladder through the urethra. After ambulation, the swabs are removed. Blue staining indicates a vesicovaginal fistula, while moisture with clear fluid indicates a ureterovaginal fistula. Taking pyridium orally on the day of the test will turn the urine orange, clearly distinguishing

it from the methylene blue-stained bladder fluid and enhancing the diagnosis of a ureterovaginal fistula.

Intravenous pyelography is useful in noting any disruption in ureteral integrity. This makes it superior to ultrasonography for the diagnosis of urinary tract injuries postoperatively. Both imaging techniques may detect ureteral obstruction with upper tract dilation. IVPs detect most sites of urinary leakage, but may miss ureteral leakage that is immediately adjacent to the trigone. This occurs because dye filling the bladder may obscure any small leak in that area. Cystoscopy with retrograde pyelography remains the definitive test of choice for location of lower urogenital tract fistulas.

The use of a double balloon urethral catheter such as a Tratner catheter may also be of use under fluoroscopic guidance for urethral fistula. Occasionally fistulas are so small that they present as a symptom of stress incontinence. These can only be found by filling the bladder and having the patient complete a provocative maneuver such as a cough or the Valsalva maneuver.

PREVALENCE AND FREQUENCY

In the United States, estimates of urogenital fistula formation range from less than 0.5 percent of hysterectomy procedures,[19] to 10 percent of radical hysterectomies found in an early series reported by Meigs.[20] Graber et al[21] noted only 16 bladder injuries in over 800 hysterectomies, an incidence of less than 2 percent. In the largest reported series, Wharton[22] noted only 83 bladder injuries (0.5 percent incidence) in over 16,000 major gynecologic procedures. In 15 patients, the bladder was injured on entry into the abdomen. All other 62 injuries occurred while the bladder was being dissected off of the cervix or away from other organs. Sixty-five percent of the injuries occurred at benign surgery, usually in the presence of endometriosis or pelvic inflammatory disease. If injuries are noticed at surgery, they are usually closed; if not noticed, fistulas occur.

Ureteral injury occurs even more commonly in some series than bladder injuries. Daly and Higgins[23] noted an incidence of 1.5 percent in 1,093 women undergoing pelvic operations.

In developing countries, vesicovaginal and other urogenital fistulas occur at a rate of 1 to 3 for every 1,000 deliveries.[24] At least 20,000 women await repair in Nigeria alone, while as many as 200,000 may be waiting across Subsaharan Africa.[24] When one considers the social isolation and ongoing human suffering associated with fistulas, this must be viewed as a medical disaster. Even after successful closure of the fistula (in 85 to 95 percent), over 60 percent of patients who have had obstetric fistulas are left with a number of problems, including foot drop or leg contractions from sciatic nerve injury, amenorrhea, vaginal atresia, stress urinary incontinence, and dyspareunia.[5] Since most victims are adolescents, these disabilities are often lifelong. The overall effect of the urogenital fistula problem in the developing world is immense.

MANAGEMENT OF FISTULAS

Gynecologic High Vaginal Vault Fistula Posthysterectomy

Tancer[2] recently reviewed 126 cases of genitourinary fistulas. Of these, 91 percent (110) followed surgery, with the abdominal hysterectomy for benign disease being the most common procedure. Tancer states that most of these vesicovaginal fistulas develop high in the vaginal vault. Using a partial colpocleisis, or Latzko technique, Tancer successfully closed these fistulas on the first attempt in 92 percent of the cases.[2,25] The nine patients whose fistulas failed to close on a first attempt were successfully closed on the second attempt, using the same operative technique.[2]

As shown in the Figures 39-1 to 39-4, the author prefers to first identify the typically small posthysterectomy fistula with a lacrimal duct probe. The fistula is then dilated with

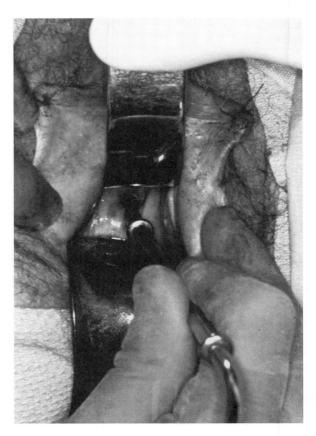

Fig. 39-2. Fistula tract dilated to make it more operable.

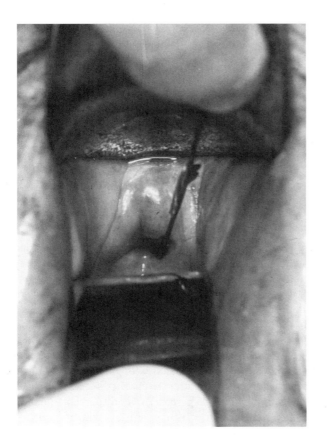

Fig. 39-1. Pinpoint vesicovaginal fistula following gynecologic surgery. Tract identified with lacrimal duct probe.

regular Hanks dialators up to a size 10 or 12. This allows insertion of a small pediatric Foley catheter into the fistula tract. Inflating the 3 to 5 ml catheter balloon allows the surgeon to place traction on the fistula and thus draw the vaginal cuff near the introitus, making vaginal dissection easier. In the Latzko dissection, a vaginal mucosal incision is made around the fistula, and then vaginal epithelial flaps are raised and removed in a wide circle around the fistula tract.[25] The catheter is then removed and the tract may be removed or inverted into the bladder with closure. Multiple layers of sutures (using 2–0 or 3–0 absorbable sutures) are placed in a transverse interrupted fashion with an imbricating technique to facilitate closure without tension. Sutures at the lateral edges of the fistula are placed just beyond, and above and below, the fistula edges. The second layer utilizes transverse U-shaped sutures that actually tie even further beyond the lateral edges of the fistula tract. Longitudinal or vertical suture lines are usually best avoided, since these may bring ureters too close to the midline and facilitate ureteral kinking, tissue ischemia, obstruction, and even further fistula formation. Likewise, circumferential pursestring sutures are usually avoided since tissue ischemia at fistula edges may occur.

Occasionally, in the repair of high vaginal vault fistulas,

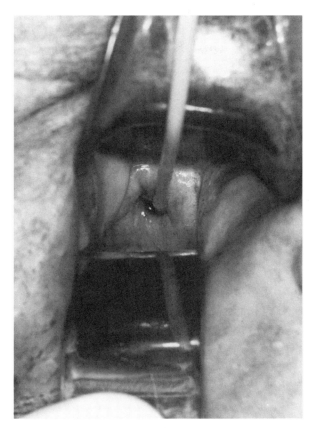

Fig. 39-3. Pediatric Foley catheter inserted into fistula tract to pull fistula into easier operating field. Incision is made immediately outside of the fistula tract, through vaginal epithelium.

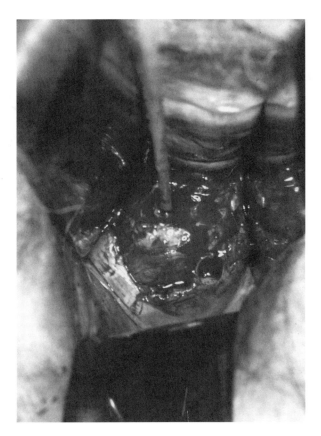

Fig. 39-4. Widely excised vaginal epithelium, leaving fascial and bladder layers ready to close in multiple layers.

the cul-de-sac, or pouch of Douglas, is entered. This may actually aid and improve repair rates. The posterior peritoneum may be raised from the pelvic floor as a flap and used as a third or fourth layer in the Latzko closure. The vaginal epithelium must be carefully reapproximated to close the cul-de-sac after this repair.

Other causative factors contributing to fistulas high in the vaginal vault include those secondary to radiation necrosis or to a long obstructed labor with cesarean hysterectomy. These are usually larger and have a great deal more fibrosis and tissue scarring. If the vaginal repair approach is undertaken, an early technique that was first developed by Maurice Collis of Ireland in 1861,[26] and later refined by Makenrodt in the 1880s, may be considered.[27] In this technique, vaginal flaps are raised away from the bladder. However, these flaps are preserved to be used in the final closure layer. Many times new tissue sources will be brought into this repair. The Martius graft, or labial fibrofatty tissue graft, is most commonly used to reinforce repairs even high in the vaginal vault.[28] Gracilis muscle grafts are also used on occasion.[29] These grafts lend strength, support, and sealant to the fistula closure.

Urologists usually prefer the abdominal approach for all genitourinary fistulas. This dates back to the earliest such repairs as described by Trendelenburg in the 1890s.[30] Some prefer the transvesical route of repair, with a separate closure of vagina and bladder.[31] All of these routes allow interposition of omental tissue as an added layer between bladder and vagina[32] (Fig. 39-5). Generally, when the fistula is especially high in the vault, the transvesical route becomes the preferred approach of most general surgeons.[1]

Obstetric Fistulas

Obstetric fistulas are usually classified according to their anatomic location (Fig. 39-6). Each type is repaired by a different method.

Suburethral or Juxtaurethral Vesicovaginal Fistulas

Suburethral or juxtaurethral vesicovaginal fistulas are the most commonly seen obstetric fistulas in Ghana and Nigeria. These are found at the urethrovesical junction. If total urethral transection with retropubic fixation of the fistula has

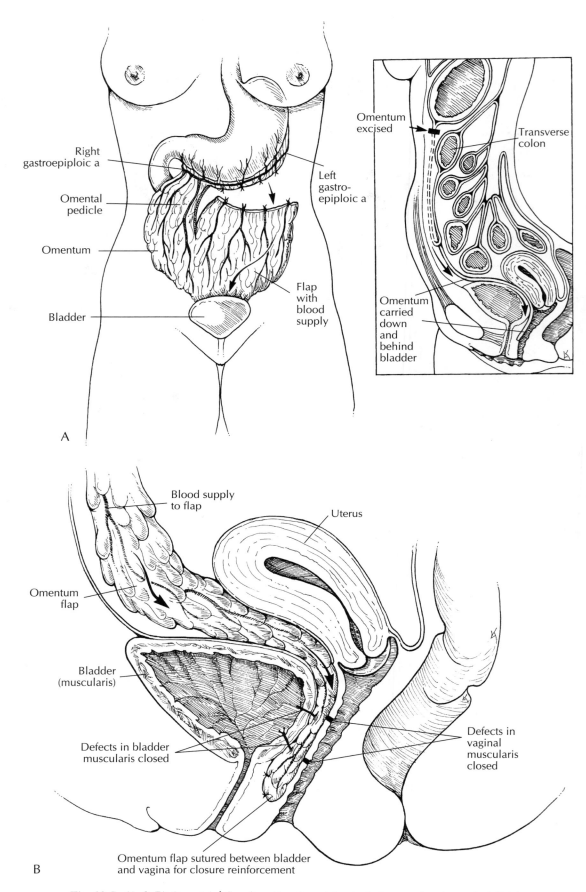

Right
gastroepiploic a

Omental
pedicle

Omentum

Bladder

Left
gastro-
epiploic a

Flap
with
blood
supply

Omentum
excised

Transverse
colon

Omentum
carried
down
and
behind
bladder

A

Blood supply
to flap

Uterus

Omentum
flap

Bladder
(muscularis)

Defects in
vaginal
muscularis
closed

Defects in bladder
muscularis closed

Omentum flap sutured between bladder
and vagina for closure reinforcement

B

Fig. 39-5. (A & B) Omental J-flap for adjunctive abdominal closure of vesicovaginal fistula.

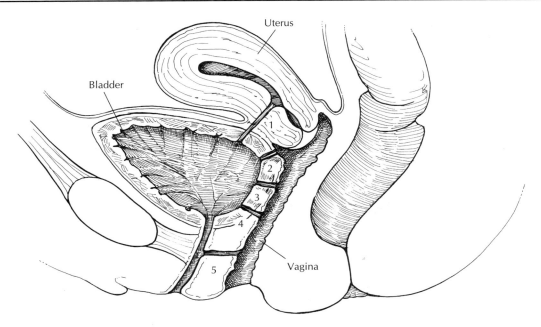

Fig. 39-6. Anatomic types of obstetric fistulas: 1, vesicocervical fistula; 2, Juxtacervical vesicovaginal fistula; 3, Midvaginal vesicovaginal fistula; 4, Suburethral vesicovaginal fistula; 5, Urethrovaginal fistula.

not occurred, the repair is one of simple vaginal tissue mobilization with a layered closure, giving a 95-percent successful closure rate. When retropubic fixation of fistula edges has occurred, anterior bladder wall mobilization through the space of Retzius (entered vaginally) is required to bring bladder wall edges to the severed urethra. Martius graft placement may improve closure rates in such instances, but patients develop type II stress urinary incontinence in at least 10 to 20 percent of these repairs.[33,34]

Midvaginal or Massive Vesicovaginal Fistulas

Midvaginal or massive vesicovaginal fistulas are also common in West Africa. These require wide tissue mobilization into the paravaginal spaces bilaterally to facilitate closure of the bladder. When the fistula is 4 cm or more in diameter, if direct closure of vaginal mucosa is attempted, this routinely leads to vaginal stenosis, or gynatresia. Efforts to preserve vaginal depth by using full-thickness Martius skin grafts to close vagina have helped in lessening the postrepair stenosis rates[35] (Fig. 39-7).

Juxtacervical Vesicovaginal Fistulas

Juxtacervical vesicovaginal fistulas are those that are found directly above or adjacent to the anterior cervical lip. If the cephalad edge of the vesicovaginal fistula is not visible vaginally, the repair is best accomplished by a combined vaginal and abdominal approach, with insertion of an omental graft

between bladder and cervix.[32] Success rates approach 100 percent in most series.

Fistulas With Total Urethral Loss

Fistulas with total urethral loss remain difficult to manage. Repair methods include mobilization of vulvar and labial tissue to create a neourethra.[36,37] When scarring is especially severe, the author prefers mobilization of anterior bladder wall through the vagina, and utilizing an anterior bladder wall flap to create a urethra, as described by Tanagho[38] (Fig. 39-8). Elevation of the newly formed urethrovesical neck is required to lessen the rate of type III stress urinary incontinence associated with this repair, even when fistula closure has been successful.[39]

Gynecologic Urethrovaginal Fistulas

The urethrovaginal fistula in the developed world most often follows urethral diverticulum repair attempts, anterior repairs, and forceps rotations. These are usually readily closed by wide mobilization into lateral periurethral spaces and layered closure. Vertically placed layers, when possible, lessen the chance of urethral shortening postoperatively. Careful dissection of distinct tissue layers will allow closure in a fashion that does not place suture lines directly over one another. Martius graft placement is simple and often helpful in the repair of these fistulas (Fig. 39-9).

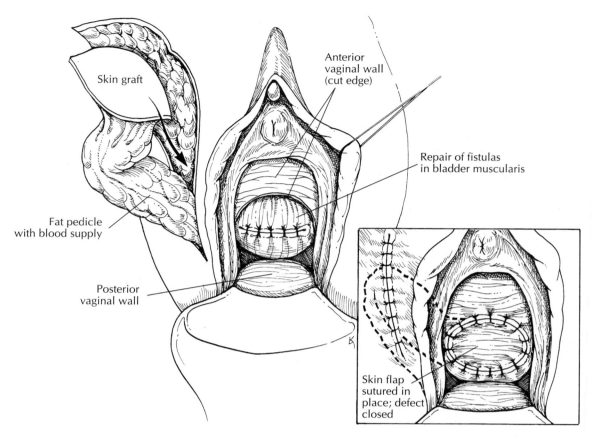

Fig. 39-7. Putting a full-thickness Martius graft in place to preserve vaginal depth.

Ureterovaginal Fistulas

Anatomy

The repair of ureterovaginal fistulas requires an approach and technique that will both restore normal function of the ureter and close the fistulous defect. The ureter is not a passive tube that drains urine into the bladder from the kidney. The intraoperative hallmark of a functioning ureter is its peristaltic waves. This is a result of its basic anatomic design. The ureter consists of three layers. Its innermost layer is the epithelial mucosal tissue consisting of transitional cells. The middle layer, which is responsible for peristalsis, is composed of longitudinal, circular, and spiral fibers. The outer layer is composed of an adventitial sheath composed of collagen, elastic, and nonmyelinated nerve fibers, which protects and supports the blood vessels both within and around the ureter. The outer layer is sometimes referred to as Waldeyer's sheath.[40]

Because of the anatomic location of the bladder and kidneys, the ureters must traverse a distance usually running from the superior aspect of the abdomen to the inferior portion of the pelvis. Divided by the pelvic brim, the ureter has two portions: the pelvic and the abdominal. Both portions are usually of equal length and measure 12 to 15 cm in the adult. Originating from the renal pelves, lateral to the first lumbar vertebrae, the ureters course inferiorly along the anterior border of the psoas muscle to the pelvic brim. As the ureter passes under the uterine artery, it is only 1.5 cm lateral to the cervix at the level of the internal os. Passing through the cardinal ligament, the lowest 1 to 2 cm of the ureter can be palpated vaginally just medial to the vaginal apex. Attempts to control heavy bleeding from the vaginal cuff with large sutures are a common cause of ureteral injury. Above the pelvic brim, the ureter is loosely attached to the parietal peritoneum and moves with the peritoneum during blunt dissection. When looking for the ureter, either abdominally or in the pelvis, the underside of the peritoneum should be inspected.

Running the length of the abdomen and the pelvis, the ureter takes advantage of many different blood supplies. Varied sources of perfusion add a protective shield to the ureter if injured. The most important aspect of ureteral blood supply is its unpredictable source. Eighty percent of all ureters have a single artery that runs its entire length. This artery usually originates from the renal artery but it may also be supplied by the aorta and ovarian, iliac, uterine, middle hemorrhoidal, superior vesicle, and vaginal arteries. Twenty per-

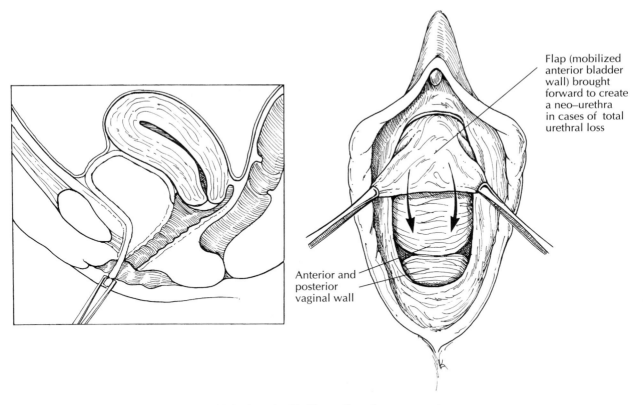

Flap (mobilized anterior bladder wall) brought forward to create a neo-urethra in cases of total urethral loss

Anterior and posterior vaginal wall

Fig. 39-8. Anterior bladder wall used as a neourethra.

cent of ureters do not have a single vessel running their course. These ureters are supplied by an anastomosing network of small vessels supplied by the major vessels named above. Care must be taken during dissection of the ureter not to compromise its blood supply. Above the pelvic brim, dissection should be done with a lateral approach. In the pelvis, the approach should be taken anteriorly. These simple methods will greatly enhance the preservation of the ureteral blood supply.[41] Disruption of the ureteral blood supply may lead to the loss of peristalsis, segmental dilatation, and eventual fistula formation after a delay of days or weeks.

Surgical Approach

After the diagnosis of a ureterovaginal fistula is made, the timing and method of repair must be considered. Recently, some authors have advocated an aggressive approach to fistula repair at the time of its discovery.[42,43] Previous thought has centered around immediate repair only when the fistula was discovered within 3 to 5 days of the initial operative procedure. In this author's experience, the timing of the repair is probably less important than the selection of the proper procedure. Schlossberg[44] demonstrated in the animal model that after ureterotomy, healing of the mucosa is complete after 3 weeks, and that smooth muscle bridging is com-

plete by 6 weeks. If the ureter is allowed to develop extensive fibrosis, angulation, or poor smooth muscle regeneration, peristalsis may fail to return. This finding argues favorably for an immediate and direct repair of the fistula, whenever possible.

When the presence of pelvic infection or other pelvic pathology prevents a direct surgical approach, radiology-assisted percutaneous nephrotomy will allow temporary urinary drainage until a ureteral repair can be undertaken safely.

One exception exists to this rule: if it is possible to pass a stent across the fistula site, spontaneous healing of a small lesion may occur. This endourologic management requires placement of a ureteral stent for at least 4 to 8 weeks. Such an approach has been successful in 7 of 16 women since 1980 in Kursh's series.[45] During the first 7 days after ureteral stents are placed, it is advisable to have separate transurethral catheter placement for bladder drainage to prevent any ureteral reflux.

In most posthysterectomy ureteral injuries, a simple ureteral reimplantation is the most effective repair. Most vesicovaginal fistulas from gynecologic surgery are usually very close to the bladder and this facilitates reimplantation. The initial identification and dissection of the ureter in the pelvis is the obvious initial step. Because of recent postoperative healing, the best place to start may actually be above the

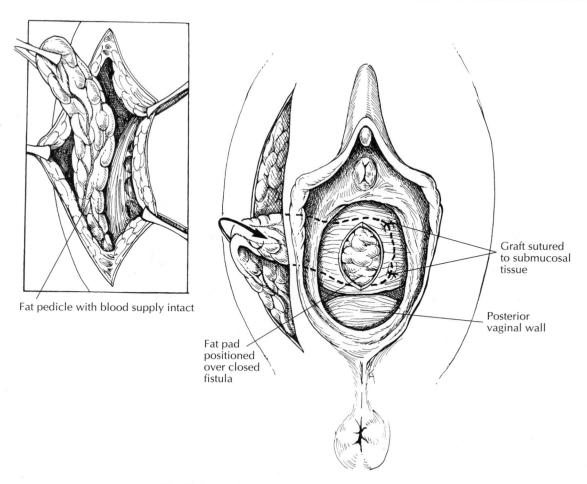

Fat pedicle with blood supply intact

Fat pad positioned over closed fistula

Graft sutured to submucosal tissue

Posterior vaginal wall

Fig. 39-9. Martius graft, using fibrofatty labial tissue.

pelvic brim. This can be done by mobilizing the colon medially from the pericolic gutter. Paying close attention to the ureteral blood supply, the ureters can be traced downward to fistula site.[4]

The ureter is often dilated from partial or total obstruction. The site of the fistulous tract may not be easily seen in the presence of periureteral fibrosis. Dissection can be very difficult. If a surgical impasse is reached, the most viable aspect of the ureter should be tagged with a 2–0 or 3–0 absorbable stay stitch at its proximal end. The distal portion of ureter, close to the fistula, should be ligated and cut.

The bladder should be incised in a transverse fashion to facilitate reimplantation under direct visualization. The transverse incision also allows for the development of a Baori flap if necessary. This would allow reimplantation of an injury as high up as the pelvic brim. If the bladder must be mobilized to give it extra length for reimplantation, perivesical fibrofatty tissue can be excised from the bladder serosa. This excision of fibrofatty tissue is done on the contralateral side of the ureteral injury. Bladder mobilization of this type allows for later stabilization with a psoas hitch.[48] The psoas hitch is usually performed by attaching mobilized bladder serosa to the psoas muscle with interrupted permanent sutures, on the same side as the ureteral injury.

After the bladder and the noninjured ureter are mobilized, a transverse opening into the dome of the bladder is made. The ureter is now ready for reimplantation. The distal end of the injured (and tagged) ureter is pulled into the bladder through a separate stab incision near the trigone. Approximately 1 to 2 cm of ureter should be pulled through this incision. The end of the ureter should be spatulated and 3–0 absorbable sutures should be used to anchor this ureter to the bladder mucosa. Keeping the reanastomosis tension free is of paramount importance. The serosa of the reimplanted ureter should be sutured to the outside serosa of the bladder. This should be done close to the reimplantation site. Stents are not always used in the reimplanted ureter but might be helpful if there appears to be tension on the suture line, a present pelvic infection, or a question of ureteral viability.

The psoas hitch can compliment the strength of the repair by stabilizing the bladder. This is done by using 2–0 nonabsorbable suture to cover the repaired ureteral site with the bladder. Several stitches will attach bladder serosa to the psoas muscle on the same side as the injury. This will also decrease the chance that the ureter will retract out of the bladder. A drain should be placed next to the reimplantation site to minimize any peritoneal irritation from possible urine leakage.[47] To decrease any chance of ureteral reflux or bladder distention, a suprapubic or transurethral bladder catheter should be left in place for 14 to 21 days.

End-to-end or side-to-end anastomoses of ureteral segments carry a relatively high ureteral stenosis rate, whether or not stents are used. However, for the rare injury above the pelvic brim, this may be the only option (rather than percutaneous diversion). End-to-end anastomoses are performed by spatulating the ends to make the suture line circumference as large as possible. Usually 4–0 or 3–0 absorbable sutures are used, and a watertight closure is achieved in one layer. A Penrose drain, coming out of the overlying skin, is usually placed to divert any escaping urine away from the peritoneal cavity. If stents are used, they are usually removed in 2 to 4 weeks, but this may be delayed if follow-up IVP studies show continuous leakage.

Ureteral lacerations, like small bowel laceration, are repaired by suturing the ureter in the opposite direction of the laceration. This preserves the circumferential size of the ureter where it was lacerated, thus avoiding a suture method that would lead to ureteral stenosis. Ureteral stents are usually inserted for 2 to 4 weeks.

POSTOPERATIVE CARE

Many controversies still exist about postoperative care. Most surgeons treat any vaginal repair attempt like any other vaginal surgery, and provide perioperative antibiotic prophylaxis. Most surgeons in developing countries provide antibiotics for urinary antisepsis for as long as catheter drainage is maintained. Some prefer suprapubic drainage, although most prefer transurethral drainage. For the very small gynecologic fistula in a well-nourished American, 3 to 5 days of catheter drainage after closure, or until microscopic hematuria clears, is probably adequate. For large obstetric fistulas or radiation fistulas, 14 to 21 days of drainage is preferred.

One thing on which all fistula surgeons agree is the need to have adequate systemic or local hydration to ensure constant bladder flushing. This prevents any clotting of blood and blockage of the catheter, which leads to bladder distension and disruption of fistula repair suture lines. Whether this is achieved by intravenous fluid, intermittent catheter flushing with small amounts of normal saline, or copious amounts of oral intake, its importance cannot be underestimated.

TIMING CONSIDERATIONS

The traditional teaching in fistula surgery was to delay at least 8 to 12 weeks after the onset of leakage before attempting any repair. This was meant to give the tissue time to recover from whatever traumatic event had resulted in a fistula. It was designed as a plan for the large obstetric fistula. In reality, it often requires 8 to 10 weeks at a minimum for tissue inflammation to resolve after the infection and tissue necrosis that accompany prolonged obstructed labor. However, with the small gynecologic fistula, extensive infection and tissue necrosis is uncommon. Therefore, early repair attempts (within 1 to 2 weeks of leakage) that include excision of the fistula tract have become more common.

O'Quinn[48] studied early repair attempts, with and without systemic steroids. She found that overall leakage days were reduced by attempting early closure of fistulas, even if the successful closure rate was slightly less than that achieved by delayed repairs. Collins[49] had also championed the immediate repair approach for postsurgical genitourinary fistula. Recently, Waaldijk[50] has even published promising results with the early repair of obstetric fistulas in Nigeria.

UNUSUAL ASPECTS OF UROGENITAL FISTULAS

When sutures are placed into the bladder lumen, it is not uncommon for bladder stones to form. These may grow to be several centimeters in diameter. Removal to control infection may have to be done even transvesically long after a successful fistula closure.

The use of electrocautery through the cystoscope may be helpful in closing very small vesicovaginal fistula tracts of less than 0.5 cm in size. Falk and Orkin[51] first reported the use of cystoscopic electrocautery in 1957 to successfully treat of 10 vesicovaginal fistulas (all less than 3 mm in diameter). Kursch[52] noted the successful closure of 10 of 14 patients with fistulas 2 to 3 mm in diameter, or less. The theory is simple. The cautery destroys the fistula tract lining, leaving the bladder and vaginal tissues to reseal during 2 to 4 weeks of indwelling catheter drainage. This technique should be attempted on very small fistula defects, but is not helpful on any larger fistulas.

Finally, urogenital fistulas may be more complex than first imagined. Suprapubic catheter placement, when done blindly, has resulted in leakage of small bowel contents into the bladder, giving the ''green urine sign'' on postoperative rounds. Immediate bowel resection and separate bladder repair is required. Colovesical fistulas have been reported with diverticulitis, severe endometriosis, and as a result of third-world obstetric trauma. Abdominal repairs with resection of injured bowel areas, as well as excision and repair of bladder fistula tracts, are usually necessary to ensure closure.

REFERENCES

1. Lee RL, Symmonds RE, Williams TJ: Current status of genitourinary fistula. Obstet Gynecol 72:313, 1988
2. Tancer ML: Observations on prevention and management of

vesicovaginal fistula after total hysterectomy. Surg Gynecol Obstet 175:501, 1982

3. Judd ES: The operative treatment of vesicovaginal fistulae. Surg Gynecol Obstet 30:447, 1920

4. Waaldijk K: The surgical management of bladder fistula in 775 women in Northern Nigeria. Benda BV, Nymegen, 1989,

5. Elkins TE: Surgery for the obstetric vesicovaginal fistula: a review of 100 operations in 82 patients. Am J Obstet Gynecol 170:1108, 1994

6. Ahmad S: Urinary fistula in gynaecological practice in north west frontier province (Pakistan). In the Proceedings of a Vesicovaginal Fistula Conference. Lahore, Pakistan, December 10, 1988

7. Elkins TE: Maternal mortality and morbidity in the developing world: personal reflections and a profession's commitment. Women's Health Iss 2:146, 1992

8. Fitzpatrick CC, Elkins TE: Radiation-induced vesicovaginal fistulas. p. 407. In McGuire E, Kursh ED (eds): Female Urology. JB Lippincott, Philadelphia, 1994

9. Droegemueller W et al: Principles of radiation therapy and chemotherapy in gynecologic cancer. p. 719. In: Comprehensive Gynecology. Mosby–Year Book, St. Louis, 1987

10. Bright TC, Peters PC: Ureteral injuries secondary to operative procedures: report of 24 cases. Urology 9:22, 1977

11. Higgins CC: Ureteral injuries during surgery: a review of 87 cases. JAMA 199:118, 1967

12. Mendez R, McGinty DM: The management of delayed recognized ureteral injuries. J Urol 119:192, 1978

13. Elkins TE: When should ureteral stents be used in benign gynecologic surgery? Curr News Gyn 1:1, 1994

14. Shore ND, Bragg KJ, Sosa RF: Indwelling ureteral stents. Semin Urol 5:200,

15. Grainger DA, Soderstrom RM, Schiff SF: Ureteral injuries at laparoscopy: insights into diagnosis, management, and prevention. Obstet Gynecol 75:839, 1990

16. Symmonds RE: Ureteral injuries associated with gynecologic surgery. Clin Obstet Gynecol 19:623, 1976

17. Zoubek J, McGuire EJ, Noll F, DeLancey JOL: The late occurrence of urinary tract damage in patients successfully treated by radiotherapy for cervical carcinoma. J Urol 141:1347, 1989

18. Moir JC: Personal experiences in the treatment of vesicovaginal fistulas. Am J Obstet Gynecol 71:476, 1956

19. Mann WJ, et al: Ureteral injuries in obstetrics and gynecology training program: etiology and management. Obstet Gynecol 72:82, 1988

20. Carlton CE: Injuries to the ureter. Urol Clin North Am 4:33, 1977

21. Graber EA, O'Rourke JJ, McElrath T: Iatrogenic bladder injury during hysterectomy. Obstet Gynecol 23:267, 1964

22. Wharton LR: Methods of preventing injury to the ureters and bladder during gynecologic operations. Ann Surg 143:752, 1956

23. Daly JW, Higgins KA: Injury to the ureter during gynecologic surgical procedures. Surg Gynecol Obstet 67:19, 1988

24. Waaldijk K: Vaginal fistula in Northern Nigeria. Int J Urogynecol

25. Latzko W: Postoperative vesicovaginal fistulas: genesis and therapy. Am J Surg 48:211, 1992

26. Collis MH: Further remarks upon a new and successful mode of treatment for vesicovaginal fistula. Dublin QJ Med Sci 31: 302, 1861

27. Mackenrodt A: Die operative Heilung grosser Blasenscheidenfistein. Zentralbl Gynakol 8:180, 1894

28. Elkins TE, DeLancey JOL, McGuire EJ: The use of modified martius graft as an adjunctive technique in vesicovaginal and rectovaginal fistula repair. Obstet Gynecol 75:727, 1990

29. Garlock JH: The cure of an intractable vesicovaginal fistula by use of a pedicled muscle graft. Surg Gynecol Obstet 255: 255, 1928

30. Trendelenburg F: Uber Blasenschneiden—fisteloperationem and Über Beckehochlagerung bei operationen. Samml Klin Vortr 355(chir. no. 109):3373, 1890

31. Mack WF: Urologic complications of pelvic surgery. Br J Urol 41:641, 1969

32. Kiricuta I, Goldstein AMB: The repair of extensive vesicovaginal fistulas with pedicled omentum: a review of 27 cases. J Urol 108:724, 1972

33. Hassim AM, Lucas C: Reduction of the incidence of stress incontinence complicating fistula repair. Br J Surg 61:461, 1974

34. Schleicher D, Ojengbede OHA, Elkins TE: Urodynamic evaluation of patients after successful closure of vesicovaginal fistulas. Int J Urogynecol 4:262, 1993

35. Margolis T, Opparo-Addo J, Seffah J, Elkins TE: Use of a full thickness Martius graft to restore vaginal depth in patients with large obstetric fistulas. Obstet Gynecol 84:148, 1994

36. Hamlin RHJ, Nicholson EC: Reconstruction of the urethra totally destroyed in labor. BMJ 2:147, 1969

37. Symmonds RE, Hill LM: Loss of the urethra: a report on 50 patients. Am J Obstet Gynecol 130:130, 1978

38. Tanagho EA: Bladder neck reconstruction for total urinary incontinence: 10 years of experience. J Urol 125:321, 1981

39. Elkins TE, Ghosh TS, Tagoe GA, Fort D: Transvaginal urethral reconstruction from tubularized anterior bladder wall in the repair of obstetric fistulas. Obstet Gynecol 79:455, 1992

40. Guerriero WG: Ureteral trauma. In Guerriero WG (ed): Management of Acute and Chronic Urologic Injury. Appleton-Century-Crofts, E. Norwalk, CT, 1984

41. Guerriero WG: Ureteral injury. Urol Clin North Am 16:237, 1989

42. Witters S, Cornelissen M, Vereecken R: Iatrogenic ureteral injury: aggressive or conservative treatment. Am J Obstet Gynecol 155:582, 1986

43. Hoch WH, Kursh ED, Persky L: Early, aggressive management of intraoperative ureteral injuries. J Urol 114:530, 1975

44. Schlossberg SM: Ureteral healing. Semin Urol 5:197, 1987

45. Kursh ED: Ureteral injuries. p. 337. Kursh ED, McGuire EJ (eds): In Female Urology. JB Lippincott, Philadelphia, 1994

46. Harrow BR: A neglected maneuver for ureterovesical implantation following injury at gynecologic operations. J Urol 100: 280, 1968

47. Boari A: Contributo sperimentale alla plastica dell' uretere. Atti Acad Sci Med Nat Ferrara 68:149, 1894

48. O'Quinn AG, Degefu S, Batson HK et al: Early repair of vesicovaginal fistula following preliminary corticosteroid. Presented at the Society of Pelvic Surgeons, New Orleans, November 1984

49. Collins CG, Pent D, Jones FB: Results of early repair of vesicovaginal fistula with preliminary cortisone treatment. Am J Obstet Gynecol 80:1005, 1960

50. Waaldijk K: The immediate surgical management of fresh obstetric fistulas with catheter and/or early closure. Int J Gynaecol Obstet 45:11, 1994

51. Falk HC, Orkin L: Nonsurgical closure of vesicovaginal fistulas. J Obstet Gynecol 9:538, 1957

52. Kursh ED: Etiology, evaluation, and endoscopic management of vesicovaginal fistulas. p. 359. In Kursh ED, McGuire EJ (eds): Female Urology. JB Lippincott, Philadelphia, 1994

CHAPTER FORTY

MANAGEMENT OF RECTOVAGINAL FISTULAS AND THE DISRUPTED ANAL SPHINCTER

MARC R. TOGLIA
THOMAS E. ELKINS

Anal incontinence, the involuntary loss of flatus or feces, is rapidly gaining recognition as a condition that occurs more commonly than previously thought.[1-3] It occurs most frequently in multiparous women and has its highest incidence in adults over the age of 65. Recent studies have estimated that 7 to 11 percent of healthy adults will admit to incontinence of gas or feces.[4,5] In a survey of 249 female residents in three extended care facilities in the Indianapolis area, 50 percent admitted to incontinence of stool.[6] Unfortunately, the symptoms of anal incontinence are frequently underreported by patients and commonly unrecognized by clinicians. The emotional, psychological, and social problems created by this condition can be both devastating and debilitating.

The most common cause of anal incontinence in healthy women is related to obstetric trauma. Recent investigations have highlighted the role that occult anal sphincter and denervation nerve injuries occurring at the time of vaginal delivery play in the etiology of anal incontinence.[7,8]

Rectovaginal fistula and chronic third- and fourth-degree lacerations are probably the most commonly recognized cause of anal incontinence seen in an obstetrician/gynecologist's practice. (See the box in *Nonobstetric Causes of Anal Incontinence* for other causes.)

ANATOMY AND PHYSIOLOGY

Clinical management of problems associated with the anal canal and lower rectum requires a thorough understanding of both the anatomy and physiology of this area as well as the functional changes that occur as a result of vaginal delivery. Anal continence is a complex mechanism that requires both intact anatomy and appropriate neuromuscular function. The sphincteric musculature is composed of two striated muscles; the puborectalis portion of the levator ani and the external anal sphincter, and the smooth muscle of the internal anal sphincter. Unlike most other striated muscles, the puborectalis and external anal sphincter maintain a constant resting tone that is proportional to the volume of the rectal content and relax at the time of defecation. Both of these muscles contain a majority of type I (slow twitch) muscle fibers, which are ideally suited to maintaining a constant tone over time. Each muscle group also contains a smaller proportion of type II (fast twitch) fibers, which allow them to respond quickly during sudden increases in intra-abdominal pressure.[9,10] These muscles are both innervated through the pudendal nerve arising from the S3 and S4 nerve roots.

Continence of solid stool is maintained primarily by the action of the puborectalis. This muscle originates from the pubic bone on either side of the midline, and forms a U-shaped sling that cradles the rectum. The constant resting tone of the puborectalis pulls the anorectal junction anteriorly, creating an approximately 90-degree angle between the anal and rectal canals (Fig. 40-1). This angulation is readily palpable on rectal examination as a resilient muscular shelf that pulls the rectum anteriorly towards the symphysis during voluntary contraction. Sir Alan Parks proposed that this

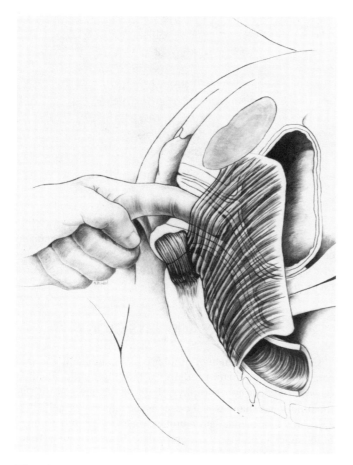

Fig. 40-1. Lateral view of the external anal sphincter and levator ani muscles showing palpation of the medial border of the levator ani muscle (puborectalis-pubococcygeus portion). Note the approximately 90-degree angle between the anal canal and the axis of the rectum. (From Toglia and DeLancey,[1] with permission.)

acute angulation creates a "flap-valve" effect in which increased intra-abdominal pressure compresses the anterior rectal wall against the pelvic floor and that this mechanism was critical to the maintenance of anal continence.[11,12] However, subsequent physiologic and radiologic studies have failed to demonstrate that such a mechanism exists[13,14] and successful surgical restoration of anal continence does not appear to depend on the restoration of this angle.[15,16] Therefore, the importance of this mechanism is questionable.

Continence of gas and liquid stools is maintained by the internal and external anal sphincters. This anal sphincter complex is nearly cylindrical as it encircles the anal canal and, measured in the midline, is 18.3 mm thick and 28.0 mm long[17] (Fig. 40-2). It is critical that clinicians realize that 54 percent of the anterior thickness of the sphincter is attributable to the internal anal sphincter. The anatomic and functional importance of the anterior component of the sphincter complex, particularly with respect to the internal anal sphincter, is often underappreciated in most anatomy and gynecologic textbooks but is critical in the proper repair of obstetric sphincter lacerations as well as in the surgical correction of anal incontinence.

The internal anal sphincter is a thickened, downward continuation of the circular smooth muscle layer of the colon and is innervated by sympathetic nerves from the presacral complex. Unlike the external anal sphincter and puborectalis muscle, the internal anal sphincter is not under voluntary control and its function is mediated largely by reflex arcs at the spinal cord level. At rest, the anal canal is kept closed by the constant tonic activity of both the internal and external sphincters. Physiologic studies have shown that the internal anal sphincter is responsible for 75 to 85 percent of the resting tone of the anal canal.[18,19] As the intestinal content passes into the rectum, the internal anal sphincter relaxes reflexively to allow the upper anal canal to "sample" the contents and to discriminate between solid, liquid, and gas. Once the intestinal contents have been determined, the internal anal sphincter contracts again to augment rectal closure. Thus, it is currently believed that continence at rest (particularly for liquid stool and flatus) is the responsibility of the internal anal sphincter, whereas continence during sudden distension of the rectum is maintained principally by the external anal sphincter.

Anal sensation is also thought to play a critical role in the normal continence mechanism. Sensory receptors located both within the anal canal[20] and within the levator ani muscles[21] are important in detecting the presence of stool in the rectum as well as determining the degree of rectal distension. The upper anal canal is also capable of distinguishing between solid, liquid, and gaseous forms of stool. Sensory feedback from these areas is important in coordinating the activities of the sphincteric musculature, permitting the anorectum to perform the remarkable task of allowing flatus to pass downward through the anus while preserving continence of liquid and solid stool.

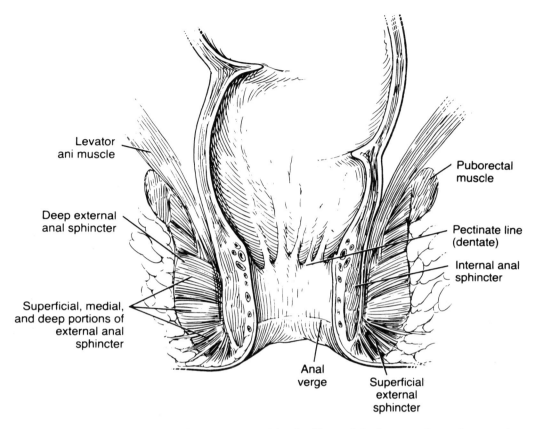

Fig. 40-2. Internal and external anal sphincters, separated by the fibers of the levator ani muscles, seen in coronal section. (From Lee,[81] by permission of the Mayo Foundation.)

VAGINAL DELIVERY AND INJURY TO THE ANAL CONTINENCE MECHANISM

New insights into the changes produced by vaginal delivery on the anal continence mechanism have been gained in the past 10 years. Vaginal delivery can damage the continence mechanism by direct injury to the internal and external anal sphincter muscles[7] or damage to the motor innervation of the pelvic floor,[22] or both.[23] Injury to the sensory innervation is also thought to occur.[24]

Injury to the continence mechanism is much more common following a uncomplicated vaginal delivery than previously recognized. Symptoms suggestive of mechanical or neurologic injury such as fecal urgency and incontinence of flatus or liquid stool, may be present in up to 13 percent of women following their first vaginal delivery.[7] Unrecognized structural injury to the internal and external anal sphincter has been shown to be present by anal endosonography in 30 percent of women following their first vaginal delivery.[7] Studies have also documented that there is a transient decrease in the strength of the internal and external anal sphincters following a vaginal delivery. Cornes and colleagues[24] and Haadem and associates[25] each reported that a reduction in both the maximum anal resting pressure and maximum voluntary contraction of the external anal sphincter occurs in the immediate postpartum period compared to women who underwent cesarean delivery.

Neurophysiologic studies have reported that uncomplicated vaginal delivery can initiate a denervation injury to the motor innervation of the pelvic floor.[22,23,26] These authors have theorized that injury initiated at the time of childbirth may progress over time and present as anal incontinence after many years, especially after the menopause. More recent studies, however, have reported that structural damage is more likely to be associated with symptoms than are neurologic factors.[7]

NONOBSTETRIC CAUSES OF ANAL INCONTINENCE

Although obstetric trauma is a leading cause of anal incontinence in women, it can also result from a variety of other conditions. Sphincter trauma leading to anal incontinence may be related to operative or accidental injuries such as impalement or pelvic fractures. Surgical procedures such as colpoperineorrhaphy, rectovaginal fistula and anal fissure repair, hemorrhoidectomy, and therapeutic anal dilation can

Causes of Fecal Incontinence

- Normal pelvic floor
  - Diarrheal states
    - Infectious diarrhea
    - Inflammatory bowel disease
    - Short-gut syndrome
    - Laxative abuse
    - Radiation enteritis
  - Overflow
    - Impaction
    - Encopresis
    - Rectal neoplasms
  - Neurologic conditions
    - Congenital anomalies (e.g., myelomeningocele)
    - Multiple sclerosis
    - Dementia, strokes, tabes dorsalis
    - Neuropathy (e.g., diabetes)
    - Neoplasms of brain, spinal cord, cauda equina
    - Injuries to brain, spinal cord, cauda equina
- Abnormal pelvic floor
  - Congenital anorectal malformation
  - Trauma
    - Accidental injury (e.g., impalement, pelvic fracture)
    - Anorectal surgery
    - Obstetrical injury
  - Aging
  - Pelvic floor denervation (idiopathic neurogenic incontinence)
    - Vaginal delivery
    - Chronic straining at stool
    - Rectal prolapse
    - Descending perineum syndrome

(From Madoff et al,[3] with permission.)

rectovaginal fistula formation and radiation proctitis may result in neurologic or mechanical damage to the rectum. Occult spinal cord injury or disease is another important cause of incontinence and is typically associated with an intact but weak external anal sphincter. Distinguishing between high and low spinal lesions requires sophisticated neurophysiologic studies.

Rectal prolapse is another important cause of anal incontinence. Most patients with rectal prolapse are women, and approximately half of them experience incontinence.[30] Uterine prolapse has been reported to commonly coexist with rectal prolapse.[31] Rectal prolapse may involve only the anal and sometimes rectal mucosa, or it may involve the protrusion of the full thickness of the rectal wall through the anal orifice. Prolapse of the mucosa only is considered to be part of the spectrum of hemorrhoidal disease and does not progress to complete rectal prolapse. The etiology of complete rectal prolapse is incompletely understood, but is thought to be related to progressive intussusception of the rectum. On examination, the anus appears patulous and gaping, with the full thickness of the rectal wall appreciated on digital examination (Fig. 40-3). Anal incontinence secondary to rectal prolapse is currently thought to be the result of pelvic floor denervation produced by the prolapse, and not vice versa.[32] The primary treatment for symptomatic rectal

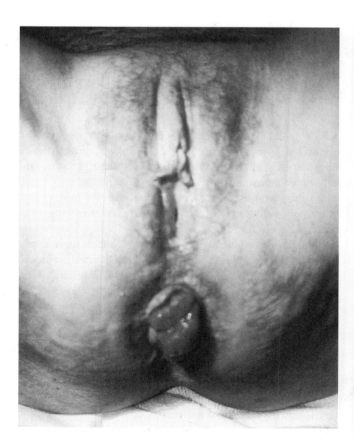

Fig. 40-3. Prolapse of the rectal mucosa in a 53-year-old woman.

all cause subsequent anal incontinence. A difficult hysterectomy, particularly those done for carcinoma of the cervix, endometriosis, or pelvic abscesses may also result in an injury to the rectum. Among elderly and institutionalized individuals, overflow incontinence secondary to fecal impaction is a leading cause of incontinence.[27,28] Diabetes can be associated with an autonomic neuropathy that can affect the internal anal sphincter and can produce incontinence, particularly with diarrheal states.[29] Radiotherapy can be associated with prolapse is surgical. Numerous approaches have been described[33] but are beyond the scope of this discussion. The common goal of these procedures is to achieve fixation of the rectum to the sacrum by means of postoperative fibrosis or rectopexy.[33] Patients with symptomatic rectal prolapse should be referred to an experienced colorectal surgeon.

EVALUATION

Clinical Examination

In the majority of cases, an adequate evaluation of the sphincteric mechanism can be gained from careful attention to the history and physical examination.[1,3] Anorectal symptoms must be specifically addressed by the clinician, as patients seldom offer this information voluntarily. As with any medical history, it is important that the patient describe her problems in her own words initially. It is important to ask specific questions regarding the onset, duration, and frequency of incontinent episodes. The patient should be asked whether the incontinence is related to solid, liquid, or gaseous forms of stool, as well as whether incontinence is accompanied by fecal urgency or the inability to tell when the rectum is distended or contracting. Fecal urgency (the inability to delay defecation) and urge incontinence are hallmarks of injury to the external anal sphincter. Incontinence to flatus and liquid stools is typically related to a dysfunction of the internal anal sphincter or a rectovaginal fistula. Incontinence to solid stool is related to dysfunction of the puborectalis muscle or the external anal sphincter, or both.

The anal continence mechanism is readily accessible to evaluation, and obstetrician/gynecologists are expertly skilled in pelvic and rectal examinations. A careful inspection of the perineum, vagina, and distal anal canal should be the starting point of any examination for anal incontinence, followed by a simple neurologic examination to test for the intactness of the motor component of S2–S4. The anal wink, bulbocavernosus, and cough reflex all test the integrity of the motor innervation of the external anal sphincter. Sensation over the inner thigh, vulvar, and perirectal areas should be tested for symmetry by light touch and pinprick.

The integrity of the external anal sphincter and puborectalis can be evaluated by observation and palpation of these structures during voluntary contraction. When a patient is asked to contract her rectum, two motions should be present. First the external anal sphincter should contract concentrically and the anus should be pulled inward. These actions should also readily be appreciated on rectal examination. The firm and resilient muscular sling of the levator ani should be readily palpable posteriorly as it creates a 90-degree angle between the anal and rectal canals. Voluntary contraction of this muscle pulls the canal and the examining finger anteriorly, toward the pubic bone. Pudendal neuropa-

thy is heralded by an external anal sphincter that is intact but has a weak resting tone as well as weak voluntary contraction. Pudendal neuropathy affecting the puborectalis muscle can be recognized if the anorectal angle is obtuse and if there is a palpable weakness with voluntary contraction.

Rectal sensation is difficult to test for on examination and must be inferred from the history. Conscious perception of rectal distension results in a reflex contraction of the external anal sphincter in order to preserve continence. Patients who experience incontinence because of impaired rectal sensation fail to contract the external anal sphincter during periods of rectal distension or contraction. Seepage of fecal contents promptly ceases once the patient perceives the leakage or distension through voluntary contraction of the external anal sphincter.

Diagnostic Testing

Sophisticated diagnostic testing for evaluating the anal continence mechanism are currently being used in clinical and physiologic research, but are cumbersome to perform and not widely available to the practitioner. In most patients presenting with anal incontinence, neurophysiologic and manometric measurements of anorectal pressures are probably unnecessary before attempting a surgical repair. The most frequently used physiologic tests are electromyography, anal manometry, anal endosonography, and cinedefecography.

Electromyography has been used to evaluate the integrity of external anal sphincter innervation following a traumatic injury, as well as to document the presence of pelvic floor neuropathy.[34] Electromyography is the study of the electrical activity produced by the depolarization of muscle membranes and the resulting action potential. Both concentric-needle and single-fiber myography have been used to help determine and measure sphincter innervation. Denervation injury is accompanied by subsequent reinnervation of the effected motor unit, which can be measured by fiber density. Thus, EMG studies provide indirect evidence of prior neurologic injury by measuring the amount of reinnervation. Patients with anal incontinence secondary to pudendal neuropathy often demonstrate prolonged motor unit potentials or increased fiber density indicative of nerve damage.

Motor nerve conduction studies can be used along with electromyography to assess nerve function. These studies are performed by stimulating the axon and measuring the speed that it takes for the action potential to reach the muscle supplied by that nerve. The delay between stimulation and the response is called the nerve latency. A noninvasive technique for measuring the pudendal nerve terminal motor latency has been developed by Swash and Snooks.[35] A nerve stimulator is mounted on an examination glove at the fingertip, and the electrostimulus is applied rectally over the pudendal nerve at each ischial spine and recorded at the external anal sphincter. Prolongation of the pudendal nerve terminal motor latency is indicative of damage to the pudendal nerve[36] (Fig. 40-4).

Anal manometry can be used to evaluate the function of the different components of the anorectum under physiologic conditions. A variety of catheters and techniques are avail-

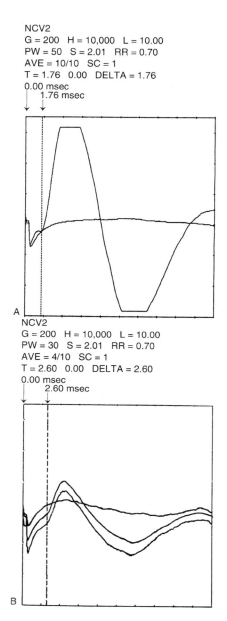

NCV2
G = 200   H = 10,000   L = 10.00
PW = 50   S = 2.01   RR = 0.70
AVE = 10/10   SC = 1
T = 1.76   0.00   DELTA = 1.76
0.00 msec
      1.76 msec

A

NCV2
G = 200   H = 10,000   L = 10.00
PW = 30   S = 2.01   RR = 0.70
AVE = 4/10   SC = 1
T = 2.60   0.00   DELTA = 2.60
0.00 msec
      2.60 msec

B

Fig. 40-4. Pudendal nerve motor terminal latency (A) before and (B) after delivery. The normal mean and standard deviation is 2.1 +/− 0.2 msec. G, gain (amplitude [V]; H, high-frequency filter setting (Hz); L, low-frequency filter setting (Hz); PW, pulse width of stimulus (msec); S, sweep speed (msec); RR, repetition rate per second; SC, scale; AVE, number of averaged stimuli; T, time to receptor of L1, cortex; Delta, difference in the two times. (From Benson,[82] with permission.)

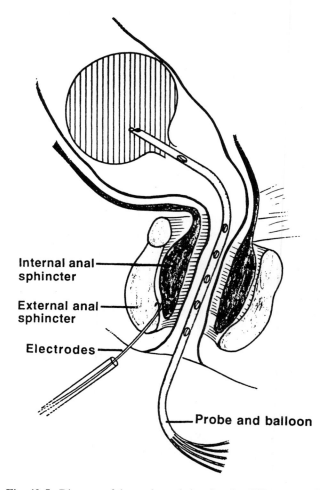

Internal anal sphincter

External anal sphincter

Electrodes

Probe and balloon

Fig. 40-5. Diagram of the anal canal showing the different muscle components and probes used to measure pressure in multiple sites in the anal canal, and the electrical activity of internal anal sphincter and external anal sphincter. (From Benson,[82] with permission.)

able to measure the pressures generated by the anal sphincters both at rest and during maximal voluntary contraction (Fig. 40-5). Resting anal pressure is mostly a reflection of the resting tone of the internal anal sphincter, and defects of this structure have been inferred from the measurement of a low resting anal pressure.[37] Anorectal pressures measured in the lower anal canal during maximal voluntary contraction reflect external anal sphincter function. Anal manometry can be used along with other clinical information to help identify the pathophysiologic mechanism of anal incontinence.

Anal endosonography is a recently introduced technique that allows for the accurate imaging of both the internal and external anal sphincter. This technique was developed at St. Marks Hospital in England and has provided much insight into the investigation and management of anal incontinence. A specially designed 360-degree sonographic probe is housed within a plastic cone approximately the diameter of

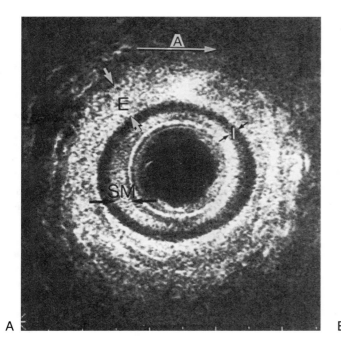
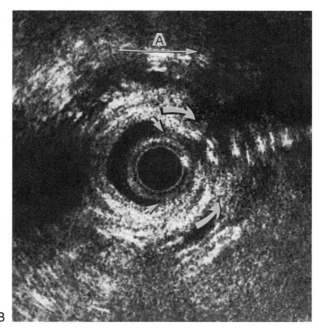

Fig. 40-6. (A) Anal endosonography in a healthy 24-year-old woman with an intact anal sphincter. Anterior (A) is to the right. The submucosa (SM) appears as a white ring outside the bright hyperechoic ring of the plastic cone that covers the probe. The internal anal sphincter (I) appears outside this ring as a densely hypoechoic ring. Outside this, the external anal sphincter (E) appears as a heterogeneous thicker ring muscle. **(B)** Anal endosonography in a 26-year-old woman with fecal incontinence after vaginal delivery. Small arrows indicate a disruption of the internal anal sphincter for half of its anterior circumference. Large arrows indicate a defect in the anterior quarter circumference of the external anal sphincter. In the middle of this defect the small white marks radiating out are an acoustic shadow of no significance. (From Kamm,[2] with permission.)

a finger. Structural abnormalities of either the external or internal anal sphincter can be readily identified by this technique. This technique has proven to be especially useful in the investigation of anal sphincter injury following vaginal delivery, as previously discussed (Fig. 40-6). Anal endosonography has also been critically evaluated in terms of its ability to identify abnormal anatomy and correlate with symptomatology. It is likely that anal endosonography will have an important role in the future investigation and management of anal incontinence.

SURGICAL REPAIR

The surgical management of anal incontinence remains a significant challenge for the obstetrician/gynecologist. Reconstructive surgery for anal incontinence should aim at restoring the continuity of both the external and internal anal sphincter. In addition, attention should be directed to establishing a thick perineal body and rectovaginal septum, as muscular support between the anterior anorectum and vagina is extremely limited. The results of such meticulous techniques will also result in a lengthening of the anal canal and

the restoration of a functional high pressure zone within the anal canal.

In some patients with an obtuse anorectal angle and evidence of pelvic floor neuropathy, it may be necessary to perform a retrorectal levatorplasty—the Parks postanal repair.[38] This operation was designed by Sir Alan Parks as a means of correcting anal incontinence in patients with neuropathy of the pelvic floor and the external anal sphincter. In this procedure, access to the levator ani muscles is gained through an incision posterior to the anus, with dissection carried out into the intersphincteric space. Once the levator ani and external sphincter muscles are exposed in this fashion, they are plicated in the midline using nonabsorbable suture. Although this operation was initially thought to be effective by restoring the anorectal angle and supporting the pelvic floor, there is little evidence to support this hypothesis. However, the procedure does effectively lengthen the anal canal and improves voluntary squeeze pressure, and has been shown to be effective in treating anal incontinence.[39] This procedure is typically reserved for patients who have evidence of a significant pelvic floor neuropathy and intact sphincteric musculature. A description of this technique is published elsewhere.[39]

Primary Repair of Third- and Fourth-Degree Obstetric Laceration

Obstetric trauma is certainly the most common cause of anal incontinence in women. Obstetric vaginal and perineal lacerations are classified as follows:

- *First-degree lacerations* involve the posterior vaginal fourchette, perineal skin, and vaginal mucosa only
- *Second-degree lacerations* extend into the fascia and musculature of the perineal body, which includes the deep and superficial transverse perineal muscles as well as fibers of the pubococcygeus and bulbocavernosus muscles
- *Third-degree lacerations* extend through all these structures and involve some or all of the fibers of the external anal sphincter
- *Fourth-degree lacerations* involve both the external anal sphincter as well as the rectal mucosa

The above classification system is far from perfect as it does not consider the involvement of the internal anal sphincter, which is obviously disrupted in all fourth-degree lacerations. The frequency with which this structure is disrupted in second- or third-degree lacerations is unknown.

Anal incontinence following the primary repair of third- and fourth-degree obstetric lacerations has previously been thought to be uncommon. However, recent studies have reported that incontinence to flatus and stool and fecal urgency occurs in 42 to 48 percent of these women.[8,25,40–42] There are several possible explanations for this surprisingly high incidence of symptoms. Early observations held that the suturing of an actively contracting muscle could lead to subsequent partial dehiscence during the ensuing weeks of healing. Others have hypothesized that childbirth may initiate a denervation injury to the pelvic floor that may result in malfunction of the continence mechanism.[43] More recently, Sultan and colleagues[8] reported on the outcome of primary repair of third-degree obstetric lacerations in 50 women. They found that 85 percent of women suffering a third-degree laceration had a persistent anal sphincter defect detected by anal endosonography despite primary repair at the time of delivery. Most of these defects involved both the internal and external anal sphincters and were associated with symptoms of fecal urgency and incontinence to flatus and liquid stool. Interestingly, motor nerve conduction studies were not significantly different between women with symptoms of incontinence and those without symptoms. These authors concluded that the primary repair of a third- or fourth-degree obstetric laceration is often inadequate and that postpartum anal incontinence is caused by persistent mechanical sphincter disruption rather than pudendal nerve injury, as had previ-

ously been thought. This new information should be a cause for our specialty to re-evaluate our technique for primary surgical repair.

It comes as no surprise that the standard repair of third- and fourth-degree obstetric lacerations may be inadequate. First, the basic tenets of repair surgery mandate the following: good exposure and lighting, adequate anesthesia, and the proper tools and assistance. The authors argue that one or more of the above is frequently missing in the labor and delivery room at the time of primary repair. Secondly, the internal anal sphincter can be difficult to identify. Located between the external anal sphincter and the anal mucosa, it is obviously disrupted in all patients with a fourth-degree laceration and probably in the majority of patients with a third-degree laceration. There is also evidence to suggest that unrecognized injury to the sphincter complex occurs in as many as one-third of women during a vaginal delivery and may be associated with symptoms of anal incontinence.[7] A thorough examination with good exposure and adequate anesthesia will allow the clinician to identify this layer as a thick, dense, white layer that is typically retracted from the anal mucosa. Standard obstetric textbooks tend to present an oversimplified description of the repair of a third- and fourth-degree laceration. Most simply recommend the identification and plication of the severed ends of the external anal sphincter with two or three interrupted, absorbable sutures.[44,45] The findings of Sultan and associates[8] clearly indicate that such a repair technique is often inadequate as it is frequently associated with persistent sphincter defects and symptomatology.

The authors cannot overemphasize the importance of repairing the internal anal sphincter. Physiologic studies have outlined its importance in anal continence and recent investigations have shown that internal anal sphincter defects are commonly associated with symptoms of anal incontinence postpartum. The authors strongly agree with Aronson et al[17] that the goal of sphincter repair (either primary or secondary) should be the reconstruction of a muscular cylinder that is at least 2 cm thick and at least 3 cm long. Such a repair would result in a more anatomically and functionally correct anal canal. To our knowledge, a detailed description of such a repair, which emphasizes the reconstruction of the internal anal sphincter, has not been described elsewhere.

The authors currently recommend that the primary repair of third- and fourth-degree lacerations take place in the labor and delivery operating suite (Fig. 40-7). Saddle block or epidural anesthesia is preferable, although pudendal block may also be sufficient in some individuals. A vaginal pack may be placed to prevent postpartum uterine bleeding from obscuring the field. A self-retaining retractor such as a Gelpie or Weitlander may be used if an assistant is not readily available. A multilayer closure is the goal of the repair. The first layer consists of reapproximation of the anal mucosa using either a running nonlocking or interrupted sutures of either 3–0 or 4–0 chromic or a delayed absorbable suture

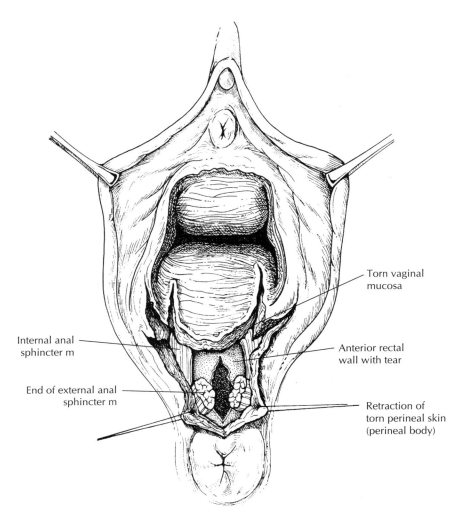

Torn vaginal
mucosa

Anterior rectal
wall with tear

Retraction of
torn perineal skin
(perineal body)

Internal anal
sphincter m

End of external anal
sphincter m

Fig. 40-7. Fourth-degree obstetric laceration. Note the retracted ends of the external anal sphincter and the retracted ends of the internal anal sphincter, which lies above and is intimately attached to the anal mucosa.

(Fig. 40-8A). The next layer should consist of the reapproximation of the internal anal sphincter over and inverting the first layer (Fig. 40-8B). The authors prefer to use a delayed absorbable suture such as polyglactin for this and all subsequent layers. This layer is often retracted laterally and appears as a thickened, white, shiny tissue that some clinicians refer to as perirectal fascia. The third layer should consist of an end-to-end plication of the disrupted external anal sphincter and capsule using interrupted or figure-of-eight sutures (Fig. 40-8C). The authors attempt to place at least four or five of these sutures, but are not opposed to placing more if it is possible. It may be necessary to sharply mobilize either sphincter in order to get a more complete and tension-free anastomosis. Although the authors currently use a 2–0 delayed absorbable suture for this layer, it is worth considering using a permanent suture such as Ethibond for this purpose. Although some clinicians advocate an overlapping sphincteroplasty as apposed to an end-to-end anastomosis,[46,47] this is probably unnecessary. The intervening recto-vaginal fascia and puborectalis fibers should then be approximated over this, followed by a repair of the subcutaneous tissue (including Colles fascia) and epithelium of the vagina and perineum (Fig. 40-8D & E).

The efficacy of prophylactic antibiotics in this setting is unproven, and is probably unnecessary as the rate of infection following repair of a third- or fourth-degree laceration is extremely low. Postoperatively, the patient should be managed with stool softeners and a low residue diet to reduce stool frequency and volume for 4 weeks.

Early Repair of Episiotomy Breakdown

Episiotomy infection and dehiscence are an uncommon but important postpartum complications. An episiotomy infection is heralded by fever, wound tenderness, and a purulent discharge, and these patients typically present 6 to 8 days following a delivery. In a retrospective review of more

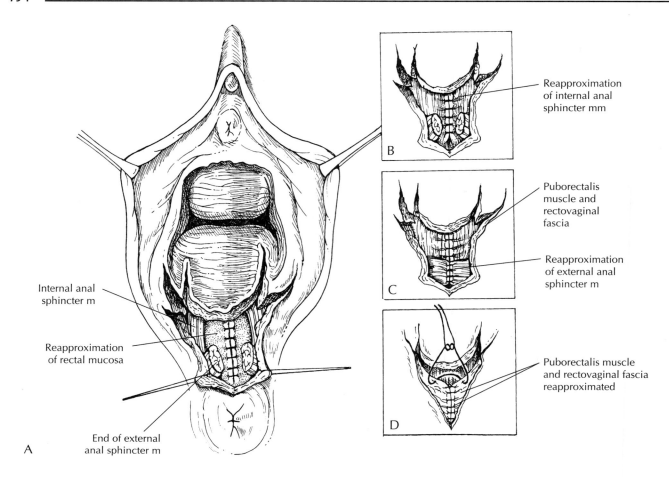

Fig. 40-8. Layered primary closure of a fourth-degree obstetric laceration. **(A)** The anal mucosa is first closed with a running or interrupted layer of 4–0 delayed absorbable suture. **(B)** The retracted ends of the internal anal sphincter are reunited with a running layer of 3–0 delayed absorbable suture. **(C)** An end-to-end anastomosis of the external anal sphincter (EAS) is accomplished using four or five interrupted 2–0 delayed absorbable sutures placed through the capsule of the EAS. **(D)** The rectovaginal fascia and puborectalis fibers are approximated with a running 2–0 delayed absorbable suture. *(Figure continues.)*

than 7,000 deliveries in which a median episiotomy was performed, Harris[48] reported an 11.6-percent rate of third- and fourth-degree extensions that resulted in a 0.1-percent incidence of rectovaginal fistulas, 29-percent incidence of poor sphincter tone, and a 0.1-percent incidence of episiotomy infection.

Traditional teaching has held that should a primary episiotomy repair fail, a second attempt should be deferred for a minimum of 2 to 3 months,[49] presumably to allow sufficient time for revascularization of the wound edges and to allow for the formation of scar tissue, which may be of value in the reanastomosis of the torn sphincter. This approach commits the patient to an extended period of physical, social, and sexual disability because of continuous incontinence. However, little data exist to support such management.

Recently, there have been several reports in the literature regarding early repair of episiotomy dehiscence and this cu-

mulative experience has been summarized.[50] Hankins and colleagues[51] reported their experience with early repair of episiotomy dehiscence in 31 women. Clinically evident infection was present in 12 patients. In all patients, aggressive wound debridement and cleansing on an inpatient unit were undertaken until the wound was free of exudate and was covered with healthy granulation tissue. Patients with evidence of wound infection were also treated with intravenous antibiotics during preoperative wound preparation. Surgical repair was performed when the wound was free from exudate. Satisfactory results were obtained in 94 percent. Two women developed small rectovaginal fistulas that required a second procedure. Other authors have reported similar results.[52–54] The overall success rate in these series ranges from 87 to 100 percent.

A protocol for early repair of episiotomy dehiscence has recently been reported.[50] Once the diagnosis of episiotomy

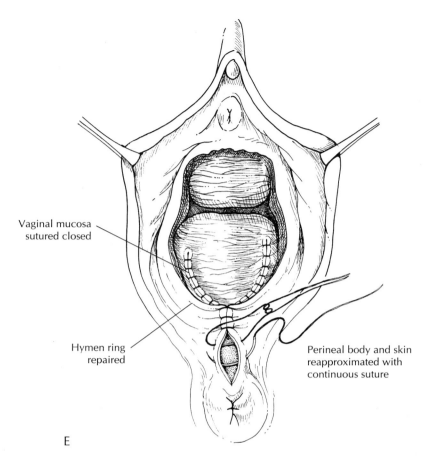

Vaginal mucosa
sutured closed

Hymen ring
repaired

Perineal body and skin
reapproximated with
continuous suture

E

Fig. 40-8 *(Continued).* **(E)** The vaginal mucosa and perineal skin are reapproximated with a continuous stitch of 3–0 delayed absorbable suture.

dehiscence has been made, a careful inspection of the wound should be performed to look for evidence of infection. The wound should be promptly debrided and suture fragments removed using intravenous analgesia or regional anesthesia if necessary. Subsequent wound care should consist of scrubbing the wound twice daily with a povidone-iodine impregnated scrub brush. If needed, 1-percent lidocaine jelly or intravenous sedation can be used to lessen the woman's discomfort. Sitz baths should be performed several times daily. A single broad-spectrum antibiotic, such as a second-generation cephalosporin, can also be used in this preoperative phase, at the physician's discretion. In the patient with a clinically evident cellulitis, a more aggressive antibiotic regimen will probably be necessary. Secondary repair is performed when the wound surface is free from exudate and covered by pink granulation tissue. On average, it will take 6 to 8 days of aggressive wound care before repair can be attempted. A bowel preparation (described later in this chapter) should be administered before the repair attempt.

There are several advantages to early repair of episiotomy dehiscence as compared with the traditional delayed repair.

Prolonged fecal incontinence and loss of sexual function are avoided. Reduction of these two important causes of puerperal morbidity may potentially decrease the risk of litigation, and subsequent hospitalization and additional surgical procedures that are associated with a delayed repair are avoided. Disadvantages of this approach are as follows:

1. It commits the patient to prolonged hospitalization early in the postpartum period, which could interfere with breast-feeding and maternal-child bonding
2. It is possible that some episiotomy dehiscences may undergo satisfactory spontaneous closure with less aggressive therapy
3. Some early attempts at repair may still fail and there may be need for subsequent surgical procedures

Currently, sufficient clinical experience exists to advocate early repair of episiotomy dehiscence. The authors hope that the excellent results described in these series will encourage others to try and report additional experience with this approach.

Repair of Chronic Third- and Fourth-Degree Lacerations

Chronic third- and fourth-degree lacerations occur either because of unrecognized obstetric trauma or breakdown of a primarily repaired laceration. Women who suffer from a chronic third- or fourth-degree laceration present complaining of incontinence to gas and liquid feces. These women rarely complain of incontinence to solid stool because the puborectalis mechanism is typically intact. In patients with a chronic fourth-degree laceration, the perineal body is nonexistent and the rectovaginal septum is attenuated (Fig. 40-9). The external anal sphincter is almost always disrupted anteriorly, a defect that it readily palpable.

Patients with a chronic third-degree laceration have a thinned but intact perineal body, in which is contained the separated ends of the external anal sphincter. The anal skin typically has a dovetail appearance, in which the radial distribution of the skin creases caused by its attachment to the external anal sphincter is absent anteriorly (Fig. 40-10). On digital palpation, the sphincter defect is easily palpable anteriorly. With voluntary contraction, constriction of the separated end of the external anal sphincter will create a dimpling in the perianal skin. Absence of this dimpling suggests significant neurologic injury to the sphincter and should warn the clinician that simple anastomosis may not completely cure the incontinence. Some surgeons prefer to utilize electromyographic studies of the sphincter muscles before any repair attempt is undertaken in order to more accurately predict which repairs will be functionally as well as anatomically successful. However, complete functional success is rarely predictable with any preoperative studies, and sphinc-ter electromyography studies are not widely available. All patients should be counselled preoperatively regarding our inability to predict functional success preoperatively.

Complete third- or fourth-degree lacerations may be approached through either a midline (transphincteric) or transverse incision. The separated edges of the external anal sphincters are typically located at the 2- to 3-o'clock and 9- to 10-o'clock position; within the perianal skin (Fig. 40-11A). The ends of the sphincter should be grasped with Allis clamps and mobilized by sharp dissection with Metzenbaum scissors (Fig. 40-11B). If the ends of the sphincter are difficult to identify or densely scarred, a needle tip muscle electrostimulator may be useful in identifying the contractile tissue of the external anal sphincter. The tip of the electrostimulator probe is touched against the edges of the tissues thought to belong to the external anal sphincter and a small electrical stimulus is applied. If the tip of the transducer is in contact with viable sphincter muscle, the entire sphincter should visibly and palpably contract.

The rectal mucosa should then be mobilized from the rectovaginal septum and vaginal mucosa. Lateral dissection should reveal the retracted ends of the internal anal sphincter. Wide mobilization at each tissue plane will allow for easy approximation without significant tension and inversion of the previous layer. Repair from this point forward is similar to that described previously for a primary repair of an obstetric laceration (Fig. 40-8). After reapproximating the rectal mucosa and internal anal sphincter in separate layers, the divided ends of the external anal sphincter should be united in the midline with interrupted delayed-absorbable or permanent suture. A number 2–0 suture should provide adequate tensile strength as well as minimize knot size. The most

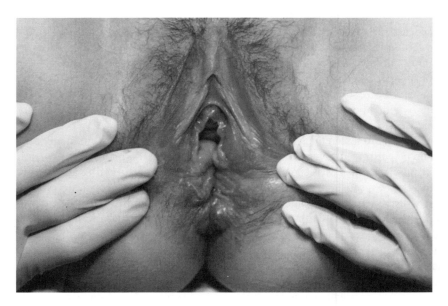

Fig. 40-9. A 23-year-old woman with a chronic fourth-degree laceration who presented with complaints of incontinence of liquid stool and gas, but not solid stool. The rectal mucosa is visible posteriorly. Note how the puborectalis keeps the rectum and posterior vaginal wall compressed against the anterior vaginal wall to maintain continence of solid stool.

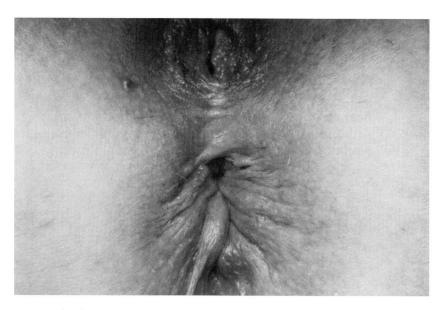

Fig. 40-10. Appearance of an intact perineum with an underlying separation of the external anal sphincter, demonstrating the dovetail sign in a patient with a chronic third-degree laceration. Note the absence of the anal creases anteriorly. (From Toglia and DeLancey,[1] with permission.)

cephalad and inferior suture should be placed first, and at least four sutures (preferably five) should be used to reunite the ends of the external anal sphincter. Although many general surgeons advocate an overlapping sphincteroplasty, the authors prefer a simple but meticulously performed end-to-end anastomosis.

Further support of the anal canal is provided by approximating the puborectalis in the midline, followed by reapproximation of the subcutaneous tissues of the vagina and perineum. These important layers will also take tension off of the underlying suture lines. Finally, the vaginal mucosa and skin overlying the epithelium should be reapproximated with either continuous, nonlocking, or interrupted sutures. The end result of the surgical repair should be the reconstruction of an adequate perineal body, a thickened rectovaginal septum, and an intact cylindrical sphincter complex that is approximately 2 cm wide and 3 cm long. The anus should easily admit one finger following the procedure, but the skeletal muscle paralysis induced by the anesthesiologist may leave the anal canal weak in tone.

Some clinicians have advocated using the Warren flap procedure when repairing a chronic third- or fourth-degree laceration (Fig. 40-12). This procedure interposes a triangular flap of vaginal mucosa mucosal flap between the rectal lumen and the primary suture line of the external anal sphincter.[55] As noted by Tancer et al[56] it should be remembered that this operation was designed during the preantibiotic era when the purpose of the flap was to prevent feces from soiling the suture line, which was braided silk. The Noble procedure, advocated for the repair of the complete perineal laceration, involves mobilizing the retracted anterior anorectal

wall and pulling it through to the anal orifice and repairing the external anal sphincter over this. The mobilized anterior anorectal wall is then sutured to the perianal skin.[57] Again, the main objective of this procedure was to prevent infection of the suture lines by fecal seeding postoperatively. Corman[58] described an alternative approach to the chronic third-degree laceration that allows for reconstruction of the perineal body. A cruciate skin incision is made across the attenuated perineal body and the skin and subcutaneous flaps are developed laterally. After the fistulous tracts are excised and the divided ends of the sphincter are reunited, the skin flaps are transposed in order to reconstruct the perineal body.

Rectovaginal and Anovaginal Fistulas

Rectovaginal and anovaginal fistulas commonly result from obstetric trauma. In underdeveloped countries, approximately 85 percent of rectovaginal fistulas are related to birth injuries. Many of these fistulas are the results of pressure necrosis of the rectovaginal septum secondary to compression by the fetal head during prolonged labor. In the United States, obstetric trauma remains an important cause of rectovaginal fistula. Many fistulas occur following an unsuccessful primary repair of a third- or fourth-degree laceration or from unrecognized injury at the time of vaginal delivery. Episiotomy infections, although uncommon, can also result in the formation of a fistulous tract. Rectovaginal fistulas may also occur following difficult hysterectomies, especially those performed for severe endometriosis with involvement or obliteration of the cul-de-sac, as well as surgical procedures involving the posterior vaginal wall, perineum, anus,

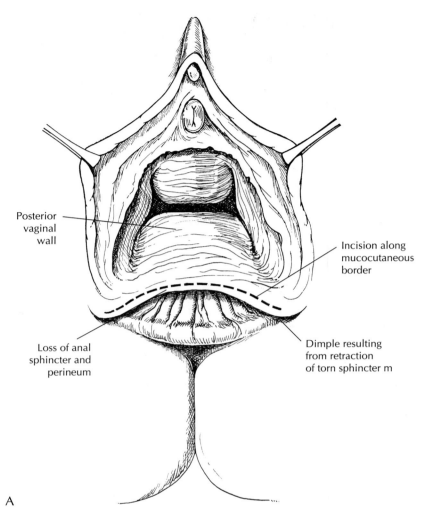

Posterior
vaginal
wall

Incision along
mucocutaneous
border

Loss of anal
sphincter and
perineum

Dimple resulting
from retraction
of torn sphincter m

A

Fig. 40-11. Layered closure of a complete third-degree perineal laceration. **(A)** A transverse incision is made at the junction of the vaginal and rectal mucosa and extended laterally to expose the retracted ends of the external anal sphincter. *(Figure continues.)*

and rectum. Inflammatory bowel disease is another important cause of rectovaginal fistulas in women.

Women suffering from anovaginal or rectovaginal fistulas present with complaints of uncontrollable passage of gas or feces from the vagina. A malodorous vaginal discharge and fecal soiling of the undergarments are also common complaints. Symptoms may be more common with loose bowel movements. Occasionally, a small fistula may be asymptomatic. It is important to inquire about fecal urgency and fecal incontinence associated with urgency as this often suggests that the external anal sphincter is disrupted as well.

Most anovaginal and rectovaginal fistulas of obstetric origin are located in the lower third of the vagina and are typically located just inside the introitus and are readily apparent on physical examination. Located close to the midline, the velvet-like red rectal mucosa may be evident. There is often

a tenting of the anal mucosa, which is palpable on rectal examination and the rectovaginal is thinned at this location.

It is critical that the clinician evaluates the entire sphincteric mechanism in women with a rectovaginal fistula to exclude coexisting causes for incontinence such as a disrupted anal sphincter. Although concomitant sphincter injury has been reported to exist in 8.3[59] and 32 percent[60] of women presenting with rectovaginal fistulas, the authors suspect that concomitant internal or external sphincter injuries (or both) exist far more frequently when the location of the fistula is within the distal 3 cm of the anal canal, since anatomic and physiologic studies have demonstrated that this is the normal length of the sphincter complex. Failure to recognize and repair such a sphincter injury may result in continued incontinence following a successful fistulectomy.

Fistulas resulting from operative trauma, malignancy, or

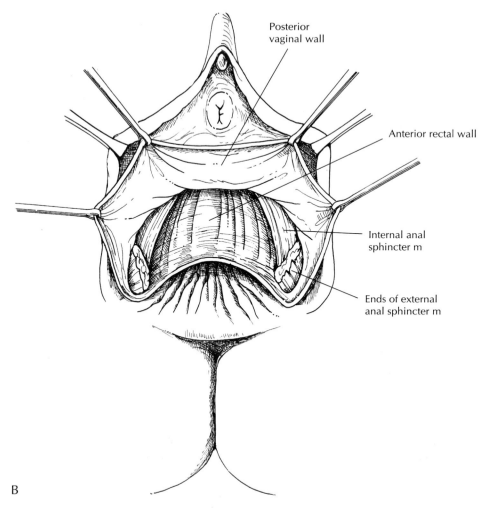

Posterior
vaginal wall

Anterior rectal wall

Internal anal
sphincter m

Ends of external
anal sphincter m

B

Fig. 40-11 *(Continued).* **(B)** The ends of the internal anal sphincter are identified and sharply mobilized if necessary. Repair from this point is identical to that described for a primary repair of a fourth-degree laceration.

inflammatory processes can occur anywhere along the rectovaginal septum. Rectovaginal fistulas that occur following abdominal hysterectomy are often located close to the apex of the vagina.

Small, pinpoint fistulas can, on occasion, be difficult to locate. The use of magnification such as a colposcope may be valuable. Lacrimal duct or silver wire probes can also be used to assist in identifying the fistula tract. A few drops of methylene blue dye can be mixed with lubricating gel and massaged into the anterior rectal wall. Alternatively, an enema consisting of warmed saline and a few drops of methylene blue dye can be instilled into the rectum using a genitourinary syringe. Others have recommended using peroxide instilled rectally, since it will not stain the tissues.[61] Proctoscopy may also be useful in visualizing the fistulous tract from the rectal side. When confronted with a high rectovaginal fistula, a barium enema may sometimes be helpful in

delineating the location and level of communication of the fistula (Fig. 40-13).

Classification of Anterior Perineal and Rectovaginal Defects

In 1980, Rosenshein and associates[62] proposed an anatomic classification of perineal and rectovaginal defects designed to assist with clinical management (Table 40-1). Others have proposed a modification to their classification.[49] Baden and Walker[63] have proposed a grading system for vaginal defects that includes the anterior perineum and posterior vaginal wall. Common to all of these classification systems is that obstetric trauma most commonly results in injury to the distal one-third of the vagina and the anorectum. Fistulas that occur within the first 3 cm from the anal orifice and are below the dentate line are called anovaginal fistulas. Fistulas cephalad to the dentate line are truly rectovaginal.

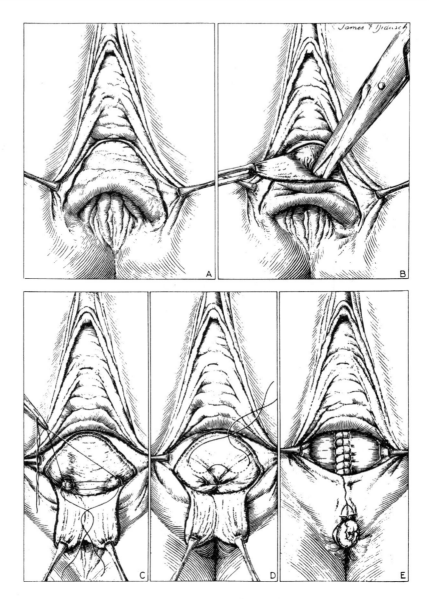

Fig. 40-12. Warren flap procedure for complete third-degree laceration. **(A)** Line of incision, outlining flap of vaginal mucosa. **(B)** The flap is dissected free and turned back. **(C)** The flap is retracted downward. The ends of the sphincter are delivered and are sutured with delayed absorbable sutures. **(D)** The sphincter ends have been united, and the puborectalis muscles are approximated in the midline with 0 delayed absorbable sutures. **(E)** The vaginal incision has been closed with a continuous lock stitch that is continued subcuticularly over the perineum. The margins of the flap are included in the continuous suture, which may create a peaked appearance, temporarily, to the perineal skin. If redundant, it may be trimmed. (From Thompson,[49] with permission.)

Surgical Repair Methods

The basic principles essential for the successful fistula repair include

1. Wide mobilization of the adjacent tissue planes
2. Complete excision of the fistula tract
3. Multilayered closure, which reapproximates broad tissue surfaces without tension

4. Proper timing of the repair

The surgical techniques are easy to learn and certainly belong in the armamentarium of every obstetrician/gynecologist.

Most obstetric and traumatic fistulas are amenable to early repair. Although some investigators have advocated waiting 3 to 6 months to repair these fistulas, the authors agree with Hibbard[64] that the decision of when to operate should depend

Causes of Rectovaginal Fistulas

- Obstetric causes
  - Failed primary repair
  - Episiotomy infection
  - Unrecognized injury
  - Prolonged labor with pressure necrosis
- Traumatic causes
  - Hysterectomy
  - Posterior rectal wall, perineal, anala, or rectal surgery
  - Irradiation
  - Endometriosis
- Neoplastic tumors
  - Carcinoma of the rectum, vagina, cervix, and endometrium
- Inflammatory disease
  - Crohn's, diveticulitis, perirectal, or pelvic abscess
  - Systemic lupus
  - Tuberculosis, lymphogranuloma venereum
- Other
  - Vaginal or rectal trauma
  - Leukemia, aplastic anemia, agranulocytosis
  - Congenital (e.g., imperforate anus)

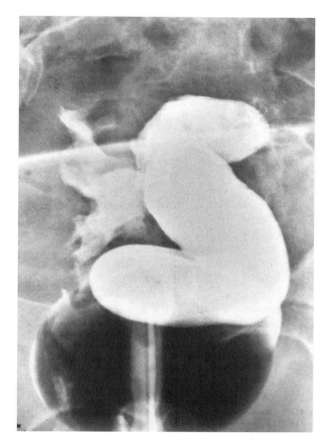

Fig. 40-13. Barium enema illustrating a rectouterine fistula in a 66-year-old woman referred from a nursing home because of a foul-smelling vaginal discharge.

on the status of the involved tissue rather than an arbitrary period of time. One disadvantage of this approach is that some small fistulas may undergo spontaneous closure. Surgical repair should be deferred until there is resolution of any local cellulitis, inflammation, or induration. If wound infection is present, aggressive wound care, including sitz baths, should be performed as well as a 10- to 14-day course

Table 40-1. Classification of Rectovaginal Septal Defects

Type	Description
I	Loss of the perineal body not associated with a fistula (chronic third- and fourth-degree laceration)
II	Loss of the perineal body associated with a fistula in the lower third of the vagina
III	Fistula involving the lower third of the vagina with an intact or attenuated perineum
IV	Fistulas involving the middle third of the vagina
V	Fistulas involving the upper third of the vagina

(Adapted from Rosenshein,[62] with permission.)

of a broad-spectrum oral antibiotic. Institution of a low residue diet will decrease the frequency of bowel movements and possibly prevent continuous seeding of the wound with liquid stool. In addition, this may also restore some degree of fecal continence. These patients should be examined weekly and repair should be performed when all gross evidence of infection, induration, and inflammation has subsided. Preoperative preparation of the rectum is discussed in detail in a later section.

Repair techniques vary significantly with the type and etiology of the fistula. The authors prefer to use delayed absorbable sutures such as polyglactin or polyglycolic acid instead of chromic catgut in the repair of these fistulas for several reasons. First, the tensile strength is maintained longer and the knot is more secure. In addition, smaller-diameter sutures of delayed absorbable material are stronger than comparable catgut and knot size is also smaller. Tissue reaction is also less with delayed absorbable suture. There may be a role for the monofilament delayed absorbable and permanent sutures in these repairs, but so far, the authors

Types of Rectovaginal Fistula Repairs

- Simple fistulectomy and drainage (for fistula-in-ano)
  - Transvaginal or transrectal approach
  - Latzko technique
- Layered closure with excision of the fistula tract
  - Transphincteric approach (episioproctotomy)
  - Transverse transperineal (Thompson, Emory University)
- Sliding flap advancements
  - Warren procedure
  - Noble procedure
  - Anterior rectal wall advancement
  - Endorectal advancement flap
  - Internal anal sphincter segmental advancement
  - Endorectal pull-through
- Transabdominal repair
  - Mobilization and layered closure with or without interposition of the omentum
  - Bowel resection procedures with or without interposition of the omentum
- Split flap technique
- Adjuvant procedures
  - Martius graft (bulbocavernosus transposition)
  - Modified Martius graft (labial fat pad)
  - Rectus abdominis muscle
  - Omental interposition
  - Gracilis muscle graft
  - Sartorius muscle graft
  - Gluteus muscle

have been satisfied with the results using polyglactin and polyglycolic acid.

Simple Fistulectomy

Small rectovaginal fistulas that are secondary to obstetric or traumatic causes are often amenable to repair by simple fistulectomy either by a transvaginal or transrectal approach. An incision is made around the fistula, which will allow both for the complete excision of the fistulous tract as well as mobilization of the vagina, rectum, and rectovaginal septum to allow for a tension-free closure (Fig. 40-14 A & B). The surgeon's nondominant index finger can be inserted into the rectum during the procedure to assist in the repair. Sharp mobilization of the vagina and rectum in a circumferential fashion should be accomplished first, by providing traction and countertraction on the edges of the fistula (Fig. 40-14C).

Once these tissue planes are widely mobilized, the entire fistulous tract is excised, along with any adjacent scar tissue (Fig. 40-14D). The edges of the "new" surgical fistula should contain fresh, viable tissue. The edges of the anterior rectal wall are then inverted, either by placing a pursestring suture or, as these authors prefer, by placing interrupted submucosal stitches of 3–0 or 4–0 delayed absorbable sutures (Fig. 40-14E). The most cephalad and most distal sutures should be placed at least 5 mm above and below the fistula. A second layer of suture (2–0 delayed absorbable) is then placed in the muscularis of the anterior rectal wall to invert and take tension off of the first suture line (Fig. 40-14F). This layer should begin and end approximately 5 mm above and below the initial suture line.

The pararectal fascia or puborectalis muscle is then approximated to provide a third layer of closure (Fig. 40-14G). If deemed necessary, a modified Martius graft discussed in detail below can be interposed before this step. Finally, the vaginal mucosa is approximated with a continuous 3–0 suture (Fig. 40-14H). Meticulous care must be taken to ensure complete hemostasis and closure of all potential dead space. A small vaginal pack soaked in a dilute betadine solution may be placed and serves as a "wick" to absorb any seepage from the wound during the first 18 to 24 hours postoperatively.

Transphincteric Approach

Anovaginal and low rectovaginal fistulas that are the result of obstetric trauma frequently require reanastamosis of the external and internal anal sphincters and reconstruction of the perineal body and rectovaginal septum. Often, only a bridge of perineal skin exists intact in these women (Fig. 40-15). In such a patient the preferred approach is a midline perineal incision (transphincteric or perineoproctomy approach) with wide mobilization of the posterior vaginal wall and a multilayered closure as described for a chronic third- or fourth-degree laceration. It is important that the fistula tract be excised in its entirety as previously discussed.

Transverse Transperineal Approach

Rectovaginal fistulas located above the sphincter complex can also be approached with a transverse transperineal incision. This approach allows the surgeon to preserve the intact internal and external anal sphincter, and allows for wide mobilization of the rectal and vaginal tissue. Experience with this technique in 21 patients was recently reviewed by Wiskind and Thompson.[65] A transverse incision is made across the perineal body above the sphincter complex and dissection is carried out between the anterior rectal wall and the posterior vaginal wall to mobilize the tissues widely both laterally as well as cephalad to the fistula tract (Fig. 40-16A & B). Dissection above the fistula tract is usually quite easy as the vagina and rectum are only loosely connected above this point.

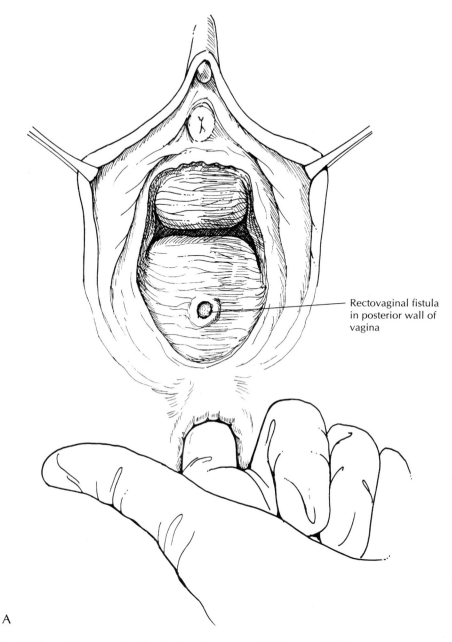

Rectovaginal fistula
in posterior wall of
vagina

A

Fig. 40-14. Repair of a small rectovaginal fistula through a transvaginal approach. **(A)** The surgeon places the nondominant index finger into the rectum to demonstrate the fistula. *(Figure continues.)*

The fistula tract is next excised as is any scar tissue surrounding the tract on both the vaginal and rectal sides (Fig. 40-16C). This is best accomplished with Metzenbaum scissors. The rectal wall defect can be closed either longitudinally or transversely with interrupted 3–0 or 4–0 delayed absorbable suture. This layer should invert the rectal mucosa without tension. Although Wiskind and Thompson[65] describe closing this and subsequent layers transversely, the authors usually prefer to close the layers longitudinally in all but the smallest fistulas (Fig. 40-16D). By closing the

rectal mucosal and perirectal fascial layers longitudinally, the anal canal is lengthened and that this may help to reestablish the "high-pressure zone" of the anal canal. Closing the vaginal mucosa and perineal body longitudinally helps avoid narrowing the vaginal introitus and also lengthens the perineal body. Other clinicians advocate closing the rectal and vaginal defects in perpendicular directions in order to avoid overlying suture lines. If one elects to close the defect in this fashion, the rectal defect should be closed transversely and the vaginal mucosa closed longitudinally, as this

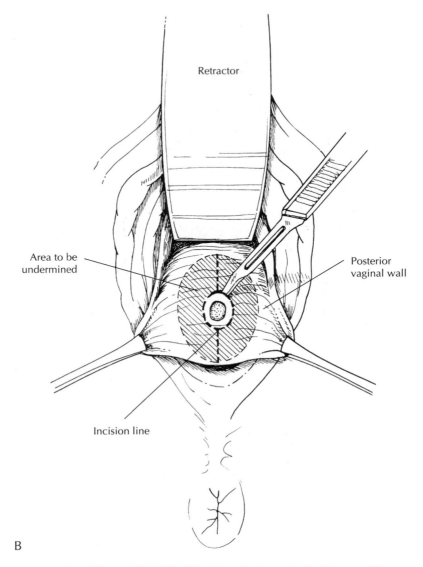

Retractor

Area to be
undermined

Posterior
vaginal wall

Incision line

B

Fig. 40-14 *(Continued).* **(B)** An elliptical incision is made about the fistula tract. *(Figure continues.)*

is much less likely to result in a narrowing of the vaginal introitus or the creation of a transverse ridge across the posterior vaginal wall, which can result in dyspareunia.

A second layer of closure is then placed into the muscularis of the rectum in the same direction as the first layer, thus imbricating the first layer and reinforcing the closure (Fig. 40-16E). The puborectalis muscles are next approximated in the midline, thus providing an additional reinforcing layer between the anterior rectal and posterior vaginal wall (Fig. 40-16F).

The subcutaneous tissues and skin of the perineal body can then be approximated with a running nonlocking closure. The skin is then closed either with interrupted mattress sutures or with a running closure of 4–0 delayed absorbable suture (Fig. 40-16G).

Transabdominal Approaches

Occasionally, a high rectovaginal fistula located near the vaginal apex will require an abdominal approach with sharp dissection of the rectum from the vagina. This is seen most often after pelvic radiation, or as a complication following pelvic surgery for endometriosis, diverticular disease, or associated with a pelvic or rectal malignancy. Occasionally, it can be seen with inflammatory bowel disease. In third world nations, this type of fistula is also seen following a prolonged, obstructed labor secondary to extended tissue ischemia and subsequent necrosis.

The transabdominal approach to rectovaginal fistulas is facilitated by the use of long instruments and retractors, such as those used in thoracic surgery. At one point in time, many clinicians advocated a diverting colostomy for any fistula

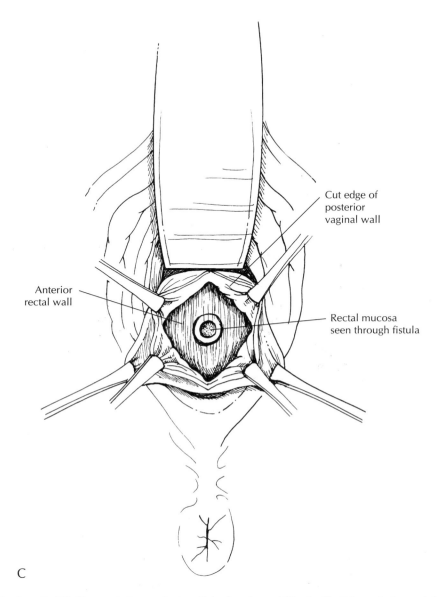

Cut edge of
posterior
vaginal wall

Anterior
rectal wall

Rectal mucosa
seen through fistula

C

Fig. 40-14 *(Continued)*. **(C)** The posterior vaginal wall is sharply mobilized off of the anterior rectal wall. *(Figure continues.)*

that lay above the peritoneal reflection. Today this is rarely necessary, given improvements in surgical technique and antibiotic therapy. When performing an abdominal closure of a rectovaginal fistula, it is imperative that the rectum and vagina be widely mobilized from the fistulous communication. This tract should then be either excised or inverted, and each organ should be closed in a multilayered fashion. Serosal dissection on the colonic side around the fistula site can be extensive, especially when closing large defects. Caution must be exercised when performing this dissection as excessive dissection can disrupt a significant portion of the blood supply to the bowel, which can interfere with successful closure and healing of the fistula. If extensive bowel ischemia is present, complete transection of the compromised segment of bowel with a colorectal reanastomosis is often preferable to a layered closure of the fistula. Occasionally, extensive bowel ischemia (e.g., radiation induced) may necessitate using a permanent diverting colostomy as the primary procedure.

Repair of the high rectovaginal fistula via the transabdominal route is best facilitated by the use of an omental J-flap, interposed between the separately closed vagina and rectum. The omental J-flap is created by first dissecting the omentum from its attachment to the transverse colon, while leaving it attached to the stomach. A J-shaped incision is then made approximately 4 cm inside the lateral border of the omentum

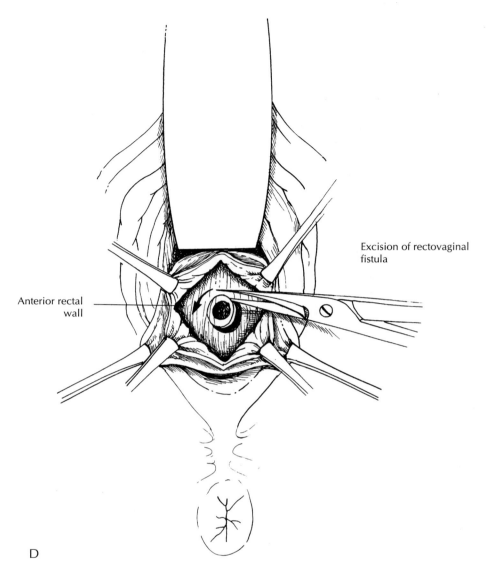

Anterior rectal
wall

Excision of rectovaginal
fistula

D

Fig. 40-14 *(Continued).* **(D)** The fistula tract is excised, including the adjacent vagial and rectal mucosa. *(Figure continues.)*

adjacent to the edge of the stomach, down past the most distal and lateral termination of the mesenteric vessels within this omental apron. This partially detached flap is then rotated down to the fistula site and sutured in place between the rectum and the vagina.

A second adjuvant procedure that has been employed successfully by the senior author, is to detach a segment of the rectus abdominis muscle and interpose it between the rectum and vagina. This provides excellent neovascularity and tissue support to the fistula repair site.

Colovesical fistulas are fortunately quite rare. They are usually associated with the same conditions and disease processes that cause the high rectovaginal fistulas discussed above. In these instances, a diverting colostomy is almost mandatory initially in order to divert the fecal stream (and

to minimize the risks of ascending urinary tract infection and renal damage), while tissue inflammation subsides.

Abdominal approaches to these types of fistulas may take one of two routes. Dissection posterior to the bladder can be used to completely dissect the bladder from the rectum. A multilayered closure of each organ, followed by an omental or muscle interpositional flap, will usually be successful. Alternatively, a transvesical approach may be attempted. In this approach, the dome of the bladder is opened and the fistula tract identified. Care is taken to identify the ureteral orifices before beginning the dissection. After identifying the fistula tract, careful dissection of the bladder serosa from the vagina and colon is done through the fistula tract within the bladder mucosa. Even with careful dissection and a multilayered closure, the failure rate is significant. For this rea-

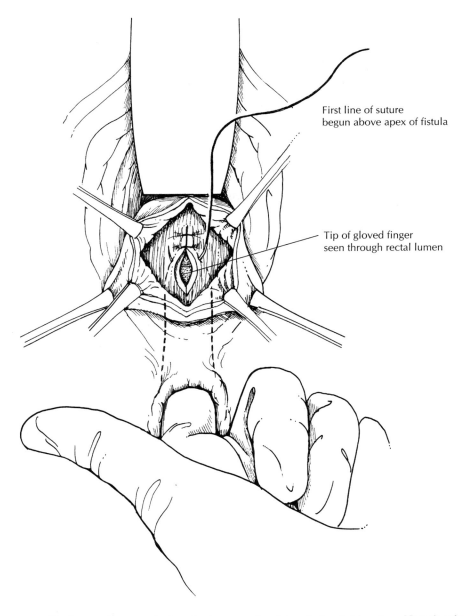

First line of suture
begun above apex of fistula

Tip of gloved finger
seen through rectal lumen

E

Fig. 40-14 *(Continued).* **(E)** The rectal mucosa is closed using a running delayed absorbable suture. Note that the suture line is begun at least 5 mm above the apex of the fistula. *(Figure continues.)*

son alone, strong consideration must be given to incorporating an interpositional flap as described above when approaching these unusual but debilitating conditions.

Adjuvant Procedures

Modified Martius Graft

The use of a modified Martius bulbocavernosus muscle or labial fat pad graft has improved the success rate in the closure of large or difficult vesicovaginal and rectovaginal fistulas by transplanting a vascular graft with healthy tissue to the repair site.[66] A vertical incision is made over the labia majora (Fig. 40-17A). The superficial fibroadipose tissue is sharply mobilized with care taken to preserve the blood supply of the graft either superiorly or inferiorly (Fig. 40-17B). For most rectovaginal fistulas, the base of the pedicle should be on the inferior border of the graft, which will allow the graft to be rotated medially without significant tension. The graft is then tunneled subcutaneously beneath the vaginal mucosa and labia minora to overlay the repaired fistula site (Fig. 40-17C). The graft should be secured at its edges with interrupted sutures of 3–0 chromic or delayed absorbable suture (Fig. 40-17D). The labial incision is repaired in two

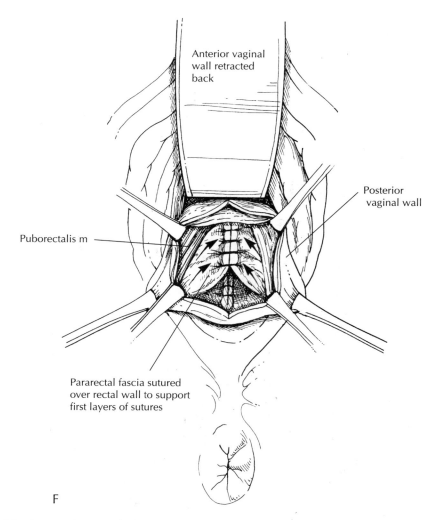

Fig. 40-14 *(Continued)*. (F) Second layer of the closure, which inverts the first layer. *(Figure continues.)*

layers (Fig. 40-17E). If the host site is particularly wet, it can be drained via a small Penrose or Jackson-Pratt drain.

The use of a modified Martius graft should be considered in patients with inflammatory bowel disease, irradiation-induced fistulas, and those that have failed previous attempts at closure. It should also be considered in the repair of rectovaginal fistulas located in the middle to upper third of the vaginal vault, where there may not be sufficient tissue to transpose between the vagina and the rectum. The labial fat pad graft provides neovascularity, fills in dead space, and enhances granulation tissue formation. It is doubtful, however, that it provides any significant structural support.

Paradoxical Incision at the Time of Sphincteroplasty

In 1937, Miller and Brown[67] proposed that a paradoxical incision be made in an inferior part of the external anal sphincter such as the 5- or 7-o'clock position, at the time of sphincteroplasty, to relieve the tension on the primary suture line. It was believed that this technique would also relieve postoperative muscle spasm, and help prevent postoperative anal stricture. It is unlikely, however, that this technique adds to the success of the repair and can be associated with unnecessary complications. Most clinicians have subsequently abandoned its practice.

Diverting Colostomy

There is little role for a diverting colostomy in the modern day approach of the obstetric, postoperative, or traumatic rectovaginal fistula, even in patients who have had multiple prior surgical repairs. However, there continues to be a role for the diverting colostomy in the management of radiation-induced fistulas, large rectovaginal defects (greater than 4 cm in diameter), and possibly some fistulas that are secondary to inflammatory bowel disease, in which diversion of the fecal stream is felt to be critical to the success of the repair.

Surgical repair of the fistula should be delayed 8 to 12

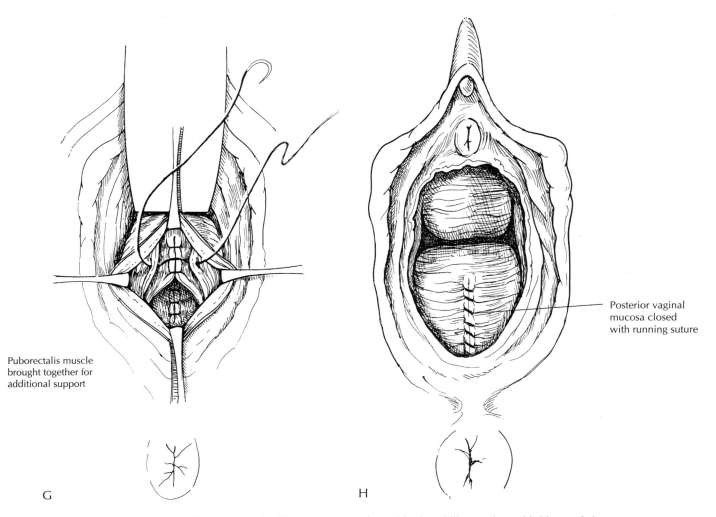

Puborectalis muscle
brought together for
additional support

G

Posterior vaginal
mucosa closed
with running suture

H

Fig. 40-14 *(Continued).* (G) The puborectalis fibers are reapproximated in the midline to give a third layer of closure. (H) Closure of the vaginal mucosa.

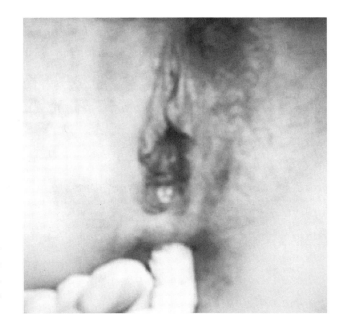

Fig. 40-15. Large anovaginal fistula hidden by a bridge of intact perineal skin and subcutaneous tissue. On excising this tissue longitudinally, it was obvious that the external sphincter was disrupted as well. Repair is carried out as described for a chronic third- or fourth-degree perineal laceration.

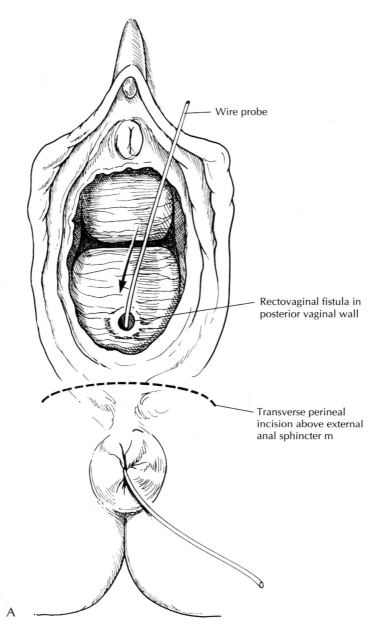

Wire probe

Rectovaginal fistula in
posterior vaginal wall

Transverse perineal
incision above external
anal sphincter m

A

Fig. 40-16. Transverse transperineal approach to a rectovaginal fistula located above the sphincter complex. **(A)** A wire probe is used to identify the fistula tract. A transverse transperineal incision is made above the sphincter complex. *(Figure continues.)*

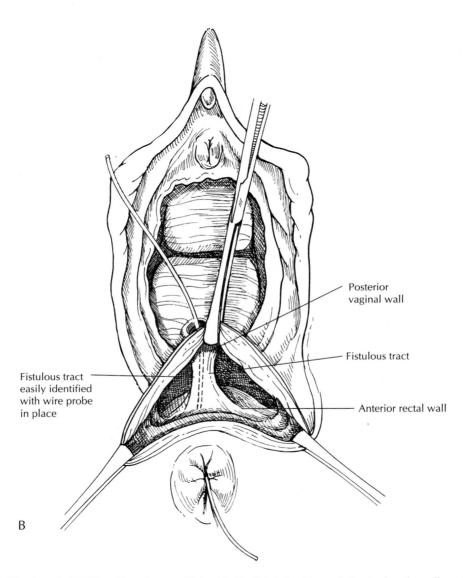

Posterior
vaginal wall

Fistulous tract

Anterior rectal wall

Fistulous tract
easily identified
with wire probe
in place

B

Fig. 40-16 *(Continued).* **(B)** Dissection above and lateral to the fistula tract is carried out using sharp dissection. *(Figure continues.)*

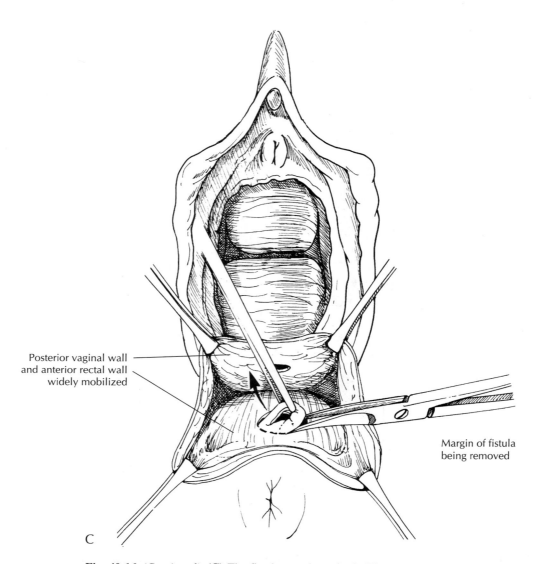

Posterior vaginal wall
and anterior rectal wall
widely mobilized

Margin of fistula
being removed

C

Fig. 40-16 *(Continued).* **(C)** The fistula tract is excised. *(Figure continues.)*

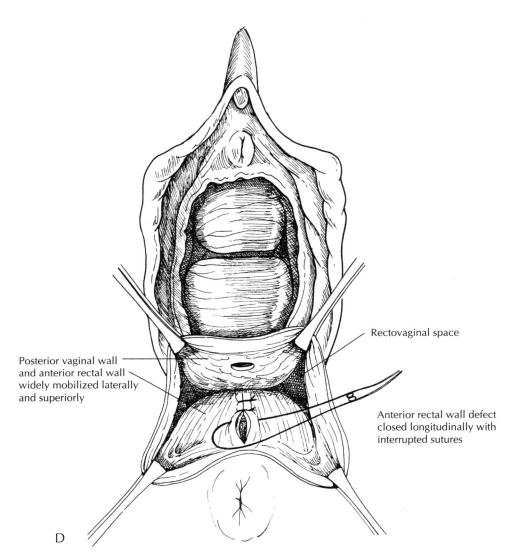

Rectovaginal space

Posterior vaginal wall
and anterior rectal wall
widely mobilized laterally
and superiorly

Anterior rectal wall defect
closed longitudinally with
interrupted sutures

D

Fig. 40-16 *(Continued).* **(D)** The anterior rectal wall defect is closed longitudinally with interrupted 4–0 delayed absorbable sutures. *(Figure continues.)*

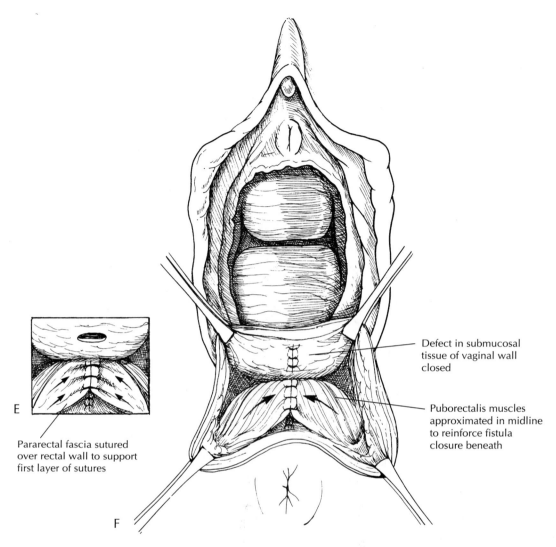

Pararectal fascia sutured over rectal wall to support first layer of sutures

Defect in submucosal tissue of vaginal wall closed

Puborectalis muscles approximated in midline to reinforce fistula closure beneath

E

F

Fig. 40-16 *(Continued).* **(E)** A second layer of closure is performed, imbricating the first layer. **(F)** The puborectalis fibers are reapproximated in the midline. *(Figure continues.)*

weeks after the colostomy until all evidence of inflammation and cellulitis has resolved. Takedown of the colostomy is usually performed 3 to 4 months after the fistula repair has been performed.

Special Considerations

Radiation-Induced Fistulas

Radiation-induced fistulas are seen with less frequency than in past years, probably as a result of the refinements in modern radiotherapy. Fistula formation following radiotherapy is believed to be the result of progressive endarteritis obliterans and tissue hypoxia. These fistulas may occur even years after the completion of radiotherapy. These fistulas may be quite large and be located high in the posterior vaginal wall. Often, they are associated with a degree of rectal stricture,

with significant perirectal fibrosis. Successful closure frequently necessitates extensive excision of the surrounding damaged tissue.

Boronow[68] reported excellent results in managing 10 patients with radiation-induced rectovaginal fistulas using a layered closure with interposition of a modified Martius graft. He stressed five steps essential to the successful closure of these fistulas:

1. The margins should be biopsied to exclude recurrent or persistent malignancy.
2. Surgical repair should be delayed at least 6 months to allow the radiation-induced damage to come to a halt.
3. A diverting colostomy should be done before the repair.

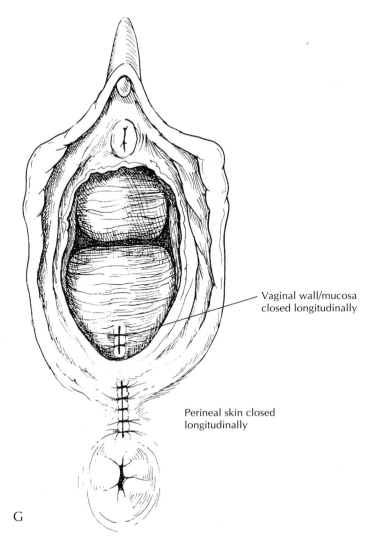

Vaginal wall/mucosa
closed longitudinally

Perineal skin closed
longitudinally

G

Fig. 40-16 *(Continued).* **(G)** The perineal body is reapproximated longitudinally with interrupted sutures to lengthen the perineal body.

4. Interposition of tissue with a new blood supply, such as a Martius graft.
5. A carefully layered closure of the fistula without tension on the suture lines.

Others have reported similar short-term success using the Martius graft. Aartsen and Sindram[69] reported initial success in closing 14 radiation-induced fistulas using a Martius graft, but noted that fistula recurred in 8 of these patients during 10 years of follow-up.

High rectovaginal fistulas caused by radiation occasionally need to be approached abdominally. After mobilizing the rectum from the vagina, all of the scarred, fibrous, and nonviable tissue should be resected from around the fistulous site. Bricker and colleagues[70] have advocated an abdominal approach for radiation-induced fistulas in which the rectosigmoid is divided and interposed over the fistula site. The

advantage of this technique is that the interpositioning flap retains its original vascular supply.

Repair of Fistulas Secondary to Inflammatory Bowel Disease

Rectovaginal fistulas associated with inflammatory bowel disease such as Crohn's disease or ulcerative colitis has always represented a challenging problem for both gynecologists and colorectal surgeons. Surprisingly, the overwhelming majority of patients who present with inflammatory bowel disease of the colon have Crohn's disease rather than ulcerative colitis. Early experience, in which the overall success rate was poor, led to a recommendation that fecal diversion with colostomy should be performed in most cases.[71] However, more recent reports suggest that success is mostly dependent on controlling the disease process itself and timing the repair during periods of remission.

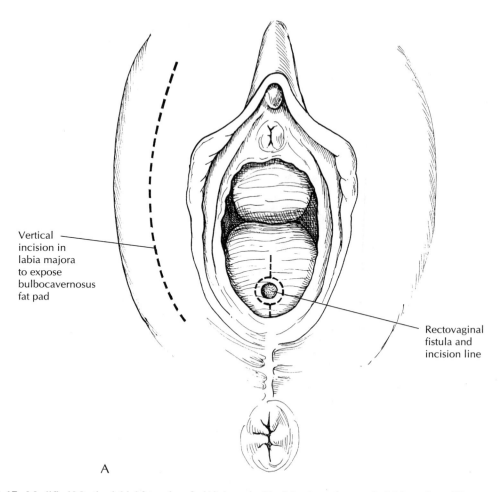

Vertical incision in labia majora to expose bulbocavernosus fat pad

Rectovaginal fistula and incision line

A

Fig. 40-17. Modified Martius labial fat pad graft. (A) A vertical incision is made over the labia majora. *(Figure continues.)*

Rectovaginal fistulas are not uncommon with Crohn's disease. In the original monograph of Crohn and Yarnis,[72] 14.2 percent of 542 patients developed perirectal fistulas and only 1.6 percent developed rectovaginal fistulas. However, a more recent study reported a 23-percent incidence in patients with Crohn's disease limited to the rectum.[73]

Rectovaginal fistulas that occur with inflammatory bowel disease may be single or multiple. A single vaginal orifice may lead to several tracts leading to the anus, and there may be microabscesses along these tracts. Some advocate injecting methylene blue through the vaginal orifice in order to identify all tracts. A tranverse, transperineal approach is often ideal in these patients as the sphincter complex tends to be uninvolved. A modified Martius graft should be considered in order to bring in additional tissue and blood supply, and to fill in the tissue defect, which may result from the complete excision of all fistulous tracts.

Most clinicians recommend that when inflammatory bowel disease is the cause of a rectovaginal fistula, surgical repair should be delayed until the bowel disease is adequately treated. It is important to realize that associated perianal disease is oftentimes responsible for many of the symp-

toms in patients with a rectovaginal fistula.[74] In one large series of 886 women with Crohn's disease, Radcliffe and associates[75] reported that 67 percent of the 90 women with rectovaginal fistulas thought that the symptoms of the intestinal disease were more significant than those of the fistula. There is also the small possibility that the fistula may spontaneously resolve once the bowel disease is under control.

Determining the optimal time to attempt local repair should be done in conjunction with a gastroenterologist. Not only should the patient's symptoms be quiescent, but there should also be no evidence of active rectal disease on proctoscopy.

PREOPERATIVE AND POSTOPERATIVE CONSIDERATIONS

There is no universal agreement in how patients should be treated both pre- and postoperatively, and it is unlikely that there will ever be any prospective clinical trials that compare different preoperative regimens.

Dietary manipulation both pre- and postoperatively

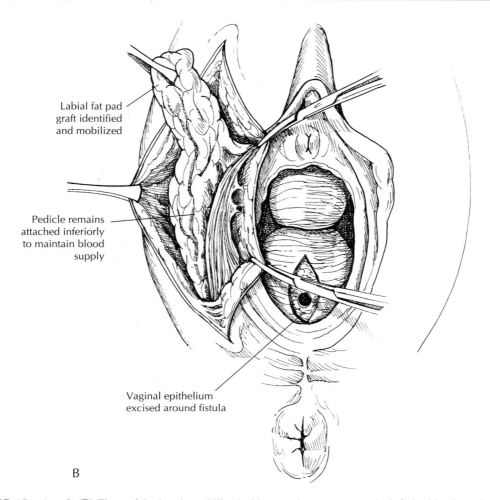

Labial fat pad graft identified and mobilized

Pedicle remains attached inferiorly to maintain blood supply

Vaginal epithelium excised around fistula

B

Fig. 40-17 *(Continued).* **(B)** The graft is sharply mobilized with care taken to preserve the inferior blood supply. *(Figure continues.)*

should be considered in all patients undergoing sphincteroplasty or rectovaginal fistula repair. The ultimate goal is to avoid fecal seeding of the wound during the procedure and to decrease the amount of stool that will pass over the repair in the first few weeks of healing. Institution of a low residue diet should be considered and should be started 1 week before the scheduled procedure. This will result in a decreased volume of stool, which will become small and hard in consistency. This will effectively eliminate seeding of the fistulous tract with liquid stool just before the intended procedure and may result in some degree of fecal continence. In most reported series, a clear liquid diet is instituted in the last 48 to 72 hours before the surgical procedure.

Mechanical bowel cleansing is also routinely recommended. Although many investigators recommend giving an oral agent such as Golytely or magnesium citrate on the day before the surgical procedure, the authors prefer to give either of these agents 48 to 72 hours preoperatively, because giving them closer to the procedure often results in a thin fecal effluent being present at the time of the repair. Either

magnesium citrate (32 oz or 2 bottles) or Golytely (4 to 6 L) can be administered at home. Tap water or Fleets enemas should be given the night before surgery (either as an inpatient or outpatient) to complete the emptying of the lower colon and rectum. A standard antiseptic surgical scrub should be performed as for any other vaginal surgery. The distal rectum and anus can be prepared for surgery in a similar fashion.

The role of preoperative antibiotics is also controversial. Early reports suggested giving an oral antibiotic bowel preparation with 1 g of erythromycin and neomycin given at 1 PM, 2 PM, and 11 PM the day before the procedure, followed by rectal irrigation with 200 ml 2 percent neomycin solution. In recent years, the use of broad-spectrum intravenous antibiotics during the perioperative period has become popular. Some investigators have suggested that no antibiotic prophylaxis is necessary.[56] A single dose of a broad-spectrum antibiotic such as cefoxitin or cefotetan given 30 minutes before the procedure is probably more than adequate in the absence of infection.

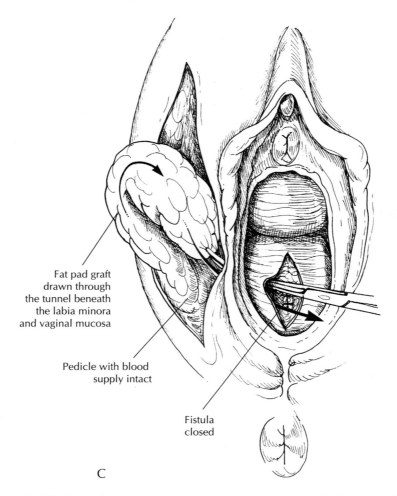

Fat pad graft
drawn through
the tunnel beneath
the labia minora
and vaginal mucosa

Pedicle with blood
supply intact

Fistula
closed

C

Fig. 40-17 *(Continued).* **(C)** The graft in tunneled subcutaneously beneath the vaginal mucosa. *(Figure continues.)*

Postoperatively, patients should be continued on a clear liquid diet for 24 to 72 hours. Ambulation should not be discouraged. A low residue diet should then be instituted for at least 3 to 4 weeks. Stool softeners are also routinely given during this period. Others have recommended high fiber diets or bulk enhancers such as Metamucil in order to create soft (yet voluminous) stool. Laxatives and enemas should be avoided. Patients should be instructed in wound care and taught how to perform Sitz baths for the first week following the procedure. A heat lamp or a blow dryer on a cool setting can also be used to keep the area dry. It is probably unnecessary to keep these patients in the hospital until their first bowel movement. Most patients can be discharged home on the first or second postoperative day, as long as they are seen within 1 week to have the incision examined. While on a low residue diet, it is common to have a bowel movement as infrequently as twice weekly.

Urinary retention is not an uncommon complication following fistula repair. It is reasonable to place a Foley catheter and a vaginal pack at the end of the surgical procedure and to remove them both on the first postoperative day. The use of antibiotics in the postoperative period is debatable and is probably unnecessary.

ADJUVANT MEDICAL TREATMENT

The primary treatment for obstetric and traumatic causes of anal incontinence is surgical repair. However, mechanical injury to the continence mechanism is often associated with nonreversible neurologic injury that may become progressive with age and the menopause. In patients with a significant denervation injury, surgical repair alone will often yield unsatisfactory results.

Conservative or medical therapy for anal incontinence includes dietary manipulation, pharmacologic management, and muscle exercises, as well as behavioral and biofeedback techniques. Dietary manipulations include a low residue diet to reduce stool bulk and frequency, and avoidance of flatus-producing foods. Pharmacologic agents such as loperamide or diphenoxylate with atropine induce constipation and can be titrated by the patient to achieve the desired effect.[76,77]

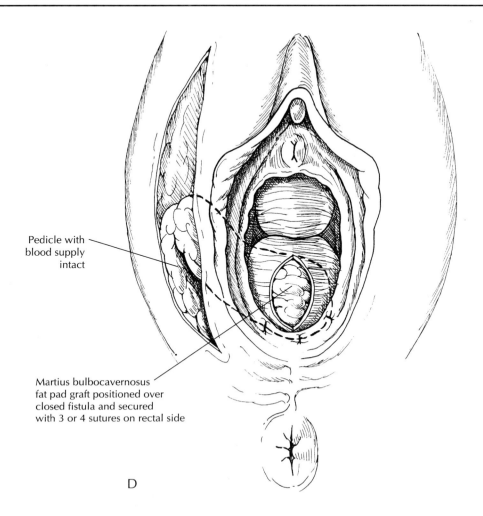

Pedicle with
blood supply
intact

Martius bulbocavernosus
fat pad graft positioned over
closed fistula and secured
with 3 or 4 sutures on rectal side

D

Fig. 40-17 *(Continued).* **(D)** The graft is secured at its edges with interrupted sutures. *(Figure continues.)*

Biofeedback training can engender a more conscious attitude in the patient with regard to sphincter function. These techniques have been shown to be effective in improving one's ability to perceive rectal filling[78] and to recognize physiologic cues that can signal impending incontinence. Any patient who has significant evidence of pelvic floor denervation should be offered a preoperative trial of biofeedback. Biofeedback training should also be offered to patients who achieve less than satisfactory results following surgical repair, as it can improve both sensory and motor function, and is often effective in improving continence in these patients.[79] Similarly, pelvic muscle exercises are also effective in rehabilitating the pelvic floor, and can be used both as the primary therapy,[80] or postoperatively to strengthen the pelvic floor muscles.

SUMMARY

Technical developments over the last decade have greatly improved our understanding of the anal continence mechanism as well as increased our ability to evaluate anal inconti-

nence. Recent scientific studies have established the functional importance of the internal anal sphincter, and have demonstrated that unrecognized and unrepaired injury to this structure is associated with significant symptoms. Refinements in surgical techniques and improvements in adjuvant therapies such as biofeedback, behavioral therapy, electrostimulation, and pharmacologic agents have enabled clinicians to offer more effective treatment for anal incontinence.

In the past, insufficient attention has been paid by obstetricians to the anatomic repair of third- and fourth-degree obstetric lacerations. Although they occur infrequently, these lacerations should be treated as a serious complication by the obstetrician/gynecologist and meticulous attention given to their repair.

The emotional, psychological, and sexual problems created by anal incontinence can be both devastating and debilitating. Many women are so embarrassed by their symptoms that they suffer needlessly for extended periods. Clinicians should therefore be aggressive in seeking out these symptoms in patients at risk. Once the diagnosis of anal incontinence or a rectovaginal fistula is made, treatment should be

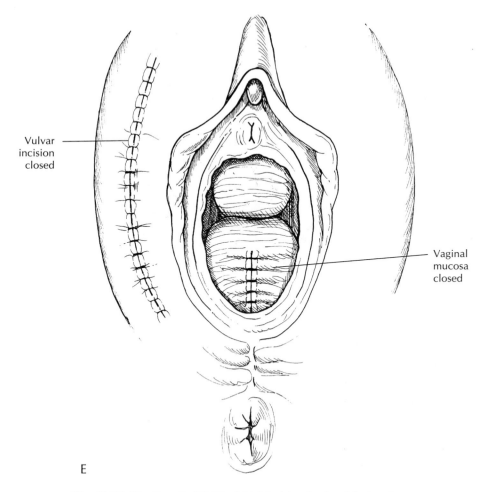

Vulvar
incision
closed

Vaginal
mucosa
closed

E

Fig. 40-17 *(Continued).* **(E)** The labial incision is closed in two layers.

initiated immediately and surgical repair should be performed as soon as it is technically feasible.

REFERENCES

1. Toglia MR, DeLancey JOL: Anal incontinence and the obstetrician-gynecologist. Obstet Gynecol 84:731, 1994

2. Kamm MA: Obstetric damage and faecal incontinence. Lancet 344:730, 1994

3. Madoff RD, Williams JG, Caushaj PF: Fecal incontinence. N Engl J Med 326:1002, 1992

4. Talley NJ, O'Keefe EA, Zinsmeister AR, Melton JL: Prevalance of gastrointestinal symptoms in the elderly: a population based study. Gastroenterology 102:895, 1992

5. Denis P, Bercoff E, Bizien MF et al: Etude de la prevalance de l'incontinence anale chez l'adulte. Gastroenterol Clin Biol 16:344, 1992

6. McClellan E: Fecal incontinence: social and economic factors. p. 326. In Benson JT (ed): Investigation and Management of Female Pelvic Floor Disorders—Investigation and Management. WW Norton, New York, 1992

7. Sultan AH, Kamm MA, Hudson CN et al: Anal sphincter disruption during vaginal delivery. N Engl J Med 329:1905, 1993

8. Sultan AH, Kamm MA, Bartram CI, Hudson CN: Third degree obstetric anal sphincter tears: risk factors and outcome of primary repair. BMJ 308:887, 1994

9. Gosling JA, Dixson JS, Critchley HOD, Thompson SA: A comparative study of the human external sphincter and periurethral levator ani muscles. Br J Urol 53:35, 1981

10. Swash M: Histopathology of pelvic floor muscles. p. 129. In Henry MM, Swash M (eds): Coloproctology and the Pelvic Floor. 1st Ed. Butterworths, London, 1985

11. Parks AG, Porter NH, Hardcastle J: The syndrome of the descending perineum. Proc R Soc Med 59:477, 1966

12. Parks AG: Anorectal incontinence. Proc R Soc Med 68:681, 1975

13. Bartolo DCC, Roe AM, Locke-Edmunds JC et al: Flap-valve theory of anorectal continence. Br J Surg 73:1012, 1986

14. Bannister JJ, Gibbons C, Read NW: Preservation of faecal continence during rises in intraabdominal pressure: is there a role for the flap valve? Gut 28:1241, 1987

15. Miller R, Bartolo DCC, Locke-Edmunds JC, Mortensen NJ:

Prospective study of conservative and operative treatment of faecal incontinence. Br J Surg 75:101, 1988

16. Miller R, Orrom WJ, Cornes H et al: Anterior sphincter plication and levatorplasty in the treatment of faecal incontinence. Br J Surg 75:1058, 1989

17. Aronson MP, Lee RA, Berquist TH: Anatomy of anal sphincters and related structures in continent women studied with magnetic resonance imaging. Obstet Gynecol 76:846, 1990

18. Sweiger, M: Method for determining individual contributions of voluntary and involuntary anal sphincters to resting tone. Dis Colon Rectum 22:415, 1979

19. Frenckner B, Euler CV: Influence of pudendal block on the function of the anal sphincters. Gut 16:482, 1975

20. Duthie HL, Gairns FW: Sensory nerves and sensation in the anal region in man. Br J Surg 47:585, 1960

21. Taverner D, Smiddy FG: An electromyographic study of the normal function of the external anal sphincter and pelvic diaphragm. Dis Colon Rectum 2:153, 1959

22. Snooks SJ, Setchell M, Swash M, Henry MM: Injury to innervation of pelvic floor sphincter musculature in childbirth. Lancet 2:546, 1984

23. Snooks SJ, Henry MM, Swash M: Faecal incontinence due to external sphincter division in childbirth is associated with damage to the innervation of the pelvic floor musculature: a double pathology. Br J Obstet Gynaecol 92:824, 1985

24. Cornes H, Bartolo DCC, Stirrat GM: Changes in anal canal sensation after childbirth. Br J Surg 78:74, 1991

25. Haadem K, Dahlstrom JA, Lingman, G: Anal sphincter function after delivery: a prospective study in women with sphincter rupture and controls. Eur J Obstet Gynaecol 35:7, 1990

26. Snooks SJ, Swash M, Henry MM, Setchell M: Risk factors in childbirth causing damage to the pelvic floor innervation. Int J Colorect Dis 1:20, 1986

27. Barrett JA, Brocklehurst JC, Kiff ES et al: Anal function in geriatric patients with faecal incontinence. Gut 30:1244, 1989

28. Wrenn K: Fecal impaction. N Engl J Med 321:658, 1989

29. Schiller LR, Santa Ana CA, Schmulen AC et al: Pathogenesis of fecal incontinence in diabetes mellitus: evidence for internal-anal-sphincter dysfunction. N Engl J Med 307:1666, 1982

30. Madoff RD, Watts JD, Rothenberger DA, Goldberg SM: Rectal prolapse treatment. p. 319. In Henry MM, Swash M (eds): Coloproctology and the Pelvic Floor. 2nd Ed. Butterworth-Heinemann, Oxford, England, 1992

31. Kupfer CA, Goligher JC: One hundred consecutive cases of complete prolapse of the rectum treated by operation. Br J Surg 57:481, 1970

32. Neil ME, Parks AG, Swash M: Physiological studies of the anal sphincter musculature in faecal incontinence and rectal prolapse. Br J Surg 68:531, 1981

33. Levin KE, Pemberton JH: Rectal prolapse: pathogenesis and management. p. 128. In Benson JT (ed): Female Investigation and Management of Female Pelvic Floor Disorders. WW Norton New York, 1992

34. Swash M: Electromyography in pelvic floor disorders. p. 184. In Henry MM, Swash M (eds): Coloproctology and the Pelvic

Floor. 2nd Ed. Butterworth-Heinemann, Oxford, England, 1992

35. Swash M, Snooks SJ: Motor nerve conduction studies of the pelvic floor innervation. p. 196. In Henry MM, Swash M (eds). Coloproctology and the Pelvic Floor. 2nd Ed. Butterworth-Heinemann, Oxford, England, 1992

36. Jones PN, Lubowski DZ, Swash M, Henry MM: Relation between perineal descent and pudendal nerve damage in idiopathic faecal incontinence. Int J Colorect Dis 2:93, 1987

37. Sun WM, Read NW, Donnelly TC: Impaired internal anal sphincter in a subgroup of patients with idiopathic faecal incontinence. Gastroenterology 97:130, 1989

38. Parks AG: Anorectal incontinence. Proc R Soc Med 68:681, 1975

39. Henry MM: Fecal Incontinence. In Benson JT (ed): Investigation and Management of Female Pelvic Floor Disorders. WW Norton, New York, 1992

40. Haadem K, Dahlstrom JA, Ling L, Ohrlander S: Anal sphincter function after delivery rupture. Obstet Gynecol 70:53, 1987

41. Sorensen SM, Bondesen H, Istre O, Vilman P: Perineal rupture following vaginal delivery—long-term consequences. Acta Obstet Gynecol Scand 67:315, 1988

42. Haadem K, Ohrlander S, Lingman G: Long term ailments due to anal sphincter rupture caused by delivery—a hidden problem. Eur J Obstet Gynaecol Reprod Biol 27:27, 1988

43. Snooks SJ, Setchell M, Swash M, Henry MM: Injury to innervation of pelvic floor sphincter musculature in childbirth. Lancet 2:546, 1984

44. Cunningham FG, MacDonald PC, Gant NF (eds): Williams Obstetrics. 18th Ed. Appleton & Large, E. Norwalk, CT, 1989

45. Gabbe SG, Niebyl JR, Simpson JL (eds): Obstetrics: Normal and Problem Pregnancies. 2nd Ed. Churchill Livingstone, New York, 1991

46. Fang DT, Nivatvongs S, Vermulen FD et al: Overlapping sphincteroplasty for acquired anal incontinence. Dis Colon Rectum 27:720, 1984

47. Browning GP, Motson RW: Anal sphincter injury. Management and results of Parks sphincter repair. Ann Surg 199:351, 1984

48. Harris RE: An evaluation of median episiotomy. Am J Obstet Gynecol 106:660, 1970

49. Thompson JD: Relaxed vaginal outlet, rectocele, fecal incontinence, and rectovaginal fistula. p. 941. In Thompson JD, Rock JA (eds): TeLinde's Operative Gynecology. 7th Ed. JB Lippincott, Philadelphia, 1992

50. Ramin SM, Gilstrap LC: Episiotomy and early repair of dehiscence. Clin Obstet Gynecol 37:816, 1994

51. Hankins GD, Hauth JC, Gilstrap LC et al: Early repair of episiotomy dehiscence. Obstet Gynecol 75:48, 1990

52. Hauth JC, Gilstrap LC, Ward SC, Hankins GDV: Early repair of an external sphincter ani muscle and rectal mucosal dehiscence. Obstet Gynecol 67:806, 1986

53. Monberg J, Hammen S: Ruptured episiotomia resutured primarily. Acta Obstet Gynecol Scand 66:163, 1987

54. Ramin SM, Ramus RM, Little BB, Gilstrap LC: Early repair of

episiotomy dehiscence associated with infection. Am J Obstet Gynecol 167:1104, 1992

55. Warren JC: A new method of operation for the relief of rupture of the perineum through the sphincter and rectum. J Am Gynecol Soc 72:322, 1882

56. Tancer ML, Lasser D, Rosenblum N: Rectovaginal fistula or perineal and anal sphincter disruption, or both, after vaginal delivery. Surg Gynecol Obstet 171:43, 1990

57. Noble GH: A new technique for complete laceration of the perineum designed for the purpose of eliminating infection from the rectum. Trans Am Gynecol Soc 27:357, 1902

58. Corman ML: Anal incontinence following obstetrical injury. Dis Colon Rectum 28:86, 1985

59. Hibbard LT: Surgical management of rectovaginal fistulas and complete perineal tears. Am J Obstet Gynecol 130:139, 1978

60. Corman ML: Anal incontinence following obstetrical injury. Dis Colon Rectum 28:86, 1985

61. Shieh CJ, Gennaro AR: Rectovaginal fistula: a review of 11 years experience. Int Surg 69:69, 1984

62. Rosenshein NB, Genady RR, Woodruff JD: An anatomic classification of rectovaginal septal defects. Am J Obstet Gynecol 137:439, 1980

63. Baden WF, Walker T (eds): Fundamentals, symptoms, and classification. p. 9. In Surgical Repair of Vaginal Defects. JB Lippincott, Philadelphia, 1992

64. Hibbard LT: Surgical management of rectovaginal fistulas and complete perineal tears. Am J Obstet Gynecol 130:139, 1978

65. Wiskind AK, Thompson JD: Transverse transperineal repair of rectovaginal fistulas in the lower vagina. Am J Obstet Gynecol 167:694, 1992

66. Elkins TE, DeLancey JOL, McGuire EJ: The use of modified Martius graft as an adjunctive technique in vesicovaginal and rectovaginal fistula repair. Obstet Gynecol 75:727, 1990

67. Miller NF, Brown W: The surgical treatment of complete perineal tears in the female. Am J Obstet Gynecol 34:196, 1937

68. Boronow RC: Management of radiation-induced vaginal fistulas. Am J Obstet Gynecol 100:1, 1971

69. Aartsen EJ, Sindram IS: Repair of the radiation-induced rectovaginal fistulas without or with interposition of the bulbocavernosus muscle (Martius procedure). Eur J Surg Oncol 14:171, 1988

70. Bricker EM, Johnston WD, Patwardhan RV: Repair of postirradiation damage to colorectum: a progress report. Ann Surg 193:555, 1981

71. Goligher JC, Duthie H, Nixon H: Surgery of the Anus, Rectum and Colon. 5th Ed. Bailliere-Tindall, London, 1984

72. Crohn BB, Yarnis H: Regional Ileitis. 2nd Ed. Grune & Stratton, Orlando, FL, 1958

73. Ritchie JK, Lennard-Jones JE: Crohn's disease of the large bowel. Scand J Gastroenterol 11:433, 1976

74. Cohen JL, Stricker JW, Schoetz DJ et al: Rectovaginal fistula in Crohn's disease. Dis Colon Rectum 32:825, 1989

75. Radcliffe AG, Ritchie JK, Hawley PR et al: Anovaginal and rectovaginal fistulas in Crohn's disease. Dis Colon Rectum 31:94, 1988

76. Hartford WV, Krejs GJ, Santa Ana CA, Fordtran JS: Acute effect of diphenoxylate with atropine (Lomotil) in patients with chronic diarrhea and fecal incontinence. Gastroenterology 78:440, 1980

77. Read M, Read NW, Barber DC, Duthie HL: Effects of loperamide on anal sphincter function in patients complaining of chronic diarrhea with fecal incontinence and urgency. Dig Dis Sci 27:807, 1982

78. Miner PB, Donelly TC, Read NW: Investigation of mode of biofeedback in treatment of fecal incontinence. Dig Dis Sci 35:1291, 1990

79. Penninckx FM, Elliot MS, Hancke E et al: Symposium: fecal incontinence. Int J Colorect Dis 2:173, 1987

80. Whitehead WE, Burgio KL, Engel BT: Biofeedback treatment of fecal incontinence in geriatric patients. J Am Geriatr Soc 33:320, 1985

81. Lee RA: Atlas of Gynecologic Surgery. WB Saunders, Philadelphia, 1992

82. Benson JT (ed): Investigation and Management of Female Pelvic Floor Disorders. WW Norton, New York, 1992

CHAPTER FORTY-ONE

PELVIC DENERVATION AND UTERINE SUSPENSION

JOHN F. STEEGE

Pelvic denervation and uterine suspension procedures have in common the intent of relieving pelvic pain. Either or both may be combined with other procedures performed toward the same end, such as lysis of adhesions or treatment of endometriosis. Likewise, either or both may be performed by laparotomy or laparoscopy. Unfortunately, they also share a long history of waxing and waning popularity, including periods of probably significant overuse. With both, it is difficult to document clinical efficacy due to subjective end points and numerous confounding variables.

Historical claims that uterine suspension by itself improves fertility have generally fallen out of favor (for a conflicting view, see Ivey[1]), while the additive role of the procedure when combined with other infertility surgery remains uncertain. This chapter focuses instead on the role of uterine suspension in the treatment of pelvic pain. Following discussion of the history, anatomy, and pathophysiology of denervation, the surgical techniques and clinical results for each approach are discussed. Uterine suspension is reviewed in the same manner. The chapter concludes with a discussion of general pain theory and research methodology as they pertain to these procedures.

PELVIC DENERVATION PROCEDURES

Background

The popularity of uterine denervation for the treatment of dysmenorrhea and other painful conditions of the pelvis has waxed and waned over almost 100 years. After a period of infrequent use, there has been recent demonstration that uterosacral interruption and presacral neurectomy can be performed via laparoscopy. Accordingly, with the advent of operative laparoscopy, both uterosacral interruption (usually by electrocautery or laser uterosacral nerve ablation [LUNA],[2] and presacral neurectomy[3] have joined the growing list of laparoscopic gynecologic surgical procedures performed.

Anatomy and Physiology

Sympathetic sensory afferent fibers from the uterus form the inferior hypogastric plexus lateral and inferior to the uterosacral ligaments, then traverse the uterovaginal plexus of Frankenhaeuser on each side before travelling cephalad to unite in the superior hypogastric plexus. The precise course of these fibers is highly variable[4] (Fig. 41-1) as they cross the common iliac vessels and ascend anterior and lateral to the aorta before entering spinal cord segments T10 through L1.

Traditional teachings maintain that parasympathetic branches from the upper vagina and cervix travel to their S2 through S4 origins partly independently and partly via Frankenhaeuser's plexus. Bonica[5] on the basis of extensive work with a variety of segmental, regional, and local blocks administered during labor, has challenged this formulation, suggesting that sacral fibers to the lower uterus and cervix are motor rather than sensory. This assertion is supported by the observation that uterosacral interruption may not add to the effectiveness of presacral neurectomy for relief of pelvic pain.

The adnexae are innervated largely by the ovarian nerves, which travel predominantly with the arterial supply of the ovaries. Although one report suggests that transection of the

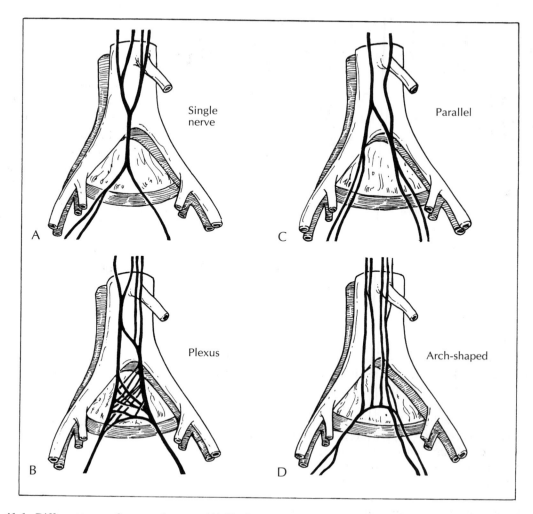

Fig. 41-1. Different types of presacral nerves. (**A**) Single nerve type, 24 percent; (**B**) plexus type, 58 percent (**C**) parallel type, 16 percent; (**D**) arch-shaped type, 2 percent.

infundibulopelvic ligament will relieve adnexal pain without compromising ovarian function,[6] subsequent corroboration is lacking. Pelvic denervation should therefore be expected to relieve only central pelvic pain.

Motor function of the lower large intestine is mediated by sacral parasympathetics and, to some extent, by sympathetic supply via the inferior mesenteric plexus. Motor function for the bladder is mediated both by sacral parasympathetics, as well as by some sympathetic output from the inferior hypogastric plexus. Given the multiple levels of enervation, it follows that partial interruption of the nerve supply to these structures may partially interfere with their function. In most instances these changes can be accommodated. The literature supports this notion in reporting constipation as a complication of presacral neurectomy in 0 to 30 percent of cases. Inhibition of bladder function, manifested by mild urinary retention, is also noted anecdotally. Neither of these complications has received either careful observational re-

porting or physiologic investigation in the form of bowel motility studies or urodynamic studies.

Another area of potential concern is sexual response. The two major components of this response are vasocongestion, thought to be primarily parasympathetically mediated, and contraction of uterine and vaginal musculature, which appears to be sympathetically mediated. Early reports on denervation procedures either did not mention changes in sexuality at all, or specifically denied adverse effect. However, these observations took place before the time when these neurologic pathways were understood. More recent reports are anecdotal at best with regard to this matter, and certainly none have undertaken serious investigation. It is curious that on the one hand, some laparoscopists are advocating supracervical hysterectomy in order to preserve cervical innervation and thereby conserve sexual response, while others are suggesting that thorough denervation of these structures does not alter sexual response.

Denervation procedures for pain relief in other areas of

the body are often followed by the re-emergence of enervation, and therefore pain. The time course for re-enervation is usually 12 to 18 months, suggesting that adequate follow-up for pelvic denervation should be at least that long. Sympathetic denervation procedures for vascular compromise of the lower extremities occasionally fail after this length of time, although the re-enervation process seems less successful in autonomic denervations than it does in somatic procedures. The literature on pelvic sympathectomy in general has reported a range of follow-up times, seldom offering a mean and uniformly failing to report the number of patients followed for over 2 years.

Surgical Technique

Presacral Neurectomy

The surgical approach to sympathectomy requires opening the retroperitoneal space in a triangular area bordered by the iliac vessels, (the interiliac trigone), with the apex of the triangle at the bifurcation of the aorta (Fig. 41-2). All retroperitoneal tissue anterior to the sacrum and iliac vessels must be excised, proceeding from the ureter on the right and to the root of the sigmoid mesentery on the left. Some sympathetic branches may emerge from between the left common iliac artery and vein.

The traditional transabdominal approach is through a midline incision, although it can be accomplished via a Pfannenstiel incision in some patients. The peritoneum is incised in midline over the body of L5 for a distance of 6 to 8 cm and retracted laterally. The bundle of fatty tissue containing nerves that lies anterior to L5 and S1 vertebrae may then be isolated by blunt dissection as a unit, taking care to isolate and avoid the middle sacral artery and vein. Proximal and distal ligatures are place around the bundle before it is excised and sent for pathologic examination. The peritoneum has traditionally been closed, but current practice would suggest that it need not be reapproximated.

The laparoscopic approach is fundamentally identical—simply being accomplished with longer instruments (Fig. 41-2). It is most often performed in conjunction with other laparoscopic procedures, which may dictate initial trocar diameter choices and placements. With the patient placed in modified lithotomy position, the presacral area may be viewed either via the umbilical trocar or through a low midline trocar, with the operator standing between the patient's legs. In the latter case, it is best to move the video monitor cephalad, so that the monitor view is from the operator's perspective. With the patient in steep Trendelenburg's position, a right lower quadrant probe is needed for retraction of small bowel, and a left lower quadrant port for a sigmoid colon retractor. The base of the sigmoid mesentery and the right ureter must be clearly identified before beginning. The root of the sigmoid mesentery takes a highly variable course across the presacral area, sometimes crossing as high as S2.

From this point on, the difficulty of the procedure depends entirely on two factors: hemostasis and bowel retraction. When extra ports are needed to accomplish retraction, the procedure can begin to look cumbersome, but when this is readily accomplished (as it usually is in the thinner patient), the procedure is much more straightforward. Similarly, the blunt dissection of the presacral tissue is more easily accomplished in the patient with less retroperitoneal fat. The author prefers to use bipolar cautery scissors, although others may prefer monopolar scissors or the neodymium:yttrium aluminum garner (Nd:YAG) laser. Kleppinger forceps should be available, although they will often not be sufficient to stabilize the venous bleeding from periosteal perforators. The bundle of fatty tissue containing the presacral nerves may be transected with cautery scissors or laser in two places, freeing the intervening tissue for removal and pathologic examination (Fig. 41-3). Again, the peritoneum need not be closed.

Despite the proximity of the great vessels to the area of dissection, reports of significant hemorrhage are very infrequent in the literature. The middle sacral artery and vein are perhaps greater hazards, as they may be obscured by fat and have a very variable course through the interiliac trigone and hence down the anterior sacrum. Presacral veins, which perforate the periosteum, are more of a problem at the S2-S3 level, which should be caudad to the main area of dissection. If such perforators are encountered, hemostasis is most easily accomplished by pressing stainless steel thumbtacks directly into the sacrum.[7] Methods are currently being developed to apply thumbtacks via a laparoscopic instrument.

Given the variability in the course of sympathetic nerves as described, it might be tempting to sever them at a higher level, where they are more concentrated, in hopes of achieving better relief of pelvic pain. However, the closer the dissection is to the inferior mesenteric artery, the greater the risk of potential bowel compromise.

Laparoscopic Division of the Uterosacral Ligaments

Current approaches to altering the uterosacral ligaments have their origins in Doyle's work.[8] Any energy source (unipolar or bipolar cautery, or laser of any type) that can be used through the laparoscope may be used to partially or completely divide the ligaments. Most surgeons have treated the ligaments over approximately 1 cm of their length, directly adjacent to the uterus, in order to interrupt the sympathetic supply to the uterus at the point where the nerve fibers are most concentrated (Fig. 41-4). Some also destroy a line of tissue between the uterosacrals, on the posterior surface of the lower uterine segment.

In many women, a substantial arterial supply follows the inferolateral aspect of the ligament, making cautery necessary for hemostasis in many instances. Before using cautery

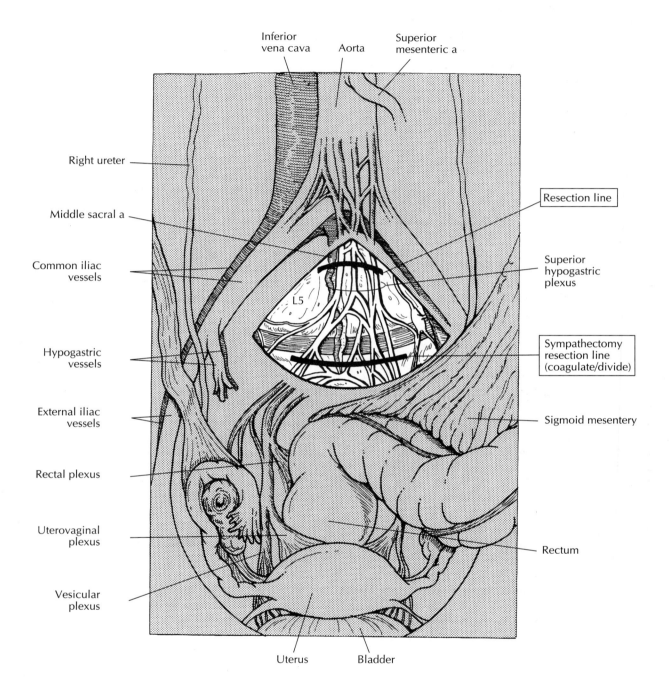

Fig. 41-2. Laparoscopic presacral neurectomy.

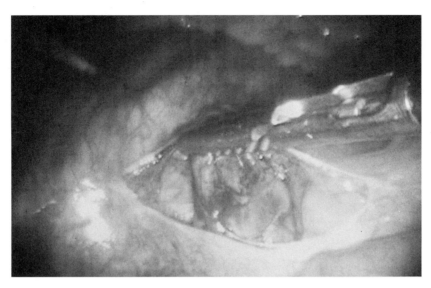

Fig. 41-3. Laparoscopic instrument grasping a presacral nerve bundle.

in this area, the operator must be certain to visualize the ureter and retract it out of the way if necessary.

Results

Presacral Neurectomy

The clinical literature includes a total of over 12,000 cases reported over the last 70 years. There is general internal consistency in the reports, in that pain relief is obtained in approximately 70 to 80 percent of women. These percentages apply to early populations of women without pelvic pathology in whom the procedure was done for dysmenorrhea alone, as well as later series, which included mixed populations of women with and without significant pelvic pathology.

With the advances in medical therapy for primary dysmenorrhea, a more current dilemma is to investigate the value of presacral neurectomy in women who are having conservative pelvic surgery for such disorders as endometriosis and pelvic adhesions. Unfortunately, the literature offering a valid comparison of conservative surgery versus conservative surgery plus presacral neurectomy is extremely limited. Candiani[9] reported a series of 71 patients with stage III or IV endometriosis, 36 of whom were randomized to conservative surgical resection only, while 35 were randomized to surgery plus presacral neurectomy via laparotomy. Careful pain assessments were performed on the approximately 50 percent of the population who reported pain preoperatively. The authors were also careful to evaluate dyspareunia as well as dysmenorrhea as separate categories. Quite dramatic improvement was obtained in both groups in the study, thus failing to demonstrate a significant additional benefit attributable to presacral neurectomy. Unfortunately,

since only a portion of the population had pain preoperatively, the total number of patients with pain who were subjected to randomization is relatively small, thus limiting the statistical power of the study. Tjaden et al,[10] after initial positive clinical experience with presacral neurectomy in conjunction with conservative resection of stage III and IV endometriosis, randomized eight women to conservative resection with or without presacral neurectomy. The four allocated to presacral neurectomy obtained good relief, while the others did not. At that point, the institutional review board mandated stopping the study, as statistical significance had been reached. The authors went on to report good results in 15 of 17 patients in a subsequent clinical series.

LUNA Procedure

There is a similar dearth of literature investigating the effectiveness of LUNA. Several clinical observational studies report significant relief of dysmenorrhea in 60 to 75 percent of patients,[11,12] while the only prospective study in the literature, done by Lichten and Bombard,[2] reports only 45 percent of patients treated with LUNA to have persistent relief of dysmenorrhea 1 year after the operation. In fairness, it would seem that the laparoscopic procedure currently done most often is not as extensive a denervation as that devised by Doyle[8] and may therefore be expected to have less good results.

It might be argued that if the question of benefit remains unsettled, the presacral neurectomy and LUNA should still be performed in view of the apparently low incidence of complications. However, ureteral injuries are reported anecdotally with an unknown frequency following the LUNA procedure, and two cases of uterine prolapse were reported to occur soon after the same procedure.[13] A more extensive

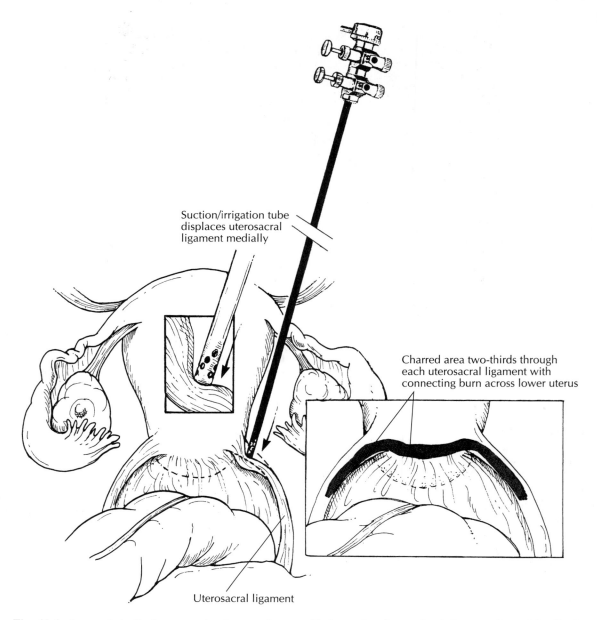

Suction/irrigation tube
displaces uterosacral
ligament medially

Charred area two-thirds through
each uterosacral ligament with
connecting burn across lower uterus

Uterosacral ligament

Fig. 41-4. Approach to the laparoscopic uterosacral nerve ablation, using the suction-irrigator to better identify the uterosacral ligament.

clinical follow-up of the LUNA procedure would be a substantial addition to the literature.

By the same token, potential bladder, bowel, and sexual complications of presacral neurectomy need to be examined on a far more rigorous basis than they have been in the past, and on a large series of patients.

While the LUNA procedure is apparently of some demonstrable value and is relatively safe to perform, the laparoscopic presacral neurectomy involves considerably greater hazard and should remain the province of the more experienced operative laparoscopist. Clinicians should continue to choose patients carefully, rather than simply including pre-

sacral neurectomy as part of a surgical laparoscopic procedure with several components.

UTERINE SUSPENSION PROCEDURES

Background

It has often been said that the existence of multiple treatments for the same problem usually suggests that all the treatments are imperfect. Perhaps this should be applied to pelvic support surgery in general and uterine suspension pro-

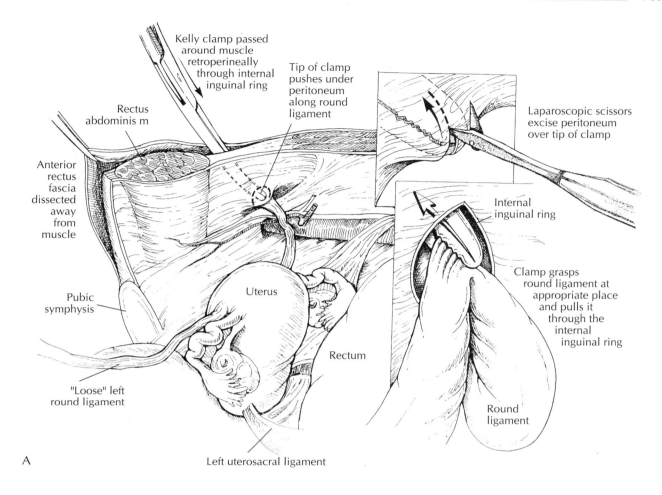

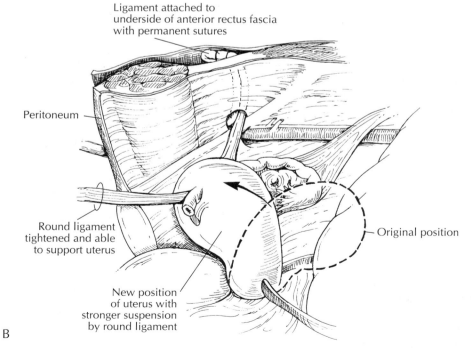

Fig. 41-5. (A & B) Modified Gilliam uterine suspension.

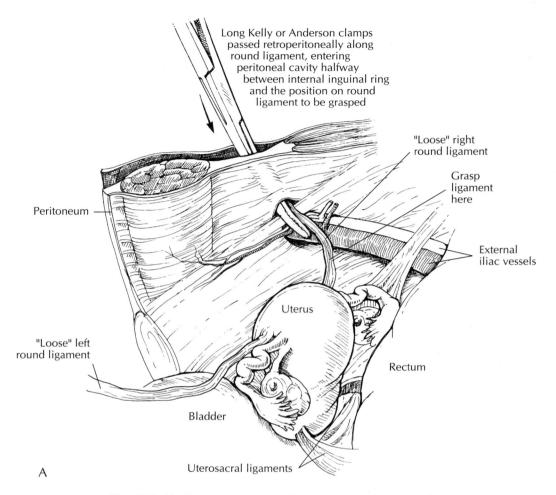

Long Kelly or Anderson clamps passed retroperitoneally along round ligament, entering peritoneal cavity halfway between internal inguinal ring and the position on round ligament to be grasped

"Loose" right round ligament

Grasp ligament here

External iliac vessels

Peritoneum

Uterus

Rectum

"Loose" left round ligament

Bladder

A

Uterosacral ligaments

Fig. 41-6. (**A–C**) Laparoscopic modified Gilliam uterine suspension.

cedures in particular. In fairness, the proliferation of techniques may have more to do with the need for very long-term follow-up for proper evaluation; new techniques appear before old ones are well evaluated.

This discussion, focuses on those procedures that lend themselves to performance either by laparotomy or laparoscopy, and on some newer procedures that attempt to reestablish good pelvic support without sacrificing the uterus.

Anatomy and Physiology

The pathophysiology of uterine retroversion remains unclear. Up to 15 percent of women have a retroverted uterus as a variation of normal anatomy, hence the debate concerning whether uterine retroversion should be held responsible for symptoms in anyone. Although the problem is essentially unstudied, the clinical impression held by many is that symptoms arise in the individual who has a combination of at least two of the following: uterine retroversion, foreshortened bony pelvis, petite stature, pelvic pathology such as adhesions or endometriosis, constipation, diminished sexual

response, pelvic congestion syndrome, and a sexually anatomically mismatched partner.

It would seem apparent that uterine retroversion may be attributed primarily to the round ligaments; either they are too weak or too long, or both. For example, after a pregnancy, a previously anteverted uterus may become retroverted. Alternatively, the uterus may be retroverted lifelong, as a variation of anatomy. Recent work by Benson et al[14] suggests that pelvic neuropathy may contribute substantially to loss of pelvic support in general, and that transvaginal dissection may cause further deterioration of pelvic innervation. Applying this logic to the problem of postpartum uterine round ligament and uterosacral ligament changes that may result in new uterine retroversion would imply that shortening (operating on) these damaged ligaments would not provide long-lasting improvement. By contrast, it is feasible that the uterus may be retroverted in some women due to congenitally elongated round ligaments of normal strength. If lifelong uterine retroversion becomes symptomatic due to some other condition, uterine support surgery may be additive when combined with a procedure directed

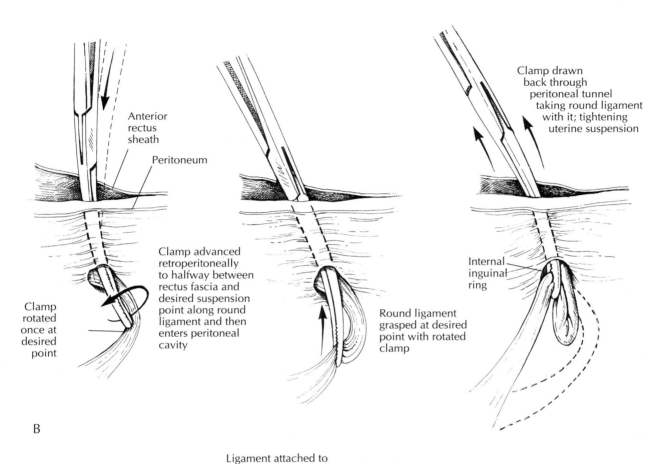

Anterior rectus sheath

Peritoneum

Clamp rotated once at desired point

Clamp advanced retroperitoneally to halfway between rectus fascia and desired suspension point along round ligament and then enters peritoneal cavity

Round ligament grasped at desired point with rotated clamp

Clamp drawn back through peritoneal tunnel taking round ligament with it; tightening uterine suspension

Internal inguinal ring

B

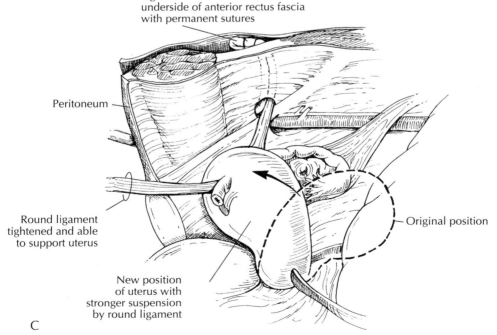

Ligament attached to underside of anterior rectus fascia with permanent sutures

Peritoneum

Round ligament tightened and able to support uterus

New position of uterus with stronger suspension by round ligament

Original position

C

Fig. 41-6 *(Continued).*

toward any additional pelvic pathology (e.g., endometriosis). Variation in patient mix may be responsible for the varying opinions of different authors regarding the value of uterine suspension procedures. The measurement of outcome in terms of pain relief following uterine suspension procedures may require stratification along these lines.

Surgical Technique

Modified Gilliam Suspension

The modified Gilliam suspension is perhaps the most widely utilized[15] (Fig. 41-5). The midportion of the round ligament on each side is brought up through a puncture in the rectus fascia lateral to the rectus muscle, and attached with permanent sutures to the underside of the fascia. Traditionally performed via a transverse abdominal incision, the same result may be readily accomplished laparoscopically. Steptoe[16] was the first to report a laparoscopic technique, followed by Smith et al,[17] reporting on pelvic pain, and Candy,[18] on dyspareunia.

A somewhat simpler method is to approach the round ligaments via bilateral 2-cm incisions directly over each internal inguinal ring, and pass a long Kelly or Anderson clamp retroperitoneally along the round ligament to a point halfway between the point of entry in the rectus fascia and the desired point of suspension along the round ligament (Fig. 41-6). The clamp then enters the peritoneal cavity and is rotated to grasp the round ligament at the desired point. The ligament is then drawn back through this retroperitoneal tunnel and attached to the underside of the rectus fascia with permanent suture. Care must be taken to suture to the cephalad side of the fascial incision in order to avoid entrapping the nearby ilioinguinal and ileohypogastric nerves.

The modified Gilliam approach carries with it the appeal of not leaving behind any intraperitoneal sutures or foreign bodies. Slightly faster methods of improving uterine position by shortening the round ligaments include plicating them with a running permanent suture in accordion fashion or placing a Fallope ring on each round ligament.

Balde-Webster Suspension

In the Balde-Webster suspension, each round ligament is brought through a perforation in the mesosalpinx and sutured to the posterior aspect of the uterus. Although this suspension could certainly be performed laparoscopically, the approach has not been reported.

Suture plication of the uterosacral ligaments may be both additive to any of the above procedures in terms of achieving uterine anteversion, and preventative in terms of reducing the chance of an enterocele developing in the future. In any approach, care must be taken to avoid creating sharp angulations in the course of the fallopian tubes.

Results

A careful search of the medical literature has failed to reveal any significant follow-up study of uterine support surgery. Textbook descriptions generally suggest that the uterus will resume a retroverted position either over time or following subsequent childbirth, but more precise descriptions are not available.

GENERAL PAIN THEORY

The Cartesian theory of pain perception suggested that dedicated pain fibers carried pain signals from the periphery to the brain. Pain was believed to be proportional to tissue damage or stimulation. Virtually all current theories of pain perception suggest that peripheral signals be termed *nociceptive,* with the term *pain* being reserved for the central process of recognition of peripheral nociceptive signals. Downregulation or upregulation of signals may be under the control of higher centers in the brain and impinge on the spinal cord directly, and multiple biochemical modulators may exist in the spinal cord, all of which serve to substantially alter the impact of aberrant sensory signals from the periphery. Thus, information travels in two directions between brain and spinal cord. Add to this the impact of individual experience, cultural and personal expectations, and personality, and one has a most complex mechanism responsible for recognizing and interpreting pain.

In many instances of chronic pain, the intensity of the pain bears little or no relationship to the amount of tissue damage. The development of a ''chronic pain syndrome,'' psychologically and behaviorally defined, may significantly influence the outcome of gynecologic surgery performed to relieve pain.[19]

Early manuscripts regarding pelvic denervation would occasionally attribute failure to psychiatric causes (otherwise undefined), but virtually none of the literature undertakes any form of behavioral or psychiatric evaluation. Given the chronic and debilitating nature of the pain experienced by women usually subjected to denervation procedures, multiple variables become relevant.

Given the level of neurologic redundancy in the pelvis, it seems unlikely that any procedure will result in complete and total denervation. Hence, some afferent, and probably nociceptive signals will no doubt persist in many circumstances. The factors listed may serve to augment the impact of such persistent nociceptive signals, thus accounting for instances of partial or complete failure of the procedure.

METHODOLOGIC CONCERNS

Recent reports of pelvic denervation were well reviewed by Vercellini.[20] Unfortunately, almost all reports continue to be either observational or retrospective nonrandomized

---

Relevant Variables for Studies of the Treatment of Pelvic Pain

- Demographic factors
  - Age
  - Race
  - Ethnic group
- Pain characteristics
  - Location (central versus lateral)
  - Duration (dyspareunia, daily menstrual)
  - Severity
- Psychological disorders
  - Affective disturbance
  - Premorbid psychological baseline
  - History of sexual abuse
  - History of domestic violence
- Behavioral impairments
  - Work patterns
  - Home responsibilities
  - Recreation
- Sexual function
  - Baseline sexual function
  - Alterations in sexual function before treatment
  - Partner factors
- Gynecologic assessment
  - Extent of pelvic pathology
  - Prior medical and surgical treatments
- Study characteristics
  - Prospective/retrospective
  - Randomized
  - Duration of follow-up
  - Type of surgical procedure
  - Concommitant medical, behavioral, or psychological treatments

---

combination of a verbal descriptive scale,[24] and a true linear analog scale without anchors placed in various sections of the scale

2. Psychological variables, such as mood disturbance and anxiety disorders should at least be systematically noted, if not psychometrically assessed. In studies, psychometric instruments or structured psychiatric interviews may yield diagnostic categories that may be stratified or included in multivariate analyses

3. Sexual abuse histories should be noted

4. For an investigator or clinician to comment on possible changes in sexuality associated with pelvic surgery, a careful baseline sexual history is needed. Ideally, any recorded sexual dysfunction should be characterized and data on sexual frequency should be prospectively collected

Finally, technology is currently available to accurately describe bladder and bowel contractility and diagnose dysfunctions. These methods should be used preoperatively and postoperatively to more carefully evaluate the impact of denervation on these autonomic functions.

SUMMARY

Given the ambiguous nature of the available data regarding the success and complications of the LUNA, presacral neurectomy, and uterine suspension, clinicians at present are left to use their best judgement in each individual case. At the present time, the author uses the LUNA procedure on occasion, but is careful to leave the lateral third of each uterosacral ligament intact to guard against prolapse. Since the author rarely operates on someone with absolutely no pelvic pathology (less than 10 percent of laparoscopies), it is very difficult to assess the impact of the LUNA. If further reports of prolapse associated with the LUNA procedure appear, switching to a laparoscopic version of the Doyle procedure may be advisable.

At present the author performs laparoscopic presacral neurectomies quite rarely. The benefits of the presacral neurectomy are sufficiently established to mandate use of the procedure when doing extensive resection of endometriosis. Since the author tends to see patients with a complex mix of physical and psychological factors in their pain, it is advisable to reserve the presacral neurectomy for those cases of purely central pelvic pain in which all other reasonable treatment methods have been exhausted, including psychotropics and psychotherapy. In general gynecologic (non-pain-clinic) practice, there is a common tendency to overuse surgical methods in general, and neuroablative procedures in particular. In the future, when considering a presacral neurectomy, it may be useful to first perform laparoscopy under local anesthesia and use local anesthetic to block the presacral nerves, thus evaluating the independent impact of the pro-

studies. Virtually all series include a mixture of patients with various degrees of organic pathology. Sample sizes are limited, and follow-up is highly variable. Furthermore, pain is usually reported on the basis of a very simple nonvalidated categorical scale.

The literature on the long-term efficacy of uterine suspension procedures is similarly lacking both quantitatively and qualitatively.

Review of the variables relevant to pain suggests that the surgeon should address the following areas before proceeding with surgical treatment of the patient's pain:

1. Location, duration, and severity should be systematically recorded. Severity is perhaps best rated by a

posed neurectomy. Although this will not separate the effect of resection of central pelvic endometriosis from the effect of the block, it would at least evaluate the degree to which the organic component of the pain may originate from areas not supplied by the presacral nerves.

Uterine suspension is another procedure that the author performs on only very selected cases. It has proved valuable in about 15 cases in which a petite woman with a foreshortened pelvis and a retroverted uterus seemed to have inescapably deep dyspareunia. In most cases of uterine retroversion, counseling about the adjustment of positions during coitus provides sufficient relief. Success of the surgery has been good, at least until the next pregnancy or until concomitant pathology progresses to the point that extirpative surgery is needed.

REFERENCES

1. Ivey JL: Laparoscopic uterine suspension as an adjunctive procedure at the time of laser laparoscopy for the treatment of endometriosis. J Reprod Med 37:757, 1992

2. Lichten EM, Bombard J: Surgical treatment of primary dysmenorrhea with laparoscopic uterine nerve ablation. J Reprod Med 32:37, 1987

3. Perez JJ: Laparoscopic presacral neurectomy. J Reprod Med 35:625, 1990

4. Elaut L: The surgical anatomy of the so called presacral nerve. Surg Gynecol Obstet 23:581, 1932

5. Bonica JJ: The Management of Pain. 2nd Ed. Lea & Febiger, Malvern, PA

6. Brown OD: A survey of 113 cases of primary dysmenorrhea treated by neurectomy. Am J Obstet Gynecol 57:1053, 1949

7. Timmons MC, Kohler MF, Addison WA: Thumbtack use for control of presacral bleeding, with description of an instrument for thumbtack application. Obstet Gynecol 78:313, 1991

8. Doyle JB: Paracervical uterine denervation by transection of the cervical plexus for the relief of dysmenorrhea. Am J Obstet Gynecol 70:1, 1955

9. Candiani GB, Fedele L, Vercellini P et al: Presacral neurectomy for the treatment of pelvic pain associated with endometriosis: a controlled study. Am J Obstet Gynecol 167:100, 1992

10. Tjaden B, Schlaff WD, Kinball A: The efficacy of presacral neurectomy for the relief of midline dysmenorrhea. Obstet Gynecol 76:517, 1990

11. Daniell JF: Fiberoptic laser laparoscopy. Baillieres Clin Obstet Gynecol 3:545, 1989

12. Sutton C, Hill D: Laser laparoscopy in the treatment of endometriosis. Br J Obstet Gynaecol 97:181, 1990

13. Good MC, Copas PR, Doody MC: Uterine prolapse after laparoscopic uterosacral transection. J Reprod Med 37:995, 1992

14. Benson JT, McClellan E: The effect of vaginal dissection on the pudendal nerve. Obstet Gynecol 82:387, 1993

15. Gilliam DT: Round-ligament ventrosuspension of the uterus: a new method. Am J Obstet Gynecol 41:299, 1900

16. Steptoe PC: Laparoscopy in Gynecology. E. and S. Livingston, London, 1967

17. Smith OB, Heksetm JF, Sherman RL: Laparoscopic uterine suspension. J Reprod Med 18:98, 1977

18. Candy FW: Modified Gilliam uterine suspension using laparoscopic visualization. Obstet Gynecol 47:242, 1976

19. Steege JF, Stout AL: Resolution of chronic pelvic pain following laparoscopic adhesiolysis. Am J Obstet Gynecol 165:278, 1991

20. Vercellini P, Fedele L, Bianchi S, Candiani G: Pelvic denervation for chronic pain associated with endometriosis: fact or fancy? Am J Obstet Gynecol 165:745, 1991

21. Melzack R: The McGill Pain Questionnaire: major properties and scoring methods. Pain 1:277, 1975

CHAPTER FORTY-TWO

SURGICAL TERMINATION OF PREGNANCY

LEE P. SHULMAN
FRANK W. LING

Uterine evacuation is an integral part of obstetric and gynecologic care. Even those obstetrician-gynecologists, family practitioners, and surgeons who do not perform elective pregnancy terminations are frequently called on to provide uterine evacuation procedures to women presenting with nonviable fetuses or hydatidiform moles. Regardless of a practitioner's ultimate decision to offer pregnancy termination, the ability to perform first- and second-trimester uterine evacuation procedures is integral to providing safe, effective, and appropriate obstetric care.

Although the vast majority of surgical pregnancy terminations performed in the United States are for elective indications, the techniques used for all uterine evacuation procedures are fundamentally the same. This chapter reviews the surgical techniques used for uterine evacuation in first- and second-trimester viable and nonviable pregnancies, the safety of these procedures, and the management of complications.

GENERAL OVERVIEW

Physicians performing any uterine evacuation procedure should obtain a comprehensive patient history, irrespective of the indication for the procedure. Preoperative counseling, including a thorough review of the risks of the surgical procedure, is then provided, and a signed informed consent obtained from all patients. A complete physical examination is performed before the procedure. Information concerning the patient's hematocrit and Rh status is obtained, and other tests may be warranted according to the individual's past medical or surgical history or indication for the procedure.

Liberal use of preoperative ultrasonography should be considered in cases of discrepancies between uterine size and gestational age questionable fetal viability, and possible abnormal intrauterine contents (e.g., hydatidiform mole). In addition, use of concurrent intraoperative ultrasonography should be considered in cases of abnormal cervicouterine architecture (e.g., uterine fibroids, cervical constriction) or abnormal intrauterine contents (e.g., hydatidiform mole).

Included in the preoperative counseling is a review of the risks and benefits of the various analgesia options. Local analgesia (e.g., paracervical block) is usually sufficient for most first-trimester procedures, with spinal, epidural, or general anesthesia being used according to patient wishes, gestational age, and indication for procedure.

DILATION AND EVACUATION

Dilation and evacuation (D and E) refers to the opening of the uterine cervix before the evacuation of intrauterine contents by a variety of surgical and nonsurgical methods. In most cases, other than the skill and expertise of the operating surgeon, the primary factor in choosing a particular surgical technique is the content and volume of intrauterine tissue. As such, dilation and evacuation procedures are utilized throughout the first and second trimesters of pregnancy, as well as for most nonviable pregnancies of comparable gestational ages. The surgical techniques used for such evacuation procedures can be divided into three main categories: (1) very early uterine evacuation, or menstrual extraction; (2) suction curettage for first- and early second-trimester preg-

---

Pertinent Patient Information to be Obtained Before Uterine Evacuation

- Age, gravidy, parity
- Last menstrual period or other indication of gestational age
- Indication for procedure
- Any problems with current pregnancy
- Past medical and surgical history
- Past gynecologic history
- Outcome and problems in all previous pregnancies
- Allergies
- Drug/medication use

---

nancies; and (3) extraction procedures reserved for second-trimester procedures.

Nonsurgical techniques for uterine evacuation by labor induction using systemic (e.g., intravaginal prostaglandins) or intra-amniotic (e.g., saline, prostaglandins) abortifacients are not reviewed in this chapter. However, practitioners who use such nonsurgical methods must be prepared to use surgical techniques of uterine evacuation in cases of retained products of conception; retained placenta is a relatively common occurrence following labor induction methods. In addition, appropriate resuscitation or surgery in cases of hemorrhage, sepsis, uterine rupture, or perforation must be readily available for patients undergoing uterine evacuation by labor induction.

Menstrual Extraction

Interruption of pregnancies before 42 days following the last menstrual period can be achieved by the so-called menstrual extraction method, also known as menstrual regulation or minisuction curettage. This surgical technique was initially reported in the early 1970s, at a time when legal abortion was not uniformly available throughout the United States.[1,2]

Operative Procedure

Menstrual extraction is optimally performed within 2 weeks of a missed period. The procedure should not be performed later than 7 weeks' gestation, as this increases the risk for incomplete abortion, infection, and hemorrhage.[3] A narrow

cannula (e.g., Karmen cannula, Fig. 42-1) is guided through an undilated endocervical canal into the uterine cavity. In women who present with constricted cervical canals, minimal cervical dilation may be necessary to successfully introduce the cannula into the uterus; such dilation should thus be considered if the cannula cannot be easily passed into the uterine cavity. A 50-ml syringe is then attached to the Luerlock end of the cannula and the products of conception are aspirated by 20 to 30 rapid depressions of the syringe plunger. After aspiration, the catheter is removed under continuous maximum negative pressure.

Aspirated contents are then placed in a Petri dish containing a small amount of sterile water or saline in order to view the aspirate for placental tissue. Absence of such tissue may indicate incomplete abortion, ectopic pregnancy, or a more advanced gestation. Appropriate diagnostic measures (e.g., ultrasound, serial human chorionic gonadotropin (hCG) assays, serum progesterone assay) should be initiated on failure to obtain placental tissue. Rh-immune globulin should be administered to all unsensitized Rh-negative patients undergoing menstrual extraction. In addition, consideration of prophylactic antibiotics (e.g., tetracycline) is warranted either before or following menstrual extraction. Patients should be informed that passage of small amounts of tissue and blood via the vagina can be expected following menstrual extraction. Physicians should be contacted if the patient begins to bleed heavily or develops fever or abdominal pain.

Complications

In the 1980s, unfavorable experience with menstrual extraction led most obstetrician-gynecologists in the United States to abandon this procedure. Because menstrual extraction is performed so soon after a missed menstrual period, one problem was that the procedure was unwittingly performed on many nonpregnant women (27 to 59 percent).[4,5] Another problem was that failure rates from incomplete abortion or a continuing viable pregnancy were 10 to 11 percent.[3–5] Moreover, operative complications (e.g., infection, hemorrhage, uterine perforation) were similar to first-trimester suction curettage.[6] Many of the potential advantages of menstrual extraction over first-trimester suction curettage were thus negated, and with the widespread availability of suction curettage, menstrual extraction was, for the most part, abandoned.

Nonetheless, the procedure is still performed by some physicians in the United States and is utilized in some developing countries where few other resources are available or where hospital-based or ambulatory pregnancy termination is not readily available.[3] Although the original technique described in the 1970s did not utilize concurrent ultrasonography, a recent study by Caspi and colleagues[7] demonstrates the benefits of concurrent ultrasonography for menstrual extraction, with decreased rates of complications compared to

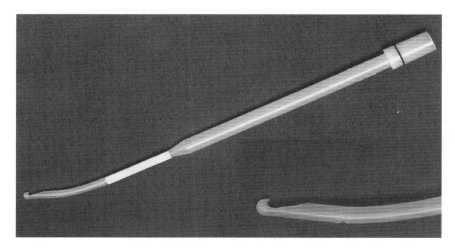

Fig. 42-1. Karmen cannula used for menstrual evacuation. Note curved tip of cannula (insert).

conventional menstrual extraction techniques. However, renewed interest in menstrual extraction will invariably depend on issues such as cost-benefit analysis and the feasibility of training practitioners in this surgical technique.

Suction Curettage

Suction curettage is the most commonly used method for pregnancy termination in the United States today.[3,8] The procedure is usually performed between the 7th and 13th menstrual weeks and does not require hospitalization except in high-risk cases (e.g., patient with a bleeding disorder). Unlike menstrual extraction, suction curettage usually requires cervical dilation.

Operative Procedure

Dilation

The endocervical canal can be manually dilated using instrument sets having progressively increasing diameters (e.g., Pratt dilators, Hegar dilators) (Fig. 42-2). Alternatively, synthetic dilators (e.g., Dilapan (polyacrylonitrile), Lamicel gnesium sulfate sponge), or the seaweed, *laminaria japonicum* (laminaria)), can be used. These osmotic dilators serve to gradually dilate the endocervical canal by absorbing cervical moisture. This uptake in water and the resulting expansion of the dilator produces both a softening of the cervix and dilation of the endocervical canal to 2 to 3 times the original diameter. Another benefit of dilation using osmotic dilators is the release of endogenous prostaglandins that "soften" the cervix and further facilitate the dilation process.[9] However, unlike manual dilation that is performed immediately before evacuation, use of osmotic dilators requires a period of time, depending on the specific dilator, before dilation is accomplished and evacuation can be performed.

Schulz and colleagues[10] showed that procedures utilizing laminaria resulted in a fivefold reduction in cervical lacerations when compared to manual dilation. Our clinical experience indicates similar dilating efficiency between Lamicel and laminaria, with Lamicel tents resulting in adequate dilation in a shorter interval (4 to 6 hours) than laminaria tents (12 to 14 hours). Antiprogesterone agents such as RU-486 and systemic prostaglandins have also been shown to be effective in promoting cervical dilation for uterine evacuation[11] and may facilitate manual and osmotic dilation.

Anesthesia

If manual dilation is used to dilate the cervix, placement of a paracervical block is appropriate before dilation; xylocaine *without* epinephrine is one agent commonly used. If laminaria or synthetic dilators are used, a paracervical block can be deferred until their removal. Some operators add synthetic vasopressin (Pitressin) or other vasoactive substances to the injectable anesthetic to reduce intraoperative blood loss, although the safety and efficacy of this practice is, as yet, not determined (Koplic L, personal communication, 1990). The paracervical block is placed by injecting approximately 3 to 5 ml of anesthetic agent into the cervical mucosa at the 4- and 8-o'clock positions (Fig. 42-3). Before injecting, negative pressure should be placed on the syringe to assess whether the needle is within a blood vessel; if blood returns on negative pressure, the needle should be removed and replaced in a different area of the cervical mucosa. Regardless of the anesthetic or vasoactive agent used, vasovagal syncope, or "cervical shock" can occur after administration of a paracervical block. Although the patient may appear to have had a seizure, vasovagal syncope is self-limited and is differentiated from seizure activity by bradycardia, rapid recovery, and lack of a postictal state. Atropine can be used to treat such a patient or can be added to the administered anesthetic agent to prevent vasovagal syncope.[12]

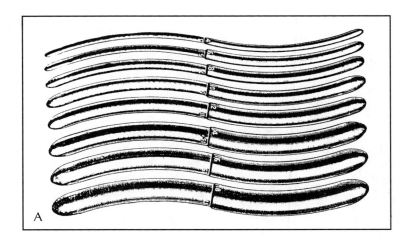

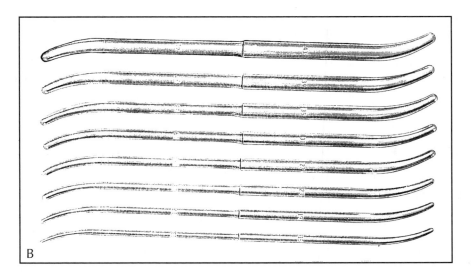

Fig. 42-2. (A) Hegar dilators. **(B)** Pratt dilators.

Curettage

Once dilation of the endocervical canal has been achieved, a nonflexible curved suction curette (Fig. 42-4) is inserted into the uterine cavity; this insertion is done without suction being applied. Choice of suction curette size is dependent on gestational age. At the authors' center, the size of the suction curette usually equals the gestational age (in weeks) of the pregnancy. For example, a #8 suction curette (8-mm diameter) would be used to evacuate a 8-week (menstrual weeks) size uterus. A transparent polyethylene tubing connects the curette to the collection vessel once the curette is within the uterine cavity. Suction is then applied using an aspiration device (e.g., Model VH-II Aspiration Machine, Berkeley Bio-Medical Engineering, Inc., Berkeley, CA). The curette is rotated on its axis with little motion along the longitudinal axis of insertion during tissue aspiration; this reduces the likelihood of instrument perforation of the uter-

ine fundus (Fig. 42-5). When no further tissue can be aspirated, the curette is withdrawn under continuous suction. A metal curette may then be used to gently curette the endometrial cavity to verify that all products of conception have been removed. The sharp metal curette used for this purpose should be the largest curette that easily passes through the cervical canal. If products remain within the cavity after sharp curettage, suction curettage is repeated.[13]

Postoperative Care

All products of conception are sent to the pathology department for evaluation. Following the procedure, patients are monitored for 30 minutes for hemorrhage or changes in vital signs. Women who are Rh-negative and unsensitized should receive 300 μg Rh-immune globulin following the procedure. Prophylactic antibiotics (eg., doxycycline 100 mg or-

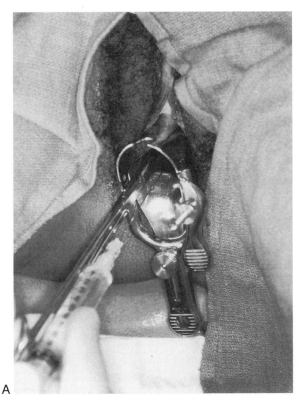

A

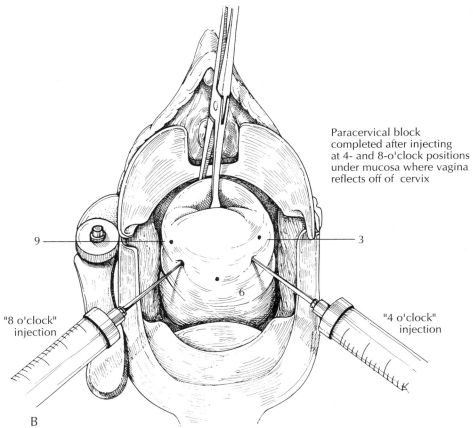

Paracervical block
completed after injecting
at 4- and 8-o'clock positions
under mucosa where vagina
reflects off of cervix

9 —————— 3

6

"8 o'clock"
injection

"4 o'clock"
injection

B

Fig. 42-3. (A) Placing a paracervical block at the 4-o'clock position of the cervix under direct visualization. **(B)** Illustration showing close-up of block placement.

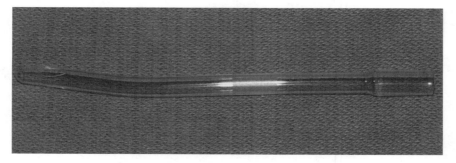

Fig. 42-4. Nonflexible curved #10 suction curette (10-mm diameter) used for suction curette.

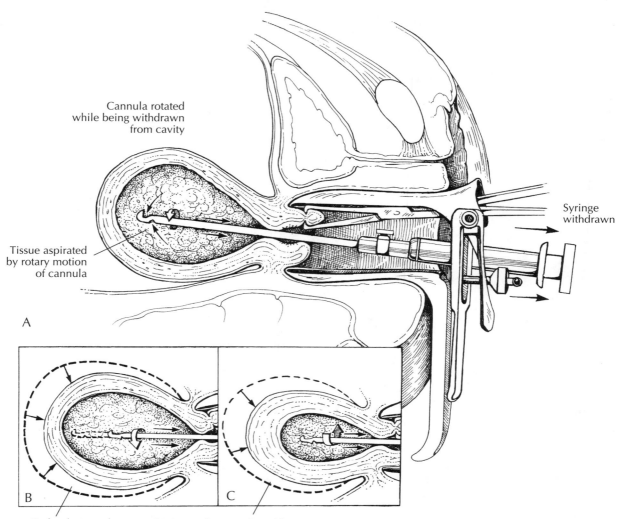

Cannula rotated while being withdrawn from cavity

Syringe withdrawn

Tissue aspirated by rotary motion of cannula

A

B

C

Body of uterus decreases in size as tissue aspirated from uterine cavity

Fig. 42-5. (A–C) Rotation of the suction curette. Little rotation should occur when the instrument is near the uterine wall, to avoid perforation.

ally, twice daily for 10 days) are effective in preventing infection[14,15]; accordingly, at the authors' center, all patients receive a 10-day regimen of tetracycline or doxycycline. Methylergonovine maleate (Methergin) is effective for decreasing postabortal bleeding resulting from uterine atony and helps prevent development of hematometra.[16] To decrease the incidence of this complication, the authors give patients a 5-dose regimen of 0.2 mg methylergonovine maleate to be taken orally every 4 hours beginning immediately after completion of the procedure.[13]

Complications

Immediate

Complications resulting from suction curettage can be categorized as being either immediate or delayed. Immediate complications include hemorrhage and uterine perforation. Postabortal hemorrhage may result from cervical laceration, uterine perforation, or uterine atony. Reducing the risk of cervical laceration can be achieved by use of cervical osmotic dilators (e.g., laminaria, Lamicel)[17] or careful manual dilation. The specific location of a uterine perforation, a complication more significant in the gravid than in the nongravid uterus, determines the extent of hemorrhage and expression of symptoms. A fundal perforation may go undetected as there is likely to be minimal bleeding, whereas a lateral uterine perforation may lacerate uterine blood vessels, resulting in immediate and profuse hemorrhage. In addition, a broad ligament hematoma may also develop as result of a lateral perforation and present as a delayed complication manifest by diffuse lower abdominal pain, pelvic mass, or maternal fever. The type of analgesia may also impact on the risk of postsuction hemorrhage. A study by Peterson and colleagues[18] found an increased risk of cervical laceration, uterine perforation, and uterine atony in women undergoing first-trimester suction curettage with general endotracheal anesthesia. However, Hakim-Elahi et al[19] found no increase in morbidity in women undergoing suction curettage with general anesthesia using methohexital.

The evaluation of a patient in whom uterine perforation is suspected depends on the presenting symptoms and the instruments used at the time of the suspected perforation. If the perforation occurred before the application of suction curettage, the patient would be observed for a period of approximately 1 hour for signs of hemorrhage, characterized either by profuse bleeding per vagina, change in vital signs (tachycardia, hypotension), or development of a broad ligament hematoma. If none of these signs or symptoms are demonstrated, the patient is discharged home and contacted within 24 hours. If any of these signs or symptoms are subsequently demonstrated, consideration of abdominal exploration is warranted. If the potential perforation occurred after the application of suction curettage, consideration of exploration is usually warranted. If abdominal contents are aspi-

rated into the suction curette, immediate exploratory laparotomy should be performed. Even if no intra-abdominal contents have been aspirated after a suspected perforation following the application of suction, consideration of abdominal exploration is still appropriate as intra-abdominal organic trauma may have occurred that could result in delayed, but severe, complications.

The extent and severity of the woman's symptoms will usually dictate whether laparoscopy or exploratory laparotomy is utilized. Generally, the more severe the symptoms, the more likely that hemorrhage resulting from perforation has occurred, necessitating exploratory laparotomy and repair of the uterine rent and possibly other proximal maternal structures. However, practitioners must be ready to utilize either laparoscopy or laparotomy depending on the events leading to the suspected perforation as well as the patient's own history and physical evaluation.

Immediate postoperative pain without overt bleeding via the vagina may indicate development of hematometra. Hematometra (also known as uterine distension syndrome or postabortal syndrome) usually presents with complaints of dull, aching lower abdominal pain, possibly accompanied by tachycardia, diaphoresis, or nausea. The onset is usually within the first hour after completion of the procedure. Pelvic examination reveals a large globular uterus that is tense and tender. Treatment requires immediate uterine evacuation, permitting the uterus to contract to a normal postprocedure size. Administration of intramuscular methylergonovine maleate (0.2 mg) is then given to ensure continued contraction of the uterus.[13]

Delayed

Delayed complications of suction curettage may be defined as those complications occurring more than 72 hours after the procedure. These occur in approximately 1 percent of cases and include fever, infection, hemorrhage, and retained products of conception, either separately or in combination.[19,20] Retained products of conception may present as postabortal bleeding, fever, midline pelvic mass, or pelvic-abdominal pain. Ultrasound can facilitate the diagnosis of delayed postabortal complications; regardless, any evidence of retained products of conception (e.g., enlarged uterus with fever or bleeding) should prompt the physician to consider suction curettage to complete evacuation of the uterus.

Many delayed complications should, in theory, be preventable. Careful examination of the tissue obtained by suction curettage can signal an unsuccessful or incomplete uterine evacuation procedure resulting from an ectopic pregnancy or retained intrauterine contents. Failure to obtain a sufficient volume of tissue necessitates an ultrasound examination. If an intrauterine pregnancy or remaining products of conception are visualized, consideration of concurrent ultrasound guidance to facilitate completion of the procedure is warranted. Women with suspected ectopic pregnancies should be monitored carefully with serial human chorionic gonadotropin levels. Although surgical interventions (e.g., salpingectomy, salpingostomy) have traditionally been used to treat ectopic pregnancies, nonsurgical regimens using methotrexate have been used with success.[26]

Summary

Overall, suction curettage is a safe and effective method of pregnancy termination. Hemorrhage, cervical laceration, and uterine perforation occurred in 1.1 percent of 42,598 suction curettage procedures performed at 8 weeks' gestation in a 1973 series reported by Tietze and Lewit.[20] These complications were even less frequent (0.06 percent) in a series of 170,000 consecutive cases reported by Hakim-Elahi et al.[19] The marked difference in complication rates between the two studies may reflect ongoing operator experience; Tietze and Lewit[20] published their report at a time when legal abortion was just beginning to become available in the United States with relatively few experienced physicians available to provide suction curettage. Hakim-Elahi et al[19] described the long-term experience of three large Planned Parenthood abortion clinics in New York City from 1971 (when abortion became legal in the state of New York) through 1987; most of the procedures were performed by experienced obstetricians. In this same study, the authors reported that only 1 in 1,405 cases (0.07 percent) required hospitalization because of incomplete abortion, sepsis, uterine perforation, hemorrhage, inability to complete procedure, or combined (intrauterine and tubal) pregnancy. In addition, minor complications such as mild infection, incomplete abortion requiring resuction in an ambulatory setting, cervical stenosis or laceration, or convulsive seizure resulting from administration of local anesthetic occurred in 1 of 118 cases (0.84 percent).[19]

Surprisingly, complication rates for suction curettage performed before the seventh week are apparently higher than for procedures performed between weeks 8 and 10.[3,20] Presumably this reflects difficulty in completing uterine evacuation as result of the small volume of the intrauterine contents, a problem commonly encountered with menstrual extraction. Conversely, suction curettage performed after the 13th week is technically more difficult and results in a higher rate of complications because of the larger volume of intrauterine contents. Finally, the setting at which the procedure is done does not appear to affect morbidity. Castodot[3] reported that suction curettage procedures performed in an outpatient setting resulted in low rates of morbidity and mortality, comparable to procedures performed within a hospital setting.

With regard to maternal mortality, suction curettage has the lowest maternal mortality rate of any surgical pregnancy termination method. In fact, the reported death rate is far less than the national maternal mortality rate of 9 per 100,000 live births.[12,22] Hakim-Elahi et al[19] reported no maternal deaths in 170,000 consecutive first-trimester suction curet-

tage procedures. The above-cited studies, as well as studies by other investigators[6,23,24] indicate that first-trimester suction curettage is the safest method for surgical pregnancy termination; second-trimester techniques of extraction, intra-amniotic instillation of abortifacients and hysterotomy or hysterectomy all carry higher mortality rates (Table 42-1).

Second-Trimester Extraction Procedures

In the United States, extraction is the most common technique used for second-trimester pregnancy termination.[8] Extraction has the lowest mortality rate of all second-trimester pregnancy termination procedures (Table 42-1) and comparable morbidity to other second-trimester techniques.[12] Second-trimester extraction procedures can be performed in an ambulatory setting, unlike those procedures that are dependent on initiation of uterine contents; accordingly, extraction procedures are less expensive to perform than labor induction techniques.[25] The psychological benefits of a rapid, outpatient method have also been documented. Kaltreider et al[26] reported that 30 patients undergoing second-trimester extraction experienced less postoperative pain, anger, and depression than 20 women undergoing labor induction methods. In addition, second-trimester extraction requires less time to complete than labor induction methods.[27] Despite the benefits of outpatient second-trimester extraction procedures, many physicians that provide obstetric and gynecologic services do not provide this procedure, either because they have not been trained in this technique or because of a misconception that labor induction methods are safer than extraction[12] (Table 42-1). Although labor induction methods do require less physician interaction with the uterine evacuation process than surgical extraction of the intrauterine contents, labor induction methods utilizing systemic or intra-amniotic abortifacients are not necessarily safer than extraction for second-trimester uterine evacuation.

Operative Procedure

Dilation

Second-trimester extraction requires dilation of the cervix. Although careful manual dilation can achieve sufficient cervical dilation to allow uterine evacuation in many cases, this technique carries a significantly increased risk of cervical laceration, hemorrhage, and unsuccessful uterine evacuation as a result of the need for more extensive dilation of the cervix due to the increased volume of intrauterine contents.[10] The preferred technique employs osmotic dilators, with many physicians using laminaria tents for second-trimester extraction procedures. Proper use of laminaria tents requires leaving them in place 12 to 18 hours to achieve optimal cervical dilation, thus necessitating a 2-day procedure; however, patients can be sent home following insertion of the laminaria tents. Alternatively, synthetic dilating devices

Table 42-1. Legal Abortion Death Rate[a] in the United States From 1972 to 1982

Procedure	Gestational Age (wk)						Total
	≤8	9–10	11–12	13–15	16–20	≥21	
Suction curettage	0.5	1.0	1.8	NA	NA	NA	0.8
Extraction	NA	NA	NA	3.6	9.5	10.4	5.1
Instillation	NA	NA	NA	5.0	10.9	11.7	10.1
Hysterectomy/hysterotomy	NA	48.2	33.1	62.6	80.9	115.1	44.8
Total	0.5	1.1	1.8	4.3	11.1	11.8	1.6

[a] Death rate is number of maternal deaths per 100,000 procedures.
(From Atrash et al,[22] with permission.)

(e.g., Lamicel, Dilapan) that achieve safe and optimal dilation within 6 to 8 hours can be used so that the entire procedure can be completed within 1 day.

Anesthesia

As with suction curettage, general anesthesia should be avoided, if possible, as it increases maternal morbidity and mortality.[28] Depending on the setting for procedure and the desires of the patient, systemic analgesics (e.g., nasal or intravenous butorphanol [Stadol]), morphine sulfate, nonsteroidal anti-inflammatory drugs (NSAIDs) such as ketorolac tromethamine (Toradol) or flurbiprofen (Ansaid), or epidural analgesia can be used for safe and effective analgesia in most cases. As with suction curettage, many practitioners administer a paracervical block, with or without a vasoactive agent, following removal of the cervical dilators and before uterine evacuation if general anesthesia is not used. Physicians should be aware of the infrequent maternal side effects observed with paracervical blocks (see the section, *Suction Curettage*). Accordingly, certain cardiac disorders (e.g., cardiac arrhythmias) may be relative contraindications to paracervical analgesia. In addition, the authors begin all patients on prophylactic antibiotics at the time of cervical dilation, and antiemetic and antianxiety medications are provided as needed.

Evacuation

Products of conception are evacuated using instruments specifically designed to extract intrauterine contents at this stage of gestation. The authors prefer either the Sopher (Fig. 42-6) or Bierer ovum forceps, although several other ovum forceps (Clemetson, Peterson, Barrett, Sanger, Moore, Forester, Van Lith, Kelly placental forceps) are applicable for uterine evacuation at this stage of pregnancy. Concurrent ultrasonography is also helpful in facilitating uterine evacuation.[29,30] Although ultrasound guidance is not essential for safe and successful uterine evacuation, we find that it often expedites the evacuation procedure, particularly in problematic cases such as when patients have severe uterine anteversion or anteflexion or uterine fibroids.

Curettage

After the products of conception have been evacuated, suction curettage is performed to remove any remaining tissue. The physician must examine the specimen to verify that all products of conception have been removed. Following second-trimester extraction, the authors observe patients for excessive bleeding via the vagina or changes in vital signs. Patients are instructed to expect some lower abdominal cramping, bleeding via the vagina (comparable to menstrual flow in volume), and possibly low-grade fever. Severe manifestations of these signs and symptoms may presage serious complications and require immediate evaluation by a physician. To prevent uterine atony, the authors provide patients with a 5-dose course of oral methylergonovine maleate (0.2 mg) started immediately after the procedure and continuing every 4 hours until completed. Rh-immune globulin (300 μg) is administered to unsensitized Rh-negative patients. The authors also personally contact patients by telephone 24 to 48 hours following the procedure, and arrange postoperative visits 2 to 3 weeks later.[13]

Complications

Uterine Perforation

The major complication of second-trimester dilation and evacuation is hemorrhage resulting from uterine perforation. As with suction curettage, severity of symptoms depends on the location and extent of the uterine perforation. Lateral perforations involving laceration of the uterine artery or vein are most dangerous because of the possibility of profuse hemorrhage. Other causes of hemorrhage include cervical or vaginal laceration, uterine atony, retained products of conception, or coagulopathy (apparently secondary to release of tissue thromboplastin into the maternal venous system during second-trimester extraction). Although ultrasound guidance, postoperative methylergonovine maleate and careful inspection of products of conception will reduce the incidence of intraoperative and postoperative hemorrhage, complications will invariably occur. Operators must be prepared

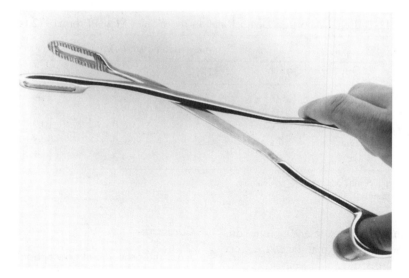

Fig. 42-6. Sopher ovum forceps used for dilation and evacuation procedures.

to administer necessary resuscitation maneuvers needed to stabilize such patients and manage their complications.

Infection

Infection is another serious complication that may occur after second-trimester extraction procedures. Antibiotic prophylaxis is effective in decreasing febrile morbidity in both first- and second-trimester uterine evacuation procedures.[14,5] Frequently, postoperative infection is the result of retained products of conception. If there is any evidence of retained products of conception, suction curettage should be performed to complete evacuation of the uterus. Ultrasonography may be particularly useful in the evaluation and treatment of such patients.

Summary

When performed by an experienced physician[31] second-trimester extraction carries significantly lower morbidity rates than those methods requiring labor induction or surgical procedures (i.e., hysterotomy, hysterectomy)[12,22,32–35] (Table 42-1). Kafrissen et al[34] compared the safety of 9,572 extraction procedures with 2,805 instillation procedures using an instillate composed of prostaglandin $F_{2\alpha}$ and urea. All procedures were performed between 13 and 24 weeks' gestation. Serious complications (fever of 38°C or more, hemorrhage requiring blood transfusion, or performance of unintended surgery as result of an abortion-related incident) occurred in 0.49 percent of patients undergoing extraction procedures compared to 1.03 percent of patients undergoing prostaglandin/urea procedures. Of all complications evaluated, only uterine perforation occurred more frequently in the extraction group. Among women undergoing abortions through the 15th menstrual week, Robins and Surrago[33]

found that 400 patients undergoing surgical extraction had a lower frequency of complications (i.e., blood loss requiring transfusion, cervical laceration, retained products of conception, fever, vomiting, and diarrhea) than 112 patients undergoing labor induction abortions by intravaginal prostaglandin suppositories.

However, similar rates of morbidity are observed when one compares extraction procedures to labor induction methods performed during the 17 to 20 gestational week interval. Peterson and colleagues[36] reported that the rate of unplanned hospitalizations resulting from extraction at 13 weeks was 0.6 percent, but was 1.4 percent at 20 to 21 weeks. Kafrissen et al[34] determined the relative risk of serious complications comparing extraction to prostaglandin/urea instillation abortions performed at 17 to 20 weeks' gestation to be 1.0. Thus, extraction performed later in the second trimester appears to result in morbidity rates similar to labor induction techniques. Choosing the best technique for second-trimester uterine evacuation will depend on the indication for uterine evacuation, availability of skilled personnel, and the advantages of extraction (e.g., outpatient procedure, less expensive to perform) compared to other second-trimester uterine evacuation techniques.

With regard to maternal mortality, second-trimester extraction is as safe for the woman as having a normal pregnancy and delivery,[37] a statement that cannot be made about other second-trimester pregnancy termination techniques. The Joint Program for the Study of Abortion (JPSA III) showed extraction to be associated with the lowest maternal death/case ratio when compared to instillation techniques or hysterotomy/hysterectomy[22,35] (Table 42-1). Maternal mortality rates associated with extraction procedures, as with maternal morbidity, increase with the gestational age at which the procedure is performed, and become similar to that of instillation procedures later in the second trimester.[35]

The authors believe that in addition to safety, the other benefits of extraction procedures (e.g., low cost, shorter time interval to complete abortion, lesser psychological stress for the woman) make extraction the preferred method for most second-trimester uterine evacuation procedures.

Those physicians who elect to use labor induction methods (e.g., intra-amniotic or intravaginal prostaglandin) after detection of fetal demise or for other pregnancy termination indications must be able to provide sharp and suction curettage or manual uterine evacuation using ovum forceps. Retained placenta or other products of conception occur relatively frequently following labor induction methods; inability to complete the uterine evacuation in a timely fashion could result in serious complications resulting from hemorrhage or infection. Determination of which evacuation method to use following an incomplete second-trimester extraction procedure is based on the gestational age of the pregnancy, the amount of tissue remaining within the uterus, and the operator's own judgment as to the best method for completing the procedure.

HYSTEROTOMY AND HYSTERECTOMY

Although hysterotomy and hysterectomy were commonly used techniques for uterine evacuation before the 1970s, they have essentially been abandoned as techniques for uterine evacuation because of high rates of associated maternal morbidity and mortality[38] (Table 42-1) and the ready availability of less invasive techniques. Hysterotomy refers to the removal of the fetus through an incision in the uterus, whereas hysterectomy refers to the removal of the pregnancy by removing both the uterus and the fetus as a single unit. In both cases, a midline abdominal incision from the umbilicus to the pubis is made and extended to the abdominal cavity. If a hysterotomy is to be performed, a vertical incision in the midportion of the uterine fundus is made and extended to the caudal portion of the uterus. Myometrium is then carefully dissected until the amniotic cavity is reached. At this point, fetus and placenta are manually removed and the uterus is carefully checked for remaining products of conception. The uterus is then closed in at least two layers; abdominal closure is performed in the same fashion as exploratory laparotomy. If a hysterectomy is to be performed, it is accomplished in essentially the same manner as a hysterectomy for an enlarged uterus. Surgeons should be mindful of the potential increased risk of intra- and postoperative hemorrhage because of increased vascularity resulting from pregnancy.

These procedures result in the highest rates of morbidity and mortality among first- or second-trimester uterine evacuation procedures (Table 42-1). However, there is bias in these data; frequently, less invasive second-trimester extraction procedures were not available, either because of a lack of skilled practitioners or the advanced gestational age of the pregnancy. In addition, only the very ill patient would be offered these procedures in the belief that such women would not be able to tolerate the 20 to 30 hours of labor needed for a nonsurgical uterine evacuation procedure utilizing intra-amniotic or systemic abortifacient agents. Accordingly, such patients would be expected to have higher complication rates regardless of the method used to terminate the pregnancy. Recently, a report by Bowers and colleagues[39] demonstrated the applicability of second-trimester extraction procedures for critically ill women requiring pregnancy termination between 20 and 24 weeks' gestation.

Hysterotomy is now justified only in rare cases in which systemic or intra-amniotic abortifacients have failed to terminate the pregnancy *and* no physicians skilled in performing second-trimester extraction procedures are available. Hysterectomy may be justified in very rare instances when the need for termination is accompanied by cervical, uterine, or ovarian pathology (e.g., cancer). However, the author's have not encountered such a need in over 15 years of clinical practice.

SPECIAL CASES

Fetal Demise

The uterine evacuation procedure and postoperative care provided to women carrying a nonviable embryo or fetus is essentially the same as that provided to women undergoing first- or second-trimester pregnancy termination. The exact type of evacuation procedure is determined by the estimated gestational size as determined by menstrual history, bimanual pelvic examination, and ultrasonographic biometric and gestational sac measurements. In those patients for whom the length of time of fetal demise is unknown, blood tests such as the pathrombin time/partial thromboplastin time (PT/PTT), fibrinogen, or fibrin split products are necessary to detect disseminated intravascular coagulopathy (DIC) and may prevent life-threatening complications arising from the coagulopathic state that can develop as result of a nonviable fetus remaining within the uterus.

Fetal Abnormalities

Chorionic villus sampling (CVS) and advances in high-resolution ultrasonography, especially endovaginal ultrasonography, allow first-trimester prenatal diagnosis of many fetal abnormalities. Accordingly, for those women who are carrying fetuses with abnormalities detected in the first trimester and who elect to terminate their pregnancy, suction curettage is the uterine evacuation technique of choice in most cases. However, maternal serum analyte screening for fetal neural tube defects and Down syndrome,[40] as well as most ultrasonographic evaluations[41] and genetic amniocenteses, are performed during the second trimester. Thus, the need for second-trimester uterine evacuation techniques remains because most fetal abnormalities are still not detected until the second trimester.

Although extraction is the most commonly used method of second-trimester pregnancy termination in the United States, the technique most commonly used for second-trimester pregnancy terminations performed after detection of fetal abnormalities is labor induction, either by intravaginal insertion of prostaglandin suppositories or by intra-amniotic instillation of abortifacient agents (e.g., saline, urea, prostaglandin).[42] A recent but informal survey of the seven prenatal diagnostic centers participating in the United States Collaborative Chorionic Villus Sampling Study found that most second-trimester genetic pregnancy terminations at these, and presumably many other perinatal centers, continue to be performed by labor induction methods.[43]

Despite the obstetric advantages of second-trimester extraction compared to labor induction, geneticists appear reticent to recommend extraction when women elect to terminate pregnancies after detection of congenital abnormalities. Perhaps this bias reflects a perceived inability to consistently confirm prenatal diagnoses following this procedure, as confirmation of prenatal diagnosis is essential for providing accurate genetic counseling in the future. The authors' experience[44–46] has demonstrated successful and consistent confirmation of prenatal diagnostic results by evaluation of products of conception obtained by second-trimester dilation and evacuation. Successful and consistent confirmation of prenatal diagnoses following extraction procedures requires pathologists, geneticists, and practitioners who have expertise in evaluating fetal tissue and who can utilize ultrasound and other surgical methods to obtain appropriate fetal tissues for confirmatory analyses. Although recovery of an intact fetus may occasionally be required to confirm a specific prenatal diagnosis, the authors believe that dilation and evacuation can be offered to most women electing to terminate a pregnancy because of fetal abnormalities. Avoiding a prolonged labor for these patients may also be of some potential benefit.

Hydatidiform Mole

Unlike most indications for first- and second-trimester pregnancy terminations, uterine evacuation following detection of hydatidiform mole should be performed within a hospital. All such patients should have ample blood product replacement (e.g., 4 to 6 U of packed red blood cells) readily available before uterine evacuation. Suction curettage should be used to evacuate the uterus, even when intrauterine volume is consistent with a second-trimester gestation. In cases of large (uterus of 12 weeks size or more) intrauterine volume, consideration of concurrent ultrasound guidance is warranted. Intravenous oxytocin and methylergonovine maleate should be judiciously used to prevent excessive hemorrhage during and immediately following the procedure. All postoperative women should be provided with antibiotic prophylaxis and a Methergin regimen to prevent infection and hemorrhage.

REFERENCES

1. Goldsmith S, Margolis AJ: Aspiration abortion without cervical dilatation. Am J Obstet Gynecol 110:580, 1971
2. Karman H, Potts M: Very early abortion using a syringe as a vacuum source. Lancet 1:1051, 1972
3. Castodot RG: Pregnancy termination: techniques, risks and complications and their management. Fertil Steril 45:5, 1986
4. Atienza MF, Burkman RT, King TM et al: Menstrual extraction. Am J Obstet Gynecol 121:490, 1975
5. Hodgson JE: A reassessment of menstrual regulation. Stud Fam Plann 8:263, 1977
6. Hodgson JE: Major complications of 20,248 consecutive first trimester abortions: problems of fragmented care. Adv Plann Parent 9:52, 1975
7. Caspi B, Appelman Z, Manor Y et al: Early pregnancy termination: an improved technique for 'menstrual regulation' with ultrasound assistance. Adv Contracept 8:349, 1992
8. American College of Obstetricians and Gynecologists (ACOG): Methods of midtrimester abortion. ACOG Technical Bulletin 109, 1987
9. Uldberg N, Ulmsten U: The physiology of cervical ripening and cervical dilatation and the effect of abortifacient drugs. Baillieres Clin Obstet Gynecol 4:263, 1990
10. Schulz KF, Grimes DA, Cates W Jr et al: Measures to prevent cervical laceration during suction curettage abortion. Lancet 1:1182, 1983
11. Darney PD, Dorwand K: Cervical dilation before first-trimester elective abortion: a controlled comparison of meteneprost, laminaria and hypan. Obstet Gynecol 70:397, 1987
12. Stubblefield PG: Pregnancy termination. p. 1303. In Gabbe SG, Niebyl JR, Simpson JL (eds): Obstetrics: Normal and Problem Pregnancies. 2nd Ed. Churchill Livingstone, New York, 1991
13. Shulman LP, Elias S, Simpson JL: Induced abortion for genetic indications: techniques and complications. p. 721. In Milunsky A (ed): Genetic Disorders and the Fetus: Diagnosis, Prevention and Treatment. Johns Hopkins University Press, Baltimore, 1992
14. Burnhill MS, Armstead JW: Reducing the morbidity of vacuum aspiration abortion. Int J Gynaecol Obstet 16:204, 1978
15. Levallois P, Rioux JE: Prophylactic antibiotics for suction curettage abortion: results of a clinical controlled trial. Am J Obstet Gynecol 158:100, 1988
16. Sands RX, Burnhill MS, Hakim-Elahi E: Post-abortal uterine atony. Obstet Gynecol 43:595, 1974
17. Atienza MF, Burkman RT, King TM: Forces associated with cervical dilatation at suction abortion: qualitative and quantitative data in studies completed with a force-sensing instrument.

p. 343. In Naftolin F, Stubblefield PG (eds): Dilatation of the Uterine Cervix. Raven Press, New York, 1980

18. Peterson HB, Grimes DA, Cates W Jr et al: Comparative risk of death from induced abortion at ≤12 weeks' gestation performed with local versus general anesthesia. Am J Obstet Gynecol 141:763, 1981

19. Hakim-Elahi E, Tovell HMM, Burnhill MS: Complications of first-trimester abortion: a report of 170,000 cases. Obstet Gynecol 76:129, 1990

20. Tietze C, Lewit S: Joint Program for the Study of Abortion (JPSA): early medical complications of legal abortion. Stud Fam Plann 3:97, 1972

21. Stovall TG, Ling FW, Carson SA et al: Nonsurgical diagnosis and treatment of tubal pregnancy. Fertil Steril 54:537, 1990

22. Atrash HK, MacKay T, Binkin NJ et al: Legal abortion mortality in the United States: 1972–1982. Am J Obstet Gynecol 156:605, 1987

23. Nathanson BN: Ambulatory abortion: experience with 26,000 cases (July 1, 1970 to August 1, 1971). N Engl J Med 286:403, 1972

24. Hodgson JE, Portmann KC: Complications of 10,453 consecutive first-trimester abortions: a prospective study. Am J Obstet Gynecol 120:802, 1974

25. Crist T, Williams P, Lee SH et al: Midtrimester pregnancy termination: a study of the cost effectiveness of dilatation and evacuation in a free-standing facility. North Carolina Med J 44:549, 1983

26. Kaltreider NB, Goldsmith S, Margolis AJ: The impact of midtrimester abortion techniques on patients and staff. Am J Obstet Gynecol 135:235, 1979

27. Grimes DA, Hulka JF, McCutchen ME: Midtrimester abortion by dilatation and evacuation versus intra-amniotic instillation of prostaglandin F2a: a randomized clinical trial. Am J Obstet Gynecol 137:785, 1980

28. Stubblefield PG: Midtrimester abortion by curettage procedures: an overview. p. 277. In Hodgson JE (ed): Abortion and Sterilization: Medical and Social Aspects. Academic Press, San Diego, 1981

29. Hornstein MD, Osathanondh R, Birnholz JC et al: Ultrasound guidance for selected dilatation and evacuation procedures. J Reprod Med 31:947, 1986

30. Darney PD, Sweet RL: Routine intraoperative ultrasonography for second trimester abortion reduces incidence of uterine perforation. J Ultrasound Med 8:71, 1989

31. Cates W, Schulz KF, Grimes DA et al: Dilatation and evacuation procedures and second-trimester abortions. The role of physician skill and hospital setting. JAMA 248:559, 1982

32. Robins J, Surrago EJ: Early midtrimester pregnancy termination: a comparison of dilatation and evacuation and prostaglandin-induced abortion. Obstet Gynecol 48:216, 1982

33. Robins J, Surrago EJ: Early midtrimester pregnancy termination: a comparison of dilatation and evacuation and intravaginal prostaglandin F2a. J Reprod Med 27:415, 1982

34. Kafrissen ME, Schulz KF, Grimes DA et al: Midtrimester abortion—intraamniotic instillation of hyperosmolar urea and prostaglandin F2-alpha vs. dilatation and evacuation. JAMA 251:916, 1984

35. Grimes DA, Schulz KF: Morbidity and mortality from second-trimester abortions. J Reprod Med 30:505, 1985

36. Peterson WF, Berry FN, Grace MR et al: Second-trimester abortion by dilatation and evacuation: an analysis of 11,747 cases. Obstet Gynecol 62:185, 1983

37. Rovinsky JJ: Abortion on demand. Mt Sinai J Med 51:12, 1984

38. DeCherney AH, Schwarz RH, Drobney H: Infection as a complication of therapeutic abortion. Pa Med 12:49, 1972

39. Bowers CH, Chervenak JL, Chervenak FA: Late second trimester pregnancy termination with dilation and evacuation in critically ill women. J Reprod Med 34:880, 1989

40. Phillips OP, Elias S, Shulman LP et al: Maternal serum screening for fetal Down syndrome in women less than 35 years of age using alpha-fetoprotein, hCG and unconjugated estriol: a prospective 2-year study. Obstet Gynecol 80:353, 1992

41. Rosendahl H, Kivinen S: Antenatal detection of congenital malformations by routine ultrasonography. Obstet Gynecol 73:947, 1989

42. Rayburn WF, Laferla JJ: Mid-gestational abortion for medical or genetic indications. Clin Obstet Gynecol 13:71, 1986

43. Jackson LG, Zachary JM, Fowler SE et al: A randomized comparison of transcervical and transabdominal chorionic-villus sampling. N Engl J Med 327:594, 1992

44. Shulman LP, Ling FW, Meyers CM et al: Dilatation and evacuation is a preferable method for midtrimester genetic termination of pregnancy, letter. Prenat Diagn 9:47, 1989

45. Shulman LP, Ling FW, Meyers CM et al: Dilation and evacuation for second trimester genetic pregnancy termination. Obstet Gynecol 75:1037, 1990

46. Shulman LP, Ling FW, Meyers CM et al: Dilation and evacuation for second-trimester genetic pregnancy termination: update on a reliable and preferable method. Am J Gyn Health 5:30, 1991

CHAPTER FORTY-THREE

DIAGNOSIS AND SURGERY OF BENIGN AND MALIGNANT DISEASES OF THE BREAST

CLAIRE M. CARMAN

As obstetrics and gynecology becomes recognized as a primary care specialty, the gynecologist can anticipate becoming more involved with the management of benign and the diagnosis of malignant breast disease. As a result, within the past decade there has been an increasing awareness of the need for breast disease to be an integral part of residency training in obstetrics and gynecology, so that residents who have completed their training demonstrate an understanding of screening, evaluation, and management of breast disease.

To lay the groundwork for both the practicing and resident physician, this chapter presents an overview of the management of breast problems. With an emphasis on patient self-screening and the multitude of treatment options available to patients today, it offers guidelines for a directed history and physical examination and indications for mammography, biopsy, and referral to breast surgeons.

EPIDEMIOLOGY

Breast cancer is the most common malignancy and the second most common cause of cancer deaths in women in the United States.[1,2] The most commonly investigated risk factors for the development of breast cancer include a positive family history, a history of certain types of benign breast disease, a variety of individual reproductive factors (menopausal status, age at menarche, parity, and age at first full-term pregnancy). The strongest association has been demonstrated to be a positive family history, with the risk being greater when the history involves a first-degree relative (mother, sister) than a second-degree relative (grandmother, aunt)[3]. Further studies have shown that certain recognized benign pathologic processes (i.e., atypical lobular or ductal hyperplasia lobular cancer in situ [LCIS])[4] and reproductive factors may further increase the risk of developing cancer in a population already at risk. In addition, some reproductive factors have an effect on risk that is independent of a family history of the disease.[5] Most distressing of all, however, may be the study of Seidman et al,[6] who have shown that more than 70 percent of breast cancer cases cannot be explained by established risk factors, indicating a continued need for adherence to the screening recommendations of the American Cancer Society.

The assessment of a patient's risk of developing breast cancer is multifaceted and not rudimentary. For instance, some risk factors, such as LCIS, completely negate the influence of other factors. The presence of two risk factors in the family history plus atypical hyperplasia (AH) carry far more risk than each factor independently. Risk factors are age dependent and not static over a patient's lifetime. As a patient ages, concurrent causes of death must be considered.

Based on data collected by the Surveillance, Epidemiology and End Results program of the National Cancer Institute, the incidence of breast cancer increased 32.5 percent between 1980 and 1987, with a less dramatic increase between 1987 and 1989.[7,8] The initial large upward trend has been attributed by several investigators to increased detection of breast cancer, especially of localized cases and small tumors, which is a result of an increase in public education, self-examination, and mammography use. The subsequent slight downward trend in number of new cases has been attributed to the universal acceptance of screening methods that increase detection of small or localized tumors.[7-10]

Although mortality rates for breast cancer have not decreased over the same time frame, survival times have increased.[7,8] This trend is also believed to be a result of detec-

tion at earlier stages of disease that are more responsive to treatment.[7,8] It is hoped that with the continued and more widespread acceptance and use of cancer control efforts, mortality rates will also eventually decline.

SURGICAL ANATOMY OF THE BREAST

The breasts are modified sweat glands located between the superficial and deep layers of the superficial pectoralis fascia (Fig. 43-1). The glands are composed of 15 to 20 lobes that are subdivided into lobules and acini. The lobules are connected to the nipple by ducts that dilate into ampullae as they converge onto the nipple. Several minute ducts then extend to and open into the nipple (Fig. 43-2). The nipple is surrounded by darker pigmented skin called the areola. Two glands that secrete lubrication for the nipple are located within the areola: montgomery glands (accessory areolar glands) and sebaceous glands (Fig. 43-3). The glandular and ductal tissues are surrounded by fat and fibrous septa, called

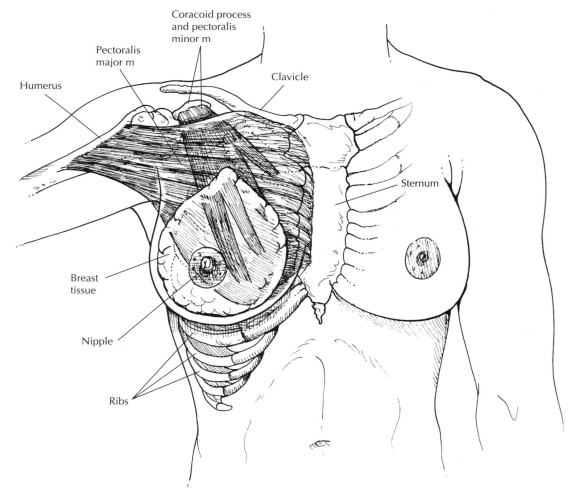

Fig. 43-1. Position and structure of the breast.

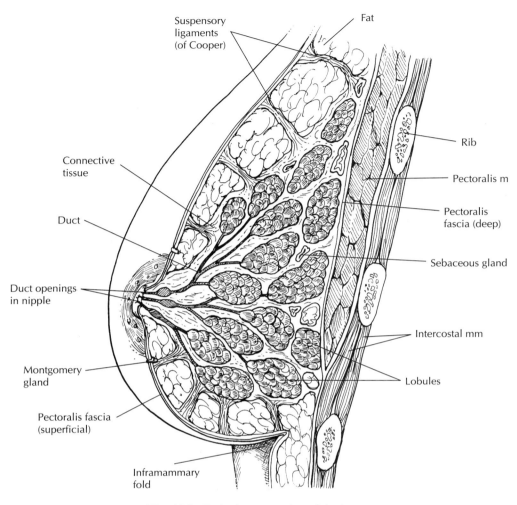

Fig. 43-2. Sagittal cross-section of the breast.

Cooper's ligaments, which attach superficial fascia to the skin (Fig. 43-2).

Figure 43-4 illustrates the blood supply and lymphatic drainage to the breasts. The principal blood supply to the breast is derived from the internal and mammary and lateral thoracic arteries. The three major pathways of lymphatic drainage from the breasts are the transpectoral, internal mammary, and axillary. The axillary nodes are divided into three levels. Level I lies to the lateral border of the pectoralis minor muscle; level II lies behind the pectoralis minor muscle; and level III is located medial to the medial border of the pectoralis muscle (Fig. 43-4). Axillary lymph node dissections of levels I and II are done for breast cancer staging.

Sensory innervation of the breast is supplied primarily by the lateral and anterior cutaneous branches of the second through sixth intercostal nerves. During surgery, caution should be used to preserve two nerves in the axilla: the long thoracic nerve of Bell (nerve to the serratus anterior muscle) and the thoracodorsal nerve (nerve to the latissimus dorsi muscle) (Fig. 43-4). The long thoracic nerve passes posterior

to the axillary vessels, and emerges on the chest wall in the medial portion of the subscapular fossa. Lying superficial to the deep fascia that overlies the anterior serratus muscle, the long thoracic nerve provides a posterior limit to the axillary dissection of the deep fascia. Injury to this nerve results in "winging" of the scapula and loss of shoulder power. The thoracodorsal nerve passes behind the axillary vessel, makes a medial approach to the subscapularis vessels, and then crosses anterior to these vessels to enter the medial surface of the latissimus dorsi muscle. As the nerve passes through the axilla it courses through the level I lymph nodes. Although injury to the thoracodorsal nerve is not associated with significant cosmetic or functional defects, if possible, it also should be identified and preserved during surgery.

DETECTION

All women should be educated by their primary care physician and gynecologist about the importance of breast self-examination as a means of detecting breast cancer.[8] In addi-

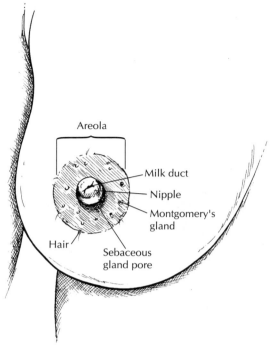

Fig. 43-3. Superficial nipple areolar anatomy.

Table 43-1. Staging AJCC Clinical Staging System

TNM

T—Primary Tumor
  T0 No evidence of primary tumor
  T1s In situ carcinoma
  T1 <2 cm
  T2 2–5 cm
  T3 >5 cm
  T4 Tumor any size with direct extension to chest wall or skin
N—Regional lymph node
  N0 No lymph node involvement
  N1 Cancer in axillary lymph node
  N2 Axillary node positive cancer matted
  N3 Supraclavicular node
M—Metastasis
  Mx Presence of distant metastases cannot be assessed
  M0 No distant metastases
  M1 Distant metastases (includes metastases to epsilateral supraclavicular nodes)

(From Blandt and Copeland,[18] with permission.)

tion, in 1993, the American Cancer Society reaffirmed its stated guidelines for routine mammograms as an important diagnostic tool for detection of breast cancer.[11] These guidelines, intended to apply to asymptomatic women of average risk, are age specific. For women between the ages of 20 and 40 years, a breast self-examination is recommended monthly and a clinical breast examination every 3 years. For women aged 40 to 49 years, a breast self-examination is recommended monthly, a mammogram every 1 to 2 years, and a clinical breast examination every year. Finally, for women who are 50 years and older, a breast self-examination is recommended every month, and both a mammogram and a clinical breast examination are recommended annually. In addition, the author recommends a clinical breast examination with the annual pelvic for women between the ages of 20 and 49 years.

EVALUATION

Radiologic Imaging of the Breast Mass

Radiologic imaging is an important step in the evaluation of breast lumps. It is important that the patient be referred to a facility that is accredited by the Food and Drug Administration (FDA); patients should be instructed to look for the accreditation certificate. In addition, the author recommends that each mammogram be interpreted by a radiologist who has received additional training in the interpretation of mam-

mograms. There are two different types of mammograms. One is a screening mammogram that is a four view mammogram of asymptomatic women. These mammograms can be performed within 15 to 30 minutes and do not require the presence of a radiologist. The second type is a diagnostic mammogram that does require the presence of a radiologist. A diagnostic mammogram is ordered when a patient notices a mass on self-examination or a change in her screening mammogram is noted and further evaluation is indicated. Special mammographic diagnostic techniques such as cone compression and magnification may be used, as well as ultra-

Table 43-2. Stage Grouping

Stage	TNM Grouping
0	Tis, N0, M0
I	T1, N0, M0
IIA	T0, N1, M0
	T1, N1,[a] M0
	T2, N0, M0
IIB	T2, N1, M0
	T3, N0, M0
IIIA	T0, N2, M0
	T1, N2, M0
	T2, N2, M0
	T3, N1, M0
	T3, N2, M0
IIIB	T4, any N, M0
	Any T, N3, M0
IV	Any T, any N, M1

[a] The prognosis of patients with stage N1a disease is similar to that of patients with stage pN0 disease.

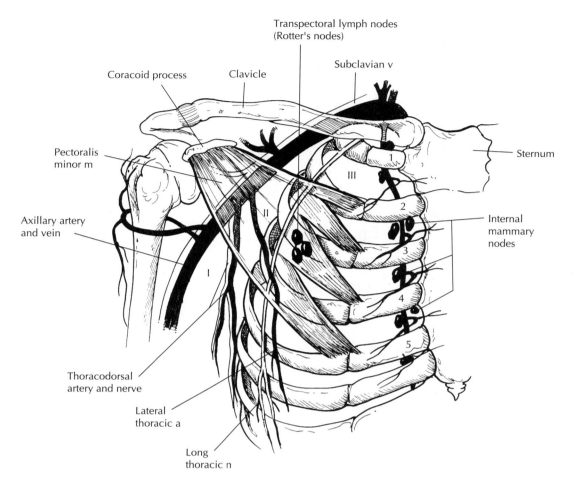

Fig. 43-4. Blood supply and lymphatic drainage of the breast (see text for details).

sound. The coned compression technique involves the use of a smaller paddle to spread out an area of tissue with more compression. This is useful to determine whether an area in question represents a distortion, overlapping tissue, or a true mass (Fig. 43-5). Magnification is beneficial for closer evaluation of areas of calcification and the margins of masses (Fig. 43-6). Frequently, these work-ups require additional time and should be scheduled appropriately.

Ultrasound is an effective adjunct to routine mammography. If a patient presents with a palpable mass or a well-defined lesion on mammogram, an ultrasound can differentiate between a cystic and a solid lesion. Many patients are under the false assumption that an ultrasound can be an alternative to a screening mammogram. This author explains to them that ultrasound is only used to differentiate between solid and cystic masses, and is not appropriately used as a screening tool. If the ultrasound demonstrates the mass to be a simple, asymptomatic cyst, no further treatment is needed. If the ultrasound demonstrates the mass to be solid, a needle biopsy may performed or a surgical biopsy recommended. Recently, 14-gauge core needle biopsies have been done as well as needle aspiration biopsies.

Neither light scanning (diaphanography and transillumination) nor thermography are recommended as screening or diagnostic tools for breast cancer detection or evaluation. Studies done to date using these imaging modalities are either limited in size or show unacceptable sensitivity and/or specificity results.[12]

For most patients, the radiologic examination should be performed before the physical examination by the breast surgeon. When a patient makes an appointment to evaluate a breast lump, and she has had a mammography, she should be instructed to bring her films and a copy of the radiology report to her first office visit. In cases in which the patient has not had a radiologic examination, and she is within the American Cancer Society guidelines for receiving a mammogram, she should be instructed to make an appointment for one before seeing the breast surgeon. At this point, the physician's office can guide the patient by either making the appointment for the patient, being specific about the type of images to be done, or directing the patient to a recommended facility and instructing her to point out the lesion to the technician before the imaging procedure. In cases in which the patient is younger than 35, the surgeon should examine

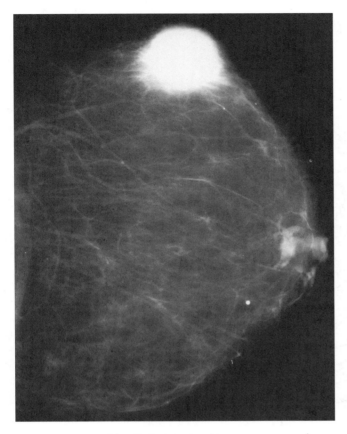

Fig. 43-5. Spiculated mass.

the patient before the radiologic examination, and make a recommendation depending on the level of suspicion. When a diagnosis of cancer is made, the traditional TNM staging system determined by the American Joint Committee for Cancer Staging (AJCC) is used as outlined in Tables 43-1 and 43-2.

History

A detailed patient history is an important component of the initial evaluation of a breast mass. The patient should first be questioned regarding breast self-examination and how the lump was discovered. The following questions should then be asked: how long the mass has been present, whether it has increased or decreased in size since it was first detected, whether it is associated with her menstrual period and/or changes in size during her menstrual cycle, and whether it is movable or painful. Answers can help make a preliminary diagnosis. Benign masses are usually moveable, may be painful, and change in size with the menstrual cycle. By contrast, a mass that is not painful and appears to be fixed is suggestive of a malignancy.

The patient should also be asked to recall whether or not she has had previous breast masses. If the response is affirmative, inquire whether they were biopsied, what the diagno-

sis was, and how they were treated. It is helpful to obtain a copy of the pathology report from any previous masses whenever possible.

Because there is a well-known increased risk of breast cancer in women who have a positive family history,[3,4] a detailed family history is meaningful. Paternal and maternal relatives who have had breast cancer, the age at diagnosis, and the age and cause of death should be noted. The number of women in the family tree who have had breast cancer is of consequence, as well as the incidence of associated cancers such as ovarian or colon cancer. Finally, whether the other family members who have had cancer were treated with chemotherapy and/or radiotherapy is a consideration, as it might influence the way the patient views her treatment options.

"Fibrocystic Disease"

During the course of taking a patient's history, it is not uncommon for her to mention a history of "fibrocystic disease." "Fibrocystic disease" is unfortunately not a diagnosis, but rather a loosely used term that refers to a number of breast conditions, ranging from normal physiologic changes to precancerous conditions, including the minor tenderness, swelling, and lumpiness most women experience during or before their periods; mastalgia (severe breast pain), cyclical or noncyclical, which interferes with the patient's normal life; infections and inflammations; discharge and other nipple problems; unusual nodularity; and dominant lumps, such as cysts, fibroadenomas, and atypical hyperplasia. Only cysts, fibroadenomas, and atypical hyperplasia are potential surgical problems. Unfortunately, however, many physicians still recommend abstinence from caffeine and other "folk remedies" for the condition, despite the lack of well-designed scientific studies to support these theories. It is therefore important to follow such a statement with a careful inquiry regarding the source and symptoms of this diagnosis, reassuring the patient that what has been labeled a disease is more likely the result of normal female physiology.[13] The best reassurance for women is always the demonstration, through careful screening, that there is no suspicion of malignancy in her breast.

Physical Examination

After the history is complete, a physical examination of the breast should be accomplished in both the sitting and lying positions, observing for external as well as internal changes. (Fig. 43-7). Externally, the skin is observed for any edema (peau d'orange), erythema, or retraction. If the nipples are inverted, the history of the inverted nipples should be documented. In the sitting position, any asymmetry, bulging, nipple retraction, or skin changes should be noted (Fig. 43-7A). The patient should raise her hands above her head, press her palms together, and lean forward, to aid in visualiz-

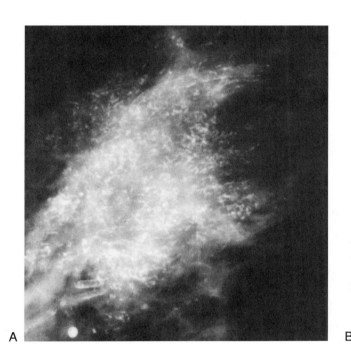

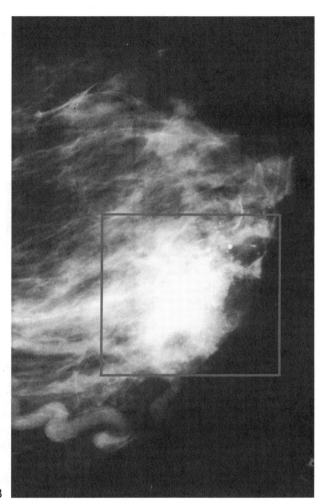

A   B

Fig. 43-6. **(A)** Magnification of **(B)** clearly demonstrating microcalcification of ductal carcinoma in situ (DCIS).

ation of the inferior pole (Fig. 43-7B). In addition, if the patient's breasts are pendulous, having her stand up and lean forward improves the view of the underside of the breasts. She is then instructed to place both palms on her hips and press in, to tighten the pectoralis muscle (Fig. 43-7C). This action tightens the Cooper's ligaments, and accentuates any dimpling that may be present. While the patient is still sitting, the superior poles of both breasts are palpated lightly in a downward sweeping motion (Fig. 43-7D), and then palpated for enlargement of supraclavicular, infraclavicular, and axillary lymph nodes (Fig. 43-7E).

Finally, the breasts are examined with the patient in a supine position, palpating each side both separately and simultaneously for comparison (Fig. 43-7F & G). The physician moves from one side of the table to the other, to determine if switching sides leads to an altered perception of an area of prominence. When palpating for the mass, it is important to carefully cover the entire area of the chest containing breast tissue, extending from the clavicle to the sternum, down to the lower rib, and lateral to the latissimus dorsi.

If a dominant mass is palpated, its position in the breast is noted (by its position on the clock) and measured. Other characteristics that should be documented are whether the mass is smooth, firm, rubbery, well demarcated, easily moveable, ballotable, tender, or attached to the chest wall or the skin. Malignant masses tend to be firm, irregular, fixed to either the skin or fascia, and not moveable when palpated. Benign lesions tend to be softer, smoother, and have more regular borders than malignancies, and are easily moveable. The measured size is then correlated to what has been seen on the mammography or ultrasound. It should be noted, however, that masses seen on the mammogram may not correlate to the area of palpation, or a mass may be palpated that is not noted on mammogram. In both these cases, a thorough evaluation of the mass is still indicated.

Also, the costochondral junction of the peristernal area and anterior axillary lines should be checked by pressing down on the ribs. This often elicits tremendous pain that is indicative of costochondritis, a source of breast pain easily treated with nonsteroidal anti-inflammatory agents. Because pain is an uncommon symptom of breast cancer, many physi-

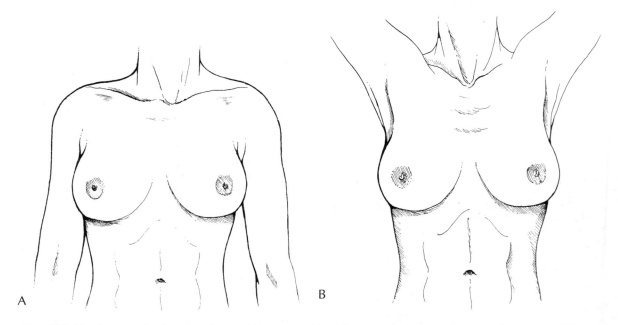

Fig. 43-7 Physical examination of the breast. **(A)** Arms at side. **(B)** Arms raised to visualize lower breast pole. *(Figure continues.)*

cians and patients have the misconception that if a mass is tender, it is benign. There are exceptions to the typical presentation, however, and all true masses should be completely evaluated.

The presence or patient report of nipple discharge should be evaluated. Most women will exhibit some discharge when their nipple is squeezed; the discharge is usually normal. Caution is warranted on physical examination, therefore, as many times women and/or their physicians will squeeze the nipple to see if there is a discharge, which may be an unnecessary, anxiety-provoking procedure. Although nipple discharge is a common complaint, the significance is variable depending on the nature of the discharge, and the physician must distinguish between physiologic and pathologic nipple discharges. Physiologic discharges are usually nonspontaneous, multiductal, and bilateral, and the color can range from clear and serous to a thick, green opalescence.

Some women are prone to discharges. Discharges are more common during puberty and menopause. Newborns may exhibit a discharge, known as ''witch's milk,'' that is the result of a normal hormonal process. In addition, some medication causes a nipple discharge, including birth control pills, antihypertensive medications, major tranquilizers, and H_2 blockers. Another instance will be the case of a pituitary adenoma that presents as a spontaneous, milky discharge, or galactorrhea. The prolactin levels and thyroid levels should be checked, and the patient referred to a neurosurgeon or endocrinologist.

There are instances when a nipple discharge is a legitimate concern. In patients who present with a spontaneous, persistent, and unilateral discharge, usually out of one duct, the presence of intraductal papilloma, intraductal papillo-

matosis, intraductal carcinoma in situ, or cancer would be suspicious. Approximately 4 percent of all cases of spontaneous, unilateral nipple discharges are cancerous. When a nipple discharge meets this description, evaluation for occult blood should be done. The author does not usually perform a Papanicolaou smear, as it shows only plasma cells and is rarely diagnostic of a carcinoma. If the nipple discharge is spontaneous, unilateral, and from one duct, regardless of whether it is demonstrated to be hemoccult negative or positive, a ductogram is done. A ductogram is performed with a radiologist, and involves injecting methylene blue and radiographic dye through a catheter into the duct, to map out the duct involved. A biopsy is then performed to dissect out the duct filled with blue dye, and the specimen is sent to pathology (Fig. 43-8).

Fine Needle Biopsy

For those patients in whom a mass is palpated or an asymmetry is noted on physical examination, a fine needle biopsy (FNB) is indicated. This simple procedure can be done in the office on the initial visit. After a brief explanation of the procedure, the breast is prepared with a cleansing solution of alcohol or Betadine. Although local anesthesia is not necessary for this procedure, the author prefers to use it, as many women who have had previous aspirations perceive those doctors who do not offer it to be unconcerned about the pain they are causing the patient. For this purpose, the author uses an infiltrate of 1-percent lidocaine hydrochloride into the skin over the lesion.

To perform the aspiration, the author uses a Cameco holder with a 10-ml syringe and a 21-gauge needle (Fig. 43-

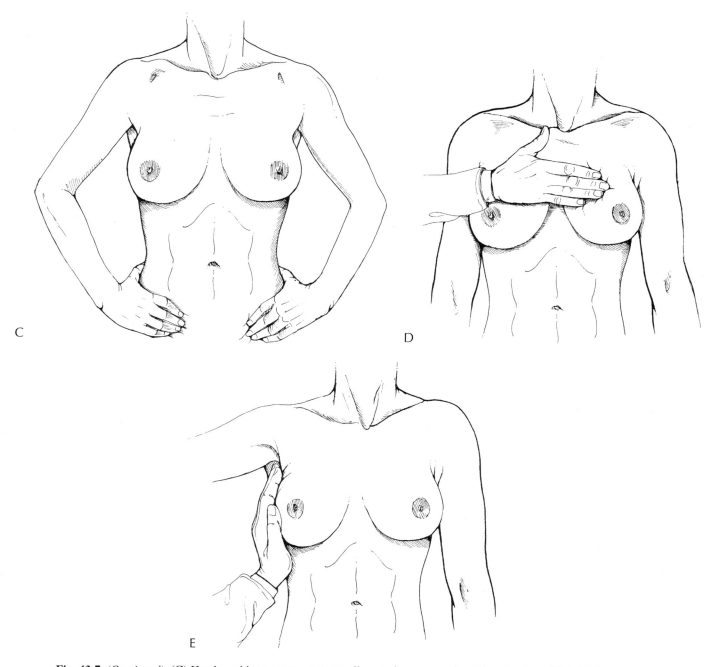

C

D

E

Fig. 43-7 *(Continued).* **(C)** Hands on hips to contract pectoralis muscle, accentuating skin retraction. **(D)** Initial breast palpation with patient in sitting position. **(E)** Examination of axilla. *(Figure continues.)*

9). This helps to accomplish a uniform aspiration, and reduces the strain on the surgeon's hand during the procedure. The needle is inserted into the mass, and suction is applied. Using a twisting motion, the mass is entered 10 to 20 times, or until there is enough fluid or material to fill the hub of the needle (Fig. 43-10). Once there is a small amount of tissue in the syringe, the suction is released, the needle is removed from the breast, and pressure is placed on the FNB site to prevent formation of a painful hematoma. The tissue

is immediately placed on two slides for smears, with an assistant standing by to apply the cytology fixative. The hospital cytopathologist is consulted regarding preference for specimen preparation. After the slides are prepared, the cytosol fluid is aspirated into the syringe to wash off any remaining cells, and sent to pathology for preparation of a cell block.

If, during the aspiration, a large amount of blood comes out, the procedure is immediately aborted by withdrawing

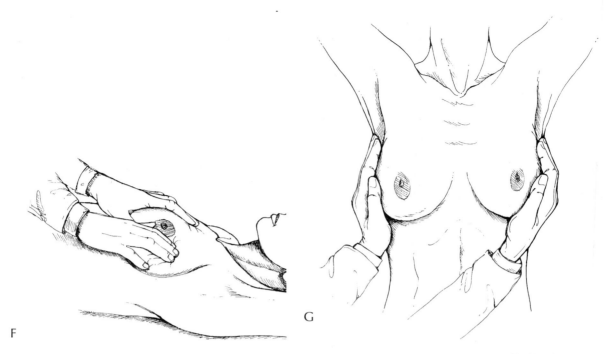

F

G

Figure 43-7 *(Continued).* **(F)** Palpation of breast in supine position with ipsilateral arm raised. **(G)** Simultaneous palpation of each breast to assess symmetry.

the needle and applying direct pressure to the mass. Depending on the physician's opinion about the potential diagnosis, the aspiration may be attempted from a different angle or the patient scheduled for an open biopsy. After the procedure, the patient is sent home with a written statement about the possible outcome of the biopsy (benign, malignant, or nondiagnostic) and its significance, as well as a reminder that definitive results will not be available for 2 to 3 days.

Follow-up on the results will vary between patients. A benign lesion frequently hugs a needle, while a malignant lesion may feel gritty. If the mass feels gritty during the aspiration, and the patient has a positive family history, even if the results were benign, an excisional biopsy is indicated. If the breast tissue hugs the needle during the aspiration, and the area feels like physiologic nodularity, the area simply is re-examined in 2 to 3 months.

All areas of suspicion need follow-up regardless of the results of the FNB. Patients are requested to attend classes on breast self-examination, and the importance of their participation in the observation period is impressed on them. If, during this time, the patient says the area has changed, or it does not go away, a surgical biopsy is indicated. It should be noted, however, that these areas frequently are the result of hormonal changes, and will resolve. In those cases in which the result of the fine needle aspiration was malignant, the author has the patient return to the office the next day to begin her education about breast cancer and discuss her treatment options, thus eliminating the need for a surgical biopsy.

Aspiration of a Cyst

If the ultrasound imaging and physical examination of the patient lead the physician to conclude that the mass is simple cyst (Fig. 43-11), and it is not bothersome to the patient, aspiration is not necessary. In cases in which a documented cyst is painful to the patient, the author will aspire it. If it does not, based on ultrasound, appear to be simple cyst or it has an intracystic solid component (Fig. 43-12), biopsy is indicated.

The breast is prepared for a cyst aspiration using the same techniques and rationale as described above for a fine needle aspiration. If a 7-megahertz ultrasound is available in the office, it can be used to direct the cyst aspiration. The color and opacity of the fluid that is aspirated should be noted. Clear, straw-colored, cloudy, or green fluids are normal for a cyst. The decision to send all specimens to cytology is controversial.[14] The author discards all fluid unless it is bloody, or the patient has a strong family history of breast cancer; these cases are sent to cytology. After the cyst is aspirated, the area around the lesion should be examined for an underlying or residual mass, and the findings clearly documented. If a residual palpable mass is noted, it should be biopsied.

In cases in which the fluid was sent to cytology, the patient will be given the pathology results as soon as they are available. In all cases, a follow-up is scheduled 3 months after the procedure.

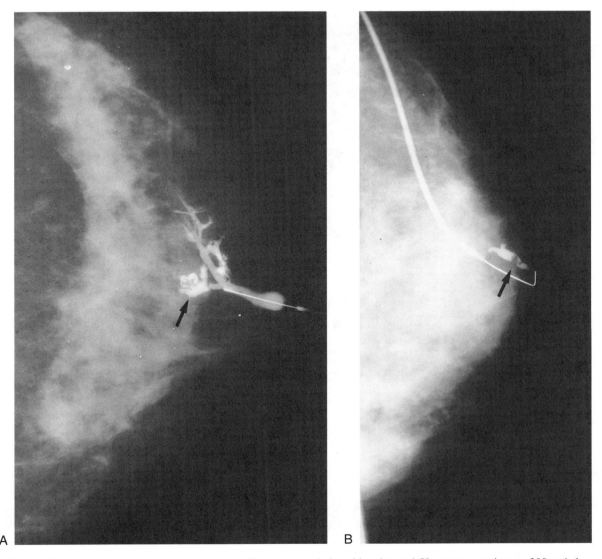

A   B

Fig. 43-8. A ductogram containing, by volume, 50 percent methylene blue dye and 50 percent omnipaque 300 ng/ml, helps to show the orientation of the breast duct. (**A & B**) An intraductal papilloma (arrow) is demonstrated.

Excisional Biopsy

Excisional biopsy is indicated for all dominant masses, unless proven to be a simple cyst. In cases in which the fine needle aspiration or aspiration of a cyst was suspicious, or a residual or underlying mass was noted, an excisional biopsy is also indicated. In those cases in which an excisional biopsy is indicated, it should be scheduled as soon as possible. Pre- and postoperative instructions are written at the time the biopsy is scheduled and read to the patient. A prescription for pain medication is also given, with instructions to have it filled preoperatively.

All excisional biopsies are done in the hospital, so that pathology can immediately process the specimens and, if the biopsy reveals a malignancy, the tissue can be properly processed for prognostic markers. The procedure is illus-

trated in Fig. 43-13. It is important, when planning an incision for a biopsy, to be aware that there is always the possibility of further surgery on the breast for either a partial or modified radical mastectomy. The incision should be made over the mass, to avoid contaminating a tunnel of tissue in the event that the mass is malignant. In addition, when planning the incision, it is important to keep in mind that women's clothing often allows exposure of the skin on their breasts in the triangular area between the shoulders and the xyphoid. To make the scar more cosmetically acceptable, the incision should therefore be in the least visible area. In the superior pole of the breast, the incisions should be parallel to the areola. Below the breast, radial incisions are acceptable; however, the triangular area between the shoulders and the xyphoid process should be avoided whenever possible (Fig. 43-14).

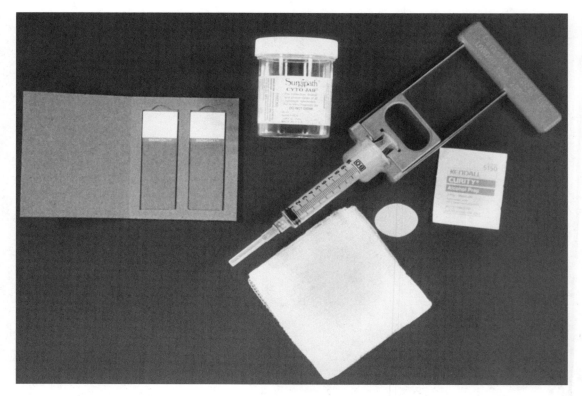

Fig. 43-9. A Cameco holder with a 10-ml syringe and a 21-gauge, 1.5 in needle is typically used for fine needle aspiration.

With rare exceptions, this procedure is accomplished under local anesthesia, with or without intravenous sedation (0.5 to 2 mg midazolam hydrochloride). After the mass is outlined with a sterile marking pen and the incision is drawn, the area is injected with 1 percent lidocaine with epinephrine. The patient will be able to feel a touch or any pulling sensation, and she should be instructed to alert the physician if she experiences any sharp pain, so that more lidocaine can be infiltrated. The author also prefers to keep the patient's face visible, to be aware of pain or discomfort in her facial expressions that she is not vocalizing.

The mass is then removed using scalpel or scissors. If it is difficult to adequately grasp the mass with clamps, the author places a 3–0 nylon suture for purposes of retraction. Electrocautery is avoided when removing the mass because it can cause a burn artifact, making it difficult to evaluate for the presence of cancer at the margins. After removal of the mass, it should be oriented for the pathologist. In the event that the specimen is cancerous, this also allows the surgeon a means of determining where more tissue needs to be resected, if the cancer is close to or involving a margin of the specimen. For this purpose, a long suture is placed in the lateral and a short suture in the superior aspect of the specimen, and a notation is made regarding the location of the mass (e.g., upper right quadrant, 1 o'clock, 2 o'clock).

The uncut specimen is submitted to pathology for evaluation of margins, and if found positive for cancer, hormone receptors and prognostic factors are evaluated. The biopsy is not sent for frozen section because these are not conclusive; and this author does not use that information to begin definitive treatment, but rather, waits to final pathology results, which are available in 24 to 36 hours.

The breast tissue is not closed, especially on the inferior pole. If the underlying breast tissue in the inferior pole is closed, it appears acceptable when the patient is lying down in the operating room, but leaves an unsightly, puckered appearance when she stands up (Fig. 43-15). The dermis is closed with absorbable suture. The epidermis is closed with a subcuticular running Proline that is removed one week after the procedure. Mastisol, steristrip, and a sterile pressure dressing are applied. The patient is taken to recovery, and discharged after her vital signs stabilize.

Needle Localized Breast Biopsies

Due to the widespread use of screening, suspicious lesions that were detected on mammogram often require biopsy before they are large enough to palpate. This requires sending the patient to the mammography suite before the biopsy for

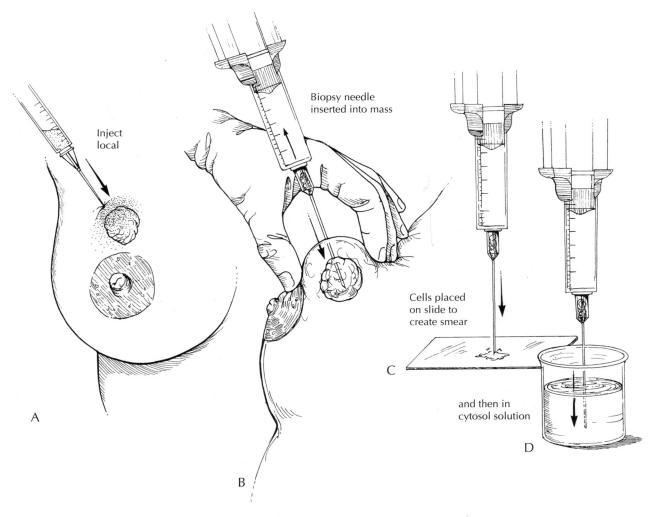

Inject
local

Biopsy needle
inserted into mass

Cells placed
on slide to
create smear

C

and then in
cytosol solution

D

A

B

Fig. 43-10. (A–D) Fine needle aspiration technique.

needle localization of the area of concern. The author explains this procedure to the patient in detail before scheduling.

This procedure involves positioning the patient in the mammogram machine. The skin is cleansed and anesthesized, and a thin wire is placed through the skin to localize the area of concern. To avoid the possibility of creating a pneumothorax, the wires are frequently placed tangential to the chest, instead of directly perpendicular to the lesion, and enter the skin far from the area to be biopsied.

The patient is then brought into the operating room, and prepared for surgery as described above for an excisional biopsy. When the wire has been inserted far away from the lesion of concern, a stiffening cannula is used to help determine the location of the wire tip (Fig. 43-16). The stiffening cannula is inserted over the wire, and using palpation and movement of the stiffener, the end of the localizing wire in area of concern is detected (Fig. 43-17). It is not always necessary to incise at the precise location where the wire

has entered the skin, and continue down along the wire, since the wire often is inserted in a visible location far from the area to be biopsied. An incision is made directly over the lesion, dissecting to the area of concern. A flap is raised to the wire, the cannula is removed, and the wire is gently pulled into the wound. The stiffener is replaced, and the dissection is continued along the stiffening cannula until the area to be biopsied is reached, usually at the base of the cannula. A benefit of the cannula is that it is not sharp like a needle, which could rip a glove and puncture the surgeon's finger. It also makes it more difficult to inadvertently cut the localizing wire and comes in assorted lengths for different lesion depths. The wire and area of concern are then sharply dissected free, oriented as described for an excisional biopsy specimen, and sent to radiology to verify that the microcalcifications or the mass of concern are present within the specimen. If the area of concern is present in the specimen, it is then sent to pathology. If the mass is not present within the specimen, the surgeon may attempt to remove

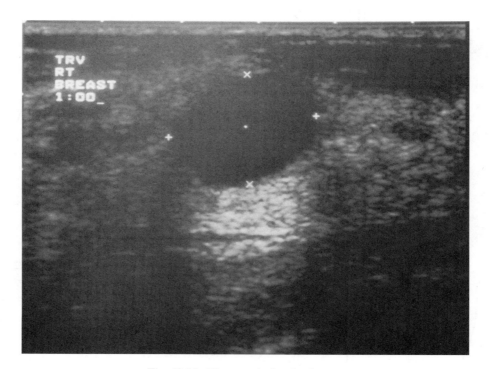

Fig. 43-11. Ultrasound of a simple cyst.

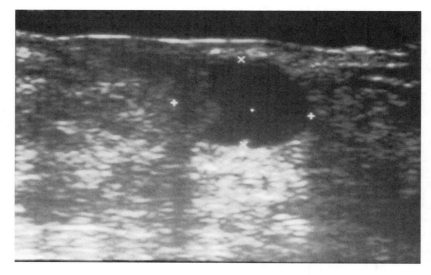

Fig. 43-12. Ultrasound of an intracystic mass.

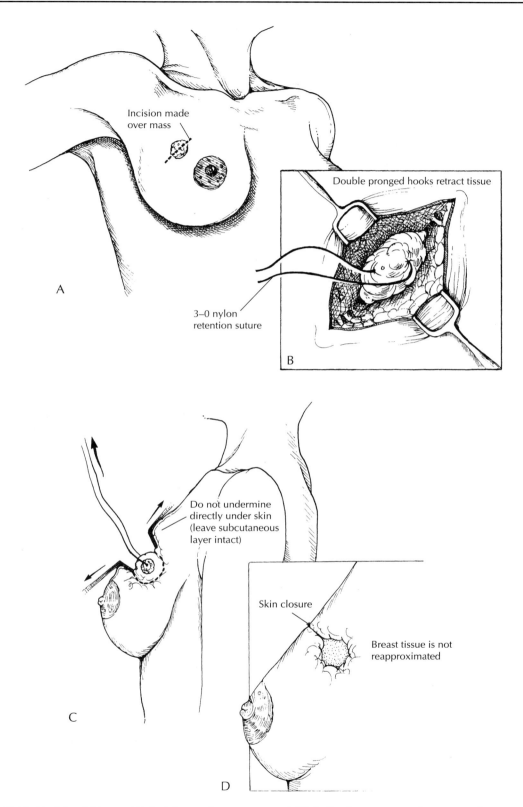

Fig. 43-13. Excisional biopsy. **(A)** Incision made over mass and **(B)** 3–0 nylon suture used as a retraction suture. **(C)** Undermining is avoided and the subcutaneous layer left intact. **(D)** Skin closure. *(Figure continues.)*

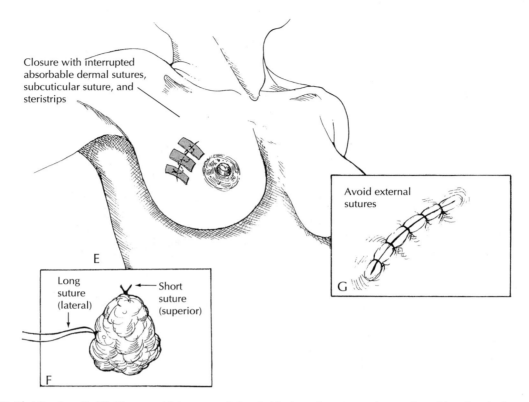

Fig. 43-13 *(Continued)*. **(E)** Closure with interrupted absorbable dermal sutures and a nonabsorable subcuticular suture with steristrips. **(F)** Biopsy is oriented with a long suture laterally and short suture superiorly. **(G)** External suture is avoided because it could leave suture marks for a poor cosmetic result.

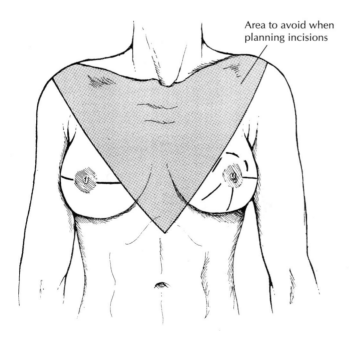

Fig. 43-14. Direction of biopsy incisions.

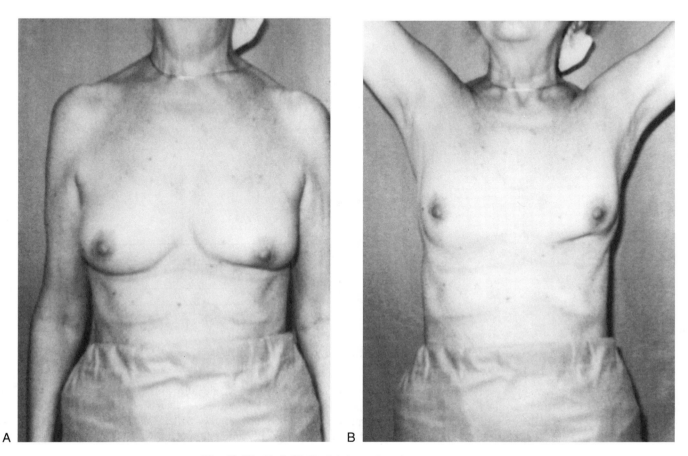

Fig. 43-15. (A & B) Unsightly puckered appearance.

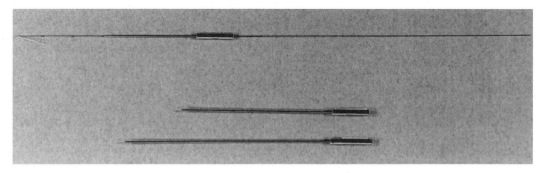

Fig. 43-16. Standard Kopans biopsy wire with different length stiffening cannulas. (Courtesy of Ranfac Corporation, Avon MA.)

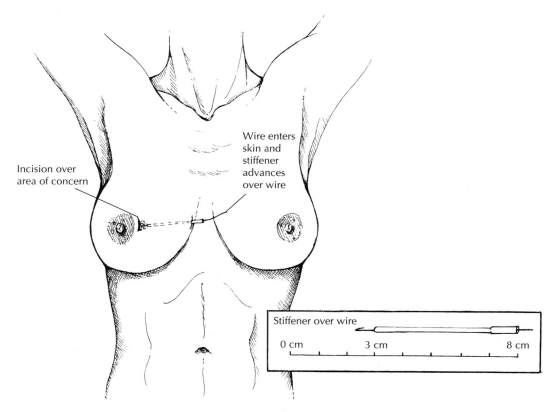

Fig. 43-17. Use of stiffeners to locate the area to be biopsied.

more tissue and process it as above. However, if this is not possible, another mammogram is scheduled in 4 to 6 weeks to determine whether the area of concern is still present. If it is, another mammogram localization for biopsy will be performed. The patient is informed of this unlikely possibility before the procedure.

Stereotactic Breast Biopsy

Stereotactic breast biopsy is an x-ray guided method for localizing and sampling breast lesions that were discovered on mammogram and are considered to be suspicious for malignancy. The technique uses digital mammography to image the lesion, which is sampled with a 14-gauge core biopsy needle. This avoids the surgical incision and alteration of the breast tissue. Over the past 15 years, its use in sampling small, nonpalpable breast lesions has been investigated in multiple series, and shown to have a sensitivity of 90 to 95 percent for breast cancer detection.[15]

The use of steroetactic breast biopsy is becoming more widespread. However, indications for its use are not well defined to date. Currently, the most common applications for stereotactic breast biopsy are for diagnosis of mammographic lesions that are most likely benign (in patients who are too anxious to wait for 6-month follow-up), and for diagnosis of malignancy in highly suspicious lesions (thereby avoiding biopsy and allowing a one-step procedure). The indications for the use of stereotactic breast biopsy operator dependent. The author believes that its use should be limited to surgeons and radiologists who have been trained in the technique and have had good clinical correlations from the results. Patients should also be informed that this technique, although avoiding the scar in the breast, only samples the lesion and does not completely excise it.

Ultrasound-Guided Biopsy

An ultrasound with a 7.5 MHz transducer may also be used to identify nonpalpable solid lesions that are initally found on mammogram. The area over the mass is cleansed and anesthetized with 1 percent lidocaine. A small skin nick is made with an #11 blade to allow the 14-gauge core biopsy needle (or 22-gauge needle to do an FNB) to pass easily into the breast tissue.

Under ultrasound visualization of the needle passing into the lesion is possible. When using a fine needle, the method used is similar as previously described for a palpable mass. When a core biopsy is done, the 14-gauge spring load needle is used to take five to six cores of the lesion. The wound is closed with a small steristrip and a bandaid. Presure is held to prevent hematoma.

Pathology results are available in 48 hours. An open biopsy is avoided if pathology is benign. If the results are malignant, an open biopsy is also avoided and planning for definitive treatment can begin.

TREATMENT OPTIONS

Education about breast cancer is of primary importance after a patient has been diagnosed with the disease. Treatments are divided into two major categories: local treatment of the breast itself and systemic treatment of the entire body (chemotherapy). The author believes that it is also important to include a third treatment: emotional support.

Emotional Support

A good starting point for emotional support is local breast cancer support groups. Where necessary, patients are referred to social workers to help them work out any family circumstances that need attention. An alternative approach for patients who do not feel comfortable in groups is found in a book by David Spiegel, Living Beyond Limits (Random House, New York, 1993).

Because many patients have had cancer for 6 to 10 years before diagnosis, they should be counseled that they have time to learn about the disease and seek second opinions regarding treatment options. Furthermore, they should be advised that it is no longer considered necessary to immediately perform surgery to prevent spread of the tumor, as it is well known that a tumor confined to the breast is not fatal, but that it is metastatic disease that is the ultimate cause of death.

Local Treatments

The local treatment options are partial mastectomy with axillary node dissection and radiation, and mastectomy with or without immediate reconstruction. A partial mastectomy is also called a lumpectomy, a wide excision, a segmental mastectomy, and a quadrantectomy. Many people are confused by the multiple names given to this procedure; the author prefers to use the term partial mastectomy, as listed in the Current Procedural Terminology (CPT) codebook.

Partial Mastectomy With Axillary Node Dissection

The National Cancer Institute stated in 1992[1] that, in the stages I and II of disease, a partial mastectomy with axillary node dissection is preferable to a mastectomy. This author has found that the ability to do a partial mastectomy is limited by the ability to remove the tumor with a 1- to 2-cm margin of normal tissue, and still maintain a cosmetically appealing breast. By contrast, in women with large pendulous breasts who actually would benefit from a breast reduc-

tion, the author has performed a partial mastectomy in conjunction with breast reduction and postoperative radiation. This enables the successful removal of large tumors in a woman with large breasts, and preserves symmetry with good cosmetic result.

More than 90 percent of the author's patients who undergo this procedure are treated as outpatients. All patients are seen preoperatively by a radiation therapist who explains the risks and benefits of radiotherapy, and helps to determine whether the patient is a suitable candidate for conservative surgery. The radiation therapist offers the patient a second opinion regarding her treatment choices, and this author always offers the patient the option of seeing another surgeon for a second opinion.

Tunneling through breast tissue to remove a carcinoma can present a problem to radiation therapists, in terms of providing boost doses. For this reason, the incision should be made directly over the carcinoma in a partial mastectomy. The same incisions should be used as described for a biopsy, with the tumor excised through an incision over the tumor. The tumor is removed in such a way that it is completely surounded by fat or breast tissue (Fig. 43-18). A wider excision may be made if a prior biopsy indicated a positive margin.

The mass should again be oriented for the pathologist with suture tags (short for superior, long for lateral), and the entire uncut specimen submitted to pathology for inking of margins. The author calls pathology department preoperatively to request an alert if any margins are grossly involved at the time of surgery. This provides an opportunity to go back and take a wider excision of a margin before closure. A portion of the tumor is also sent by the pathologist to test for hormone receptors and prognostic factors, if not accomplished at the time of biopsy.

Electrocautery should not be used to excise the mass because, as mentioned with the biopsy procedures, thermal injury makes histologic interpretation of the margins difficult to identify, and has been shown to decrease estrogen receptor concentration.[16] Once the specimen has been submitted to pathology, however, hemostasis may be obtained using electrocautery to avoid ecchymosis and hematoma.

Unless there is a large defect, the underlying breast tissue is not reapproximated, and the subcutaneous and subcuticular closure is performed without drains. If there is a large defect, the author develops flaps of breast tissue, and reapproximates them using a 3–0 absorbable suture. As with a smaller defect, the subcutaneous and subcuticular layers are then closed without drains.

The axillary dissection is accomplished via a separate transverse incision in the hairline at the base of the axilla, (Fig. 43-19). Care is taken to avoid extending the incision over the lateral border of the pectoral major muscle, which frequently leads to hypertrophy of the scar. The lateral border of the pectoralis muscle and axillary vein are then located, and dissection is continued down along the axillary

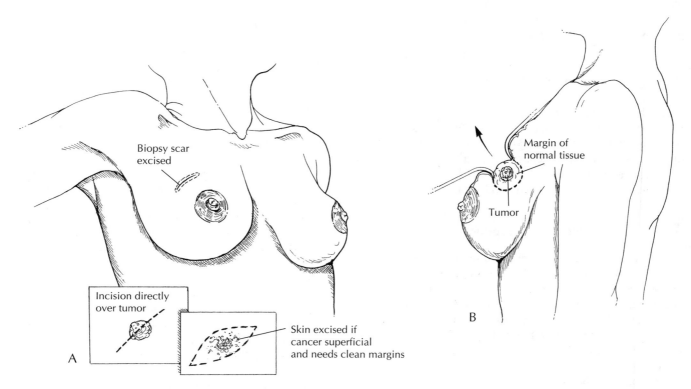

Fig. 43-18. (A) Biopsy scar excised, if present. If not, incision made directly over cancer. Skin is excised if cancer is superficial and needed for a clean margin. (B) Cancer mass with a margin of normal tissue excised or biopsy cavity excised. The amount excised is indicated by location of positive margins on biopsy.

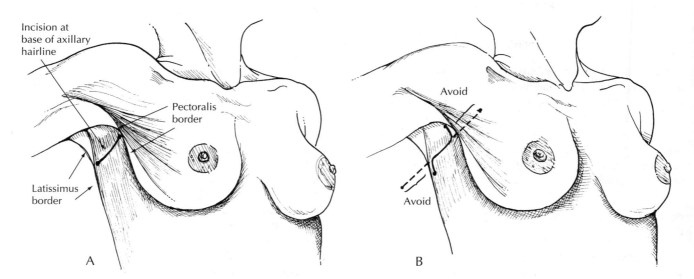

Fig. 43-19 (A) Incision made in base of axillary between lateral borders of the hairline pectoralis and latissimus dorsi. (B) Crossing the borders of the pectoralis or latissimus muscle the scar tends to hypertrophy. The incision is extended superiorly and inferiorly if more exposure is needed. *(Figure continues.)*

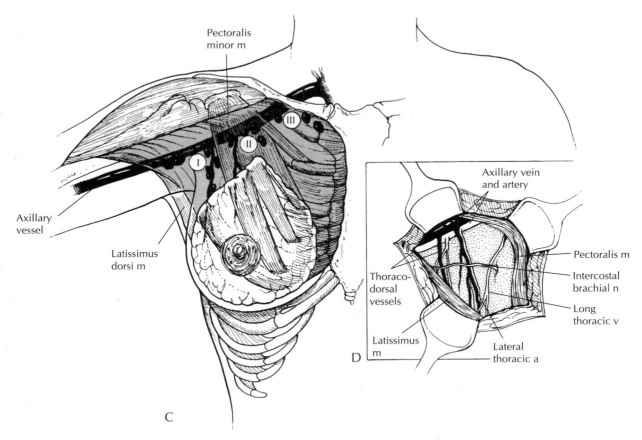

Fig. 43-19 *(Continued).* **(C)** Levels of axillary lymph nodes. **(D)** Fatty lymphatic tissue of levels I and II is removed. Superior border is the axillary view; medial border is the medial border of the pectoralis minor; lateral border is the latissimus muscle. The long thoracic vessels, thoracadorsal neurovascular bundles (for reconstruction), and intercostal brachial nerve are identified, if possible.

vein to the thoracodorsal neurovascular bundle. Slow, sharp, and blunt dissection frees the levels I and II lymph nodes from the axillary vein superiorly, pectoral minor medially, and latissimus dorsi laterally, while avoiding the intercostal brachial nerves that provide sensation to the skin of the upper posterior arm. The long thoracic and thoracodorsal nerves are identified and documented as functional and intact. After obtaining hemostasis with ties and pressure, the clavipectoral fascia is closed with interrupted absorbable suture. The wound is closed with interrupted 4–0 absorbable sutures, and the skin reapproximated with a 4–0 running subcuticular nonabsorbable suture that is removed 1 week after surgery. These closures are accomplished without drains. The wound is dressed with Matisol, steristrips, and sterile gauze.

After surgery, patients frequently want to know how many lymph nodes were removed, the assumption being that lymph nodes are discreet entities that can be removed one by one. The author explains to them that a fat pad was removed containing the levels I and II nodes; the actual number of nodes removed was a function of the extent of the dissection, the total number of lymph nodes, and how thoroughly the

pathologist has extracted the nodes from the fat pad. Often, after a patient finds out that the margins are clean or that there is no cancer in the lymph nodes, she assumes that she does not need radiotherapy. The author always emphasizes that the total chest area must be treated, either with a mastectomy or a partial mastectomy, with radiotherapy.[1]

As soon as the lymph node status, prognostic factors, and pathology are available, an appointment is set with an oncologist. Today, oncologists frequently recommend chemotherapy before radiotherapy. However, no official recommendations regarding the sequence and timing of radiotherapy and chemotherapy have been made. This is explained to the patient in a postdiagnosis discussion, and the radiation therapist and oncologist decide how they will proceed.

Radiation

Although local control can be obtained in some patients with surgical excision alone, no subgroups have yet been identified in who radiotherapy can be avoided.[1] After surgery, therefore, the remaining breast tissue is treated with radiotherapy. This treatment typically involves a total dose of up to 4,500 to 5,000 cGy over a period of 6 weeks. In addition, boost irradiation over the surgical bed has been used.

Systemic Adjuvant Treatment

Systemic adjuvant treatment of breast cancer in the form of chemotherapy and/or tamoxifen has been used to reduce the rate of recurrence. Up to age of 70, all women who have cancer in the lymph nodes are treated with some form of systemic chemotherapy. Tamoxifen is used in postmenopausal women of all ages, whereas its use remains controversial in premenopausal women. For node-negative women, an oncology consult is obtained to determine whether the risk of recurrence is greater than the risk of the treatment. The oncologist will advise the patient based on tumor size, lymph node involvement, estrogen and progesterone receptor status, and other prognostic factors.[1] The author refers all patients to an oncologist for evaluation, and encourages them to participate in the decision-making process.

Mastectomy

When women choose not to have a partial mastectomy with axillary mode dissection, or their disease is too large to remove and leave a cosmetically acceptable breast, a mastectomy is their only option. This can be accomplished either with or without reconstruction. The two basic types of modified radical mastectomy are skin sparing and nonskin sparing. The skin-sparing technique is used in cases where the patient has elected to have immediate reconstruction.

In a skin-sparing mastectomy, the nipple and areola complex are removed, leaving the surrounding breast tissue to act as a "skin brassiere," to hold in the material for reconstruction (Fig. 43-20). This preserves the normal skin and some degree of normal sensation in the chest wall as opposed to a delayed reconstruction or nonskin sparing mastectomy, in which the insensate abdominal skin must replace the removed breast skin, creating a skin paddle (Fig. 43-21).

To accomplish a skin-sparing mastectomy, an incision is typically made laterally, from the lateral aspect of the breast (to include the biopsy scar if present), and horizontally, to the nipple areola complex (that is included in the excision) (Fig. 43-22). A zig-zag incision allows for a larger opening and less trauma to the skin flap. If this opening is not large enough to remove the breast tissue, an incision can be extended vertically, at the 6-o'clock position of the breast. When performed in conjunction with a contralateral reduction, a Wise pattern,[17] an incision commonly used for breast reduction, is used (Fig. 43-23). The flaps are then elevated, dissecting the breast tissue away from the subcutaneous tissue of the skin, using either a scalpel, scissors, or electrocautery—superiorly, to the clavicle; laterally, to the latissimus dorsi; medial to the sternum; and inferiorly, below the inframammary fold. Finally, the breast mound is dissected free from the pectoral muscle, including the pectoralis fascia.

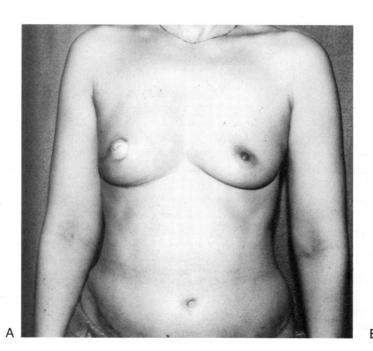
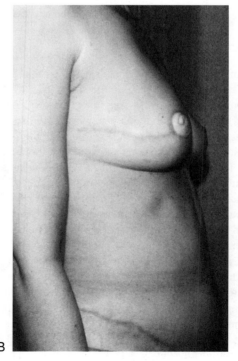

Fig. 43-20. (**A**) Skin-sparing mastectomy with free tram flap reconstruction. Note the abdominal skin in the nipple/areolar area. (**B**) Lateral view of skin-sparing mastectomy. Note scars on lateral aspect of breast and abdomen.

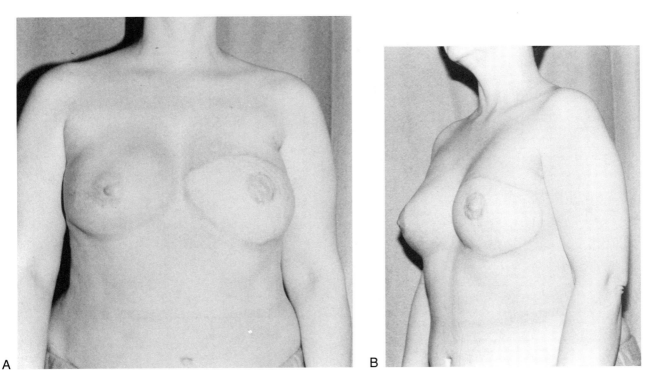

Fig. 43-21. **(A)** Delayed reconstruction with nipple reconstruction on a skin paddle. **(B)** Lateral view.

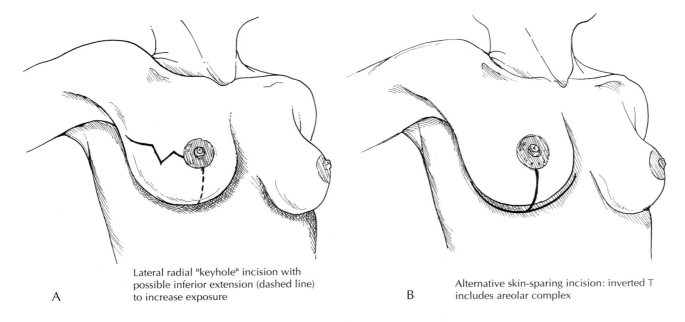

A   Lateral radial "keyhole" incision with possible inferior extension (dashed line) to increase exposure

B   Alternative skin-sparing incision: inverted T includes areolar complex

Fig. 43-22. **(A & B)** Skin-sparing mastectomy.

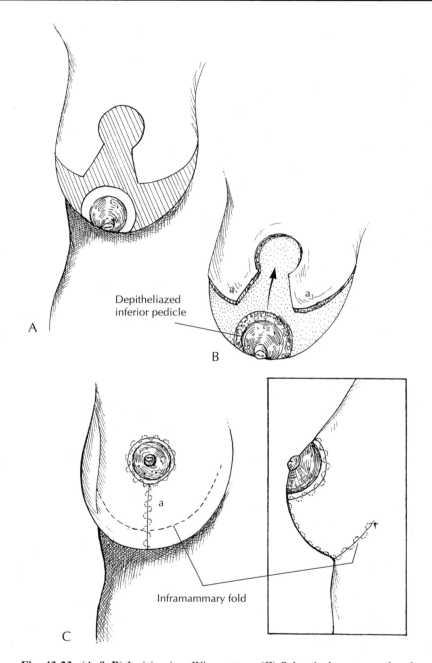

Depitheliazed
inferior pedicle

Inframammary fold

Fig. 43-23. (A & B) Incision in a Wise pattern. (C) Subcuticular sutures placed.

Next, attention is turned to the axillary dissection, which is accomplished as described above for a partial mastetomy with an axillary node dissection. Again, the thoracic and thoracodorsal nerves should be documented as functional and intact so that in the event that immediate reconstruction is planned using the latissimus or free TRAM (transverse rectus abdominis myocutaneous) flap reconstruction technique, the thoracodorsal vessels may be used for flap reconstruction of the breast. Drains are placed through a separate incision (one into the axilla, and a second under the mastectomy flap) and sutured into place with 3–0 nylon suture.

With the exception of drain placement, closure is accomplished in the same manner as described above for a partial mastectomy with axillary node dissection.

Breast Reconstruction

The issue of breast reconstruction is multifaceted, and the complexities of surgical choices and techniques are beyond the scope of this text. However, if a woman requires or chooses a mastectomy to treat her disease, she should be referred to a plastic surgeon preoperatively to learn about her reconstructive options. Because of the long-term emotional and psychosocial consequences of this disfiguring surgery, the author believes that the only reason not to have a reconstruction are that the woman is either not physically or emotionally able to tolerate the extended surgery, or she does not have insurance coverage for the procedure. The author counsels patients that immediate reconstruction is an option.

The method of breast reconstruction chosen is determined by patient choice and physician counseling, and is based on the size of the mass removed, the size of the remaining normal breast, body habitus, prior surgeries, and the expertise of the reconstructive surgeon. Breast reconstruction techniques commonly used today typically involve either tissue expansion followed by prosthetic implant placement, or autogenous myocutaneous flaps. Prosthetic devices currently in use in the United States include saline implants or silicone implants (still available at some institutions in controlled trials). The most commonly used muscle flaps employed for this reconstruction include a pedicle TRAM flap, a free TRAM flap, or a latissimus myocutaneous flap. Some patients are candidates for combined procedures in which implants are placed beneath flaps. To date, this author has not experienced delayed chemotherapy due to complications with immediate flap reconstruction.

Total Mastectomy With Axillary Node Dissection

In some cases, a patient may be in the middle of high-dose chemotherapy and not feel physically able to cope with reconstruction. In other situations the patient is not healthy enough to undergo a long operation. In these situations, the patient may choose to have a modified radical mastectomy, which the author prefers to call a total mastectomy with axillary node dissection (due to the traumatic implications associated with the use of the word "radical").

In a total mastectomy, an elliptical incision is made on the breast that includes the biopsy and the nipple/areola complex (Fig. 43-24). Flaps are created superiorly to the clavicle, medially to the sternum, laterally to the latissimus dorsi, and inferiorly below the inframammary fold, removing enough skin to close the skin flaps flat against the chest wall. Excess skin is removed to ensure a comfortable fit of an external prosthesis and bra. Excess tissue, or dog ears, are removed medially and laterally as much as possible. The axillary dissection is the same as described above for a partial mastectomy with axillary node dissection. Radiation is not typically required after a total mastectomy, unless the tumor is large or adherent to the pectoralis muscle. Use of adjuvant systemic therapies are dependent on the same prognostic factors as discussed above for a partial mastectomy.

BREAST INFECTIONS

Lactational Mastitis

Lactational mastitis is most common in the first month of lactation after the giving birth to the first child. The breast becomes painful, red, and swollen. The infection should be treated immediately with antibiotics (penicillin, a cephalosporin, or erythromycin), and drainage of the breast continued either by manual pump or breast feeding.

Approximately 5 to 10 percent of cases will develop an abscess. A unilocular superficial abscess may be successfully treated by needle aspiration of the cavity, and culture- and sensitivity-directed antibiotic therapy. A deep locular abscess may require surgical incision and drainage to break down the septa.

If surgical incision and drainage are required, the incision is made in Langer's lines, and the abscess is opened. The loculations are divided, and drains are placed. Women are frequently asked to stop breast feeding at this point. However, the bacteria in the milk do not appear to harm the child. Unless the mother is put on medication that is potentially harmful to the infant (tetracyclines, aminoglycosides, sulfonamides, or metronidazoles), women can nurse safely, if they so desire. The major impediment to breast feeding is that there is continued leakage from the drain site, and there may be a cavity that makes sucking impossible from the affected breast. In these cases, the infant can nurse from the contralateral breast, and the milk can be expressed from the affected breast.

Chronic Recurring Subareolar Abscess

Chronic recurring subareolar abscess is a fairly common infectious process of the breast in which patients present with a superficial abscess associated with cellulitis. Because it is difficult to treat, affected patients need to be forewarned that there is a high likelihood of the infection returning, despite appropriate therapy.

On the initial office visit, the author anesthetizes a small area to make a cruciate incision over the abscess, and evacuates the abscess cavity to relieve pressure and alleviate pain. This is followed by local wound care with wet to dry dressings over the next several days.

Two to three days after the acute inflammatory process is resolved, the patient is brought to the operating room under heavy intravenous sedation. A crescent of skin over the abscess is ellipsed, the areola is elevated, and the surgeon explores for the sinus tract. If a sinus tract is identified, the tract that communicates with the nipple is excised, as well as all the indurated, fibropurulent tissue. The area is packed, and wet to dry dressing changes done, allowing the wound to heal by secondary intent. In cases in which the patient has a chronic, smoldering, indurated area that becomes ery-

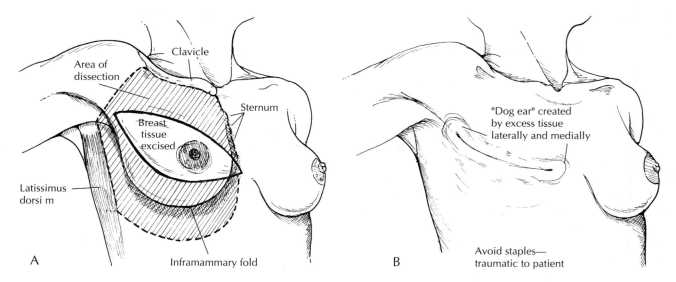

Fig. 43-24. Simple mastectomy. **(A)** Enough breast skin for a flat chest wall closure is excised, avoiding excess tissue medially and laterally. Gray area is the extent of dissection; superior to clavicle, medial to sternum, interior to below inframammary fold, lateral to latissimus dorsi. **(B)** Excess tissue medially and laterally ("dog ears") makes wearing prostheses more difficult. Additionally, avoid skin staples, as many patients find them psychologically traumatic.

thematous without frank purulence, the author tries to sharply excise the indurated area and primarily close the wound. Because the condition has a rare association with breast cancer, the tissue should always be sent to pathology for microscopic evaluation.

MACROMASTIA

Oversized breasts are termed *macromastia*. Women with macromastia often experience severe neck and shoulder pain that may be associated with headaches. They frequently develop grooves in their shoulders from the pressure of bra straps, with some experiencing numbness and tingling in their hands caused by brachial plexus compression secondary to the bra strap. Rashes commonly occur under oversized breasts from accumulation of moisture and lack of air circulation.

In cases of macromastia resulting in symptoms that interfere with activities of daily living, health insurance may pay for a breast reduction. Breast reduction is not considered a cosmetic procedure when done to reduce or eliminate symptoms. Although there are many surgical approaches to breast reduction, the resultant scar is generally around the areola, from the nipple to the inframammary fold, and along the inframammary fold.

HYPOMASTIA

Abnormal smallness of the mammary glands is termed *hypomastia*. This condition has no medical implications for the patient if left untreated. However, many women desire

augmentation for cosmetic reasons. There are several types of saline implants available today that can be placed in the breast for this purpose, as well as a number of different surgical approaches to accomplish the desired affect. A discussion of these techniques is beyond the scope of this text. Because of the recent controversy surrounding the use of breast implants for augmentation, it is important to encourage women to discuss the implications with their plastic surgeon before undergoing a corrective procedure.

It is important to note that implants decrease the accuracy of mammograms by blocking areas of tissue and obscuring the view. Women over 35 years of age should therefore have a preoperative mammogram, and any areas of concern evaluated with an ultrasound before augmentation. Women who have undergone augmentation with breast implants should have mammograms with an Eklund view to enhance visualization.

SUMMARY

With the current increase in awareness of breast cancer, women are presenting to this author's office more frequently with concerns that they have developed breast cancer, based on small changes in their breasts. By simply taking the time to explain procedures in detail and answer patients' questions, anxiety is alleviated for most women (Fig. 43-25).

Whenever it is necessary to surgically approach a patient, even for a biopsy, the author always considers the possibility that more surgery will be needed in the future. In addition, in the event that breast cancer is diagnosed, it should be kept in mind that the surgeon is just one member of a team of

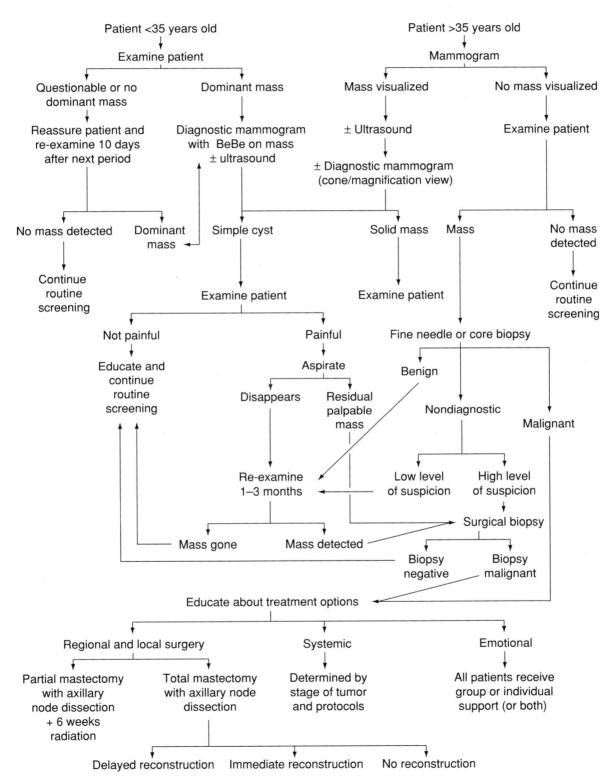

Fig. 43-25. Treatment algorithm for breast mass.

physicians treating the patient. Women are typically presented with a lot of information on which to base their decision about treatment, and cooperation between team members can also go a long way to relieve anxiety and help patients make the right choices for themselves.

Fortunately for women today, our understanding of breast cancer and the widespread use of screening are allowing for detection of disease at a earlier stage when it is more treatable. Awareness of breast cancer, and pressure to find causes and preventions continue to rise. We can only hope, for the sake of generations to come, that this trend continues.

REFERENCES

1. National Institutes of Health Consensus Development Panel. Consensus statement: treatment of early-stage breast cancer. J Natl Cancer Inst Monograph No. 11:1–5, 1992

2. Deaths from breast cancer—United States. MMWR 43:273, 1994

3. Sattin RW, Rubin GL, Webster LA et al: Family history and the risk of breast cancer. JAMA 253:1908–1913, 1985

4. Page DL, DuPont WD, Rogers LW, Rados MS: Atypical hyperplastic lesions of the female breast. CA Cancer J Clin 55: 2698, 1985

5. Anderson DE, Badzioch MD: Combined effect of family history and reproductive factors on breast cancer risk. CA Cancer J Clin 63:349–353, 1989

6. Seidman H, Stellman SD, Mushinski MH: A different perspective on breast cancer risk factors: some implications of the nonattributable risk. CA Cancer J Clin 32:301–313, 1982

7. Miller BA, Ries LAG, Hankey BF, Kosary CL, Edwards BK (eds): Cancer Statistics Review: 1973–1989. National Cancer Institute, NIH Publication No. 92–2789, 1992

8. Miller BA, Feuer EJ, Hankey BF: Recent incidence trends for breast cancer in women and the relevance of early detection: an update. CA Cancer J Clin 43:27–41, 1993

9. Garfinkel: Current trends in breast cancer. CA Cancer J Clin 43:5, 1993

10. Remington PL, Lantz PM: Using a population-based cancer reporting system to evaluate a breast cancer detection and awareness program. CA Cancer J Clin 42:367, 1992

11. Mettlin C, Smart CR: Breast cancer detection guidelines for women aged 40 to 49 years: rationale for the American Cancer Society reaffirmation of recommendations. CA Cancer J Clin 44:248, 1994

12. Bassett LW, Hendrick RE: Clinical Practice Guideline: Quality Determinants of Mammography. US Department of Health and Human Services, AHCPR Publication No. 95–0632:120, 1994

13. Love SM: The myth of fibrocystic disease. p. 76. In: Breast Book. 2nd Ed. Addison-Wesley, Reading, MA, 1995

14. Love SM, Schnitt JJ, Connolly JL, Shirley RL: Benign breast disorders. p. 21. In Harris JR, Hellman S, Henderson IC, Kinne DW (eds): Breast Diseases. JB Lippincott, Philadelphia, 1987

15. Schmidt RA: Stereotactic breast biopsy. CA Cancer J Clin 44: 172, 1994

16. Bloom ND, Johnson F, Pertshuck L, Fishman J: Electrocautery: effects on steroid receptors in human breast cancer. J Surg Oncol 25:21, 1984

17. Wise RJ: A preliminary report on a method of planning the mammaplasty. Plast Reconstr Surg 17:367, 1956

18. Blandt, Copeland: The Breast: Comprehensive Management of Benign and Malignant Diseases. WB Saunders, Philadelphia, 1991

CHAPTER FORTY-FOUR

QUALITY ASSESSMENT: A GYNECOLOGIST'S PRIMER

J. LAWRENCE COLLEY

At present, gynecologic surgeons confront not only illness and injury, but also the tumultuous transformation of their cottage industry into "big business." Payers are beginning to employ quality improvement methods that, although an integral part of business training, are not specifically taught in medical education or residency programs. Physicians are confronted with assessments, or "profiles" of their performance, and are asked by third party payers to verify their credentials with multiple hospitals and managed care organizations (MCOs). Disciplinary actions and adverse outcomes are recorded in computerized databases. Patient (customer) survey results, rather than "repeat business" are becoming the physician's benchmark for patient satisfaction. Furthermore, MCOs may expect physicians to alter their practice patterns to conform with clinical practice guidelines or utilization criteria originating from specialty societies, government, or the MCOs themselves. The purpose of this chapter is to present the gynecologist with an overview of the economic forces that are transforming health care financing and delivery. Additionally, this chapter provides exposure to quality assessment from the perspective of those who pay for medical care. (There are little or no data on gynecologic surgery, so examples are drawn from areas where such numbers are available.)

ROOTS OF ECONOMIC TRANSFORMATION

In the United States through the 1970s and 1980s, the health care sector of the economy expanded at two to three times the rate of the economy as a whole.[1] This is not a problem per se, as one should not expect all sectors of the economy to expand at the same rate. Indeed, as societies advance economically, basic items (e.g., food and clothing) consume proportionally less of their productivity and other items (e.g., consumer electronics, transportation, recreation, and advanced medical care) consume proportionally more. Health care has grown faster than the whole economy but its growth has not outstripped all other sectors. The personal computing industry, for example, has grown even faster than health care, but there is no call to restrain its growth.

Why is economic growth in other areas of the economy welcomed, while growth of the health care sector perceived as a problem? It is important to note that health care is distinguished from virtually all other goods and services in the that individuals purchase it indirectly through their insurance or prepaid health plan. Furthermore, most individuals do not choose or purchase their insurance or prepaid health plan directly, but receive an employer-sponsored plan in lieu of erstwhile monetary compensation. Employer-based coverage is so ubiquitous that it is accepted as a given, but its prevalence is attributable to the fact that the value of coverage-as-compensation is not taxed as income. The profound importance of this point cannot be overstated. The tax subsidy for employer-based coverage is the economic engine that has driven the market toward managed care and its attendant features such as quality improvement. The traditional economic paradigm for insurance as risk pooling for unpredictable large, expenses does not add value for the routine services that comprise the majority of health care spending. Women, for example, are not "at risk" of periodic examinations and Papanicolaou (Pap) smears, but instead expect to receive them. However, the natural tendency of the market to take maximum advantage of a tax break has led to coverage of low-cost and frequently utilized services.

When coverage includes services people expect to utilize, a fundamental shift in the economic paradigm occurs as a result. The customer is now paying in advance for services, not hedging against unforeseen catastrophe. When a service has already been paid for, there is no price sensitivity at the point of sale. In other words, there is no economic barrier to consumption and the customer (patient) does not care what the service costs. Both consumption (utilization) and cost (unit price) are unfettered, unless these is active management from outside the doctor/patient relationship.

It is sometimes erroneously stated that health care is not governed by the usual laws of economics, such as the law of supply and demand. However, any other sector of the economy would behave like health care if financed as such. If instead of purchasing groceries individuals purchased food insurance, they would behave differently in the grocery store. Grocers would respond appropriately by selling only the best food and charging more for it. Furthermore, if food insurance could be tax deductible as an employee benefit, most food insurance (and therefore, groceries) would eventually be purchased through employers. This untaxed sector of the economy would grow faster than the rest of the economy and would attract intelligent and creative entrepreneurs. Inexorably, the scope of employer-based food plans would expand to gain the tax advantage (e.g., by including restaurant meals). Innovative producers would create increasingly tastier, more elaborate, more convenient, and more expensive food. The more these items were made available to individuals, the more they would be consumed (i.e., supply-induced demand). This system would produce satisfied individuals, employers, and grocers for a time. But inevitably, the cost of this system would become burdensome due to the subversion of normal market restraints. Although quality would be excellent, the high price would demand perfection. The natural end to this unnatural scenario would find employers establishing prepaid food plans that limit choice, optimize nutritional outcomes, and restrain price. This fantasy scenario exactly parallels the evolution of health care financing in the United States. Managed care and its attendant quality improvement programs are a rational response to an irrational economic environment.

WHY ASSESS QUALITY

Quality assessment occurs for two reasons: to improve quality and to inform the purchasing decisions of consumers. Information about quality is used by the producer of goods or services for the purpose of *internal* re-engineering to optimize quality. Similar information is useful for the *external* projection of product attributes to the customer (as in the

Consumer Reports paradigm). As big business entities become both the producers and the purchasers of health care, one would expect the health-care industry to assimilate the prevalent big business culture of quality and value.

Continuous quality improvement (CQI) evolved in manufacturing industries, but now MCOs are adopting its methods. The essence of CQI is an ongoing cycle of measurement and optimization. Although traditional quality assurance employed a few specialists to reject inferior items at the end of production, CQI enlists the participation of all people involved in each stage of production. Thus, MCOs will look to all of their participating physicians to participate in quality improvement.

Quality assurance has long been a feature of manufacturing industries. The modern perspective of industrial quality has been profoundly changed by W. Edwards Deming, an American expatriate whose ideas influenced the transformation of Japanese industry after World War II. Because of Deming's influence, businessmen seldom speak any more of quality assurance, which emphasizes the achievement of a defined, finite, and static level of quality. The new paradigm is CQI,[2] which defines perfection as an ultimate goal (Fig. 44-1).

HOW TO VIEW QUALITY

The traditional and still valid framework for viewing quality in health care was established by Avedis Donabedian. He described quality in terms of structure, process, and outcome.[3] Outcomes are comprised of three major subsets: health outcomes, economic outcomes, and patient satisfaction. To illustrate Donabedian's structure, process, and outcome construct, it can be viewed in the context of a common gynecologic problem, the diagnosis and treatment of *Candida albicans* vaginitis.

Quality in structure consists of having at hand the physical assets necessary to address the clinical situation. Clean slides and cover slips, potassium hydroxide solution at the correct concentration, and a functional microscope are structural attributes. Quality in process relates to the physician's ability to think and do the correct things correctly. Processes include formulating the differential diagnosis, determining the need to view the "wet mount," recognizing the infectious agent, prescribing appropriate therapy, and following up as necessary. Treating empirically would not constitute a high quality process, even if it were to lead to a good outcome. The relationship between process and outcome is statistical; they are correlated, but the coefficient of correlation is not unity. In other words, in individual cases, an optimal process can result in a poor outcome, and good outcomes can (and often do) occur despite poor processes. Quality processes are those that create the best possible outcomes the greatest percentage of the time.

The relevant health outcomes in the example of diagnos-

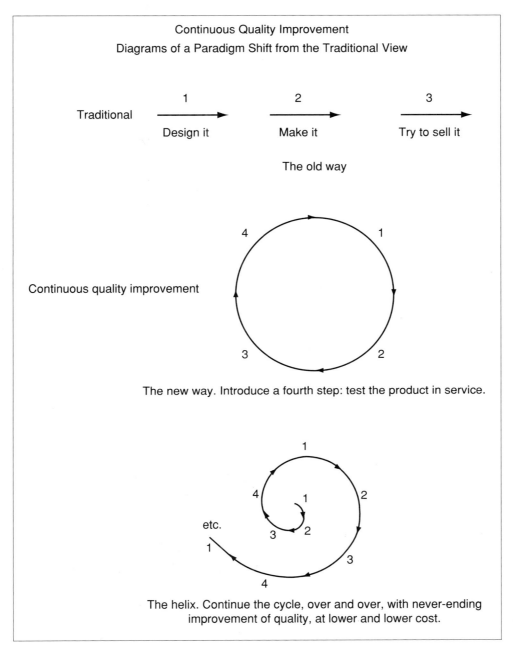

Fig. 44-1. Continuous quality improvement model developed by W. Edwards Deming.

ing vaginitis are the control of the *Candida* organism and the disappearance of the patient's signs and symptoms. An excellent health outcome contributes substantially to patient satisfaction, but other factors such as waiting times, friendliness of office staff, and cost also influence satisfaction.

Structure, process, and outcome constitute a valid conceptual framework for quality assessment in hospitals as well as in physician offices. Credentials committees, institutional review boards, infection control nurses, and tissue committees are examples of structural elements of quality in hospitals. The observation, measurement, review, and interven-

tion activities of these entities constitute process. Processes are designed to decrease the frequency of some outcomes (e.g., nosocomial infections or surgical removal of normal appendices) and increase the frequency of others (e.g., indicated mammograms or Pap smears). Many hospitals have focused on the cesarean section rate as an outcome of pregnancy and are attempting to identify and redesign processes that lead to high cesarean section rates. The American College of Obstetricians and Gynecologists has taken an interest in pregnancy outcomes, leading it to issue guidelines for primary and repeat cesarean sections. Because of customer

Table 44-1. Profile Comparing Cesarean Rates at Hospitals in the Tidewater Region of Virginia

			Cost and Length of Stay											
	Vaginal						Cesarean Section							
Hospital	No. of Cases	Average LOS	Average Hospital Charges	Average Physician Charges	Average Age	No. of Cases	Average LOS	Average Hospital Charges	Average Physician Charges	Average Age	Total Cases	Cesarean Section Rate (%)
A	69	2.58	$6,085.57	$2,394.90	28.33	25	5.12	$10,130.96	$3,116.44	29.12	94	26.60
B	143	1.85	$4,156.55	$2,698.09	27.73	28	2.75	$7,055.61	$3,155.46	30.18	171	16.37
C	22	1.55	$2,878.64	$2,012.50	25.59	2	2.50	$6,434.00	$3,370.00	26.50	24	8.33
D	198	2.07	$3,705.35	$2,419.62	28.96	49	3.73	$7,312.57	$2,621.51	31.08	247	19.84
E	132	1.98	$4,455.86	$2,489.67	31.30	45	3.38	$7,540.02	$2,933.24	30.82	177	25.42
F	29	2.07	$3,665.52	$1,834.93	28.45	15	3.67	$8,172.47	$2,239.13	29.13	44	34.09
G	287	2.08	$5,046.30	$2,573.93	29.50	86	3.55	$7,805.51	$3,011.06	30.74	373	23.06
H	48	1.85	$3,136.79	$2,060.04	28.75	16	2.94	$4,588.75	$2,172.69	27.56	64	25.00
I	17	2.00	$3,035.76	$1,958.06	27.41	5	3.00	$6,243.20	$2,086.20	27.60	22	22.73
J	45	2.29	$3,832.80	$2,527.09	27.84	21	3.86	$5,877.57	$3,408.95	30.10	66	31.82
K	5	2.60	$3,585.40	$1,800.00	25.20	2	6.50	$13,159.50	$2,394.00	31.00	7	28.57
L	814	2.22	$5,080.30	$2,670.58	30.48	353	3.72	$9,157.86	$2,852.27	30.97	1167	30.25
Total	1,809	2.13	$4,688.77	$2,555.97	29.67	647	3.67	$8,411.57	$2,866.17	30.64	2,456	26.34

Abbreviation: LOS, length of stay.

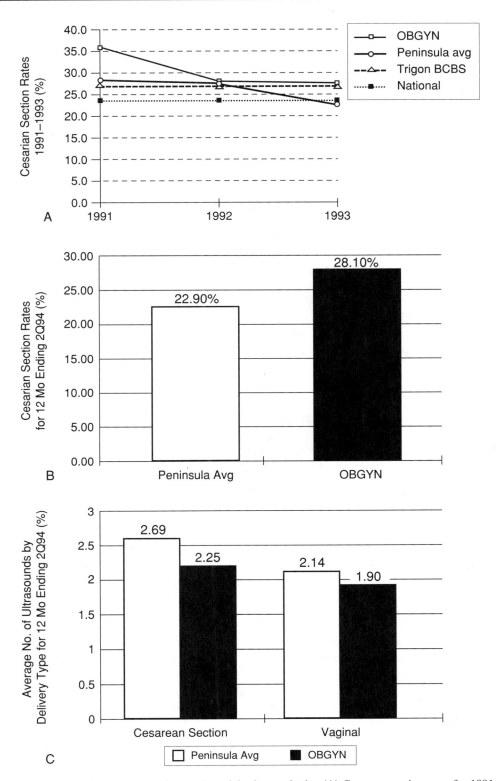

Fig. 44-2. Delivery and ultrasound rates for an obstetrician/gynecologist. (**A**) Cesarean section rates for 1991 to 1993. (**B**) Cesarean section rates for 12 months ending the second quarter of 1994 (2Q94). (**C**) Average number of ultrasounds per delivery, by type of delivery for 12 months ending 2Q94. Peninsula, a region of Virginia that includes Williamsburg, Newport News, and Hampton *(Figure continues.)*

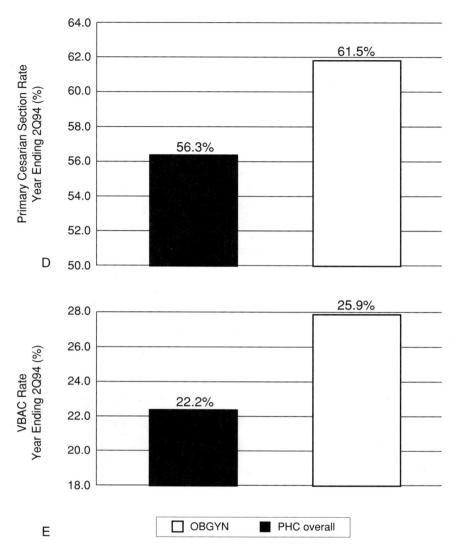

D

E

☐ OBGYN   ■ PHC overall

Fig. 44-2 *(Continued).* **(D)** Percentage of cesarean sections that are primary cesarean sections for year ending 2Q94. **(E)** VBAC (vaginal birth after cesarean) rate for year ending 2Q94 (denominator is deliveries for women with previous cesarean).

interest in cesarean rates and the simple, objective nature of their measurement, many MCOs are also emphasizing mode of delivery as a key outcome of pregnancy (Table 44-1 and Fig. 44-2).

Most clinicians will recognize the inherent value of quality assessment for the purpose of quality improvement. Most will also recognize the significant potential for careless or superficial quality measures to cause harm. An institution or a doctor may have a high cesarean section rate for reasons other than practice pattern variations. Some patient populations may be more prone than others to complications that call for the performance of cesarean sections. The populations of different geographic regions may have different attitudes toward care or expectations about the outcomes of care that influence their choices. Furthermore, it is not clear what

the optimal cesarean section rate should be in a given population. Therefore, we should consider cesarean section rates and other outcome measures in the context of severity of illness, geography, and other factors. The remainder of this chapter describes specific methods health services researchers and outcomes researchers have devised to measure quality. The author also examines variations in practice patterns as a result of predisposing factors.

CASE MIX, SEVERITY, AGE, AND SEX

Some variation in economic and clinical outcome is explained by differences in the age and sex of the patient. Using straightforward matrix algebra one can adjust data for these differences. After variation attributable to age and sex is removed, variation attributable to case mix and severity remains. Simply stated, case mix refers to a patient population's illnesses, injuries, or pregnancies, and severity refers to how sick the patients are. Clearly, case mix and severity are related to one another, that is, they are codependent, not independent variables. For example, the diagnosis of influenza implies greater severity than does the diagnosis of rhinovirus. Although some variation in severity remains within diagnostic categories (i.e., some cases of influenza are worse than others), diagnosis-driven case mix adjustment methods explain much of the variation in severity and severity-related outcomes. Various systems (e.g., Medis Groups) can explain some residual variation due to severity after case mix adjustment.[4] Some (e.g., Disease Staging) incorporate the concept of comorbidity (e.g., asthma would complicate and make more severe a case of rhinovirus).[5] Some adjustments for comorbidity are imbedded in most case mix systems.

The case mix adjustment method most familiar to clinicians is Diagnosis-Related Groups (DRGs). Fetter et al[6] empirically derived DRGs by evaluating hospital data using multivariate regression techniques to identify groupings of diagnoses (and occasionally age, sex, procedures, and other factors) that predict variation in resource consumption. Note carefully that DRGs were developed to predict economic, not clinical, outcomes. For example, the DRG for acute myocardial infarction with patients discharged alive has a higher "weight" than does the DRG for infarction patients who die in the hospital. This is because patients who die in the hospital from infarctions usually expire early in their hospital admissions and therefore have shorter stays and consume fewer resources. In this example, sicker patients have lower DRG weights than less sick patients. For another example, compare chemotherapy admissions to maternity episodes. Cost and DRG weights may be similar, but chemotherapy entails a higher probability of adverse health outcomes.

Generalizing from these examples, the reader can see that DRGs are much better suited to evaluating varying hospital costs than to evaluating differences in mortality (as reported annually by the Healthcare Financing Administration) or other health outcomes. Aggregate or average weights across DRGs have great value for predicting cost variations, but much less value for predicting clinical outcomes. To use DRGs for evaluating clinical outcome variations, one must look within a single DRG and not across the spectrum of DRGs. Just as critically, DRGs are appropriate for analysis of inpatient data only.

Predictive models for ambulatory data have been longer in development than DRGs because outpatient data are more diverse. Recently, two competing proprietary systems, Ambulatory Care Groups (ACGs) and Clinical Complexity Index (CCI) have matured to the point of practical application in the marketplace. Like DRGs, these algorithms have significant explanatory value for variations in resource con-

sumption. Both ACGs and CCI are as effective for explaining variation in resource consumption among ambulatory services as DRGs are for inpatient services.[7] The objective measure of a case mix or severity system's effectiveness at predicting cost variations is the coefficient of variation (R^2). The coefficient of variation measures the "goodness of fit" for the least squares regression line describing cost as a function of case mix or severity weight. If a model produces an R^2 value of 0.35 when costs are plotted as a function of case mix or severity weight, then the model is colloquially described as explaining 35 percent of the variation in cost. DRGs, ACGs, and CCI each explain between 30 and 40 percent of variation in resource consumption. DRGs leave residual variation attributable to age and sex; ACGs and CCI incorporate full age and sex adjustment. After adjustment for age, sex, case mix, and severity, the remaining variation is attributable to physician practice patterns (the measurement investigators usually want to isolate) and patient propensity to consume.

EPISODES OF CARE

To analyze patterns of cost, utilization, process, and outcomes, health services researchers sometimes cluster services into logical groupings called *episodes*. To create an episode, one brings together information relating to a service (e.g., hospitalization or surgery) or an illness to create a meaningful unit for analysis. The concept is best explained by example. If an MCO wants to evaluate and manage the cost of hysterectomies it needs to look at whole hysterectomy episodes, not just subsets such as hospital services or surgeon's services. Linking all information related to a hysterectomy creates a hysterectomy episode of care; this would include information about the surgeon, assistant surgeon, anesthesia, pathology, consultant, hospital, laboratory, radiology, and pharmacy. Clustering claim data into episodes enhances insight into process, efficiency, and value. An episode approximates management of a patient "problem." An MCO might wish to compare the cost of hysterectomy when performed by different gynecologists. One surgeon may have a relatively high professional fee but may avoid unnecessary testing and drugs that increase hospital cost. That surgeon may work quickly and precisely, minimizing anesthesia and operating room time and shortening postoperative hospitalization. Comorbidities may be more prevalent in one physician's practice than in another's. Looking only at the professional fee would create an incomplete and potentially misleading picture. At a higher level, episodes can facilitate the evaluation of health plan design and its relationship to utilization and cost. An excellent example is Keeler and Rolph's[8] analysis of Rand Health Insurance Experiment data using painstakingly constructed episodes. The use of episodes permitted the investigators to separate demand-induced utilization from physician-directed utilization and to separate utilization from episode cost. Plan design (e.g., health maintenance organization (HMO) versus fee-for-service and deductibles versus first dollar) was found to influence the initiation of episodes much more than the cost of episodes.

Methods for episode creation and analysis are much less standardized than are case mix and severity methods. As described in the health services research literature and as applied in the managed care setting, episode algorithms are highly variable and tailored to specific purposes. Some episode algorithms are based on conditions (e.g., pregnancy) and others are based on services (e.g., delivery). Methods also vary with respect to time cutoffs (e.g., 9 months for pregnancy versus several days for delivery) and how exacerbations of chronic or progressive illnesses are characterized (e.g., whether chronic pelvic pain with periodic exacerbations is one episode or several). When considering episode data in a managed care context the clinician should be aware that episode algorithms are more likely to be ''homegrown'' than the leading case mix and severity systems, and are less likely to be extensively validated. Only recently have episode algorithms become commercially available, and these are not yet extensively used. Therefore, clinicians may wish to formulate their own impressions of the face validity of the methods used. If a clinician is to assume financial risk of the management of episodes, it is critical to understand what is and is not grouped into those episodes.

REGIONAL VARIATION ANALYSIS

Also known as *small-area analysis,* regional variation analysis is the study of geographic differences in patterns of care. John Wenneberg, M.D. is widely regarded to be the pioneer of regional variation analysis.[9] Wenneberg observed three- and fourfold variations in major surgery rates (including hysterectomy) for residents of Boston as compared to New Haven. Differences in patients' age, sex, race, illness burden, severity, appropriateness, and cultural attitudes failed to explain these large differences in procedure rates.

Large geographic variations in procedure rates are often driven by differences in physician practices, which are rooted in medical education and training.

At Trigon Blue Cross Blue Shield, the author uses regional variation methods to identify practice pattern variations within Virginia. Physicians participating in our quality improvement program use these data to identify areas for guidelines development and application (Tables 44-2 and 44-3). When considering regional variation data, clinicians should remember that for most procedures the optimal utilization rate for a population is not known. Determining whether relatively high utilization is too high or whether relatively low utilization is too low requires expert judgment and discretion; the author and collegues consult panels of clinicians to interpret results. That outcomes and appropriateness do not always correlate with variations in utilization challenges us to narrow the range of clinical options we accept as appropriate and to refine the way we define and measure appropriateness.[10] The increasing prevalence and increasing specificity of national guidelines for clinical practice may narrow the range of options that are considered to be appropriate and may diminish geographic variations in practice patterns.

CREDENTIALS AND PROFILES

Many insurers and MCOs now require specific credentials and profiles from physicians to assess eligibility for network participation. Trigon Blue Cross Blue Shield, for example, predicates network participation in obstetrics and gynecology on board certification (or eligibility to sit for the boards), hospital privileges, unrestricted licenses (medical, drug enforcement agency, state pharmacy), malpractice insurance, and lack of felony convictions. Also considered are disciplinary actions, malpractice history, and age-, sex-, and severity-adjusted economic profiles. To the extent possible, outcome information (e.g., patient satisfaction, cesarean section rates) are incorporated into the data set.

Hospitals, group physician practices, independent practice associations, physician hospital organizations, and MCOs all have an interest in the credentials of physicians and in

Table 44-2. 1993 Regional Variation Within Virginia[a]

Region	Vaginal Deliveries	Cesarean Deliveries	Total Deliveries	Cesareans (%)
Blue Ridge	12.4	4.3	16.6	25.7
Lynchburg	7.9	2.7	10.5	25.4
Northern VA	12.4	3.3	15.6	20.9
Peninsula	12.7	4.1	16.8	24.3
Richmond	12.8	5.2	18.0	28.9
Roanoke	13.1	4.8	17.9	26.9
South Hampton Roads	11.8	3.8	15.6	24.2
Southwest VA	10.6	5.0	15.6	32.0

[a] Delivery rate comparison (deliveries/1,000 female policyholders).

Table 44-3. Regional Variation Within Virginia[a]

Region	Dilation and Curettage	Abdominal Hysterectomy	Vaginal Hysterectomy	Total Hysterectomies
Blue Ridge	13.3	3.4	2.4	5.8
Lynchburg area	11.2	3.9	1.6	5.5
Northern VA	14.1	3.4	1.5	4.9
Peninsula	12.5	4.1	3.5	7.6
Richmond	13.9	4.0	1.8	5.8
Roanoke	14.2	4.7	2.3	7.0
South Hampton Roads	12.9	3.3	3.2	6.5
Southwest VA	14.9	5.8	1.9	7.7

[a] Number of procedures per 1,000 female policyholders.

profiles, or measurements, of physicians' processes and resultant outcomes. Hospital quality assurance activities have long included verification and assessment of staff physician credentials. Credentials such as board certification or experience with specific procedures determine staff privileges and are important for both structural quality and liability risk management. Today, insurance companies, managed care companies, integrated health systems, and hospitals profile and assess the credentials of their networks and staffs. Physicians understand why they need to assess the credentials of new associates or partners joining their group practices and can therefore understand why integrated health systems must do the same.

In contrast to credentialling, profiling to measure performance is much less stereotyped in its methods. At Trigon Blue Cross Blue Shield the author and colleagues use the proprietary Peer-A-Med system from Equifax as one tool for profiling physicians. Using claim data, patients are assigned to physicians with an attribution algorithm and age-, sex-, and severity-adjusted variations in cost and utilization are measured on a per patient basis. The system uses CCI to adjust for severity.[11] For each physician's assigned patients, the system assesses direct services (for which the physician is paid) and indirect services (for which hospitals, laboratories, consultants, and so forth are paid) (Fig. 44-3). Economic profiles report gross utilization and dollar volume rates for major categories of services (e.g., laboratory, radiology) and report greater detail for procedures of particular interest, which vary by specialty. In addition to profiling for economic variations, profiles for other attributes, such as provision of preventive services, consistency of follow-up after hospitalization, and patient satisfaction are done. Networks are profiled in batches by specialty and geographic region. Therefore, the profiles are designed to permit comparisons to peer group averages.

Profiling methods and applications vary significantly from one managed care company to another. Some companies apply explicit limits in variation to determine a physician's initial or continuing eligibility to participate in networks, but others do not. Some directly link profiles to

incentive payments while others do not. Most companies expect profiles to increase average efficiency and decrease variations in practice patterns through heightened physician awareness of peer group average practices and most efficient practices. To the extent that specialist or hospital profiles are made available to primary care doctors, those profiles can produce more informed referral decisions. Profiles can provide management information for clinicians, who are the ultimate managers of care in a good managed care system. Profiles also can and will be used by MCOs to determine eligibility for network participation.

Clinicians will need to consider profiles from different companies according to their merits. Important considerations include patient selection, sample size, patient attribution, physician peer group identification, and adjustment for age, sex, and severity. It is important to pay particular attention to the identity of one's peer group. Some of the largest statistical variations seen in our early profiling efforts at Trigon were attributable to individuals limiting their practices to the subspecialty areas of the specialty within which they were grouped.

OUTCOMES RESEARCH

Outcomes research is the measurement of patient outcomes as they occur in the natural clinical environment, as opposed to the laboratory environment of an investigation protocol. Outcomes research emphasizes effectiveness rather than efficacy, "ultimate" outcomes (those that patients actually experience) rather than intermediate outcomes, and quality improvement rather than quality assurance. The practical application of outcomes research today is limited to some progressive managed care companies in a few focused areas of clinical practice. However, many researchers expect advancements in information systems and primary data sources such as universal computerized medical records to produce an explosion in outcomes research applications, with revolutionary implications for the practice of medicine.

TRIGON BLUE CROSS BLUE SHIELD PROVIDER PRACTICE PROFILE
GENERAL MEDICINE–TIDEWATER REGION–POINT OF SERVICE CLAIMS INCURRED IN 1994

SAMPLE A	DIRECT	INDIRECT	OVERALL
Patient Count	42	18	42
Relative Clinical Complexity Index	0.95	1.04	0.81
Expected Average Cost Per Patient	$220	$1,414	$887
Actual Average Cost Per Patient	$210	$2,237	$1,169
$ Difference	($9)	$823	$282
% Difference	-4.3%	58.2%	31.7%
Standard Deviation From Mean % Difference	0.06	2.62	1.82
Rank (1 represents the lowest % difference)	33 of 63	63 of 63	62 of 63

PROVIDER REFERRAL SUMMARY*
*PROFESSIONAL SERVICES ONLY

	PROVIDER	PEER GROUP
% Of Patients With Referrals		
Calculation Method: Total patients with specialist claims	43%	66%
Total primary care patients		
% Of Total Dollars		
Calculation Method: Total specialist dollars allowed	61%	65%
Total primary care & specialist dollars allowed		
% Of Total Services		
Calculation Method: Total specialist services	26%	48%
Total primary care & specialist services		

SELF REFERRAL SUMMARY*
*PROFESSIONAL SERVICES ONLY

	IN NETWORK		OUT OF NETWORK	
	PROVIDER	PEER GROUP	PROVIDER	PEER GROUP
Total Patients	12	2785	2	432
Total Dollars Allowed	$1,650	$726,850	$186	$100,516
Total Services	19	9036	2	860
Average Dollars Allowed Per Patient	$137	$261	$93	$233
Average Services Per Patient	1.58	3.24	1.00	1.99

COST AND UTILIZATION PERFORMANCE
% DEVIATION FROM PEER GROUP AVERAGE

$/PAT   ENCS/PAT   SVCS/PAT
58 32   29 -9 0   16 -22 -17 -4

DIRECT   INDIRECT   OVERALL

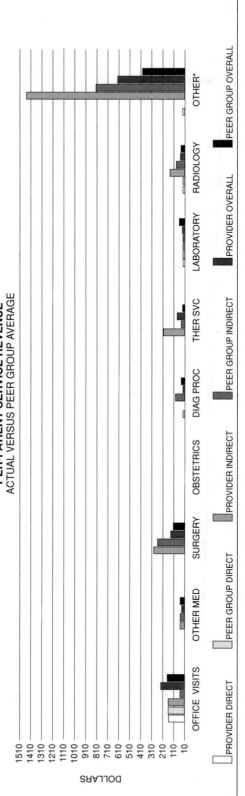

PER-PATIENT SERVICE REVENUE
ACTUAL VERSUS PEER GROUP AVERAGE

OFFICE VISITS — OTHER MED — SURGERY — OBSTETRICS — DIAG PROC — THER SVC — LABORATORY — RADIOLOGY — OTHER*

PROVIDER DIRECT — PEER GROUP DIRECT — PROVIDER INDIRECT — PEER GROUP INDIRECT — PROVIDER OVERALL — PEER GROUP OVERALL

*"Other" includes allergy and mental health svcs, and for indirect and total analysis, also includes all facility svcs.

Fig. 44-3. Trigon Blue Cross Blue Shield provider practice profile.

Traditional clinical research is about outcomes, but it is not outcomes research. Traditional clinical research measures efficacy, a term that describes optimal results produced under highly controlled and idealized conditions. In the traditional clinical trial, precise protocols govern the selection of patients, the delivery of care, the setting in which care is delivered (usually tertiary care centers), and the censure of data relating to patients who for various reasons may not be evaluable with respect to specific outcomes. The results of these controlled experiments are often generalized, without appropriate consideration of their generalizability. Even after efficacy is demonstrated, effectiveness in clinical practice outside the research setting remains unknown. Outcomes research is designed to fill this void by measuring effectiveness outside the research setting. This is important for managed care and indeed for the practice of clinical medicine, because effectiveness in practice may vary significantly from the theoretical maximum effectiveness or efficacy. Effectiveness, unlike efficacy, may vary considerably from doctor to doctor or hospital to hospital. The outcomes emphasized in outcomes research are those that are experienced by patients, ultimate rather than intermediate outcomes. Normoglycemia in gestational diabetes is an example of an intermediate outcome, since patients are usually oblivious to hyperglycemia except at extreme values. However, babies that are large for gestational age are examples of ultimate outcomes. The degree to which it is appropriate to focus on intermediate outcomes depends on how tightly correlated they are with ultimate outcomes.

Outcomes research employs administrative data (e.g., insurance claims), other large computerized data bases (e.g., cancer registries and vital statistics such as birth and death

registries), and specialized survey instruments to assess outcomes. Although lacking the clinical richness of medical records, such data sources yield the power of very large numbers and long longitudinal time frames. A noteworthy example of useful clinical information from claims data is Wennberg's study of prostate surgery outcomes from Medicare data.[12] Using subsequent claims for treatment of complications to identify clinically significant sequellae (e.g., incontinence, impotence) and using the end of Medicare eligibility to identify death, the researchers inferred significantly higher complication rates than were known from the traditional efficacy literature (which reports experiences of relatively small numbers of patients treated at medical centers, often lost to follow-up after a few weeks). A powerful method of assessing outcomes in large populations is to complement administrative (e.g., claim) information with data from standardized, externally validated survey instruments. The SF-36 (short form with 36 questions) health status survey instrument is particularly noteworthy.[3] Developed by John Ware as an abstract from a longer instrument, the SF-36 is extensively validated in the peer reviewed literature and is reliable and reproducible. Serial measurement of health status (Fig. 44-4) can detect a change in health status, which is a proxy for outcome. Health status is predictive of both clinical and economic outcomes and is therefore useful for comparing populations and health plans to one another.

The SF-36 is a generic health status instrument that is applicable across most conditions (e.g., medical, surgical, mental health, acute, chronic), both sexes, and most ethnic groups. A variety of standardized instruments exist for more detailed study of specific conditions or procedures. Many of these instruments are available from the Health Outcomes

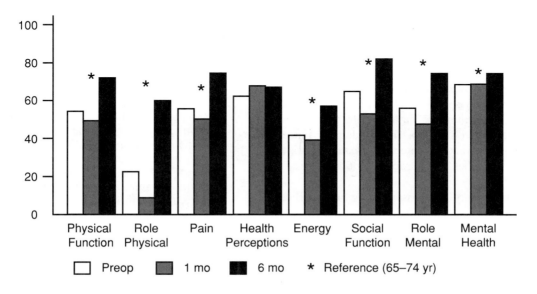

Fig. 44-4. Diagram of a change in SF-36 scores as a result of cardiac surgery showing that surgery restores health status to approximately normal levels. This demonstrates that the coronary artery bypass (CABG) procedure enhances quality as well as quantity of life. SF-36, short form with 36 questions.

Institute. As noted earlier in this chapter, patient satisfaction is an important outcome. An MCO gains obvious market advantage from having network physicians that satisfy customers (patients). At Trigon Blue Cross Blue Shield, satisfaction is measured with scaled sections from the Group Health Association of America survey instrument.[14] Survey data may be used to measure customer satisfaction with health plans or insurance products. Surveys may also be used to measure patient satisfaction with physician practices. Some MCOs assess patient satisfaction with individual doctors, and many physicians welcome the information. However, surveying to permit scientifically valid comparisons between physicians is expensive. Many MCOs will use nonrandom sampling methods and will sample too few patients to yield statistically significant results. Physicians should interpret results in light of sampling methods and response rates for particular companies, and when contracting with managed care companies, doctors must understand how patient satisfaction will be measured.

The goal of outcomes research is to increase effectiveness by measuring outcomes and identifying opportunities for improvement. Outcomes research promises to be an integral part of CQI in clinical medicine. To optimize outcomes by re-engineering processes we must first have a method of measuring the outcomes. That method is outcomes research.

THE GUIDELINES MOVEMENT

Clinical guidelines, or practice parameters, are familiar to most clinicians, but for completeness and because of the current emphasis on guidelines they are reviewed briefly. The National Cancer Institute, American College of Physicians, American College of Obstetricians and Gynecologists, the Rand Corporation, and many other professional, academic, and research organizations have produced guidelines for decades. Guideline sets now number in the thousands while sources of guidelines number in the hundreds and include many, if not most, specialty societies. Influential newcomers include various specialty societies, the Academic Medical Center Consortium, and the Agency for Health Care Policy and Research (AHCPR). The federally funded AHCPR is sponsoring patient outcome research teams to develop condition, rather than procedure-oriented guidelines[15] (Fig. 44-5).

Guidelines vary greatly in philosophy (e.g., appropriateness versus necessity), methodologic underpinnings (e.g., objective evidence versus consensus), orientation (e.g., procedure versus condition), and format (e.g., algorithm versus text).[16] Many managed care companies, hospitals, and physicians are optimistic that guidelines will increase the prevalence of best clinical practices and reduce the extreme variations in practice patterns now found across regions. Some hope that guidelines will also lower cost. This author considers that hope to be wishful thinking, since guidelines are

---

Example of a Text Guideline From the American College of Obstetricians and Gynecologists

- Procedure
  - Cesarean delivery (74 all; subcode dependent on which type of procedure is used)[a] (CPT codes: 59510 [global service], 59514 [delivery only], or 59515 [delivery and postpartum care only])
- Indication
  - The major single indication is lack of progress (failure to progress). Reasons for lack of progress include: disproportion (653), primary uterine inertia (661.0), secondary uterine inertia (661.1), other and unspecified uterine inertia (661.2), prolonged first stage (662.0), prolonged labor, unspecified (662.1), and prolonged second stage (662.2)
- Confirmation of indication
  - No change in either dilation of cervix or descent of presenting part after at least 2 hours of active labor following completion of the latent phase
  - Active labor is defined by
    - Cervix dilated to at least 3 cm in nullipara or 4 cm in multipara
    - Contractions at least every 2 to 3 minutes
    - Strength of contractions at least 50 mmHg internal pressure as measured by intrauterine catheter or inability to indent fundus on palpation
- Action prior to procedure
  - Rupture membranes
  - Institute oxytocin when progressive cervical dilation and descent of presenting part fails to occur in the active phase because of poor uterine contractility
  - Obtain anesthesia consultation and evaluation
  - Type and screen blood sample
  - Monitor fetal heart rate (by electronic fetal monitoring or auscultation) immediately before preparation of abdomen
  - Request that qualified personnel be in attendance for resuscitation and care of newborn
  - Perform vaginal examination just before surgery to reconfirm lack of progress

---

[a] Unless otherwise stated, *each* numbered and lettered item *must* be present.

(From American College of Obstetricians and Gynecologists,[16] with permission.)

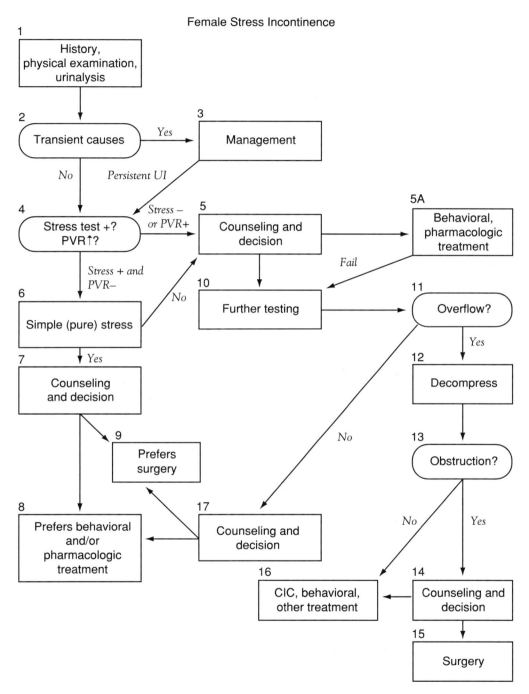

Fig. 44-5. Example of algorithm guideline from the Association for Health Care Policy and Research (AHCPR). UI, urinary infection; PVR, postvoid residual. (From U.S. Department of Health and Human Services.[15])

generally created to improve quality and cost effects are serendipitous. A few guidelines may decrease cost, but many will increase cost or be cost-neutral. However, the market will accept marginal cost increases for improved outcomes as long as those outcomes are perceived by patients (customers) to be important and are measurable.

Clinicians and managed care companies alike will need to choose from the multitude of guidelines to follow. As most clinicians know, many guidelines from "authoritative" sources disagree with one another. A useful approach is to regard areas of universal concurrence (e.g., advising mammograms for women age 50 and over) as necessary care and areas of substantial disagreement (e.g., advising mammograms for women ages 35 to 49) as care that is appropriate but not necessary. Trigon pays claims for screening mammograms in women under the age of 50, but does not consider the absence of such screens to constitute a quality problem (i.e., these mammograms are appropriate but not necessary).

Of all areas of initiative in quality improvement, guidelines are probably the most important to clinicians. Knowledge of authoritative guidelines related to one's specialty can impart liability protection; ignorance of those guidelines can impart liability exposure. Many people in the guidelines movement, including those from organized medicine, hope that practicing within guidelines will provide an affirmative defense against malpractice claims. There is some promise that this hope might be realized but there is insufficient case law to make a prediction at this time.

REPORT CARDS

Many clinicians have heard or read about "report cards" designed to inform consumer decisions about the purchase of health care. Although some physicians may view individual profiles as report cards, the term is generally meant to apply to assessments of organizations. Notably, the HEDIS (Health Plan Employer Data and Information Set) report card is intended to help employers to evaluate health plans.[17] HMOs will issue report cards according to HEDIS prescription for group purchasers to consider when choosing coverage. Clinicians should know that many of the quality improvement and data reporting initiatives of MCOs are driven by direct marketplace demands. The National Committee for Quality Assurance (NCQA) has established standards for HMO quality and data reporting (HEDIS). Analogous to the Joint Commission on Accreditation of Health Care Organizations (JCAHO), the NCQA is a private sector organization and compliance with its standards is voluntary. However, these standards may become de rigeur (as with JCAHO accreditation) if the marketplace continues to embrace them. Large group purchasers are beginning to make explicit reference to NCQA standards in their requests for proposals from prepaid health plans. Those areas placed under close scrutiny by HEDIS will be points of emphasis for MCOs, which will in

---

HEDIS 2.5 Quality of Care Measures

- Childhood immunization rate
- Cholesteral screening
- Mammography screening
- Cervical cancer screening
- Low birth weight
- Prenatal care in first trimester
- Asthma inpatient admission rate
- Diabetic retinal examination
- Ambulatory follow-up after hospitalization for major affective disorder

---

Abbreviation: HEDIS, Health Plan Employer Data and Information Set.
(From National Committee for Quality Assurance,[17] with permission.)

---

turn make them points of emphasis for network physicians. If a given standard is required of an HMO, then the HMO will consider physician compliance with that standard as part of quality evaluation in selecting participating physicians.

SUMMARY

Medicine is in the midst of a revolutionary market transformation, an inevitable result of collective financing. What was once a cottage industry is becoming big business. Big business players in the health care arena will apply quality assessment and quality improvement techniques modeled after those that have been successful in the manufacturing sector. These methods represent new challenges and new opportunities for physicians.

REFERENCES

1. Council of Economic Advisers: Economic Report of the President and The Annual Report of the Council of Economic Advisers. United States Government Printing Office, Washington DC, 1995
2. Deming WE: Out of the Crisis. Massachusetts Instutute of Technology, Cambridge, MA, 1986
3. Donabedian A: Evaluating the quality of medical care. Milbank 44:166, 1966
4. Brewster AC, Karlin BG, Hyde LA et al: MEDISGRPS: a

clinically based approach to classifying hospital patients at admission. Inquiry 22:377, 1985

5. Gonnella JS, Hornbrook MC, Louis DZ: Staging of disease: a case-mix measurement. JAMA 251:637, 1984

6. Fetter JL, Hin Y, Freeman JL et al: Case mix definition by diagnosis related groups. Medical Care, suppl. 2, 18:1, 1980

7. Handy BM, Phelps CE, Mooney C et al: A comparison of three methods of case mix adjustment in physician level analyses of practice variations. Med Decis Making 12:332, 1992

8. Keeler EB, Rolph JE: The demand for episodes of treatment in the health insurance experiment. J Health Econom 7:337, 1988

9. Wennberg J, Gittelsohn A: Small area variations in health care delivery. Science 182:1102, 1973

10. Wennberg JE, Freeman JL, Shelton RM, Bubolz TA: Hospital use and mortality among Medicare beneficiaries in Boston and New Haven. N Engl J Med 321:1168, 1989

11. Perkins NAK: Case-Mix Adjustment of Physician Practice Profiles Using Claims Data. Doctoral dissertation, University of Rochester, Rochester, NY

12. Wennberg JE, Roos N, Sola L et al: Use of claims data systems to evaluate health care outcomes: mortality and reoperation following prostatectomy. JAMA 257:933, 1987

13. Ware JE, Jr, Sherbourne CD: The MOS 36-item short-form health survey (SF-36). I. Conceptual framework and item selection. Med Care 30:473, 1992

14. Davies AR, Ware JE Jr: GHAA's Consumer Satisfaction Survey and User's Manual. Group Health Association of America, Inc., Washington DC, 1991

15. US Department of Health and Human Services, US Public Health Service: Urinary Incontinence in Adults: Quick Reference Guide for Clinicians. AHCPR Publication Number 92-0041, p. QR10. Agency for Health Care Policy and Research, Rockville, MD, 1992

16. American College of Obstetricians and Gynecologists: Quality Assessment and Improvement in Obstetrics and Gynecology. American College of Obstetricians and Gynecologists, Washington, DC, 1994

17. National Committee for Quality Assurance: Health Plan Employer Data and Information Set (HEDIS) Version 2.5. Washington, DC, 1993

CHAPTER FORTY-FIVE

MEDICOLEGAL ISSUES

CLIFFORD A. RIEDERS

OBSTETRIC MALPRACTICE STATISTICS

According to Medical Malpractice Verdicts Settlements & Experts, between July 1994 and July 1995 there were a total of 81 obstetric/gynecologic medical cases reported. The largest numbers were for hysterectomies, totaling 18. Fifteen of those were negligently performed, and 3 were consent issues. The next leading area of malpractice actions in this specialty was related to laparoscopic tubal ligations, totaling 13. The largest number of these related to failure to sterilize (6), followed by various complications primarily involving puncture or laceration wounds. Complications attributed to abortions and failure to diagnose breast cancer total 7 each. Failure to diagnose as a general topic came next, with a total of 6, which included ectopic pregnancies and disease processes such as colon cancer and colitis. Next comes abnormal papanicolauo smear interpretations, with 5 occurrences either for improper or no follow-up. Those associated with rectovaginal fistula repairs, complications from diagnostic laparoscopy and/or laparotomy, and ectopic pregnancies each total 4. The remainder were attributed to 3 for endometriosis, 2 for birth control issues and dilation and curettage procedures, ending with 1 each for hysteroscopy, laser conization, failure to examine breasts, fibroid cysts, and vaginal growths.

INFORMED CONSENT

In spite of many fears concerning informed consent cases, as one can see, there are less of those than many people believe. There have been suggestions that informed consent cases may begin to focus on potential loss of sexual response, or theoretical protection against heart disease, as issues necessary to be included in discussing certain procedures.

Even if informed of the risk of injury, such as ureteral or bladder trauma, the plaintiff may argue that the injury resulted from improper surgical technique or inadequate skill. If intraoperative recognition and repair are done, and explained to the patient and her family postoperatively, liability is minimized. When injuries are detected late in the hospital course, with resulting corrective procedures or consultations, then both surgical technique and postoperative care will be questioned. Attention to the patient's complaints postoperatively, and appropriate documentation and evaluation are mandatory. If there are complications, ideally they should be recognized early and dealt with promptly, with consultation as needed. In these situations, the operative report will usually be read in great detail. It behooves surgeons to read their operative notes prior to signing them, to correct errors that, on the stand, can be very embarrassing. Also, if abnormal anatomy was identified during surgery or problems encountered such as dense adhesions or difficulties with dissection, this should be included in the operative report. Hurried, extremely brief notes can hamper a subsequent defense.

A physician is bound to disclose risks that reasonable persons would consider material to their decision of whether to undergo treatment. In many states, informed consent does not apply to hospitals, but to only individual doctors and only applies to surgery. That is not true, of course, in all states. The patient should be informed with appropriate literature; some doctors are experimenting with videotape. Should a doctor talk about all possible effects without number, and therefore, risk omitting something, or should the informed consent be general? This is where one must rely on one's knowledge, skill, and experience. The patient must be frankly and honestly told about all risks and whether they are major or minor. A doctor is charged with a duty to explain not only the operation itself, but also the seriousness of the procedure, its risks, complications, and alternatives.

Some states have adopted a prudent patient standard in informed consent cases. In such states, the standard of care is not what a reasonable medical practitioner would have done in the situation, but whether the physician disclosed those risks that reasonable persons would have considered material to their decision whether to undergo treatment.

COMMON INJURIES RESULTING IN MALPRACTICE SUITS

Fistulas involving the bladder or ureter, or both, frequently lead to malpractice suits alleging improper surgical technique. Injury to the ureter and bladder are venial sins, but failure to recognize them a mortal sin. Attention to anatomy and absence of haste are all that can be recommended.

Failed sterilizations are also a common source of suit. Wrongful life and its attendant cost may be argued. However, the alleged malpractice is improper surgical technique. Documentation of the adequacy of the procedure and an emphasis on potential failure when obtaining consent help with the defense.

Operative laparoscopy has led to a number of suits involving bowel injury during dissection of adhesions, trochar injuries to bowel and vessels, and ureteral injuries during laparoscopically assisted vaginal hysterectomies. In all these situations, one can expect the deposition to focus on establishing the surgeon's credentials, with specific attention to where the techniques were learned, number of prior procedures, and familiarity with the specific procedure involved. Proper credentialing for laparoscopic surgeons greatly aids

with the defense. Although rare, the severity of bowel and urinary tract injuries suggests they be mentioned while obtaining consent. As with any complications, delay in recognition usually leads to increasing patient injury and allegations of negligence.

Use of saline injection by syringe, open insertion when appropriate, or other techniques to help insert the initial trochar safely should be carefully detailed in the operative report. Injuries occurring from insertion of second or third trochars are difficult to defend, since controlled entry under direct visualization is the standard of care. Excessive force and uncontrolled entry with subsequent organ injury is difficult to defend. Laparoscopic repair of bladder, bowel, or other organ is feasible, but should not be attempted unless the surgeon is experienced in the technique. Lack of prior experience will be brought out in depositions before trial.

Ureteral injuries from stapling devices is assumed to be due to failure to identify the ureters prior to firing. Documentation of ureteral identification is necessary in the operative report.

Extension of electrical burn is seen less frequently than in the past, perhaps due to better instrumentation. Again, documentation of care in avoiding normal tissues is needed to defend these cases.

Laparoscopic equipment failure and resulting patient injury is a potential defense. However, equipment failures should be properly documented according to routine hospital protocol, and the offending instrument saved—not discarded. The manufacturer will obviously seek documentation of device failure, while discarding the instrument or failing to follow proper protocols raises questions about the surgeon's veracity.

If video recording of a procedure is done, the film should not be erased or destroyed. Doing so raises serious questions about the surgeon's credibility. Whether filming every procedure is warranted is a moot point, with good arguments for and against routine video recording.

The key to avoiding lawsuits is careful attention to the patient and operative technique. Communication is vital, both with the patient and her family and with legal counsel. Detailed records must be maintained and kept intact. When sued, the surgeon must approach the case thoughtfully and carefully, with communication with the attorney. Understanding the legal process as outlined should lessen uncertainty and make the extreme length of the process, often measurable in years more understandable.

GENERAL OVERVIEW OF MEDICAL MALPRACTICE

This chapter is written from the viewpoint of an experienced attorney familiar with litigating cases against gynecologic surgeons. From this perspective, recurrent errors have become evident—errors of medical judgment and errors of common sense wherein physicians unfamiliar with the legal terrain have tripped themselves up with errors of commission and omission.

There is no question that medical costs are rising and that fear of liability is clearly a perceived factor in this rising cost. In 1990, the United States spent 12 percent of its gross domestic product on health care. This amount greatly exceeds the sum spent on national defense or education. The United States Congressional Budget Office estimates that health care spending will increase to 18 percent of the gross domestic product by the year 2000. It has been argued that medical liability, or the threat of liability, greatly contributes to these health care expenses.[1]

Medical malpractice is frequently touted as a problem for health care practitioners. Although this is not the place for debate concerning the value of medical malpractice suits or their effect on practitioner and patient alike, there are some basic facts related to litigation that every physician should understand and that will help that physician protect against medical malpractice suits. To say that defensive medicine is a culprit as a consequence of lawyers filing too many suits, or that medical liability is simply unfair to the honest practitioner, permits self-delusion, which will only cause more litigation. The facts are that in virtually every profession today the practice of "business" is as important as the profession itself. Self-referral is a prime example of the current and growing encroachment of commercialism on medical practice.[2] Joint ventures and free-standing medical services may generate more income for physicians than their primary medical practices. The point is that health care professionals have to recognize the perceived economic impetus on the part of the medical profession to perform diagnostic tests and to keep the patient coming back. Second, physicians and health care providers have to realize that there really is such a thing as medical malpractice, and that it is more than the horrific cases in which a drunk surgeon operates on an innocent patient. By now, the informed reader will be aware of the Harvard Medical Practice Study, which found that in New York state hospitals in 1984 there were more than 27,000 negligent adverse events, including 7,000 deaths and almost 900 cases of permanent disability.[3] This involves only in-hospital negligence. This large volume is against the preserved backdrop that doctors, understandably, do not like to report on other doctors, and that there are peer review shield laws in many states that prohibit medical malpractice from coming to light. The National Practitioner Data Bank is not yet available to health care consumers; but this is one of the great sources of reported medical malpractice incidents being developed.

The other item that health care professionals must come to recognize is that, as attorneys specialize and become more adept at handling medical malpractice cases, the number of cases is declining. In other words, better trained lawyers bring fewer cases (even though the number of medical malpractice cases may even be increasing in some regions). The

Harvard Medical Practice Study opined that only 1 in 8 negligently injured patients ever brings a claim. According to Deborah Hensler, who wrote a study titled *Compensation for Accidental Injuries in the United States,* only 1 in 10 injured consumers seek compensation from the tort liability system. Studies from such centers as RAND and even the American Medical Association corroborate these drops in medical malpractice claims.[4,5]

> The claim frequency for all physicians is 7.7 claims per 100 physicians in 1990, as compared with 7.4 per 100 in 1989. While the claims rate did increase between 1989 and 1990, that increase was not statistically significant. In general, the results indicate a leveling off of the claims rate in contrast to the increases of the early- and mid-1980s.[6]

Frequently, the question is asked, "How often do plaintiffs win?" Surveys show that juries nationwide have become "markedly tougher on people who sue doctors, insurance companies, and other deep-pocket defendants, siding less often with plaintiffs." This according to research published in *The New York Times,* citing Jury Verdict Research, a legal publishing firm in Horsham, Pennsylvania. According to *The New York Times:* "From 1961 to 1991, a plaintiff's chances of prevailing at trial in personal injury suits changed remarkably little, never rising above 63% or falling below 57% in any year. Then came the drop to 52% in 1992." It has been observed that the change is most noticeable among middle-class jurors. Jurors also seem to be offended by lawyer advertising. "In medical malpractice cases, which involve some of the largest awards, the winning rate dropped to 31% in 1992 from 48% in 1989." The change seems to be carrying through, even after compilation of the latest figures.

Once we shift the focus from complaints about lawyers, greedy claimants, and an inhospitable legal system, we can then honestly, and with integrity, look at how physicians might reduce their odds of dealing with a medical malpractice situation.

Precisely what constitutes medical malpractice? How does a bad result differ from malpractice? The 50 states have different laws on medical malpractice and many states are now governed by specific statute. Generally, however, physicians have a duty to conduct themselves as a reasonable physician would act. This concept is sometimes referred to as the "standard of care." A physician has the obligation to attend and treat a patient, to consult as appropriate, to maintain records, and to advise a patient of any risks that may be involved in the treatment.

In a very general way, the following elements must be proven in a medical malpractice case:

1. The physician did not possess and employ the required skill and knowledge or
2. The physician did not exercise the care and judgment

of a reasonable person in like cases *and* that the injury complained of either

Resulted from the failure on the part of the physician to possess and employ the required skill and knowledge, or

Resulted from failure to exercise the care and judgment of a reasonable person in like circumstances

In some states, the theory of gross negligence or negligence giving rise to punitive damages may be applicable. In a very general way, most states will not permit punitive damages absent intentional conduct or conduct that is so flagrant that it grossly deviates from the ordinary standard of care. Many states utilize a concept called *sovereign immunity* to protect doctors who work for, or are employed by, the state.

In most states, the question is one of whether due care has been exercised, and expert testimony of a physician familiar with the same field as the physicians who are being sued is necessary. In virtually all states it is a requirement that medical testimony be given to a reasonable degree of medical certainty. In such states, the testimony by a physician who testifies against a defendant must state, to a reasonable degree of medical certainty, that the defendant acted without due care of a reasonable physician in the position of the defendant and that such act or failure to act increased the risk of harm. It may then be a question for the jury as to whether the increased risk was a substantial factor in producing the harm.

In most states, the ''two schools of thought'' doctrine is applicable. Where competent medical authority is divided, a physician will not be held responsible, if, in the exercise of the physician's judgment, the physician has followed a course of treatment advocated by a considerable number of recognized and respected professionals in the given area of expertise. This test may be stated differently in more conservative states. Usually, the burden of proving that there are two schools of thought falls with the defendant. In those states that subscribe to this doctrine, it is typically stated that once an expert states the factual reasons to support the claim that a considerable number of professionals agree with the treatment employed by defendant, there is sufficient evidence to warrant an instruction to the jury on the ''two schools of thought'' doctrine.

The doctrine of *res ipsa loquitur* may be available to the plaintiff. Under this doctrine it may be inferred that harm suffered by the plaintiff is caused by negligence of a defendant when

- The event is of a kind that ordinarily does not occur in the absence of negligence
- Other responsible causes, including the conduct of a plaintiff and third persons, are sufficiently eliminated by the evidence
- The indicated negligence is within the scope of the defendant's duty to the plaintiff

If *res ipsa loquitur* is permitted to be proven, expert medical testimony is only necessary to indicate that the injury would not have occurred without negligence, when there is no fund of common knowledge from which a lay person can reasonably draw the inference or conclusion of negligence. In so-called obvious cases, expert testimony may not be necessary at all. A clamp left behind may be such a case.

In most states, it is necessary for a plaintiff in a malpractice case to prove causation. This is a cause-and-effect type of relationship. Some states permit a finding of negligence where the negligent conduct of a doctor increases the risk of harm to a patient. This is a very complex area of the law. Suffice it to say, however, that some states hold that once a plaintiff has demonstrated that a defendant's acts or omissions have increased the risk of harm to another, such evidence furnishes a reason for the fact-finder to go further and find that such increased risk was in turn a substantial factor in bringing about the resultant harm; the necessary causation will have been established if the jury sees fit to find cause in fact. In so-called increased risk of harm cases, a medical opinion need only demonstrate with a reasonable degree of medical certainty that a defendant's conduct increased the risk of harm sustained. In many states, it would then be up to the jury to decide whether the conduct was a substantial factor in bringing about the harm.

Finally, some states hold that a physician or surgeon is the ''captain of the ship'' and is responsible for the conduct of others. Again, this is a complex doctrine and is applied differently in different jurisdictions.

FOURTEEN SIMPLE PRINCIPLES FOR MALPRACTICE AVOIDANCE

Oddly, the ways for physicians to decrease their chances of being sued are rather simple but work with astounding success. Physicians should

1. Spend more time with patients to explain problems, obtain informed consent, and listen to their concerns
2. Make sure they have adequate staff, who are both sensitive and empathetic, whether as receptionists or registered nurses
3. Attend continuing education classes, and ensure that the physician assistants, registered nurses, and young physicians on staff attend regularly
4. Have a system to be sure that they have documented records, especially for matters such as referrals to other specialists and phone calls in and out
5. Read all the records made by others pertaining to the care being given, whether made by a medical student, an attending, a nurse, a diagnostician, or other; if somebody makes a record, there is a reason

for so doing and physicians have an obligation to read it

6. Be the first one to tell the patient rather than the last one (if something goes wrong) (the physician should talk to the patient before the patient talks to a lawyer)

7. Although often under high stress, never be rude or insulting to a patient; even a nasty or "off-the-wall" patient should be treated politeness and dignity

8. If having a problem with drugs, alcohol, or emotional problems, get help from one of the help groups that exists for the medical profession; doctors under stress themselves are perhaps the greatest source of medical malpractice claims

9. Be sure the informed consent procedures are really *informative* and always document the information given patients

10. Take complete and proper medical histories, and make sure the staff does the same

11. Avoid functioning where not completely competent and confident; with new modalities such as laser or laparoscopic surgery, physicians should progress from didactic training to inanimate and animal models, and then to graded, supervised patient procedures; before undertaking a new procedure, physicians should be sure the training is adequate and that they have assisted others in performing the same procedure and be honest with patients when discussing their experience with new procedures

12. Do not be corrupted by a patient or other professionals; just because a patient may demand a certain procedure, does not mean a physician must do it; if one does not believe something is right for a patient, tell them and politely dismiss that patient

13. Not turn away emergencies once they have become the attending physician or the physician for the patient

14. Make sure they have an adequate system for handling patients when unavailable

As indicated, physicians can discourage lawsuits by establishing a rapport with their patients, not rushing their patients, talking to them, and following the other principles outlined. It is vital for physicians to spend time with their patients to get to know them and to let them know the physician, to not rush them and to answer their questions, to provide a thorough explanation of the planned surgery, and to get enough feedback to be sure that the patients understand the risks. The benefits of a good bedside manner should not be forgotten. The time lost in exercising good "bedside manner" will probably save vast increases in insurance premiums. Good staff attributes that deal with people, the need to attend continuing medical education courses, and very importantly, the need to read entries and respond to all entries are crucial. Too many doctors do not read the entries of others or disavow that they are even bound by entries made by the doctors and nurses with whom they work. This is outrageous and can cause great embarrassment to a doctor in a lawsuit situation. The need to inform the patient (and sometimes the hospital risk management division) of bad outcomes cannot be ignored. Sometimes things do go wrong and the doctor is better off if this is admitted it up front. Common sense and good public relations such as given above can do more to decrease medical malpractice claims than anything else.

LITIGATION VERSUS SETTLEMENT

It is frequently asked when a doctor should fight a case and go to trial or settle. This is often a difficult decision, because many physicians enjoy the right to instruct their carriers as to whether they will permit a settlement. Some doctors demand a settlement, even though they should not settle, because they do not want the expense or aggravation of going to trial. Other doctors will unreasonably fight a case when it should be settled. This will often create an adversarial situation between the doctor and the insurance company-appointed lawyer. Sometimes the insurance companies and state insurance guaranty funds will put pressure on physicians, indicating that if they refuse to settle, they may be dropped for further coverage or may have to pay an "excess" verdict out of their pocket. An excess verdict is where there is insufficient coverage to pay the full amount of any verdict.

A case can be settled during trial or even postjudgment. This occurs with some frequency in the so-called hard to call cases. This also occurs with an increasing degree of frequency in bifurcated cases. Such cases are those in which the liability of the doctor is tried first with no jury decision on damages until it is decided that the physician or hospital (or both) has done something that violates the standard of care.

Some of the considerations in deciding whether to go to trial or to settle a case are as follows:

1. Ego. Physicians should sit back and really think about whether they are merely hurt because their medical competency has been questioned. It is not a question of a physician's worth as a human, but rather whether a jury has a substantial possibility of being convinced that the physician has done something wrong.

2. Rely on the advice of respected professionals. To paraphrase Abraham Lincoln, lawyers' stock and trade is their judgment. Physicians should spend some time with the lawyer to understand their view and not hesitate to ask for the presence of personal counsel at any such meeting. Sometimes lawyers and firms will even be willing to have another partner or associate sit in on a meeting where it is decided whether to go to trial or settle.

3. Consider the location (urban or rural). In some places, jury verdicts are simply more possible than in others. The risk is going to be greater in certain metropolitan areas than in many rural areas, although that is not an absolute determination by any means. Some rural jurors can take a very populous view and be very angry at the amount of money they think doctors earn.

4. Consider the cost. There are costs not only to the insurance company, but also personally. The physician will be out of the office, and presumably losing money from the practice. Even if working for a hospital or group, an earning loss may occur because of an inability to see patients.

5. Consider the value of the claim and the amount of available insurance. If there is a reasonable claim for $1 million and that is the limit of insurance the physician may want to consider whether there may be a "excess" verdict problem. Many doctors do carry umbrella insurance these days, but that is not always the case. (An "excess" problem is where there is insufficient coverage to pay the verdict, and the plaintiff can come after the physician's personal assets.)

6. Consider whether the position of the insurance company attorney may be different from the adjuster who works for the insurance company. If the insurance company-appointed lawyer and the insurance adjuster differ, the physician may want a personal attorney involved to express concerns to the insurance company.

7. Remember that bad things happen to good people, and even the best predictions of experts can go awry. There is a certain amount of uncertainty in the jury process, regardless of how strong or weak a case may be.

8. Ask the lawyers or insurance company for the results of other similar cases in the location. Many municipalities and states keep good computer records about verdicts or settlements by type of case, age of the people involved, and the like. That information is readily obtainable from a variety of sources, and will provide some guideline.

9. If questioning whether one is responsible, physicians should not hesitate to speak with the experts chosen by your attorney or people within your profession. Some lawyers will be reluctant to have the physician speak with a hired expert because of fear that in cross-examination such conversations may be revealed. If your lawyer (with whom you should check first) does not want you to speak to the experts hired, ask the attorney if there is someone else to consult in the medical field, such as a respected or trusted colleague. Again these conversations may come up on cross-examination, depending on your state, and therefore always check with the attorney before you do this.

There are other considerations as well, but the best advice is to be deliberate, consider all the facts, rely on the advice of counsel, and speak to respected colleagues, if that is advisable (after consultation with your counsel). By all means, do not let ego get involved; do not let anger at the "system" or at "plaintiffs" result in an irrational decision; and do not develop an unreasonable fear of agencies and organizations to whom settlements are reported. If one has made a mistake, that is why one has insurance.

Another very important point that must be made is that physicians should to examine their own record. Even within specialties, there is a broad difference as to lawsuit indicators. For example, there are certain surgeons who get sued all the time, and some who never get sued. Is the difference public relations? Is the difference that some surgeons will take the riskier or tougher cases? There are no good studies to answer these questions, but it is certain that some professionals get sued more than others. Physicians who find themselves facing a high number of lawsuits, even for their specialty, should talk to the peer review people at their hospital or colleagues at another institution, or reconsider the level of continuing education they are receiving.

DO'S AND DONT'S OF MALPRACTICE AVOIDANCE

Finally, there are some basic do's and dont's:

1. Do not change or alter records. This may be very tempting, but it will probably be discovered and this will really blow any defense out of the water, not to mention creating punitive damages. This happens more than it should, and it is very crucial that it not occur.

2. Do not say anything to anybody, unless and until you talk to your attorney.

3. Notify your carrier immediately of any claim or any *potential* claim.

4. Do not go wild trying to "get the facts straight" by speaking with other involved physicians and nurses. This will likely come out in depositions and looks very bad. Let the chips fall where they may.

5. Do not try to control every aspect of the case, including the attorneys. The attorneys who defend these cases are usually highly specialized.

6. Do not try to play lawyer in your deposition with the plaintiff's lawyer. You may be a great doctor, but it is unlikely that you are as good a lawyer as plaintiff's counsel.

7. In trial, it is okay to be concerned, but do not have the countenance of being angry and arrogant.

8. When questioned, remember that whether at deposition or trial, it is not a debate. This is not a debating society. It is your job to try to understand the ques-

tions and be forthcoming. If you do not understand a question, say so. Never guess.

9. Be careful about suggesting experts to your lawyers who are personal friends and could be undermined in cross-examination.
10. Do read the medical literature relevant to the alleged malpractice.
11. Do show respect for the parties, the attorneys, the judge, the jurors, and the system.
12. Before you get sued, do make sure that you have adequate coverage and adequate umbrella coverage. From the plaintiff lawyer's point of view, when should a case be pursued? Obviously, there must be enough damages to justify the cost of bringing a case or there must be some significant principle involved in the event that damages are not sufficient.

Any good plaintiff's lawyer will need to review medical records and is entitled to them. Many states have a patient bill of rights that require that records be produced. Speak with your attorney if you have any questions about what is or is not part of the record. The charge for records should not be outrageous and doctors should not give their patients a hard time getting records, since, that alone, may often make a patient suspicious. Most lawyers obtain an informal outside review before they file a case, and in some states, such a review (formal and informal) is actually required. In some states, an intent to sue or a summons without a complaint may be filed to prevent the statute of limitations from expiring. Often, such cases are not pursued, and again, in that process, the doctor and insurance company should be cooperative. The case may very well go away.

As explained, an expert witness is somebody who has the right to render a judgment on the quality of care offered. Although some states require that the physician be in the same specialty as the defendant, other states are a bit more lenient and simply require familiarity with the general area.

DEPOSITION AND TRIAL

Probably the most important part of a case for most people is preparing for the deposition. There are many rules on this and you should talk to your attorney. Most importantly, be truthful, do not be evasive, and do not ramble. Do not play lawyer and do not engage in needless trivial arguing with the attorney. This is not a contest to see who can be more clever, or who knows more medicine. Answer questions truthfully and briefly. Do not volunteer unasked information or attempt to educate your adversary. Be prepared. Read the records, speak with your lawyer, and make sure you are familiar with the literature. Look at the complaint that has been filed, your answer, any written answers to questions, and whatever else is in the file that you can access. An educated witness is a good witness. The records should be

intact and unaltered. If an error is made, the proper incident report should be filled out and whatever forms the state, licensing body, or insurance companies may require. This is one way to prevent or keep down punitive damages.

The following are the events that lead to a trial:

1. Examining whether the case exists by gathering records, talking to witnesses, and talking to experts
2. Obtaining an informal or a formal expert report, if necessary
3. Filing an intent to sue, or in some cases, a complaint
4. Formal discovery such as depositions, examinations before trial, independent medical examinations, exchange of written questions, and the like
5. The obtaining of further expert reports
6. Sometimes a second wave of discovery, based on information learned from depositions
7. Sometimes requests for admissions in which one party or another admits or waives a particular position
8. Pre-trial conference, such as a meeting with the judge, and deciding on all the procedural matters
9. Trial preparation
10. Jury selection
11. The trial itself

COMMON TYPES OF NEGLIGENCE LEADING TO LAWSUITS

The following is a summery of recent lawsuits and the specific nature of the negligence in order to be specific as to those areas which a practitioner needs to be aware:

1. *Improper rectovaginal fistula repairs and informed consent for same.* These repairs can lead to infectious process or impair the operation of other organs. It is important that the patient understand the consequences of the fistula repair, the necessity thereof, and the implications.
2. *Vaginal growth not properly diagnosed.* Needless to say, depending on the type of growth, its chronicity, and the possibility that it will develop into a carcinoma are all areas of great concern. There is a variety of diagnostic testing, not to mention invasive views, which ought to be explored, or at least discussed, with the patient.
3. *Leiomyoma leading to a hysterectomy.* Sometimes surgery need not occur at all. When it is necessary to do that surgery, the consequences of not doing it must be carefully explained to the patient, as well as the risks thereof.
4. *Hysterectomies.* This speaks for itself. The author and colleagues often see hysterectomies that involve damage to other organs, such as the ureter. Inconti-

nence can occur with hysterectomies, but perhaps the greatest area of liability concerns the tangential hormonal consequences. Women, even properly educated, are seldom prepared for the sequelae to a hysterectomy. There is much debate, which most patients are well aware, concerning whether there are too many hysterectomies performed in this country or too few. These issues need to be explored and thought about. The surgery needs to be carefully planned and all attendant organs well visualized.

   A. Negligently performed
       i. While pregnant
       ii. Creating vesicovaginal fistula
       iii. Instances of damaging a ureter
       iv. Suffering a pulmonary embolus
   B. Informed consent. Informed consent must not only be by virtue of a specific form itself, but the doctors', as well as anesthesiologists', own consult or progress note should reflect when and where informed consent was given and the nature thereof.

5. *Dilation and curettage.* These procedures are often necessitated by an ongoing disease process, as well as a variety of other reasons. Failure to perform could result in sterility or other serious effects. A proper understanding of the procedure, what it entails, and its consequences or failure must be carefully explained to the patient.
   A. Pelvic inflammatory disease caused by the procedure and thus in turn creating a need for hysterectomy

6. *Abortions,* complications of
   A. Infections
   B. Cerate lacerated cervix
   C. Requiring laparotomy secondary to misread pathology report
   D. Negligent performance of abortions, leading to uterus repair

7. *Laparoscopic tubal ligations* resulting in
   A. Nicked bowel, or parts thereof
   B. Iliac artery lacerations
   C. Failure of sterilization
   D. Hematoma

8. *Diagnostic laparoscopy or laparotomy* leading to
   A. Peritonitis
   B. Bowel perforations
   C. Failure to remove both ovaries when indicated

9. Although this is somewhat covered by 7 and 8 above, *trocar injuries,* especially with regard to consent and lack of control of the instrument.

10. *Ectopic pregnancies* leading to
   A. Rupture
   B. Complete hysterectomy
   C. Removal of fallopian tubes bilaterally

11. *Breast cancer not diagnosed.* As every practitioner knows, breast cancer diagnosis is a major issue, and sometimes is not in the hands of the obstetrician. There are many attendant diagnostic potentialities. For example, cytopathologists may be involved, as well as radiologists and other experts. It is the role of obstetricians/gynecologists to be sure that they are aware of the latest diagnostics, the patient's history in this regard, and what means are available further to develop a differential diagnosis.

12. *Failure to diagnose nonmalignant breast disease*

13. *Unnecessary removal of organs,* such as ovary

14. *Failure to diagnose ectopic pregnancy*

15. *Endometriosis*
   A. Unnecessary surgery performed
   B. Not diagnosed

16. *Laser conization leading to bleeding requiring hysterectomy*

17. *Hysteroscopy—failure to diagnose bicornate uterus*

18. *Complications of uretal bladder diagnosis*

19. *Laser injuries.* See 15, above. This can be because of instrument difficulties, but more often because of lack of training or use where not appropriate.

The above is certainly not intended as a complete list of all possible problems, but those events which most customarily lead to problems.

SUMMARY

The prudent practitioner, with an eye toward the law, could practice medicine without fear of lawsuits. True, anybody can be the subject of frivolous misconduct by another. This can take the form of a lawsuit or any other unkind cut that one human is capable of delivering to another. The best way to avoid malpractice is not to live in abject fear of it, but rather to understand the system, be attentive to ones patients, and treat all humans with the respect one would like to receive.

REFERENCES

1. United States Congressional Budget Office: Economic Implications of Rising Health Care Costs. 1. October 1992.
2. Relman AS: Self-referral—what's at stake? New Engl J Med 327:1522, 1992.
3. Harvard Medical Practice Study: Patients, doctors, and lawyers: malpractice injury litigation and patient compensation in New York. 11-1, 1990
4. 55 RAND Institute for Civil Justice, 1991
5. Study on Medical Malpractice Reform. American Medical Association, Chicago, IL, 1992
6. Socioeconomic Characteristics of Medical Practice, Medical Professional Liability Claims Premiums, 1985–1990. 2–3

INDEX

Page numbers followed by f *indicate figures; those followed by* t *indicate tables.*